JOURNEY THROUGH
THE ORIENT

JOURNEY THROUGH
THE ORIENT

Text and photographs by

MARTIN HÜRLIMANN

Introduction by Sacheverell Sitwell

A STUDIO BOOK

THE VIKING PRESS · NEW YORK

Weidersehen mit Asien

© 1959 ATLANTIS VERLAG AG ZURICH

Journey through the Orient

© 1960 THAMES AND HUDSON, LONDON

TRANSLATED BY ISOBEL NEILSON

PUBLISHED IN 1960 BY THE VIKING PRESS, INC.

625 MADISON AVENUE, NEW YORK 22, N.Y.

LIBRARY OF CONGRESS CATALOG CARD NUMBER: 60-8515

TEXT PRINTED BY JARROLD AND SONS, NORWICH, ENGLAND

PLATES PRINTED BY IMAGO AG ZURICH, SWITZERLAND

Contents

Contents

Introduction

THIS BOOK is of double interest to the public because in addition to its splendid array of photographs in colour and in black and white it is the début of Dr Hürlimann as the writer of the text accompanying his camera upon its travels. It is in fact his first full-length text, and there is every reason to think the reading public will not be disappointed in him. He has long been known, internationally, as one of the world's foremost commentators with his lens, but now he appears for the first time as the mind behind the camera.

At the first of many dips the page opens at a pilgrim in his mushroom-shaped straw hat, staff in one hand, begging-bowl in the other, standing in front of a long line of charabancs. Behind him a young woman dressed like an air hostess leads along a group of small boys in school uniforms. It is a commentary upon the divided soul or dichotomy of present-day Japan. And turning the pages we come to one of the most beautiful of Hürlimann's colour plates; a village scene during the boys' festival in Japan with two small boys walking under a green bamboo pole from which float great streamers in the form of more than life-size fish, paper fish twice as big as the small boys, and with their scales marked white on black and white on red. What beautiful photographs there are, too, of processions of Shinto priests under the tall cryptomerias at Ise! They resemble some esoteric, outdoor performance of *The Magic Flute*.

But we must turn to the beginning of the book which is in Beirut, where there is indeed a tinge of disappointment for we only see a demonstration of students and the gimcrack modern buildings, whereas Beirut with all its brazen modernity has more to offer in the way of Oriental costume than either Cairo or Istanbul. But we are removed at jet speed to India, a subcontinent that most exactly suits

Hürlimann's camera. I have to admit that the Taj Mahal does always look to me a little hunched or narrow-chested. The pair of little cupolas to either side of the dome have no room to show their character, and I cannot admire the four 'lighthouse' minarets built of white marble bricks. The giant Qutb Minar, rising in five storeys to nearly two hundred and fifty feet with corbelled balconies, is another matter altogether. It looks what it is, a tower of victory, expressed in masculine thirteenth-century language. How curious, in parenthesis, that a tower almost the twin to the Qutb Minar should have been discovered in Afghanistan and photographed for the first time, not more than a couple of years ago.

There are photographs contrasting the homeless street dwellers of Delhi and the lotus-tanks of Lutyens that stretch in front of his pink sandstone, 'Elgarian' imperial buildings, and then we find ourselves at Chandigarh, the new capital of the Punjab which is being built to Le Corbusier's plans. The contrast is extreme, and might not in the end be entirely to Le Corbusier's credit for his section of cement honeycomb, but with squared instead of hexagonal cells, and his 'ratelier' elevations begun to look slum-ridden and poverty-stricken while they are still new. How much more proper to the teeming Indian population are the ghats of Benares with their crowded steps leading down to the Ganges! Sadhus and fakirs smeared with ashes are non-suited to cement cubbyholes.

The main interest of this book however is Hürlimann's China, approached by way of Hongkong. Here, preluding with a lateen-sailed boat on a choppy sea only a few yards from the stark office buildings, is Chinatown, the historic Chinatown of the past, for it is evidently extinct in China, Hongkong thereby assuming to itself a picturesque importance that it never had before. But Macao, the Portuguese settlement only a few hours' sail away, Portuguese since 1557, for more than four centuries, must be the original and authentic Chinatown with its mingling of Jesuit church façades built by Japanese converts, its opium dens, and memories of the poet Camoens. In comparison, the street scenes in Hongkong are but street scenes in Peking from *Aladdin*, or any other Victorian pantomime.

And so to the real China, where the polychrome buildings of the Forbidden City come alive under Hürlimann's camera. Their colour may even be enhanced by the plainness of the blue boiler-suits which have taken the place of national costume. So marked is the recent improvement in colour printing that in certain of the photographs of Peking, not having been myself to China, I seem to recognise what I assume to be the peculiar, pale light of Central Asia, only having encountered it in person at Meshed in Persia, where it is extremely visible, but not at Isfahan. Such in all probability is the pale sunlight of Bokhara and Samarcand. This special quality of light is most evident in the pictures of the Red Gate, and of the Great Wall of China winding away into the hills. The mass of the Forbidden City must be imposing in scale and it is certainly impressive and formidable in plan, but is it not, in fact, ugly in detail? The double page in colour of dragons in tilework has the ugliness and monotony of thousands of years of similar work, whether in the profiled scenes on Egyptian temples, or among the winged, man-headed bulls of Babylon and Persepolis. And the more than life-size bronze lion is just that little bit too 'Chinese', which is the fault of nearly everything accomplished under the Manchu emperors, including the dragon-writhing, cloud, and wave-laden imperial robes at the Victoria and Albert Museum. The story would be different could there but be photographs of the China of a thousand years ago.

By-passing the Japanese section that we looked at first we arrive at the pictures of Siam. Here, for some aesthetic reason difficult to determine, tawdriness and bad taste come into their own and do not give offence. The two huge figures of temple guardians which are of the lowest class of sculpture, in fact they are scarcely sculptures at all and only of circus, fun-fair standard, are yet of genuine fairy-tale effect. They have pagoda headdresses and the winged shoulders of the Royal ballet dancers, and are greatly enhanced by the red-tiled temple behind them with its tilted eaves and cobra finials, the front of the gables being scattered all over with rose-coloured flowers upon a bright yellow ground. Pictures of the *klongs* (canals) of Bangkok are picturesque even if they try not to be, and there follow Buddhist monks in glorious saffron robes, and a wonderful fruit and flower market of the sub-tropics. So ends this picture-book by a famous photographer of our day. It is only sad, as always, that the camera was not invented several hundred years ago. Had that been so, the revolution in painting would have come earlier. But then because of the very presence of the camera, there would have been less to photograph for Dr Hürlimann. On the other hand, now he has made his début as a writer, we may think regretfully of the many missing pages from his pen.

I think the reader will enjoy the writing of this great photographer. That it is a special kind of talent, I, who have never taken a photograph in my life, would be the first to agree. And as in the case of one or two other of his confrères the gift in question has sharpened his observation and helped him to achieve a style. One closes the last page of his text with real regret for on the strength of this alone he is one of the acutest observers of our time. Something of an Asian specialist but, also, an encyclopaedist traveller all over the world, and with things to say on everything that he has seen.

SACHEVERELL SITWELL

Asia Revisited

THE READER of this book is invited to accompany a photographer on a journey undertaken at the rapid pace of our time. We travel by air, covering on an average two thousand miles between stops, and every time we land we encounter a different culture and yet another race in this largest of continents, which emerges from several thousand years of history into the present transformation of the world.

Asia is the seat of ancient cultures. Its population constitutes easily half the human race; its peoples, religions, and customs are of a bewildering variety, representing every stage of civilisation and social system from theocratic absolutism to uncompromising Marxism. But today all have to come to terms with the laws of technical progress; every race is involved in the world-wide struggle between the great powers and their ideologies.

In the Near East, where the noble cultures of pre-Christian centuries have been surveyed in their entirety only in the past few decades through new discoveries from the highlands of Anatolia to the delta of the Indus, the followers of the prophet Mohammed established their kingdoms and the palaces of their rulers with fire and sword, with religious zeal, and with great artistic sense: in the region of the North Indian rivers we see, in the triumphal monuments and tombs of the conquerors and in the fairy-like palaces of the Mogul emperors, the most Oriental and perhaps most beautiful products of this art, which is precluded from fashioning any likeness of God and instead displays the whole wealth of its inventiveness in architecture and ornamentation.

In India the stern—though already here somewhat tempered—monotheism of the West confronts the polytheism of the Hindu religions and their profusion of images. Their proclivity towards the transcendental works to prevent the peoples who live between Adams Bridge and the rampart of the Himalayas from achieving large-scale political organisations of any duration; they have become all too easily the victims of usurpers who penetrate the north-western passes or come from across the sea. But the places of pilgrimage from the Lingam of Ramesvaram in the extreme south to the snow-covered abode of Shiva, with their lofty towers and innumerable idols, are distinctive signs of a national community in which even the bewildering diversity of races and tongues merges.

The religious genius of India radiated powerfully eastwards; it put its stamp on the culture of the Indo-Chinese kingdoms and Indonesia; and with the image of the Buddha, the prince's son who achieved enlightenment through renunciation and meditation, it gave Asia as far as the Japanese Archipelago one of the great symbols of human faith.

The awareness of history among the Chinese forms a sharp contrast to the prevailing disdain in which the so-called forces that shape history are held by the peoples of India. The East Asian is not a dreamer who considers this life as merely a passage-way between the great mysteries of existence in the other world; he is a realist; he addresses himself in this world to the permanence of things. He does not cremate his dead but erects tombs which defy the passage of time; his ancestors accompany him through his daily life; family ties ensure the stability of the State. The Tsin race lent the emerging society a formative impulse equalled only in Rome—the creation of a script whose characters denote not sounds but concepts, and an adherence to moral principles handed down from legendary times and codified most effectively by Confucius—which made possible the impressive unification of the largest continuous mass of people known to history. One after another, neighbouring regions were absorbed into this cultural community by a process which does not yet seem to have come to an end. In speaking today of 600 (or is it already 650?) million 'Chinese' we acknowledge an historical achievement which far surpasses the ephemeral splendours of even the greatest dynasties, an achievement equal to the entire Greek-Roman-Christian culture of the West.

How different does this Asia appear today when the 'colonialism' of the Western empires has acquainted her with new ways of life, and young nationalism strives in a much more radical way to become part of the new universal culture? We may catch a glimpse of the answer.

This was my fourth journey to Asia.

In 1922–3, as a student, I travelled through Indonesia, China, and Japan. My second visit in 1926–7 started from Ceylon, and from there I travelled over Adams Bridge to the mainland and for seven months wandered through the subcontinent, from the Shiva and Vishnu relics of the Dravidic South over the mountains of the Deccan to the populous valleys of the Indus, Ganges, and Brahmaputra; from the oldest Christian mission stations on the Malabar coast to the tea gardens and Lama temples of Darjeeling. I sailed in a houseboat through the fields of blossoming lilies in the Kashmir valley. Finally I reached the kingdom of Nepal, at that time strictly barred to strangers, and was the guest there of the Maharaja Chandra of the family of the Rana, who had for a generation ruled as an enlightened despot. I took photographs of the magnificent monuments, and the poor villages of the undernourished millions, from which poured a steady stream of pilgrims to the holy places.

On the return journey through the deserts and oases of the Near East I got to know the young States of Iraq, Syria, and Lebanon, where British and French garrisons were still more or less visible, and in Turkey I came across an already largely disillusioned East which was trying under the stern guidance of Kemal Ataturk to come to terms with the machine age.

After a brief stay in Europe I undertook in 1927–8 my third journey to Asia, which was particularly directed to the Southern Buddhist lands. From Ceylon I went first to Burma and its hinterland; at that time you could travel there for days peacefully, through woods and by log-canoe on the rivers to the various tribes, under the protection of the British, which was embodied in a single British official for a whole group of small Shan States. To the east was the independent kingdom of Siam, and, closely allied to it in culture but ruled by a French resident minister, the kingdom of Cambodia, seat of the splendid ruins of Angkor. Finally, after passing through the rest of what was then French Indo-China, I re-entered territory influenced by Chinese culture, crossing the viaducts of the Yunnan railway, an admirable achievement of French engineers, into one of the most southerly pro-vinces of the Middle Kingdom. There Chinese colonialism had just, and none too soon, completed the assimilation of the foreign races to the superior Tsin society.

At the time of these travels, the spell of the East was almost unbroken. Heavily veiled Mohammedan women and men wearing the red fez mingled with the Christian population in the streets of Beirut; brassware and other products of native handicrafts glittered in the bazaars. Sacred, pitifully lean cows wandering about freely were a conspicuous feature of the Indian street scene, even in modern cities like Bombay; the Sadhu smeared with ash and the Hindu beggar-monk embodied the ascetic ideal of the country, which was studded with temples and idols; and the whole nation seemed to be on a constant pilgrimage to the holy places. In Bangkok, Hongkong, and Peking rickshaw coolies ran panting and puffing through the streets with their small vehicles; in the twilight of the temples incense burnt faintly before golden Buddhas; people still drove across the country in two-wheeled carts drawn by a pair of ponies in double harness, just as the great Kung Fu-tse used to travel; and ideas about Eastern wisdom and the Western zeal for research could be exchanged over bowls of delicious food in old, renovated eating-houses; no provision about a national language impeded an amicable understanding among scholars and art-lovers.

Europeans and Americans moved self-confidently and safely through this world of natives; men in sun-helmets admired the picturesque customs, bought idols and magical implements for ethnographical collections and noted down legends and proverbs. Warships of the great powers anchored in the most important seaports; the commercial houses of the white people sustained foreign trade, and behind the bejewelled native potentates representatives of the protecting power worked the levers of policy.

There was only one major exception: while the continental Asians allowed their kingdoms to collapse into anarchy and apathetically accepted white supremacy, or else got helplessly caught up in blind xenophobia, a number of resolute men in the Land of the Rising Sun recognised the signs of the time; in 1868 they overthrew the medieval Shogunate and in the name of the young Emperor Meji inaugurated the age of reform. The hasty adoption of Western technology enabled Japan to repulse her Russian rival on the coast of the Pacific at the beginning of the 20th century, and be admitted to the exclusive club of the colonial powers.

After the Second World War the political map of Asia altered radically. French and British occupation forces disappeared from the Near East. The kingdoms and republics in the former dominions of the Ottoman Sultan, deprived of foreign help, are still struggling for existence as nations, united only in their hatred of the 'imperialists'. In the decisive step towards independence the British-Indian Empire became divided into a Mohammedan and a Hindu State, so much stronger have religious feelings proved to be than the precepts of geo-graphy, economics, and politics. New States also came into being in Ceylon, Burma, and the Malay Peninsula; the colonial kingdoms of the Dutch East Indies and French Indo-China have been dissolved, Korea has achieved a precarious independence, and in place of the political vacuum which arose in the

Middle Kingdom after the decline of the Manchu dynasty there is the monolithic block of 600 million strictly organised workers and peasants; while in Formosa, which was colonised by the Chinese and occupied for fifty years by the Japanese, the Kuomintang Government, expelled from the mainland, steadfastly hopes for a change of fortune. In Siam the absolute monarchy has been replaced by a constitutional monarchy; generals govern instead of princes, and the kingdom has since been called Thailand, the land of the free. Japan, stripped of her overseas possessions, must look for outlets for her products, on which she depends, in the free competition of world markets; in the meantime the military caste has played out its great game; the Tenno no longer appeals to the prerogatives of his divine descent.

The world has become more hard-headed. 'Tractors instead of prayer-wheels' is the catch-phrase; the aspirations of the new ruling class are directed towards planning and socialism, religious traditions are being jettisoned as irksome ballast, but monuments and other national art objects are receiving all the benefit of zealous care combined with scientific methods. The code of Western civilisation, whether in a capitalist or a Communist form, is being applied as faithfully as possible.

Flying in 1958 is a comparatively comfortable affair for the European who has the necessary travellers' cheques at his disposal. He may no longer be greeted so deferentially as 'Sahib' and 'Master', and he must share his comforts with people of other races—at least with those who belong to the political and economic *élite*—but there are hotels with air-conditioned rooms, and restaurants with every possible speciality. Car travel has reduced the risk of sunstroke, so that sun-helmets have become a curiosity. Airports give an impression of endless prosperity and technical routine, with an ever-present, polite, and efficiently functioning civil service. With a pleasant feeling of security one can go on a conducted tour and see, as if in a film, strange temple customs, gay market scenes, and primitive huts, in the comfortable assumption that zealous officials co-operating with all sorts of national and international institutions will soon manage to achieve technical and social progress in these places too.

Even the Iron Curtain loses much of its terror for the politically naïve traveller once he has succeeded in slipping through it. In my case this adventure was effected very simply: I went to the Chinese Embassy in Berne for a visa, waited a few months for an answer and had already given up hope of getting it when, just a day before my departure, I received the permit and quickly had my passport stamped. This stamp with its two puzzling letters enabled me to cross this frontier as easily as others, with just as polite though perhaps slightly stricter officials. And on the other side there were again comfortable hotels, not as gleaming with the chromium of American credit as in the West but yet of good middle-class standard; there was, it is true, a travel service which was run by the State—but conducted tours are not, after all, the invention of Communists.

The collection of photographs in this book is the fruit of a return to Asia lasting three months. I travelled for exactly eleven weeks, from 5 March to 12 May, 1958, a breath-taking venture with hardly a pause for reflection. I broke my journey in Beirut, Karachi, and Bombay, went aboard again in Calcutta, used the stop at Hongkong for an excursion to Peking, and saved up the visit to colourful Bangkok for the return journey from Japan to Europe. This, then, is a personal report, a snapshot of this vast territory at a decisive phase of its history, in the perspective provided by my previous journeys.

Once again we see everywhere the heritage of great civilised nations with their imposing achievements; compared with this their share in 20th-century civilisation seems for the present very modest. Pilgrims still throng the steps down to the sacred Ganges, a pious clapping of hands still echoes through the tranquil groves of the Shinto shrines. But the intellectuals look to Marx and Lenin for guidance, and elsewhere for dollars, to master the problems crowding in upon them; industrialisation cannot come quickly enough for them. Centuries of delay are to be made up for by dams, afforestation, and new methods of agriculture. The days of feudalism are numbered, and in the last colonies the suitcases are already packed.

The Lebanon

THE AIRCRAFT took off from Geneva at midnight and wheeled round towards the Alps; beneath us was a pale landscape of rock and snow; a tiny warm light flickered from a valley; then the landscape retreated, the plain of the Po stretched out in the darkness, the view was confined to the moonlit wings of our machine. The lights were put out, the seats clamped back; the night passed without one being aware of it.

We were heading for a bright streak in the clouds; flying east, we were an hour nearer the dawn; the Mediterranean now lay clear beneath us, to the left appeared land with snow-capped mountains, then an island—was it Cyprus? The coast ahead was scarcely visible, yet already our aircraft was coming in to land over parched Asian soil.

I used the landing at Beirut for a two days' break on my flight to Tokyo. As we drove through the bare, hilly country and approached the city the first concrete blocks of flats appeared, with broad windows and verandas facing the sea, some not yet finished and flanked by huge Coca-Cola advertisements. The palace is in this district too—a prosaic group of buildings put up in 1948 for the Third General Conference of UNESCO. A palm tree and a few figures in flowing Arabian garb were the only signs of the Orient.

From my hotel, one of the several smart new hotels of the Lebanese capital which would look the same in Caracas or anywhere in the world, it is still a good half-hour's walk along the sea front to the old town. Today Beirut has about half a million inhabitants, more than a quarter of the country's population. Superficially at least the American way of life seems to have been accepted. Beirut is a kind of open port for the Near East, in which it is apparently still possible to do good business; goods from abroad are easy to obtain; skyscrapers with lifts are springing up in the old quarters like mushrooms; there are amusement arcades for the sailors of all nations.

The young people go about in blue jeans, and only a few men wear the fez which thirty years ago was common enough; hardly any women are veiled.

Like Christianity Islam seems to have lost much of its impetus; the non-religious 'left', Arab nationalists, the resentment against the great powers, the young people with Western education hungry for recognition, status, and power—all these have become more violently bitter than the former religious fanatics.

To demonstrate how precarious the situation of this State was in March 1958 —two processions of demonstrators (schoolchildren and students) marched past me when I was in the centre of the town; they linked hands and hoisted on to their shoulders some of their comrades, who shouted party cries fanatically; they were chanting their slogans rhythmically and you needed only to understand one

Pages 21–26 BEIRUT

21 The Mediterranean coast with the Dove Grottoes.

22, 23, 26 top New buildings on the waste land above the rocky shore to the west of the city and harbour.

24, 25, 26 below Two long processions of demonstrators—schoolchildren and students —passing through the old town. They shouted pro-Arab slogans in chorus and carried pictures of President Nasser (25). In dress and features the inhabitants of this Mediterranean city were very little different from those on the European shore. The schoolgirls' uniforms (25) remind one of French styles.

Pages 27–28 FLIGHT FROM BEIRUT TO KARACHI AND BOMBAY

27 After crossing the Persian Gulf we flew over the desolate mountains on the Persian coast. At about 16,000 feet it was only rarely possible to take satisfactory photographs of the mist-shrouded landscape.

28 Between Karachi and Bombay huge cloud formations parted to give a glimpse of the Indian peninsula of Kathiawar.

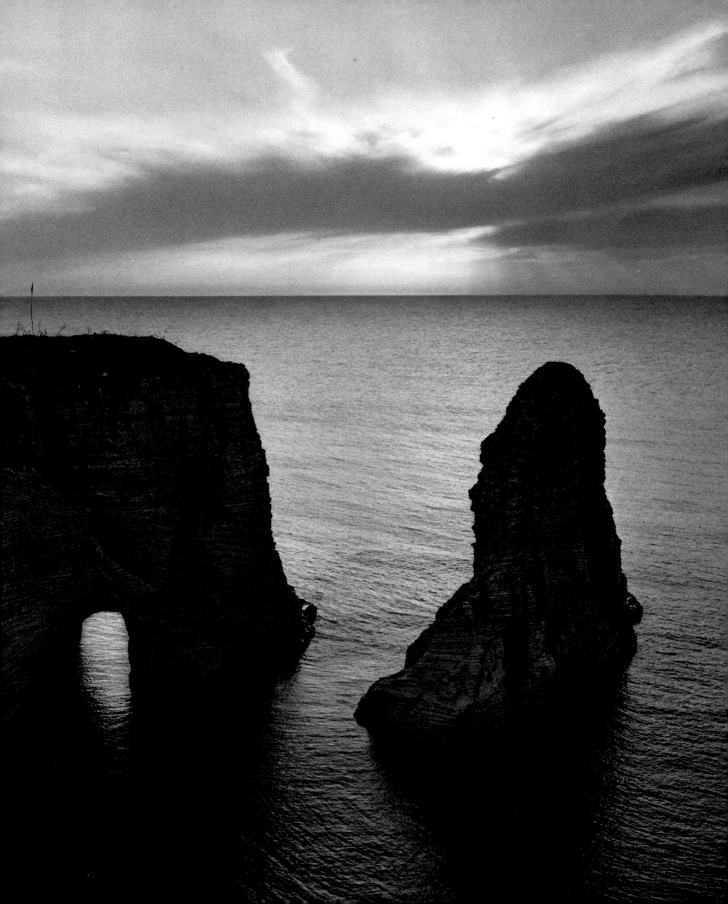

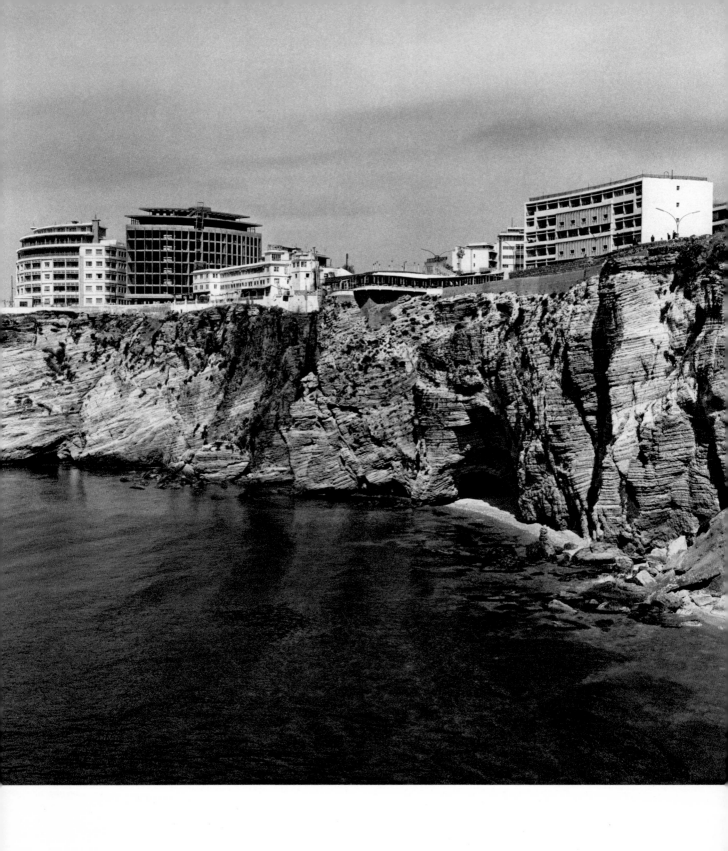

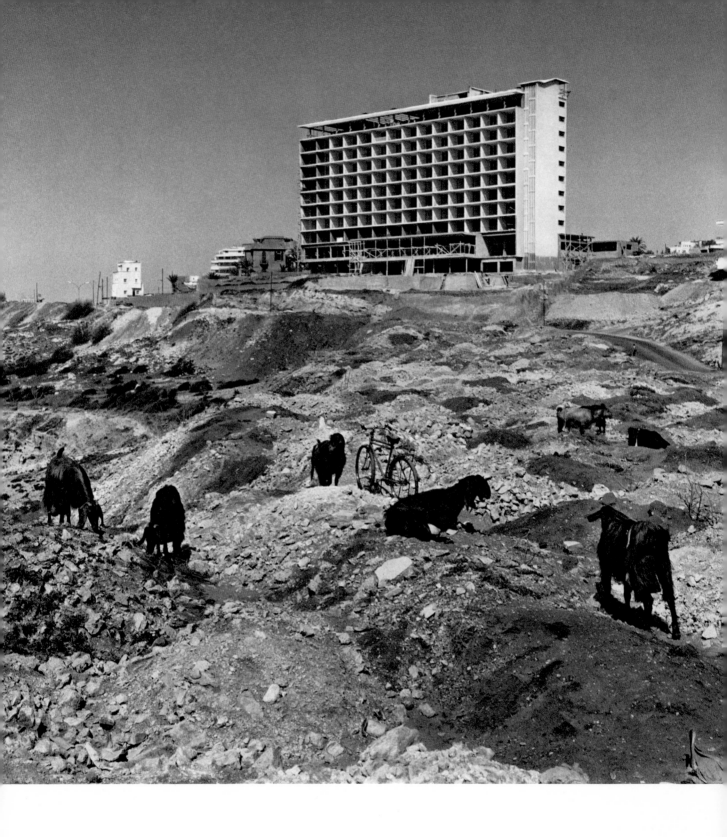

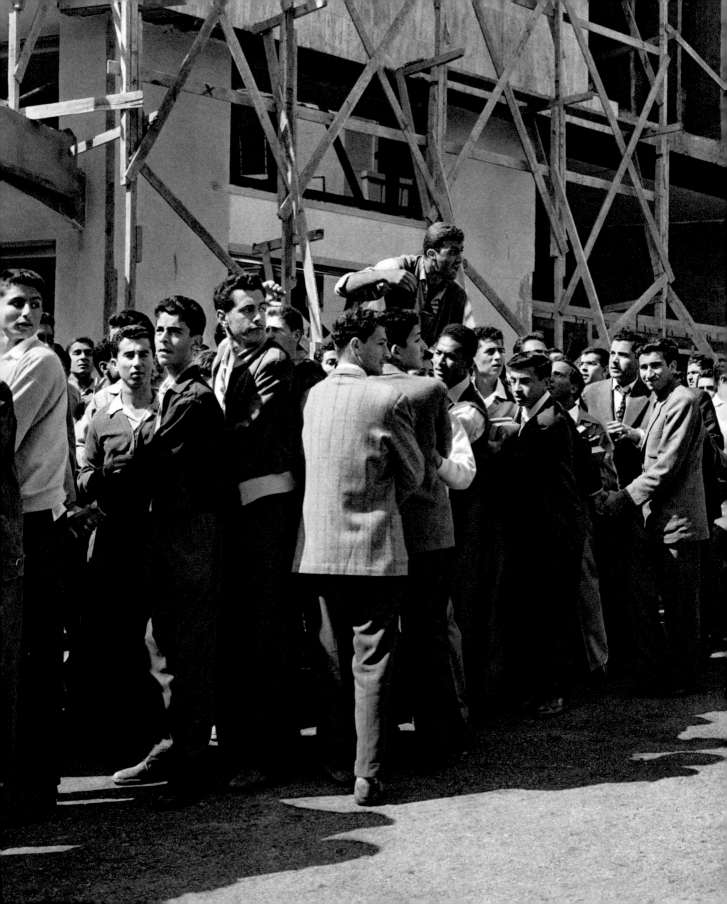

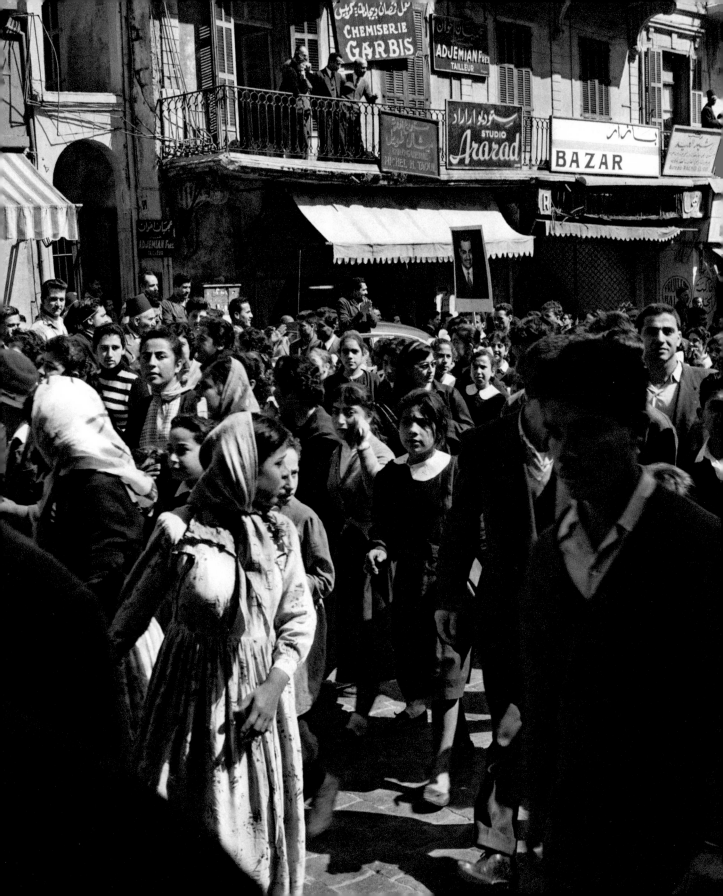

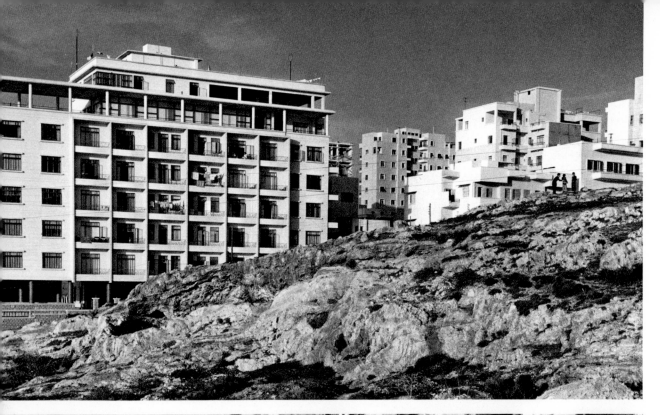

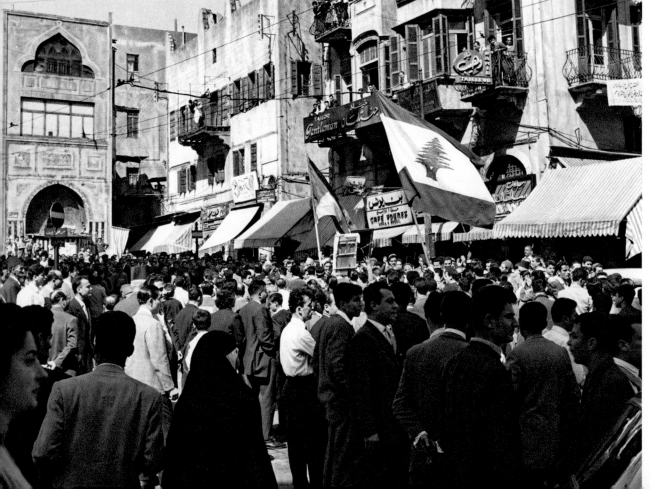

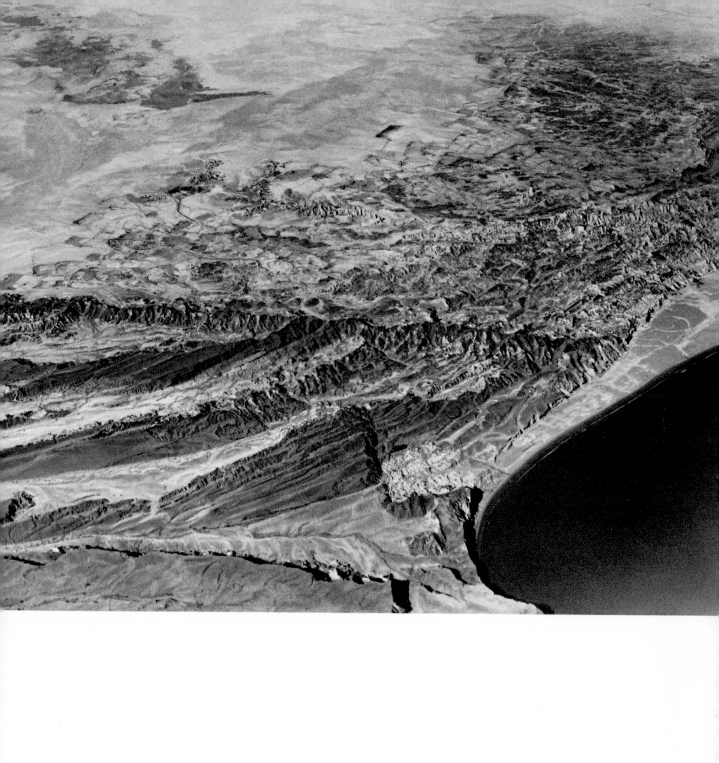

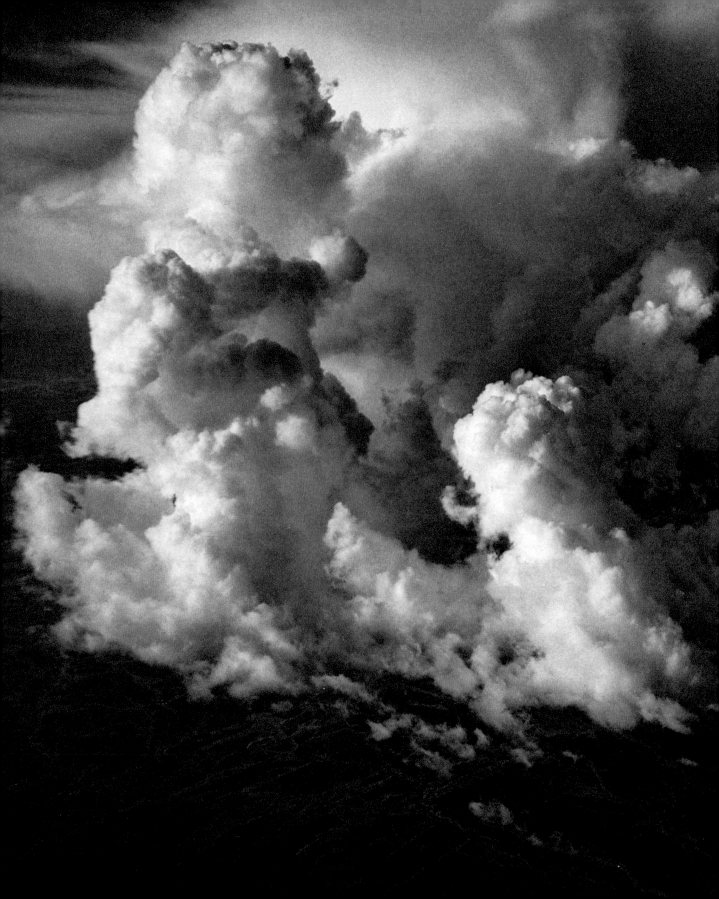

word to know what it was all about: 'Nasser! Nasser! Nasser!' Portraits of the grinning, bull-necked Egyptian were carried like icons.

Who sees those faces knows that no appeal to reason would change their opinion; they batten on hatred—and have we not ourselves recently, in the heart of our European culture, experienced such loud-voiced processions of demonstrators with the same type of fanaticism?

At midnight, when I left the hotel in Beirut to continue my journey on the next plane from Geneva, the cool sea-breeze had become hot and stormy, the desert wind in which one could scarcely stand. There was still a great deal of activity in the waiting-room of the airport: Beirut is one of the most important junctions in the East. It was soon past the time of departure and the Lebanese stewardess offered refreshments as is customary when there are delays. A child cried, his mother dozed, and his father rocked another child in his arms; three dark-skinned, impressive Indonesians (looking like relations of Sukarno) sat in a corner, and a group of Saudi-Arabians, some in flowing burnouses, others in European dress, were deferentially greeted; then whole families appeared, the women stout and half-veiled, interspersed with Mecca pilgrims on their way to Ruad. Finally, the Lebanese girl in uniform explained in barely intelligible English that in the sandstorm our aeroplane had been unable to find the runway and had gone on to Damascus—perhaps it would come back for us here, otherwise we would be driven to Damascus, three hours away over poor roads. But Damascus is in Syria, with its own entrance regulations. The windows rattled in the storm unceasingly—but still aeroplanes landed and took off. I occupied the night by reflecting on the political scene, at the beginning of this Eastern journey.

The Night at the Airport

None of the modern Near Eastern States came into existence through a national movement. There was no historical tradition as for instance in Finland or the

States Succeeding the Ottoman Empire

Baltic States. No real, integrated whole resulted from the competing claims of the colonial powers and their ideologies, of the League of Nations, and of the native dynasties. The case of Egypt was different: here was a geographical and a centuries-old political entity—as well as an agglomeration of population. On the other hand Nasser's rule does not rest on a world historical tradition, such as Hitler had at his disposal in the enormous potential of German efficiency. The repeated miserable failure of the Egyptian military forces against Israel would in any other circum-stances have meant a devastating political defeat, and the drive of the Arabs towards unity, the resentment of their semi-Europeanised intellectuals, and the ambition of their colonels would have petered out without result.

Where does the 'historical' claim to a given country begin and end? Is the last conqueror in the right? Or the one before the last? The farmers who tilled the land or the nomads who have let it run to waste? There is almost no country in the world which is still inhabited by its indigenous people and where sooner or later some usurper has not legitimised a claim to the territory, and then after him another—the Angles, Saxons, and Normans in England, the Helvetii, Romans, and Alemanni in Switzerland; the Poles, Russians, and Germans in East Prussia, and so on. All of them are in the right, or none.

The Role of Religion

Religion is still powerful enough to lead to the foundation of new States like Israel and Pakistan; and Islam, the militant religion *par excellence*, is still a strong link between peoples. As a place of pilgrimage Mecca has not gone out of fashion any more than Rome and Lourdes and Benares. And yet, can all the activity about the holy places, although publicised by modern methods of communication and propaganda, disguise the fact that secularism is gaining strongly everywhere? Do not even the Olympic Games and the art festivals of our age lack the dedica-tion to which they owe their origin? And is not the anti-religion of Marxism-Leninism, the conquering faith of our age, followed by its believers through all twists of expediency in blind enthusiasm according to the directives of the Pontifex Maximus of the party?

The Muslim League has split into fragmentary parties, for whom the Islamic character of Pakistan is far less the guiding principle that it was for Jinnah, the founder of the State. Jawaharlal Nehru, who no longer wants to be called Pandit, stands far removed from Hinduism as a religious community in our sense of the word; his thinking is secular, directed towards socialist planning. In the Jewish State the parties which are guided by the Old Testament and the Talmud form a minority. Kemal Ataturk, with his resolute disestablishment of the Church, has anticipated a development which has got hold of the whole of the East. The Muslim Brotherhood in Cairo no longer prospers under the rule of Nasser, the pilgrim to Mecca. But all this does not alter the fact that the Islam of the Arab peoples is a factor with which their leaders must reckon, and which the atheist Pontifex of Moscow knows how to exploit with the help of his Mohammedan subjects.

At about four o'clock in the morning a smart young man in uniform appeared and explained in Swiss-German that our Douglas aircraft was to take off again from Damascus at daybreak and, if possible, pick us up at seven. At five we breakfasted, at six the aircraft landed, at seven o'clock we were in the air flying due east.

Flight over Deserts and Oilfields

The delay had one advantage in that the eight-hour journey to Karachi would be in daylight. As we were flying at about 16,000 feet the landscape disappeared in a haze. At that height photographs through the cabin window are not worth taking, but if you happen to have a geologist on board you can learn a great deal from the view.

At lunch our attention was drawn to a notice on the menu that no alcohol could be served over Saudi-Arabian (Sunnitic) territory. For hour after hour we flew over the Syrian-Arabian desert near the frontier of Saudi-Arabia and Iraq: beneath us yellow, sometimes rather reddish sand, with a network of veins branching out, drawn by occasional streams; no vegetation, no houses, as far as the eye could see. But from the starboard side we could see a broad track which we followed all the time; and once a small black speck was discernible on it, probably a motor-car hurrying westwards. Occasionally smaller tracks crossed the great desert road and were lost in bends between the bare shallow ranges of hills. At last we saw a settlement, a few mud huts in the cheerless desert, with no sign of water or vegetation. Soon afterwards we flew over an oil station with its own runway. Another motor-car on the track. And now pools of oil appeared among the dry sand and stones. Soon after we could see the clear blue sea; we had crossed the Arabian peninsula and were flying along the southern shore of the Persian Gulf; on the right land, sea, and pools of oil interlaced. A town is situated here which has grown rich from oil: Bahrein.

Pakistan

WE HAD TO put our watches forward three hours to get the correct time in Karachi. The loudspeaker announced that we would reach the capital of Pakistan after six o'clock in the evening, and that the weather there was fine—glancing out of the windows at the cloudless blue sky one could not imagine anything else!

We crossed the cape which separates the Persian Gulf from the Gulf of Oman, and came down to a town by the sea, spread out between sand and mud. There was scarcely anything green; it was a desert town with extensive suburbs—if one can call these huts suburbs; when flying low we saw that many of the buildings had not even roofs. Since 1939 Karachi has been developed by the English from a fishing town, to become the great port of the Indus delta. Before the war it had about 300,000 inhabitants; today one and a half million people live there, and the former provincial capital is now the capital of a nation of eighty millions.

How different the Indians are from the Arabs, Jews, and Turks of the Near East. *Karachi* We had imagined ourselves entering a Mohammedan country, and we did indeed pass mosques and see the people at the filling-station engrossed at prayer time regardless of traffic. But the first thing anyone returning to this country notices is the strong unique atmosphere of India; the gazelle-like charm of the fleet-footed crowds in flowing white robes, the soft expression of their eyes. A fiercer facial-type is not unknown: President Mirza-Iskander, the strong man of Pakistan, is one of these—neither are genial pashas—some of these also can be found in the govern-ment ranks. But all share the dreamy gaze of the great Indian family.

Since my last stay thirty-one years ago, Karachi has changed astonishingly little in spite of the fact that its population has increased eight-fold. It is true there are new, many-storeyed office buildings, but no more than in any other European town. The public buildings in the centre, such as the High Court, the parliament buildings, and the technical college are built in late classical English Colonial style; the museum treasures from the Mohenjodaro, Gandhara, and Mogul era, are stored in a Victorian Gothic palace. My hotel stood in 'Victoria Street'—you find English street-names everywhere.

Pakistan is a poor country; the growth of its capital was not planned, people simply flocked to it, among them hundreds of thousands of refugees who left India at the time of the partition in 1947 and who have not yet been absorbed into the economy of the country. For large-scale urban development both money and ideas are obviously lacking—that is, everything needful except people.

The Troubles of a Young Nation

It is worth noting that in the middle of our materialistic century the religious conviction and persuasive power of one man, Mohammed Jinnah, and his friends were able to provide the initiating force of a powerful new State in defiance of all the rules of geography and political economy, an entity that owes its existence solely to the people's confession of faith in the prophet Mohammed. There could be no stronger proof of the power which religion still has today on the Indian sub-continent. Still? Even the Islamic lands have given up many of their old religious customs; Jinnah himself was thoroughly modern, a highly educated lawyer with a distinguished bearing; the women round him wore no veil and took an active part in politics; the sister of the founder of the State is considered to be the most intrepid guardian of his spiritual heritage. Indeed a glance at the map makes us admire the courage with which the men of the Muslim League dared to unite two parts of the country which are almost cut off from each other.

The current problems of Pakistan were apparent after study of Karachi's daily newspapers. I called on the editor of *Dawn*, a morning newspaper founded by Jinnah, to discuss these problems with him. Mr Attaf Husain is probably the most influential journalist in Pakistan, a man sparkling with intelligence and eloquence. What did he think about the corruption that everyone was talking about? It was true, he replied, that there was corruption in the East; in India it was perhaps a little better because there parliamentary control prevented the worst from happening. That was why it was important for Pakistan to choose her own parliament. In Western Pakistan the owners of landed property and the officers were too powerful, but in Eastern Pakistan the elections could not be influenced so easily. The food position was so critical because land reforms could not be carried out properly, for lack of trained men to apply the modern methods for which material was available. As for industrial development, only fifty per cent of capacity was utilised.

A visit to the Parliament showed the effect of the British example. English is spoken for the most part, and the educated classes from the different parts of the country still depend on it for mutual understanding. The Minister of Finance, Amjad Ali, dressed in a European suit with a carnation in his buttonhole, answered questions good-naturedly and seriously; Mr Speaker, a venerable little man with a white beard, chimed in, while to his right and left stood two figures in old-fashioned uniforms testifying to his presidential dignity. The members, some of whom wore turbans and frock-coats, discussed excitedly the formulation of separate motions; the position of East Pakistan inevitably came under discussion. As in every democratic parliament you could feel the mutual antagonisms of the politicians; they addressed their opponents sarcastically as 'my honourable friend', and generally preserved the rules of the game as it is played at Westminster.

The Parliament of Pakistan in Session

In an outlying north-western district of Karachi, on a small hill, is the tomb of the father of the nation, 'Qaid-i-Azam', Mohammed Ali Jinnah (1876–1948).

Jinnah's Tomb and Refugee Settlements

Pages 37-44 KARACHI

37 Unlike the Arabs in the Near East, the Pakistani and Indians were usually quite willing to be photographed.

38 top One of the central points of the 19th-century colonial city is this Victorian Gothic building, built in 1865, and surrounded by public gardens. It is called Frere Hall after Sir Bartle Frere, Chief Commissioner from 1850 to 1859, and now contains a library and the national museum, with important documents of the old Sind civilisation and Gandhara art.

38 below Girls on their way to school—nowadays they are allowed much more freedom than their mothers would have dreamed of. The founders of the Moslem State did not insist upon maintaining the traditional exclusion of women from public life. The girl on the left is wearing the characteristic Punjab dress with wide trousers. On the right there are a motor-cab and a pedicab, which have replaced the rickshaw in most Eastern countries as the cheapest means of transport (*see also page 42 above*).

39 In Karachi only a few mosques remind one that this is the metropolis of a State which owes its existence to the Mohammedan creed. At the hour of prayer, even in the midst of the bustle of the modern city—here, at a filling-station—you see the faithful taking off their shoes, turning towards Mecca, and saying their prayers.

40-41 below The city of Karachi is surrounded by extremely primitive settlements of Mohammedan refugees from the time of the partition of India. This collection of clay and wood huts at the north-east of the city has developed into a separate 'township'.

41 top On the hill above this settlement is the temporary tomb of the 'Qaid-i-Azam', the founder of the State, Mohammed Ali Jinnah. Shoes are taken off before you step on to the shining marble floor.

42 top The view from the long Iron Bridge, which leads to the docks, towards the city, with the domed building of the Port Trust and, beside it, one of the new skyscrapers.

42 below Carts drawn by camels, with their long, easy strides, are still most commonly used for the transport of larger loads.

43 A young boy in the bazaar enjoying a cigarette.

44 A contrast typical of present-day Karachi; wherever there is still an open space in the city refugees have built their hovels—immediately beside the modern flats of the still-small privileged classes.

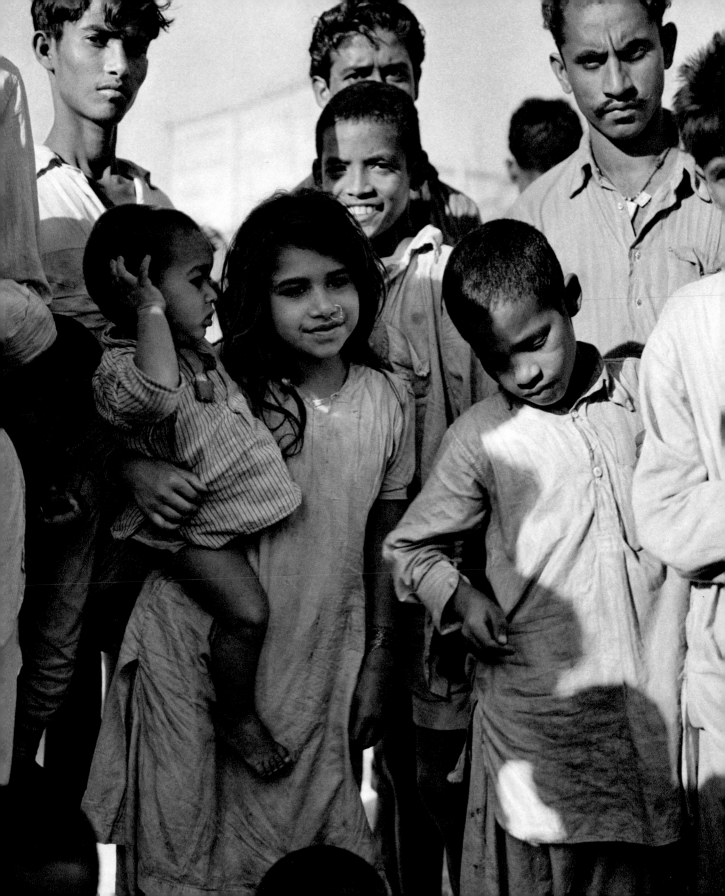

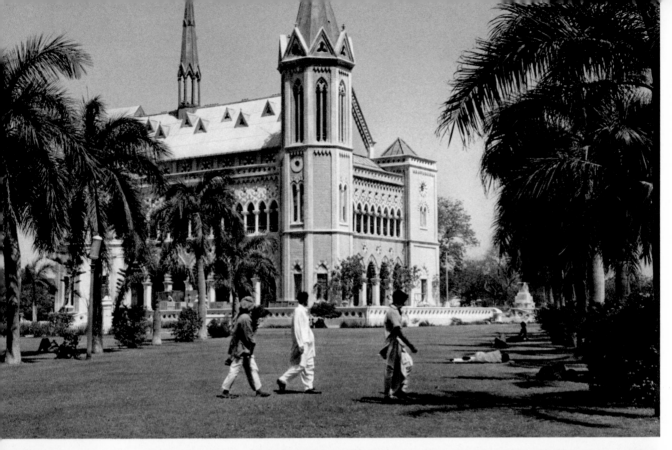

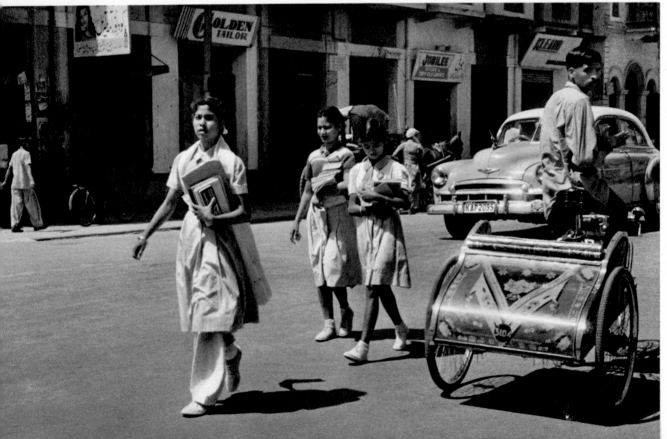

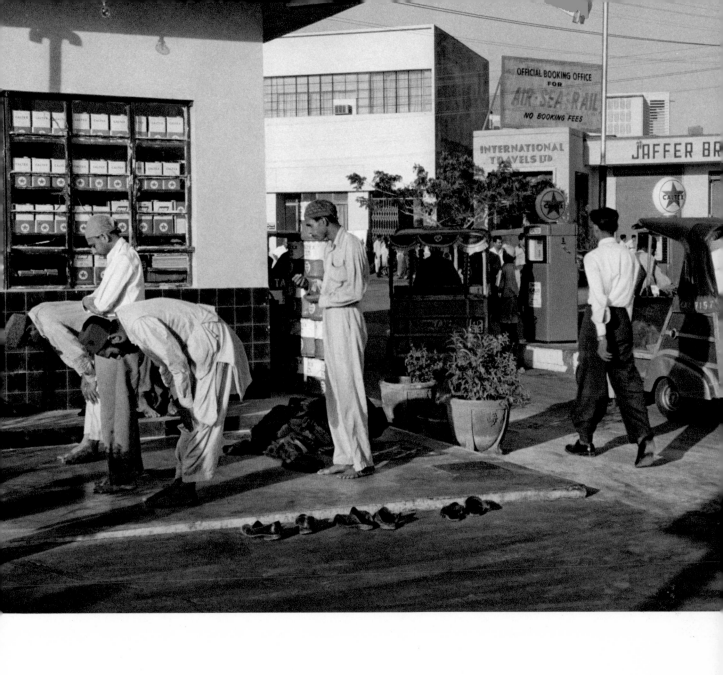

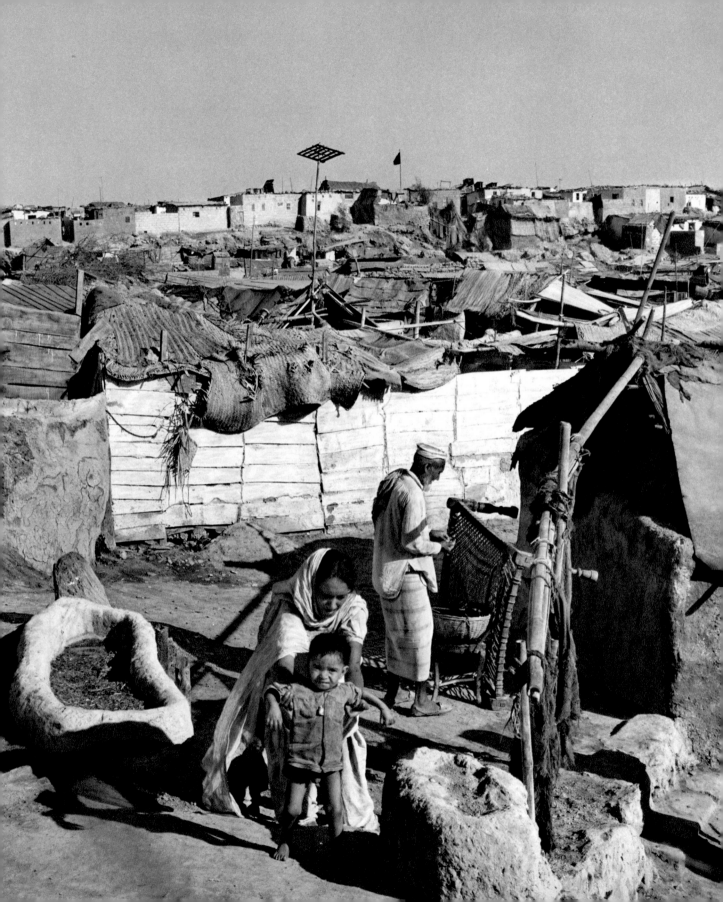

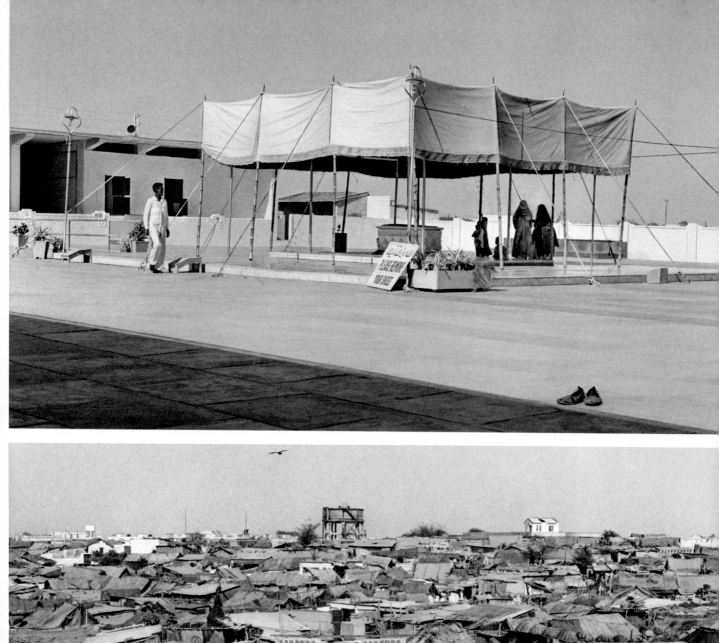
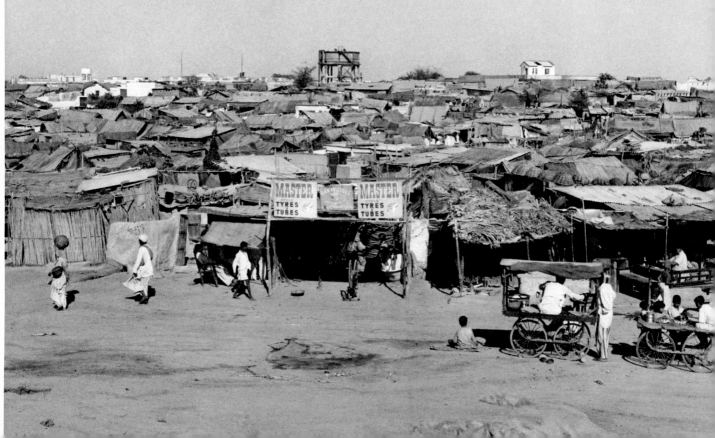

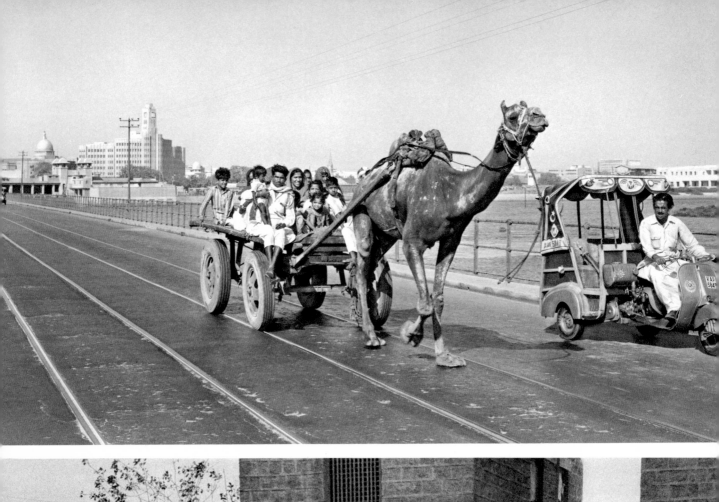
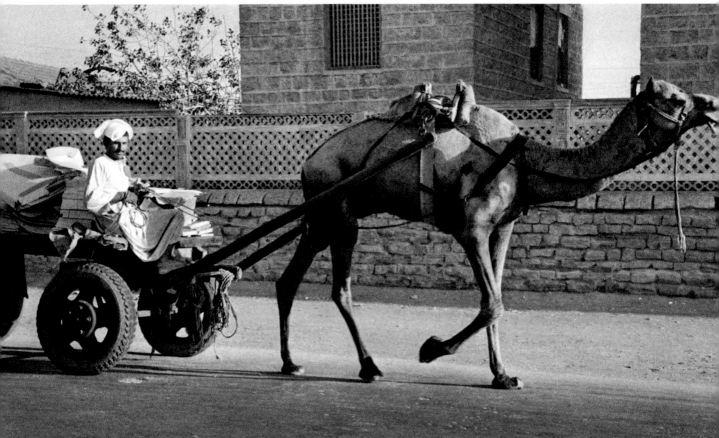

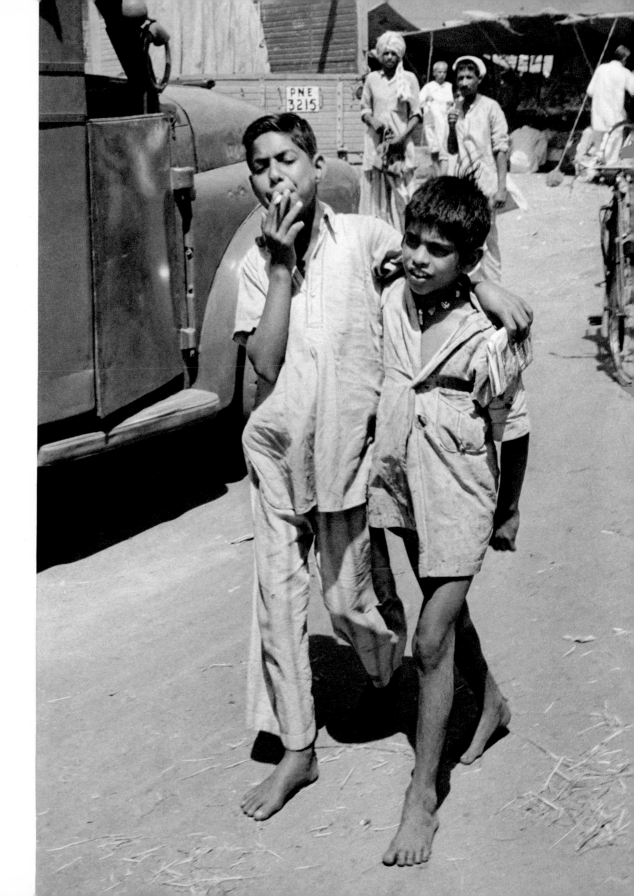

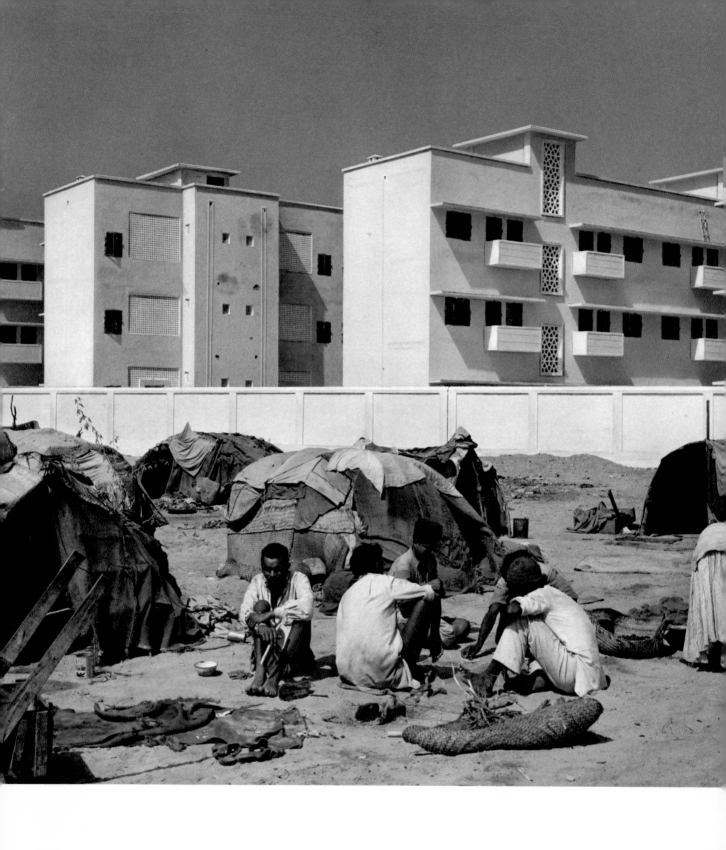

A simple sarcophagus lay under an awning in the centre of a marble platform. The provisional nature of the tomb—it is soon to be replaced by a mausoleum of bold new design—has its own pathos. Near Jinnah's memorial is the tomb of his first Prime Minister, Liaquat Ali Khan (born 1895, assassinated 1951) and next to it the tomb of Sardar Abdur Nishtar.

Looking about this place of remembrance and dedication the visitor is very conscious of the gravity and indeed the tragedy of the situation in which the young nation finds itself after the premature deaths of its two most important leaders. In the valley there lies a town of makeshift mud and wooden huts, where thousands of refugees live and work with their hands, pursue their trades and produce children. And this is not Karachi's only refugee settlement, it is even one of the most comfortable. In other districts farther off they are much more primitive; all degrees of misery are to be found among hundreds of thousands of people driven away from their homeland. More than six million Moslems with few possessions streamed from India to Pakistan when in 1947, on the departure of the British, the quarrels between Moslem and Hindu blazed up anew; and on the other hand some five million Hindus sought a new home in India—many of whom have yet to find it.

India

THE THREE AND A HALF HOUR flight from Karachi to Bombay—by far the shortest single stretch of this East Asian line—took me from one city to another, and it was as if I came from the house of the poor man to that of his rich cousin, from a province into the great world. The customs and passport formalities—which as in other airports were carried out very politely and speedily—reminded us that we were entering a new country.

The Republic of India is, it is true, very far from being a rich country—on the contrary, there is an enormous amount of poverty among the peasants. But there is also a good deal of wealth; an urban middle class of government employees and intellectuals moves along the broad pavements of the towns, and a current of optimism, vitality, and a proud idealism flows everywhere amid Oriental fatalism and dreamy humdrum habit.

Bombay: the Gateway of India   Bombay, the most Westernised city in India, is a trading town developed by the British since the end of the 19th century, on a group of islands, with an ideal natural harbour and huge docks, warehouses, and banks. Here is the chief field of activity of the Parsi, that small but extremely energetic group of disciples of Zoroaster who play a dominant role in the economy of the country, and during the British occupation were pioneers of industrialisation. Thirty years ago Bombay already had a population of one million with an improved, modern administration. The green hills round about free it from the problem of water scarcity, and the fresh sea-breezes make the climate bearable, especially for the favoured inhabitants of the spit of land called Malabar Hill.

The drive from the airport took us eighteen miles through different parts of the town with again and again new glimpses of the sea. On the stretch of country between the port and Back Bay, in wide squares and avenues and surrounded by lawns, rose splendid Victorian buildings; and in the south-west, since my last visit a new district had been built around Church Gate Street. Here my hotel was situated, air-conditioned and very elegantly furnished, but with the utmost economy of space and the first traces of neglect. Close by was the elegant office of Swissair, where at night the passers-by could admire a decorative fresco by Hans Erni on the rear wall of the illuminated room. Then row upon row of concrete blocks, flats, all kinds of offices, a huge new government building, large oil concerns. Some of the best groups of buildings are designed by English and American architects in the style which makes cities uniform all over the world; even the German Democratic Republic has put up its own skyscraper there for its trade mission.

The cows which used to wander about freely, forming an essential part of the Indian street scene, are banned from the centre of Bombay—the English would never have dared to enforce such a measure!—and even the ox-carts and rickshaws had disappeared from my district. Motor-cars rush along the new long white Marine Drive and in the evening people stroll along the broad promenade while the lights of modern comfort shine over the shore.

In the official tourist office an elegant Indian lady presided, very matter-of-fact, an efficient manageress—but when she rose one glimpsed between her short bodice and her skirt the light brown skin of the Ajanta frescoes. I was given a qualified guide to show me round the town—a bespectacled young woman who wore a light freshly laundered *sari* and spoke faultless Oxford English, learnt at her college. We visited different parts of the town by taxi; the hill near Government House where from the parks and gardens you could see the coast and the mass of houses, the 'Gateway of India'—where the resigning Viceroy used once to make way for his successor as he landed, and where, in the poor quarters, the people are herded together in poverty. The spread of industrialisation has increased the flow of people to the city; after the census of 1941 there were one and a half million inhabitants here; today there are said to be three and a half million. Numerous cinemas advertised the latest products of the Indian film industry on enormous posters; today India competes with the United States and Japan as the greatest annual producer of films; many of these, based on legendary as well as realistic material, are shown only for a few days.

In the stores are sold products of individual Indian regions, the local handicrafts—pictures, textiles, metalwork, and carving. Unfortunately these are more reminiscent of the feebler Soviet products or the cuckoo-clocks and wooden bears of the Bernese Oberland than of the magic of mysterious old bazaars and curiosity stalls.

Diplomatic Cocktail-party — I was lucky enough to be invited to one of the many cocktail-parties at which foreigners and prominent Indians meet. Bombay is a dry city and even tourists can indulge in alcohol only by special permission. The splendid ice-cold drinks served at the consulate were therefore all the more enthusiastically appreciated. Old acquaintances turned up who had come up in the world since I had last seen them. An Indian diplomat spoke with mocking wit of his experiences in Peking, about which he had written a book. A lady in a specially magnificent *sari* and with a kind and noble face heard with delight that in the past I had met her and her brother Jawaharlal's father, the Pandit Motilal Nehru. The Swiss Ambassador and representatives of the Basle Chemical Industry were there, celebrating the opening of a new factory.

Industrialisation — The Indian Government is prepared to devote some of its socialist enthusiasm to speeding up the production of goods that until now have had to be imported. The Indians accuse the British rulers of having prevented the formation of a native industry in order to keep the monopoly of this large market for their textile factories in Lancashire; now they must catch up and become economically independent. The foreign capitalist is invited to co-operate in developing new undertakings with his experts, and to provide fifty per cent of the capital. He would receive a share of the profits which he could transfer abroad. But in ten years the industry must be completely in Indian hands with Indian staff. Will this work? After all, industrialisation was not bought or stolen by the Europeans: it is the product of centuries of development; without people like Galileo, Descartes, and Newton there would be no science faculties, for these too are a product of the mind, of the European mind. Can one simply take over the end-product and graft it on to a different kind of society? There is no analogy in world history which helps us to answer that question—the technology which unified the world is something which was never there before; we must first learn how it is to be mastered.

Again and again you hear that it takes two or more Indians to do the work of one European. It is not that the Indian is ungifted—the *élite* dazzles us with its intellect and you find talents here of the most varied kind. But they base their economic reconstruction, and indeed the whole life of the nation on European ideas. The Indians are prudent enough not to lay all the blame on foreigners but to be self-critical. The efficiency of European versus Indian workers is openly discussed in the newspapers; bonus schemes are introduced to improve output.

Taking Over from the Europeans

The Hindustani Machine Tools Factory in Bangalore was constructed with the help of the firm of Bührle at Oerlikon near Zürich; in the first period (1955) the output of a Swiss worker was four times that of an Indian worker. The introduction of higher bonuses for production has now had such good results (writes *The Statesman* in Delhi) that a ratio of 1 to 1·7 between the Indian and Swiss worker has been reached; indeed a few picked workers from Bangalore (on a kind of Indian *stakhanovite* system) almost equalled the average individual production at Oerlikon. Nehru has claimed that: 'As long as the factory was controlled by foreign [i.e. Swiss] experts, nothing good came of it; but since the foreigners have gone and some of our capable people have taken command, astonishing progress has been made.' If this is true, then since my visit an amazing change must have taken place in India and my opinion of the efficiency and character of the people will need to be revised.

Flight from Bombay to Delhi   The Indian airlines as well as the great network of railways were at our disposal to cover the wide stretches of the subcontinent between Adams Bridge and the Himalayas. A 'Viscount' brought us to the capital of India in two and a half hours, during which time we were looked after by two young Indian women in graceful, colourful clothing.

The desert stretches far inland and threatens to overwhelm the country until the main period of the monsoon makes the fields green and fills the temple and village pools again. It was the period of drought and the country below us was yellow

Pages 51–54   BOMBAY AND ELEPHANTA

51   On the small island of Elephanta in the Bay of Bombay seven cave temples were hewn out of the rock, probably about the middle of the 8th century. The largest is dominated by the colossal Trimurti, one of the most imposing Hindu works of art. The group, twenty feet high, represents Shiva, prince of the gods, in a three-fold statue as Brahma the creator (centre), Rudra the destroyer (left), and Vishnu the preserver.

52   In the busy city streets.

53 top   From the promenade of Marine Drive, where people stroll in the evening, you can see ships lying at anchor in Back Bay.

53 below   To the north of the city high, modern office blocks and tenements extend farther and farther towards the tongue of land called Colaba.

54   A large public laundry.

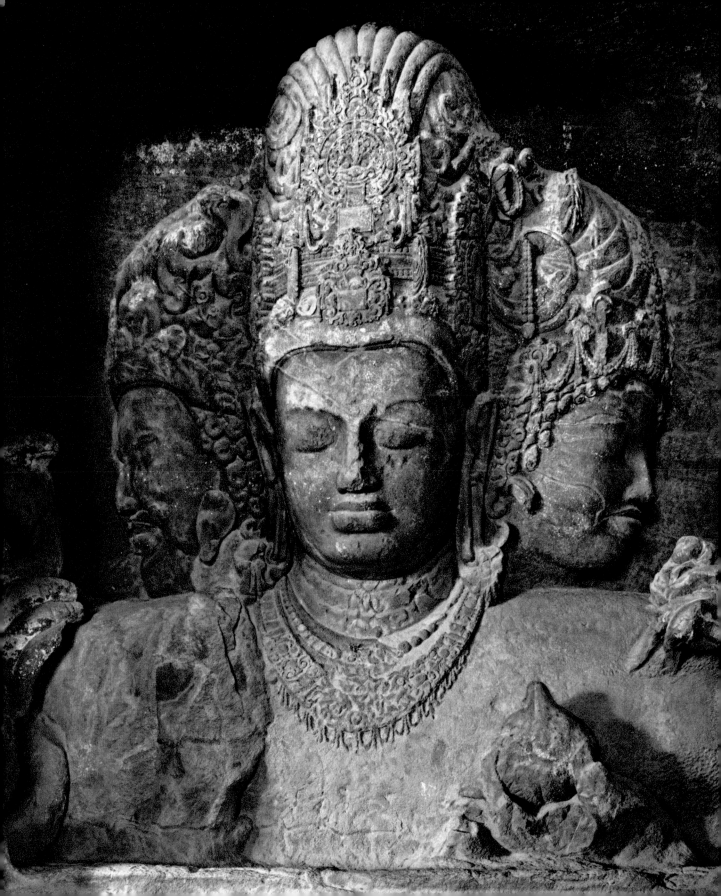

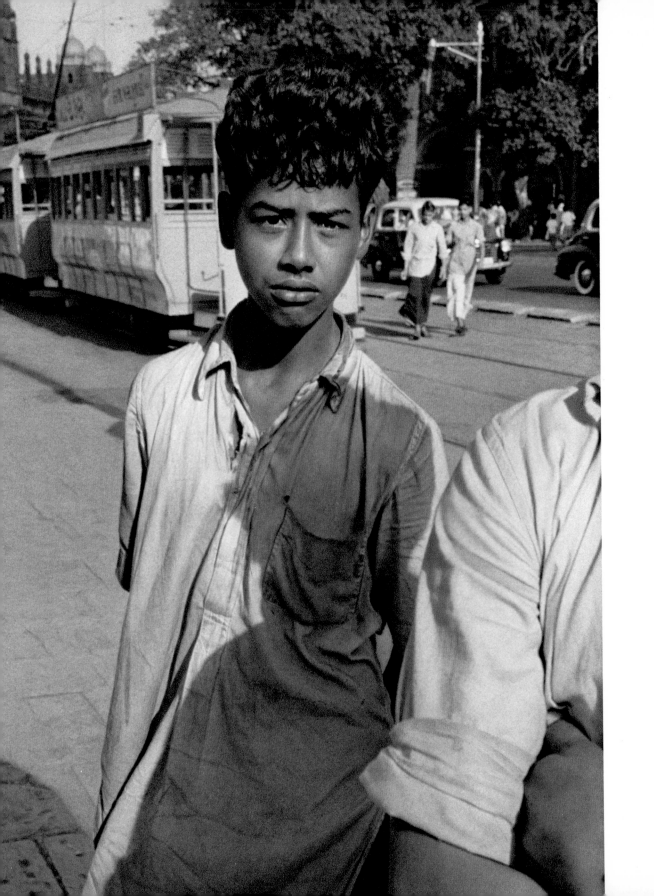

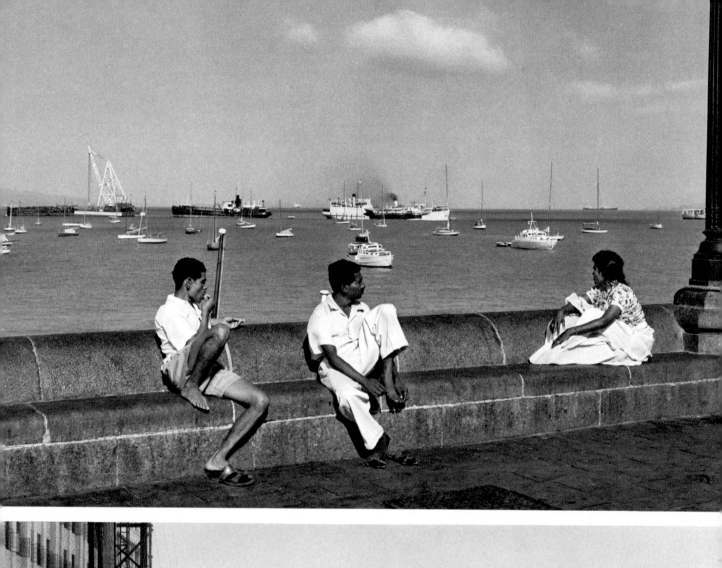
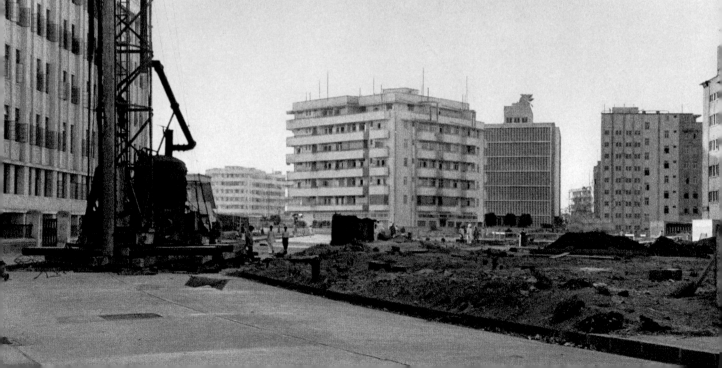

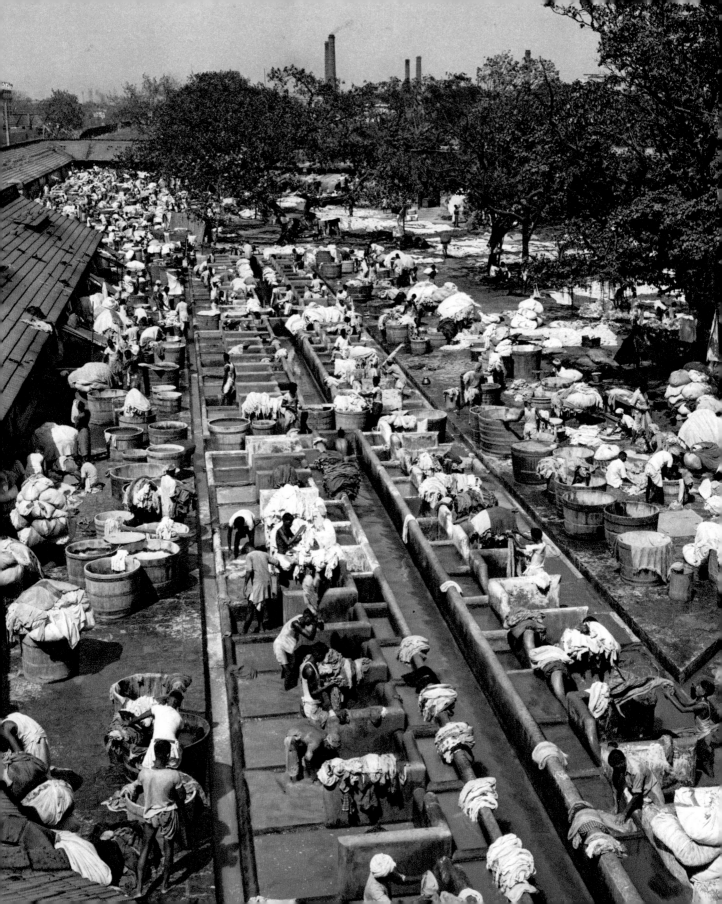

and parched, with dried-up river-beds, bare mountain ranges, and here and there a village. About half-way between Bombay and Delhi it became more densely populated; two small reservoirs appeared between the slopes, and straight across the valley and mountains ran strange thin lines as if someone had covered the land with fine pen-strokes, or as if forces from inside the earth had made the surface tremble.

The city, lying like a throne in the north of the country, with the upper course *The Three Towns* of the sacred rivers and the Himalayas behind it and the huge triangle of the *of Delhi* Deccan in front, has been the residence of many of the mightiest rulers of India. The Ashoka pillars recall the rule of the Buddhist apostle Emperor in the 3rd century B.C., and the city of 'Indraprastha', described in the Mahabharata as the seat of the Pandavas kings, is said to have been there. The oldest preserved buildings date back to Hindu princes of the Middle Ages; but Delhi became important as a place of residence only with the Mohammedan conquerors who, in the footsteps of Alexander the Great, again and again penetrated from the north-west into the Indus and Ganges regions. Scattered over twelve miles lie the ruins of the fortresses, palaces, mosques, and tombs erected by these powerful warriors.

Kutb-ud-din and his son-in-law and successor Altamsh built the 200 foot high *Old Delhi* tower of Qutb Minar in Lalkot, inscribed with texts from the Koran, in about 1200. The mosque Kussat-ul-Islam, begun by them, was completed about 1300 by Ala-ud-din of the Khalji dynasty. The founder of the Tughlak dynasty, Chias-ud-din (1320-5), had a domed castle erected as a tomb near the mighty walls of the fortress of Tughlakabad; another Tughlak, Firoz Shah (1351-88), moved the citadel to Firozabad. In the days of Humayun, the second Mogul ruler of India, the walls, battlements, and gates of Purana Kila were built; his more

important rival the Afghan Emperor Sher Shah (1540–5) built there the decorative mosque of Kila Kona.

Delhi during the   Delhi proper is the capital of the later Mogul emperors, situated to the north of
Mogul Period   the fields of ruins; it was founded by Shah Jahan in 1637, and the palaces and
gardens inside the red walls of the fort and the great mosque date back to him—a
group of red sandstone and white marble buildings which are among the finest
examples of Islamic architecture. Here, in 1857, lived the ninety year old shadow-
Emperor Bahadur when the great Indian Mutiny broke out, and the rebels were
for a short time buoyed up with false hopes of an independent India with the great
Mogul at its head. In 1877 Disraeli had his queen proclaimed Empress of India
in this historic place.

Delhi as the Residence   When I stayed in Delhi in 1927 the population was almost as much Moham-
of the Viceroy   medan as Hindu. At the great Friday prayer-meeting the broad courtyard of
Jami Masjid was filled with believers kneeling together. You felt that you were
in an Islamic stronghold, and no one then imagined that India was to be divided.

But at that time Delhi was also a stronghold of British power. Between the
Ajmir Gate and the domed Tomb of Safdar Jang, where in the 18th century the
Maharaja-astronomer Jai Singh II of Jaipur had erected one of his observatories
—buildings reminiscent of Cubist sculpture, English town-planners and architects laid out 'New Delhi', with great avenues, squares, and a shopping centre, on
the typical English plan—and the crowning group of government buildings with
the Viceroy's palace. In 1927 the work was incomplete; the dome over the residence
of the all-powerful Proconsul had not yet been built, but both the government
office buildings were almost finished. The round, pillared Parliament building had
just been opened, and under the shadow of the Viceroy's right of veto quite a
spirited parliamentary life was emerging. In one of the new small whitewashed

villas of Members of Parliament I met the great Conservative Hindu leader Pandit Malavia and his friend Birla, the manufacturer who founded a magnificent Vishnu temple for the new town. Inaccessible to ordinary mortals lived the representative of His Britannic Majesty, guarded by tall Sikhs in splendid uniforms. Very occasionally His Excellency, wearing a sun-helmet and a long grey frock-coat, might be glimpsed at the races, or perhaps at some garden-party.

Their parliamentary pupils became fully fledged more quickly than the founders of New Delhi suspected; and after the Delhi of the great Mohammedan Moguls and of the English Viceroys the Indian Delhi finally took shape, the seat of the central authorities of the Federal Republic, filled with the dynamism of the first purely Indian State for more than a thousand years, and one of the political and spiritual centres of our times.

In 1958 I stayed at an enormous palace of a hotel, architecturally a combination *At the Ashoka Hotel* of a modern skyscraper and the palace of a Rajputani prince. It was built with government money for the 1956 UNESCO Conference and named after the great Emperor Ashoka, who is often referred to because he represented an Indian dynasty. This was the Ashoka Hotel in New Delhi, 'the most comfortable and sumptuous in the East'. The Swiss manager who had formerly seen to its comforts had already been replaced by an Indian. All the rooms were air-conditioned and had refrigerators for alcoholic and other drinks: in Delhi no alcohol is served in public, but except on Thursdays and Fridays you can take drink to your room, including beer brewed in India. The spacious halls of the hotel had thick carpets and comfortable arm-chairs; in the greenish-blue swimming-pool genuine and imitation film-stars were splashing about.

The dining-room was interesting; a large mural depicted an Indian sky, where Rama and Sita were enthroned in the midst of a host of heavenly musicians; on a platform beneath a live orchestra had taken up its position: in the front the players of picturesque old Indian instruments with long necks, at the back the members of a European *salon* orchestra. They played a kind of Indian light music with a European touch, an obviously new *genre* with a delicate sound all its own. Old favourites like Viennese waltzes, although faultlessly played, still had something of the sleepy singsong rhythm of the East. The audience was made up of much the same kind of people as you meet travelling by air and was certainly quite different from that of previous decades: there were sometimes parties of European tourists but the majority were representatives (half of them Asian) of various organisations: of governments, commercial combines, unions; delegates to peace and other congresses; turbaned Sikhs, almost black-skinned Dravidians, Singhalese, Burmese, Indonesians, and mysterious Chinese who might equally well have been capitalists from Singapore or commissars from Peking. The Prime Minister of Rumania was also in Delhi at the time—he looked exactly like a Prime Minister of Luxembourg or Norway and was received just as warmly with the same words and handshakes.

The Ashoka Hotel stands in the new diplomatic quarter, which was only just being built. The modern American Embassy was still under construction, and at that time there were mainly open fields round about, in which here and there between the new buildings one of the old tombs or a ruin or a poor hut appeared.

Page 59 AGRA
The Taj Mahal seen from the entrance-gate (*see also Page 89*).

Pages 60–61 OLD DELHI
The triumphal tower Qutb Minar dates from the time of the first Mohammedan rulers who lived in Delhi; on the ground floor is inscribed the name of Kutb-ud-din (1206–10), on the upper floors that of Altamsh (1211–35); in 1368 Firoz Shah Tughlak added the marble to the upper parts and crowned the whole with a dome which was destroyed by an earthquake in 1803. The huge red sandstone tower, richly decorated with inscriptions, is now about 230 feet high.

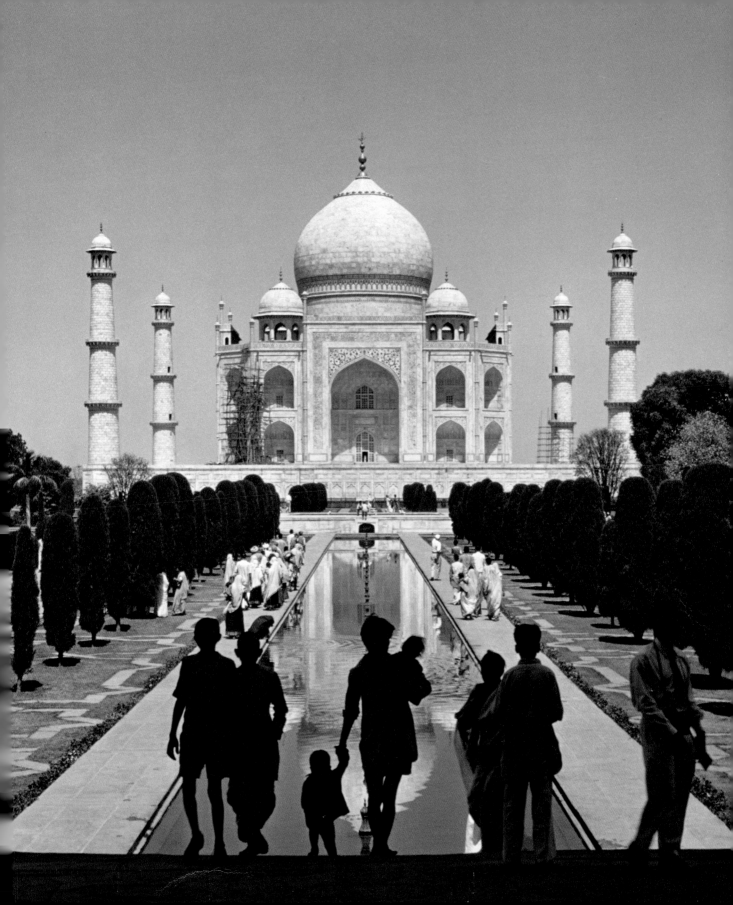

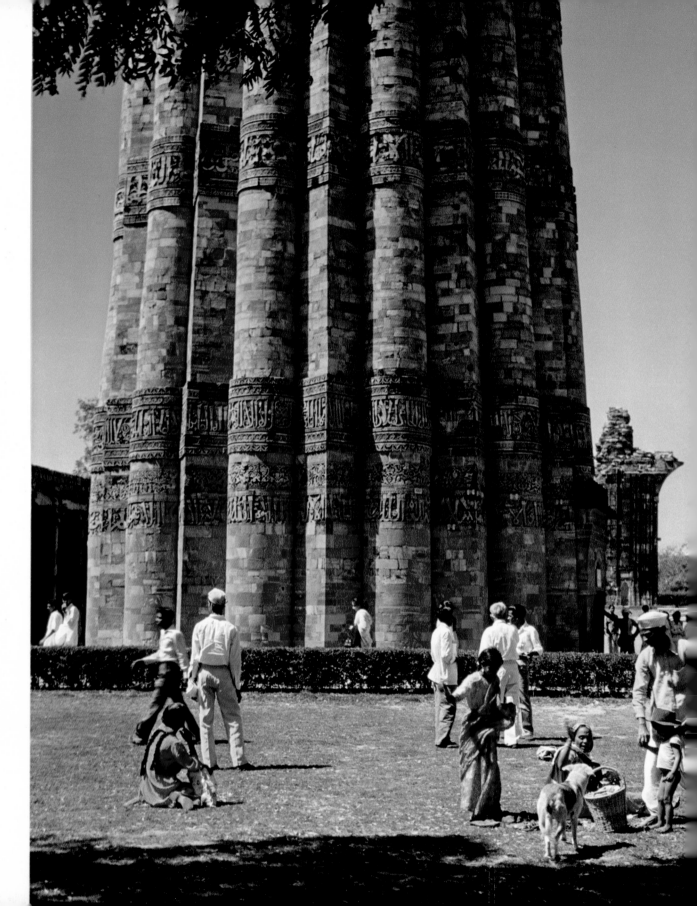

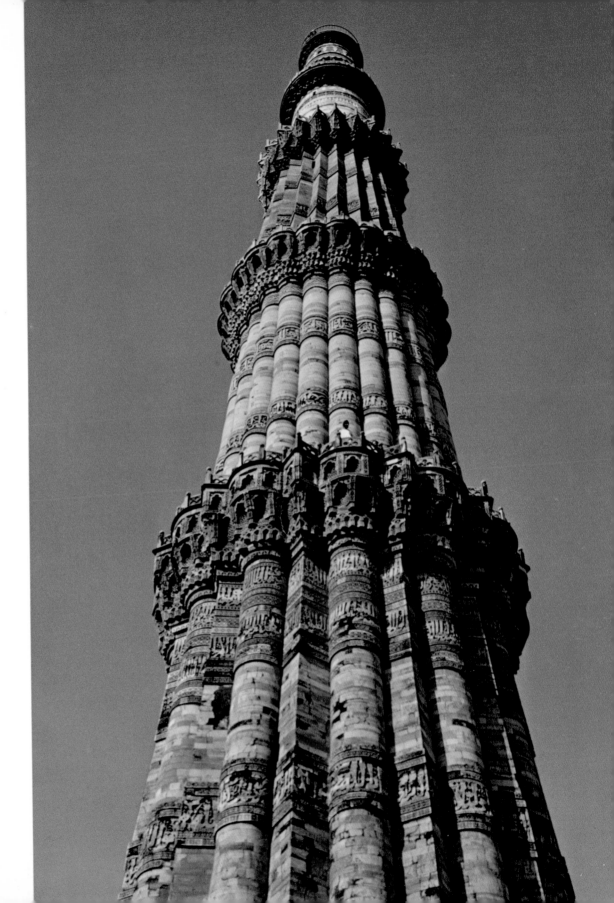

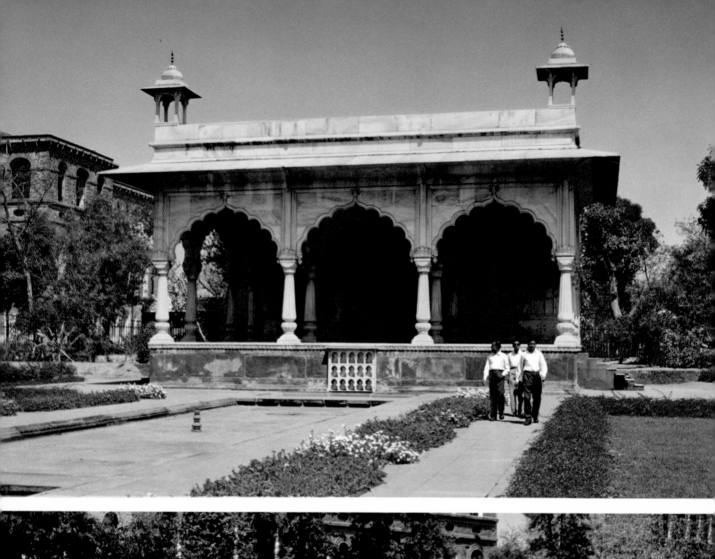
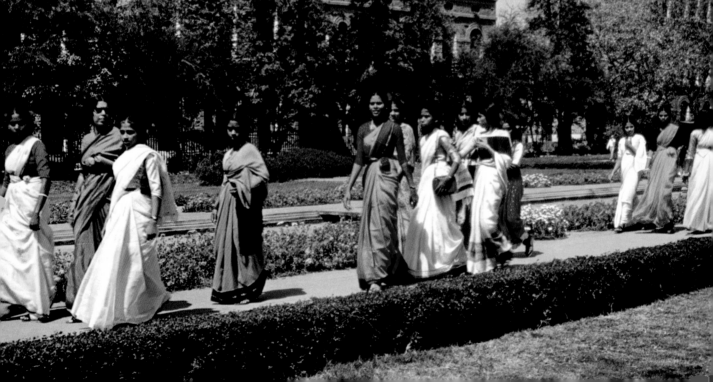

A distinguished small white *palazzo* could be identified by the papal coat of arms on the gable as the seat of the Nuncio.

Of all the places which I revisited after a long interval none had changed quite so much as Delhi. For technological civilisation had marched on, as in every large city, with its asphalt surfaces and traffic signals; and although the size of its population was far below that of Calcutta and Bombay, it formed a real centre of these two most numerous peoples of the globe united in one State. Here various aspects of past and present were sharply confronted; the problems of India and of our time were manifested in the towns and villages which formed Delhi, and we met all this too in these fascinating people who had broken out of their former dreaminess, and were making fiery speeches, carrying on profitable businesses, and were full of concern and bold ideas. I will try here to sum up my impressions of a week's stay and sketch a hasty circular tour of the town.

A Circular Tour of the Indian Capital

At the Viceroy's palace, which is now the official residence of the President of the Republic, we met a procession of the guard, mounted, wearing brilliant red uniforms and armed with lances. On the ground floor, a museum had been built round the central hall, exhibiting magnificent examples of Indian sculpture from other parts of the country—particularly from the district of Muttra which is rich in Buddhist finds. The importance of the palace was emphasised by an order prohibiting photographs of any part of it, but permission from the Embassy not

Page 62 DELHI FORT

In 1639 Shah Jahan erected the Red Fort in Delhi, which had been neglected by his two predecessors, and had the imperial residence built, with its gardens, courtyards, State-rooms, and pavilions. The Hayat Bakhsh (life-giving garden) with the white marble Bhadon pavilion is thronged with crowds of visitors, for the most part from the schools and offices of the capital.

only removed this obstacle but also gave me the opportunity to visit the State-rooms on the first floor.

There were mirrors, wood-carvings, carpets, and precious ornaments in plenty, many of them gifts from the wealthiest maharajas; the splendour of the European New-Renaissance period was combined with the magnificence of the Indian princes; on the walls of the long banqueting hall hung golden-framed portraits of viceroys wearing the Order of the Garter. As we prepared to go into the Mogul garden, laid out with colourful flower-beds at the back of the palace, the President, Dr Rajendra Prasad, wearing the white Gandhi cap, went by accompanied by two men.

With its red sandstone and commanding white dome the palace was reminiscent of Mogul architecture; it is not without dignity. Less imposing were the two large adjoining symmetrical buildings of the secretariat, which flanked the broad

Pages 65–68 DELHI

65 From the square in front of the Red Fort one steps on to the broad street Chandni Chauk, the main street of the city.

66 top Indra Chauk (formerly Connaught Circus), with its neo-Classical buildings on the London model, is the centre of the commercial district of New Delhi.

66 below The Parliament buildings were opened on 18th January 1927, four years before New Delhi became the place of residence of the Viceroy. The architect, Sir Herbert Baker, combined a neo-Classical colonnade with elements of Indian architectural style at the main entrance and in the windows.

67 Rajghat, the place where Gandhi was cremated after his assassination, is for the Indian a shrine where he walks barefoot to affirm his affection for and gratitude to the Mahatma with gifts of flowers.

68 top One of the capital's imposing buildings, the Ashoka Hotel. This was built at government expense to the south of the government buildings, in a district where new diplomatic quarters are springing up.

68 below The Congress building, Vigyan Bhawan, is one of the new structures in New Delhi in which Indian architects are successfully developing their own architectural style. The first important event here was the meeting of UNESCO in 1956.

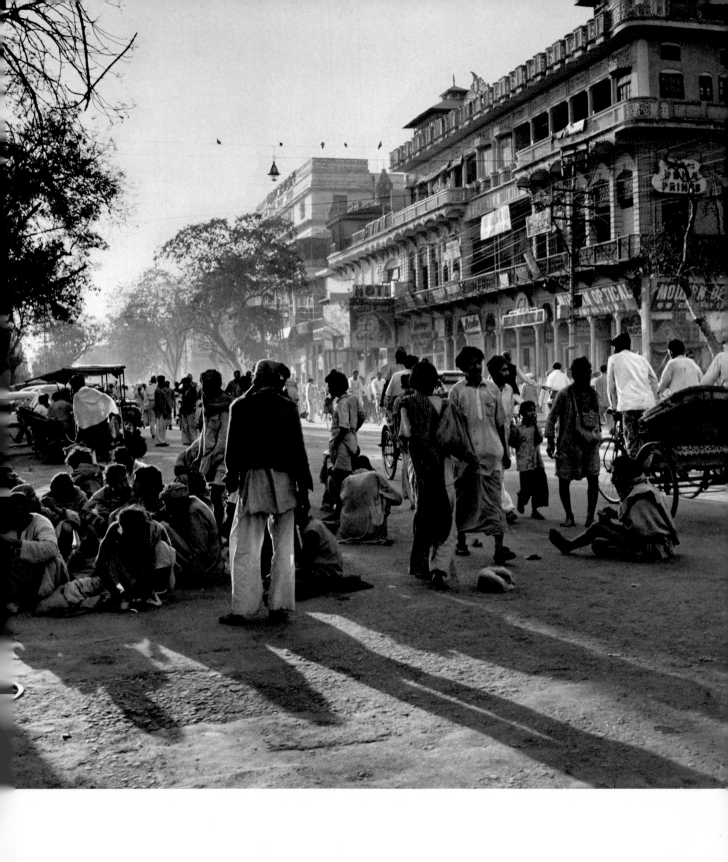

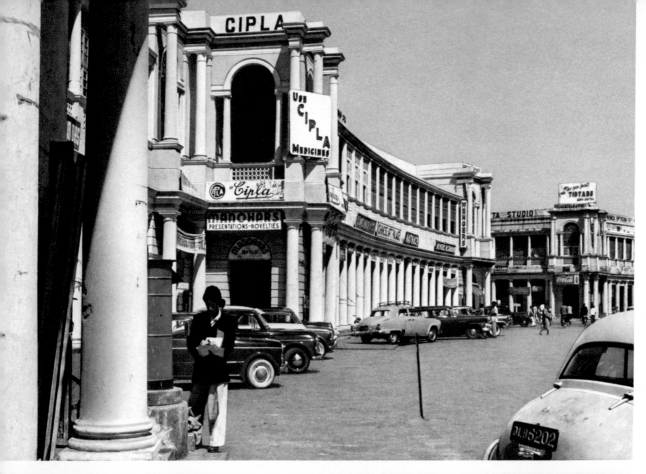

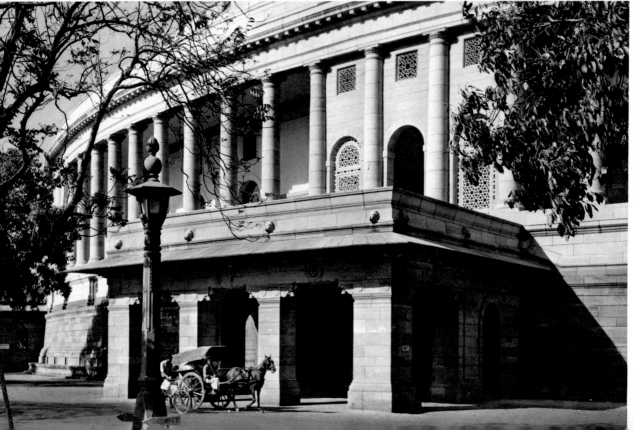

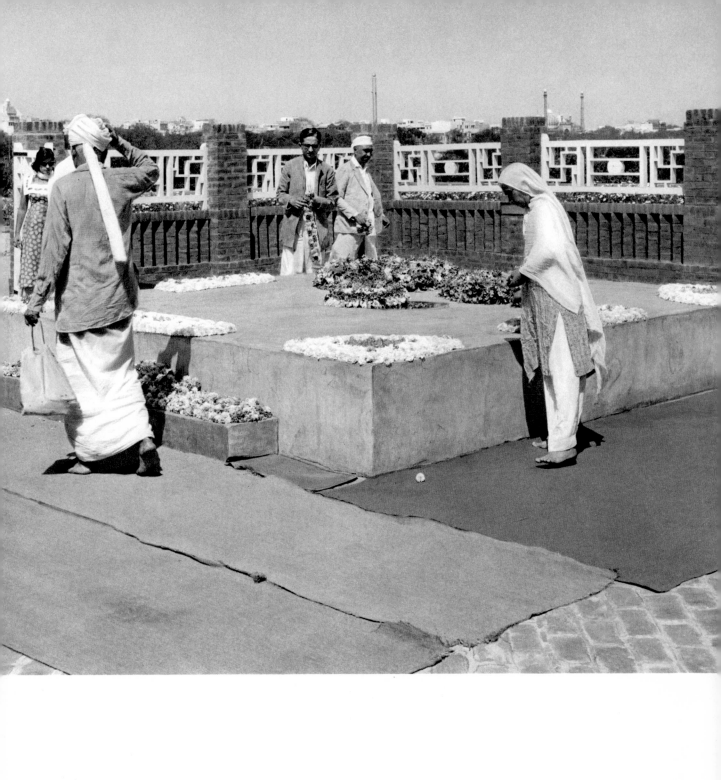

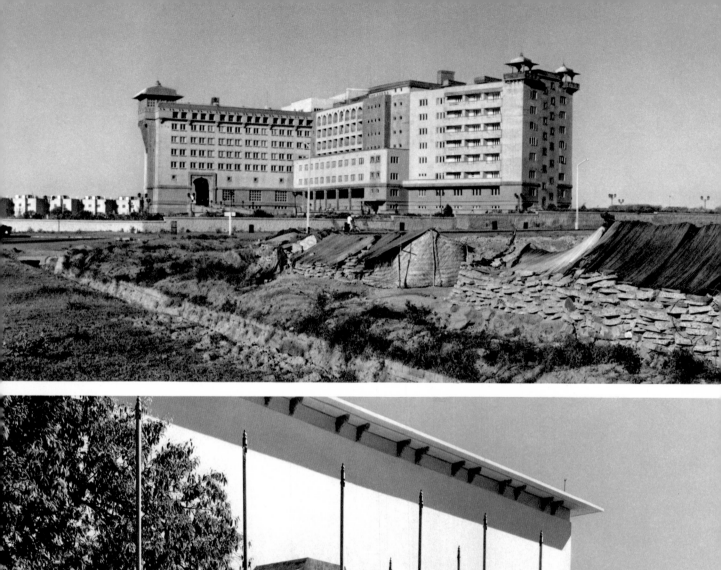

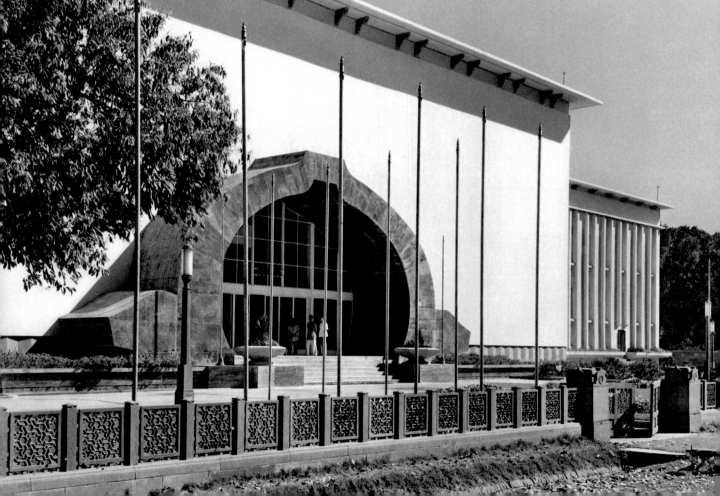

eastern entrance. The axis extended several miles eastwards—on the lawns to the right and left were the recently constructed buildings of two Ministries—and ended with the great white triumphal arch of the war memorial and the George V monument. Under a stone canopy stood the Emperor, with crown and sceptre and a train several yards long hanging down over the pedestal. The Indians, like the Pakistanis, were in no particular hurry to celebrate their 'seizure of power' by blotting out memories of their former masters; they apparently believed that there was still enough time to do that. Thus there are still today in New Delhi, Queen Victoria Road, Wellesley Road, Lady Willingdon Park and so on.

I also visited the parliament building adjoining the secretariats. Its division into Chamber of Princes, Council of State, and Legislative Assembly had, of course, lost its former meaning since the abolition of the Chamber of Princes. In the assembly which meets now, the Speaker no longer wears a wig and the English secretaries on the government bench have made way for the former opposition, but otherwise nothing has changed much in thirty-one years. If nothing specially interesting was going on there were fewer members present than visitors. The debates are still carried on in English when it is important that all the representatives, speaking different languages, should be able to understand. (This was already the case with the meetings of the National Congress in the 'twenties. The speeches were given in Hindi, Bengali, Tamil, and so forth, but the transactions of the Commissions were carried out in English.) A gentleman was reading an apparently dull speech in Hindi, to which no one seemed to listen. An elderly man in long white coat and puttees, and with a carnation in his button-hole, sat down in the empty first row, examined a sheaf of documents and left without having given the speaker a single glance: it was the Prime Minister. When the Hindi speech was finally over even the speaker left the room without showing any interest in the wisdom of the speech following. But perhaps this happens in the parliaments of other countries too.

The activity of the new town was concentrated round Connaught Place (now named Indra Chauk). Crowds of civil servants would leave their offices (built in London Classicist style and richly decorated with posters) in the evening and go home to one of the new housing estates. Elegant restaurants and shops of every kind offered the amenities of a comfortable way of life, but on closer inspection one or two small deficiencies could be found in the picture. For example, in Delhi there were excellent newspapers and magazines in English, but I could find no useful guide-book to the town and the wealth of its monuments; there was no town plan half as good as the 1914 Indian *Baedeker*: foreign newspapers were almost unobtainable, and even in our luxurious hotel they had to explain in the

Pages 71–73 NEW DELHI

71 Birla Mandir was built by Jugal Kishore Birla, one of the leading industrialists in India, in honour of the deity Lakshmi Narayan, and it is open to Hindus of all creeds and castes. The architecture follows the style of the famous medieval shrines in Bhubaneswar (Orissa).

72 top On the hill of Raisina, Rashtrapati Bhavan, built by Sir Edwin Lutyens as the Viceroy's palace, forms the western end of the axis which leads past the government buildings to the war memorial. The red and white of the sandstone is reminiscent of the colouring of Mogul buildings. The roof of the central dome is of copper. Nowadays the central reception-rooms on the ground floor are used as a museum of Indian—especially Buddhist—art.

72 below From the first floor of the Presidential palace you look over the carefully tended gardens, laid out in the style of the Mogul parks.

73 top With drums beating, the guard of the Head of the State passes one of the corner towers of the walls surrounding the grounds of the Presidential palace.

73 below The buildings of the Secretariat and the Presidential palace, designed by Sir Herbert Baker, form the heart of the capital of the British-Indian Empire. The coming and going of officials from the surrounding Ministries forms the lively foreground reflected in the ornamental pools.

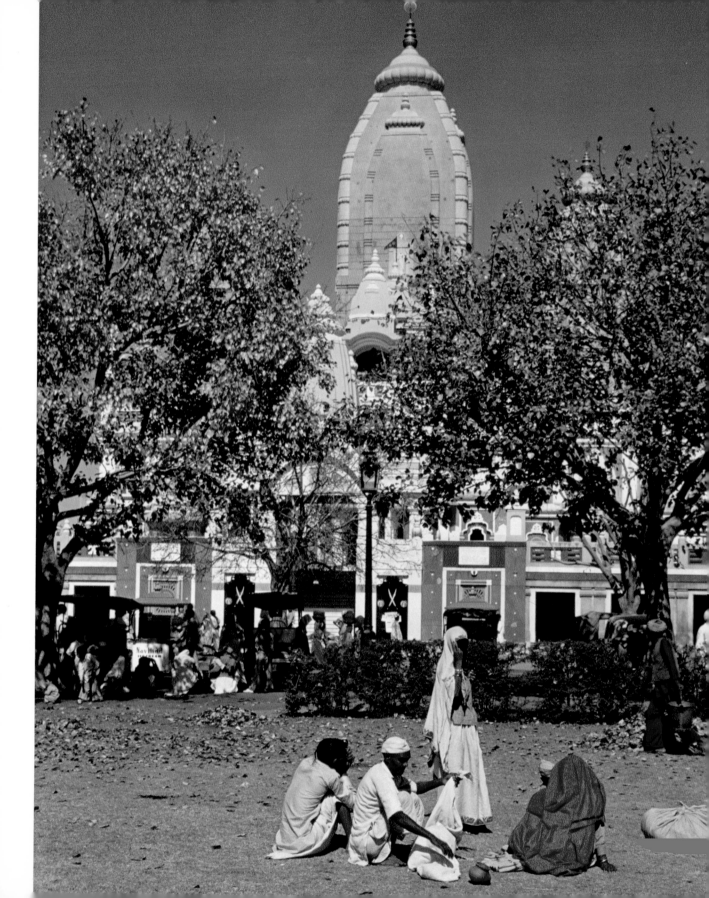

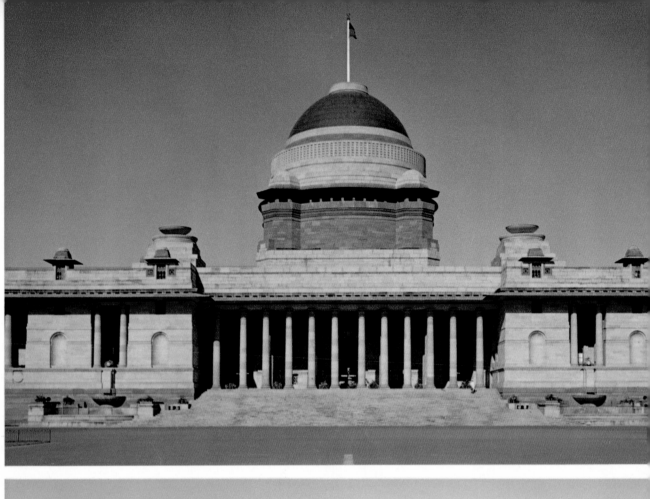

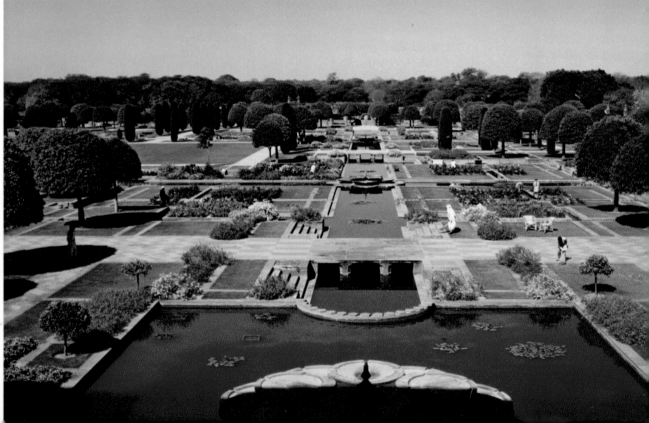

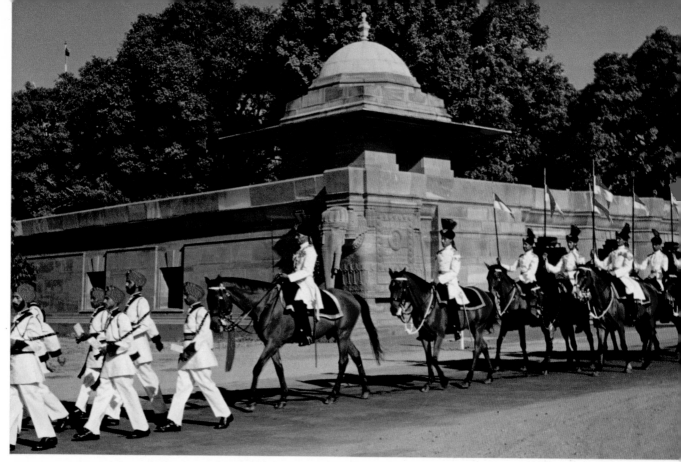

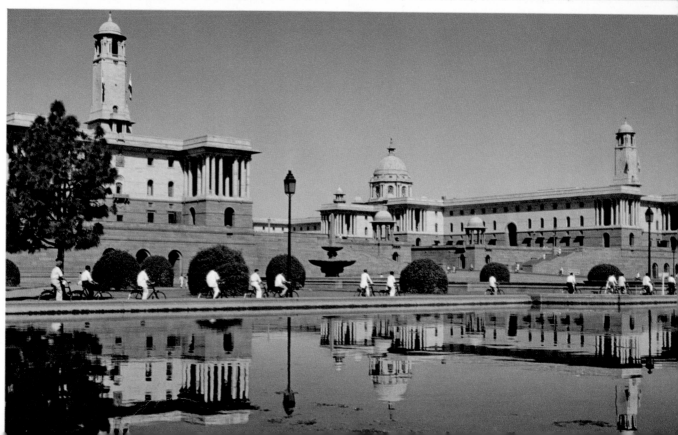

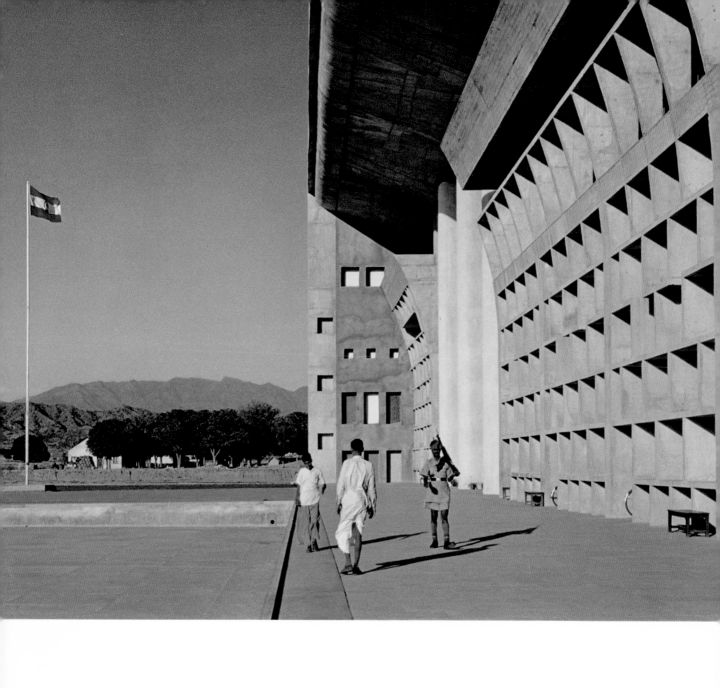

camera shop that Ektachrome films were unobtainable—for there was no foreign currency for these and other things.

Through one of the old gates I went out of the city of civil servants into the 'real' Delhi. Here trade went on as in the past; the street was filled with two-wheeled ox-carts, fast 'pedicabs' (pedal-propelled rickshaws), *tongas* drawn by ponies; sacred cows wandering around; women, seldom seen in New Delhi, thronged the streets of the bazaars; steam drifted from kitchens; children ran about on their way from school. Sometimes in the bustle you still met the solitary Sadhu, proclaiming the eternal Hindu message of renunciation. The court of the great marble mosque, though still used for worship, had become rather quiet. The Sikh temple, Gurdwara Sisanj, in the historic street Chandni Chauk, had a much livelier congregation. Here in 1675 Teg Bahadur, the ninth Guru of the Sikhs, suffered a martyr's death. On the pavement stood a marble well, in which the faithful washed their hands and feet before climbing the steps of the shrine past the huge bearded gatekeeper.

On our circular tour we have seen the Delhi now in ruins, the new official Delhi, and the Delhi of the people; but the picture would be incomplete without some mention of the Delhi of poverty, the refugees and casteless. Like Karachi, Delhi has its homeless—not as many and there is not the same degree of poverty, but the individual fates of those affected by the separation of the States are not less hard in Delhi than in Karachi. Their presence there in the affluent surroundings of an industrious bureaucracy is a constant reminder of how much there is still to do to lead such a huge community out of lethargy and fatalism into joyful creative work—or should I say: out of the hope for the blissful beyond into the illusions of paradise on this earth?

Page 74 CHANDIGARH
The west front of the Palace of Justice designed by Le Corbusier, looking towards the Siwalik mountains.

On the Jumna river which flows past the eastern part of the city is Rajghat, the place where Mahatma Gandhi, the father of the Indian nation, was cremated according to Hindi custom after his assassination by one of his countrymen (on 30th January 1948). A path through a garden led to a low platform, where shoes were taken off as in holy places throughout the whole of the East. There was a quiet coming and going there, a reverent greeting with folded hands, and the flowers of great and small fell on the monument.

The Buildings of the Mogul Period

The fabulous Mogul Age buildings of red sandstone and beautifully veined marble, surrounded by the luxuriant blossom of their gardens and mirrored in the canals and lakes, are curiously remote from the realities of Western Europe. We imagine them peopled with the figures from the delightful pictures of the miniature-painters—the turbaned nobles, beautiful women, groups of musicians in the moonlight, parties riding to hunt tigers on elephant-back, groups of jewel-encrusted courtiers surrounding the *padi-shah*, high enthroned, at the great Durbar. This was the ultimate refinement of the court art developed in Persia and carefully screened from its background of the hungry millions in their miserable hovels, gathering up their last strength for pilgrimages to the holy places, which alone linked them to the great family of Indian peoples despite all differences of race and language.

Pages 77–79 NEW DELHI

77 In Parliament Street between the Parliament buildings and Connaught Place, new buildings are constantly going up. The scaffolding is made of wood in the traditional manner, but the façades of concrete and imitation stone could be in any city in the world.

78 Delhi, too, still has its refugee settlements dating from the partition.

79 In the new generation growing up—at least in cities like Delhi—India's illiteracy has been overcome.

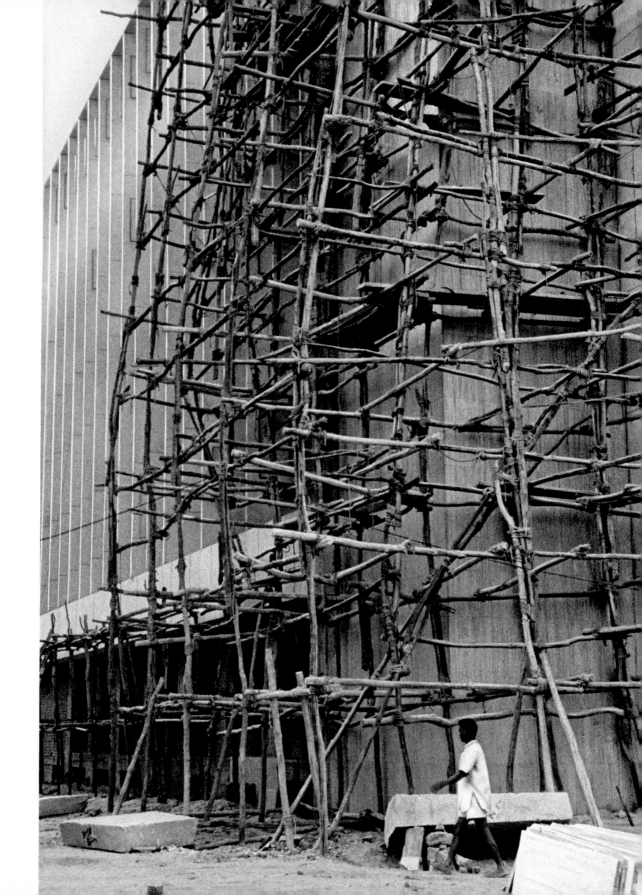

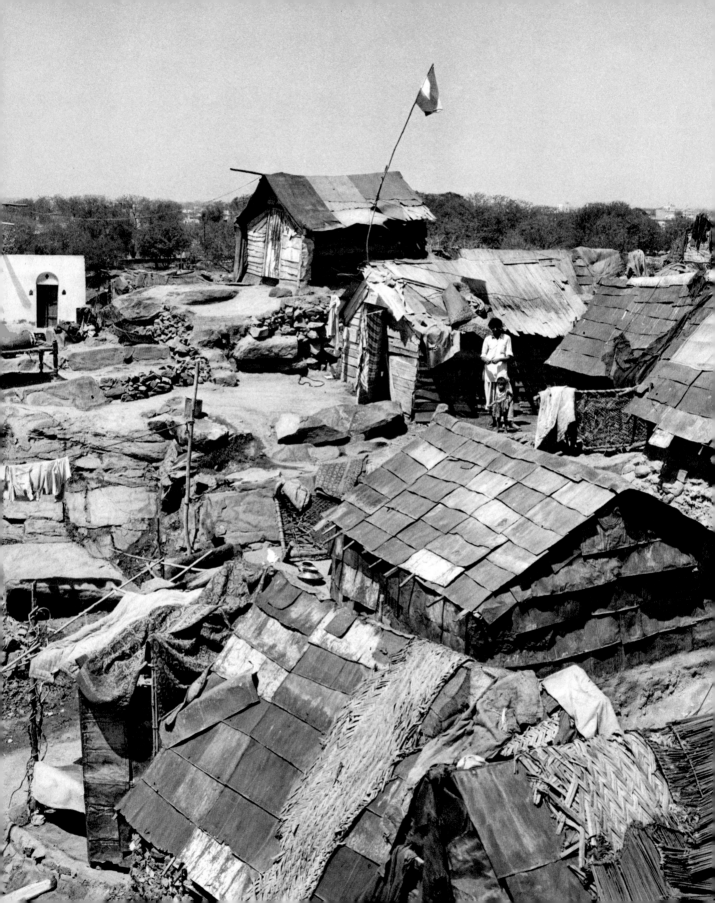

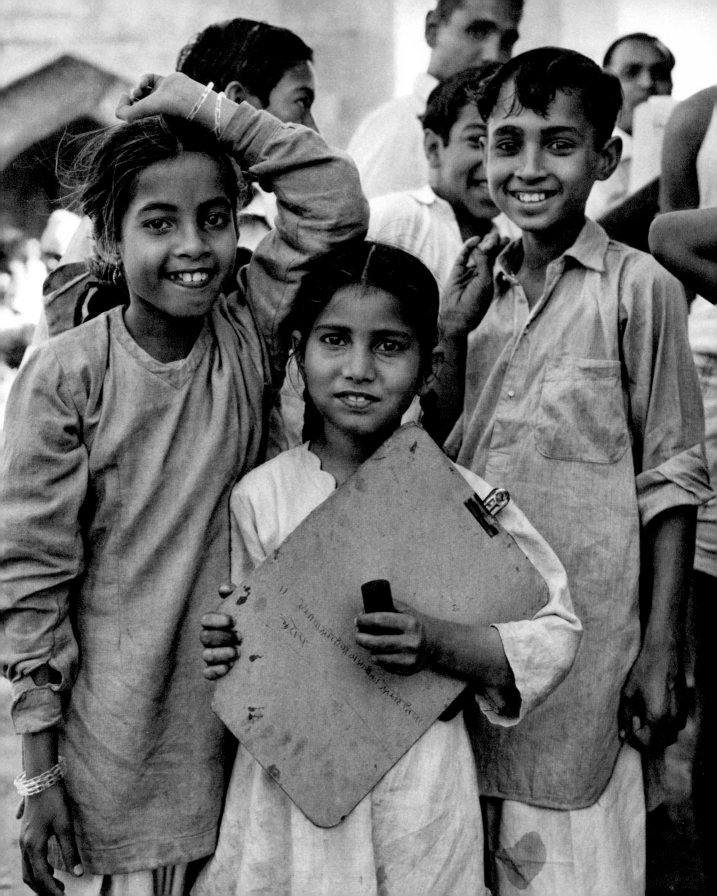

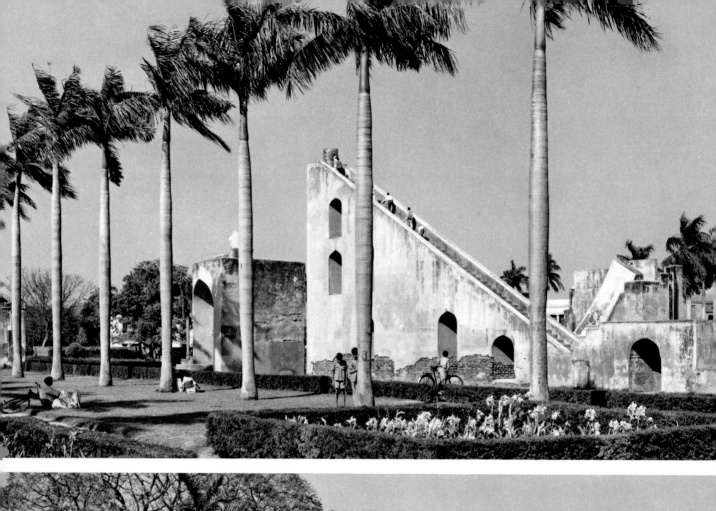

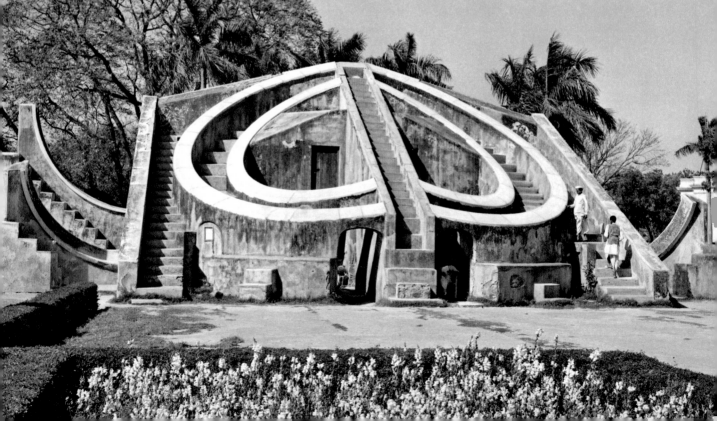

In a three-hour train or car journey you reach the most famous sight for tourists in the environs of the capital: the fort of Agra and the Taj Mahal.

It was worth going by road. Huge milestones, at intervals of about three miles, marked the old army road connecting the two capitals of the Mogul emperors and leading north-west to Lahore and over the Khyber Pass to Kabul in Afghanistan, the original seat of the dynasty. Ox-carts still went along the paths by the side of the asphalt highway, their wheels sinking into the sand. A solitary rider on a camel seemed to have lost his way on the old caravan routes and to have stumbled into our era. Even wild animals were not driven into the desert by the traffic. A jackal ran across the road, green parrots flew about in the trees, peacocks strutted over the fields, and on some of the trees perched vultures, waiting motionless all day long to pounce on a carcass. Occasionally troops of monkeys crouched at the edge of the road like small boys mischievously awaiting a chance to pilfer something with their long arms. At one stop three jugglers with tame bears were waiting for patrons; girls walked to the wells with jugs on their heads, slim and shy as gazelles; in front of the camera they quickly hid their faces with the hems of their dresses.

Shah Jahan married Arjumand Bano Begam, the daughter of one of the richest noblemen. The Prince, who already had two children of an earlier marriage, was devoted to her with a love and fidelity astonishing in a man who was so inconsiderate and dissolute; Mumtaz Mahal (Ornament of the Palace), as she was now called, presented him with one child after another and died giving birth to the fourteenth at the age of thirty-nine. A tomb of unusual beauty was to honour her memory, and thus there was built in a garden on the bank of the Jumna river,

Page 80 DELHI
Surrounded by the streets of New Delhi is Jantar Mantar, the observatory built in about 1725 by the Maharajah Jai Singh II of Jaipur. The largest of the instruments constructed for the observation of sun and stars is a 55-foot-high sundial.

Pages 83–85 OLD DELHI

83 One of the most recent and best-preserved monuments in Old Delhi is the tomb of Safdar Jang, Nawab of Oudh, who died in 1753. It can be seen from far off, and is the last of the large, domed tombs of the Mogul era.

84 At the site of Indraprastha, the legendary foundation of the Pandavas, rises Purana Kila, 'old fort', the seat of Sher Shah (1542–5). It stands on a hill surrounded by ramparts, and one enters it through a huge gateway.

85 The courtyard of the mosque Quwat-ul-Islam, which was built with pillars of destroyed Hindu temples and founded about the same time as the Qutb Minar (*see pages* 60–61). The Iron Pillar, in the centre, is one of the most venerable monuments of ancient India, dating from the fourth century; a six-line inscription in Sanskrit names the Gupta king Chandra and the deity Vishnu. The monument was probably first brought from Bihar to its present position by a later ruler.

Pages 86–89 AGRA

86–87 The Pearl Mosque (Moti Masjid), which stands in the grounds of the imperial palace, was founded in 1646–53 by Shah Jahan. With its hall of prayers of grey and blue streaked marble it is one of the most noble creations of Mogul architects.

88 Sayings from the Koran inscribed on white marble adorn the huge gateway of red sandstone, dating from 1648, through which visitors enter the grounds of the Taj Mahal, and which gives them the classical view (*page* 59) of the famous tomb.

89 The domed Taj Mahal rises on a 20-foot-high platform. Beneath the outer dome, which rises to a height of 185 feet, a second and plainer dome forms a ceiling over the interior with the symbolic sarcophagus of Mumtaz Mahal and her husband Shah Jahan, later placed beside her; the real graves are in the vault underneath. The outer walls are inlaid with fine ornamental work of precious, brightly coloured stones, with letters, abstract patterns, and plant motifs. The people standing on and under the platform give some idea of the building's monumental proportions.

Page 90 THE TOMB OF AKBAR IN SIKANDRA

From the top of the pyramid-shaped monument you can see the red sandstone entrance surrounded by four marble minarets. Akbar, who died in 1605, had himself started to lay out the grounds; his son Jahangir had the monument erected in all its splendour for his feared and admired father, and in the course of the work altered the plans. In 1691, during the reign of Aurangzeb, the tomb was broken open by rebellious peasants; they pillaged the interior, which was adorned with gold, silver, and previous stones, and flung the bones of the Emperor into a fire.

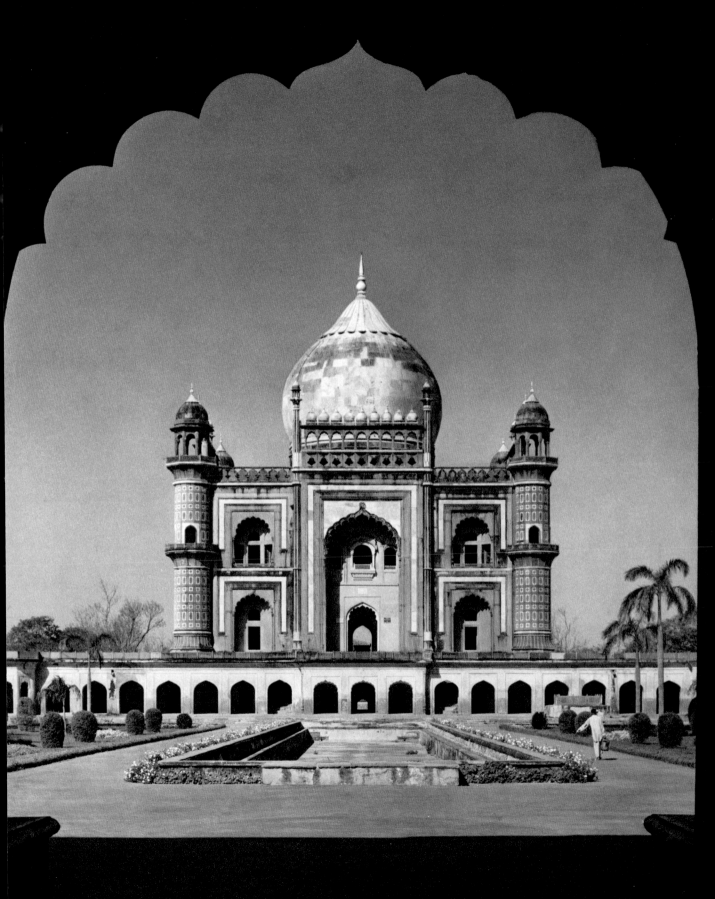

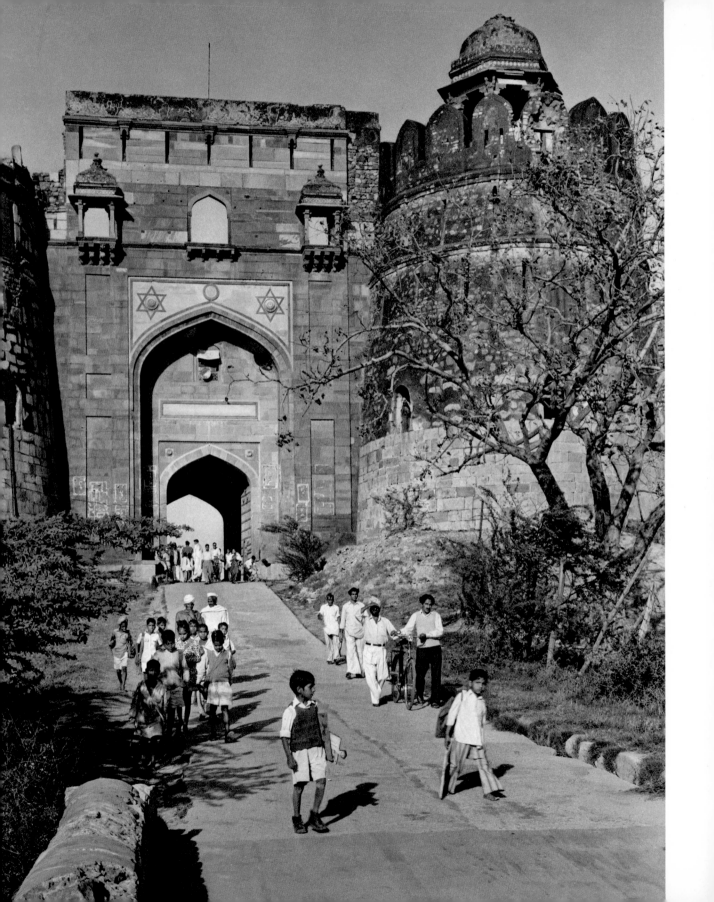

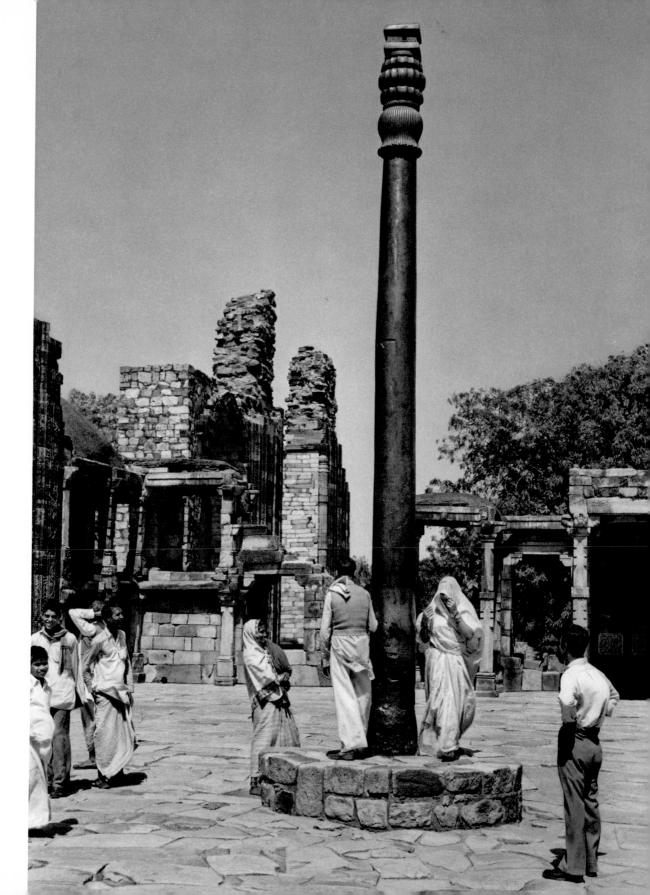

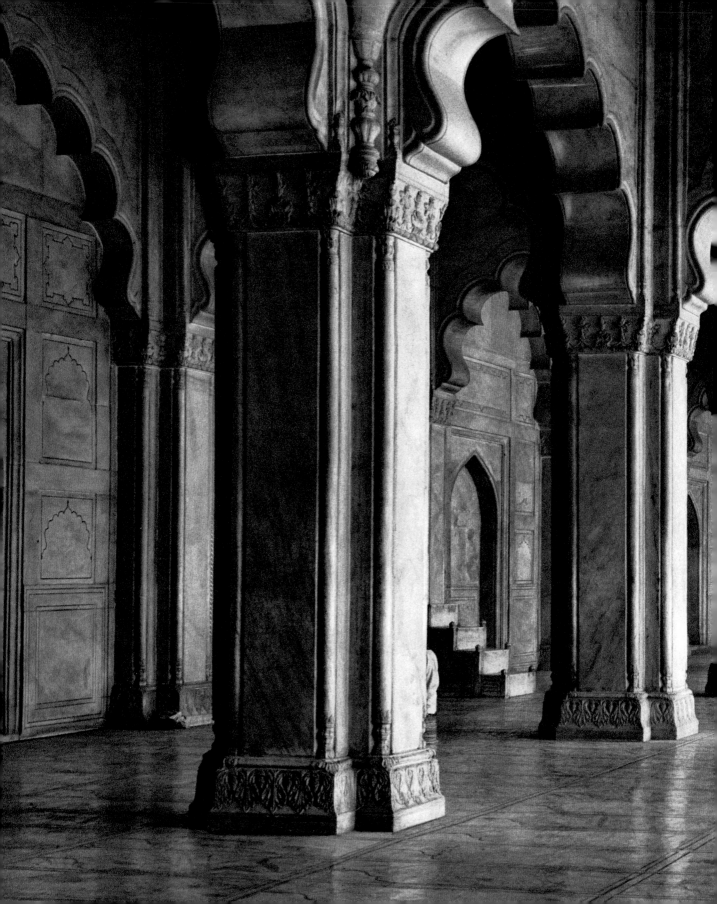

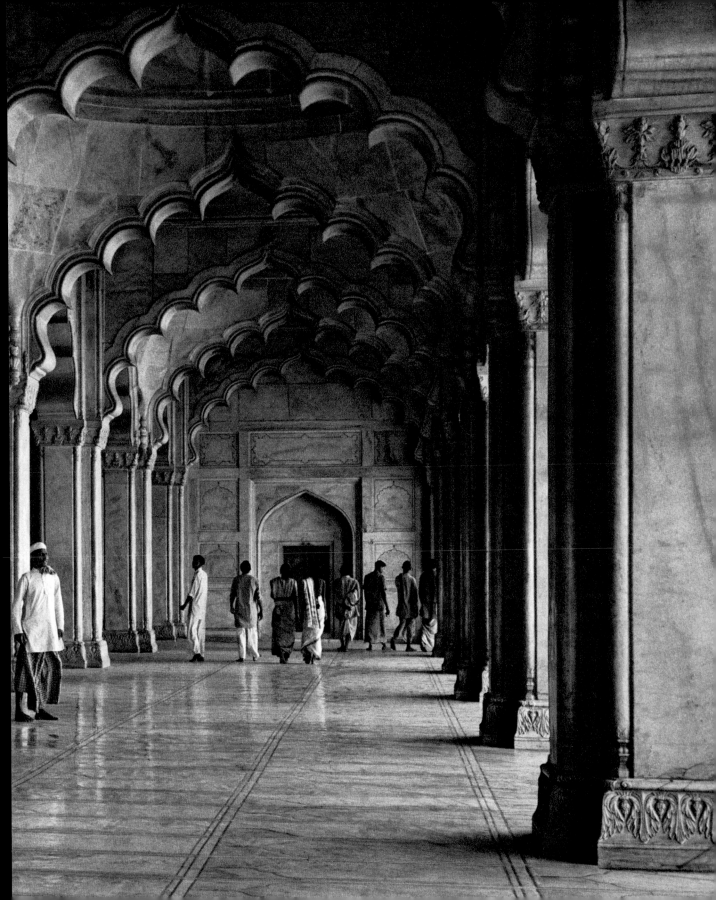

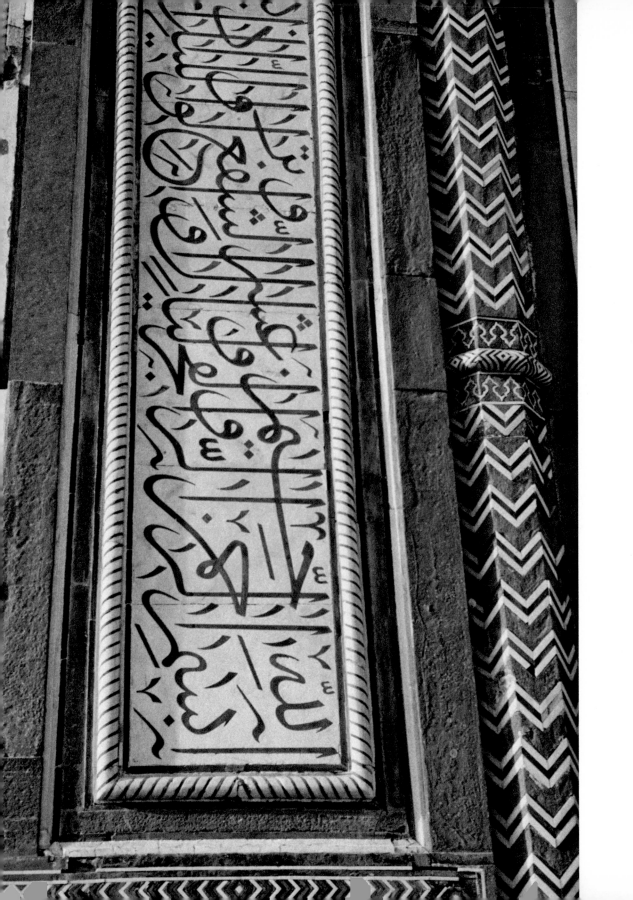

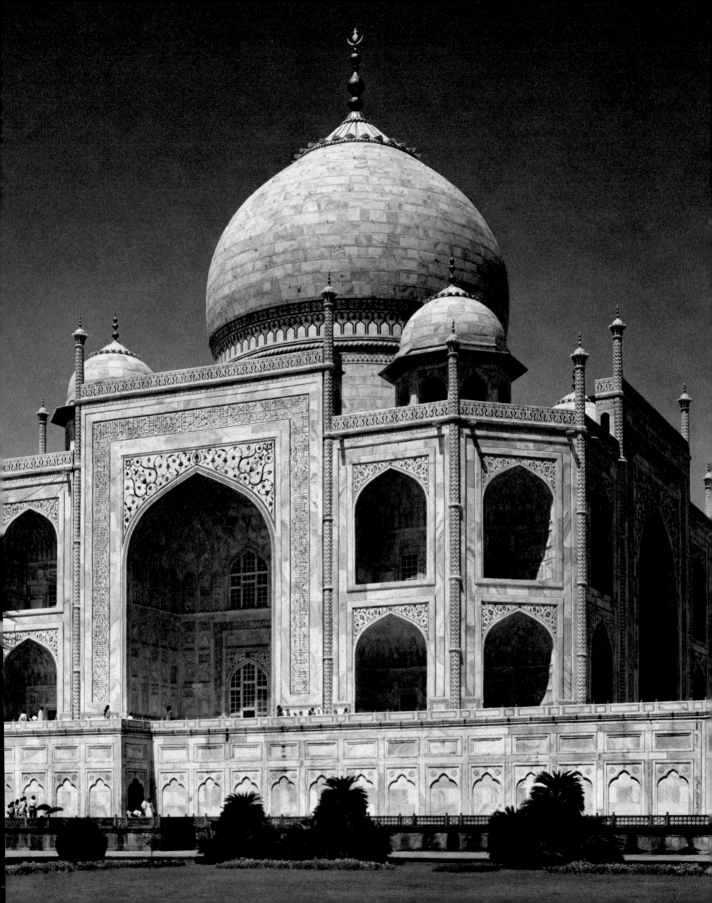

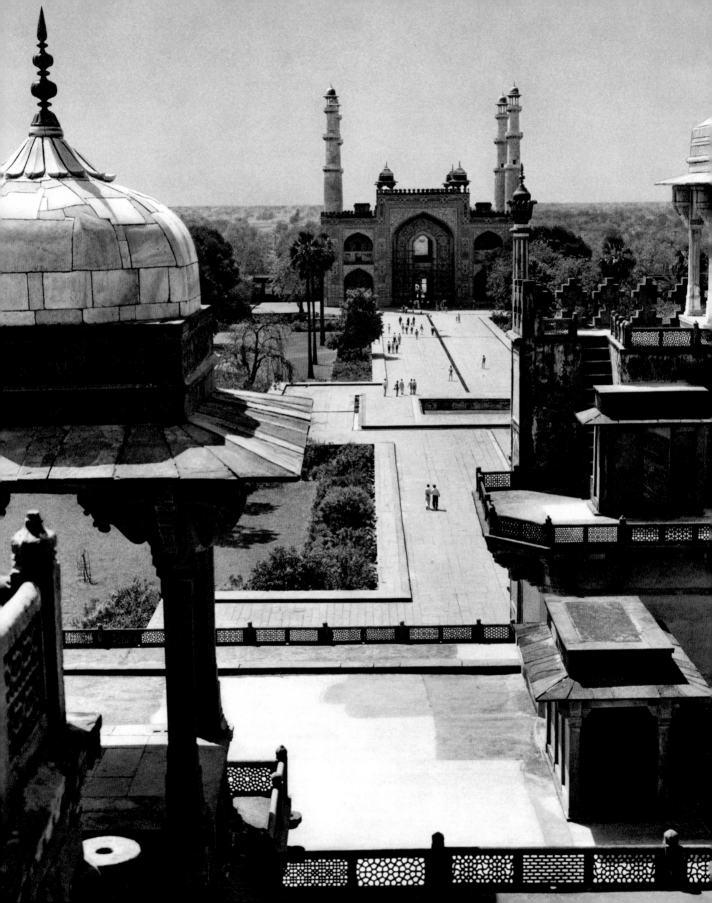

within sight of the palace at Agra, the fairy-like marble building of the Taj Mahal, with the curved cupola that never fails to impress the visitor by the faultless nobility of its lines and the majesty of its proportions, even if miniature copies and sentimental postcards have made him sceptical.

Most of the palace buildings admired today in the fort of Agra are the work of Shah Jahan: the dream-like Pearl Mosque, for instance; and during his temporary move to Delhi the series of reception-rooms, summer-houses, and mosques were built. Shah Jahan loved luxury; even a dreadful famine in the fourth to fifth year of his reign did not prevent him from increasing the treasures kept in the cellars of the palace at Agra; the famous jewel-studded peacock throne, which was taken to Persia in the 18th century, was built at his instructions.

To be the builder of a city was once the ambition of great rulers, particularly the strong founders of dynasties, who left their capital city to future generations as a reminder of the foundation of the State. Thus we see the great Constantine taking mighty strides far beyond the frontiers of ancient Byzantium, delineating with his spear the borders of the new Rome, and planting into the earth, as a sanctified centre of his Empire, Christian relics and heathen relics of the god of his city. India, into whose vast regions so many empires were drawn—and subsequently swept away again by the restlessness of its gods and the peoples obeying them—is particularly rich in such monuments to ephemeral secular power. *Founders of Cities*

Delhi itself reveals a whole conglomeration of seats of ancient dynastic powers, not to speak of the fact that in the midst of its ruins, its mosques, towers of victory, and mausolea, the English built New Delhi as an enduring monument to the British Raj in India. At the same time the Dominion of Australia received its new capital, Canberra.

The zeal for planning of British imperialism has today been surpassed by that of ambitious socialist nationalists. Uninhibited by sentimentality or traditions they are determined to make full use of technology, which has a beauty of its own, to serve the people, who have been freed from the bonds of kinship, class, and caste.

Even in our over-populated and urbanised Europe the rapid development of communications and amenities generally have been urging us towards a new form of the city. But not even the destruction of the Second World War allowed us to throw off the burden of the past; and everywhere what exists forms a fine mesh of consideration for rights of possession, of cost, of ancient cultural tradition, and habit.

The underdeveloped territories find it much easier to realise their urge towards total renewal. Therefore let us go out towards the young nations of the Orient, who are such fervent believers in planning. They too have their traditions, it is true, but why should we be concerned about them, since we are promising them in return the realisation of one of the great dreams of mankind—the New City, which belongs to the people, a place for work and peace instead of a fortified castle of some lord with its quarters for his slaves—the New Atlantis, Utopia.

The Soviet Union ought by rights to be an Eldorado for town-builders, especially in its Asiatic dominions. New towns are being christened as on the production-line system, and in addition new cities are being built. There is plenty of land. Geological, technological, and economic knowledge can be employed here without consideration of local customs. The stroke of a pen in Moscow can set whole tribes in motion, and completely change the face of the landscape. Yet what one sees and hears of the newly founded Communist towns in Siberia is scarcely different from the *bourgeois* pomp which one can admire equally well in the Stalinallee in Berlin; and in Moscow itself the 19th-century type of building, magnified to colossal proportions, has long since won its victory over the steel and concrete poetry of Le Corbusier. Long, wide avenues alone are not enough. It is one of the ironies of world history that artists are still finding a more rewarding field of activity under socialist city-planners in capitalist or semi-capitalist countries, than in States under proletarian dictatorship.

The representatives of 'functional' architecture today naturally look down on the architects of New Delhi; the eclecticism of British academicians can also be considered as a legitimate expression of colonialism, which is taboo today. Le Corbusier himself was more objective than his followers when he wrote: 'For two centuries the English trained up no Indian architects, but erected English, Scottish and . . . Tuscan buildings in the tropics. New Delhi (inspired by the Tuscan style), the capital of Imperial India, was built by Lutyens more than thirty years ago with extreme care, great talent and indeed very successfully. The critics can say what they like but any successful creation wins respect (at least from me).' This judgment too commands respect.

Its author himself had his first opportunity to realise his architectural visions, for which neither Paris nor his native Switzerland had any use, in India. A group of intellectuals led by Nehru had come into power who were ready to experiment with typical achievements of the spirit of the technical age, and they called on the leading light of modern European architecture—Le Corbusier. Thus once again it was European influence, once again a kind of colonialism.

The Buildings of New Delhi

Was there no Indian architectural tradition to meet the task? In the eighteenth century the famous Maharaja-astronomer, Jai Singh II, built his new capital, Jaipur, according to old rules, on a large scale, and it was as modern in appearance as his Cubist observatory buildings. Were the British really solely responsible for the fact that since then there had been no 'Indian' architecture? Although architecture is certainly, more than any other art, dependent on external circumstances, on the patrons, on the régime, are we not confusing cause and effect if we say that it is the fault of the imperialists? Where were the painters, sculptors, authors, scholars of this great people of ancient culture? India's great men in the Victorian period were Swami Dayanand, Ram Mohan Roy, Ramakrishna, and Vivekananda— and all the other sages and ascetics, in whom Hinduism was renewed again and again; and in the primeval forest of their ideas there was also a living architecture: temples which grew up like tropical plants, profusely adorned and hung with tinsel, monumental staircases and palaces at sacred watering-places, gleaming whitewashed or gaily coloured towers and terraces beside the crumbling buildings of yesterday.

Chandigarh

The great building commission which independent India had to allocate was the new capital of the Punjab, Chandigarh. The 'partition', the division of India in 1947, hit the Punjab particularly hard, for the new frontier between the Mohammedan and Hindu States went straight through the middle of this former province. Lahore, until then the capital, went to Pakistan; the neighbouring Amritsar, which with its golden temple was the Mecca of the Sikhs, to India. For all that, the State of Punjab in the Indian Republic still comprises a huge territory and has a population three to four times as large as that of Switzerland.

As a site for the new capital the government acquired a large area of flat land at the foot of the Siwalik mountains, not far from the former Viceroy's summer seat, Simla. In February and March 1951 Le Corbusier, as adviser to the Ministry, drafted the general plan. Two senior civil servants, P. N. Thapar and P. L. Varma, energetically supported its immediate execution; the good will of the Prime Minister was a powerful protection from adverse criticism.

Le Corbusier's Plan

The 'anatomy' of the city was to comprise among other things the head, the trunk, the veins, and the feet. The head: the State buildings, of which the Palace of Justice and the great government buildings—the Secretariat—have already been built; the parliament buildings and the governor's palace ('Raj Bhawan') are to follow. The trunk: sector 17 with public buildings such as the town hall, police headquarters, museum, and library. The feet: the industrial area in the south-east, screened off from the residential districts by a green belt. The veins: a network of streets canalising slow and fast traffic (at least on the plan). Out of a total of thirty sectors twenty-four were reserved for houses: here great scope was allowed for the needs of the inhabitants and the imagination of the architects; socialist ideas were not apparent in the thirteen different categories of house; the differences between the grandest and the simplest districts were a reminder of the old class and caste system. Each sector was a little town in itself, a rectangle of about three-quarters of a mile, in which up to 15,000 people could be housed.

The Sukhna Cho, one of the two rivers which encircle Chandigarh, was dammed up to make a reservoir for the dry season. For the rest, a dozen wells with pumps fetched precious water from a depth of 250 feet and transformed the dry ground into a landscape-garden. The first buildings were to provide accommodation for 150,000 inhabitants; later half a million people would be housed in Chandigarh.

One of the chief architect's closest collaborators was his cousin Pierre Jeanneret; he designed a great part of the already completed residential districts. From 1951 to 1954 Maxwell Fry and Jane Drew from England were the most important members of the team, which also included a number of Indians. As the civil servants responsible for the building programme had almost all studied at the University of Oxford, people spoke of an Oxford Programme. British influence in Chandigarh was thus hardly less noticeable than in New Delhi, even if it was that of a generation which preferred to look to Montparnasse rather than to Florence; civilisation in India is still based on the British way of life.

The 'Oxford' planners of Chandigarh are filled with a holy zeal for the building of what should become a guiding beacon for their country, and the example of Chandigarh should teach future architects of India. The town which Nehru has called 'a symbol of India's freedom from her traditions' receives the newcomer without a triumphal arch. My car passed between dry fields, then through the geometrical 'arteries' of the new town, to the sectors where a few houses appear over low walls, and where the two-storeyed Mountview Hotel came into sight.

I was lucky enough for my visit to coincide with that of the architect who is building all over the world. Even at the age of seventy, Charles Jeanneret, known as Le Corbusier, manages to fly from his headquarters in Paris to India for a few weeks, in order to take a look at the progress of his creations there.

In the hotel I was met by one Mr Singh, a prosperous businessman with a typical Sikh beard, who scarcely let me out of his sight during my visit to the Punjab, looking after me with tender care. He took me first to the Architects Office of the town, a single-floored temporary building. A young architect gave us information with typical Indian courtesy. In this man I saw in its most likeable form that sense of mission which has helped the Congress Movement over so many difficulties already. These people are convinced that they are on the right lines. They are ready to learn, but from their own experience and mistakes; they

Pages 97–102 CHANDIGARH

97 In the entrance hall of the Palace of Justice, which is open to the west, the parties talk with their solicitors during a pause in the proceedings.

98 Le Corbusier, the chief architect of the new capital of the Punjab, explains to visitors to his office the general layout of the city with its different sectors.

99 A courtyard in the Palace of Justice with a staircase on the right.

100 The central part of the east front of the government buildings erected by Le Corbusier, with the main entrance just before it was completed.

101 top The huge concrete structure of the Secretariat (seen from the Palace of Justice) stands by itself in a broad area of ground which will be laid out as a park.

101 below A Junior Secondary School, architect Pierre Jeanneret.

102 top Prefabricated houses for people of average means. The wall shutting off the living quarters from the traffic on the street had already been broken through by residents who wanted to save themselves the long detour.

102 below This housing estate for people of modest means gave the 'peon' a home as he had not previously known it, and a decent one even by European standards.

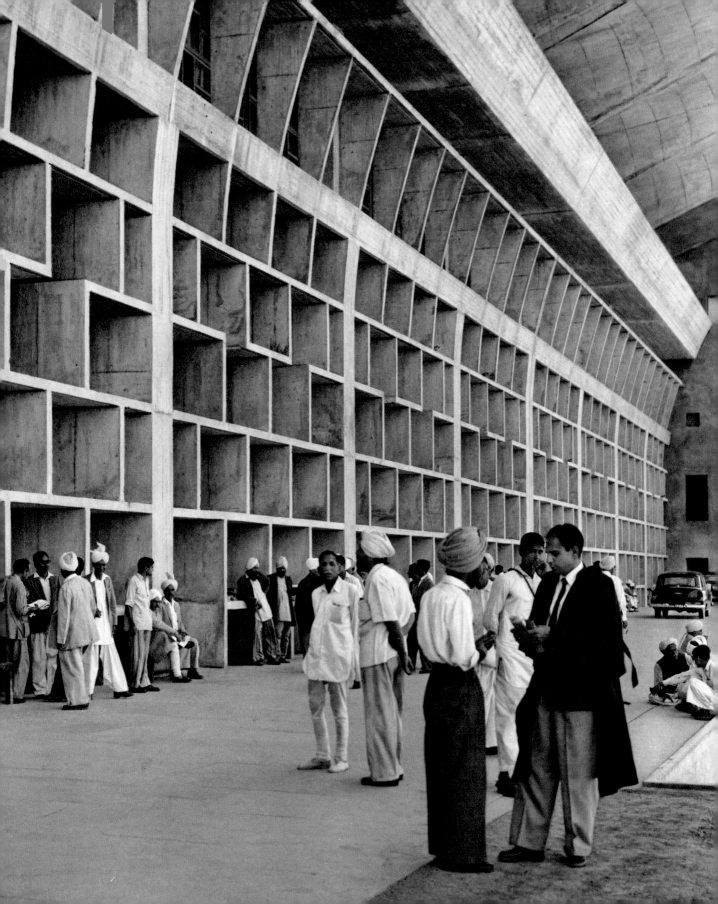

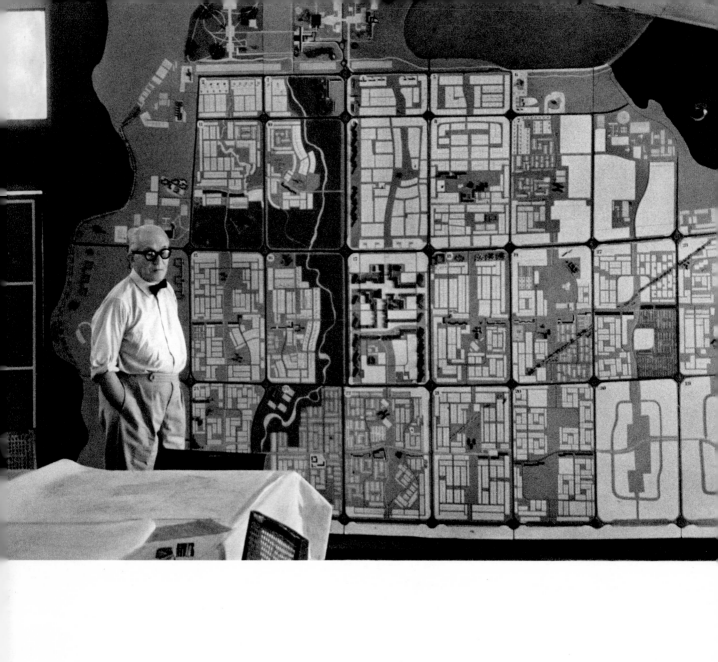

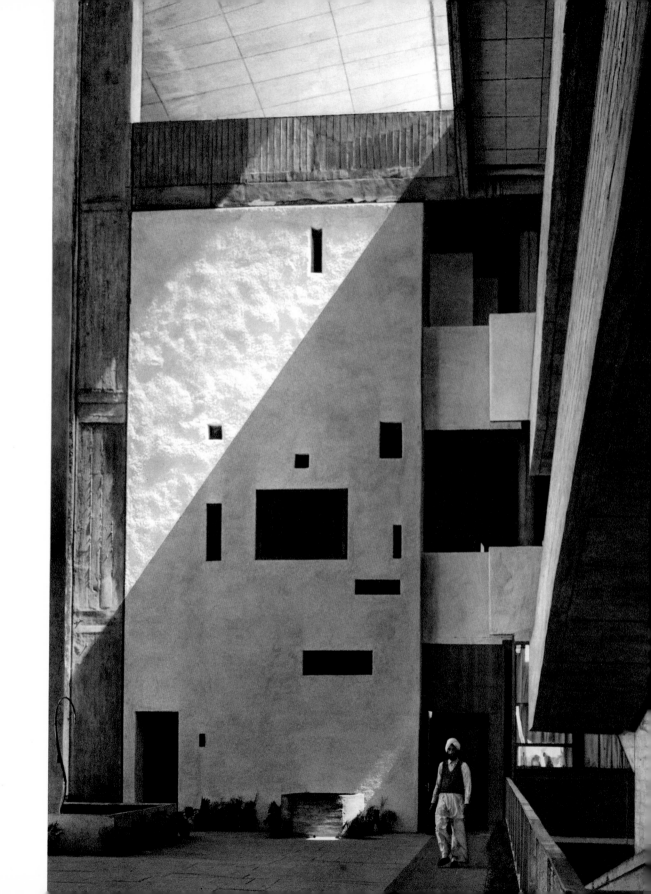

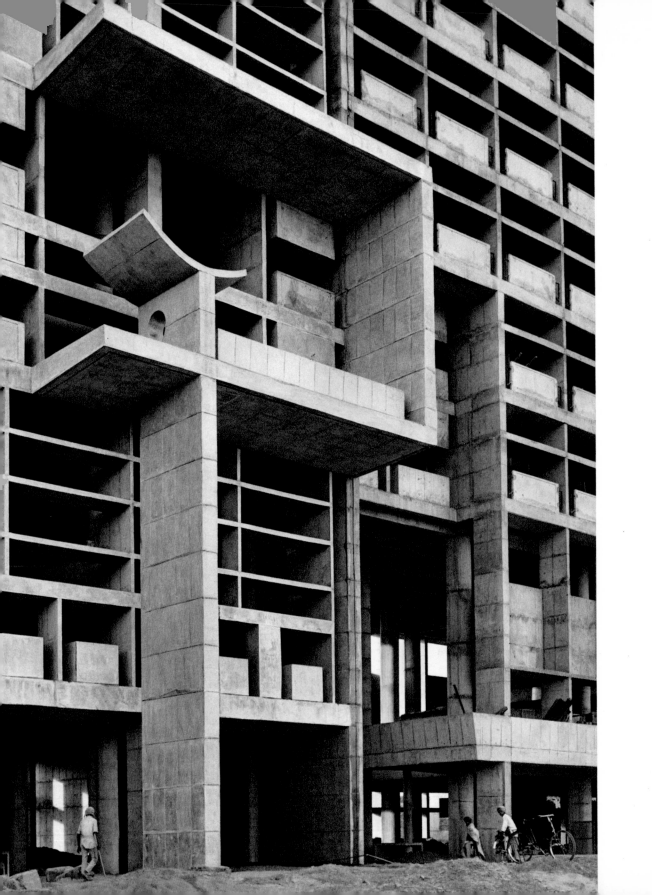

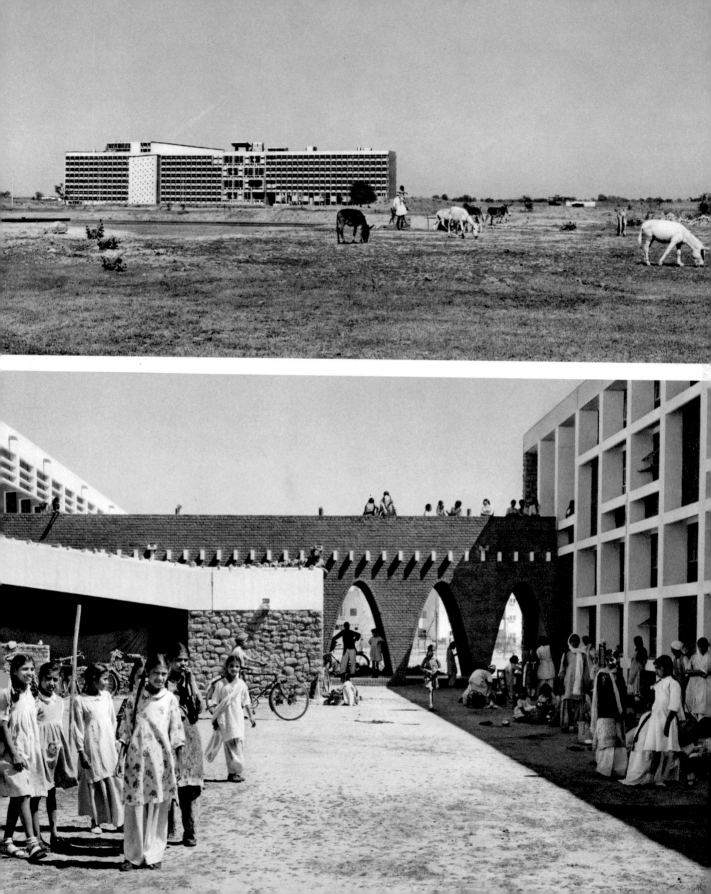

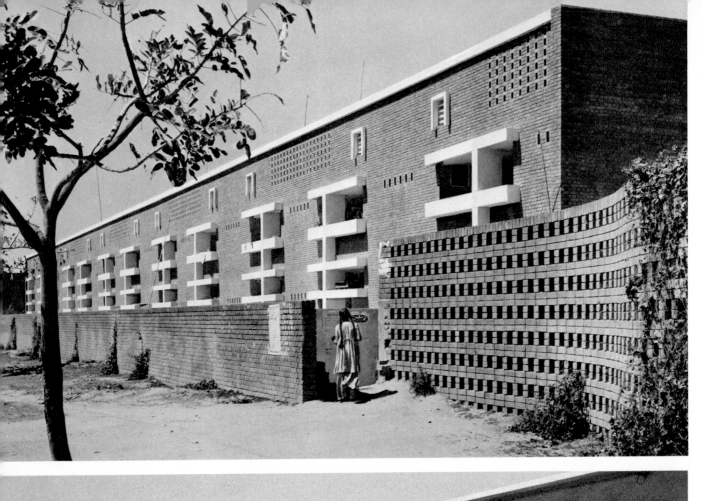

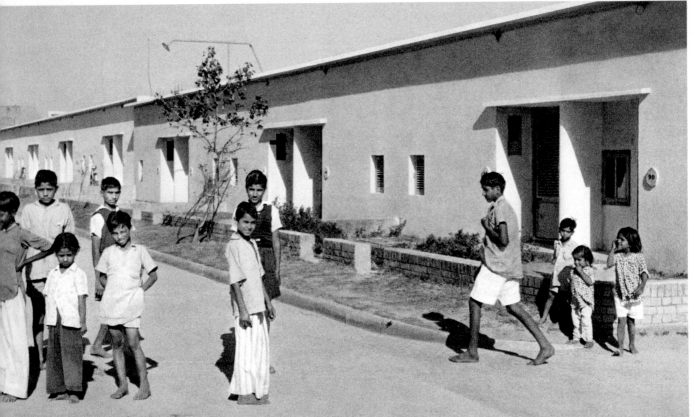

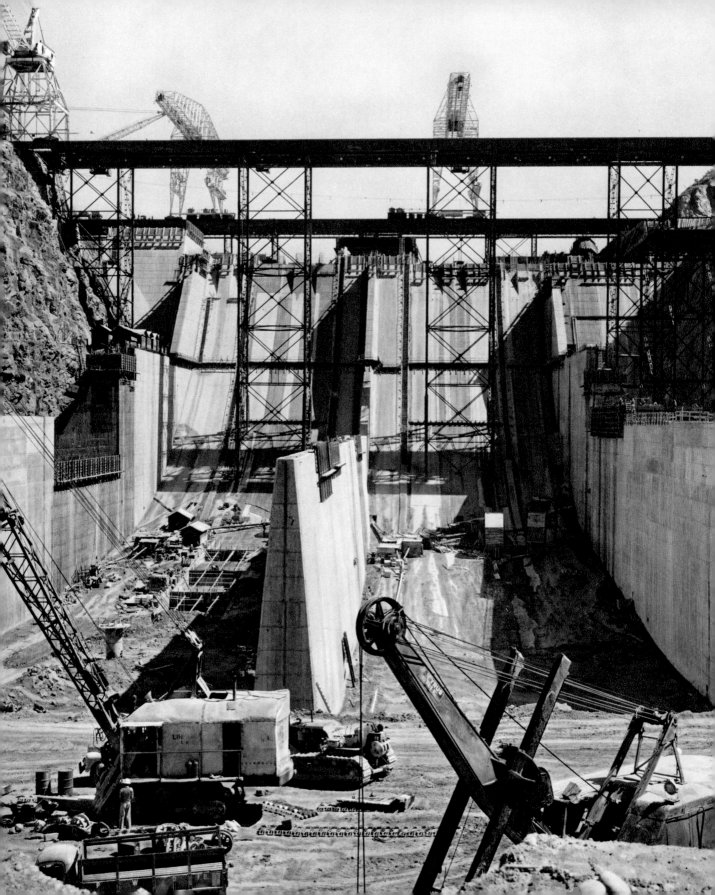

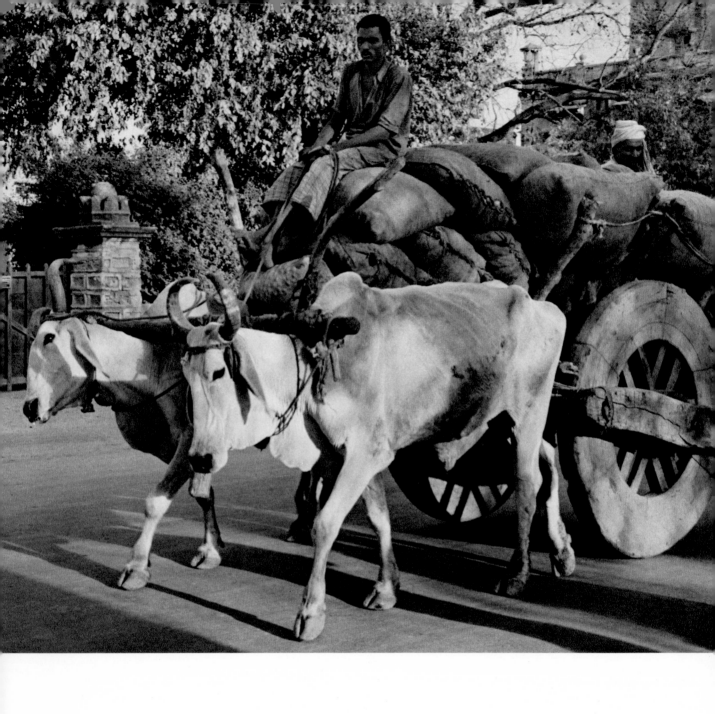

have a deep distrust of advice from outsiders, even when these have gone through the same process of learning, or derive their knowledge from comparable history.

Le Corbusier is the *guru*, the sage and teacher whose spirit is omnipresent. He is surrounded by the veneration which Indians are accustomed to vouchsafe their great men, a characteristic mixture of easy cameraderie and humble devotion. I was to meet the master himself in the afternoon. It was like going to an audience with the head of government.

The World's Greatest
Architect

Meanwhile, I took the opportunity to make a circular tour which gave me some first impressions of the new town. Above all I longed to see Le Corbusier's own capital buildings. The Palace of Justice was already in use: the outer frame looked like a chest of drawers and the body of the building consisted mainly of concrete cubes; its numerous open passages let in the fresh breeze from the mountains; from the courtyard a ramp led to the upper floors. Lawyers went in and out with briefs under their arms, as in England, or stood talking to their clients. (Indians make excellent lawyers; their eloquence—in politics also—can be compared to that of their French colleagues.)

The Capital Buildings of
Le Corbusier

The court-rooms which one entered from the western hall had on their rear walls huge tapestries designed by Le Corbusier. They were very brightly coloured and an effective decoration; their themes were abstract, some of them symbolic figures resembling serpents. These certainly represented contemporary design, to a

Page 103 THE BHAKRA DAM
The great wall of the dam nearing completion. Behind it the waters of the river Sutlej will form a lake some sixty miles long.

104   A two-wheeled cart drawn by two white oxen is the classical means of transporting goods in India. You meet it everywhere on the highroads and occasionally even in the towns.

Parisian they could not be more traditional, but they looked oddly out of place in a country where all the iconography is centuries-old and where every figure has a symbolic significance—not least the serpent. Some of the tapestries, it was said, had already been removed by the judges.

A wide stretch of waste ground separated the Palace of Justice from the government buildings, which were double the size. Women workers with baskets of sand on their heads were helping with the final stages of the construction before the arrival of the army of civil servants.

The enormous mass of concrete had been imaginatively ordered by the deliberate pencil of the artist and divested of its heaviness. But the beauty of texture of the rough walls requires imagination from the spectator in order to bear comparison with the shimmering beauty of the Mogul buildings in red sandstone and marble.

Residential Quarters

Scattered round different sectors were to be found the one- two- and three-storeyed houses which interpreted the style of Le Corbusier more or less freely and were to serve as models for further construction in the town. There were schools, institutes, and communal buildings; the glass house of the government printing works was designed by Le Corbusier himself. There were rows of houses confined to the essentials for the 'peons', the class of the population which had previously lived in conditions scarcely fit for human beings. Well-tended gardens surrounded the villas of the ministers, managers, and other comfortably off people.

Between these two extremes are eleven types of house for the middle classes. The idea of the one-family house, even on a modest scale—the idea that 'my home is my castle', dear to both Indians and Englishmen—has won the day with the 'Oxford' team in preference to the giant blocks of flats which the master has created in Berlin and Marseilles. Only when bureaucracy is unhindered, for instance in a secretariat, do we find Le Corbusier's concrete beehive.

At the appointed hour I was back at Le Corbusier's headquarters. Very soon

I found myself alone with the architect, looking at the bespectacled face of a man of lucid mind whose taut, intelligent features had a slight air of weary scepticism: a prophet of the technical era with clear eyes fixed on a far-off goal.

Le Corbusier did not seem quite clear about what benefits were to be expected of such a visit; either you had read his writings and therefore knew what was what; or you had not read them, in which case there was no need to visit him. He became enthusiastic, however, when we talked of the social ideals which influenced all he did.

In India one has to manage with little money. But it was a matter of prime importance—Le Corbusier's colleagues and the responsible ministers knew that. Above all, the Prime Minister in Delhi knew it: his generous confidence made possible all that was being done there.

I glanced at the large sheets of sketches covering the table. What was he working on at the moment?—on plans for the dam at Bhakra, an especially absorbing task. Neither France nor Switzerland had asked him to carry out that kind of project.

What do the first inhabitants of Chandigarh say about their town? Even here there is opposition and one can hear all kinds of criticisms among the paeans to the new age. Problems of climate, which received great consideration in the planning of new town buildings, were not all solved. The problem of reducing the heat of the day to a bearable level and of making the most of the cool of the night had always existed in India and had been solved satisfactorily. Some mistakes had now been made in the planning of rooms and staircases—patterns of life could not always be directed from the drawing-board. The partitions around sectors which were to keep pedestrians away from through-roads had already been broken through in some places.

The private decoration of houses is generally in striking contrast to the building-style, and shows this as something imposed from outside. Only the future can show which style will survive. The great designer, however in tune he is with humanity, always attempts to force man, with his customs and habits, into his own mould, to sacrifice him to some extent to an ideal of humanity. But where would we be without the innovators, men of daring, experimenters in the field of social and technical accomplishments?

Aperitif with my Guide

On the evening before I left Chandigarh my friendly Sikh guide invited me to his house for an aperitif. He had previously lived in Lahore and, like most of his fellow-believers, had sided with India. He had also invited one of the leading personalities in the administration, a Hindu. The three of us sat on a sofa in the drawing-room, and except for the picture of Gandhi on the mantelpiece, the scene might have been in England. While we talked and drank Indian beer a daughter of the house appeared and offered delicious pastries and other delicacies. There were no introductions or greetings even when a second and third daughter and finally his wife herself appeared. One daughter wore a becoming *sari*, the others were dressed in a shirt-blouse and baggy trousers. They did not touch any of the food but joined easily in the conversation. They spoke faultless English which they had learnt at college—the youngest was still attending a school in Simla run on British lines and was sorry that my youngest son did not yet know enough English to be her pen-friend.

The administrator had important commissions to allocate, and Mr Singh well-founded hopes. The political ideology of these men conformed to present-day orthodoxy: Gandhi was to them the beloved father of the nation; Nehru, the irreplaceable. People were proud of the independence they had won but did not bear the British any grudge. The Indian civil service—the backbone of the State—won its prestige at the time of the British administration, and, when corruption is discussed, it must in fairness be admitted that the Governor-Generals built up with an astonishingly low expenditure an excellent administrative machine. It would, of course, be unjust not to admit that the tasks of the young republic by far surpass those which engaged the vice-regal government. And it must also be said that parliamentary government has since then proved itself much more viable in India than in any other Asian country, because the members are waging successful warfare against every misuse of economic resources, even if the Minister responsible for it belongs to the all-powerful Congress Party: thus to his regret Nehru had recently to let the Minister of Finance go—one of the pillars of his government.

Nowadays, people regard the erection of a dam as the most conspicuous sign of victory over the hostile elements—a symbol of freedom from want and of national independence; the dam would prevent flooding, provide power to turn the wheels of industry, and store water to irrigate the parched land. India has its dam; this when it is completed in 1960 should have the highest walls of any in the world. 'The Bhakra Nangal project is something enormous, something overpowering, something which rouses you when you see it. The gigantic work undertaken in Bhakra is today the symbol of India's progress!' Jawaharlal Nehru's words greet school parties and other crowds of visitors who come in buses and special trains to see the great undertaking in the Siwalik mountains to the west of the Himalayas. It is very satisfying for independent India to reach American record figures.

To assess the importance of the Bhakra Dam you have to keep in mind the centuries-old problem of the country's water-supply—a problem whose solution became even more pressing with the rapid increase in population. Water is considered sacred in India; the water of the temple and village pools and of the great rivers is a source of life during the long period of drought, until the summer monsoon brings for a short time an abundance of rain. The supplying of water is

The Highest Dam in the World

therefore a much more important function of this dam than the generation of power. Irrigation canals can be run from the dammed waters of the Sutlej near Bhakra to the neighbouring Federal States; 6,424,860 acres of land would be brought under the plough and a further 3,459,540 acres would be decisively improved by irrigation. The project was conceived in 1908 and taken up in earnest during the Second World War. The beginning of the work coincided with the assumption of responsibility by the national government of Nehru.

At the Bhakra Dam   In a two-hour drive from Chandigarh we reached the Bhakra-Hidal Canal and the barrack-like town of Nandal. The various stages of construction were explained to us—the cement brought direct from the mountain, the cooling plant, and the system of tunnels. We climbed inside the mine-like dam and went up to the level of the future lake—it will be about sixty miles long. Photographs were strictly forbidden!

The complicated machinery of the plant was supplied by fifteen nations. The construction board was directly responsible to the government; it employed some 300 Indian engineers and twenty-two foreign experts, mostly Americans, but also Germans and Japanese. An American specialist received 4,000 rupees a month, the Indian engineer on the other hand only 300.

Page 111 THE SIKH SHRINE IN DELHI

In the Chandni Chauk, the main street, Aurangzeb had the ninth Guru of the Sikhs, Teg Bahadur, publicly beheaded; on the spot rises Gurdwara Sisanj, the main Sikh shrine in the capital. At the door, which is guarded by a strong, bearded custodian, there is a constant coming and going; on the left one of the faithful touches the threshold with his forehead.

112 Siesta during the hottest time of the day in a municipal park.

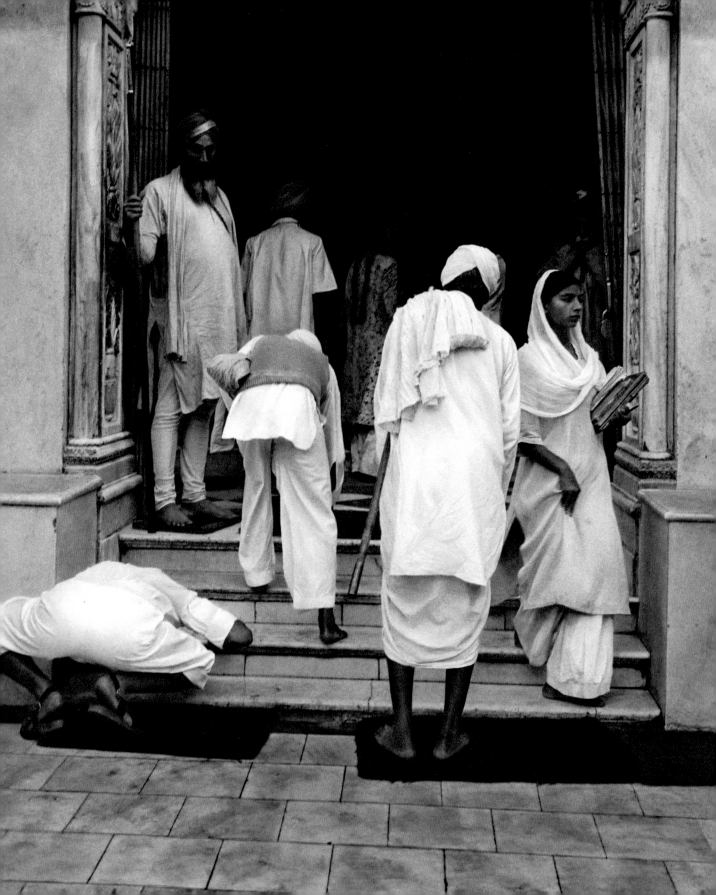

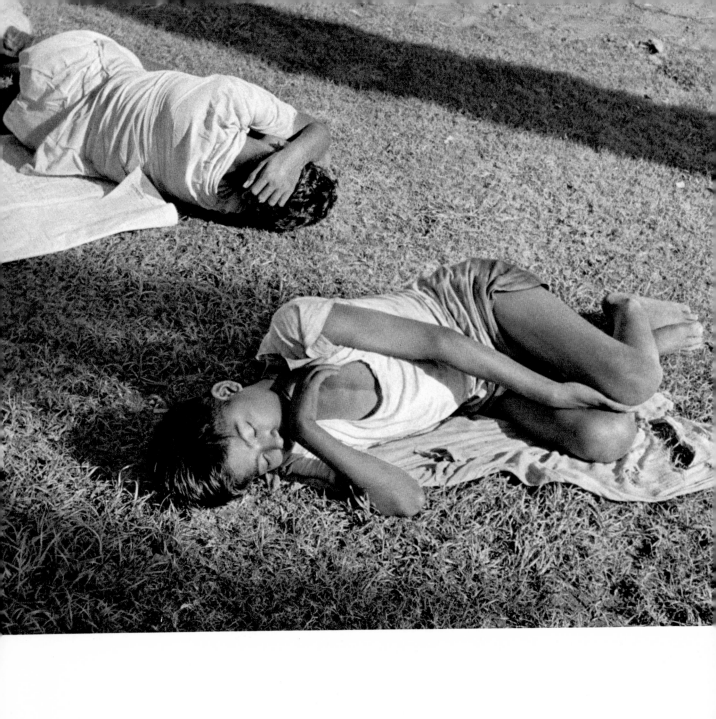

On the way back to Chandigarh from the Bhakra Dam we passed through Anandpur, the town founded in 1665 by the ninth Guru of the Sikhs, Teg Bahadur. From far off the gleaming white temple welcomed us; it is surpassed in importance among sacred Sikh shrines only by the gold temple in Amritsar. I had to go and see it.

Anandpur, a Sikh Shrine

With my friends I underwent the ceremony of washing the feet and stepped barefoot on to the polished marble flagstones of the shrine. Inside the temple there was an atmosphere of matter-of-fact cheerfulness. What the Bible is to Protestants, and the Koran to Mohammedans, the Granth is to Sikhs, and their devotion is confined to the veneration of this Holy Book and to the absorption of its wisdom.

From a small bookstall in front of the temple I bought a bundle of booklets printed in English. These, written by Jeja Singh, M.A., explained the significance of the shrine, and gave an account, suited to the Western mind, of the Sikh doctrine. This doctrine might well have been taken from the popular writings of a theosophist, and much of it could easily be absorbed into the ethical code of a good Christian.

When India was divided and the frontiers were drawn right through the middle of the Punjab, the home of most of the Sikhs, they sided with India and those from Pakistan territory became an asset to the new State. The statesmen in Delhi succeeded in harnessing the special energy of these people to the various tasks of the republic; they still make the best soldiers in the Indian Army, and you come across them particularly in the Punjab, but also in Delhi, in all kinds of important and less important posts, since there is a pressing need for reliability, lucidity, and the power of decision. That they cling stubbornly to their own Gurmakhi script, made sacred by the Granth, is one of the many problems with which schools in India today have to contend. Now and then a demand is heard for the reappearance of a Sikh State, and what today seems distant and visionary might suddenly

The Position of Sikhs in the New India

develop into a powerful movement if the Indian Federation were to prove itself too weak for the tasks it has undertaken.

Back in Delhi I met another Sikh, Dr Kushwant. He belonged to the intellec- tual *élite* of the capital and edited the newspaper *Jojana* for the Ministry of Infor- mation and Broadcasting—which did not however prevent him from expressing his personal views freely.

A Visit to Sardar Kushwant Singh

I got to know Sardar Kushwant Singh in an unusual way—unusual to us, that is. When I called on him to deliver greetings from London he immediately invited me to have breakfast with him next day at eight o'clock. His library— English for the most part, although I discovered in it also a row of books by Gide and other contemporary authors—would have done credit to any European editor, and the breakfast served by his charming wife came up to the highest British standards. His eighteen-year-old son who had just taken his final school examinations had breakfast with us wearing his dressing-gown. Once again I realised how important a common language is for mutual understanding and what English means for our relations with India and for Indians among them- selves.

Indian Villages

During my first journey to India my companion and friend, Professor Hans Wehrli, never tired of drawing my attention to the importance of Indian villages. We visited many villages then—in the extreme south, in the Deccan, in Bengal, Orissa, and Assam, in the valleys of the Ganges and Indus. There were the houses of the Brahmin, and, some distance away, the huts of the casteless—poor dwellings inhabited by undernourished people. What is the Indian village like today, after ten years without foreign rule?

The leading intellectual class, which originated among the Brahmin and higher castes, had not forgotten in its burst of industrialisation that India was primarily a land of villages and that its future depended far less on the few large towns than on the hundreds of thousands of villages with their peasant inhabitants. The movement to reform the villages, organised as 'Community Projects' and the 'National Extension Service', has in its purest form the idealistic fervour of the movement for freedom.

I was able to visit some villages in the Punjab as well as in the neighbourhood of Delhi. In both districts the 'Community Projects' had made great progress, so that some model villages such as Shamaspur not far from Delhi, already existed with new, practical buildings (which still looked modest enough compared with European villages), a village hall where technical instruction was given, the new communal water-tap, and the school.

Community Projects

All this was very encouraging, despite one's mental reservations about these show-piece villages, and precisely because they rejected all superfluous show. It is a matter-of-fact world in which religion, although not deliberately opposed, takes a back seat. The zeal for planning of the socialists is at work, their materialism softened by the humility of the Indian towards what will always remain beyond proof.

The most difficult problem—the overcoming of the caste system and the acceptance of the 'untouchables' or 'scheduled castes' as full members of the community—was solved in Shamaspur in an extremely bold way: a Harijan (untouchable) was the village chief: his expression registered pride and a sense of responsibility and also the melancholy of this country, the tragedy of a centuries-old social order of inequality before God and man.

An 'Untouchable' as Village Chief

In the illustrated brochures which gave visitors some idea of the enthusiasm for the reform of the Indian village, there was a great deal of talk about planning and organisation, about the shaking-off of foreign rule, about social progress and the poor villagers but nothing was said about the problem of the 'untouchables', which still exists. Only now can a free India dare to reform the foundations of its social order—which were of religious origin—in the spirit of a newly won humanity. Here, too, the Mahatma showed the way to the nation.

Propaganda for Birth Control

Posters had been put up on the walls of the village hall giving practical instruction in words and pictures like a kind of school primer. One of the most widely circulated posters showed on the left a happy, well-dressed family with three children, on the right a poverty-stricken family with seven children; the moral: learn about birth-control!

A co-operative organisation for the cultivation of the country is indispensable. Indian land is only a third as productive as that of other countries; to give the extra yield so urgently needed not only more irrigation plants are required but also new methods of cultivation and new energies, to rescue the villagers from under-nourishment and debility. Many millions of dollars from America's capital surplus were put at India's disposal; but at least as important as financial help is the training of the native population.

The few model villages are only tiny specks in the whole picture, and if you visit a village at random off the beaten track, usually the picture now is no different from that of thirty years ago. Even in Delhi you cannot work magic.

117 top Anandpur in the Punjab with its perfectly preserved temple, next to the Golden Temple of Amritsar the most important Sikh shrine. The buildings were destroyed in the 18th century by the Moguls and rebuilt in the following century.

117 below Peasants' ox-carts on a country lane.

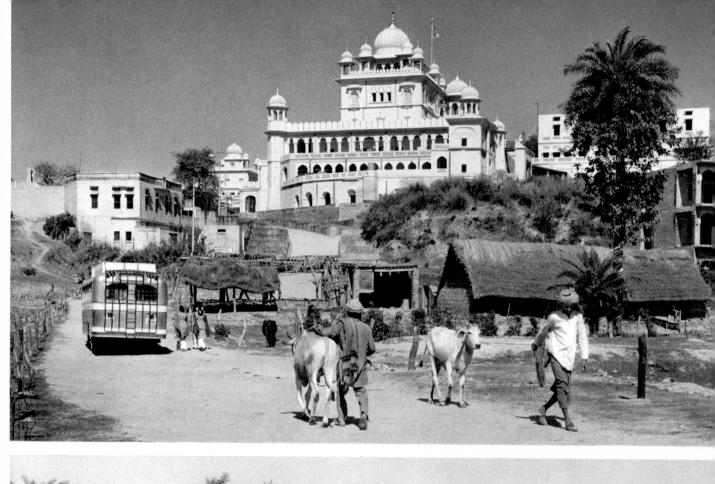

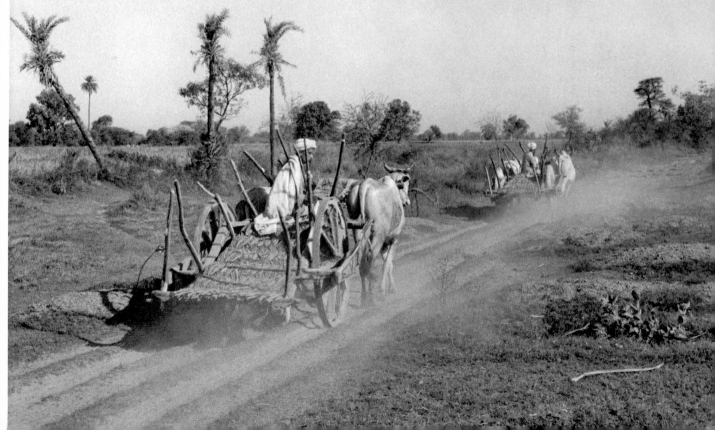

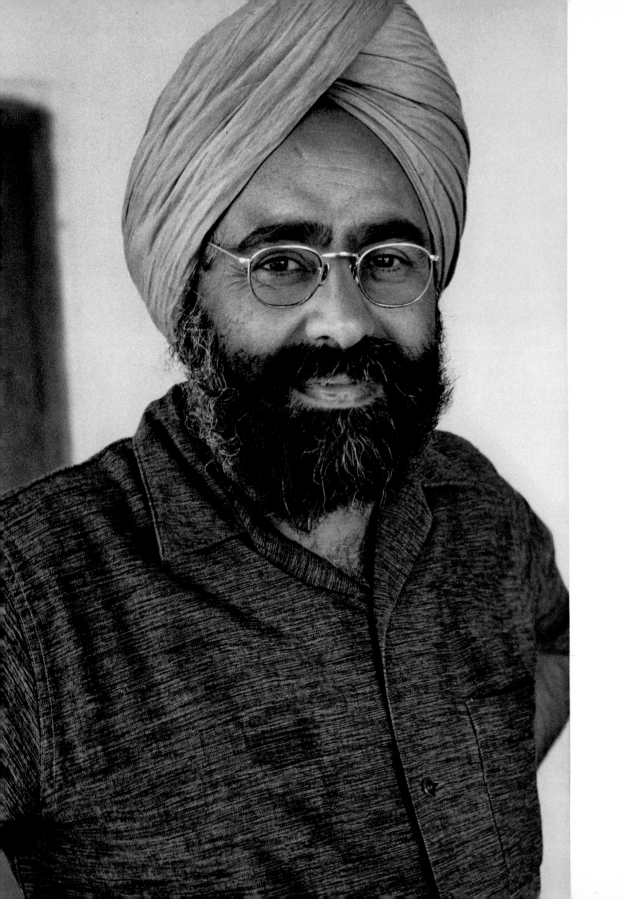

The 'Community Projects' and the 'National Extension Service', which is concerned more with expansion than with an intensive programme, cover today about a quarter of the Indian villages; in the second five-year plan they are to extend over the whole of India.

On my return from Chandigarh our Ambassador, who had taken an interest in my keen desire to meet Nehru, had good news for me, the Prime Minister was expecting me on Monday at four o'clock. I had never looked forward to an interview so eagerly.

Tea with the Prime Minister

An official led me through the bustle of the Parliament building to the room which had been the Prime Minister's study for eleven years. In the ante-room I was received by his Private Secretary and after a few minutes was face to face with the Prime Minister. He asked me to be seated but seemed to be in no hurry to talk. He was dressed in white, as when I saw him in Parliament a few days before, with a fresh red flower in his button-hole, but without the Gandhi cap.

Nehru has an unbelievably fine head, sensitive yet manly, somewhat morose and melancholy. His expression is genuine: he does not pose.

I had been warned that while sometimes Nehru is communicative, asks questions, and is a good listener, in other moods he is a strange and silent man. (He has been known to sit through a dinner-party at an Embassy without addressing the Ambassador's wife who was his charming and intelligent neighbour.)

He did not seem communicative that day. I made the odd remark in the hope that he would take it up; I had been struck by the fact that there was no hurry

118 Sardar Kushwant Singh, editor of the newspaper *Jojana* in Delhi, combines with his Sikh faith a cosmopolitan culture; he was an instructive guide on my visit to villages in the neighbourhood of the capital.

to change the names of the streets, whereas there were countries where the same street was renamed with every change of régime, two or three times in ten years. It impressed me that the Indians were so generous. 'We have even left the monument to the King—which George is it, now, V or VI?' said Nehru. 'What do you think of it, by the way?' 'It is certainly no great work of art.' 'It is horrible,' he confirmed, and for the first time his face lit up in an extremely engaging smile. Then he relapsed into his monumental silence.

I realised that he was not prepared to make once again a general comment about the fate of India, about Communism, and so on, and that neither would I learn from him anything new about Kashmir. When he asked how long I had been there and what kind of impression I had, I answered that naturally a great many of the impressive things one saw were being discussed in the newspapers and elsewhere: the dam, the villages, and so on; there was nothing particularly new to say about them. What was remarkable to me, a continental European, was that independent India kept of her own accord to the English model in so many ways.

Nehru and Birth-Control   As Nehru made no comment, I risked a rather delicate subject. I had read the newspaper report of his latest speech in which, referring to conditions in China, he supported birth-control as a check on the alarming increase in population. On the same day Krishna Menon, one of his most important colleagues, had made a speech in which he made fun of the advocates of birth-control. Nehru's laughter showed me that the ice was broken, and only now in conversation did his face show that famous charm which Macmillan found so irresistible on his recent visit to Delhi. Menon had only made fun of certain subsidiary features, but birth-control was the official policy. Nehru himself was incessantly advocating it, because it was a necessity for India. On the other hand, given the primitive condition of the people of India, only very simple means could be effective. In Calcutta a pill had been made which was apparently suitable.

I wanted to know if there was any objection on religious grounds to this propaganda, as in Christian countries the Roman Catholic Church in particular declared itself inexorably against it. Nehru replied that in fact the Roman Catholics in India, and only they, had protested; and even if they formed only a tiny minority of the population they still played a considerable role; the bishops themselves had vigorously presented their case to him. On the other hand, there was no opposition, at least no organised opposition, from the Hindus; perhaps they had not fully grasped all the issues. Meanwhile, however, birth-control was inevitably becoming a part of modern life.

I tried to sound him further. The scholarly Vice-President Radhakrishnan had just declared in a speech in New York that religions were moving towards unification, as was possible on a philosophical plane—but I felt that this way of thinking was limited to the educated. What about the villagers, by contrast: would the decline of religion or its forms, which in India—as elsewhere—keeps pace with the growth of technical civilisation, not leave a vacuum, to be filled by Communism with its materialistic dogmas as the only alternative? It was an interesting question, Nehru conceded. In the 19th century Europe had experienced its industrial revolution and had changed without renouncing its spiritual traditions. How a correspondingly industrialised India would behave he could not foresee. Communism had also changed: present-day Russia was no longer the Russia of Lenin and Stalin, and it was changing still. And Communism in China was of yet another kind. He, Nehru, had been deeply impressed on his visit to Peking by the fact that several thousand years of history still overshadowed the present.

As far as religion was concerned, Hinduism could not be called a religion at all: it taught no dogmas as for instance Islam did. In Hinduism, freedom of thought prevailed; a man who denied God could just as well be a Hindu as one

Nehru and the Hindu 'Dharma'

who prayed to God. But every Hindu has his 'Dharma', his inner law which he has to follow, and this could be very different for different people; it was not even the same all the time for each individual. Today the old social customs of Brahminism, especially the caste system, were out of date. But the Hindu could more easily than members of the Jewish, Christian, and Mohammedan religions assimilate many of the findings of modern science with his traditional conceptions. His mythology accustomed him to think in terms of millions of years and thus the geological eras were immediately comprehensible to him; the creation had not happened at a particular point in time, as in Christianity, so that he had had no need to revise his views about it.

We had finished our talk. I took my leave, thanking him warmly for the time

Pages 123–126 VILLAGES IN NORTH INDIA

123 On the highway between Delhi and Agra we met women gracefully carrying copper pots on their way to the well.

124 top In one of the small villages which we visited, between Delhi and Chandigarh, they still build bee-hive huts.

124 below In the dark room of her clay hut an old woman sits at her spinning-wheel. In spite of Gandhi's unremitting efforts for this ancient Indian cottage industry, which even the poorest and weakest can engage in, there is apparently uninterrupted development in India in the direction of mechanisation and urbanisation—and Indian factories are springing up to compete with Lancashire factories.

125 In one of the villages in the neighbourhood of Delhi, at which it had already been possible to realise the 'Community Project', we were greeted by a former Harijan, or 'untouchable', raised to the position of head of the village by his fellow-villagers. The 'untouchables' or outcasts, were a large section of the population with which contact was formerly considered to be sinful for the Hindu-caste, and which was segregated in special quarters.

126 In a village in the Punjab we came across an assembly of school classes; the pupils had gathered here from round about to take their examinations.

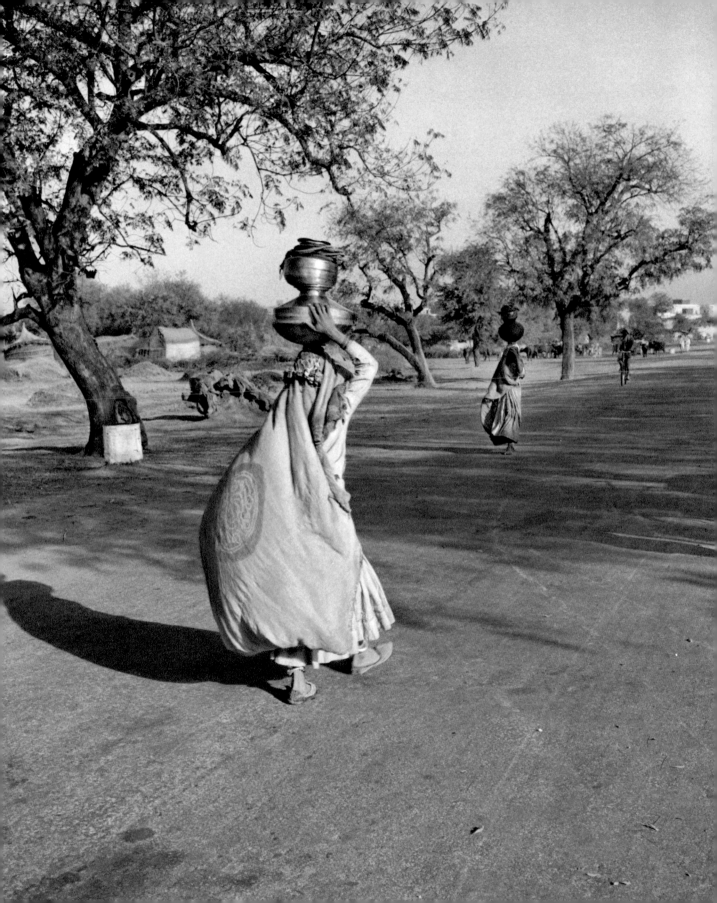

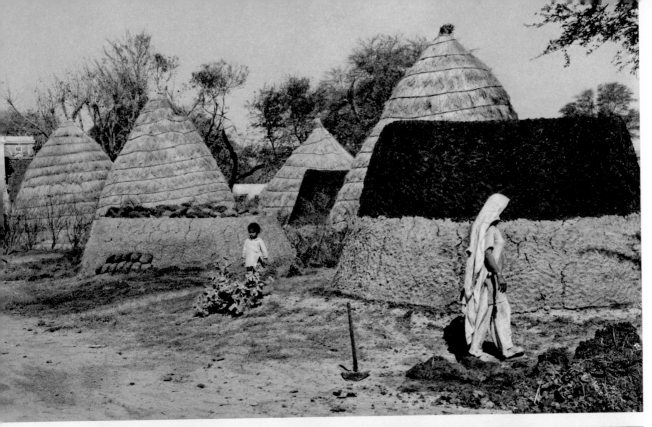

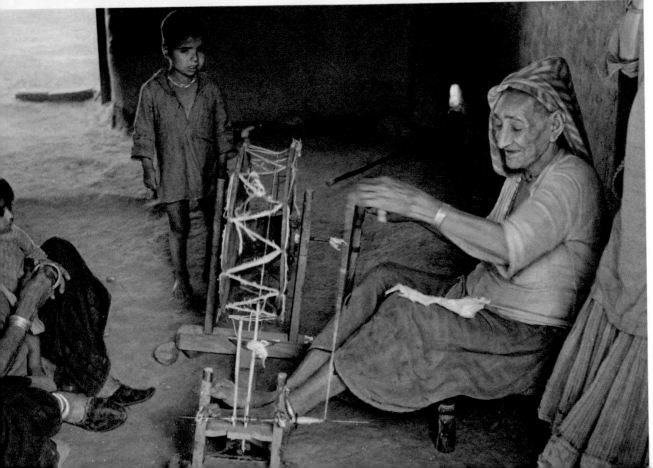

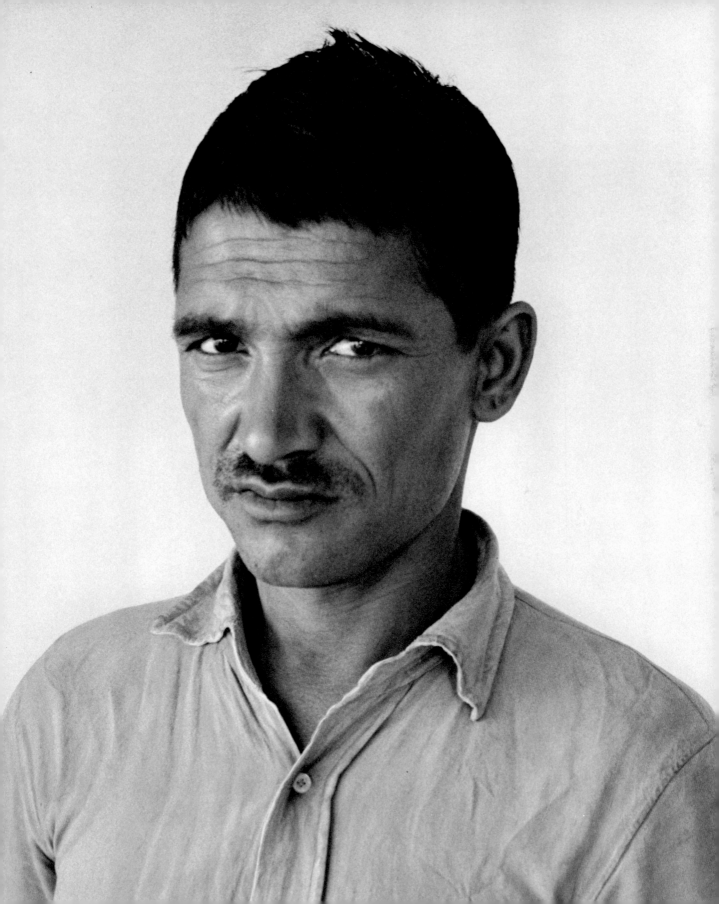

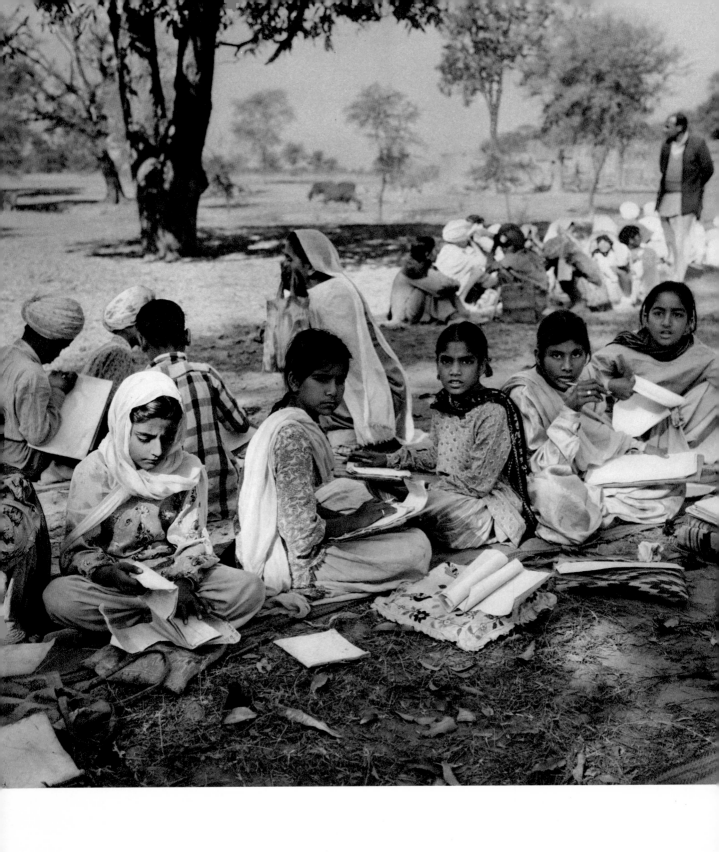

he had spared me. Although I had brought my camera with me, I could not bring myself, after all, to photograph this wonderfully impressive head.

Who are the men to whose hands Nehru can confide the rudder of the ship of State when he has grown weary? Does his daughter Indra, the present President of Congress, represent a third generation of the Nehrus coming up to assume responsibility? The halo of the champions of independence is beginning to pale, and a fresh impetus is needed to persuade the whole, many-faceted nation to accept a political leader. The people are easily gathered to see a famous man, but these masses are different masses in Bombay, Calcutta, Trivandum, Madras, Srinagar—and perhaps one day their leaders will be equally different. Perhaps already today we should look for the true leaders of the Indian people not among ambitious parliamentarians but rather among the men who, as genuine disciples of Gandhi, are devoting themselves outside party circles to the social and moral rebirth of India—men like Vinobha Bhave, who is carrying his message of land reform from meeting to meeting, spurred on simply by a spontaneous impulse of solidarity.

In Memory of British India

The nation which today is called India is very largely the creation of the British; it was they who unified the country militarily and administratively; they who transmitted the democratic maxims and principles upon which the present-day Republic rests. I myself felt a strong reaction when I saw India again after this interval: in the 'twenties I was full of enthusiasm for the Indian freedom movement; the arrogance which many British were still displaying in their clubs and the harshness of the police actions which culminated in the blood-bath of Amritsar seemed to me reprehensible; I was perturbed too by the views of some of my countrymen, to whom the superiority of the European master-race was a perfectly natural thing. Today, however, when the self-assurance of the Indians has an opportunity for full development and brings forth its own strange exaggerations, I cannot help feeling an almost anachronistic respect for the British achievement.

A Memory of Gandhi   I recall at this point my first encounter with the man the Indian nation rightly reveres as its father.

I first saw Gandhi in 1926 during the All-India Congress, which in that year was held at Gauhati on the Brahmaputra river. At that time Gandhi had kept aloof from politics for several years, and it was expected that at Gauhati he would for the first time again pronounce his views on topical political problems. In European newspapers it could be read at that time that politically Gandhi was of no account—a popular show-piece for the masses but no more. The interest which world opinion took in the Indian national movement was then so small that apart from my friend Professor Wehrli and myself the only European present was a Labour Member of Parliament from Westminster, who disappeared after the first session.

Several thousand men and women grouped according to the districts from which they came had assembled in a huge tent. The delegates wore the Gandhi cap, which India's diplomatic representatives have since made familiar the world over, and the white *khaddar* (a hand-spun and hand-woven cloth). There were bearded men from the north, bespectacled dark-skinned intellectuals from the south, representatives of all castes and classes, races and sects. Next to the box of the President were seated the members of the Central Committee, and a special space was reserved for the women delegates with their children. Towards evening lights went up, tea was served for the leaders; here and there a child was screaming in one of the boxes reserved for the women; orange peel was scattered everywhere. It was one large peaceful family. At times the deliberations themselves seemed to interest only the man who happened to be speaking and the 200 representatives of the Indian Press who were sitting in front of the rostrum.

The leaders who spoke in the opening session were mostly highly impressive individuals, with bold, proud features like Roman senators, who wore their white garments slung about their bodies like togas. There was Srinivasa Jyenger from

Madras, who that year was the President of Congress; Pandit Motilal Nehru, the leader of the Swaraj Party, with coolly observant eyes behind his spectacles, a dry speaker whose authority was felt all round him; Pandit Madan Mohan Malaviya, the Rector of the Hindu University of Benares, and the most distinguished representative of the Conservative 'collaborationist' Hindus, an elegant slight figure with a strongly-marked profile—his speech in Hindi sounded like the recital of a poem; Sen Gupta, the self-assured Lord Mayor of Calcutta; Sorojini Naidu, the last year's President of Congress, with her huge fiery eyes—author of delicate lyrical poems, but no less a master in her command of the English language as she addressed a passionate patriotic appeal to the gathering—forceful, like the mother of a Roman hero, but in personal conversation of an almost tender kindliness and a model of the *grande dame*. And finally, those representatives of Islam who were faithful to Congress: the tall, cautious, slightly nasal Abdul Kalam Azad, the only one among this group who was to assume an important position in Nehru's government in 1947, and who was to direct India's educational system for a decade; and the two fat brothers Ali, whose thunderous rhetoric was obviously taken less seriously by the assembly. Finally from the midst of all these important gentlemen there arose, treading lightly, dressed only in a dhoti and a cloth thrown over his shoulder, a spare little man. From his otherwise clean-shaven skull there dangled a thin wisp of hair as is the Hindu custom. A strong nose, broad lips beneath a small moustache; when he laughed, which he did frequently in the circle of his friends, large gaps between his teeth became visible. From all appearances an ugly little schoolmaster; and yet as one looked around over this vast assembly it was clear that only this man could be the 'great soul' of India. He had shed the magic pose of the Indian, the mystical veil in front of his eyes had been drawn aside and the light of truth radiated clearly, kindly but with commanding majesty in his gaze.

As soon as the Mahatma sat down on the speaker's rostrum, put on his spectacles

129

and pulled out a piece of paper, there was for the first time complete and utter silence in the tent. He read out slowly and clearly the resolution drafted in English on the news of the murder of the Hindu Swami Shradhanad by a fanatical Mohammedan. Then he began to speak extempore in Hindi. His clear voice penetrated the vast space without effort. He accompanied his speech with a few spare movements of his left hand, which was now holding his spectacles. He had foreseen the outrage which today shocked everyone, and Swami was to him not a martyr whose death must be lamented but a hero whose honour should be celebrated. His death was an appeal to everyone to examine his own conscience; it did not concern Swami alone but all India, covered as it was by the disgrace of the Hindu-Moslem conflict. The simplicity and directness of his speech tolerated no contradiction.

On the 'political' first day of the Gauhati Congress Gandhi kept his silence, but on the following morning in a committee meeting he intervened for the first time in years in the political discussion. Like all delegates when they are anxious to be completely understood Gandhi spoke in English. He answered directly and candidly all those who urged him to take part again in active politics. His conditions were: self-scrutiny, the overcoming of Hindu-Islamic enmity, spinning. But he also intervened in the debate on a highly topical political subject, and strangely enough this historic intervention—the only one which I heard with my own ears—was in favour of Britain. One delegate had proved that it should be made clear once and for all that the term *Swaraj* should include complete independence from Great Britain. In all probability this resolution would have been adopted, and might have greatly embittered the struggle for Indian freedom, had not Gandhi resolutely intervened. Most emphatically, almost violently he turned against those voicing anti-British sentiments. 'Certainly,' he said, 'the term *Swaraj* includes full independence, but as far as I am concerned, it presupposes at the same time close co-operation with the British people on the basis of full equality. In the meantime I have given you a very progressive programme of action: spinning.' The purpose of this appeal to spin was to enable the under-nourished peasant population to earn between harvests that small supplementary income which it needed in order to live on a human level—supplement in the way of clothes and food, but also a supplement of self-confidence, and sense of responsibility. At that time during all his extensive propaganda talks Gandhi concentrated almost exclusively on his appeal for *Khaddar*—spinning.

In the accommodation provided for the Congress leaders, on the banks of the Brahmaputra river, Gandhi occupied a hut by himself. From the early hours of the morning onwards, one could always see some two hundred people standing there, waiting in the rain, peasant-folk from the surrounding districts who were anxious to catch a glimpse of the Mahatma.

Inside the hut the only decoration, hanging above the entrance, was a small coloured portrait of the Buddha, who in the mind of the Indian of today represents not so much the founder of a religious community, a conception which nowadays exists only outside India, but rather the most eminent example of a human being of the Indian nation. Now and then a gust of wind lifted the loose window-flaps, and a stream of white light illuminated the half-dark room. All one heard was the patter of the rain. Waiting with me was Pandit Motilal Nehru, who was expecting to have an important discussion. Mrs Naidu looked in to see if the Mahatma had arrived yet, and she spoke with profound tenderness of 'this little, wonderful, great man'. Finally he himself entered, and shook my hand. Romain Rolland, who had written a beautiful biography of Gandhi, had given me a letter of introduction to him, and I briefly transmitted the greetings. He invited me to visit him at his *ashrama* should I be in the neighbourhood of Ahmedabad.

I did indeed visit him at his home, Satyagraha Ashram in Sabarmati. He lived there surrounded by a group of his most faithful helpers and their families. He was *A Visit to Satyagraha Ashram* a practical idealist, and therefore always placed more importance on the living example than on persuasion. And since India is a country of poor villages the conditions at Satyagraha Ashram were those of a poor village. Water was drawn from a deep well. An old ox who was no longer fit to do other work (for Gandhi too oxen were naturally sacred animals and must not be killed) was put on a small wheeled trolley on which he rolled down sloping rails, and thus by his weight he pulled a water-container up the deep shaft of the well. The only work he was able to perform usefully was then to walk up the slope again. With these and other little devices they tried to raise the standard of village life by making use of the existing very primitive means. In a separate room there were spinning-wheels where during the hours of physical and mental relaxation every inhabitant of the *ashrama* would spin the prescribed length of yarn from home-produced cotton, just as did the Mahatma himself, as part of his daily duties, between discussions, reading, prayer, and dealing with his unending, immense correspondence.

On arrival I called on his Private Secretary, and on this occasion also made the acquaintance of the Mahatma's wife, a quiet and modest lady. I inquired for how many minutes I could dare to detain the busy Mahatma, but once I had entered the small, bright, and simple study, I never had a chance even to look at my

Pages 133–136 BENARES

133 A pilgrim who has filled his water-vessel from the sacred Ganges sets off for his night's lodging.

134–135 Early in the morning Hindus from every district in the country throng the Ghat, the steps leading down to the Ganges, for the ritual washing and prayers.

136 On the road to the temples and bathing-places sit rows of beggars; their conduct is pleasing to God because they arouse compassion.

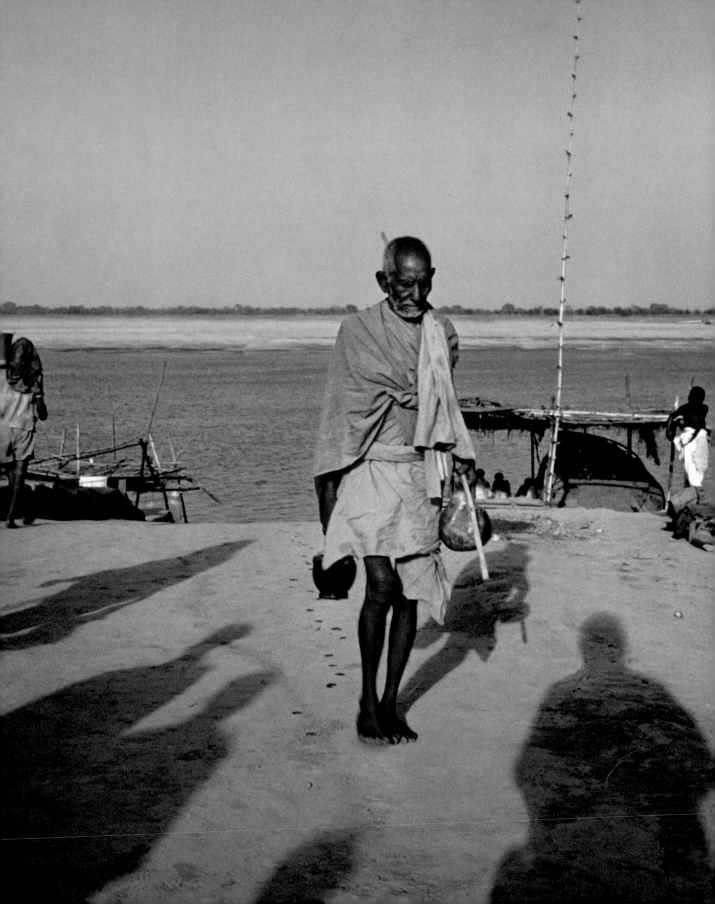

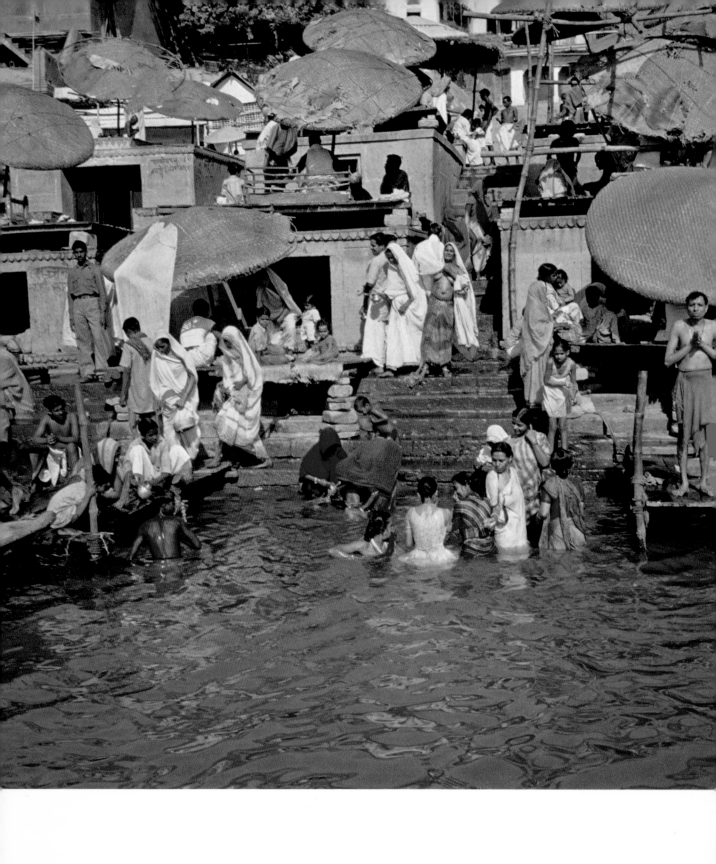

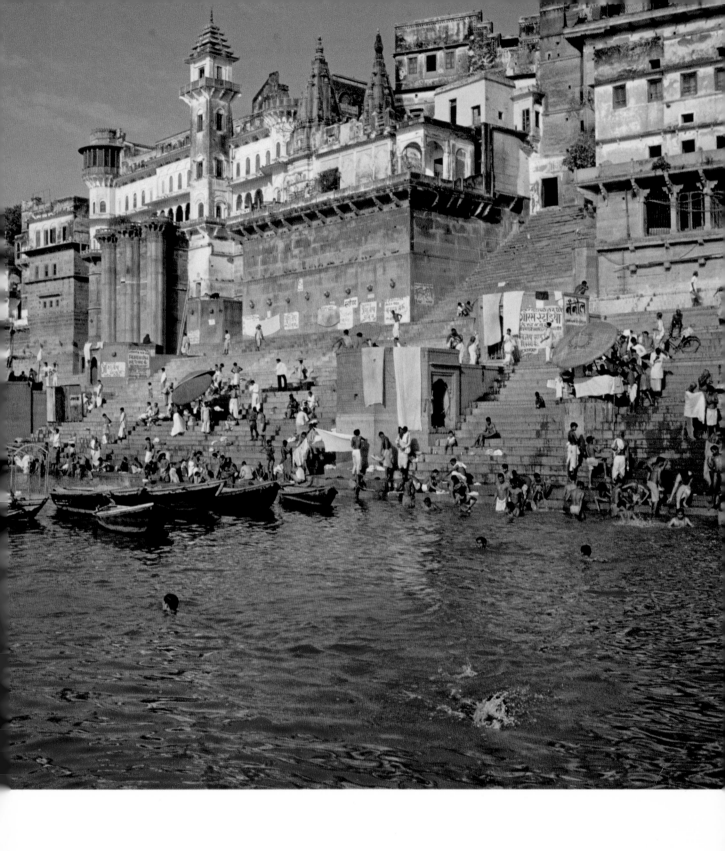

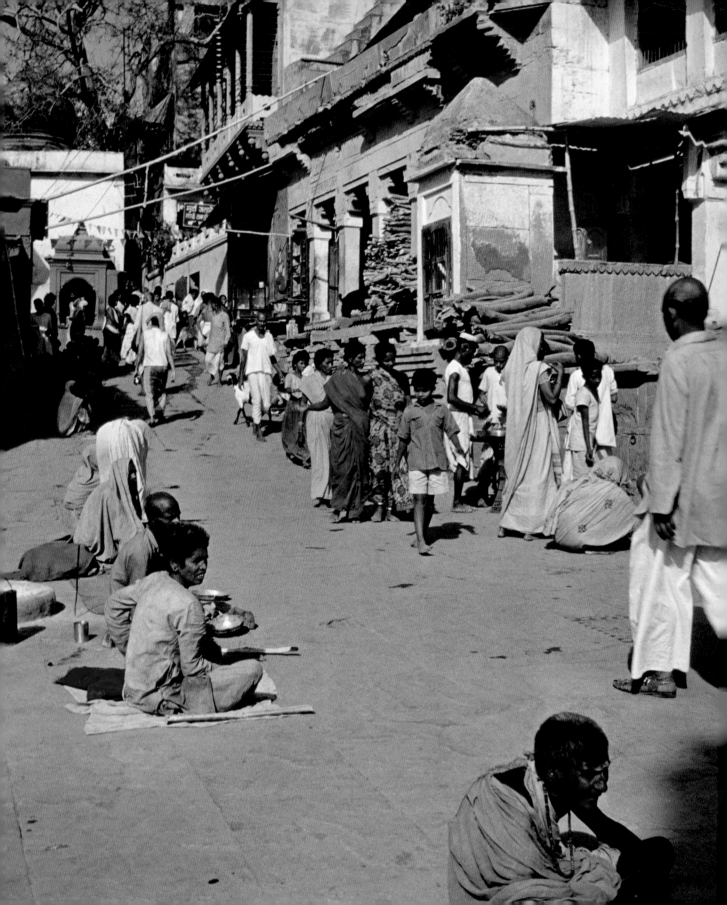

watch. Gandhi, who had been sitting on the floor on a white cushion jumped up and urged me despite my reluctance to be seated on a chair, since, as he said, I was not used to the Indian way of sitting with crossed legs. Thus I found myself enthroned somewhat ridiculously above him, but his clear, shining eyes were so friendly that all embarrassment left me immediately.

In conversation Gandhi did not lecture, he asked questions and he listened. I had to tell him of my experiences in India and he wished to hear not only of the great friendliness and hospitality that I had experienced, but also what I thought of the keeping of generous promises and reliability in general. He asked me for concrete examples, because the struggle against unreliability in his own ranks was part of his programme for an independent nation. I uttered some criticism of the all too simplifying manner in which certain Indians stress the antithesis of the materialist West and the idealist East. I remarked that outside the English-speaking area too—for example in the German-speaking area of which people in India knew so little, there existed spiritual and intellectual realities of great significance. Gandhi asked me whether in our peasant cottages Goethe was being read in the same way as were the holy ancient epics in India. 'No,' I told him, but the Bible was being read, and the Catechism. Thus, almost unawares, I started to talk and found myself involved in a discussion. Nowhere in India have I ever had a more thorough, realistic, and more candid conversation.

Before leaving Satyagraha Ashram I cast a last glance from outside through the window into Gandhi's study. There he sat, in the dusky light, all by himself, turning with one hand the spinning-wheel, while the other was forming the growing thread.

In an unusual way Gandhi answered the Biblical text: 'Be ye therefore wise as serpents and harmless as doves.' He never denied that he had been a lawyer who was accustomed to dealing with all the realities of human nature. In his book

Gandhi the Unique

The Discovery of India Jawaharlal Nehru refers humorously to the fact that the Mahatma came from Gujrat, the home of hard-bitten businessmen. The slogans coined by him, his campaigns of passive resistance, the breaking of the salt monopoly, and the boycott were not borrowed from the international arsenal of revolutionaries, but were exactly in tune with the country and the situation. He was a genius of political propaganda—and he proved that a man may be a propagandist without surrendering anything of the integrity of his conviction. He has been called a charlatan, because in the popular imagination heroes and saints are quite different; to contemporaries there is always something baffling about true originality. Gandhi could never be induced to consider his political opponent an enemy; and no people, except his own, had in him a more sincere and devoted friend than the English. His piety inspired him with tolerance towards every manifestation of godliness in man and made him hold sacred the life of every creature.

His strongest weapon was always his own physical person, which he threw into the struggle to the point of sacrificing his life. His last act of fasting, about whose outcome there was world-wide anxiety, ended with his last political victory; this he won not over alien rule but over the intolerance of his own followers, over the intolerance of politics in general. Even by his violent death at the hand of a Hindu he revealed to mankind the abyss towards which it was hastening.

To his people Mahatma Gandhi remained the leader in the fight for freedom, which had really begun only now with the assumption of independence, for the true decision was not made in the face of foreign usurpers, but in the face of his own people and its lack of a national history.

Flight from Delhi to Benares This journey to India would be incomplete without a glimpse of one of the sacred places of Hinduism. The flight from Delhi to Calcutta gave me a chance to break my journey in Benares, the most sacred of all.

The airport from which we left could be reached from the hotel in a few minutes; it lay right in the middle of the ruins of Old Delhi. Once again I got a bird's-eye view of the widely scattered monuments of the old residences, the geometrically arranged white buildings of New Delhi with the circus of Connaught Place, the old town with the Red Fort and the three marble cupolas of the great mosque, the memorial to Gandhi, and the sluggish muddy waters of the Jumna. We followed the course of the river over one of the most densely populated districts in Asia; the broad plain was covered with tiny villages with pools and wells. Scarcely a green spot could be seen, the land was thirsting for the coming monsoon. We landed first at Lucknow, the capital of the State of Uttar Pradesh with more than sixty million inhabitants. At Allahabad the almost dried-up river-bed of the Jumna joined the green waters of the Ganges: there, at the holy place on the junction of the rivers, I had once attended the Kumbh Mala feast, which took place every twelve years and to which hundreds of thousands of pilgrims streamed.

In Benares itself little seemed to have changed. From the 'Cantonment', where the hotels were surrounded by gardens of flowering trees, I went a few miles through an unimpressive new town, with its asphalt streets and cinema posters, into the old quarter.

Benares, a Place of Pilgrimage

Here there was a jam of cars and pedicabs and a stream of pedestrians; at the edge of the road a camel caravan was drawn up, and the narrow lanes were flanked by shops with brassware, silks, embroidery, and souvenirs of all kinds. A bell sounded from the temple; here and there a cow ambled among the throng of pilgrims with their brightly coloured clothes and garlands of fragrant flowers. There were Sadhus, ascetics with staves and water-containers, their skin daubed with ashes—it was often hard to distinguish between saint and charlatan—priests, beggars squatting on the ground, cripples, mangy dogs, this whole world which revolves round Shiva, the great God of destruction, creative power, and preservation.

On the way back to the hotel my guide took me to the Hindu university founded in 1916 and for a long time presided over by Pandit Malaviya, leader of the Hindu Mahasabha. It extended over several square miles and had sports grounds like English universities; both academic and residential buildings represented an attempt to combine Indian forms with the tradition of English college architecture—producing, as in the case of the recent building in New Delhi, a rather old-fashioned effect.

On the Sacred Ganges Early next day American tourists and others were sailing along the Ganges to see the unique spectacle of the river-front with its palaces, temples, and stairways (ghats) with crowds of bathers and worshippers. The believers, quite unconcerned about their neighbours and the uninvited spectators, performed their ritual practices on the steps and in the water, each one for himself alone with his God; they clasped their hands in all kinds of strange gestures, raised their arms, held their noses and dived under the water. The frontage was no longer quite the same untidy confusion of ruins and new houses as before; some ruined palaces had been demolished, and there were large gaps, cleared for development. Posters defaced some of the façades. Above all the other buildings the mosque erected by Aurangzeb rose triumphantly. But even it was not able to stifle the pulse-beat of this place of pilgrimage. The faithful streamed in, filled their containers with the sacred water of the Ganges and took it back to the far south, over Adams Bridge, as an offering to the holy Lingam of Ramesvaram, to the last of the seven holy places which bind the countries of India into a magic unit.

The macabre climax of the spectacle was reached at the burning-ghat, where a few wood-piles are almost always smoking. In the town of Shiva it is blessed to die with one's feet in the sacred waters of the Ganges; within twenty-four hours of death the corpse is carried on an open bier decked with flowers to the Jalsain ghat where the next-of-kin lights the fire. On a boat they were wrapping a dead body in a red cloth—it was an unmarried girl who was not allowed to be cremated. A heavy stone was tied to the bundle and it was lowered into the Ganges. You are confronted here with the undisguised majesty of death, in modern towns long since thrust out of sight.

Nobody can escape the momentous impact of this town of death and resurrection, this chaotic, wild, colourful, and boundless manifestation of belief in the transcendental. Does the true soul of India still dwell here, as it has done for thousands of years past? Or is even this shrine moving imperceptibly from the centre of life into the realm of ethnological curiosities and historical monuments?

After a stop at Patna, where a side-line leads to the kingdom of Nepal, which until a few years ago was closed to visitors, the old Indian Airline Dakota brought me to Calcutta, the capital of Bengal. On the banks of the muddy Hooghly, especially on the Howrah side, docks and warehouses extended for several miles. The haze from the city blended with the smoke of the factory chimneys; one missed the white quays, the blue vistas of Bombay.

The Bengali are considered a restless people. Crowds moved unceasingly over the great Howrah Bridge, and in and out of the famous temple of the Kali-Durga, where wooden stakes dripped with the blood of sacrificial goats. The sacred cows are still not banned from the street, and walk about even among the skyscrapers of the city.

In Calcutta the contrasts between the wealthy and the very poor living in over-crowded quarters are even greater than elsewhere. The turbulent city gave the British a great deal of trouble and it is even today the scene of conflicts of every kind. Calcutta was directly affected by the partition of Bengal. There are people

Calcutta: The First City of India

who dream of a reunification of Bengal, with Calcutta as the centre of a new independent Hindu-Moslem State with a population equal to that of Germany.

One evening after darkness had fallen I boarded my DC-6B at Calcutta airport, was greeted in my native Swiss-German by the stewardesses and at once provided with the latest newspapers from Europe and with food and drink. In only a few hours I had left India far behind and came under the spell of Chinese culture—and how differently this inspires us!

Pages 143–148 BENARES

On the steps of the Ghat, in recesses on the river-front, outside their primitive huts and in the bustle of the bazaars—everywhere you meet the beggar-monk, the Sadhu; one sits for hours motionless, sunk in meditation; another stands with raised arms by the river; a third makes strange motions with his hands and sacred implements—Shiva's trident, crescent, drum, and shell. Among the confusing impressions of this place of pilgrimage belong, too, the small shrine beside the road, gaudy cinema posters in the main thoroughfare; the activities of a building firm carrying out a new monumental building scheme on the river-bank, where only a little while ago the debris of a badly-built palace lay scattered about. The street with pedicabs and lean cows wandering about freely is crowded with traders and their merchandise; different again is the atmosphere in the corn-market, or in the narrow lane where fly-whisks and souvenirs are offered for sale.

Pages 149–150 CALCUTTA

149, 150 below A priest, a beggar, and a visitor in the Kalighat Temple, the most frequented Hindu temple in the capital of Bengal. It is dedicated to the Goddess Kali, wife of Shiva, after whom Calcutta itself is named.

150 top Among the sky-scrapers of the City, where the big international commercial firms have their offices, in the midst of traffic, the sacred cows still wander about.

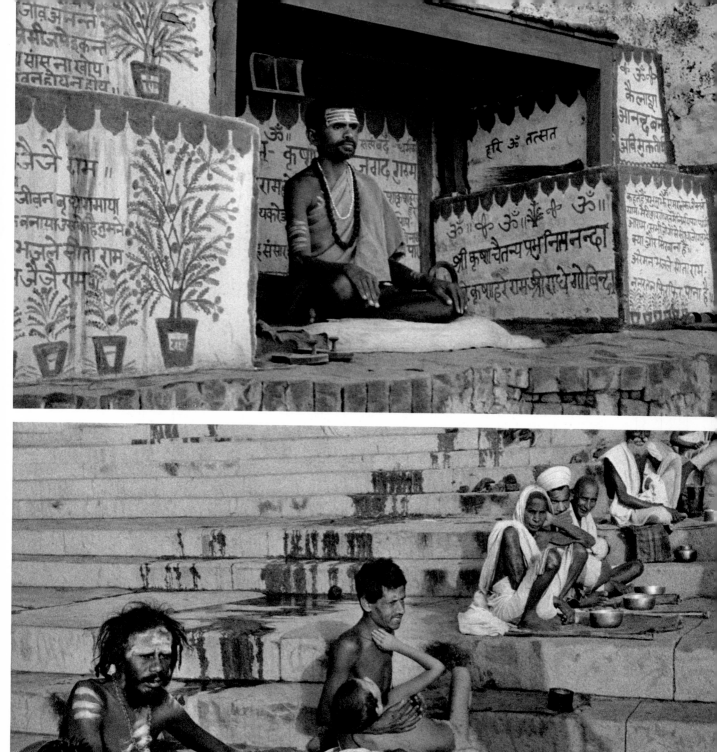

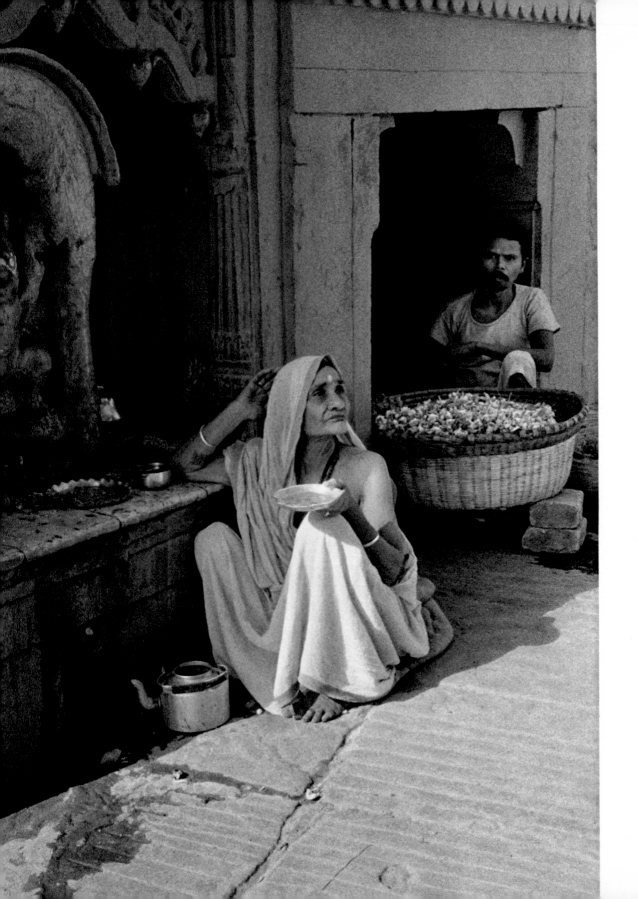

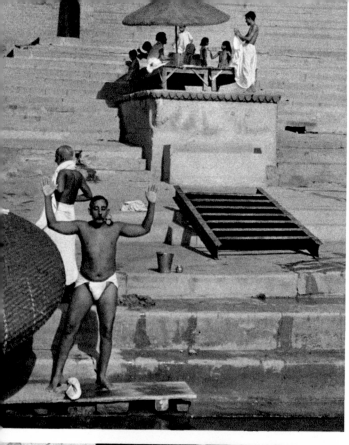
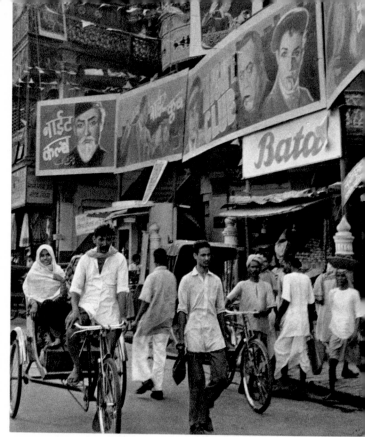
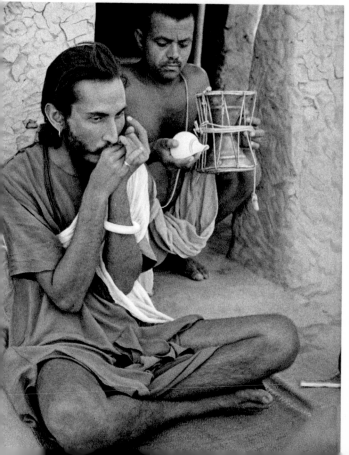
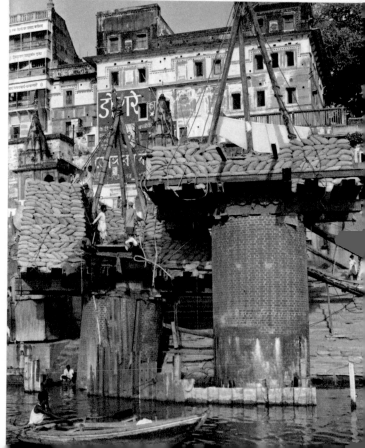

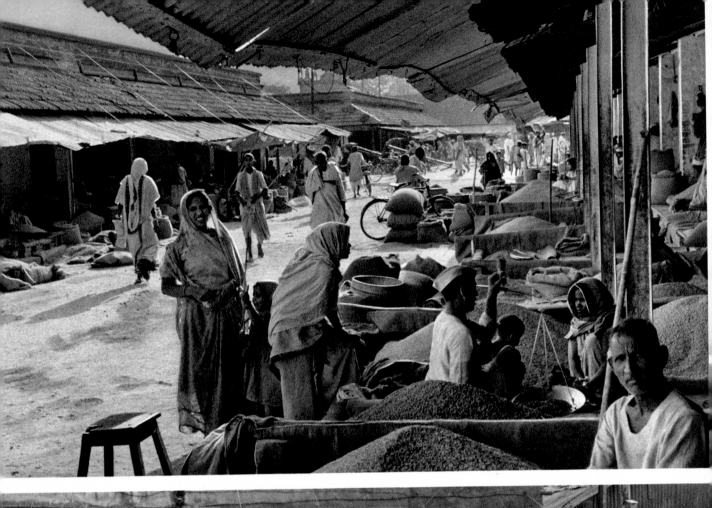
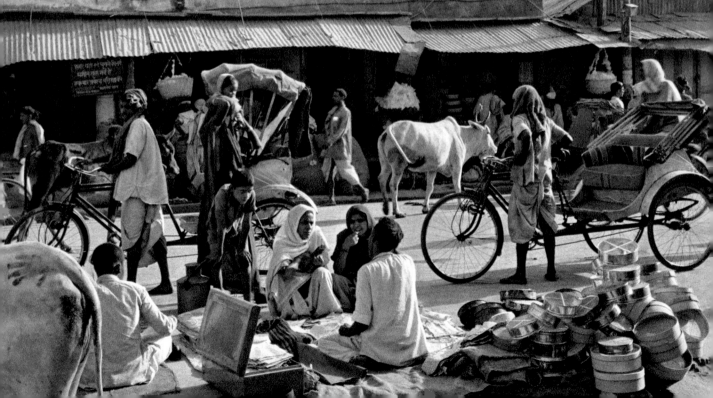

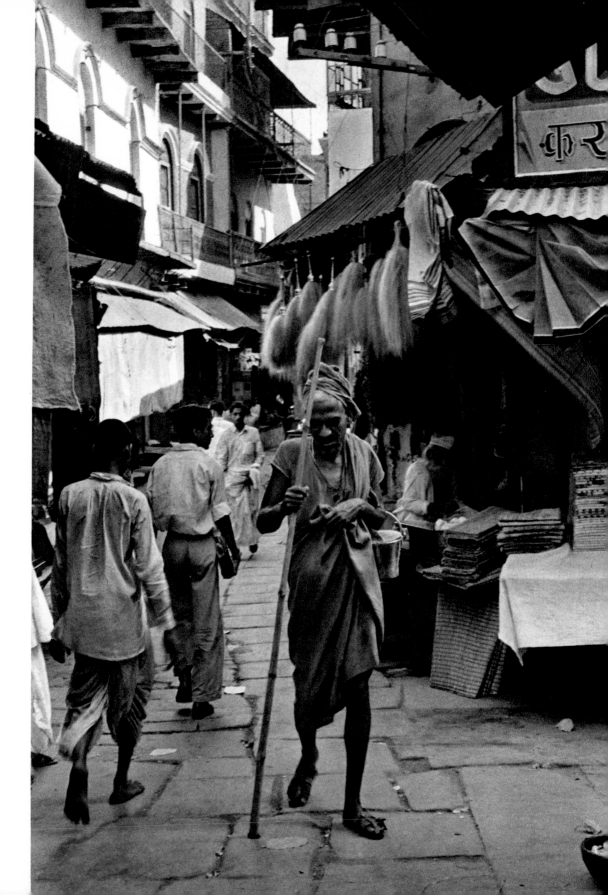

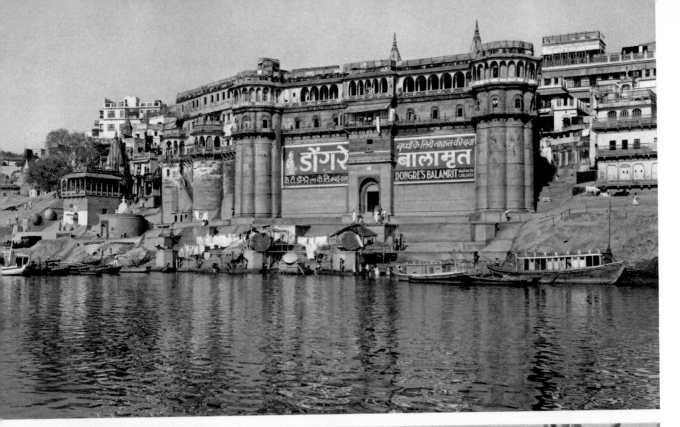

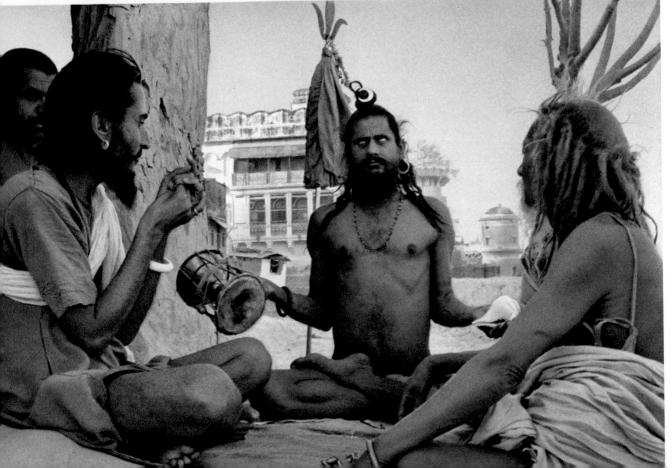

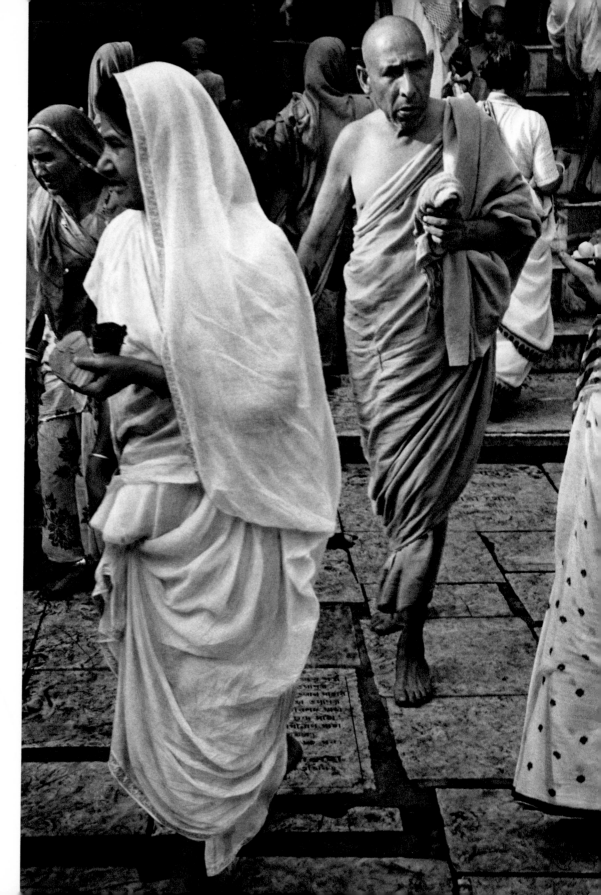

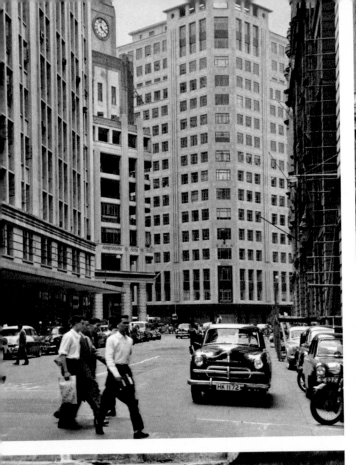
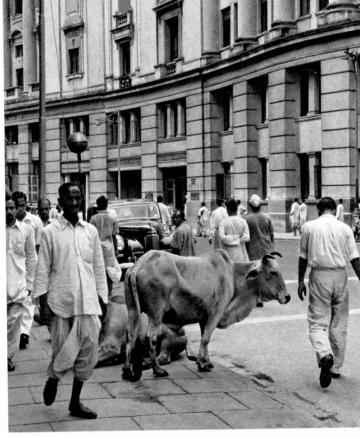
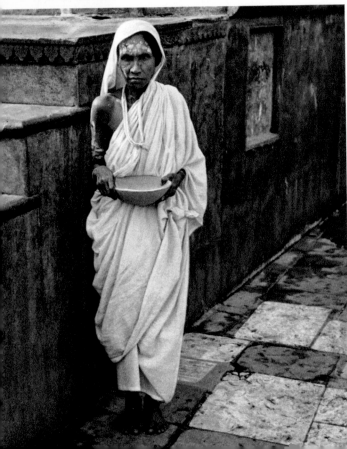
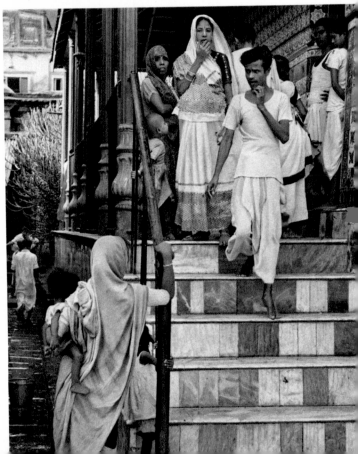

Hongkong

THE DAY was already far advanced when the first islands and fishermen's junks appeared on the surface of the sea. Macao, the small Portuguese colony, came into sight and our aircraft was already coming down from its normal height of 16,000 feet to the cluster of islands, with their mountains and bays. The approach to Hongkong was magnificent. We flew in a wide loop over the mountainous islands, the mainland coast of Kowloon, and one of the best natural harbours in the world. Between rocks and green trees, gardens and fields extended an enormous city with skyscrapers and lowly cottages, and the surface of the water was dotted with boats of every kind—pocket-battleships, large passenger steamers, and swarms of junks. We came down into this animated landscape, landing on a runway built on land reclaimed from the sea—now being enlarged to keep up with the next stage of development. Landing in Hongkong is an anxious business for a pilot; typhoons afflict this area, and sometimes the island is enveloped in thick mist, so that there is nothing to do but fly on to Manila, two hours away.

Chinese with bright faces and smart uniforms carried out a cursory passport examination, without going through our luggage. Hongkong is a free port. Even sending home undeveloped films—almost prohibitively complicated by red tape in countries like India—causes no difficulties here. You can buy everything under the sun, even Communist newspapers.

That Hongkong, geographically a tiny constituent of China, still exists as a British Crown Colony borders on a miracle, but how it exists is also a matter for wonder. It was rewarding to interrupt the flight for a week; there are few places in the world that so well repay study; and anyone who visits Hongkong just for the beauty of the scenery and the picturesque life of the people is richly rewarded.

Colonial Government Today   When the English reoccupied the country after the war there were only 600,000 inhabitants—a million had been expelled or murdered by the war-lords. By the end of 1946, however, the pre-war figure of 1,600,000 had been restored, and the influx continued, nourished by the refugees from the terror and misery of the proletarian dictatorship, but also by the natural increase of a prolific people. In 1950 there were 2,360,000 people living in the Crown Colony; today the number is probably 3,000,000.

How has the colonial government dealt with this vast over-population, without a complete breakdown? Colonies can earn no praise today; but this should not prevent us from acknowledging achievements where they really exist. Two partners have mastered the almost insoluble problem: the English, with their ability to restore order with a minimum of expenditure and force; and the Chinese with their tremendous vitality, industry, and centuries-old experience of social life. The disturbances which one occasionally reads about in the newspapers are nothing in comparison with the achievements of manufacturing, building, and organisation here.

The Refugee Settlement   Why were such a throng of people allowed in, an anonymous mass, in which even restless elements and above all the destitute felt secure? The answer is so simple that people hardly believe it any longer nowadays, but there is no other: out of humanity. But it was not only the persecuted foreigners who were deserving of humane consideration; the native population were no less entitled to protection from contamination and impoverishment by this kind of invasion. It was a dilemma similar to that which faced a neutral country like Switzerland in times of crisis, and Hongkong need not be ashamed of the comparison. The frontier was closed, but there was a constant trickle of refugees and a blind eye was turned to it. By far the greatest organising work in the absorption of refugees was carried out by the Chinese themselves in all secrecy; any of the newcomers who had an acquaintance in Hongkong was taken to a safe place.

The administration had first of all to combat hunger and epidemics; then it was a question of finding work for the immigrants who wanted neither to go farther nor to return; homes fit to live in had to be found for many thousands.

In the first stages a great deal was accomplished by private organisations, and especially by the Christian Churches. In overcoming the school problem, too, the authorities were helped by private initiative: out of 1,219 schools with 331,168 pupils, only 431 schools with 128,235 pupils are now government subsidised.

Industrialisation

More work could be found only by the creation of new industries. In a few years Hongkong, once exclusively a centre for fishing and trade, has become one of the most important industrial centres in the East. The export of consumer goods is a vital necessity for Hongkong, and the colonial rulers are less concerned with the traditional 'exploitation' in favour of British industry than with the development of a self-supporting community. In 1948 there were 1,160 factories and workshops in the Colony, which employed 60,000 workers; at the beginning of 1958, there were already 3,373 concerns with 153,033 workers registered. This development would not have been possible had there not been, as well as many industrious and skilled workmen, an influx of capital from wealthy Chinese fugitives from Shanghai and other cities.

Beside the importance of industry and trade with the free world, trade with China has generally been overrated; it is only a very small proportion of the whole.

Housing

Because of the inrush of the homeless the housing shortage became so severe that the government itself finally had to finance large new housing estates, and a

153

new department was set up —the 'department of resettlement'—to carry out the project. With the constant influx of people from China the Colony had for long been familiar with the phenomenon of 'squatters'. Squatter settlements sprang up particularly around Kowloon, wherever an open space was to be found. The huts in which families were crowded together were a constant danger not only because of all kinds of illnesses and encouragements to vice but also because of fire. On Christmas Eve, 1953, 50,000 people lost their homes through the Shek Kip Mei fire alone. This was the signal for more vigorous measures: huge six- and seven-storeyed blocks were built in the new suburbs, laid out in the shape of an H, with rooms of thirteen square yards taking five adults. Everything was restricted to essentials, the standard simpler than in Swiss and German towns, but it was a great step forward and not below the level of what China is doing for its working classes. A good 2,000 people live in a building like this; and in four new districts of this kind 103,000 people have been housed in recent years. But altogether some 300,000 Chinese are still living in the squatter settlements.

Trading Centre and Holiday Paradise The smartest district was to be found in the town of Victoria, as the original English settlement on the island is called. Here a city of skyscrapers has sprung up and building is still going on feverishly. Here is a field for private capital; the rents are enormous, for a concrete structure of this kind must pay for itself in six to seven years. One of the highest buildings was erected by the Red Chinese as their national bank—as it happens by an English architect in the conventional modern Western style. On the slopes behind the town and far along the banks among the old houses were new villas and flats for the cosmopolitan society of entrepreneurs, diplomats, and agents. From far off you could see the white pagoda of Tiger Balm

Pages 155–157 HONGKONG. In the broad harbour of Hongkong the fishing junks sail among the modern steamers and warships. Our picture shows the harbour front of Victoria.

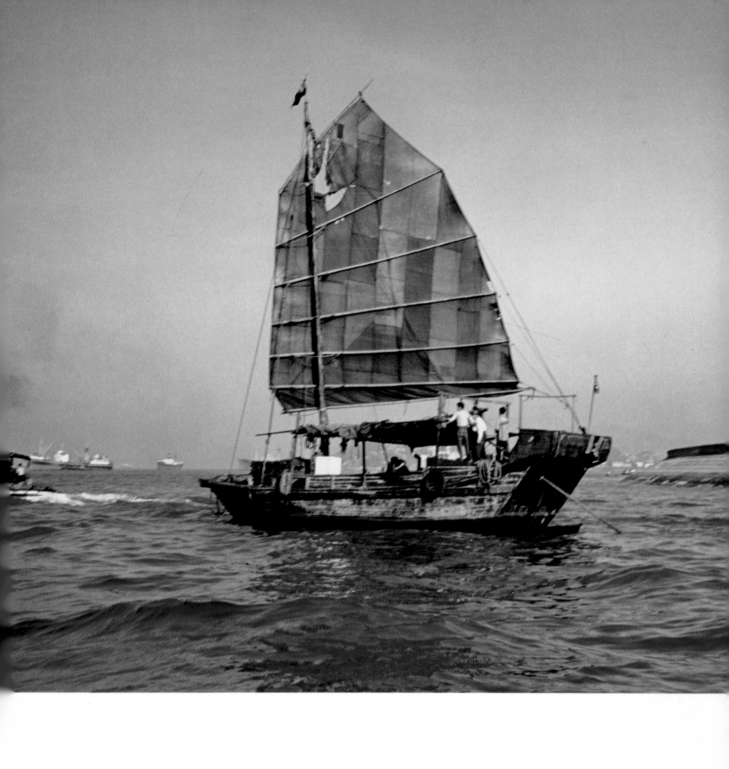

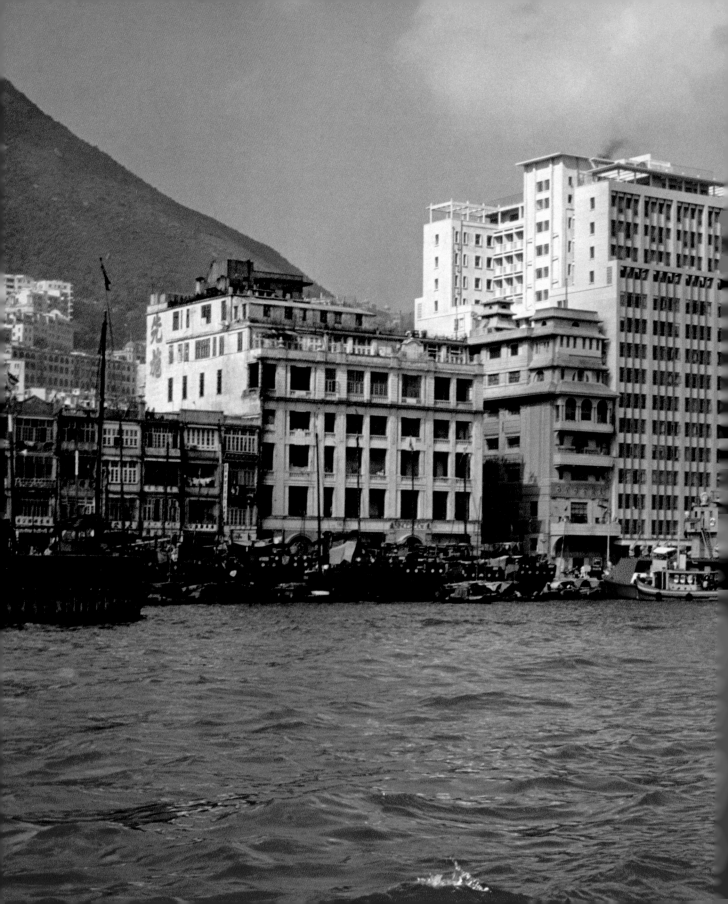

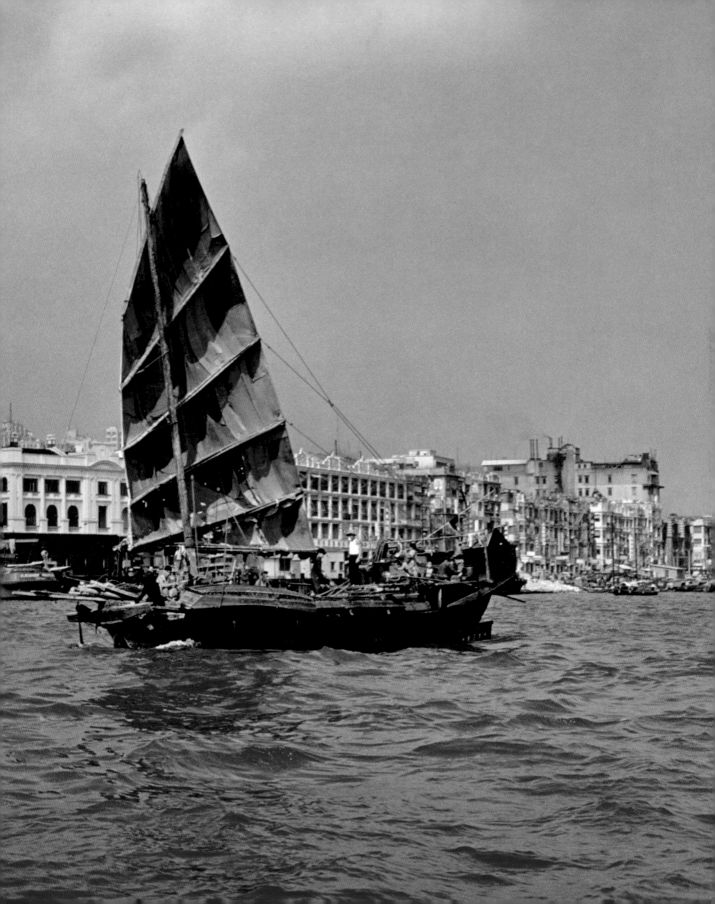

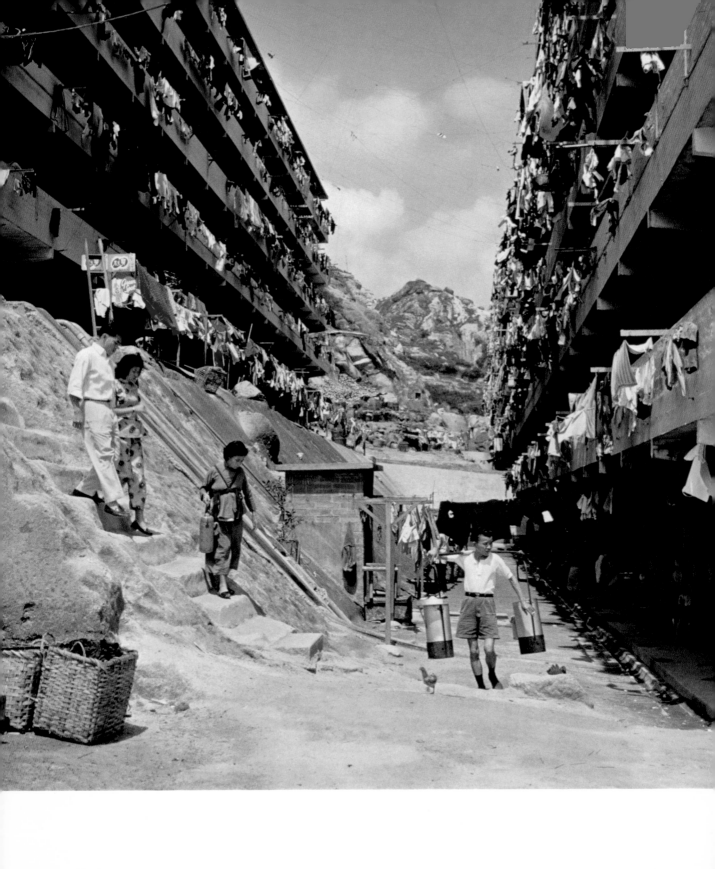

Gardens, where a Chinese Croesus built for himself a fantastic residence with a kind of waxworks of bizarre figures—it is open to the public today. Along the coast, between the fishing villages with their small fleets of junks, the sandy beach was inviting to bathers. Among the best customers of this holiday paradise are sailors from the American warships which anchor in the harbour—they spend their leave here between patrols in Formosa waters.

There are no cultural monuments to be seen in Hongkong, but the traveller has a chance to meet representatives of the most numerous people in the world and experience their explosive way of life. Without the puritanical restrictions and political directives which control life in the Chinese People's Republic, life in the British Colony develops unchecked in its various colourful ways. From the sky-scrapers of the banks and business firms, which could be situated anywhere in Europe or America, you go straight into the lively narrow streets which, by the large vertically arranged Chinese characters alone, give the impression of a permanent national festival.

Private enterprise still flourishes here in diverse forms, from the shabbiest street vendor to the rich jewel dealer, who has in front of his shop a brigand-like guard armed with an old-fashioned gun. The curiosity shops, which are banned from the streets of Peking and Shanghai, still exist here with all the gay gewgaws, imitation and perhaps sometimes even genuine Tang sculpture, laughing china idols, gaudy silk embroidery, and splendid jade jewellery. And Chinese, busy Chinese everywhere: on the pavement in rags, opulently at ease in their limousines, at the vegetable stalls and in offices; and in the midst of it all innumerable children.

A journey into the green valleys of the New Territories revealed the Chinese as peasants in the rice fields, and in vegetable gardens utilising every spot of fertile

Page 158 HONGKONG, KOWLOON. A street in a recently completed settlement for refugees from China, who had previously been homeless or else housed in the most primitive huts.

soil. Here there were still diminutive ancient towns with moats and walls and narrow, straight streets, modest replicas of those imperial residences of the Middle Kingdom which astonished Marco Polo in the Middle Ages.

And then there was that frontier where another adventure and a new world had begun—on the other side of the bridge, where the red flag of the Chinese People's Republic flutters. The train which goes on to Canton was ready; from there you can reach Peking in a day on the Chinese airline.

Pages 161–168 HONGKONG

161 In the Chinese quarter of Victoria there is a colourful market bustle, as in old Chinese towns, beneath the decorative signs. On the stalls are sold the latest products from all over the world.

162 There is a lively traffic of pedestrians in the tightly crowded business-quarter of the island town, where, as a mark of free enterprise, Chinese, British, and other capitalists have built their skyscrapers and established their businesses.

163 Quite different from the gay throng of a Chinese bazaar street is a street in this drab, forbidding residential district in a small town in the New Territories (*see page 168 below*), which for centuries has hardly changed. A Chinese dwelling-house faces the street with a blank wall: even the door gives passers-by only a glimpse of an inner wall.

164–165 From one of the surrounding hills you look over the town of Kowloon, which is on the mainland opposite the island with the older town of Victoria: in the foreground is land which has been cleared of the primitive squatter settlements of Chinese immigrants to make room for new blocks of flats; behind is one of the already-occupied housing estates of this kind erected by the government.

166, 167 In one of the steep streets in the Chinese district of Victoria children take the field when school is over.

168 The old and the new: on the shore of the island opposite the mainland these blocks of flats have sprung up in the past few years through private enterprise in connection with a new factory; the style of architecture is strictly cosmopolitan. The plate below shows the entrance to a small town in the New Territories (*see also page 163*) which has completely preserved the appearance of a medieval Chinese settlement: the town wall forms an exact rectangle with towers at the corners and a moat around it.

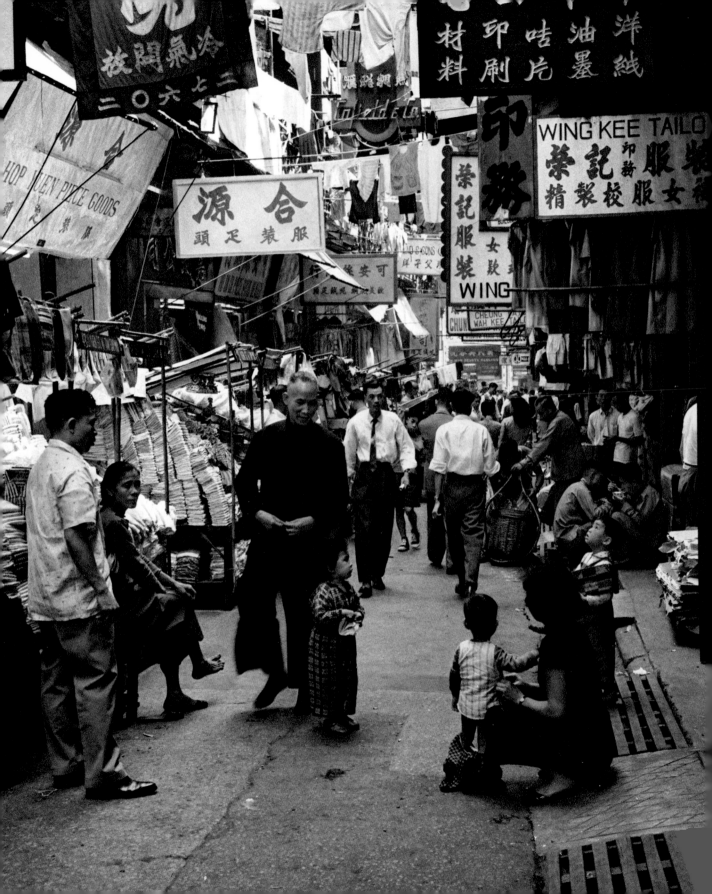

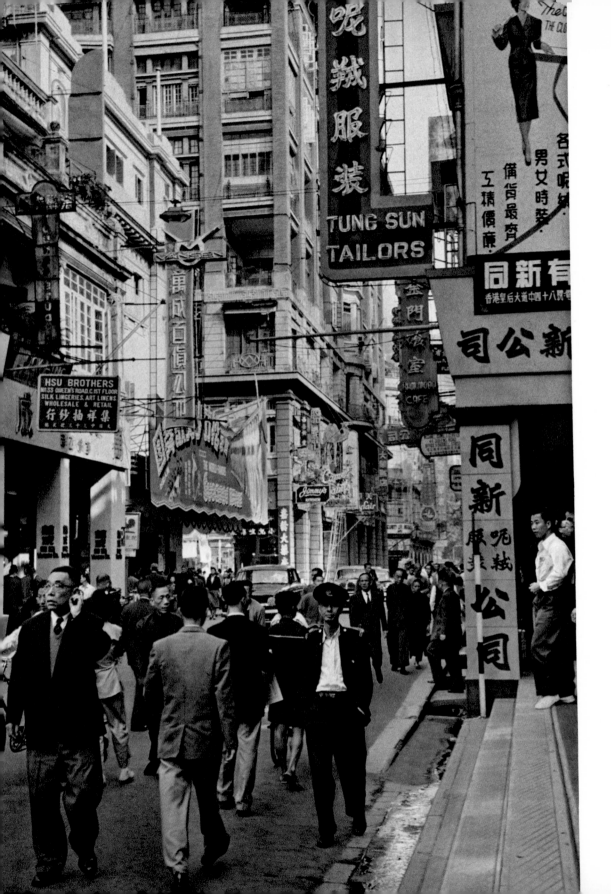

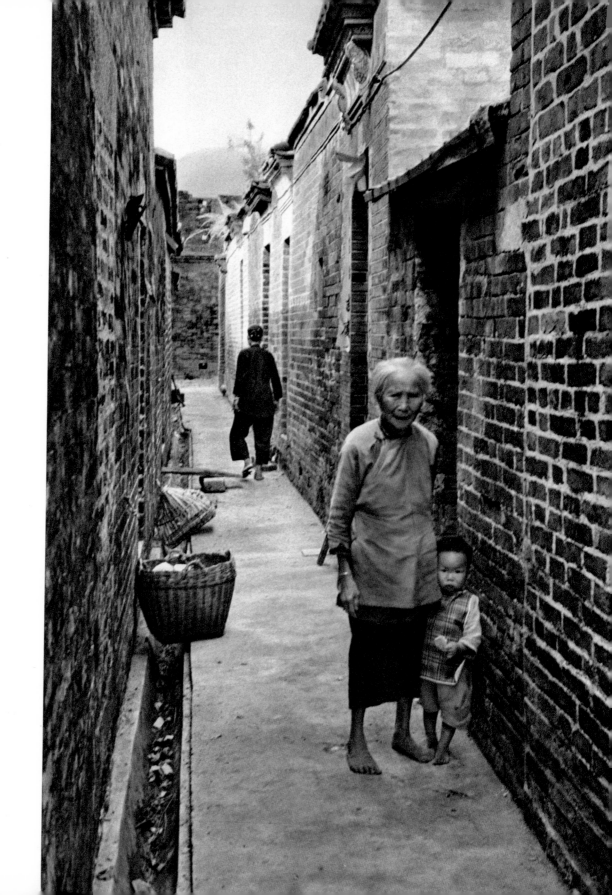

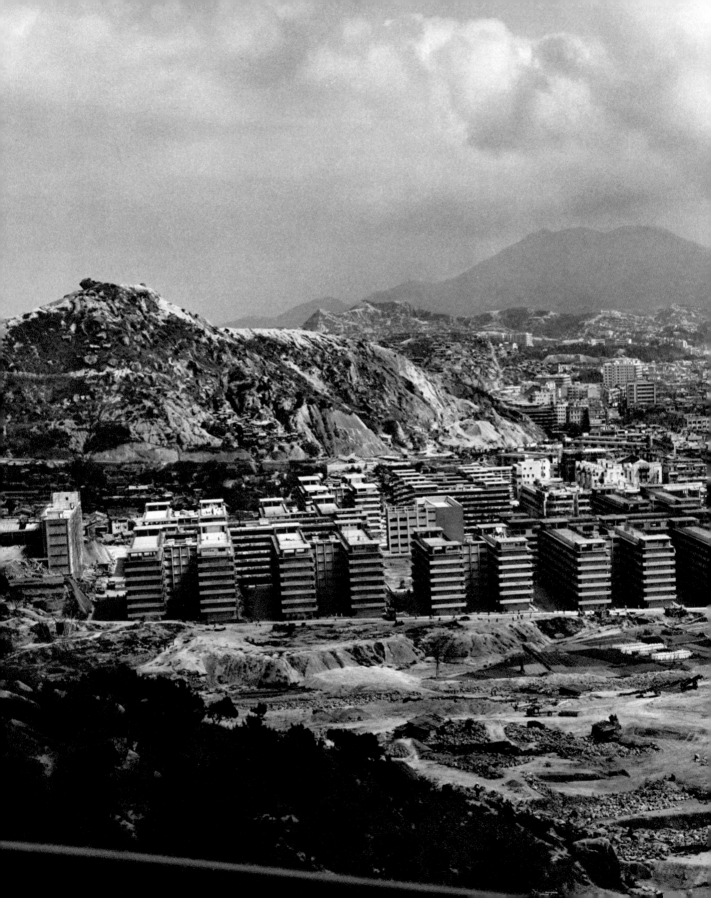

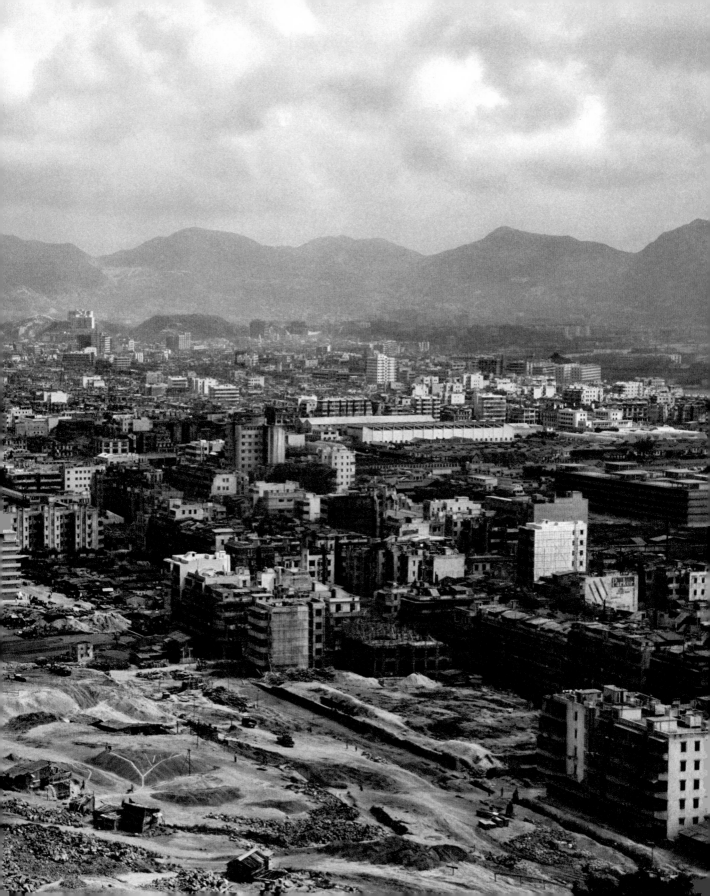

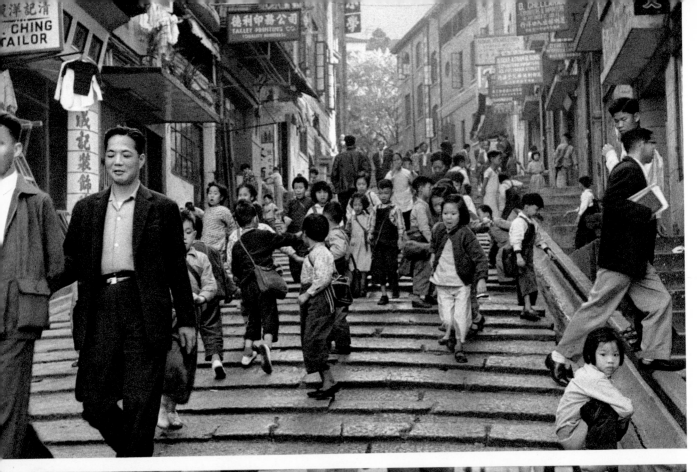
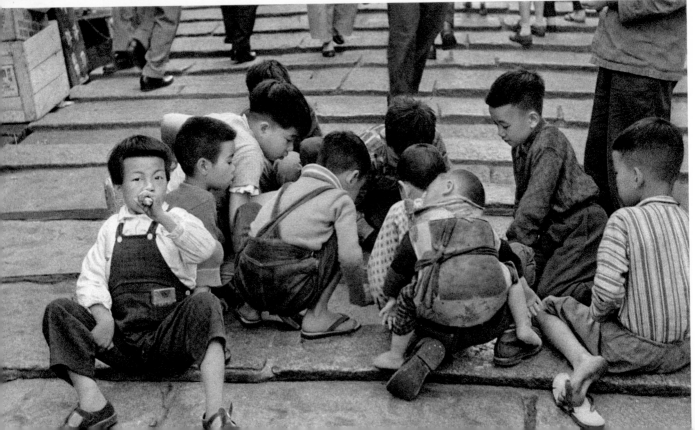

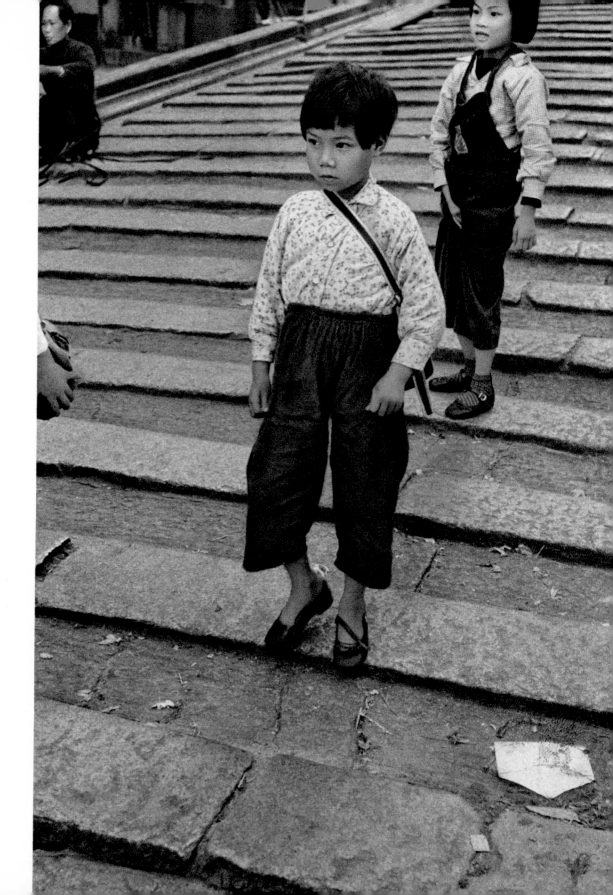

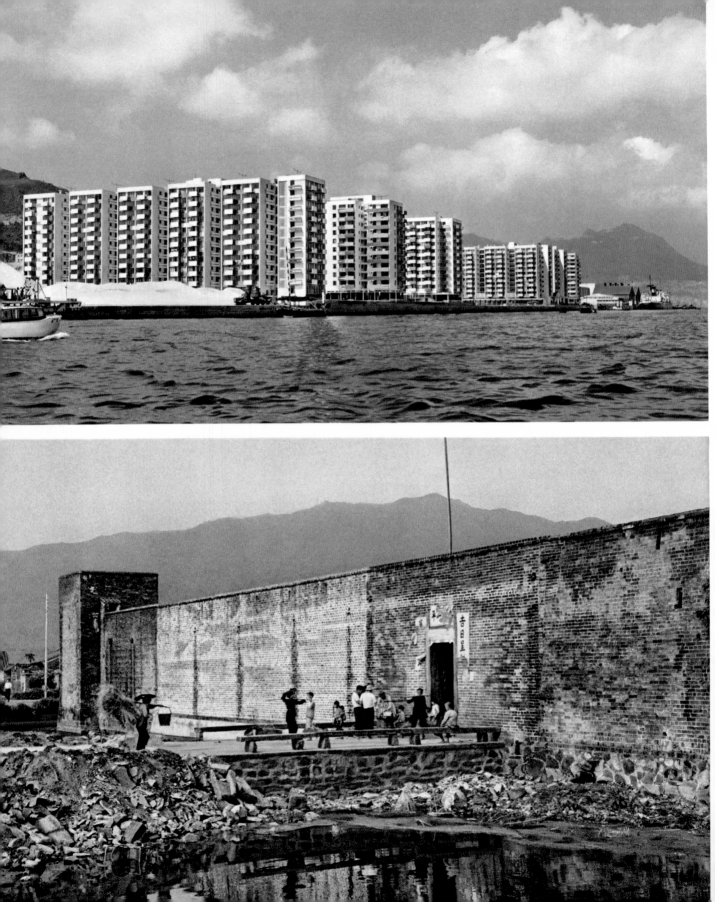

China

THE CROSSING of the Sham Chun river by the Kowloon–Canton railway is the only point at which the frontier of one of the great Western powers comes into contact with either of the two Communist States. Everything happens very peaceably in a routine manner. Passengers get off the train at Lo Wu station and hand over their passports for examination. There are no British officials in sight, the frontier examination is carried out by uniformed Chinese of the Colony.

We four Europeans had nothing to do but wait until the representative of the official Chinese travel agency got everything ready for us to cross the frontier; then we walked beside the railway track over the bridge to the station on the other side. We saw a row of Chinese queuing up with their bundles behind a railing, but we were led into a waiting-room with leather arm-chairs and greeted with hand-shakes—whether by a policeman, a customs officer, or other official was not clear. Two long questionnaires had to be filled up; I declared my photographic apparatus; the polite officials advised me also to put down my wedding-ring under 'jewels'; our money was examined and an hour later we were able to take up our reserved seats in the train. The train filled up as we waited to start. Among the passengers and railway officials we noticed for the first time people wearing white masks over their noses and mouths as a protection against germs—a sight to which one so soon becomes accustomed in Red China that in the end I forgot to photograph it.

In our carriage the passengers at once received attention: you could order for a small sum a jug of green tea, and from time to time a man came and refilled the jug with hot water; a certain amount of skill was needed to hold the lid of the jug so that when you drank the tea the tea-leaves did not also come through the slit. The railway officials busied themselves incessantly about the cleanliness of the train: the floor was swept repeatedly. During the journey, which lasted several hours, a mixed radio programme blared from a loudspeaker: booming marches, a shrill female voice, then again light music, half European, half Chinese. There was no escape, not for a minute, and the noise hammered ceaselessly into the ear-drums—how this could be borne for the journey to Peking which lasted for several days I could not imagine.

We travelled through the fertile, varied country of Kwangtung. The tillage of the rice fields was in full swing, huge oxen plodding over the damp soil; women stood ankle-deep in the water and planted the slips which are cultivated in special fields and could be seen standing close together in a bright green mass. Young men pedalled water-wheels to irrigate the land; there was activity everywhere.

Canton   At the station in Canton nothing betrayed the fact that Canton was the most restless of the thousands of towns in China. With my three Swiss travelling companions, representatives of a large industrial enterprise, I was received by an official of the travel agency: he was not only polite, as was everyone whom we met in China, but his way of expressing himself in English had something particularly gentle and kind about it—a manner which in our part of the world we would regard as the characteristic of a Christian, though there can be no doubt that the likeable young man had been tested most carefully in the orthodoxy of his Marxist-materialist beliefs. A motor-car took us to a skyscraper whose rather undistinguished entrance hardly led one to suspect that it was a hotel. Soviet Russian hotels are similar: there are no receptionists or doorkeepers; generally one comes into contact only with the staff on the floor on which one is staying, and the representative of the travel agency sees to the calling of guests, the payment of bills, and so on. From my room on the eighth floor I looked directly on to the river and heard the sirens of the steamers.

A walk along the river-bank took me to the swarm of boats on which a part of the population lived; they were just eating supper with chopsticks round their smoking stoves. Was I mistaken, or had the activity of this floating town, with its own way of life, so difficult to control, diminished? Sobriety ruled in Canton now. It is true that dirt and poverty still peeped out from nooks and crannies, from alleys and side-streets; there were still traces of those medieval odours; the sizzling of many little saucepans; that haggling in dark corners about some business deal; the high spirits of small boys, that noisy explosive temperament; you could still sense this fabric of thousands of years. But the narrow bazaar streets of yore with throngs of people and gold shop-signs, carved black furniture, heaped-up silverware, coloured silk balls, were no longer to be found. A district of neglected houses had been pulled down to make way for a 'culture park' on the model of the one in Moscow, where evening entertainments were given—films, plays, and conjuring—by the light of many gay but (since electricity is rationed) not too brightly lit lamps. The Island of Shameen, once the district of foreign consuls and business magnates, faded into the twilight; clubs, with their inter-national air of whisky-drinking comfort, were forgotten; no white man was to be seen there, unless it was a tourist who had lost his way.

We had supper on the top floor of our skyscraper hotel. The menu was inter-national, the food unexciting but irreproachable; the beer, which most guests drank with it, was brewed in China; it was not comparable to the excellent beer of the Hongkong breweries, but was just as good as that of other Eastern countries. A delegation of Russians sat at a long table: Soviet men and women seem in China particularly broad-shouldered and solid, and as if it would be unwise to joke with them, and they had nothing to joke about among themselves; like pocket-battleships with hatches battened down they moved through the Middle Kingdom. Beside them the few guests from the West, even if they are just as com-munist at heart, give the impression of being lost individualists from another planet.

Early in the morning the young man from the travel agency appeared with undiminished kindliness: he had exchanged the American travellers' cheques, paid the hotel bill, procured the air-tickets, made the hotel reservations in Peking by telegraph, and arranged for transport from the airport; with my companions— the four of us from Switzerland had been joined by a Danish businessman who lived in Shanghai—I had only to breakfast before getting into the car which was placed at our disposal to take us to the airport.

China's civilian airlines remind one of the Soviet Russian model: the passengers were principally officials, foreign (mostly Russian) expert consultants, delegations, and a few private travellers, among whom were Japanese. In the airport buildings there was less display than in Russia: there were no chandeliers, no lace covers or plush curtains; only the bust of Mao Tse-tung in one or other of the waiting-rooms called to mind the white and gold statues of Stalin. The puritanical spirit of the régime was everywhere evident, a spirit of unsentimental practicality. In civil aviation, in which only a tiny section of the population participate, the relentless loudspeaker is omitted.

From Canton four airlines radiate to Wuhan-Peking, Shanghai, Kinming, and the Island of Hanan. The line to the capital, on which we were travelling, is the most frequently used—five times a week (according to the 1958 summer time-table). The twin-engine Russian machine was similar to the civil aircraft in use in Europe in the 1930's; it gave an impression of reliability. Flying is only by daylight and evidently only in favourable weather; the flight the day before had been cancelled in view of storms reported from the centre of China—although it is quite possible that lack of passengers was the real reason for the cancellation.

During our flight covering the stretch of almost 1,250 miles to the 'northern capital', we made three stops. The first part in the early morning was the most beautiful; we flew relatively low, at about 6,500 feet, and the colourful, varied landscape of South China could be seen in relief: tracts of red earth, rice fields between the ridges of hills, industriously tilled fields and, standing out quite clearly, many small lakes and reservoirs with stretches of bare, deeply-furrowed mountains between.

The first landing-place, at Changsha the capital of Hunan, had a broad runway on which jet bombers could also land, and uninteresting reception buildings. In the waiting-room a small counter for the sale of tobacco and drinks was closed for lack of customers; on it stood a large pot with hot tea from which you could help yourself without payment.

In the centre of a round leather sofa about a dozen magazines from Communist countries were displayed, all on the model of the great Soviet Russian illustrated magazines, with gay covers depicting waving cornfields, huge tractors, dams, laughing peasant women, delegations, and important visitors shaking hands. The monthly *China in Pictures* which appeared in a Chinese and an English edition seemed to me to have the best photographs of all those propaganda publications and, thanks to the good running commentaries, made a less mono-tonous impression than the others.

There was little to be seen at Changsha: only a row of large barrack-like and apparently new buildings in the open country. Once only on this flight did a 'real' Chinese city appear: a huge, mathematically exact walled-in rectangle, like an island in an inundated territory, as if protected for ever from the inclemency of the weather and the inauspicious course of events.

Our next stop was at Wuhan—the name of the airport of the large triangle of towns, Hankow-Hanyang-Wuchang, on both sides of the Yangtse—and for the first time in years I had a chance to get some practice in the use of chopsticks. The Chinese menu was certainly better than the European fare chosen by a Russian delegation—serious, heavily built men who left the restaurant immediately with their briefcases and got into the aeroplane which was taking off for Chungking. No one understood English or indeed any European language.

On the next stage of our journey we crossed the broad, dirty-yellow river and saw something of one of the largest settlements in Asia; the great bridge, which has established direct railway communication between the two halves of China, stood out clearly; it is the pride of the nation, a stage in the opening-up of the country by means of new railway lines, roads, dams, factories.

The third stop followed in Chengchow to the west of Honan—this airport too can be used for aircraft of a type quite different from our small commercial aero-plane. At the edge of the airfield military aircraft were drawn up in a long row with their propellers and motors covered over.

The last stretch took us over the river-basin of the wild Huangho and the North Chinese lowlands, a densely built-up area where there were row upon row of villages—you could fill whole countries of Europe with them. Part of the land was under water—one of the smaller spring floods.

Arrival in Peking

The sun was already very low on the horizon behind a haze of dust when we landed at the new aerodrome in Peking. The airport had been in use for only a few weeks and some of its buildings were still unfinished. We passed a row of commercial aeroplanes among which were three with Rumanian national markings. A propellerless 'Tupolev' had just arrived from Moscow.

At once we were received by a friendly young woman, Miss Wu, who formed the short sentences of her school English slowly and correctly. The international tourist service does not provide the sort of alluring Chinese femininity that cheers the lonely traveller in the streets and on ferryboats in Hong-kong, with close-fitting gay clothes and skirts slit at the side: like most of her contemporaries of both sexes Miss Wu wore a dark blue blouse and trousers which revealed as little as possible of the human form, and was without cosmetics.

In less than an hour's comfortable journey the car of Russian make had brought us to the city—one of the huge city gates and a stretch of wall indicated behind the dust-veil of the spring evening the whereabouts of Peking.

The Peking Hotel is one of the four large international hotels in the capital. I stood in a dim, cold hall until from an invisible background the key of my room appeared and one of the 600 million Chinese took me and my luggage in the lift to my room on the second floor. My window looked on to the broad main street, running through the old city of the Tartars parallel to the wall which separates it from the so-called 'town of the Chinese'. Directly opposite were the former diplomatic quarters, which at the beginning of this century were a bastion of the foreign powers, with legations, military barracks, hospitals, clubs, and the international marine customs office. Now the widened road is lined with large government buildings.

My room was quite comfortable, whereas the old Grand Hotel of Peking had been frankly luxurious. The arms of the chair had lace covers which kept falling off and which I always carefully replaced before going out. Even the bathroom dated from the good old days; it remained untouched by the rage for reconstruction, but the mechanical parts had lasted well. In the room next to mine was a Russian technician and his family, but as a rule you met the other guests only in the dining-room.

I tried first of all to order Chinese food, but it was not provided there. The head waiter seemed to be the only person in the hotel who spoke English, although the small waitresses in their very unbecoming schoolgirls' uniforms with woollen stockings and caps understood at least a few phrases. You ordered from a menu in which a choice of dishes was given in Russian, English, and German. The cuisine was Western with a Russian touch, and you could not say it was bad; if, among the unfamiliar names, you hit on the right thing, it could even be very good, and in any case there was enough to eat. Most of the guests drank beer. The 'Tupolev' crew was also there, assembled at a round table, heavily built men to whom eating, like flying, was a serious duty in the service of the people and peace. Among the clientele were Russian delegations, officials, and experts, who sat together with the bare minimum of friendliness and conversation. Next to the Russians, Germans from East Germany formed the chief contingent. At a table beside me sat a married couple—I took their name to be Schulze, from Leipzig or perhaps even from Chemnitz. Herr Schulze scarcely ever allowed himself to smile; he was full of the dignity of a responsible civil servant; most of the time he wore a kind of uniform *à la* Stalin; Frau Schulze, by contrast, looked radiant all the time; she greatly enjoyed being able to select from such a long menu, and she smiled roguishly at the schoolgirl-waitresses, indefatigable in face of their indifference to her. Sometimes at a single table appeared a solitary guest who, to judge from his nonchalant way of smoking a cigarette and his whole behaviour, could only have come from the West; perhaps he was an enthusiastic English intellectual of the left. There he was as foreign as I.

Gradually I explored the remaining rooms on the ground floor. Through long, dim, empty halls you reached the other part of the building, where there was a post-office. There you could cover your letters with a great variety of stamps; there was a rich assortment depicting pagodas, dams, railways and ships, famous men and doves of peace. There was also a glue-pot to hand as the stamps were not gummed. In this connection it should be mentioned at once that all the letters and cards reached their European destinations promptly, those by airmail even in record time—very much in contrast to the incalculably long time taken by letters I sent home from Russia two years earlier.

In the entrance hall there were two counters: at one of them, which was seldom open, you could buy Chinese souvenirs, which would undoubtedly delight Frau Schulze; and the other, which catered for more general custom, had for sale apples, sweets, biscuits, Shanghai chocolate, and occasionally also remarkably good, fresh doughnuts.

Near the entrance behind a wooden partition with the inscription 'Information' stood as a rule two or three young people; they grinned at you cheerfully but understood not one word of what you said; if you were lucky, however, the head waiter who spoke English could be reached by the house telephone. Without Miss Wu nothing much could be done there. It was thus all the more precious to be able to get through to any number in Peking yourself by the telephone in your own room, not only to the tourist service and publicity department but also to your own Embassy, and in this world of '1984' it was comforting to be able to hear at any time through the receiver familiar Swiss-German.

Peking of the 1920's

It seemed not thirty-five years but a century since I had last stayed in Peking. I had stayed at the hotel of the Wagon Lit not far away, since adapted for some other purpose. Then there had been a proper reception-office and you could hear every European language. Among the visitors were Professor Driesch, who was guest lecturer at Peking University, diplomats, men with public and private commissions, erudite Laotse translators, and experts on Chinese art. You could meet English, Americans, Germans, and Swedes who had settled in Peking out of sheer enthusiasm for Chinese culture, and who had already penetrated the mystery of the 'spirit' walls which prevent inquisitive passers-by from looking into the courtyards of the houses from the streets. The hotel manageress looked after her Chinese boys as she did her cosmopolitan guests, and in her back room you could meet dignified old mandarins—or at least men who looked like mandarins—with long garments and caps on their heads, from which the pigtails had been cut twelve years earlier.

The foreigners who carried on gay conversations in the restaurants with the last representatives of the public world of letters, over delicious Peking duck and many other delicacies, who looked at pictures of officials of the Sung era in their *yamens*, listened to the K'in, bought Chou bronzes, and who, according to their inclination, had surrounded themselves with a generous company of kindred spirits, have all vanished. Today no foreigner from the West is allowed to live in

Peking unless he belongs to the diplomatic representation of his country. Only the representative of Reuter seems to be an exception. The tradesmen who are allowed into China live mostly in Shanghai, and if they have dealings in the capital they must put up at a hotel.

A Walk among the Blue Ants

On the evening of my arrival I went for a walk—from my avenue I turned into Wang Fu Ching Street, formerly the famous Morrison Street. Motor traffic was slight. Among the passers-by the 'blue ants' in their dark trousers and blouses and workmen's caps were more numerous than in Canton, but you still saw dignified old figures wearing long, padded coats and round caps on their heads. The traffic police with their padded, belted uniforms and round, immobile dolls' faces and stiff movements were punctilious, like automata. Some of them and one or two of the pedestrians wore white protective masks.

China Lives behind Walls

The dullness of the Peking street-scene is not entirely due to the present puritanical régime. High walls protect the private life of the city, the family, and individuals in the house and garden, and behind every entrance a special wall keeps away evil spirits who love to stare inquisitively. When the Emperor was carried out of the Forbidden City in a ceremonial procession to implore the favour of the supernatural powers at the Altar of Heaven for his people and country, the streets were not lined with cheering subjects, but all windows were closed; no mortal watched the Son of Heaven, who went in a high sedan-chair, magnificently clad, through the streets at night. Only the size of a gate and the colour of the tiles on its curved roof gave an idea of the importance of the estate lying within.

In Morrison Street

Morrison Street was naturally as open and inviting as the new Peking can be. There was a succession of commercial firms, with a department store among them; but at that time it was of course already shut and might just as well have been a government building or warehouse. Fortunately, the 'International Book-shop' was still open, so I was able to look around for a plan of the town and some useful literature. 'International' in this case naturally means 'democratic', i.e. Communist. A very good plan of Peking and its surroundings, printed in several colours with special plans of the imperial palaces, the Temple of Heaven, and the Soviet-Russian exhibition, was obtainable in a French as well as in a Chinese edition.

My first step next morning was to visit the office of the Tourist Service, as I had concocted bold plans to fulfil long-cherished desires. I wanted to visit the Lung-men caves in Honan, that imposing 6th-century museum of Buddhist sculpture; from Sian, the old imperial residence, I thought of visiting the pyramid tomb of the fabulous Shi Huang-ti and then of travelling on the recently completed railway line heading through uninhabited mountain districts to Chengtu, the capital of Szechuan; finally I could board a steamer in Chungking to see the famous gorges and rapids of the Yangtse-Kiang on the way to Wuhan.

Travel Plans

At the end of a broad road the Tien An Men, 'Gate of Heavenly Peace', with its jutting yellow roof, formed the majestic entrance to the grounds of the Imperial Palace of the Forbidden City.

The huge portrait of the leader, Mao Tse-tung, which could be seen on recent photographs hanging over the central thoroughfare, had disappeared, but strips of bright letters on a red background proclaimed the triumph of the revolution: 'Long live the Chinese People's Republic!' and 'Long live the great alliance of the peoples of the earth!' The broad assembly square in front of the gate served the same function for the party and public demonstrations as the Red Square in front of the Kremlin in Moscow. In the middle stood a stone monument. In huge gold letters, copied from Mao's handwriting, appeared the saying: 'The heroes of the people are immortal.' On the pedestal the last touches were just being put to a relief depicting scenes from the time of the foundation of the democracy—the monument was to be finished for the May Festival.

The office of the travel agency was not far away. It is a pathetic illustration of the underdevelopment of the tourist industry in the largest country in the world that on my repeated visits I never once had to wait at the only counter. Here too my fate was dependent on Miss Wu. She promised to look out by the next day the dates and tariffs—for apparently you could not simply look them up in the time-table. Meanwhile, I might get better information by calling on the publicity department of the Foreign Office. Miss Wu also advised me not to take any colour photographs, for the export of undeveloped films was forbidden and there were no facilities for developing them. This problem was to be solved at the end of my visit to China.

At the Foreign Office   I did not have to wait long in the dark entrance hall, and was led into a drawing-room with upholstered furniture and precious old porcelain vases on the

Page 181 CANTON

On the Pearl river near the Island of Shameen lies a fleet of houseboats; on the right bank opposite a manufacturing town has developed.

Pages 182–185 PEKING

182 The gate Tsien Men, which, in the central axis running from south to north, marks the transition from the Chinese city to the Manchu or Tartar city, each of them surrounded by a wall. The inscription says, 'Riding on a fiery steed let us be in the van-guard of progress. We will try our strength in the contest for progress, educate ourselves and be a match for it!'

183 In the narrow streets between the drum tower and the bell tower to the north of the Manchu city something of the atmosphere of the old Peking remains: a grandmother goes out for a walk with her grandchildren, all three in padded trousers and smocks against the cold spring winds; and fortune-tellers, who have developed their profession to a respected art in China, throw dice, look at a horoscope, and tell their fortunes to the women who listen eagerly.

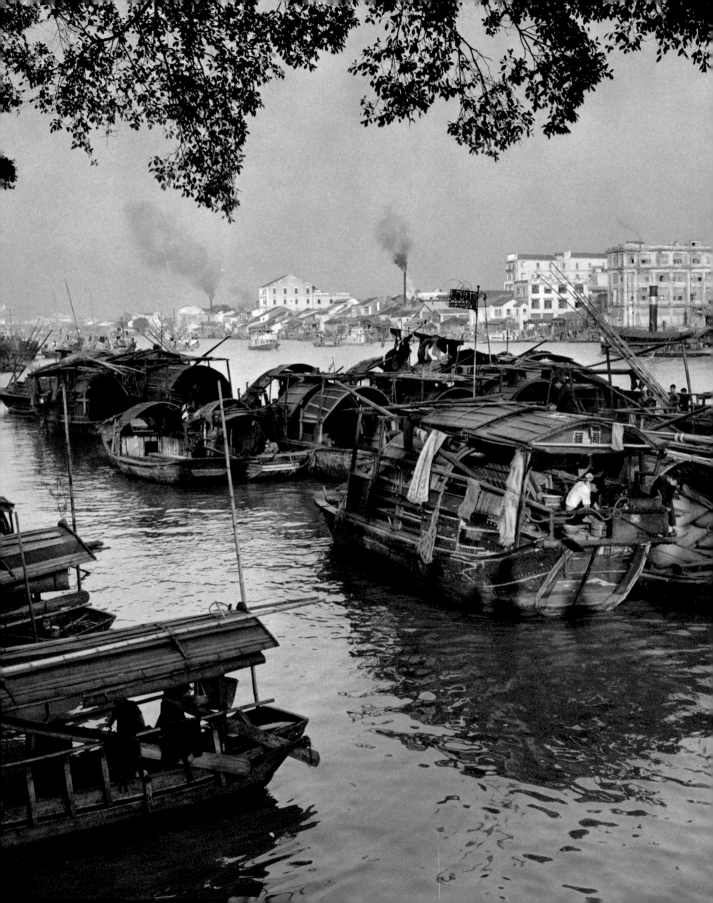

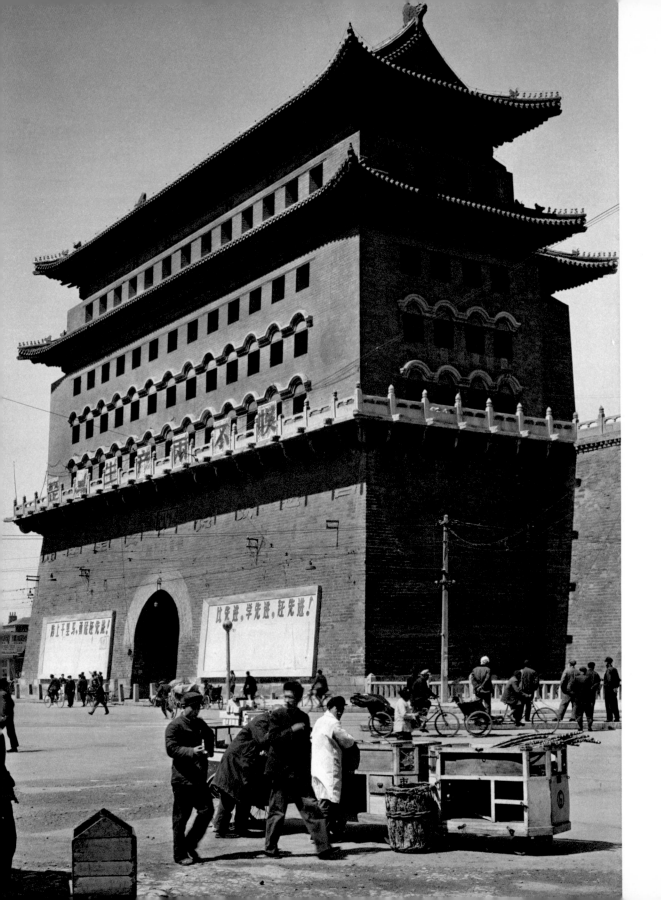

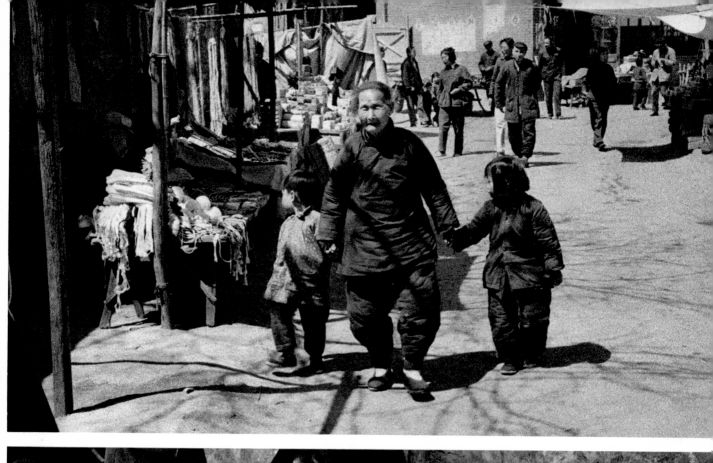

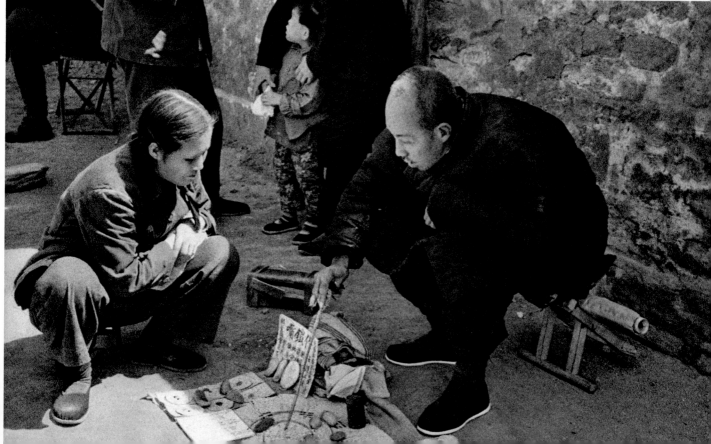

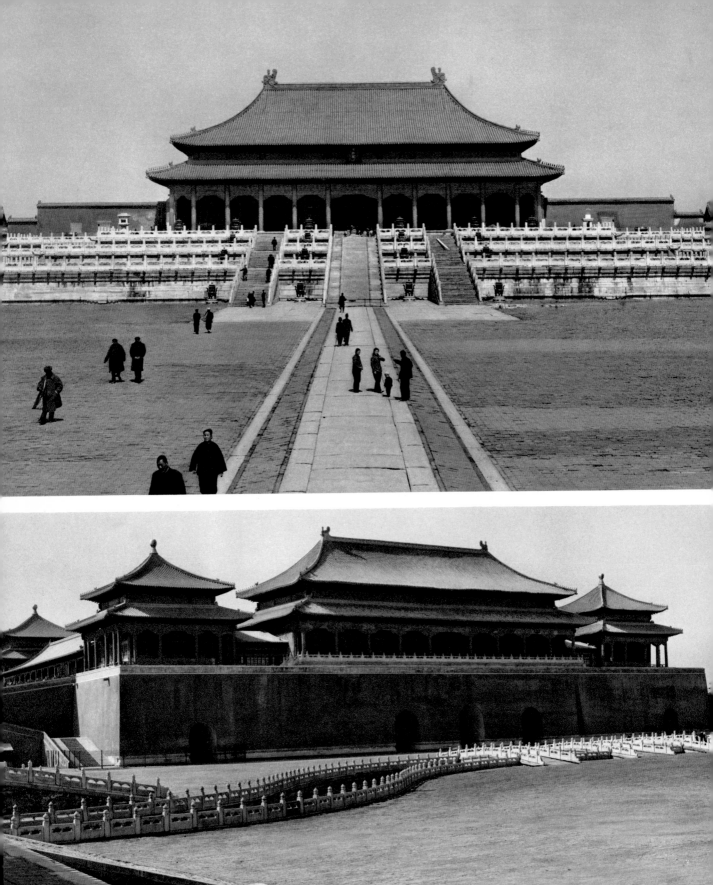

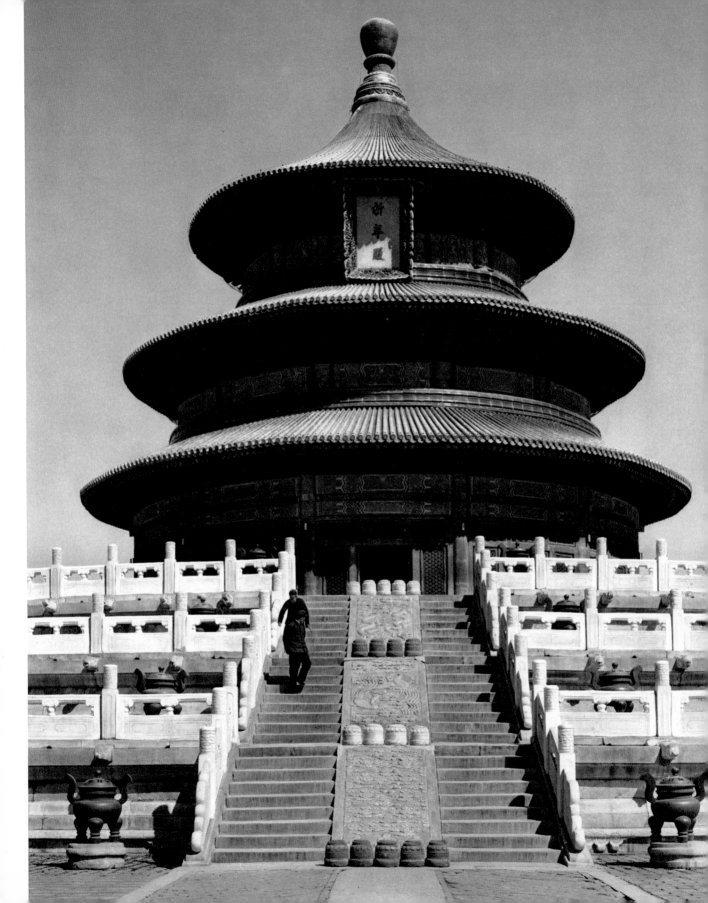

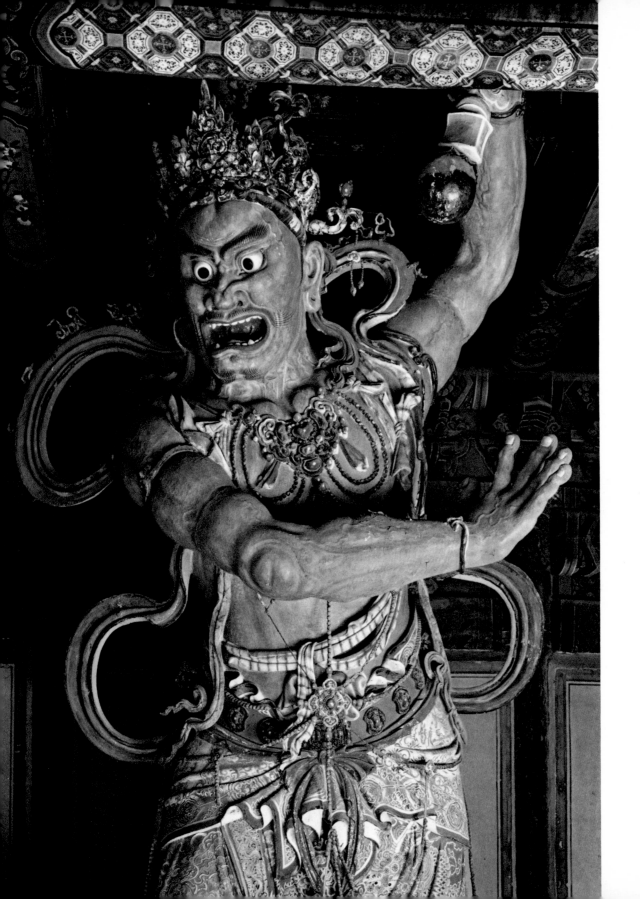

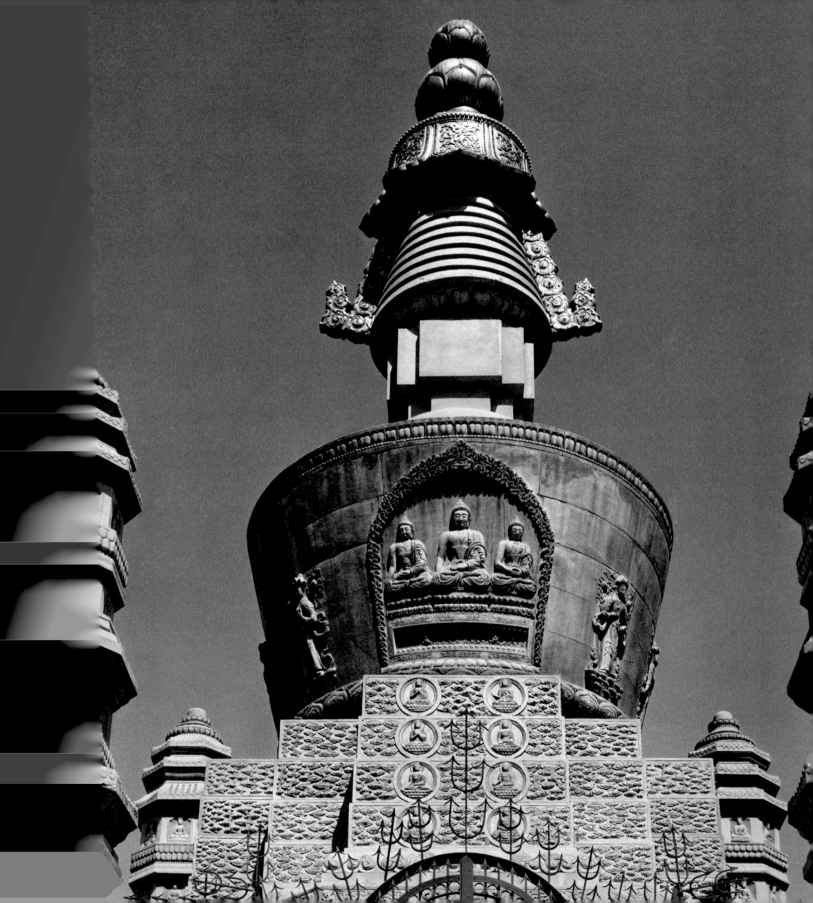

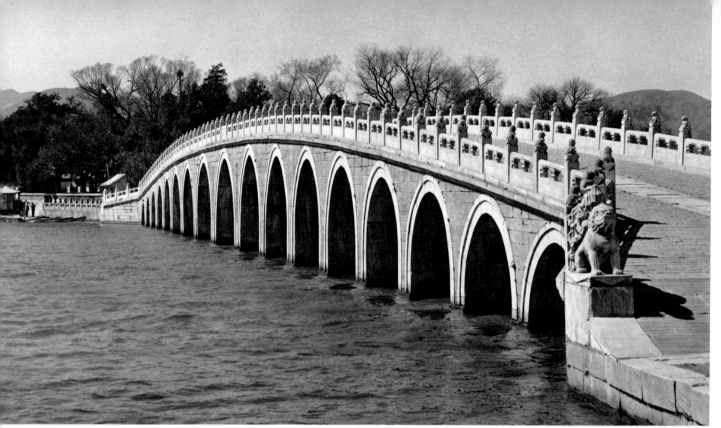

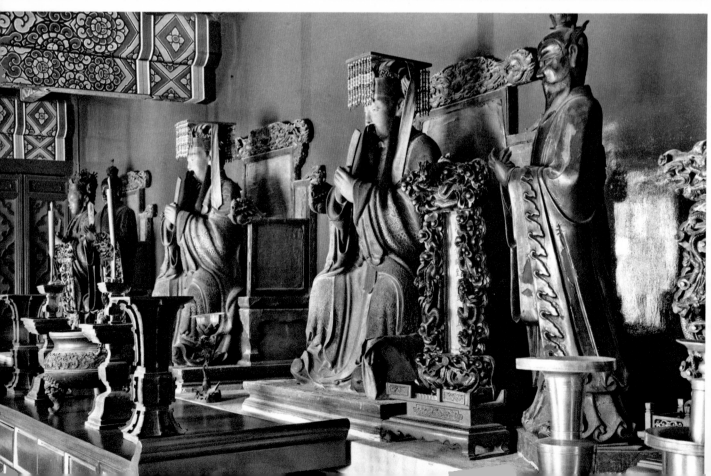

184 The Imperial Palace was built (1406–20) when the Ming Emperor Yung-lo (his dynastic name; his own name was Cheng-tsu) moved the capital of his empire from Nanking back to Peking, where the Mongol (Yuan) emperors had lived in the 13th and 14th centuries. The Manchu (Tsin) emperors took over the residence and extended it. It forms a city within a city. Visitors entering from the south by the 'Gate of Heavenly Peace' (Tien An Men, *page 197*) and the southern gate, come to the Forbidden City itself at the huge Wu Men, that is, 'Gate of the Meridian' (below), on whose upper floor a museum of history is housed today. Then comes the 'Hall of All-Embracing Harmony', Tai Ho Tien (top), with the reception-room.

185 The 'Temple of Heaven' (Tien Tan) is a group of buildings and their grounds which the Emperor used to visit at the time of his ceremonial acts of sacrifice as the Son of Heaven. The plate shows the Temple of Prayers for a Good Harvest, which rises on a terraced marble base; its triple roof is covered with blue glazed tiles. Still in the grounds of the Temple of Heaven but farther off is the smaller round building of the Imperial Vault of Heaven, and the Altar of Heaven.

186 Demon figures, such as are commonly found in Buddhist temples in China, also guard the entrance to the Temple of Azure Clouds in the western mountains near Peking.

187 Hsi Hung Sse, the 'Yellow Temple', situated outside the walls of Peking to the north, with its white marble pagoda, is one of the splendid Lama buildings built by the Manchu emperors in the capital and its surroundings in honour of their Tibetan and Mongolian subjects.

Page 188 THE SURROUNDINGS OF PEKING

188 top The park of the Summer Palace, laid out at the foot of the western mountains by the famous Dowager Empress Tzu Hsi at the turn of the last century. The bridge of seventeen arches is made of white marble; it leads to the small island with the Temple of the Dragon-King in the middle of the artificial lake of Kuenming.

188 below The Temple of the White Clouds outside the west wall of Peking has been carefully restored for visitors as a Taoist monument; the halls of prayer, which are looked after by a number of aged priests, the figures decorated with imperial emblems, the vessels, and other holy objects have all been cleaned, freshly painted and newly gilded.

window-sills. Two young men, one of whom acted as interpreter, sat down beside me and inquired what I wanted, while a small cup of green tea was served. I need hardly emphasize that even in that place, whence broadsides have from time to time been fired against the incorrigible capitalist West, the foreign guest was treated politely: I should mention here that, as also in Soviet Russia, I met on this journey through Red China only friendly, and at the worst, indifferent, people. What was less satisfactory, marring every encounter, was the difficulty of conversing with people. Conversation conducted in English with the translator of the publicity department proceeded with hardly more fluency than my conversations with Miss Wu; how different it was in India, where it was possible to discuss the most complicated political, economic, and philosophical problems with anyone in a responsible position (provided that your command of English was equal to that of the Indian you were speaking to).

The two men held out prospects of a Press pass, and handed me a questionnaire. I was then asked to tell them in good time where I wanted to travel. Two days later I received the decorative red Press pass—it was pleasant to have a pass in Chinese, even if it was of little use to me. Almost every evening now my room telephone rang and the publicity service informed me in barely intelligible English of the latest communiqués about some trade agreement or other or a peace resolution.

To make myself more easily understood I wrote down some of the things I wanted to know, and I inquired particularly about the possibility of taking photographs on my proposed journey to Szechuan. A voice on the telephone informed me one evening that photography from aeroplanes, trains, and ships was prohibited. 'Even from the Yangtse river-steamers?' Yes, even from these. This made the costly journey considerably less attractive to me. The Chinese seemed not at all anxious to make propaganda of the new railway line with its bridges and tunnels, a considerable achievement; caution and distrust predominated;

perhaps they wished to convey to me that my desire to travel went too far? So I confined myself to looking at Peking and its surroundings more thoroughly—this alone could take months.

The Lungmen-Sian-Szechuan-Yangtse journey, which for me has vanished into the realm of unfulfilled dreams was, shortly afterwards—and just as I had planned it—offered by the Foreign Office to foreign diplomats as a three weeks' excursion with a special train and everything necessary to make a good impression.

I had resolved to stick obediently to the official tourist agency and its interpreters in Red China so as not to make any false move in that planned world nor photograph anything that was forbidden. *I Become Independent*

To bring about a meeting with Mao Tse-tung would certainly have been a difficult task, although one can talk with him only through an interpreter; this fascinating personality is seldom seen and even the most famous journalists have tried in vain to get an interview.

As the tourist agency appeared little prepared for people like me—I always saw there only the polite little Miss Wu, who was already taking care of the Munich photographer, Hilmar Pabel—I struck out on my own. Reality is often different from what you imagine it to be, and even in Peking an individualist can still wander about if his visa and cheque-book are in order. It is, of course, hard to make use of taxis without an interpreter. But a row of pedicab men offered their services in front of the hotel; previously they were called rickshaw coolies and pulled the two-wheeled vehicles which they now drive with the help of a third wheel and pedals; but to all appearances it was still the same lively company as in the good old days, although rather less communicative.

I decided to place my trust in a rather elderly man—let us call him Kung; he *My Pedicab Man* knew some English and had the kind of face which inspired confidence and was stamped with the wisdom of a very old people. He demanded less than the sum Miss Wu had indicated as a probable tariff, but for all that he was not over-sensitive about tips, which were otherwise strictly taboo in Red China. As it turned out, he knew his way about Peking very much better than any taxi-driver and he guessed at once what I wanted. He became my regular companion and I generally hired his three-wheeled vehicle for the whole day. It is true that it was a slow way of going any distance, but you were also much nearer things and even had time for reflection. If it rained Kung opened up the small hood and protected me in front with an old bit of canvas; and when the wind blew icily from the northern steppes, penetrating my light summer clothes, Kung covered me with one of his padded coats, which he wore one on top of the other. Before me were his close-cropped head and sticking-out ears, and I can still hear, if I think of him, the calls ending with 'Ho' and 'Ha', with which he forced his way through the street. He seemed to know almost everyone, and whatever districts we were passing through he would greet old friends. What might he be, behind the screen of this incomprehensible language: a trusty agent of the secret police, or the head of the last, not yet liquidated, secret society, or merely a simple pedicab man? He could not be too dangerous, for it turned out that he could decipher as little as I the Chinese letters on a scrap of paper with an address, but the first schoolboy who came by solved that problem.

In the Forbidden City My first visit in old Peking was to the Forbidden City, a collection of palaces in the middle of the Tartar town. Although based on the old design of Chinese farm-buildings these acquire new majesty through their moats and rectangular walls. The southern approach to the central north–south axis made people entering the city aware of the grandeur of the imperial residence. It was a monu-mental scene with nothing grandiose about it; it inspired awe in both ruler and ruled. A broad approach road led between two parks, which surrounded the

Altar of Earth and Harvest and the Temple of the Forefathers, from Tien An Men through the south gate to the main entrance, the fortress-like Wu Men ('Gate of the Meridian'). The deep yellow of the nobly curved tiled roofs proclaimed the imperial character of the buildings. The thick red wooden pillars vanished into the shadow of the beams, in which gold and green ornaments sparkled; white marble balustrades surrounded the staircases to the halls. In the courtyard behind Wu Men a marble bridge led over the 'gold river' to the Gate of Supreme Harmony, and only when you went through this with its splendid faceted wooden roof did you see on three terraces the first and largest palace building with a double roof: Tai Ho Tien, the 'Hall of All-Embracing Harmony'. There the Son of Heaven used to sit enthroned, his face turned towards the south, receiving the delegates who brought him tribute from far and near. Two more palaces were surrounded by the same balustrades and, with Tai Ho Tien, formed the core of the imperial city: Chung Ho Tien, the square 'Hall of Perfect Harmony'—the Emperor used to rest there before going to the throne-room—and Pao Ho Tien, the 'Hall of Maintained Harmony'.

Along the central axis there was another row of three buildings similar in shape to the others, but on a more modest scale: this was the official residence of the ruler, with the 'Hall of Heavenly Purity' (Chien Ching Kung), the 'Hall of Sublime Union' (Chiaio Tai Tien), and the 'House of Earthly Bliss' (Kun Ning Kung). The most northerly part, which terminated at the Gate of Virtuous Heroism, consisted of a garden with strange miniature mountains and rocks, pavilions, statues, and trees in blossom. On both sides of the dominating central axis there extended a whole town of palaces, courtyards, arcades, temples, and small summer-houses. Collections were assigned to the various halls; bronze, porcelain, painting, especially from the time of the Manchu and the Ming, but also from earlier dynasties, evidence of a refined artistic way of life and taste for antiquities which had been indulged for many centuries.

The rooms above the southern main gate were visited by enthusiastic crowds who streamed through the museum town—these rooms alone formed a whole palace where documents of most recent history were displayed: the Opium War and the exploiting imperialists, the bearded Karl Marx as a new Confucius, the glorious movement and 'liberation' of China from all oppressors, the People's State. There was however the sober air of a schoolroom about the place. Also especially popular is the palace with the 'Hall of International Friendship', where the presents of prominent visitors are on display: Hoh Chi Minh, Sukarno, Voroshilov, Nehru, the King of Nepal, a whole gallery of Communist and neutral leaders are represented here by their gifts, from photographs with dedications to carved miniature pagodas and gold-studded ceremonial daggers—in comparison with the old imperial collection, a highly impressive show of parvenu imitations of ancient art objects.

The Last Emperor Since this rulers' seat was established at the beginning of the 15th century by the Ming emperors, at the time of their move from Nanking to Peking, no foreign visitor has managed to explore the whole of the Forbidden City. Even nowadays there is a row of courtyards—among them the one with the Lama Temple, whose roof is decorated with gilded dragons—which are not open to the public; but nevertheless there is much more to be seen now than thirty-five years ago. At that time a part of the Forbidden City was still reserved for the deposed boy-Emperor. A small princely household had been left to the last legitimate bearer of the oldest and noblest rulers' title.

However, a year later the 'Christian' General Feng Yu-hsiang suppressed this last refuge for the occupant of the dragon throne. Emperor Pu-i disappeared into anonymity with the Japanese concession of Tientsin, until in 1932 the Japanese conferred on him the ephemeral title of Emperor of Manchukuo, in order to give an appearance of independence to the satellite State they had created. Thus at one time the pale Pu-i with his blue spectacles appeared in the pages of illustrated magazines, passing through the streets of Tokyo on a State visit in the coach beside the Emperor of Japan. The last Emperor of China is still alive today. Recently the Soviet Chinese fetched him back from oblivion; they let him appear as a witness in a lawsuit; then he disappeared again into internment, where apparently they intend to keep him for the present as a museum piece, in case he should one day be useful (if only, for instance, to pose as a happy Communist gardener at a monster banquet in honour of Field-Marshal Montgomery).

The imperial grounds extend beyond the Forbidden City. Outside the north gate the central axis continues through the Ching Shan, the coal-hill formed by human hands and crowned symmetrically with several pavilions, on whose slopes the last Ming Emperor hanged himself; and to the west alongside artificial lakes stretch the gardens and buildings of the 'Winter Palace' (in contrast to the 'Summer Palace' situated outside Peking). The southern main gate of the grounds, Hsin Hua Men, naturally has its thick red doors firmly shut to the crowds of visitors and only a few initiates succeed in gaining admission; for behind it lies the residence of Mao Tse-tung, the leader of the Chinese People's Republic; his private life is shrouded in mystery; no one knows what goes on in the charming grounds behind the high walls; but no one doubts that the philosophical autocrat in the midst of his Red mandarins is as convinced of the necessity of his historical mission as were his predecessors who believed they were endowed with divine authority.

The prohibition of entry to the southern part of the Winter Palace with its famous zigzag bridge is compensated for by the opening of the park round the northern lake—Paihai. Until 1925 this part was not open to the public; since 1950 the lake has been cleared and the buildings restored; the marble bridge which leads to the island, the shining white hill-top pagoda which towers over the roofs of the many other buildings; the stately barge which carries us in comfort to the temples, halls, and resting-places on the northern shore, the splendidly coloured dragon walls, and all that has been preserved from the time of the great Manchu emperors.

The Summer Palace in the Western Mountains The artful manner in which the East Asians have been able to fit their domestic architecture and the delights of life into the harmony of nature, and to preserve it over the threshold of this century, is strikingly evident in the Summer Palace near the western mountains, some six miles from Peking. At the time of the Boxer Rising the great European powers bombarded the former Summer Palace, with its echoes of the Western Rococo style of architecture; thereupon the Dowager Empress, Tzu Hsi, had the seat restored more magnificently than ever, in the tradition of Chinese garden and palace design, with a broad artificial lake, more than a hundred buildings on its shores and, on the rising ground, halls, tea-houses, covered walks, pools, pagodas, and bridges. The impermanent wooden

Pages 197–200 PEKING

197 The square in front of Tien An Men, the 'Gate of Heavenly Peace', at the outer entrance to the Forbidden City, forms the centre of the capital. The leaders of the People's Republic watch the great parades on 1st May and other festive occasions from the battlements.

198 The central building of the three large reception-halls of the Imperial Palace, in the middle of the Forbidden City (*see also page 184*) rises from a base of three banks of white marble steps; it is the 'Hall of Perfect Harmony', Chung Ho Tien, roofed with yellow glazed tiles like all the imperial buildings.

200 Chinese in their uniform blue dress on the broad boulevard Tong Changan Kie, which runs past the Grand Hotel. The scene scarcely gives the impression that here, in the administrative centre of the city, the vitality of the largest people on the earth has found its dynamic focus.

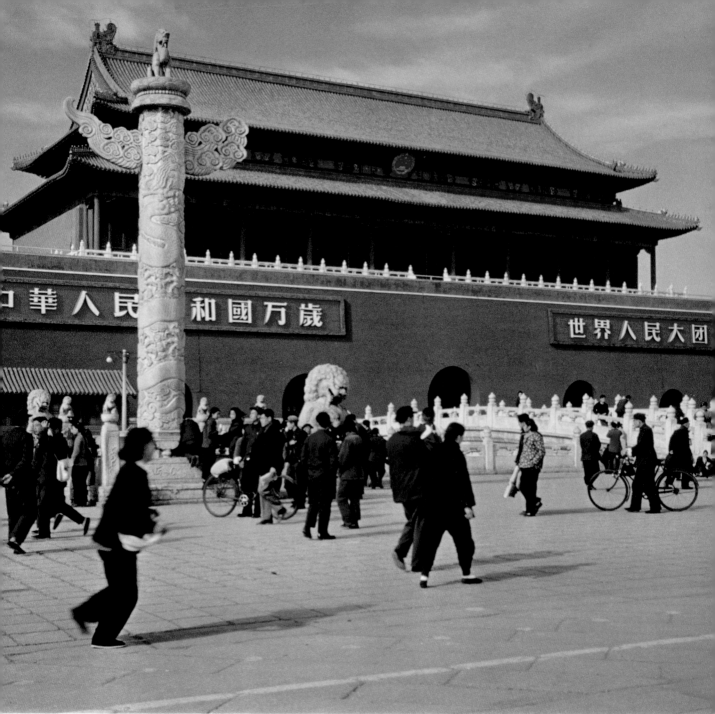

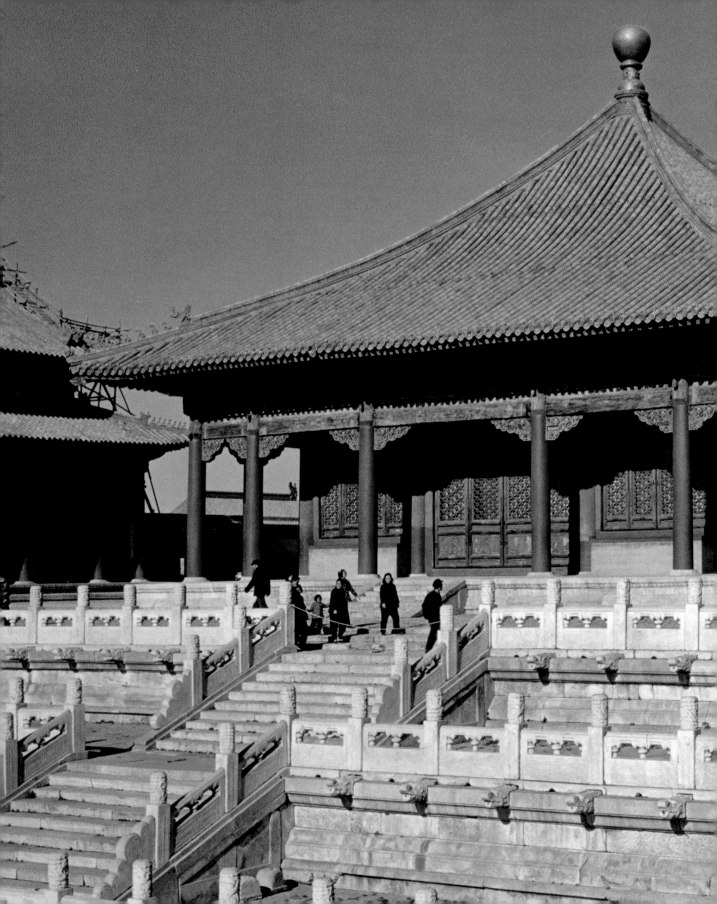

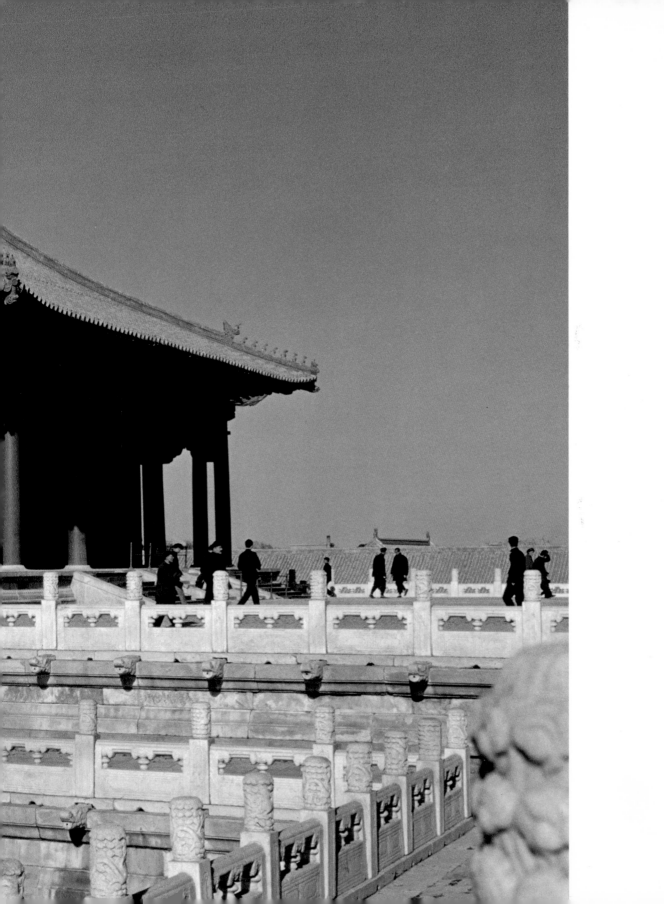

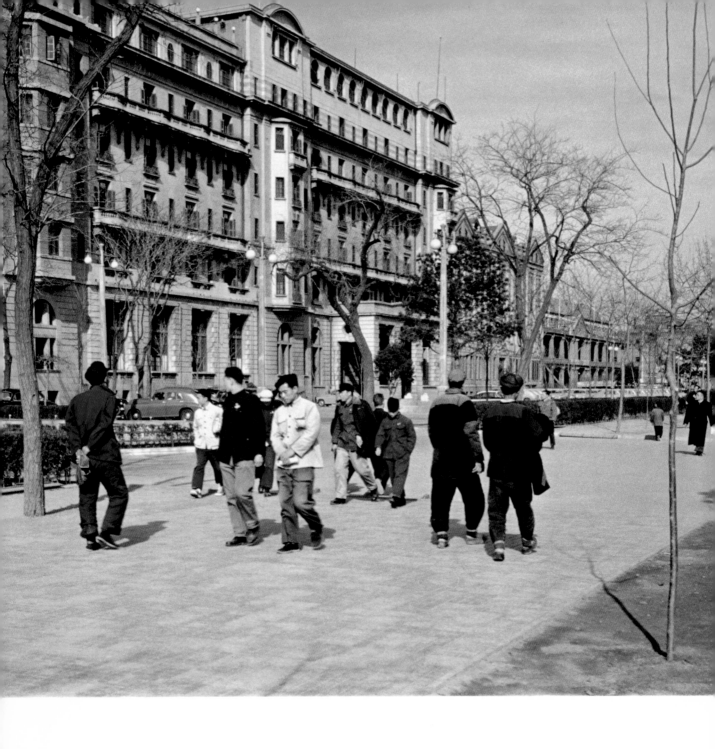

architecture with its gay magnificence of ornament is carefully looked after by the department for the preservation of old cultural monuments, and crowds of sight-seers come, particularly on Sundays, to this beautiful place near the capital.

The other buildings which provide Peking's fame as one of the greatest museums of architecture are likewise carefully cherished. Even if these palaces and shrines were erected to glorify rulers and gods who in the people's democracy have been unmasked as exploiters or myths, they were after all artistic objects created by the working people, to whom they are now given back as monuments to their inherent genius.

Lying at the southern edge of the town, and forming the largest park in Peking, are the grounds of the Temple of Heaven with their processional roads and three circular main buildings—the triple-terraced Temple of Prayers for a Good Harvest, the smaller Imperial Vault of Heaven, also with a blue roof, where the plaque with the name of the supreme god of heaven was preserved, and the marble Altar of Heaven with three flights of steps.

The Temples of the Capital

Near by is the Temple of Agriculture. While looking for the old buildings I came upon a large crowd on its way to a football match in the sports stadium, and the taxi-driver, whom I had had thoroughly instructed, was not to be persuaded to look any further for the temple, nor did anyone else seem to know anything about it. I had to call my friend Kung and the directions of the Embassy to my aid to find the altar and halls of the temple, which were on the same broad stretch of land as the sports grounds but separated from them by a wall. There the emperors used to inaugurate the cultivation of the land with symbolic rites; today it is the site of a girls' school which is accessible only with a special permit.

Ingenious 17th- and 18th-century astronomical instruments were set up on the battlements at one of the east gates; they had once been taken to Potsdam as trophies but were brought back after the First World War.

The Temple of the Ancestors, built immediately beside the Forbidden City on the model of the imperial palaces, where the memorial plaques to the emperors were set up, has been since 1st May 1950 a 'cultural palace' of the working classes and the home of Communist propaganda. Various exhibitions show the achievements of the People's Democracy and the baseness of the imperialists who are opposed to progress. In the garden in front of the main entrance stood two of those white-lacquered figures—a young Chinese worker and a girl—whose particular style is well known from innumerable examples to every visitor to Soviet Russia.

The exterior architecture of the Hall of Classics could be seen in its original colourful splendour, with gold ornaments in the timberwork. A public library had been housed in the adjacent buildings. The courtyard of the Temple of Confucius, situated beside it, with huge stone monuments to the various emperors carried by turtles, seemed by contrast very neglected. When I visited it a second time the entrance was closed—there were evidently plans to restore it in the near future.

The large Lama Temple is a special show-piece, with its succession of court-yards; its red, blue, green, and gold walls and pillars under yellow-tiled roofs; bronze censers and many figures of the Buddha in the dim light of the rooms— everything had been perfectly restored, apparently on the occasion of the visit of the Dalai Lama a few years before. Unless you met the handful of aged monks at prayer chanting in croaking unison, you could wander through the courtyards and rooms as if in a petrified forest—not a soul there and no sound except the tinkle of small bells at the roof-edges, moved gently by the wind. Once, going through the empty streets, I saw by chance through an open gate a courtyard with more Lama buildings, similarly restored in their original colours. But entry was forbidden: it was the Peking residence of the Panchen Lama, second in seniority of the ecclesiastical rulers in Tibet.

Like other Buddhist temples in and outside the town the Temple of the White Clouds, a shrine of the Taoists in front of one of the west gates, had received the attention of the restorers. Everything was spotless, ready for display—the bearded altar-figures newly painted, the freshly lacquered holy vessels on the table, gay curtains and murals; and a few old monks moved about amid this well-swept disenchantment like vigilant museum custodians.

In the Ministry of Culture, the official in charge of antiquities, a middle-aged *Research and* man with an open, intelligent face, provided over a bowl of tea, information about *Conservation* the archaeological service and the preservation of historical monuments. So far as I could gather from Miss Wu's interpreting, the Ministry of Culture had been founded in 1950 and was responsible for the organisation of museums and the care of monuments; the Council of State indicated 6,000 places which were considered worth preserving, and about 1,000 of these were being worked on, a third of them architectural monuments, the remainder tombs, and other places.

Scientific organisations such as the Research Institute for Archaeology in the Academy of Sciences, and local committees are collaborating with the central authorities. In Peking specialists are trained in the restoration of old buildings.

Up to now 124 especially valuable monuments of Chinese architecture have been restored, among them the famous temple of Confucius in K'iuh-fow. Both the Archaeological Institute and the Ministry of Culture publish periodical reports about excavations and similar work; a whole pile of these monthly journals, which the friendly man I was talking to had sent to my hotel, gave in many illustrations some idea of the enormous amount of work to be done on the research into centuries of art and culture.

On Sundays the streets of Peking were filled with sightseers; more and more *The Capital of the* people poured into the museums of the Forbidden City (for which, by the way, *People's Republic* an entrance fee had to be paid); there was an even greater throng, however, at the permanent Soviet Russian exhibition at the north-west corner of the town wall; the queue of people waiting in front of the entrance was almost as long as that at the Lenin Mausoleum in Moscow. A pavilion with a pointed tower in the style of Stalinist architecture proclaimed from afar the triumph of materialistic culture, and the people seemed eager to follow the Soviet teachers into the temple of Western civilisation.

There is as yet little to be seen of the efforts of the Communist régime to match the ancient, museum-like Peking of the Ming and Manchu emperors with a city answering their own conception of town-planning, and expressing the new people's community. A few five-storeyed blocks of government buildings differ from like glorifications of a bureaucratic conformism elsewhere only in their Chinese tiled roofs. In one of the widened main streets a skyscraper, nearly completed, promised to have an unfortunate similarity to the pyramidal skyscrapers of the new Moscow.

The Russian Model Everywhere the traveller comes across the Russian model. A few weeks before my visit the retail trade received a decisive blow. The district which was once full of stores with delicacies and porcelain, bronze and lacquer, trinkets, crystal, and silk, looked deserted—only a few shops had been preserved from the great spring-cleaning and they looked as if they had been cleared of all their goods; but no doubt they were perfectly in order—that is to say, nationalised.

Today most of the shopping is done in the public bazaars, of which there are several: there souvenirs and products of Chinese arts and crafts to decorate the drawing-rooms of the fairly well-to-do are offered for sale as well as other goods. Looking at the number of these objects displayed one concluded that there must be quite a demand for them: you could buy mass-produced plaster busts or full-length figures of Mao Tse-tung, the familiar Beethoven for the piano, or white nymphs in the style of Canova.

I met one dealer of the old school at the Embassy and he looked me up in my hotel room with a large bale of old silk. There indeed was something heartening: splendid mandarin coats, embroidery, table-cloths with gold dragons, fabrics plain or patterned in delicate colours which fifty or more years ago had been brought as tribute from Shantung to Peking, and would probably adorn a lady in far-off Europe. The salesman spoke English; he knew his customers; but his business was only apparently private: for some years now he had been working not on his own account but on behalf of a 'company', and this was nothing else but a small branch of the huge State industry.

With Miss Wu as interpreter I made a special expedition to Peking University. The block of buildings, among them a concrete water-tower in the form of a thirteen-storeyed pagoda, stands in a park outside the town wall, on the road to the western mountains. More than 8,000 students were in residence there, barely a quarter of whom were girls; they lived four to a small room with two-tier beds and one table.

A Visit to the University of Peking

With the Universities of Shanghai, Wuhan, Chungking, and Canton and the Peking Institute for Legal Studies, Politics, and Economics, the university of the capital plays a leading role in the training of the higher cadres; for it is from them that the new mandarin caste is to be drawn which will combine expert knowledge with an unshakeable belief in the doctrines of Marxism-Leninism. Most of the university had been built with American money and there were other signs from pre-Communist times of the efforts to influence the Chinese educational system from across the Pacific. When I inquired about celebrities among the professors, it turned out that none of them had acquired their scholarship in Russia but several in the United States; one had been a pupil of the Viennese historian Srbik; the Vice-Principal of the University, Shou Pei-yuan, was a former pupil of Einstein. My conversation with a very urbane professor of philosophy was unfortunately indirect for it depended on Miss Wu's English, and was thus less productive than it might otherwise have been. I asked him what had become of the history of Chinese philosophy—as consistent followers of Marx and Lenin they must find Confucius and his associates completely irrelevant, and instead must concentrate on the intellectual antecedents of Marx, the European political theorists. The professor greeted every awkward question with a radiant smile. Naturally they also studied the old Chinese philosophy. It appeared that people were not obsessed by the history of their ideology to the exclusion of everything belonging to the artistic traditions of their civilisation—faith is independent of historical considerations.

Pages 207–213 PEKING

207 The traditional, drab street scene in the residential district of a Chinese town: walls without windows give passers-by no glimpse into the houses (*see also page 163*).

208 top The style of the new administrative buildings differs from that usual in the Soviet Union only in the Chinese curved tile roofs and ornamentation on the balconies.

208 below, 209, 210, 211, 212 The Sun Yet-sen Park in the district of the former imperial gardens is one of the Peking 'culture parks', on the Soviet Russian model, where recreations and entertainments are provided, especially for the children. One Sunday we saw there an intellectual with his book; the children enjoying the chute; the flower-show; stalls for drinks and sweets; a family eating a frugal meal with chopsticks. Both grown-ups and children favour the peaked cap, which is part of the uniform dress of the 'blue ants'.

210 top left In front of the 'Palace of Culture', the former imperial Temple of the Forefathers, stands this glorification of the Chinese worker. Its naturalistic style is like that of innumerable white statues in the public parks in the Soviet Union.

210 below left. In one of the shop-windows in the main street of the Chinese city Tsien Men Takié there was a white statue of Mao Tse-tung among other ornaments for the drawing-room.

213 My almost-constant and most solicitous companion during my stay in Peking was this pedicab man.

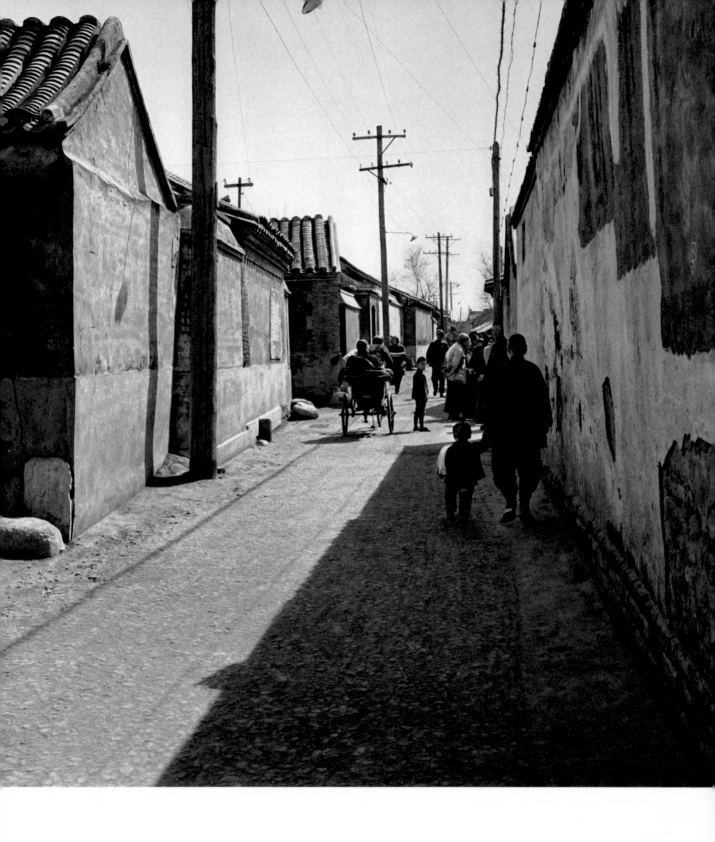

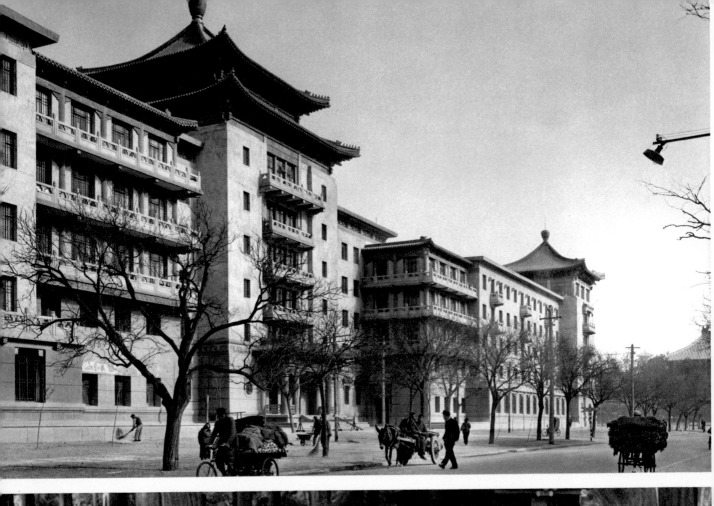

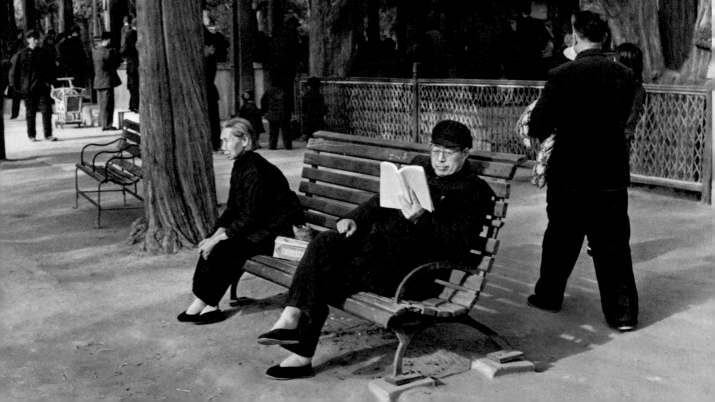

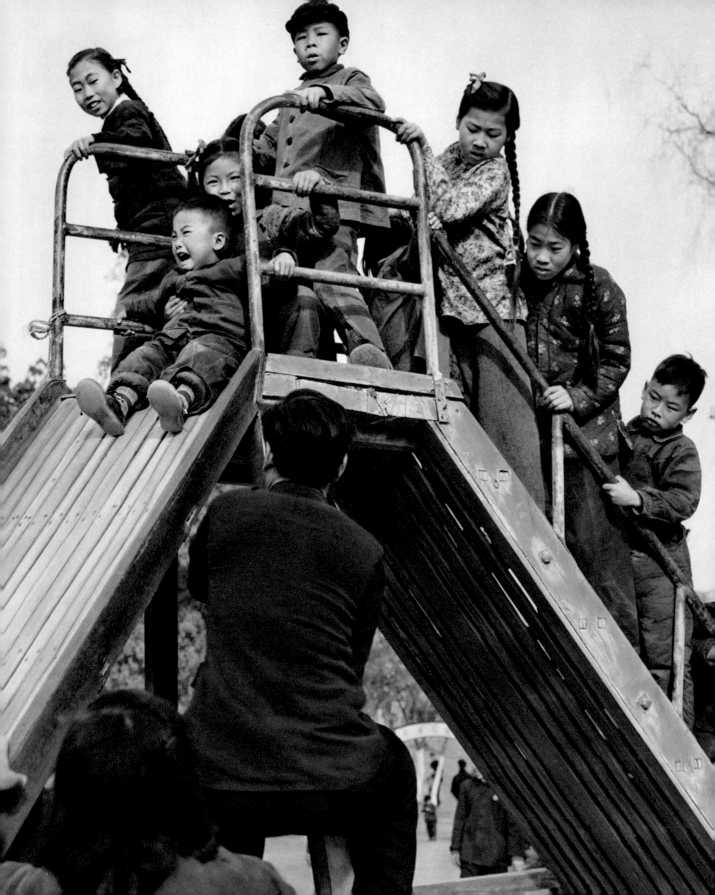

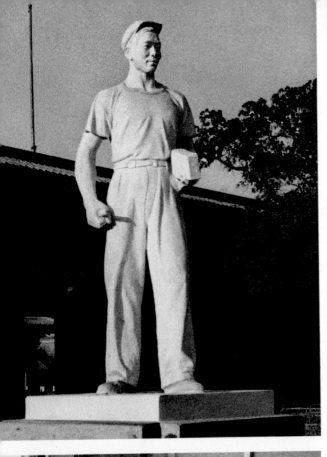
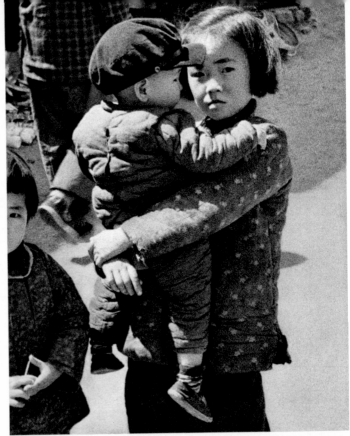
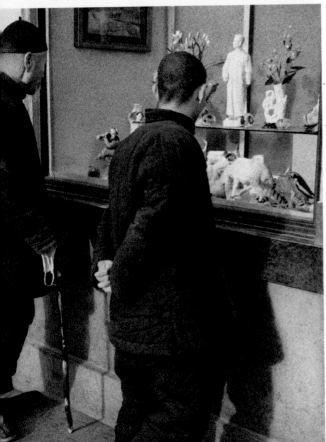
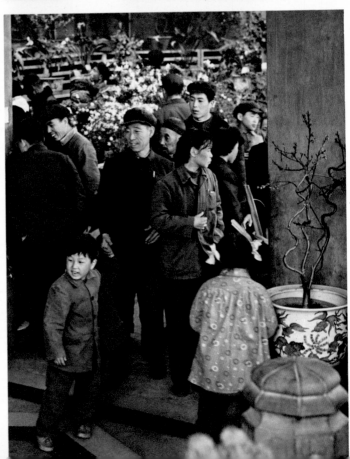

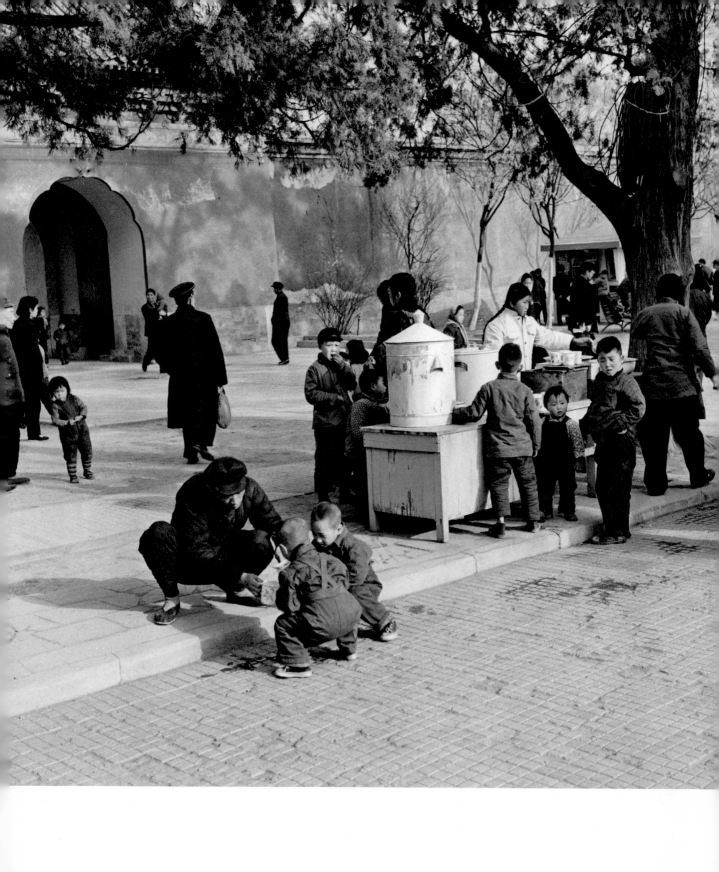

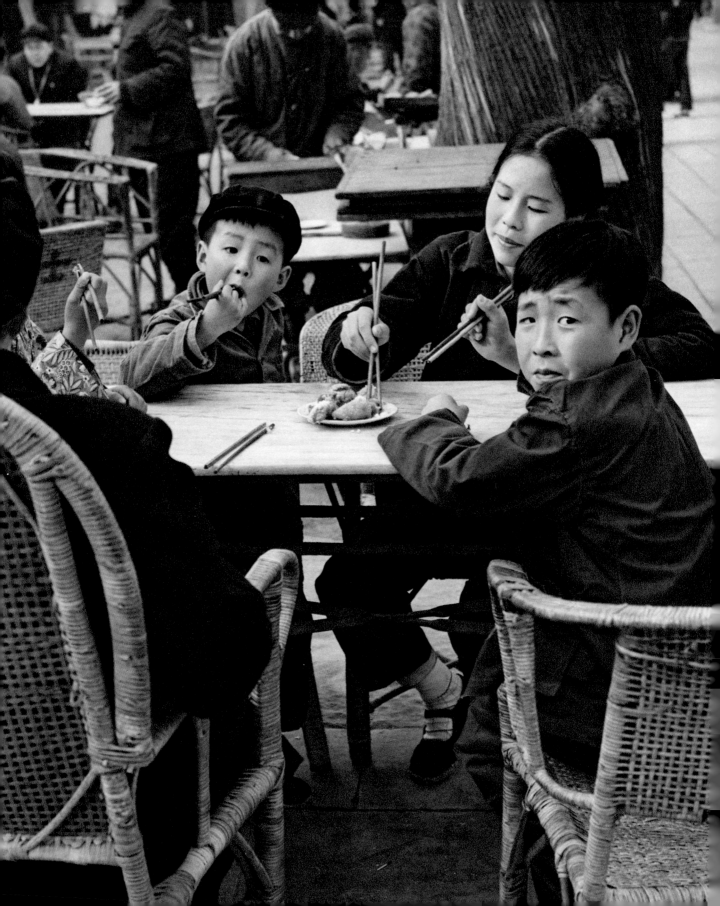

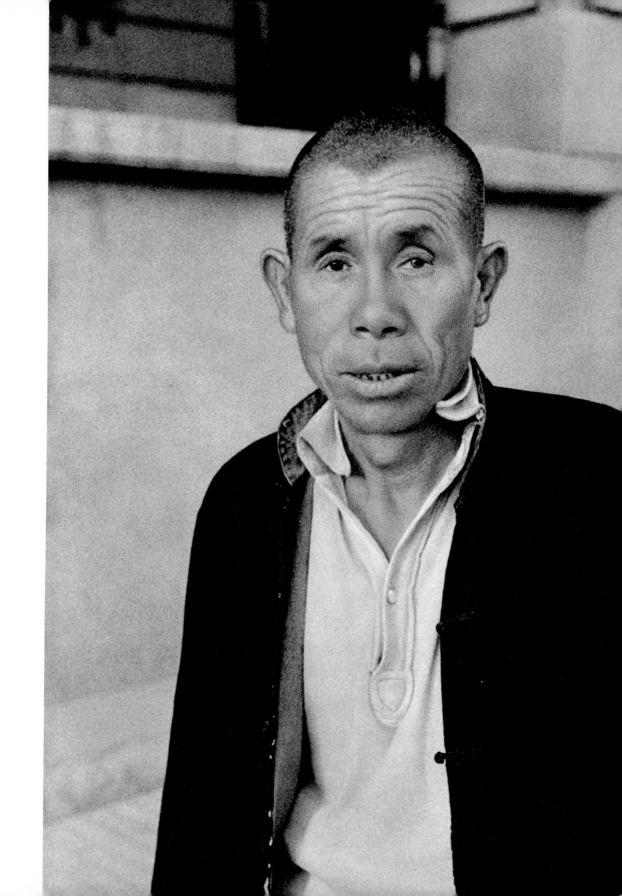

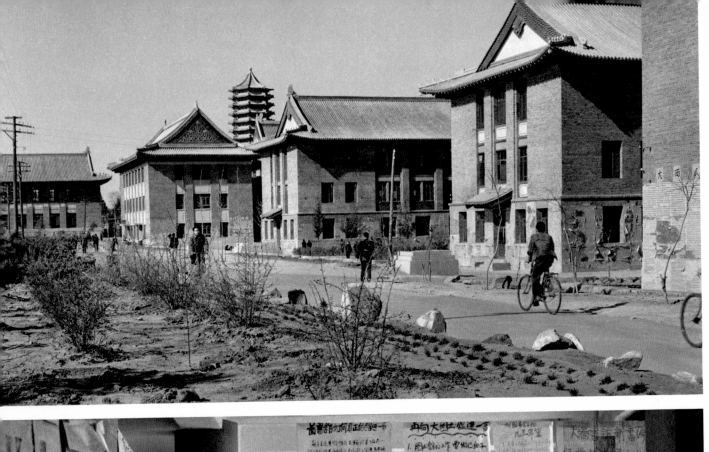

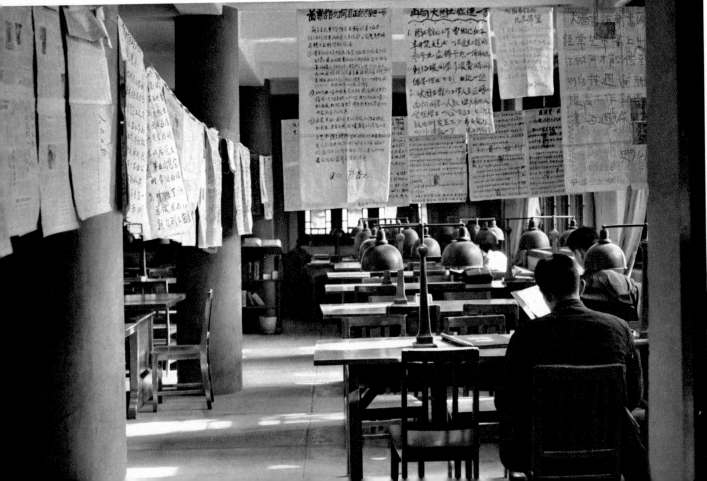

The 'culture parks' are among the most important show-pieces of the new Peking. There, on the Soviet model, every kind of entertainment is offered on payment of an entrance fee, from plays and films to flower-shows and children's playgrounds. On Sundays there was great activity, particularly in the Sun Yat-sen Park near the Forbidden City and in the zoo beside the Russian exhibition, and colour and gaiety was introduced into the monotony of blue uniforms by children, who with their stiff pigtails standing out coquettishly and gaily patterned jackets and trousers, showed the individual ambitions of their mothers.

And those children! They were the most cheerful, amusing, lively company that one could imagine! At certain times you could see among the traffic the three-wheeled miniature omnibuses in each of which eight small boys were taken by a pedicab man to the nursery school: with what high-spirited curiosity they peeped out of the windows at the world outside!

Anyone who goes to Peking to look behind the scenes and learn at first hand about things which are not otherwise to be ascertained, has a hard job before him. Even if you spoke Chinese fluently, you would have to feel your way very carefully or have old and trustworthy contacts, before you could talk openly. We often hear about the 600 million people; they form today the third most powerful piece on the chess-board of world politics and will perhaps one day be the strongest. But who are these 600 million people; what do they think? They are not ready to unburden their hearts to the few European travellers.

What Does China Think?

Page 214 PEKING

Between the city and the Summer Palace lies the University of Peking, a group of lecture rooms and residential buildings. Announcements and notices hang in the reading-room.

Here more than in other Asian countries you have to bear in mind that opinions about the general political situation and Communism are derived from an historical experience entirely different from ours. The European conception of individual rights, freedom, and democracy is the result of centuries of development; the national ethos and social responsibility are the expression of a creative process of self-realisation. Since the opening-up of sea-routes round the world the white race has appeared in Asia and Africa not only with superior technical resources —but mainly among tribes who were living, if not exactly in a state of cannibalism, in very primitive social conditions; or else, as in India, whose culture more than equals that of Europe, among a people who were incapable of creating a larger federation of states, except under the sporadically-appearing exceptionally able despots. Only the appropriation of Western ideas created the desire—and to a still uncertain degree the ability—for national self-determination.

China has a different story. Here a political system had developed which was entirely independent of the heritage of Graeco-Roman antiquity and which gave primacy to moral forces as against the arbitrariness of divine kingship; and which was therefore a true order and not the imposed regulation by the most powerful. The crisis of the dynasty and its military weakness enabled the well-equipped Europeans to inflict on the old Middle Kingdom one humiliation after another.

The American and the Russian Model

The United States confined themselves to the principle of the 'open door' and to preventing a partition of China; they gave generously from the indemnity due to them from the Boxer Rising for the education of young Chinese. Sun Yat-sen himself and innumerable students studied at universities in the United States or the universities in China established with American money; they learnt about Western civilisation in its American form, and when the Manchus abdicated a republic on the American model was the obvious solution. But the efforts of missionaries and politicians from the other side of the Pacific had little success—

the old giant did not want to wake up; he barely stirred; the way of thinking of the pampered capitalist West was not able to penetrate the family and kinship structure and the customs and secret rites of the people.

The American formula did not work; now it was the turn of Soviet Russia. To judge from experience so far its success has put in the shade everything achieved in the consolidation of the Chinese State since the rule of Kien Lung. The methods by which this has been accomplished are detestable according to the conception of present-day Western civilisation, but not unfamiliar in the history of Asia and no rarity in earlier epochs in Europe; and the liquidation of some millions of Jews by a modern European nation was not more refined. The Chinese are guided by those who know how to deal with facts. But the struggle for the soul of this great nation has not yet been concluded; it has only just begun —one can sense that from the vehemence with which it is conducted by the present rulers.

Who can look into the future? Or into the hearts of my friend Kung and his many millions of brothers? Who can know to what use the rising generations will put the instruction provided for them today?

The visitor to Peking today can learn one thing, however, and its impact is much greater when he sees it for himself: this is a nation of the present; it does not dream away its time in the Temple of the Ancestors, nor dissipate its energy on crazy notions. There is a trait of optimism and efficiency in everybody, young and old, stupid and clever, diligent and lazy, fat and thin, epicures and ascetics. Perhaps the Chinese laughs less than he used to in this barracks-like existence of the collectives, but he is still much more cheerful than, for instance, the Indian or Arab. Small errors or misfortunes are accepted with good humour, and a smile or laugh carries him through many embarrassing situations even with incomprehensible foreigners; any opportunity for fun is seized. There is, of course, often

Chinese Realism

morose, taciturn indifference in these faces, a monumental, impenetrable impartiality. This nation cannot be broken by the hardest labour; for centuries it has lived under the threat of natural catastrophes and human exploitation. Year by year millions of children with wide-awake eyes in their laughing moon faces, impudent, merry, and noisy, replace those who have become weary.

The New Dam An excursion with Miss Wu by car to the Great Wall and the tombs of the Ming emperors gave me a chance to watch the construction of a new dam in that region. A few miles from the avenue which leads to the memorial hall of the great Yung-lo and his successors, we crossed the tracks left by tractors and travelled on scarcely visible roads, among motor-lorries, through wide, dry country to a veritable battlefield; vast crowds were assembled there like swarms of ants, red flags with letters were fluttering, loudspeakers blared out their marches. Among teams of men and women who were moving earth in wheel-barrows or simply in baskets we looked for the building-site on one of the hills.

Pages 219–222 PEKING

219 At the imperial Summer Palace. The 'Bridge of the Jade Band' ornaments the western shore of the Kuenming lake.

220–221 The Wall of the Nine Dragons is one of the chief attractions of the 'Winter Palace' and Peihei Park, near the main imperial residence. One of the main motifs of Chinese art is shown repeatedly: Yang and Yin, the two dragons who embody the male and female principle, in their eternal play round the globe of perfection.

222 A lion as guardian in the first courtyard of the great Lama Temple, which was carefully restored to its original colourful magnificence by the Communist government.

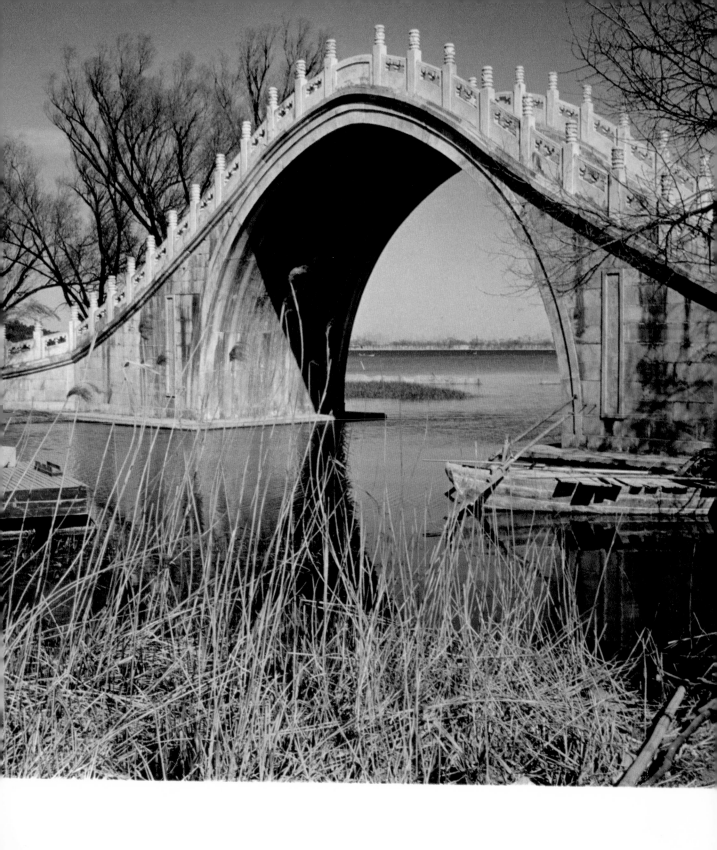

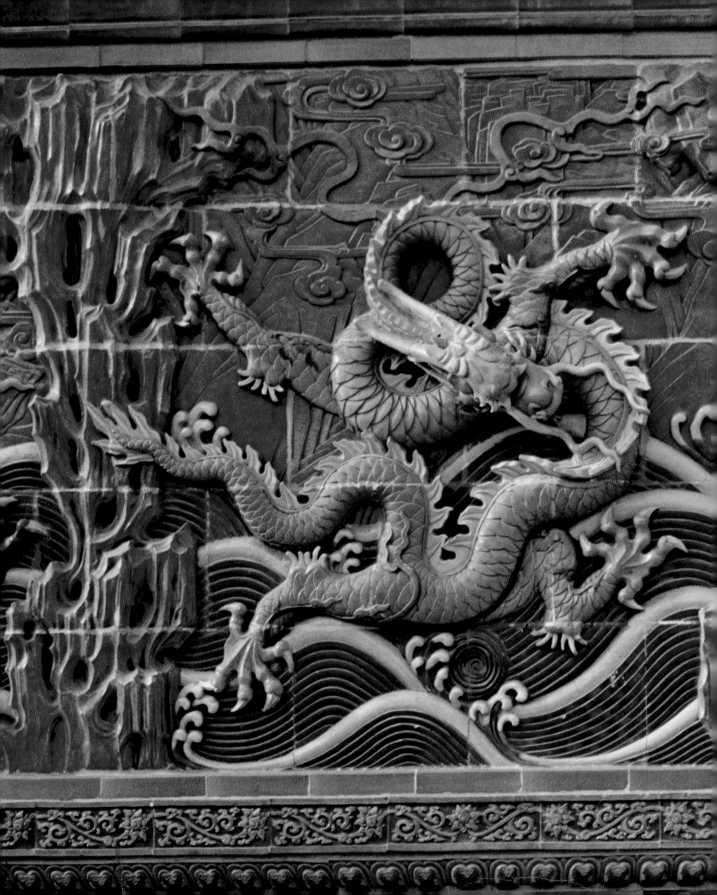

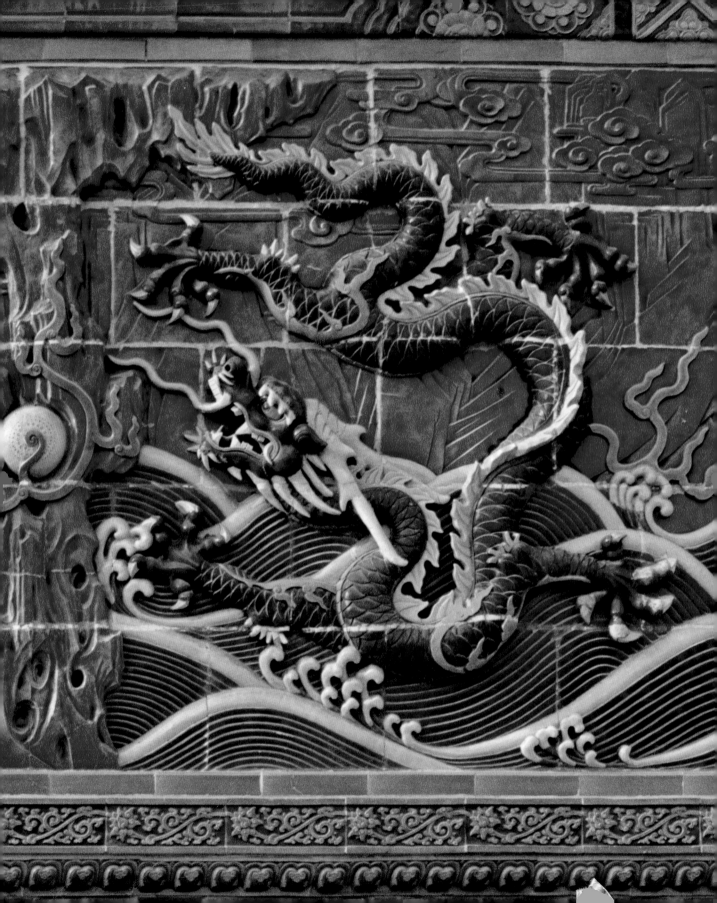

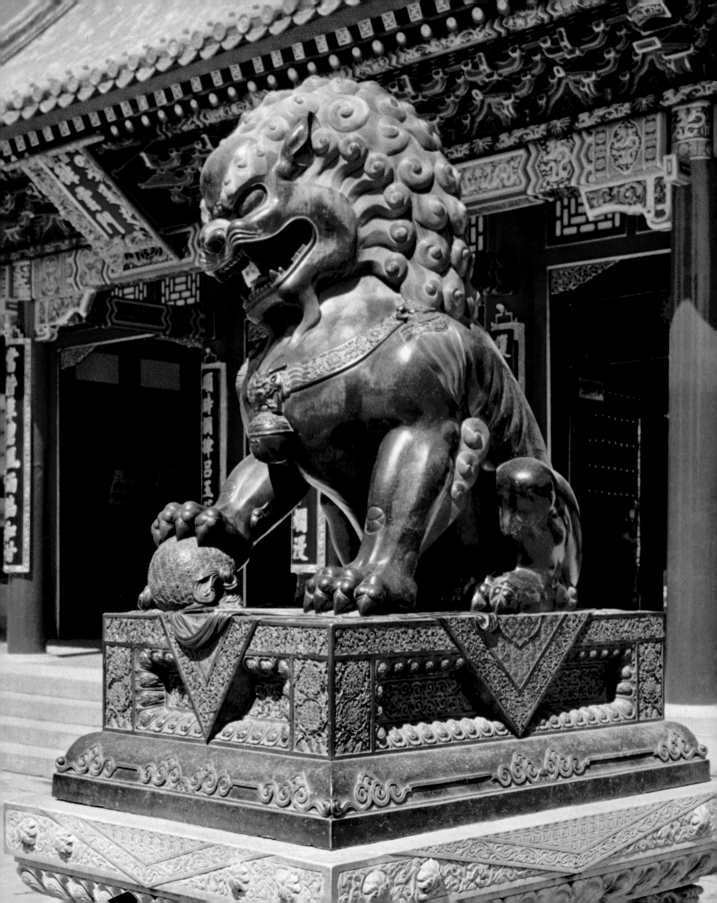

The youthful chief engineer and his assistant led us to the site of the construction of the dam. When it is completed it will make a lake three miles long and almost half a mile broad; it is one of the smaller undertakings of this kind, designed to produce new arable land. Construction had begun in January 1958 and the opening was to take place on 5th June.

Fifty-two thousand workers worked day and night in three shifts of eight hours. The army formed the main contingent. The workers were assisted by troops of school-children, civil servants, and other employees, who were drafted for ten days so as to take an active part in the national work of construction. Working methods were in some respects the most primitive imaginable, and were hardly defensible from an economic point of view; but this was not important, the necessary labour was readily available, and wages and standards of living are not discussed. It was not just a battle against the dangers of flooding and for new arable land: it was a propaganda battle too. We were in the 'year of the great leap forward'; delays of generations were to be made up for; the anvil was to become the hammer, a hammer of 600 million people.

Opera in Peking

An account of a visit to Peking could not end without a reference to the theatre. In the past few years the so-called Peking Opera has become known to people in Europe; its productions are a kind of potpourri of small one-act plays and separate dancing, acrobatic, or musical items, which are meant to make the unfamiliar acceptable to Western audiences by presenting it in small doses. But you would have to see a whole evening's play to grasp the power of expression of their diction, music, and gesticulation.

The different companies were not attached to particular theatres but appeared according to programmes and requirements on any of the Peking stages. In addition to modern propaganda plays, classical drama with episodes from China's heroic and mythical era still enjoyed great popularity. Mei Lan-fang, who for fifty years had played the parts of beautiful princesses and fairies with inimitable grace, was the highly respected head of a school of drama; but most of the women's parts which he and his rivals used to play are now being taken by actresses.

For two evenings I experienced the old China in all its fairy-tale splendour, and even the blue ants, who filled the auditorium to the last seat, looked with delight at a stage full of colour and life. You quickly became accustomed to the strained sound of the falsettos, the subtle code of gestures, the play of hands, the shaking of the long sleeves, the transition from the spoken word to the song, the exact accentuation of words, songs, and movements by percussion instruments of the small orchestra, and the ceremonious steps. The stylised expressions of grief, tenderness, and anger produced an intensity of effect in which the personality of the actor had to stand a test as stiff as in any Corneille tragedy. An extremely high standard of dancing and acrobatics is demanded from the actors, for instance in the sword dances where the hero had to prove his superiority. Scenes succeeded one another quickly. Scenery was unimportant, although nowadays, probably under the influence of the West, there is a painted backcloth; but they did not economise on the splendid costumes. In these performances tragic pathos was immediately followed by gaiety, with the recurrent themes of the sorrows of love and gallantry, evil forces and intrigues, ridiculous fancies and stupid misfortunes, treachery and true loyalty—the gamut of human passions was portrayed on that stage, as we know it only in Shakespeare.

Return to Canton   My return flight followed the route by which I had arrived. I had made my last journey by pedicab and said good-bye to my trusty companion Kung. When I asked to be allowed to photograph him before my departure his feelings seemed to get the better of him, for a strange change came over his expression; his grin disappeared and two earnest, sad eyes looked at me from a very old face.

Once again I had to spend the night in Canton in order to catch the day train to Hongkong. This time there was far more activity in the skyscraper hotel, for the international Canton fair had just been opened and many people from Hongkong were taking advantage of the easing of the visa restrictions for the occasion to glance behind the bamboo curtain.

This time I was prepared for the train with the loudspeaker. There was a tense *Back in Hongkong* moment at the frontier control, when we were again led into the room with upholstered furniture and called up individually for examination of our luggage. What would happen, in view of the ban on the export of undeveloped films, about all my photographs, in colour and in black and white, and all undeveloped? I had no document confirming the permission which had been given in Peking, but whether the presentation of my red Press pass had the desired effect, or whether they were intentionally generous, or had been advised of my arrival, at all events I was left in peace and was thus able to start out on the way back over the frontier bridge.

The British-Chinese officials did not bother about customs control. It was like home in the new railway carriage, while we passed through the smiling landscape of the New Territories. There were animated crowds on the platforms of the small stations, among them an occasional tall, lanky Englishman: the atmosphere was unmistakably that of the life of free peoples. So this then is the 'Colony'— which languishes under foreign rule?

What is the truth about China? It could not be gleaned from the streets of *Who knows the Truth* Peking; it was hidden behind a language which only a few have mastered, behind *about China?* a propaganda which only a few see through, behind a mask of caution which only a few penetrate, behind the figure 600 million which no Dr Gallup surveys.

It has become clear to the Chinese today that he can come to terms with the machine age only by a radical change of front. This was made plain to him with the necessary urgency; he believes in the man who has proved himself the strongest, he relies on the facts he sees. But what has been the significance of the Chinese family for the individual, so far? The people lived for the most part in large kinship groups, three generations together, in which a woman who did not rise to the position of mother of the family had to obey; and from young men too family communism demanded a hardly less strict discipline than the Communist State. However, we shall not know for a generation at least whether Chinese kinship is really a thing of the past; whether it is still active in the soul of the people; nor what influence the Chinese cultural heritage will have in the new forms of society.

Back in the comfortable hotel in Kowloon I was more than ever conscious of the improbability and precariousness of the situation in Hongkong: this ferry with its cosmopolitan passengers, neat Anglo-Chinese policemen, porcelain-like ladies with their coquettishly slit skirts, antique shops, bustling bazaars, villas high above the bright harbour with its warships and junks, squatter settlements,

Pages 227–229 THE MING TOMBS NEAR PEKING

At the foot of the mountain range to the north of Peking a long avenue leads to the tombs of the Emperor Kung-lo and his successors, which lie in a semicircle on the slope of the hill. Animals in pairs, representing different degrees of strength, line the road. Beside one of them stands my interpreter, Miss Wu. At one of the gateways (*see page 237 below*) a tortoise (*page 229*) as a symbol of longevity carries an inscribed stone plaque. In front of the grave-mound of Yung-lo rises a memorial hall with huge wooden pillars, on which a simple plaque commemorates the Emperor.

Pages 230–234 THE DAM NEAR THE MING TOMBS

Under the supervision of two young chief engineers, and with loudspeakers blaring, one of the many undertakings in the campaign for the technical development of the country is taking shape—sometimes by most primitive methods. Groups of men and women from every kind of office, works, and school march up with their flags. Some of the workers wear white protective masks over their mouths and noses.

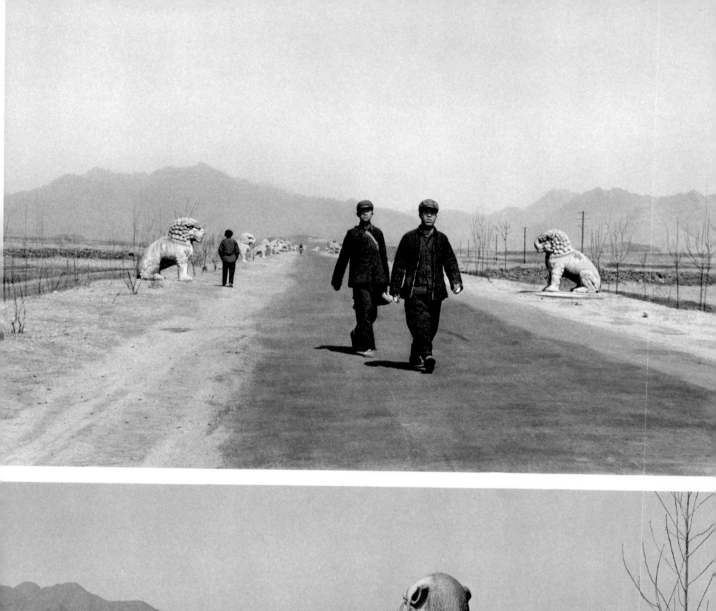
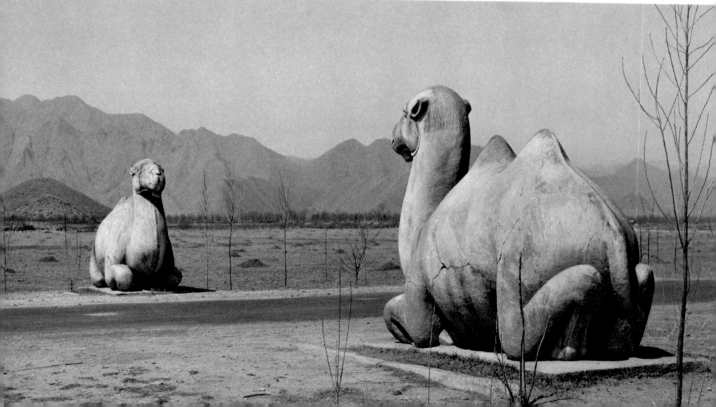

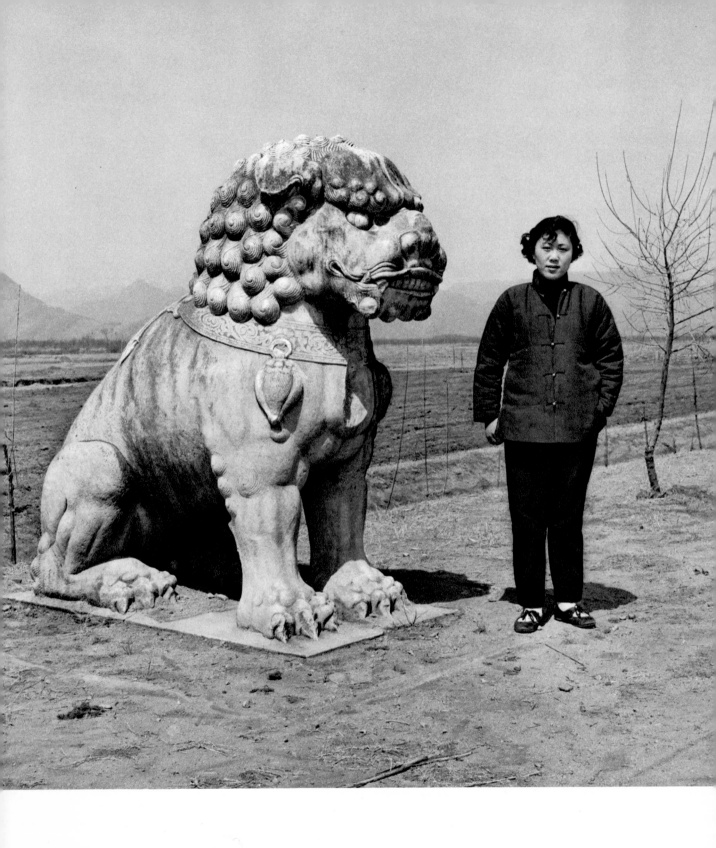

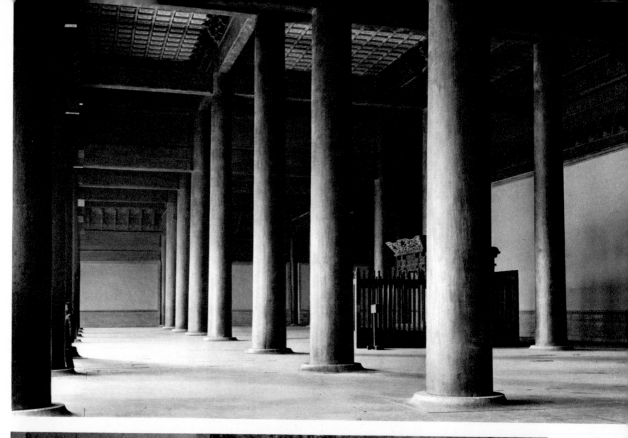

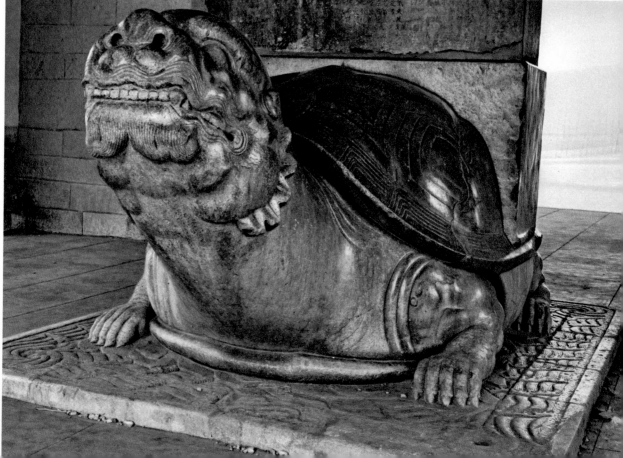

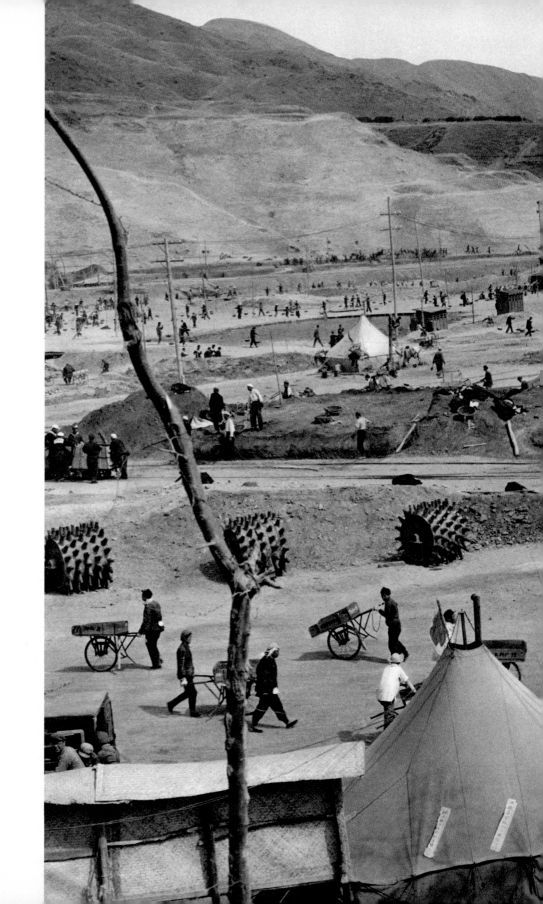

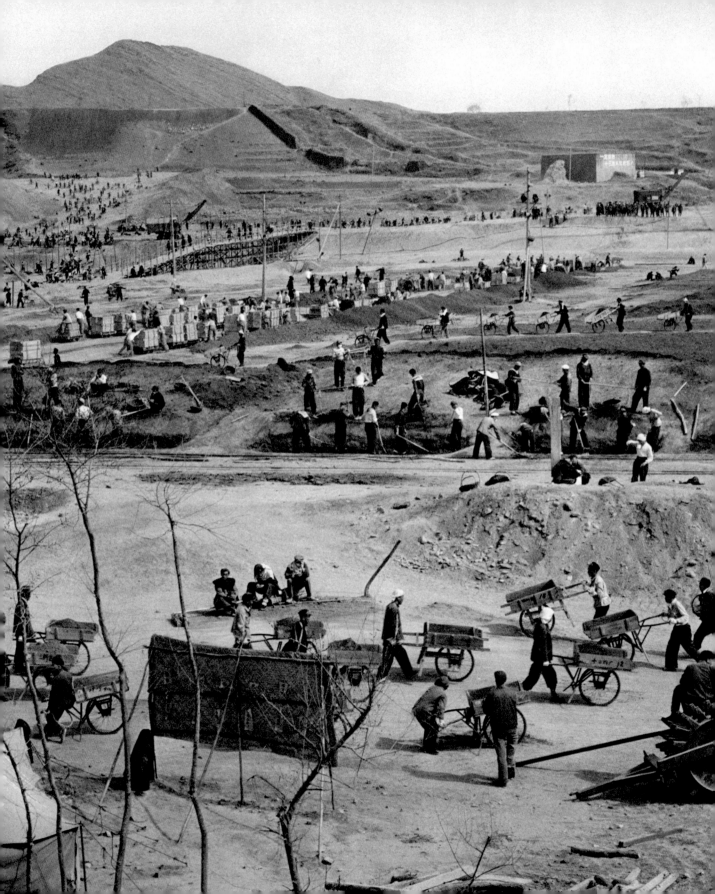

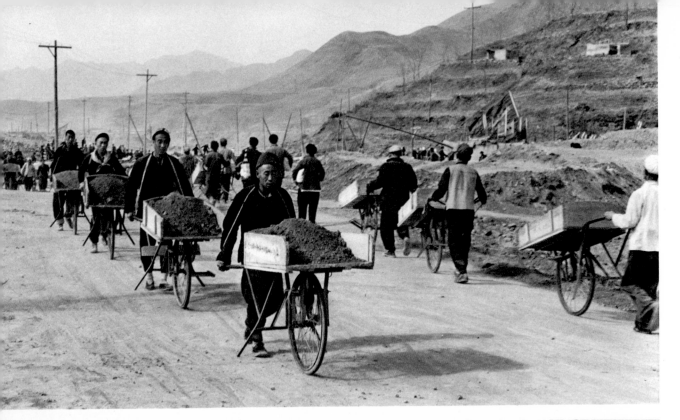

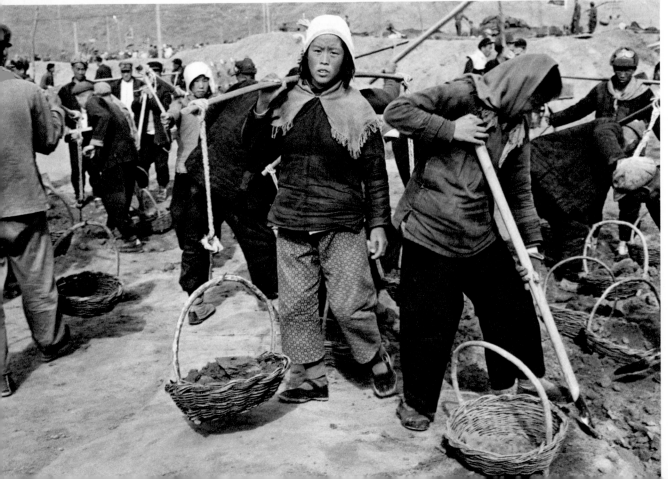

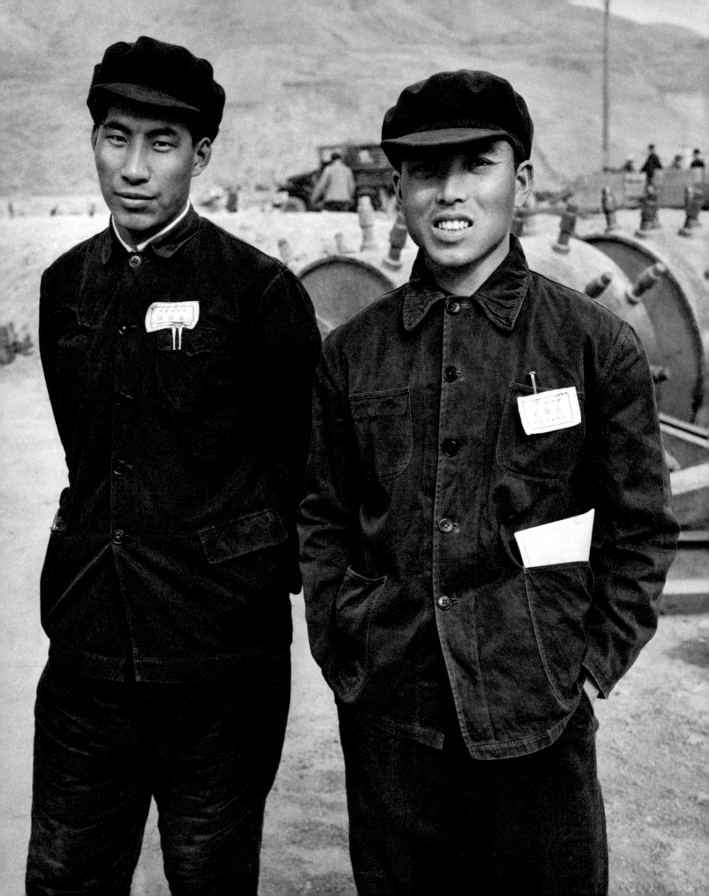

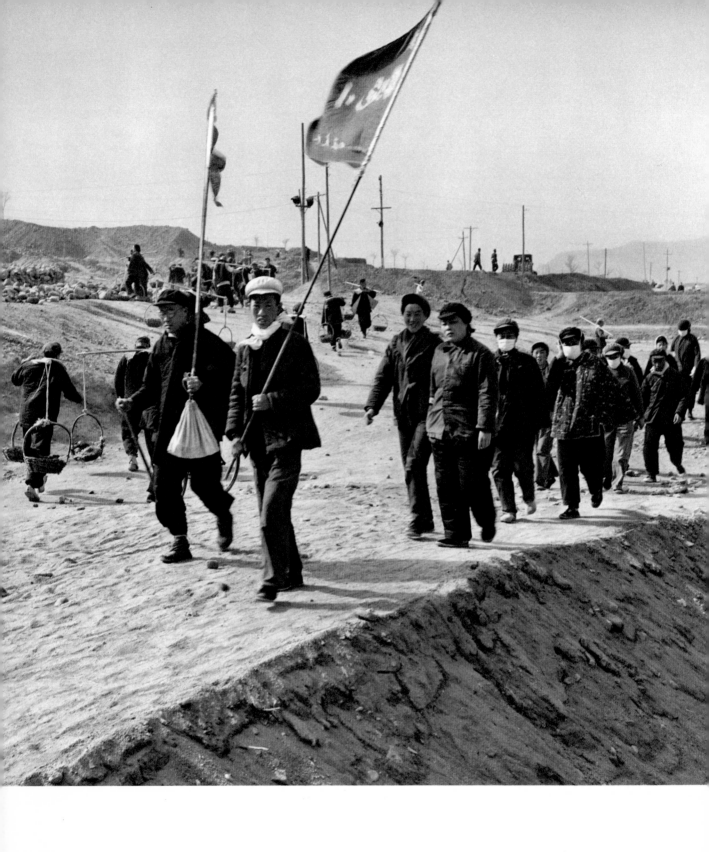

tennis courts and golf courses, sailors from every nation, assiduously fostered industries, newspapers which divulge everything so garrulously, the Governor who goes to the races. . . . How long will all this continue unchanged?

On the evening before my departure I had a visit in my hotel from a fellow-countryman who had heard through a mutual acquaintance that I had been in Peking and wanted to know what kind of impression I had formed there. He had lived for some years in South China and was now employed in the New Territories. The little information I could give him at first hand was quickly imparted, but I was eager to learn what I could from him; and while outside the last rays of the sun fell on the throng of boats in the blue bay, and lights went on and off in the white pagoda of the Tiger Park villa and in the many windows of the façades of Victoria, we sat in darkness, and I entered the Middle Kingdom once more, this time through a small side gate in its walls, and had a glimpse of one of its unvisited districts.

A Visitor Depicts China's Other Face

The Europeans whom I had met so far in Hongkong as also in China had expressed themselves either positively or else with the greatest caution and reserve about the State of Mao Tse-tung. Merchants in the British Colony accepted Communist rule as a fact which had to be reckoned with; almost all were very much impressed with the 'order', the restoration of which was considered as the greatest achievement of statesmanship.

My evening visitor surveyed world history not from the lofty heights of an office in the commercial district; he lived among the Chinese and shared their troubles; he had seen what was happening in the country and heard the news which trickled through daily from the other side of the frontier. From his dry, objective description emerged the picture of a ruthless revolution; thousands had been executed in the fields, many of them people he himself knew. Relatives, forced to be witnesses, were not allowed to bury the dead, who were left lying like vermin; at night wild animals howled, drawn from the mountains by the stench, a threat to the villages so long as the corpses lay unburied. No one who had seen it could forget it. The Chinese can wait. Millions were holding themselves in readiness for the day of retaliation. The Party knew it. The Party does not consist of the 600 or 650 million who are constantly spoken about, but is a relatively small but resolute group who must stick together through thick and thin. Carefully distributed over the country it had filled all the important positions; not for a moment could it relax its iron grip, for fear of being swept away by an outburst of repressed anger.

My visitor told me among other things about the famous extortionate interest. Formerly the peasant had been exploited by usurers. If he had no rice left to sow, he borrowed seed; six months later, when the harvest was brought in, the peasant had to give back six sacks for every one borrowed. The philanthropist was extremely indignant: 500 per cent interest for six months! Scandalous! How relieved the farmer must feel today now that he is freed from such oppression. Yet what had the farmer himself to say about it? The borrowed sack brought him a harvest of more than sixty sacks, of which he lost six. But now he has to hand over to the charitable State which has suppressed usury not 10 per cent but 90 per cent of his harvest; just the bare essentials of life are left to him.

Religious liberty exists in the Chinese People's Republic. Foreign missionaries have been eliminated as agents of imperialism, but the native priests are allowed to have their churches, mosques, and temples as long as they want to cling to such out-of-date customs. Such generosity naturally presupposes that there will be no

Page 237 THE MING TOMBS NEAR PEKING

237 top   The marble P'ailon, the outer gateway, where the long avenue begins. Its pedestals are decorated with delicate dragon reliefs.

237 below   Half-way along the avenue is the 'Great Red Gate', Ta Hung Men, with the inscribed plaque carried by a tortoise (*page 229*).

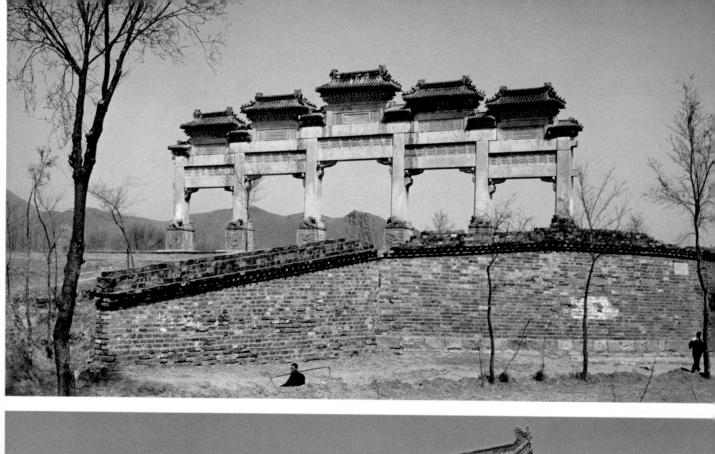

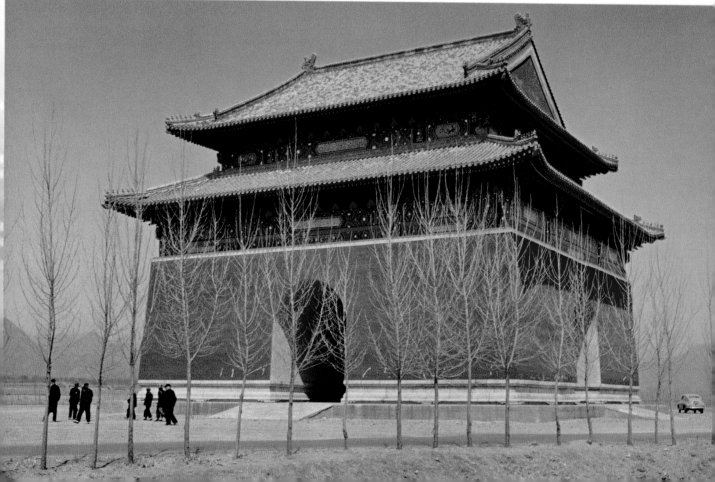

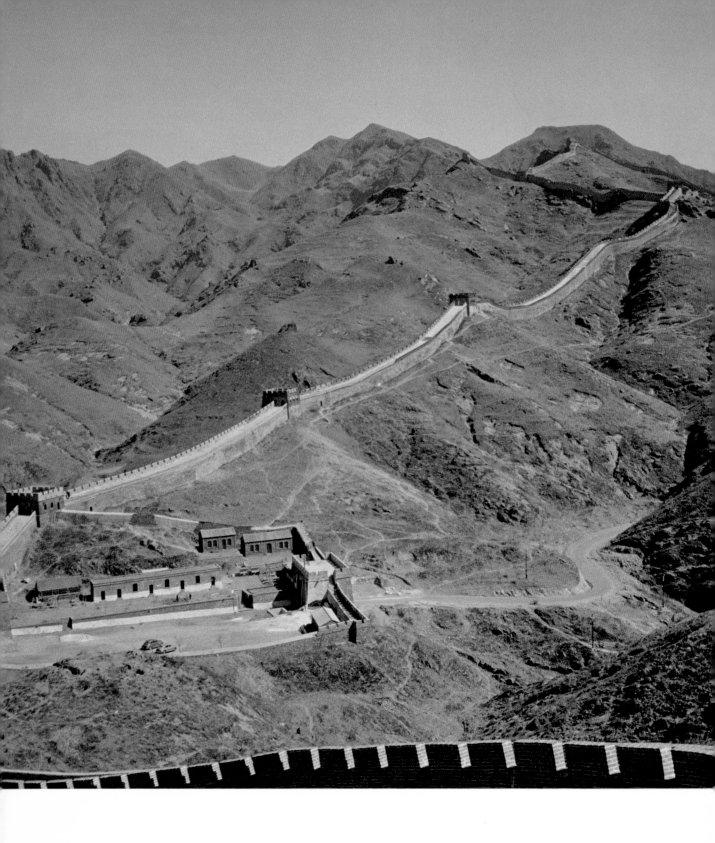

abuse of it by enemies of the people. The Roman Catholic Bishop of Canton was at that time in prison. Protestant ministers in the district had attended a training course of several weeks, in which they received instruction about the duties of a loyal citizen of the People's Republic; some refused to submit to the brainwashing and were eliminated from the course.

This, too, is the truth about China. But what is the whole truth?

Before my visitor took his leave, he suddenly put to me, out of a mutual feeling of anxiety, a question which was by no means meant to be rhetorical: 'What seems to you, a man who has been to many countries and heard many things, the most essential thing today?' I hesitated before replying: it was no time for big words; in the face of the seriousness of the situation they too easily become irresponsible, but cannot be retracted; large pronouncements already fill volumes. I had to reject the question in all modesty and humility. With that we parted. I thought for a long time about an answer which I could defend before my visitor in Hongkong and my friend Kung and the three Singh gentlemen, and now I would venture something like this: a world which no longer knows what compassion is has no room for us; therefore, let us fight for our lives!

Page 238   THE GREAT WALL OF CHINA

At the Nanka Pass the road leads to Mongolia through the wall originally built by Shi Huang-ti. With its watch-towers it extends as far as the eye can see over the bare loess mountains.

Japan

THE LAST leg of my East Asian flight took me still farther away from the tropical zone into cooler regions, into a spring with trees in blossom, into a green country, where grey days and rain made the appearance of the sun a joyous event. My hope of being able to see the famous pyramid of Mount Fuji during the flight was disappointed; the holy mountain appears as seldom as the Matterhorn; as night fell it lay somewhere in the clouds to the left of us. About seven o'clock a bay appeared with a city which was lost in the distance—at home it was then barely midday.

This is today the largest city on our planet; in 1954 Tokyo proper had already more than eight million inhabitants; together with its suburb Yokohama it now has more than ten million.

In 1868 Emperor Meiji visited the town of Edo, where since 1603 the Tokugawa Shogunate had concentrated the government of the kingdom, and gave it the name of Tokyo, 'eastern capital'. In the following year the Tenno himself moved from Kyoto to the new capital and occupied the castle of the former regents, which was surrounded by ramparts and a moat. The giddy development of Tokyo reflects the fortunes of the island kingdom since the memorable Meiji restoration.

I visited Tokyo once when I was much younger; that was in 1923, a few months before the great earthquake which reduced the capital to a heap of ruins. Much of the construction after that was destroyed during the bombing which was America's answer to the surprise attack on Pearl Harbor; 767,000 houses were destroyed and 167,000 people killed. Since then a new Tokyo has arisen, larger, more active than ever before—and it is still not nearly completed.

It is not easy to find your way about Tokyo even if you rely on one of the many small taxis—and they really are small taxis, with basic charges of 60, 70, and 80 Yen (100 Yen are about 1s. 8d.); the drivers matched their Parisian colleagues in their alarming speed. When a red light forced them to stop, they invariably brought out a schedule and whiled away the seconds totting up figures. The best thing to do was to have your destination written down in Japanese, but very accurately, because blocks of houses in different quarters sometimes have the same name and the streets are not numbered as in Europe; once you had reached the right district you generally had to look for the nearest police-station for further directions.

One part of the huge town, which had grown too quickly, still had no drainage; the water-supply was inadequate and refuse had to be removed daily in buckets. The muddy ground made the installation of pipes more difficult. Extensive residential quarters with their light, low, wooden buildings were overtopped by the watch-towers of the fire-stations. Railways through the middle of the town and underground helped to overcome the long distances.

The grounds of the Imperial Palace which was hidden behind stone walls formed as much as ever the central point of city and kingdom. To the assembly square in front of the double bridge which led to the entrance gate—which was usually closed—came omnibuses with school-children and parties of trippers; stewardesses who carried the name of their coach on a small flag accompanied their charges to the bank of the castle moat, where the inevitable group photograph was taken. There was a constant coming and going. Not far away was the curious Imperial Hotel; it had just been finished when I was last there and had survived earthquake and war; today there was talk of its having to make way soon for a skyscraper to satisfy the demand for rooms and the present value of the site.

Directly behind rose the new buildings of the city—ten storeys high on an average—like the Nikkatsu International Building, which contained the offices of four firms with which I had business (the bank, the travel bureau, Swissair, and a commercial firm), and a hotel in its upper storeys.

Not much town-planning is to be seen so far; everything had sprung up haphazardly as the enterprising spirit of financially powerful concerns wanted it. Japanese architects are very receptive towards all new trends, and, as they have innate confidence in their taste, the construction is on the whole good, and there are many out-of-the-ordinary creations. An ambitious project was taking shape in the middle of the city: a road for fast traffic was to be built in a loop through the town at second-floor level. In the completed part of it an elegant shopping-centre had been opened, while on the first floor and elsewhere there were offices and warehouses. Tenants for these were not lacking.

The main commercial area was in the Ginza, the long, broad street leading from the Shimbashi station to the north. The department stores which are usually so prominent in Japan were there; these department stores—the 'palace' of today— displayed on eight and more storeys, in rich profusion, the best of what Japan has to offer in the way of consumer goods. As a rule one floor was reserved for exhibitions, and as you went up and down the escalators you could hear from a dozen loudspeakers one of the latest international records. During a visit to Matzuja I heard a symphony by Shostakovitch, the exuberance of which re- sounded in every room, and on another occasion it was the First Symphony of Brahms, played by one of the leading American orchestras. One firm which sold printed music and instruments had its own multi-storeyed building with a music

Page 243 NARA

A school party goes through the first gate to the Kasuga shrine, about a mile away. The *torii*, which is usually built of tree-trunks and repainted in red from time to time, indicates the presence of a Shinto sanctuary; you find it both in towns and in lonely parts of the country; with its distinctive shape it has become a symbol of Japanese tradition.

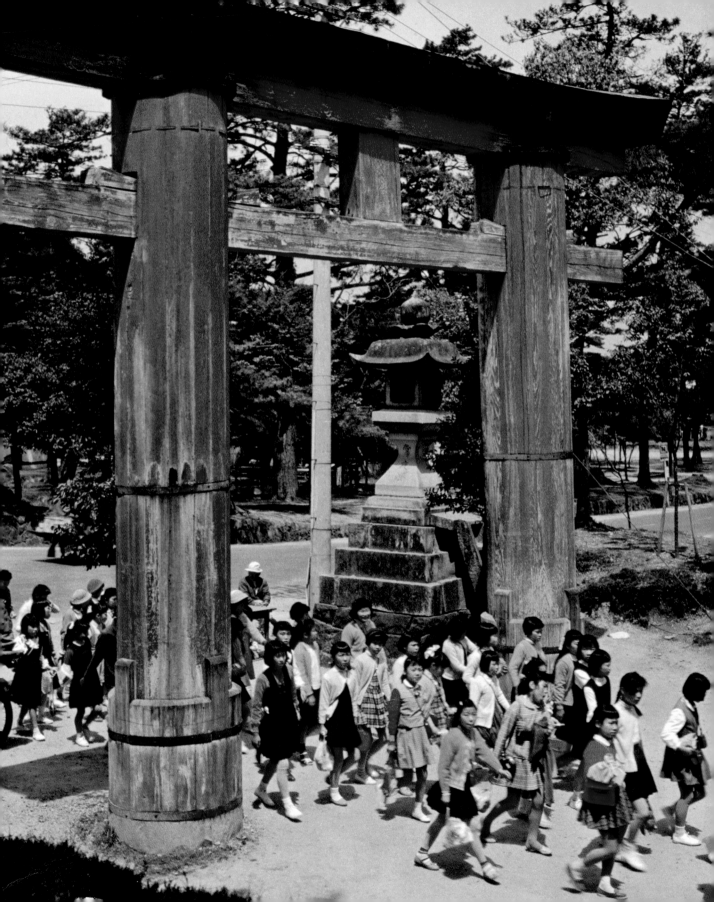

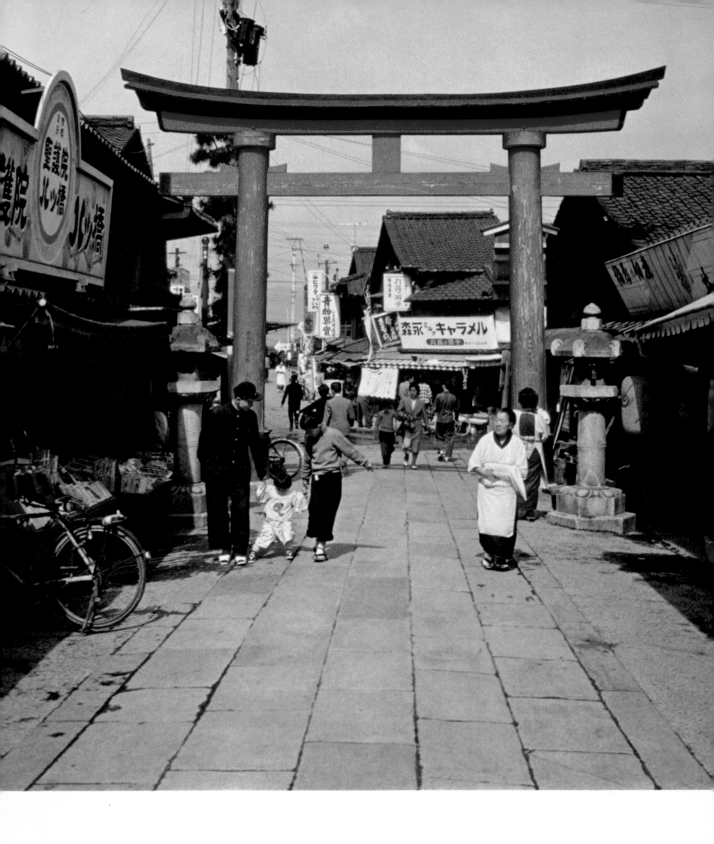

room conforming to the latest technical and aesthetic standards, with excellent pianos made by the firm itself, and with music and books including new publications in English, German, and French.

In the Ginza was the largest bookshop, which was like a department store in itself. The display on several floors was evidence of the activity of native publishing firms—their production far surpasses that of India for example and included everything from children's books to illustrated works and scientific manuals. There was a large English section, and smaller French and German sections, providing European and American—particularly scientific—publications. On the ground floor were sports goods, with golf-clubs much in evidence; and on the roof, besides a small restaurant, there were railed-off practice pitches where customers were eagerly trying out their clubs.

Golf was just then enjoying enormous popularity; the aspirations of the man in easy circumstances were embodied in the person of the week-end golfer, and even busy managers who normally sat in unapproachable state behind their office desks were to be found on the golf course if you wanted an informal talk.

Through a business matter I was able to meet a typical manager of a large *A Manager* Japanese enterprise in his office. From the friendly and accessible under-manager, who seemed prepared to give me an unlimited amount of his time, I rose to the busier and rather more reserved manager next in the hierarchy, and finally came to the ante-room of the all-powerful, where people spoke only in whispers from awe. The manager did not keep me waiting: his minutes were exactly apportioned.

Page 244 KYOTO

In the Inari suburb of the former capital of Japan a red *torii* shows that we are on the way to one of the most famous Shinto shrines in the country, Inari Taisha, distinguished by its many gates of this kind.

We sat down at a conference table and were served with a small cup of tea, but there was no superfluous conversation. He was a small man with a hard face of almost uncanny authority—he could have been one of those colonels we know from *The Bridge on the River Kwai*. He went directly at the matter in hand, and towards his goal: this was how the proposition looked to him, which was, needless to say, the way which was most advantageous to the firm; but as soon as he perceived that there was a wall where he had expected a door he was able to make a flexible readjustment.

Page 247 KAMAKURA

Among the important Shinto and Buddhist shrines in Kamakura, one of the former capitals of Japan, the Daibutsu or Great Buddha of the Kôtokuin Temple is known all over the world as one of the most sublime embodiments of contemplative Asian piety. The bronze figure, which is forty-two feet high including the base, and was originally enclosed, was cast in 1252 by Ono Gorôemon; it represents the Buddhist deity Amida with his hands in a gesture symbolising steadfast faith.

Pages 248–250 TOKYO: EVERYDAY LIFE IN JAPAN

248, 249 In front of the bridge which leads over the moat of the former Shogun castle to the Imperial Palace lies the square which is the first goal of every tourist party, especially the innumerable school parties, two of which are seen posing for the inevitable group photograph.

250 top left The Ginza, the main shopping street of Tokyo, contains the enormous building of Maruzen, possibly the largest bookshop in the world.

250 top right In the Ginza there are also department stores which are among the largest and smartest of their kind; here we look down on the ground floor of one of these with its decorations.

250 below left In a newsagent's and bookshop illustrated magazines are just as popular as scholarly works and books on modern art.

250 below right An old peasant visits the city (Kyoto).

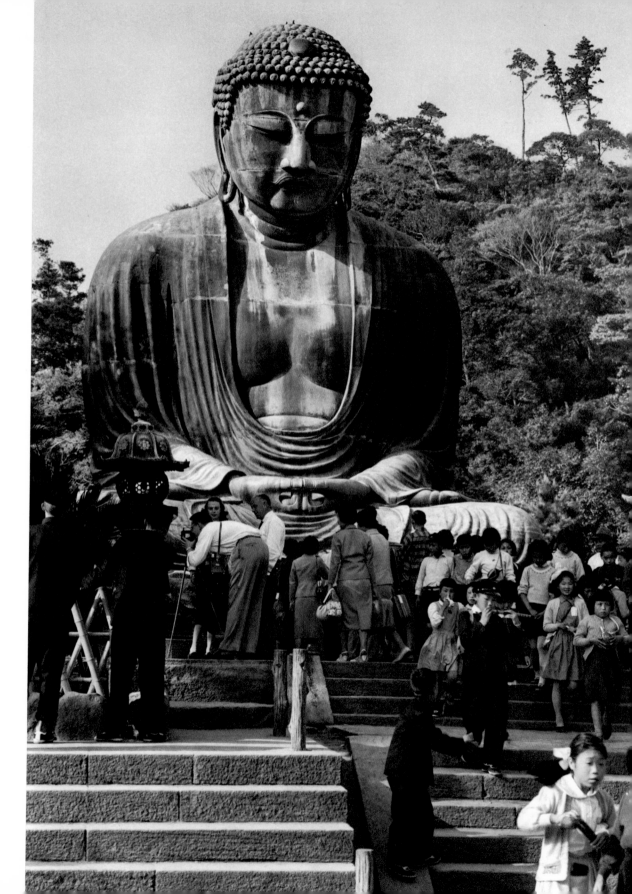

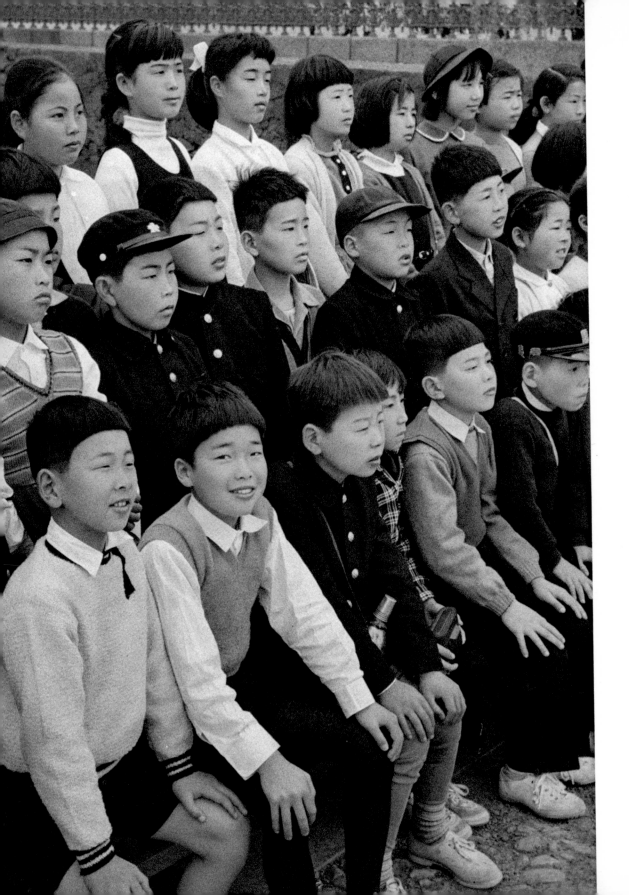

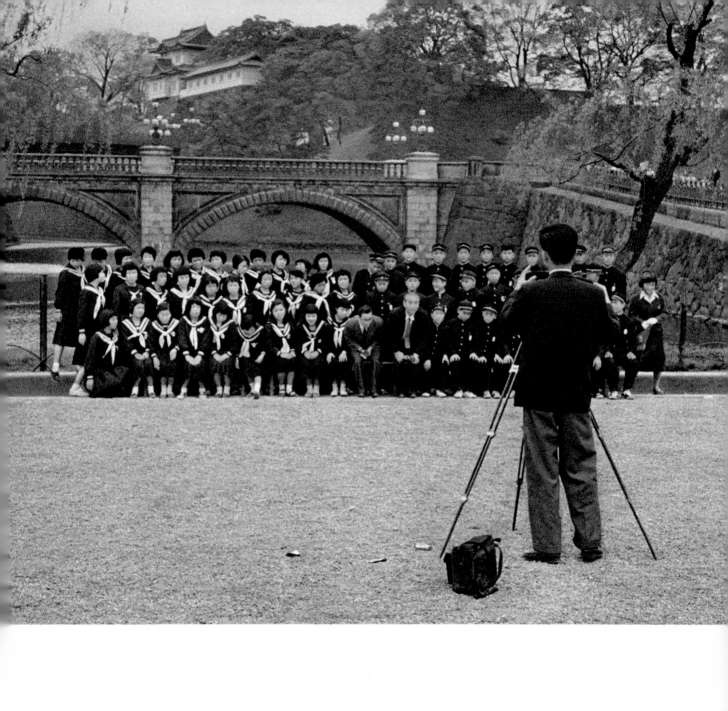

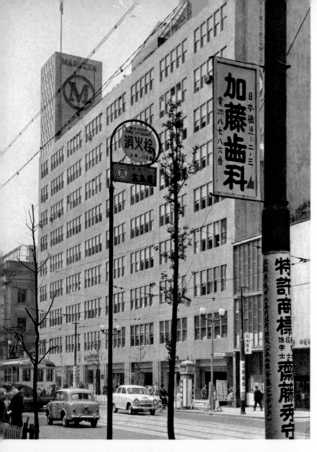

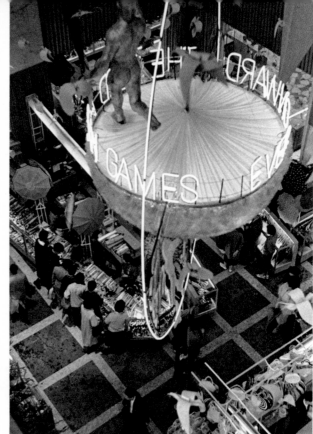

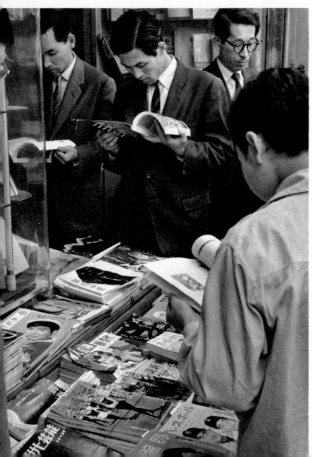

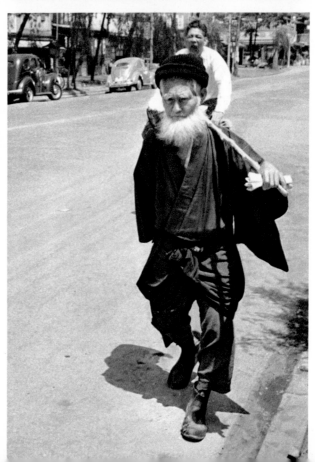

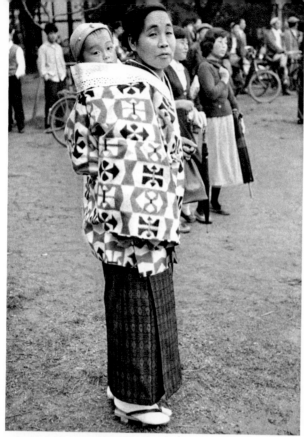
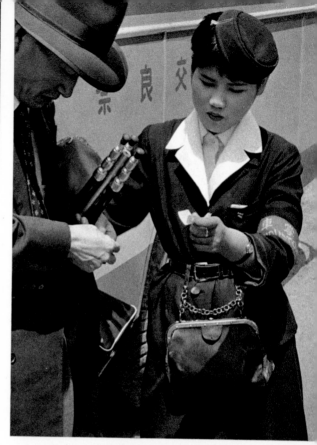
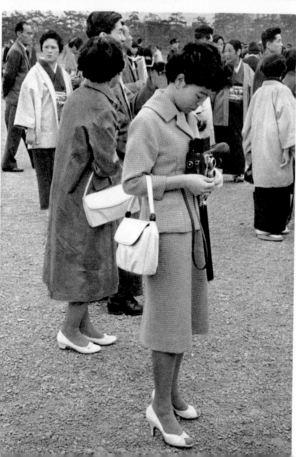
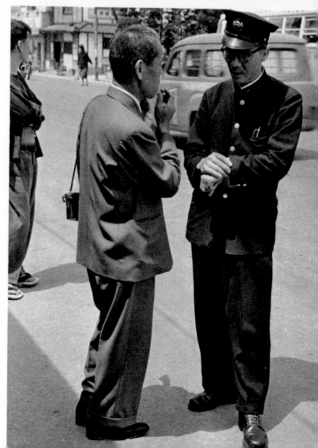

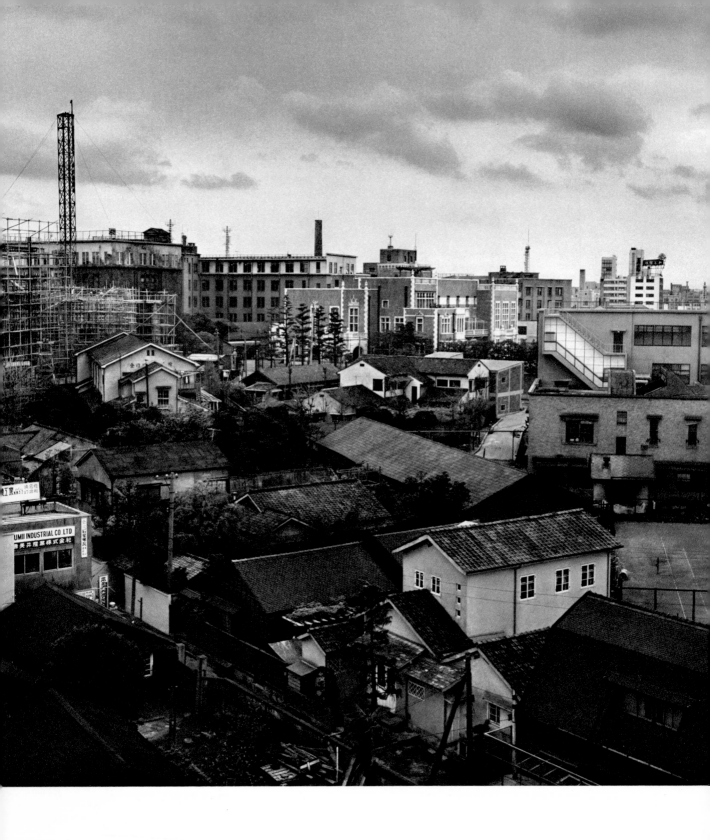

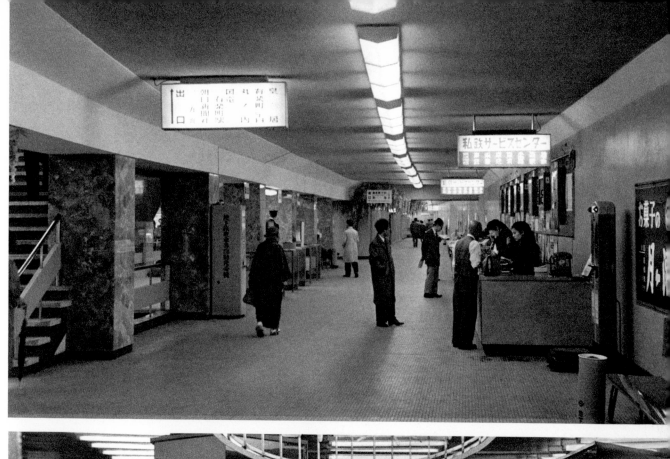

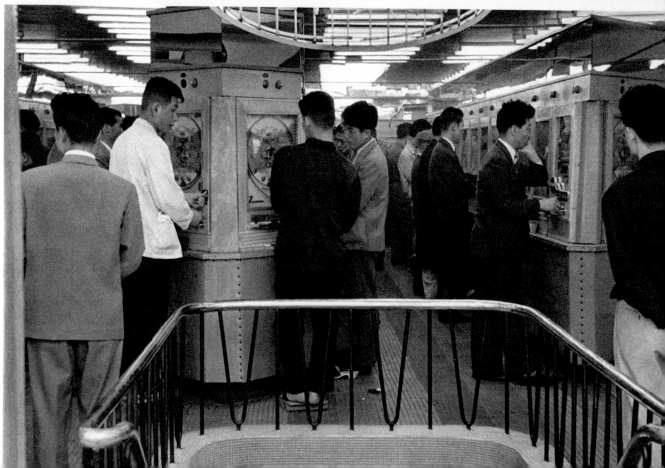

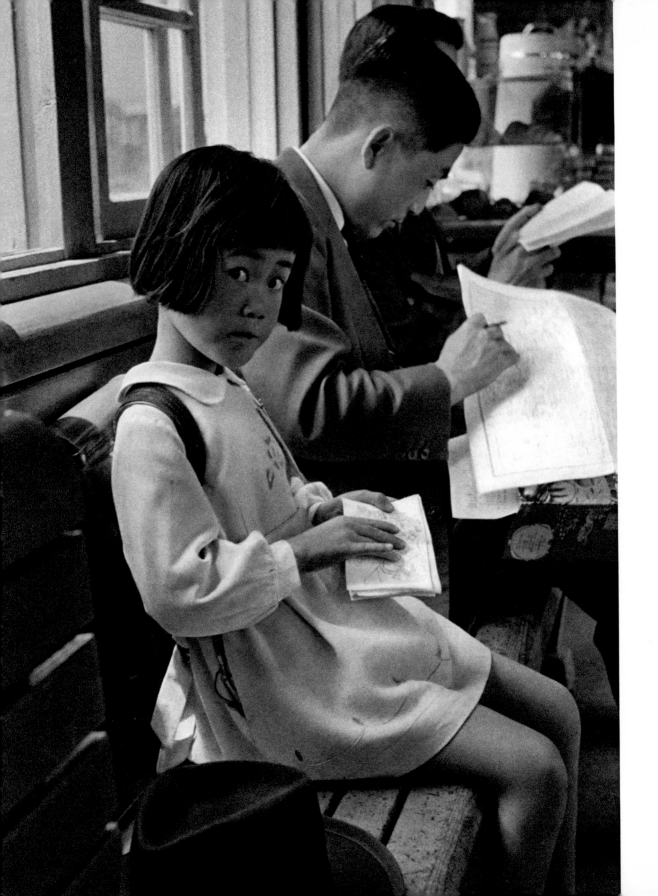

Thanks to the kind hospitality of a Japanese publishing colleague I was able to attend a garden-party given on the occasion of the annual Japanese publishers' meeting. The large garden in Japanese style, hired from a casino, had been laid out in the last century by a private individual and embellished with ancient monuments from other parts of Japan. The guests recorded their names in a register, greeted each other with a great deal of bowing, and it was soon easy to see which were the important people for whom black Cadillacs were waiting at the entrance: they strode past like princes receiving low bows, proffering gracious handshakes, and then leaving early while people of the humbler sort enjoyed themselves. In exchange for a voucher you got a snack, drinks—beer was poured

Pages 251–254   TOKYO: EVERYDAY LIFE IN JAPAN

251 top left   The larger the city the smaller the number of women who still wear the traditional kimono and wooden sandals in the street.

251 top right   Again and again you meet young girls in stewardesses' uniforms—bus-conductresses, guides on coaches, and lift-attendants—doing their job without fuss and with the utmost politeness.

251 below left   Not only professional photographers are busy in the square in front of the Imperial Palace: Japanese tourists are enthusiastic amateur photographers.

251 below right   The uniformed official is a familiar sight in the street, at stations, and on all occasions; politely but firmly he represents the principle of order, irrespective of changes in the régime.

252   The largest city in the world as seen from my hotel window: a confusion of temporary huts and quickly growing large buildings, stores, factories, and houses.

253 top   The underground railway station is smartly and efficiently designed.

253 below   Youths are the chief customers of the innumerable gaming-saloons, where the metal balls in the machines clatter all day long (Kyoto).

254   A schoolgirl waits for her bus (Nara).

out of carafes *à discretion*—and a paper hat. A very smart jazz band some twenty strong set the whole thing going.

We sat down at tables for four to six people. The publishing profession was represented there only by men; my charming female companion, Frau Mecklenburg, who owned a foreign language bookshop, was the only woman present who had anything to do with books. But, otherwise, there was certainly no lack of women: two girls were assigned to each table as companions, about half of them in Japanese, the others in European clothes, all very prettily made up and looking like film-stars. Here and there a publisher could be seen talking with animation to one of the pretty girls, but other colleagues were so engrossed in talking shop that they had scarcely a glance for the geishas who gracefully and discreetly filled up their glasses.

The Japanese Stewardess In Japan today you frequently meet young girls in the uniform of stewardesses. They conduct coach passengers to see the sights, act as bus-conductresses, work the lifts in multi-storeyed buildings, untiring in their respectfully polite directions and information, and they are employed in large numbers in department stores. There are also industrial firms which employ girls between the ages of sixteen and twenty; but the time of shameless exploitation of cheap labour is over: the self-respecting employer now sees to the welfare of his young employees; they are given some instruction in housekeeping, and are thus prepared for later married life.

Music in Tokyo I spent one evening with the cultural attaché of the German Embassy. From time to time he gave a musical soirée there, at which German and Japanese music-lovers had an opportunity to meet. On this occasion a Japanese lady singer was interpreting songs by Brahms, Hugo Wolf, and Richard Strauss; she had a perfect command of the German words, the pronunciation had been carefully rehearsed and there was not a false note; indeed it might perhaps have been less becoming to her if she had succeeded in interpreting the voluptuous sentimental music of the late Romantics any better. After the short concert I found myself in conversation with the singer's brother: he was employed in the Foreign Office but was also the music critic of one of the leading newspapers. He spoke fluent German, and you could not catch him out—he knew what had been performed at the latest music festival in Donaueschingen, what was significant in the most recent ventures of Boulez and Stockhausen, what *première* Salzburg was getting ready for. Tokyo had for long had symphony orchestras and academies of music; European musicians like the conductor Pringsheim and the violinist Pollak had already done pioneer work there decades ago. Today there is also jazz and twelve-tone music, just as there are abstract, representational, and tachist painters, and young existentialists with long unkempt hair and narrow trousers; nothing was missing in Tokyo. The Japanese seem to be more receptive to serial music than are Europeans, as they are not inhibited as we are by the powerful European tradition of tonal music.

After a rainy week—on a journey to the famous lakes of Hakone I had caught no glimpse of Mount Fuji—the weather seemed to be improving and, in the company of Mr Katsuo Fujimaki, an official guide whose knowledge of English was far exceeded by his politeness, I boarded the *Swallow* at the central station in Tokyo to visit the oldest Shinto sanctuary, the shrines of Ise. The *Swallow* was the express train to Osaka. The Japanese are rightly proud of their railways; they enjoy travelling, and travel so much by this means of transport that as well as the excellently constructed and organised network of state railways a number of private railways flourish, sometimes even serving the same places. The roads by contrast are very inadequate. In the *Swallow* the standards of cleanliness and courtesy were if possible even higher than in other trains, and you watched the delightful, ever-changing panorama from comfortable seats, through large

Journey in the 'Swallow'

257

windows. In the dining-car there was a good international menu, and flower-vases on each table contained not a few haphazardly arranged stalks, but in each case fresh flowers, carefully selected. Even the W.C. was decorated with flowers.

We travelled through a green country with mountains, rice fields, villages, and towns. Over the lightly constructed wooden bungalows bright carp-flags were fluttering in the wind, for in a few days there would be a boys' festival and a flag was hung out for every boy in the house. Almost every house had a small garden with shrubs and miniature trees; the cherry blossom was almost over but red and violet azaleas were blooming everywhere. The sea was to the left; on the right over the fields, in the delta of the Fuji river, the faint silhouette of the famous Fujiyama emerged from the clouds; even the Japanese looked up from their newspapers when the holy mountain appeared.

Pages 259–262 SHINTO

259 A steep flight of steps leads to the Tsurugaoka Hachimangu shrine, in the forest of Karnakura, in honour of the legendary Emperor Ojin (270–310), which was first erected on this spot in 1191 and last rebuilt in 1828.

260 The Naiku or Inner Shrine forms the central point of the Jingu shrines of Ise, the oldest Shinto sanctuary. Here the sacred mirror Yata-no-Kagami is preserved, the most precious object among the imperial crown jewels, which is traced back to the goddess Amaterasu, the ancestress of the Japanese nation. The shrines were last rebuilt in 1953; the position of the courtyard in the foreground alternates with the renewal which takes place every twenty years.

260 below On a day of festival (the Emperor's birthday) the Daiguji (high priest) of the Jingu shrines of Ise leads the procession of the priesthood along the avenue of cedars under one of the *torii* to the Inner Shrine.

261 The high priest leaves one of the smaller shrines of the sanctuary in the grove.

262 In the reception-building of the Inner Shrine of Ise a priest issues a document for visitors.

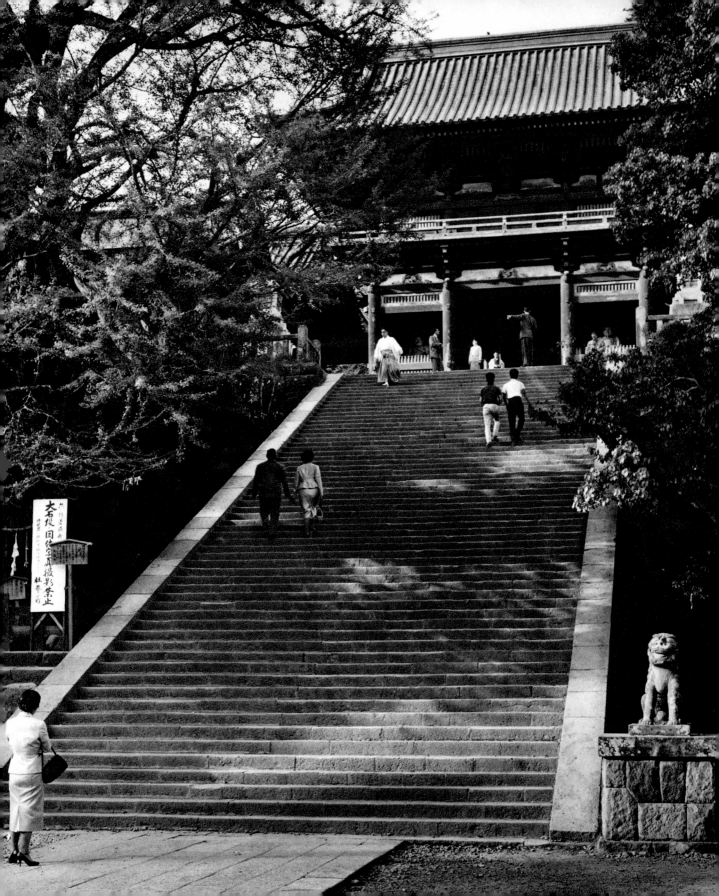

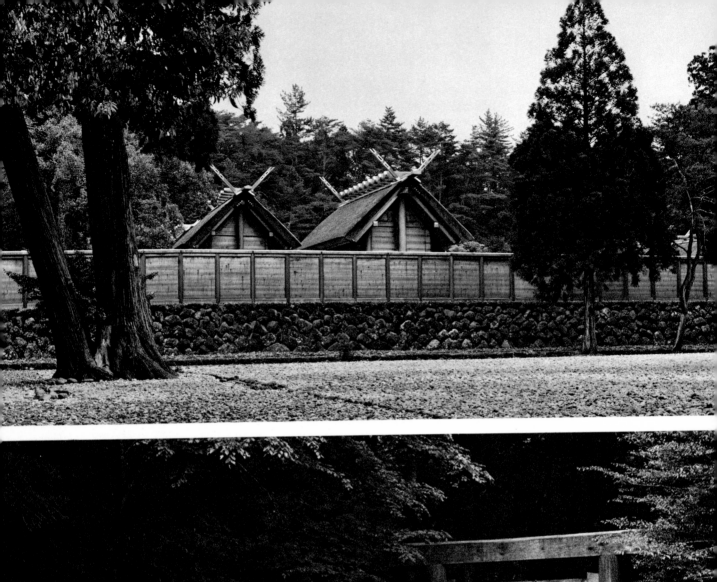
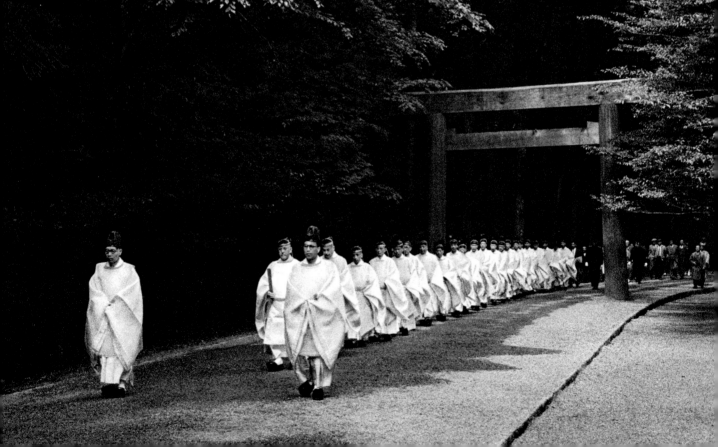

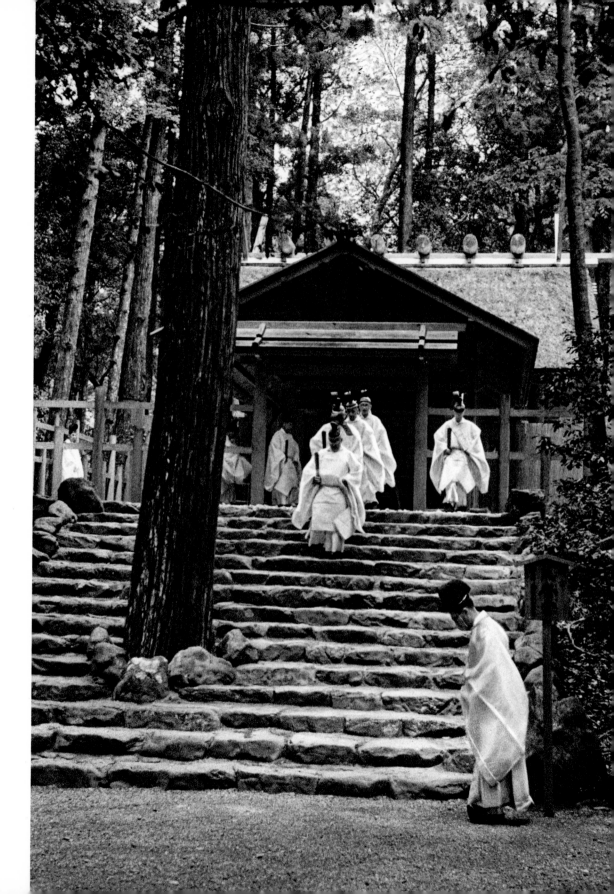

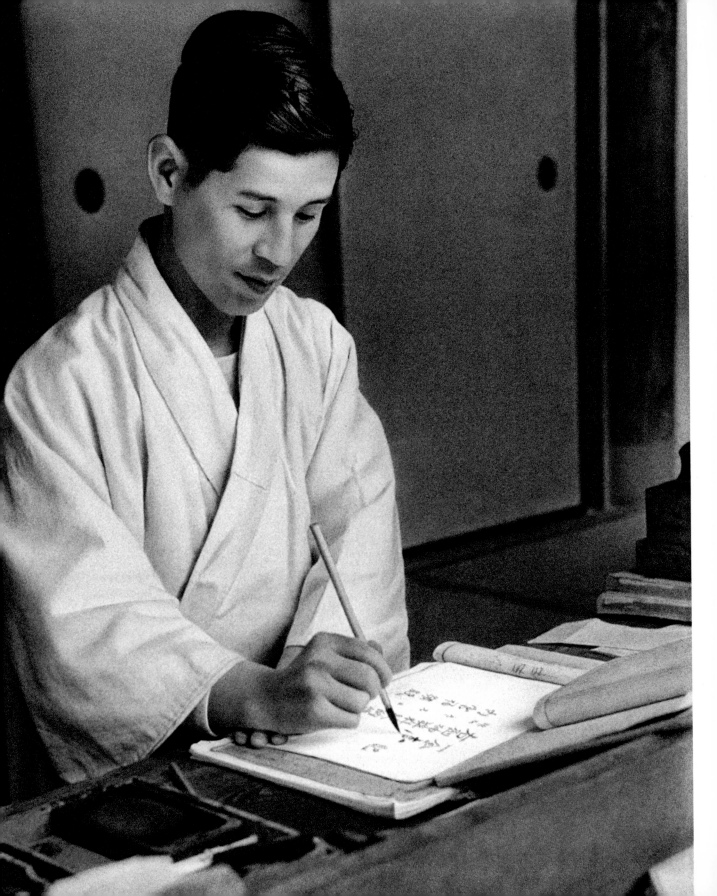

In Nagoya—a city of a million inhabitants with new multi-storeyed buildings near the station—we changed trains and got into the express *Naniwa, No. 1* of the Kintetsu Railways, which set us down one and a half hours later in Uji Yamada on the Kii peninsula. We went on by taxi to Futami-ga-ura, a well-known holiday resort by the sea. On the picturesque coast are the famous 'Husband and Wife Rocks' (Myôto-iwa), washed round at high tide. They are connected by a rope which is ceremonially renewed every year on 5th January, and symbolise the two legendary founders of Japan—Izanagi and Izanami. We got out at a Japanese-style hotel—the only kind in this town—and quite a grand one it turned out to be, for seven years ago the Emperor himself had stayed at the Asahikan Hotel. I was able to see the rooms he and the Empress occupied, in which, naturally, no other mortal has been allowed to spend the night since. At the hotel entrance shoes were exchanged for slippers, and even these had to be taken off before you entered your room. I had a bath before supper, as was the custom there: first you washed thoroughly with soap and then, when you were clean, you got into the clear hot water in the hip-bath. Afterwards you felt like a king, especially in the comfortable Japanese clothes provided—a light kimono which, like the linen, was freshly laundered for each guest and which you wore as a night-shirt, with a grey kimono over it as a dressing-gown. Similar comfortable clothes were worn by the young men whom one could see walking through the streets in clattering wooden clogs on their way to their geisha party.

Bedroom and living-room were separated from a small ante-room and veranda *In the Japanese Hotel* by sliding partitions; there was a recess with a Japanese wall-picture *(kakemono)* and a vase of flowers; a bamboo mat covered the floor; the construction of the walls and roof was visible in smooth, unvarnished wood and bamboo posts. White paper was stretched over the trellis of the sliding partitions, letting through a gentle light. In the centre stood a low varnished table. Two cushions were provided to sit on with a small stand to lean against—this was probably a concession to Western visitors who were not accustomed to sitting for hours on the floor.

I had supper here with Mr Fujimaki. We were served throughout by the same girl who scurried in and out noiselessly, brought many kinds of small dishes and bowls, poured out warm *saké* (rice wine) and saw to it that we always had enough rice. She generally sat with us at table and took part in the conversation —in Japanese, of course; my guide was very enthusiastic about her way of speak, ing, in a provincial accent which is famed for its softness. Mr Fujimaki seemed to be telling her surprising things about me, for she said with astonishment again and again 'Sôdesga!' which means 'You don't say!' The meal consisted almost entirely of sea food: two kinds of fish, cooked and raw—you dipped the small pieces of raw fish in soya sauce which always appears at any Japanese or Chinese meal; a lacquered bowl of soup which looked like an acquarium, with soft things swimming in it like algae or jellyfish; then a shell filled with other varieties of fish, and with it, naturally, the bread of the East, rice. Finally, on top of all this, baked lobster was served. After the *saké* we drank beer—beer has long been a

Pages 265–268 SHINTO

265 In the Inari shrine of Kyoto young girls, who serve for a few years in the sanctuary, were performing their ceremonial dance to the music of a temple orchestra.

266 In the Asahikan Hotel in Futami ga ura, where the Emperor himself spent the night when he last visited the shrines, rooms with every amenity in the Japanese style, including charming servants, are provided for guests.

267 On the shore at Futami ga ura stand the 'Husband and Wife Rocks', Myôto iwa; on the larger rock there is a *torii*. They represent Izanagi and Izanami, the mythical founders of Japan. At the beginning of each year the straw ropes connecting them are renewed.

268 Few of the women among the pious visitors who climb the steps through a series of *torii* to the Inari shrine in Kyoto are still dressed in Japanese clothes.

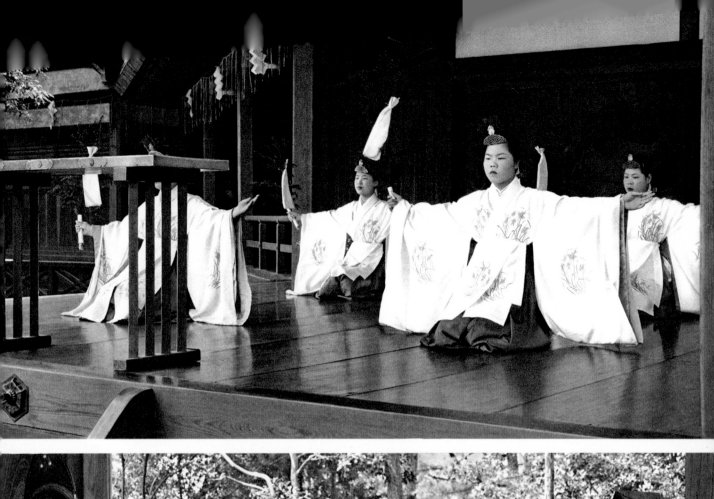
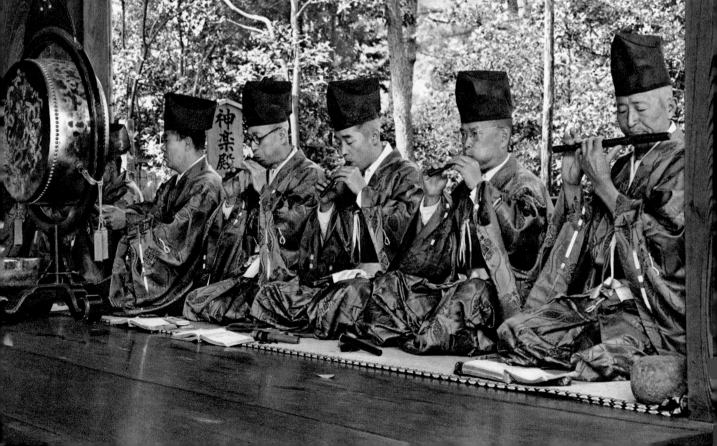

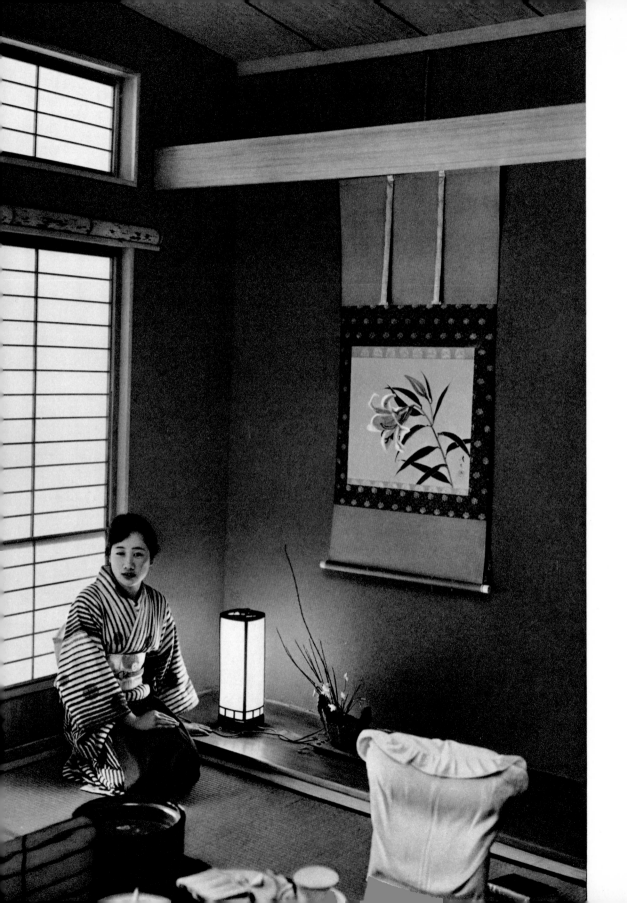

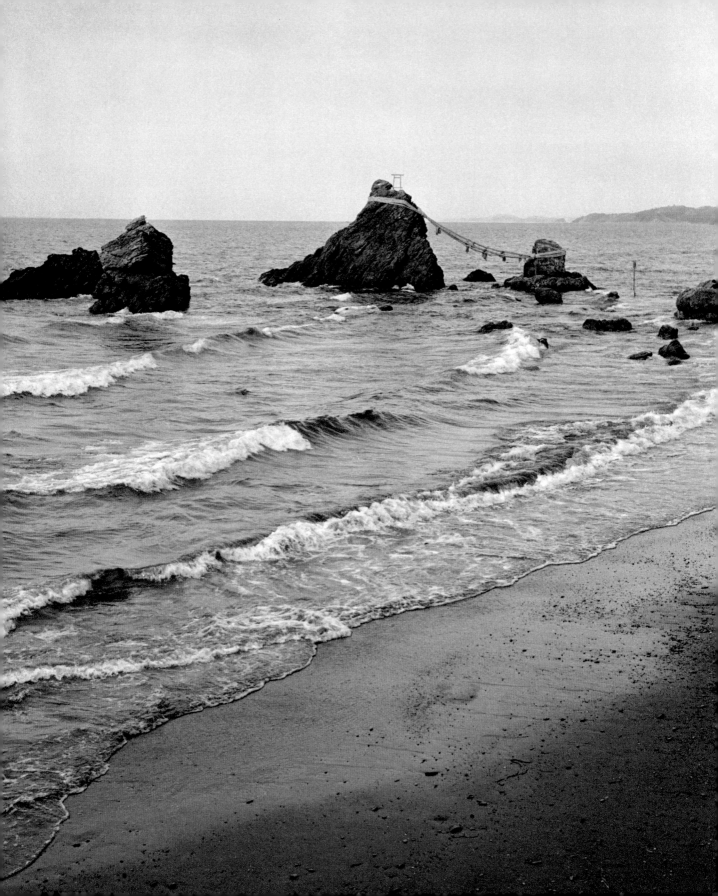

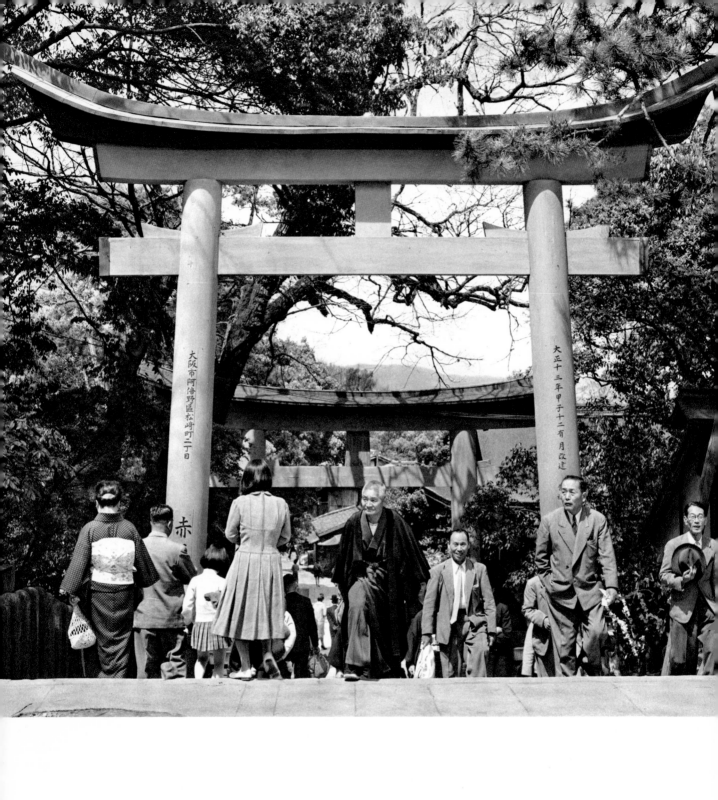

Japanese drink too; you find it everywhere in the Far East, even in places where no European has been.

When my companion had withdrawn to his own room for the night, the quaint little maid moved the table to one side, spread the bed-clothes on the floor, and finally took her leave with a last bow before closing the sliding doors behind her.

Until a few years ago no one thought of locking hotel rooms; even private houses stood more or less open; the light construction of wooden and paper partitions had for centuries reckoned without burglars. But the destitution after the last war had caused a crime-wave, so that suspicion and caution were replacing the former unconcern.

The Jingu shrines of Ise (the Shinto sanctuaries are called 'shrines' in Japan in contrast to the Buddhist 'temples') are the oldest and most venerable of the thousands of Shinto shrines which are scattered all over Japan; the crown jewels are kept there with religious rites said to be 2,000 years old. As my visit coincided with the birthday of the Emperor (29th April) I was able to see the ritual in all its dignity.

Ise—A National Shrine

After passing through the two large red outer *torii* of the Naiku or Inner Shrine the visitor went first to the bank of the Isuzu river and washed his face and hands in the crystal-clear water; then he entered the grove of majestic cypresses, several hundred years old, in whose shadow appeared the sacred buildings with their gilded roofs. The shrines were built from the wood of these trees and, apart from the topmost gilded beams on the thick thatched roofs, were without any facing or paint. Every twenty years they are rebuilt from top to bottom in exactly the same proportions and in the style which dates from before the Chinese influence. A platform covered with red gravel near the shrine marked the spot where, until 1953, the previous building had stood, and also where, in 1973, the next one will be built. Here in Japan, tradition is dependent on the loyalty of the people. No archaeological treasures can be excavated—if one generation fails, everything is lost.

The last great political crisis, when the American Proconsul hesitated about whether to permit the continuance of the Imperial House, had greatly imperilled the traditions of Ise. The Occupation government demanded that all financial contribution to the shrines of Ise by the State should cease, so that the renovation of the sanctuary due in 1949—the fifty-ninth—had to be postponed for an indefinite period. Only a nation-wide movement could ensure the preservation of this venerable symbol of continual national rebirth. An appeal by the Shinto priests was not in vain: millions responded, among them the majority of the Buddhists and also many Christians; 700 million yen were collected, and in October 1953, in the presence of a huge crowd and with all the fanfare of modern publicity, the sacred mirror, symbol of the goddess Amaterasu, was ceremonially transferred to its new home. More than two million Japanese visited the shrine in the following year.

A man in dark uniform and white gloves—he is always present at any ceremonial occasion in Japan—walked in front of the procession of white-robed priests, who were now approaching along the cypress avenue with the high priest at their head. Before reaching the main shrine the procession stopped at some of the smaller shrines. Chests made of polished wood—also renewed every twenty years—were brought out; they were opened one by one and closed again after a priest had waved a green twig over them like an aspergillum. The deep silence in the grove in which the ceremonies took place was broken now and then by thin high notes drawn from an ancient wind-instrument or by a clapping of hands, with which the attention of the goddess is entreated. It is a ceremonial ballet which takes place without words, every movement laid down by tradition. Finally the priests disappeared behind the palisade of the main shrine out of sight of the uninitiated.

How do the priests regard this cult? Do they still believe in the Sun Godhead of Amaterasu-Omikami, and that the wonderful mirror Yata-no-Kagami was really given by Amaterasu to her grandson Ninigi when she sent him down to earth to rule in her name and found the dynasty which still flourishes today? Belief in the divine origin of the Imperial House has been officially relinquished without any apparent excitement, and it is said, too, that the Shinto cult has lost its significance as the religion of the State. But my visit to Ise and to many other Shinto shrines in 1958 showed me that almost as many people as ever bow reverently in the silence of the woods and, by clapping their hands, appeal to the divinity to give peace to their souls. The luxuriance of mythology with its nature deities does not impair the sense of truth of poets and gardeners. The fresh red paint of the *torii* shines through the trees and the subdued solemnity of the religious rites has lost none of its dignity. The form lives on as an expression of veneration of everything that is inexplicable and as a sacred symbol of the nation.

Mr Fujimaki took me also to the Mikimoto Pearl Island, where in 1893 Mr Kokichi Mikimoto—immortalized wearing a bowler-hat and cape by a bronze statue—discovered how to make cultured pearls, thereby creating a flourishing Japanese export industry. A sightseeing tour of the pearl fishery was laid on. Magnificent pieces of jewellery were for sale, or for a small sum you could buy oysters which contained pearls of fine quality formed round the injected granule.

The Pearl Island

I can single out only a few of the many other sights of this visit to Japan. It is an ideal country for tourists: the long coastal stretches of the islands with their many deep bays and lakes surround a landscape of the greatest variety: the terraced slopes of the hills are covered with rice fields and woods. And there are the shrines and temples, built from the trunks of huge trees, far away in the solitude of the mountains—though you also find quiet, sacred groves with their places of devotion in the famous old towns.

My time was spent mainly in the triangle formed by the towns of Nara, Osaka, and Kyoto, which contains, except for the large urban district at the eastern foot of Mount Fuji with Tokyo, Yokohama, and Kamakura, by far the greatest concentration of Japanese cultural and economic life.

Nara   In Ise you find the national traditions of Japan which reach back unbroken from the present day to the old nature myths; by contrast, Nara with its temples is the expression of Japan's creative encounter with the greatest cultural forces of the Asian continent: the religious message of India and the established system of China.

The Western-style hotel was already a tradition here with a pre-First World War comfort: a large entrance and easy-chairs, a panelled writing-room and a garden which made you think of a European park in the Japanese style. The woods extended far into the city and between the cedars, deer grazed unconcerned among the guests.

School-children in uniform were prominent among the crowds of pilgrims to the famous temples: they seemed to be on the move all over Japan in their buses, visiting national cultural centres. Even the girls were almost all uniformly dressed in unbecoming dark-coloured sailor-suits, and you wondered how many of these plain and somewhat clumsy girls would grow up to be charming stewardesses.

Pages 273–275 JAPANESE GARDENS

273 A small farm at the foot of the Fujiyama with a well-cared-for kitchen garden.

274 In the imperial Katsura garden in Kyoto: an outing to the tea-house Shôkin-tei.

275 Two famous examples of a Zen temple garden in Kyoto attributed to the landscape gardener Sôami (died 1525): the rock garden of the Ryoanji Temple, where fine gravel represents the movement of waves on the ocean and the larger stones suggest solitary islands; and a corner of the similarly fashioned garden of the Daitokuji Temple.

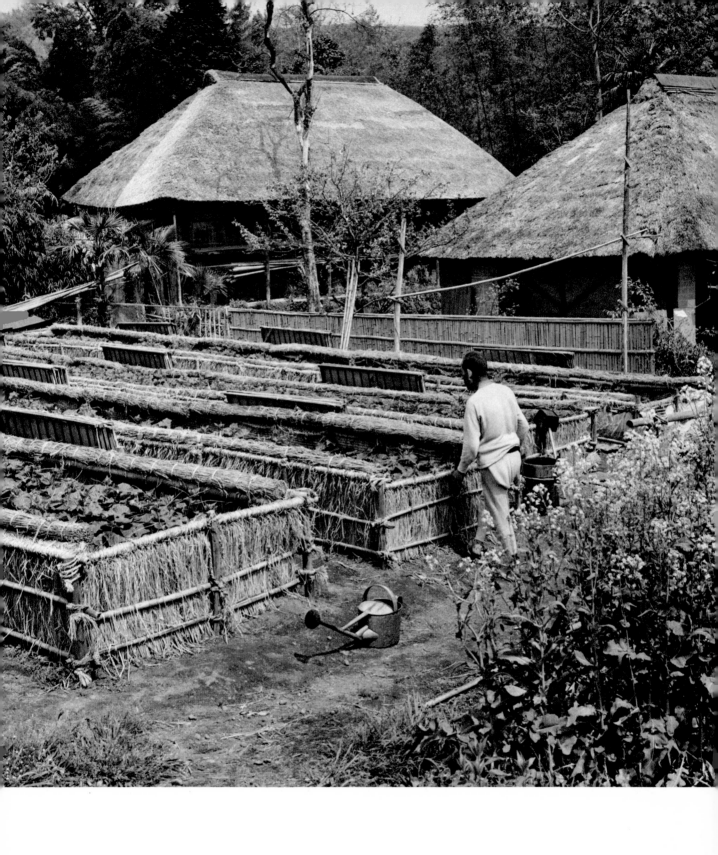

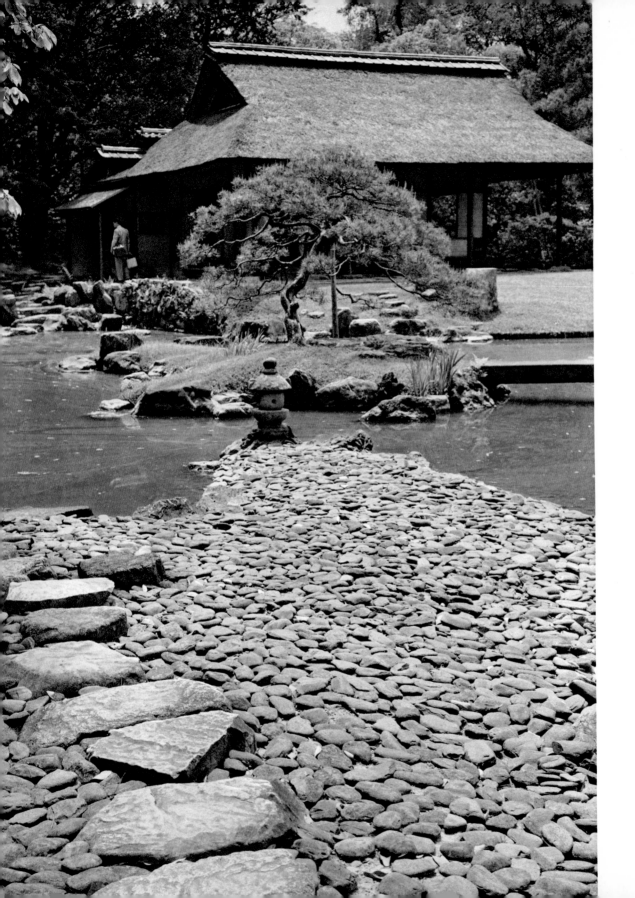

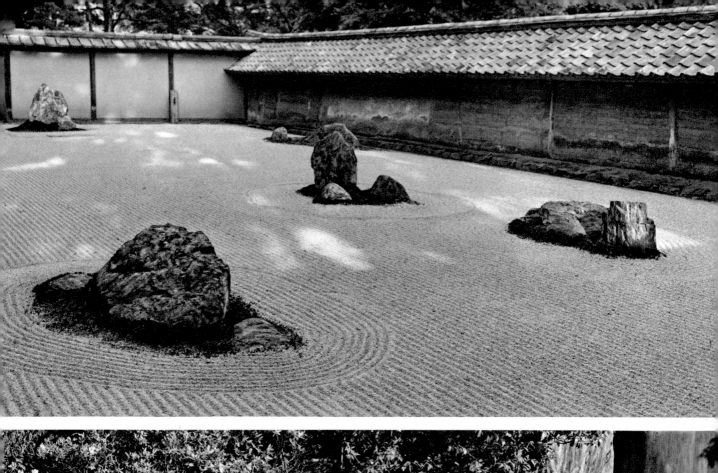
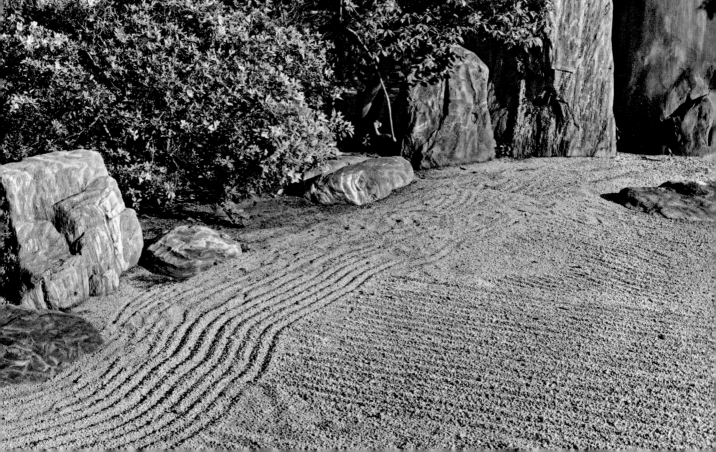

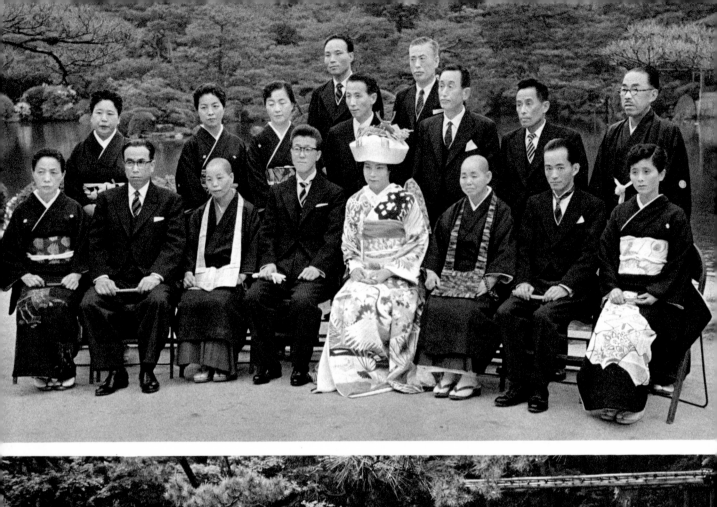

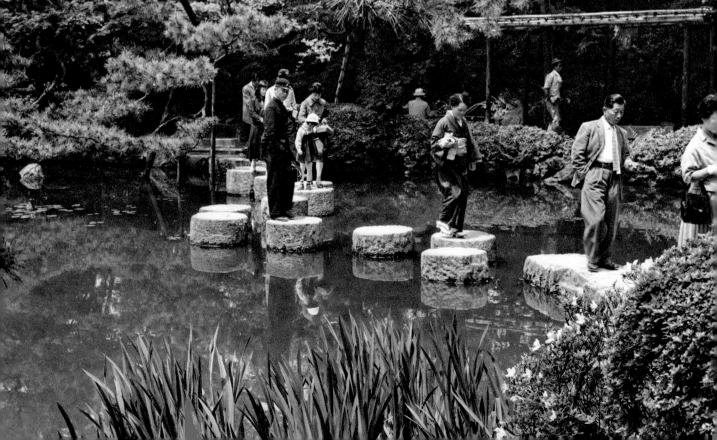

The pious wonder of the visitors to the temples and shrines—about a third of them carried cameras—might be an expression of religious emotion; but it might equally well express curiosity, or devotion to culture, or national pride. Tolerance unites the sects and forms of religion, which it must be remembered were not Churches dedicated to a particular creed in the sense of Christian dogmatism, and even included those Japanese who responded deeply to the Christian teaching of the New Testament, but who did not wish to belong to a particular Christian Church. Like the famous Daibutsu in Kamakura, the five hundred years older and even more austere 'great Buddha' in the Tôdaiji Temple of the Kegon sect is a powerful symbol of all that is still vigorously opposed to insipid materialism in the soul of Asia today. In Japan the approaches to the mysteries beyond the physical world are more ordered and more attended to than on the Asian continent. Zen-Buddhism does not make incomprehensibly mystical demands on the Western intellect; the Japanese moves about among the numerous figures of the Mahayana with a highly developed discipline and with an unerring feeling for style, as if among the gods of the Shinto cult; he experiences them as a loosely woven allegory of life, a fairyland of the soul, where poets and painters feel just as much at home as children and thinkers.

Page 276 KYOTO

276 top A wedding-party using the tea-house of the public park near the Heian shrine have taken their seats in the garden for the indispensable group photograph: the bride in ceremonial wedding-dress, the bridegroom and the other men in cut-away coats; at either side of the bride and bridegroom are aunts who belong to a monastic Order and thus have shorn heads; the rest of the women are wearing dark kimonos.

276 below In the garden of the Heian shrine, the national park in Kyoto, laid out in 1895, the pedestals from the pillars of a bridge have been used as stepping-stones over one of the idyllic pools.

In less than an hour the Nara train brought us to Osaka, a town of two million inhabitants. With its thousands of large and small factories it forms the largest industrial centre of the East. Its harbour controls 30 per cent of Japanese exports and 20 per cent of imports. Of the war damage there is now little to be seen. I stayed at the Hotel New Osaka—it had two hundred rooms with bathrooms— built in accordance with the latest international standards, with the greatest economy of space and the greatest possible comfort.

From my room on the sixth floor I looked on to the skyscraper of one of the large newspaper enterprises; one block farther away was the Osaka Grand Hotel, only just completed for the 1958 Fair. It has a panelled concert hall which can comfortably seat about two thousand people, and is one of the most elegant in the world, an example of the sure taste of the Japanese in new things as well as old; the delicate flower decorations on the wooden trellises on each side of the huge stage lent local colour to the scene.

Osaka Festival   I heard a concert given by the Leningrad Philharmonic—this is one of the many engagements by which the Osaka Spring Fair makes its claim on the festival

Pages 279–282 TOWN AND COUNTRY IN JAPAN

279   Tilling the rice fields in the Kii peninsula.

280   Posters carried at the workers' May Festival in Nara show atom bombs, a startled Mount Fuji, and demands that the Americans go home.

281   This business street in Osaka, town of two million people, has still preserved something of the gaiety of the former bazaar streets.

282   In the fishing harbour of Misaki on the Miura peninsula one of the large fishing boats puts to sea on a voyage that may last many months; a motor-boat decorated with flags leaves the harbour; and the last coloured paper streamers linking the fishermen with their relatives are broken.

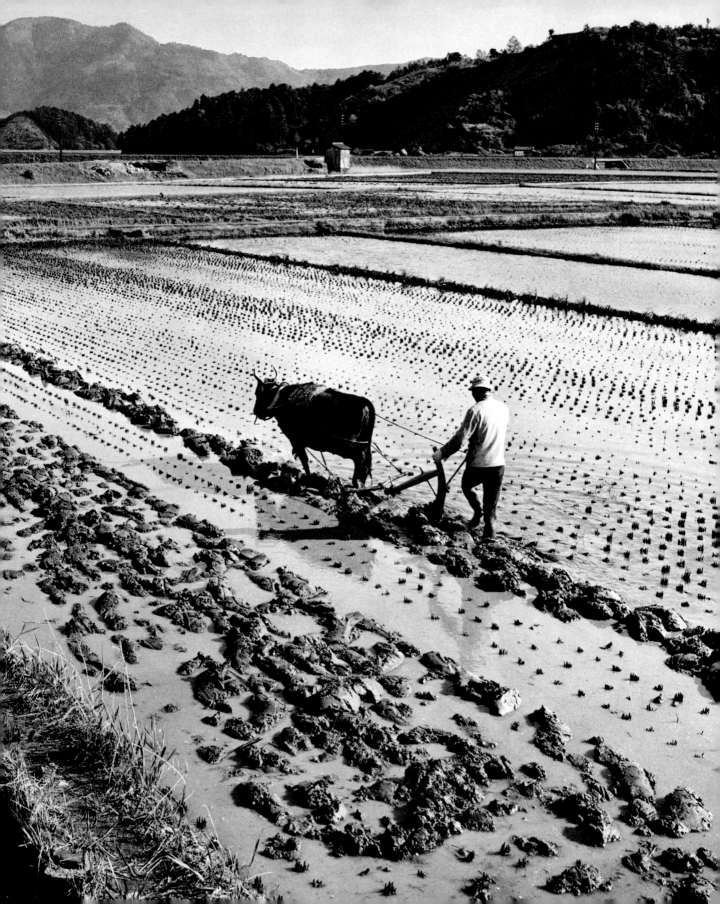

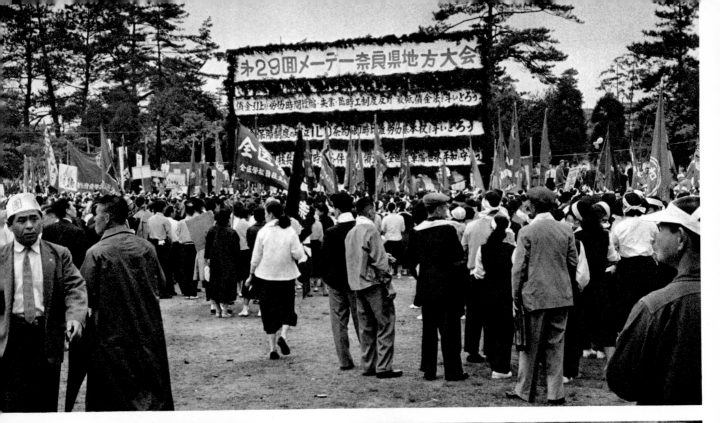

第29回メーデー奈良県地方大会

賃金引上り労働時間短縮・失業・臨時工制度反対・最低賃金法を斗いとろう

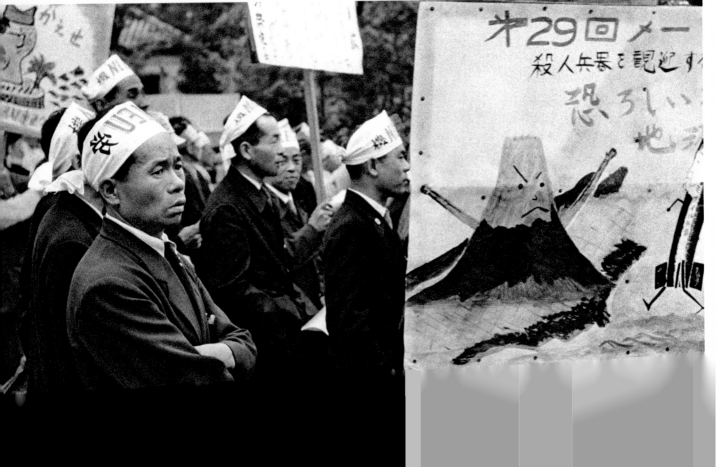

第29回メー

殺人兵器を観迎す

恐ろしい

地方

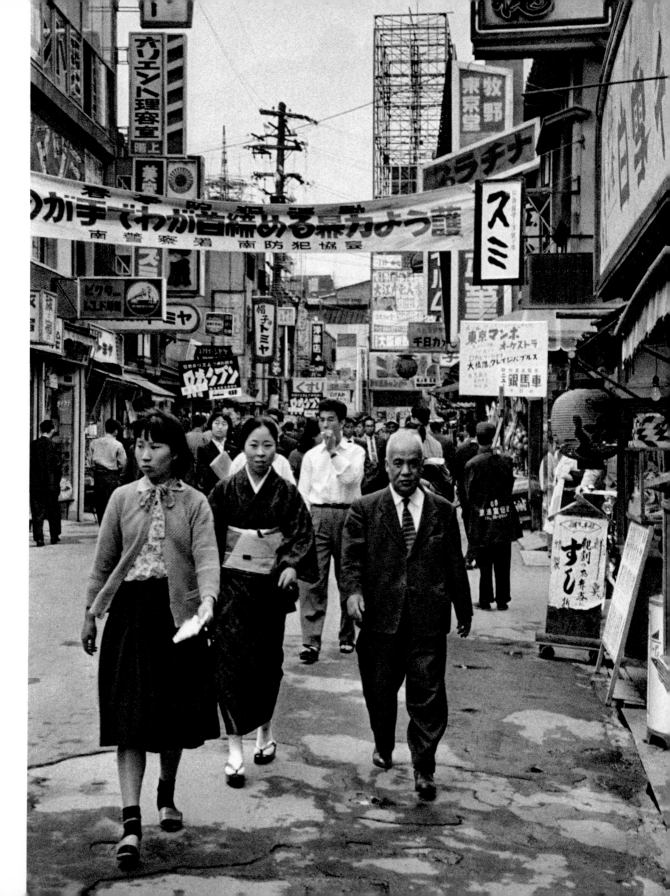

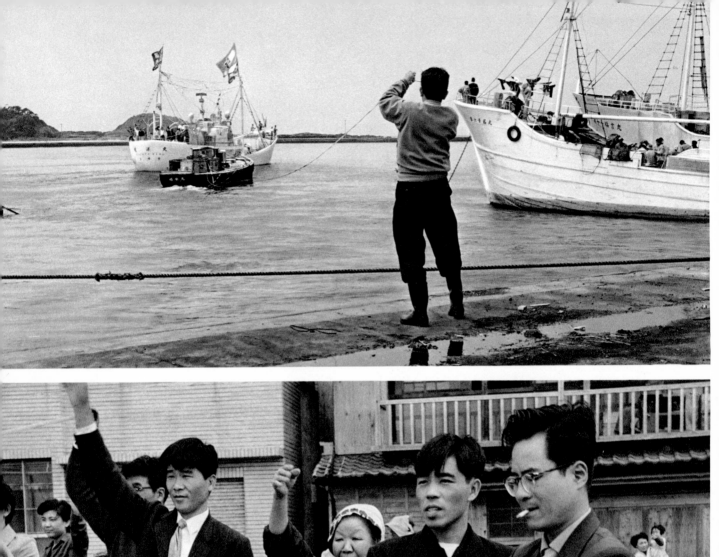
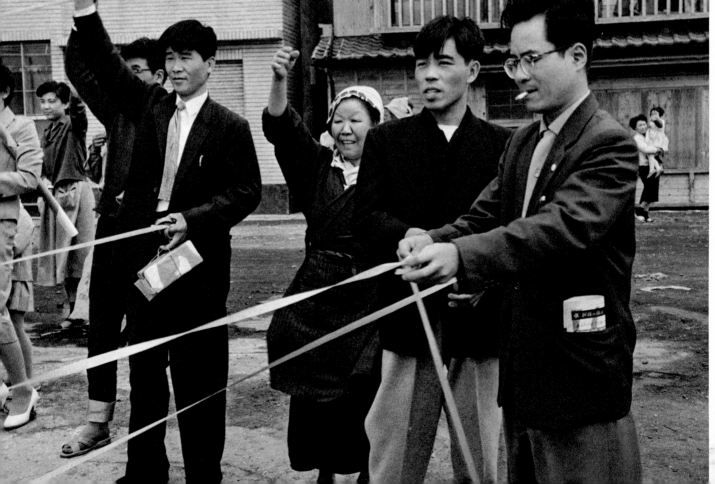

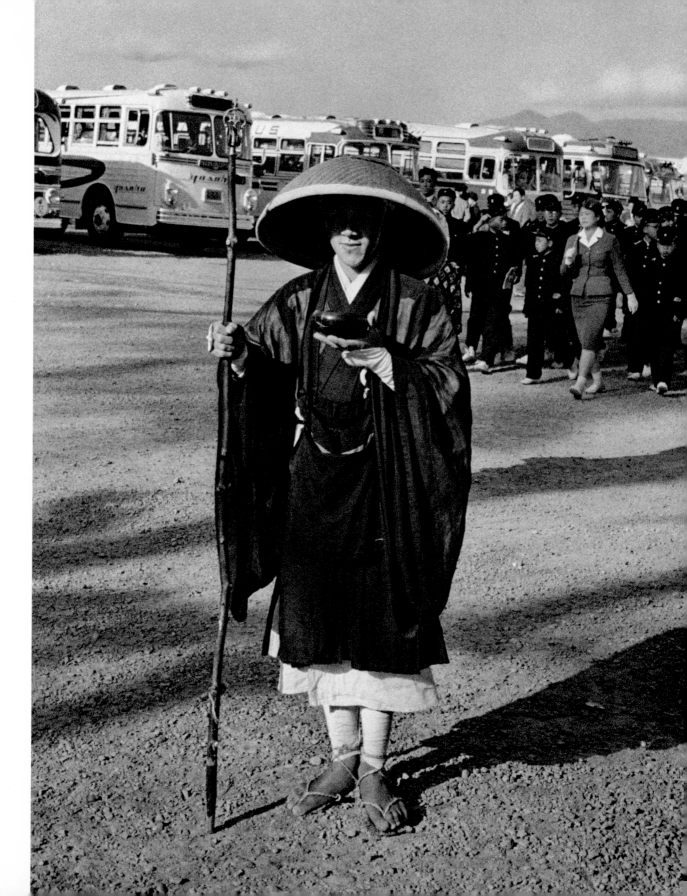

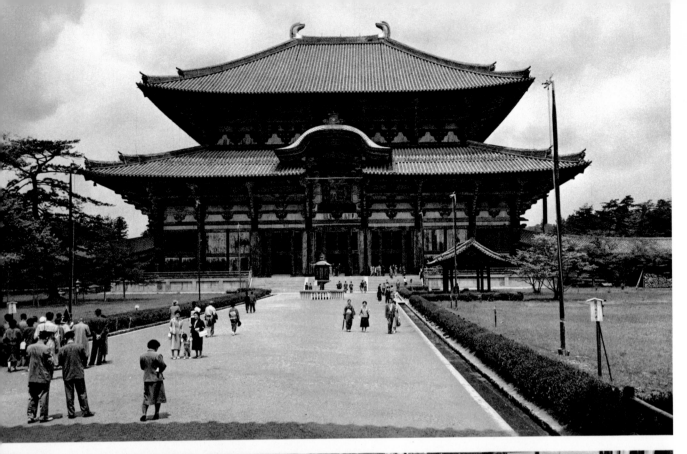

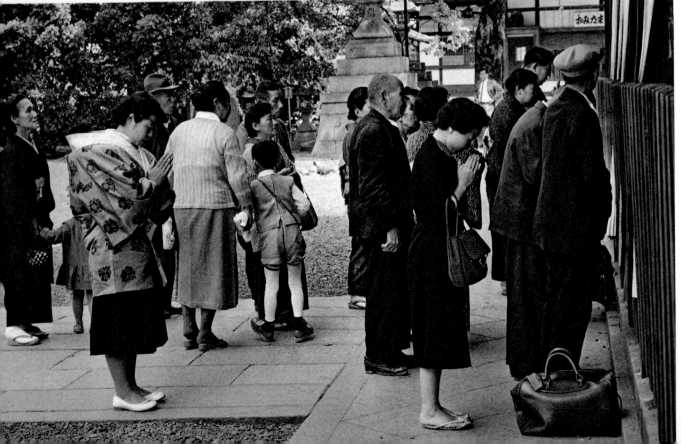

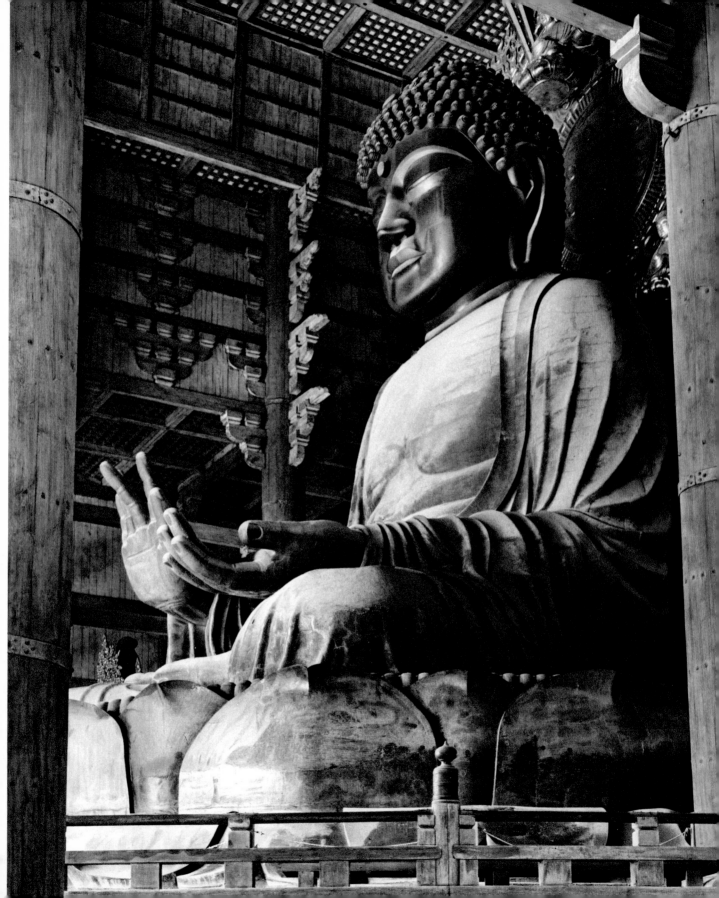

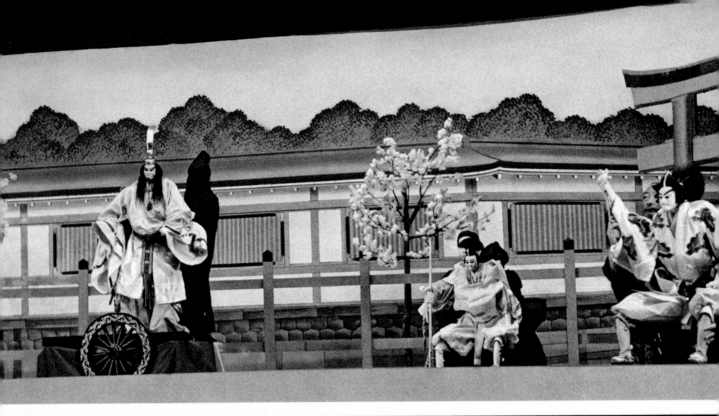

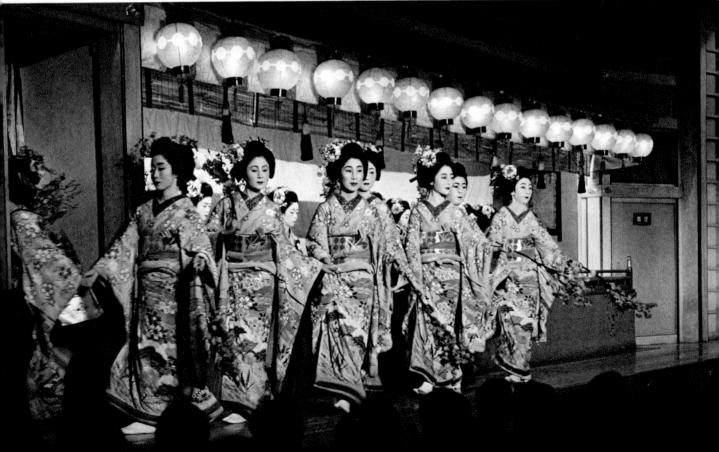

tours of the world's star performers. The Leningrad orchestra's Japanese tour was financed by one of the great newspapers. The Japanese newspapers which appear in Tokyo and Osaka are among the wealthiest and most powerful in the world. With its four provincial editions *Asahi* has a circulation of four million, *Mainichi* and *Yomiuri* not much less; two of these big three also have English editions whose circulation equals that of one of the popular Swiss newspapers. These newspapers play a very active part in Japanese cultural life as sponsors.

Pages 283–286 TOWN AND COUNTRY IN JAPAN

283 In front of one of the temples in Kyoto stands a solitary pilgrim in old-fashioned costume. He is surrounded by crowds of visitors who have arrived in coaches, conducted by stewardesses each of whom carries a small flag indicating her school or tourist party.

284 top The Tôdaiji Temple in Nara, the centre of the Buddhist Kegon sect founded in 745, was repeatedly destroyed by fire; the present building, one of the most important examples of Japanese temple architecture under the influence of China, was built in 1708. Its hall, 185 feet long, 162 feet wide, and 159 feet high, is one of the largest wooden structures in existence.

284 below Visitors to the grounds of a temple in Kyoto stop in front of the altar-rail for a brief prayer. Notice the diversity of Western and Japanese dress and footwear.

285 The Daibutsu or Great Buddha in the Tôdaiji Temple in Nara, which is even larger than the Daibutsu in Kamakura (more than fifty-two feet high and weighing 500 tons), was cast with great difficulty from a sketch by a Korean artist; it represents Buddha Vairocana with his hands in the attitude of a preacher.

286 top From a performance at the Bunraku puppet theatre in Osaka: a scene from the Sngawara Denju Tenarai Kagami, a popular 18th-century play which is about a good and a wicked minister in the 9th century. The puppets are moved by three men who, except for the heads of the main actors, are all muffled up in black. On the left side sits the formidable Minister of the Left, Fujiwara Shihei.

286 below In Kyoto the 'Cherry-blossom Dance', Miyako-Odori, performed by a company of geishas during the season of cherry blossom in April and May, is a special attraction for natives and tourists. Here a group of geishas leave by the left side-stage.

Puppet Show   Among the outstanding items in the 1958 Osaka International Festival was the joint performance of the two famous Bunraku companies. I spent more than four hours at a matinée, which was afterwards continued in an evening performance which was quite as long. Theme and form of expression of the classical Kabuki theatre are stylised in the Bunraku puppet-play to a degree extraordinary even for Japan. The excellence of the performance as a whole and the artistic competence of the actors were clearly evident even in an entirely unfamiliar language of words and gestures. This was in contrast to a production of the Siamese theatre which I was to see later in Bangkok, where in all the exotic charm and earnest endeavour was only a harmless and friendly echo of the art once practised by the King's dancers. The episode from the 9th century performed was remarkably similar to the plot of one of the 'operas' which I saw in Peking—the good minister was expelled and suffered much hardship in exile, while the wicked minister ruled; it is apparently one of the original themes of historical drama. The mime of the puppets took place on a broad stage; the figures, about half life-size, were carried and moved by three actors muffled up in black—and it was easier to fall in with the acting of this group of three than with that on the European stage of, for instance, a tenor who is too fat.

Only the main actors showed their faces—heads with immobile features as if carved out of wood. At the side, on the right, the narrator sat on a small revolving stage, his legs stretched out; the book lay open on a small desk and beside him stood a samisen player who gave the words and song a rhythmical accompaniment. The narrator did not change his position and eschewed gesticulation, so the

Page 289 KYOTO

Gay carp-flags of paper or cloth swell out in the wind all over the country for the boys' festival, Shôbu-no sekku, celebrated on 5th May; originally one flag was hoisted for every son in the house.

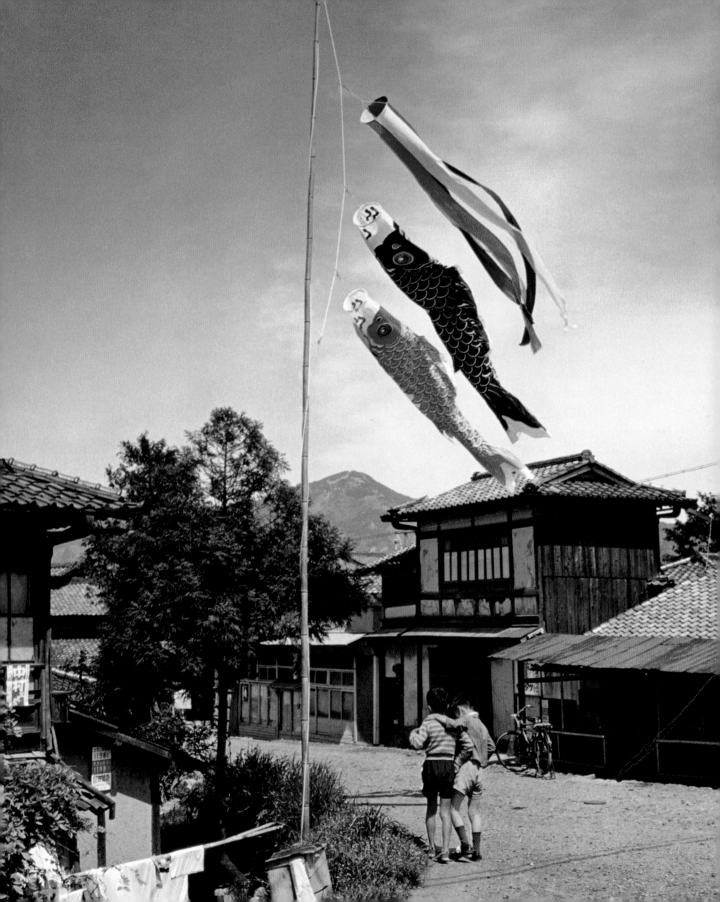

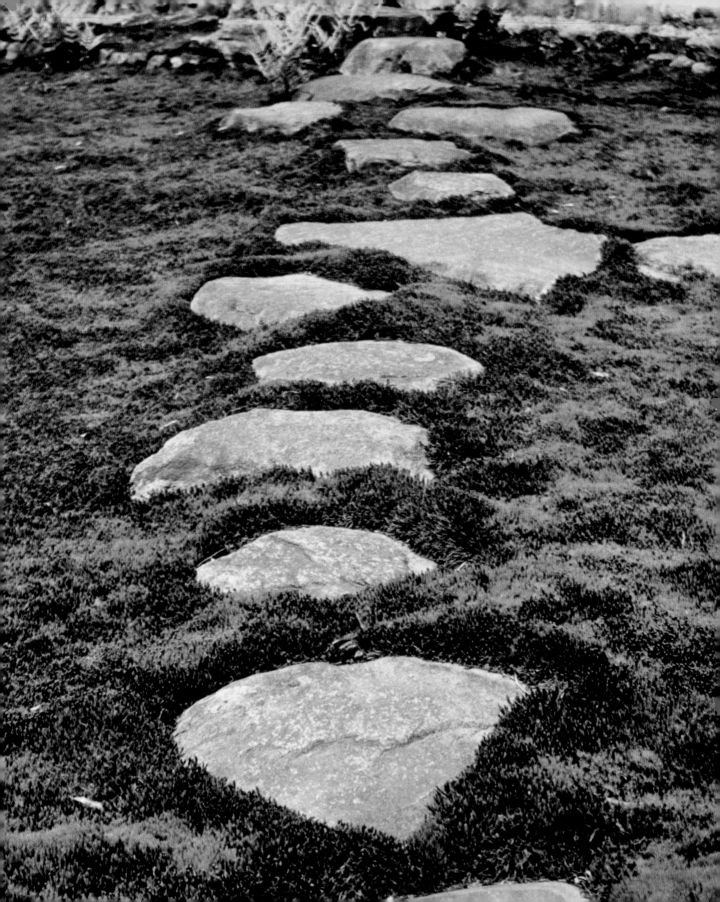

passionate force of his recitation was all the more impressive. He alone spoke the whole dramatic dialogue, intensifying it with song, which ended in laughter and sobbing. At one point the wicked minister rose and expressed his rage in a single sound which became a whole aria of demoniacal groaning. After a scene of twenty or thirty minutes the narrator was bathed in sweat; he disappeared on the revolving side-stage and the narrator of the next scene accompanied by his samisen player appeared on the new stage.

After the busy festival city of Osaka, Kyoto preserves the dignity and splendour *Kyoto* of the place where emperors lived for more than a thousand years. At the end of the 8th century, the capital, which until then had usually changed with each new ruler, was permanently established there. A broad town plan on the Chinese model with nine streets running from east to west formed Heian-Kyo 'Capital of peace', later simply called Kyoto 'Capital'. There is a profusion of temples, shrines, palaces, *torii*, statues of the Buddha, and paintings. Kyoto is still today a city of scholars and priests, of skilled crafts and the theatre, of geisha parties and dinner-parties; in every month of the year there are secular and religious festivities of some sort. Kyoto is the great museum of Japanese culture, but it keeps its vitality with a million residents and a constant stream of visitors.

In Kyoto are to be found the most famous examples of the Japanese garden. *The Gardens of Kyoto* This is the most sublime form in which the Japanese succeed in ennobling life through art. Nature itself is the model and means, and as in the buildings of Ise

Page 290 KYOTO KATSURA RIKYŪ
The garden of the imperial villa in Katsura shows the centuries-old art of the Japanese gardener in all its diversity; here are stepping-stones in a richly coloured moss-carpet.

the works of art handed down are preserved only by continual replacement. In the modern park of the Heian shrine flowering shrubs and water plants brought vivid colour into the play of grey stones, green bushes, the warm tints of the wooden tea-house, covered bridges, and water: this is the Japanese garden as we imagine it. It was visited by throngs of cheerful people, and was the ideal setting for wedding-parties. By contrast, when you strolled in the park of the imperial Katsura country-house with a uniformed guide you found an atmosphere of quiet veneration, fitting for the home of the ruler. How much more gentle and subdued everything was here than in the expansive splendour of the Summer Palace in Peking, no shrill note disturbed the harmony of stones, trees, shrubs, carpets of moss, rippling or still water, antique stone lamps, and airy wooden houses; there were no blank spaces in this landscape fashioned by artists.

A third mood is suggested by the gardens of the Daitokuji and Ryoanji temples, whose grounds are attributed to the Zen priest Sôami who died in 1525. There even the green of vegetation is excluded: finely raked sand and stones conjure up for the meditating spirit the expanse of the ocean, the eternal play of waves, the loneliness of an island, and the majesty of bare hills.

With the Fishermen of the Miura Peninsula   I spent my last days in Japan with friends in their country-house on the Miura peninsula by the sea. There are a number of fishing-villages there, not far from the old capital Kamakura and the small island of Enoshima. The Emperor has a summer villa there too. On summer days the shy, modest man, who in his nation's darkest hour bore with such courageous determination the responsibility of his high office, can be seen on the sea-shore, lightly clad and with net in hand, pursuing his scientific hobby of marine biology.

We made some purchases in the small village bazaar and at the fishmonger's, went on excursions by bus and, accompanied by a fisherman, had a shot ourselves at catching cuttle-fish and other kinds of fish. In one of the larger fishing-ports we visited a great concrete hall where huge quantities of fish are weighed and packed. The public health officers of a European country could not have found fault with anything there; Japanese hygiene is exemplary.

A magnificent cutter was putting out to sea with fluttering pennants; on deck a table was set up and covered with presents for the long journey, while from the quay people held on to their menfolk on deck with gay paper streamers, until this last link broke. They might return in a month, perhaps in six months or more, for they are allowed to come back only with a large catch; the landings must not only satisfy the home market but must leave a surplus for export; and the loss of tonnage in the war must be made up for by harder work. The fisherman with his ancient trade is one of the most industrious workers in the peaceful reconstruction of the nation: in the year of Japan's defeat the yield of 1,800,000 tons had fallen far below half the pre-war yield, but by 1955 all previous records had been surpassed and in 1957 there was a further increase of 10 per cent to 5,398,600 tons (without counting the whale catch).

Japanese courtesy, though almost proverbial, is not assumed without question. *Japanese Courtesy* A Japanese newspaper said with the self-criticism customary today that the courtesy of the Japanese was confined all to often to traditional formality and broke down in the situations of modern life, where they had to prove its intrinsic worth in the absence of a ready-made convention. The mask which Europeans are conscious of in the impassive appearance of the Japanese—in contrast, perhaps, to the more jovial expressions of the Chinese—can mislead us into thinking that Japanese courtesy is only superficial, and even into distrusting it as the attempt at deception of an exaggerated form of egoism. The Japanese smile is certainly very different from the hearty 'Hallo, old boy' and the familiar slap on the back—but do genuine and affectionate feelings need to be noisily expressed? Society did not first discover in America (or in Russia) that it is not such a simple matter to speak the truth and that some self-subordination is needed so that people can live together harmoniously.

In their theatre and sculpture the Japanese have carried the art of stylisation to a point which hardly any other civilised people has reached; their courtesy carries over this art into daily life; it restrains what is noisy and forward; it protects the handicapped, and it even invests poverty with dignity. It is not a private convention, and anyone who is prepared to accept it as a means of making life more tolerable—and perhaps also more charming—will account his experience of it as one of his most precious memories of a visit to Japan.

I can still see a little old peasant woman meeting another woman at the outskirts of a village; both bowed low as if they were ladies-in-waiting of the Empress of China. And I see the charming nods of those pretty young girls in stewardesses' uniforms and white gloves. I see the Shinto priest who offered me a bowl of green tea as it is served at the tea ceremony, and who thus bade me welcome to his country and customs. I see my publishing colleague, who was connected with me by no business of any kind but only by a chance encounter, hurrying into the hotel before my departure to bid me farewell and wave as I drove away.

Japan's Destiny   Has Japan yet found its true course? The presumption of the militarists, imbued with Samurai ideals, who wished to create a master race and carried through unscrupulous imperialism, has been crushed; the dreams of being a world power have dissolved, and the Japanese regards his role in the international theatre with

295 On the coast of the Miura peninsula stands the unpretentious tea-house in the old style which belongs to the imperial summer villa of Isshi, which the present ruler of Japan likes to visit for holidays and to study marine biology.

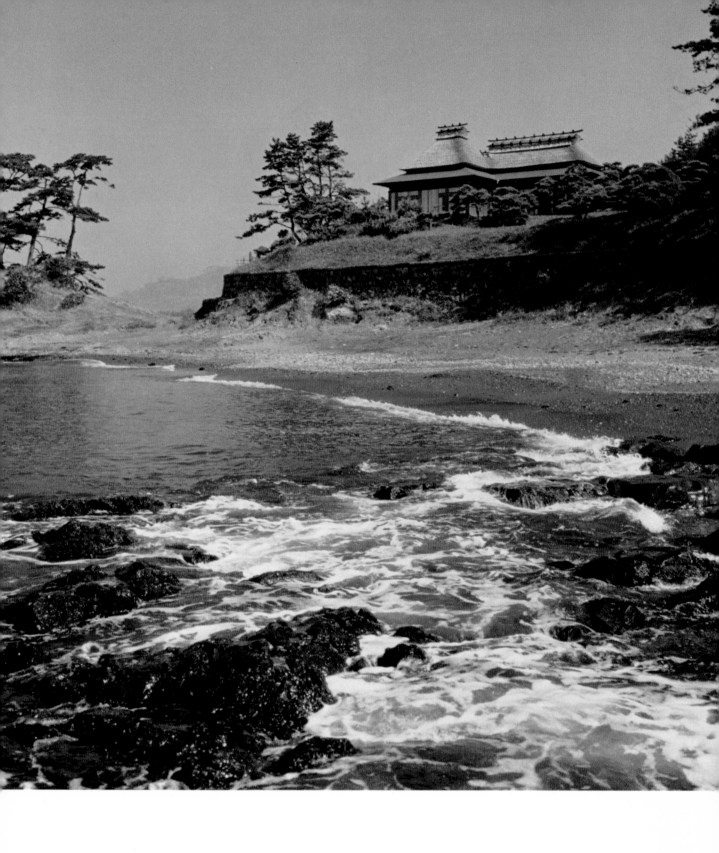

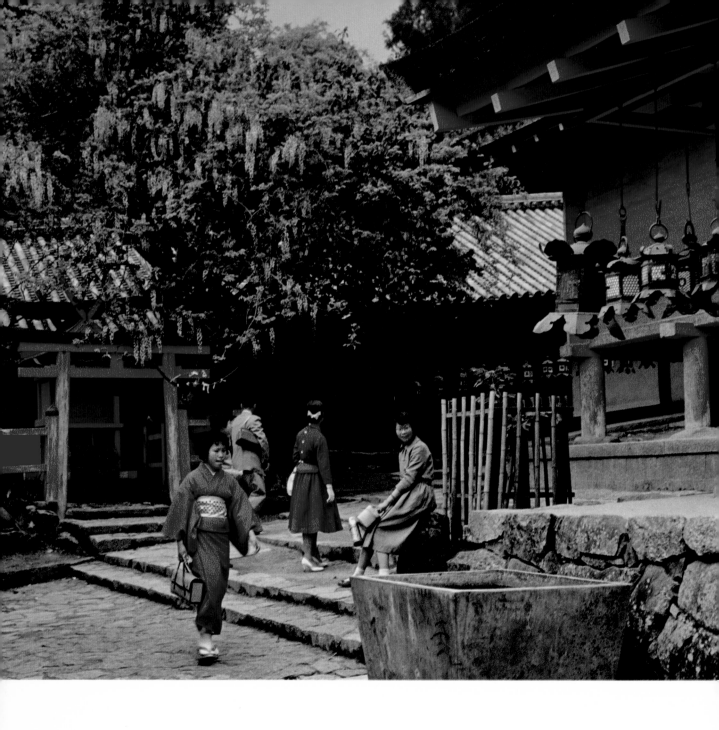

disillusionment. He looks with bated breath towards the mainland, where his huge and formidable neighbour is stretching his limbs.

We took off at midnight, the tourist class filled with a delegation of teachers from Thailand who were returning to Bangkok; in the first class was a most distinguished passenger, the mother of the ruling prince of Bhutan. The moon was reflected in the sea, but Mount Fuji remained invisible; I thought I could see a distant volcano with a thin red streak of glowing lava moving slowly down it, a very high one, since it came with us as we left the land—then I saw more clearly the wing of our Douglas with a small red streak glowing in the engine covering.

We were heading over the sea for Okinawa, Formosa, Hongkong. The day was already far advanced when we made for the runway between the hills, houses, and junks of the Crown Colony. Then flying on we crossed the South China Sea and the mountainous jungle of the Indo-Chinese peninsula, until a broad plain streaked with water-courses announced the fertile delta of the Menam and the approach to Siam's capital, Bangkok.

296   One of the Kasuga shrines in Nara at the time of the acacia blossom.

Thailand

I STILL CALL IT SIAM, but today this kingdom's correct name is Thailand. In 1932, shortly after my last visit, absolute monarchy was abolished and parliamentary government was introduced. But in the East these political terms and concepts are rarely applied so consistently and thoroughly as we are wont to apply them in Europe—and after all, they are European terms and concepts, the result of a long spiritual and political process, while for Asia they are little more than just some of the many catch-penny phrases which nowadays automatically go with participation in progress, technology, and a just distribution of wealth, and which everyone appropriates, with more or less usefulness, for his own advantage.

The absolute rule of the Royal House which in 1782 had chosen Bangkok as its residence was an enlightened despotism. It was thoroughly imbued with the mild teachings of Buddha, to whom all the splendid temples and monuments of the capital are dedicated, and it skilfully steered the ship of State through the waves of French and British colonialism, which surged on both sides. When the various territories claimed by the Thais were finally unified under a modern system of administration there were, it is true, conflicts and clashes with their

Pages 299–302 BANGKOK

299–301 On the right bank of the Menam, opposite the centre of the city, rises 240-foot-high Wat Arun with its five *prangs*. The buildings, which are richly decorated with figures made from gaily varnished tiles, remind one of the towers of the old Khmer. At the entrance to one of the halls of prayer stand two enormous guards—figures from Indian mythology.

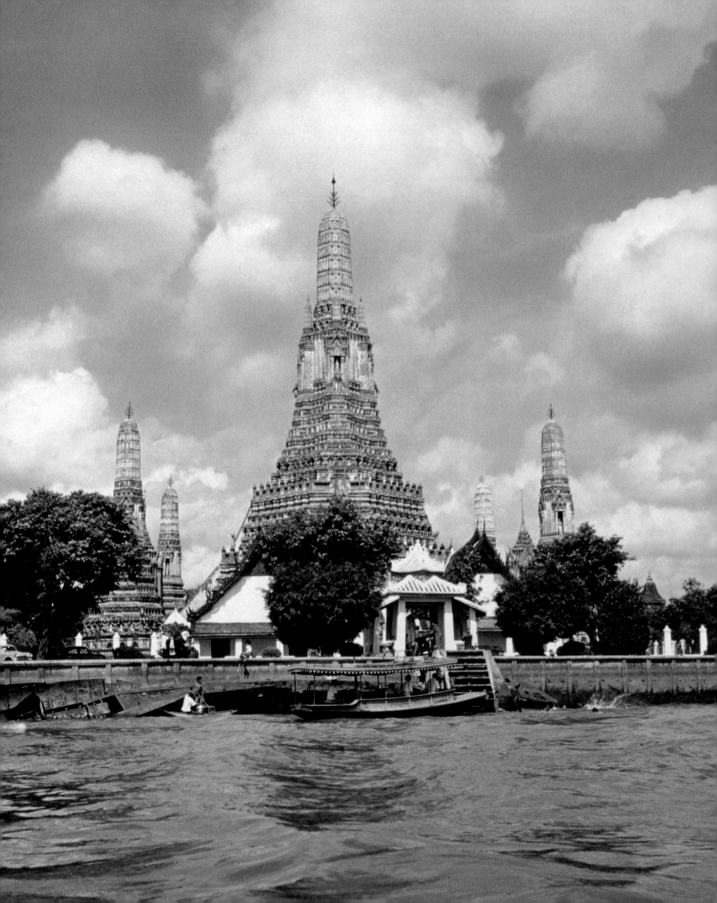

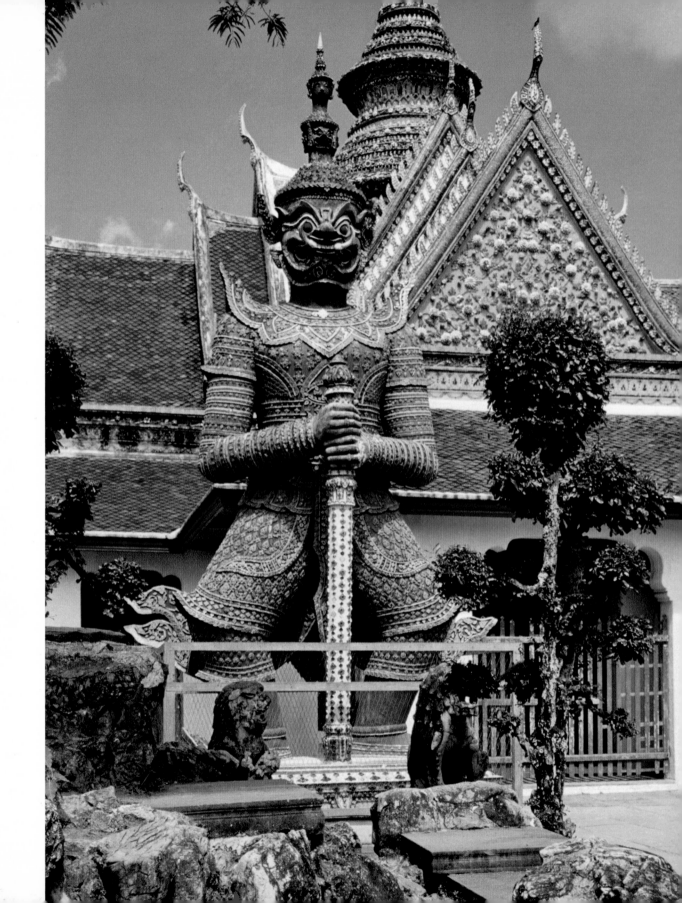

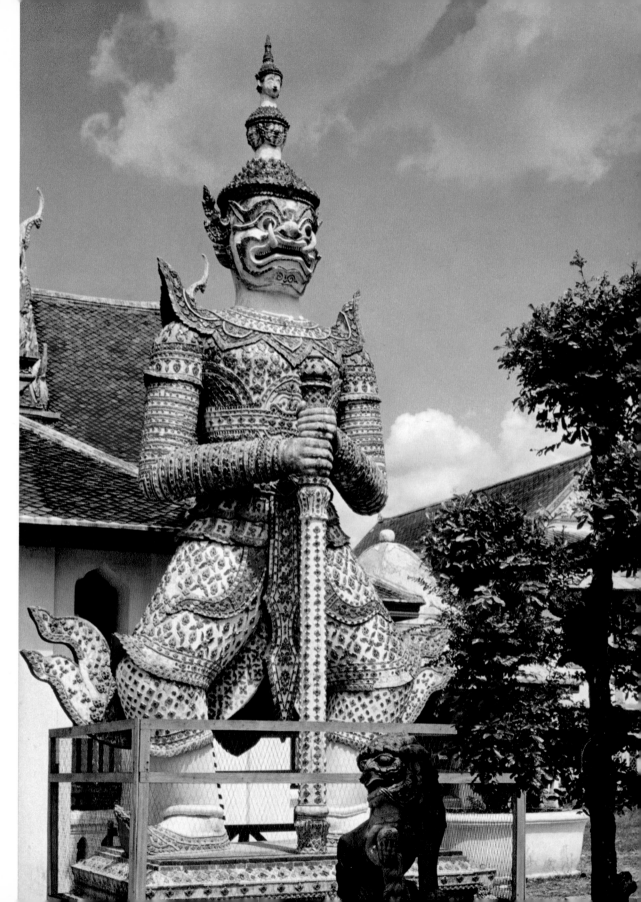

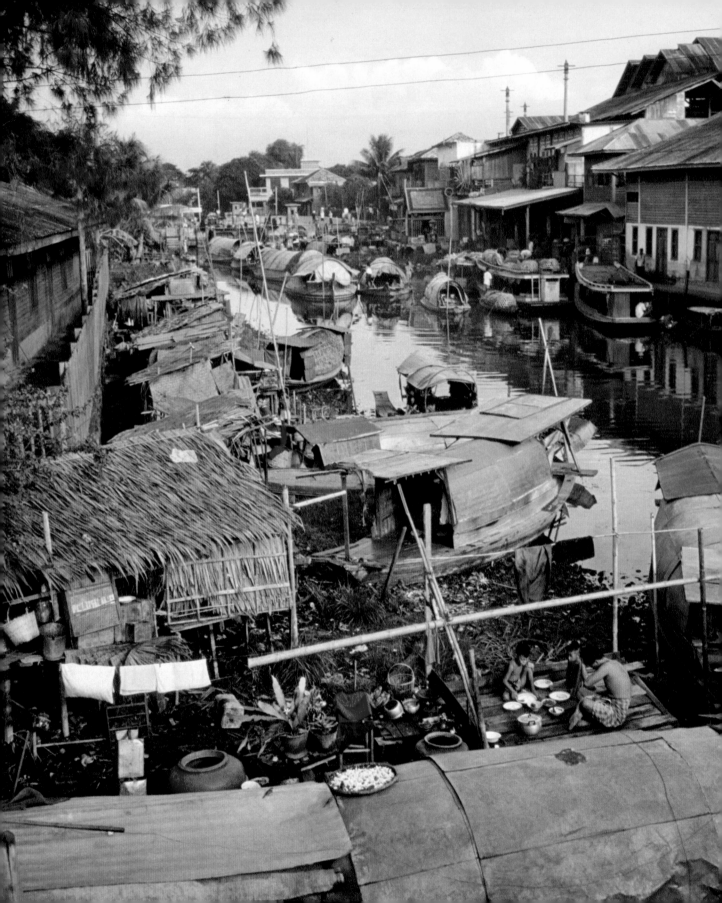

covetous neighbours: in 1893 the capital itself was threatened by the French, and in 1907 they seized the province of Cambodia, while the British added the Malayan frontier State to the Straits Settlement. But on the whole in Siam the dreaded white explorers came as friends, who gave valuable help in the development of the country. At the same time, however, there came in much larger numbers, and so to speak by the back door, the industrious Chinese from the over-populated regions around Canton, and it was they who developed the retail trade and the crafts of the royal town which was growing to become the largest city of South East Asia.

Siam is a country blessed with water. Some of its rice fields can be harvested twice a year; they not only provide enough food for its own people, but also allow an export which is distinguished by its high quality. Of the approximately 23,116 square miles of arable land about one-third is cultivated. More than half the country is covered by forests. All over the mountainous north stretch giant teak woods, and 48,264 square miles of these are under government management. A third of the world's consumption of teak is supplied by Thailand. The tin-mines are worked by Chinese labour and yield approximately 5 per cent of the world production. Other mineral deposits are still awaiting exploitation.

Since my last visit thirty years ago the population had nearly doubled to more than 20 million, but there is room for still more people in the 198,247 square miles.

At last here is a country without any seriously pressing problems, without dangerous ambitions, without the fatal heritage of resentments and dissatisfaction. British, American, Swiss, German, and other commercial enterprises are prospering here, side by side in peaceful competition; the Thai is not obsessed by the idea that he is constantly being exploited and that he must get rid of them as soon as possible; he himself benefits from them and moreover the small white colony

302 A canal (*klong*) in Bangkok with a swarm of boats.

forms a welcome balance to the expanding Chinese section of the population. Thus the tourist from the West for once does not feel obliged to display a bad conscience in this happy country.

The absolute kingdom of Siam was ruled by princes; the constitutional monarchy of Thailand, that is—the 'land of the free'—is governed by the generals. Whether they do the job differently and better the outsider dare not decide. It cannot be said that there is greater stability now, and there is still a great deal of talk about arbitrariness, corruption, loss of investments, and so forth; election promises and the rights of parliament are not observed more strictly than anywhere else in the East. From time to time there is a disturbance, when a new general puts himself in the place of a colleague; but there is no need for the world to watch this terrified, with bated breath. As long as the Thais are left to themselves the smile of Buddha will shine over them.

Picturesque Bangkok   The rainy season was imminent and the air was humid. In the morning white clouds would gather over the city; in the afternoon the sky was usually overcast, and at night the rain came down in torrents. In the cool morning the omnibuses stood ready to take us to the sights of the city. At the Menam we boarded a motor-boat to visit the 'floating market', the temples on the opposite river-bank, and the royal boats with their demon- and dragon-figures.

The picturesque East, so often robbed of its magic by motor-cars, loudspeakers, and Coca-Cola, has withstood the assault in Bangkok; here it is as enchanting as ever, and more enchanting than anywhere else. On the threshold of the Chinese cultural orbit there arose, almost in our time, as a last flower of the architectural inspiration of the religious genius of India, a splendid royal residence, of a kind which you can otherwise only imagine from ruins. All the year round the waters of rivers and canals ripple against the palm trees; lotus blossoms float in the pools; in the markets the fruits of the country are piled up—mangoes, coco-nuts, pineapples, mangosteens. Amid the traffic in this city of two million people, the monks—disciples of Buddha—still walked serenely, clad in yellow robes. Only the panting and puffing Chinese rickshaw coolies had disappeared; faster, more comfortable pedicabs were run by robust Thai lads. Neatly dressed boys and girls went to school with their satchels. Chinese children played at the sides of the streets; market-boats and cargo-boats moved along the *klongs* (canals), and boys played together by the water. Our motor-boat went along between rows of boys and when it appeared at the Wat Arun on the Menam they jumped from the paling on the bank into the river like frogs, not for money but just for the fun, so that even the discerning tourist had no cause for ironical comment.

You could wander freely about the temples and talk with the intelligent monks; and you might even meet a dainty, genuine princess working in an office. A German engineer told me how the good King Chulalongkorn himself had urged him to get on with the construction of the Siamese railway.

City of Buddhism

This whole lively, tolerant world is ruled over by the figure of the Buddha, the Enlightened One. His image, from the small figure to the huge 100-foot-high statue, dominates the grounds of all the monasteries and temples. For four centuries Siamese kings had lived at Ayuthya, but when in 1767 this town was destroyed for the second time by the Burmese, the sworn enemies of Thailand, the capital shifted to the seat of the King of Dhonburi on the Lower Menam. On the opposite bank, where Chinese had settled, Rama I, the founder of the new dynasty, established his residence in 1782, and since then the temples have sprung up, with royal patronage, which have made Bangkok one of the great art-centres of the world.

It is not so much a matter of individual architectural masterpieces—the brick buildings encrusted with ornaments, the wooden pillars, glass ornaments, gold-plating, and glazed tiles will not last for ever—but as a whole these 19th-century

307 While many of the waterways, the *klongs*, have disappeared from the Bangkok scene, in the neighbouring villages much of the market life and traffic is still to be found on them.

308 Before landing in Bangkok you see through the windows of the aircraft the fertile fields of the Menam delta, over which heavy clouds presage the start of the rainy season.

309 From the hill Wat Saket, the 'Golden Mountain', you survey the roofs of Bangkok with the magnificent temple grounds.

309 below In the middle of the broad Rajademnoen Avenue rises the 'Monument to Democracy' in memory of Thailand's transition from an absolute to a constitutional monarchy, accomplished in 1932.

310 above One of the most recent temple buildings in Bangkok, Wat Benchama bopitre, owes its name 'Marble Temple' to the use of white marble from Carrarar. The bright yellow tiles and extensive gilding make a festive frame for the Hall of Prayer and the cloisters with their many statues of the Buddha.

310 below In the hall of a monastery the monks are assembled; they are holding a religious ceremony for a family event and are now receiving flowers and fruit from the members of the family; a concession is made to modern customs by cigarettes and Coca Cola (or its equivalent).

311 Wat Po, the largest temple group in Bangkok, containing several buildings, was erected from 1793 onwards in place of an earlier temple, by the founder of the dynasty, who is buried here. The largest of the hundreds of statues of Buddha, the 'sleeping Buddha', takes up almost the whole length of one of the *wihara* (halls of prayer); the 160-foot-long figure is made of brick with a thick cement casing and is richly gilded. The Buddha is represented entering Nirvana.

312 The gold Buddha of Wat Traimitr in Bangkok. In 1956, the jubilee year of Buddhism, the huge figure was damaged in transport, and pure gold was found under a thick layer of stucco: thus, centuries after the statue had been camouflaged to protect it from enemy looting, an immensely valuable masterpiece of the medieval Sukothai period was rediscovered.

313 In the Silpakorn theatre we saw a production in classical style with the traditional princely lovers (both acted by girls here). The prince was dressed in rich, old-fashioned robes.

314–317 On the Menam and the canals flowing into it market-boats sail along and young boys bathe happily.

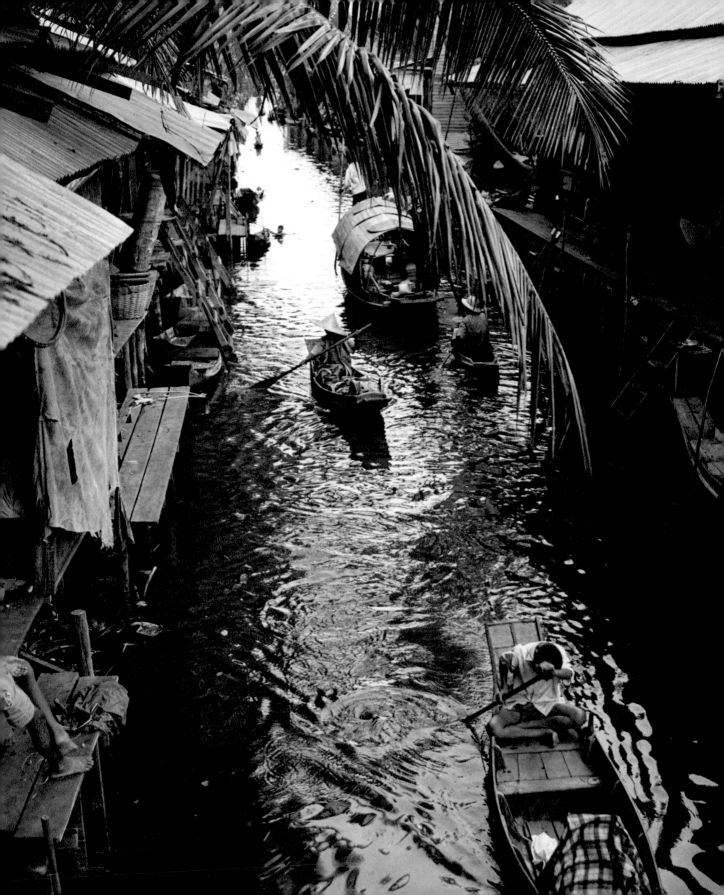

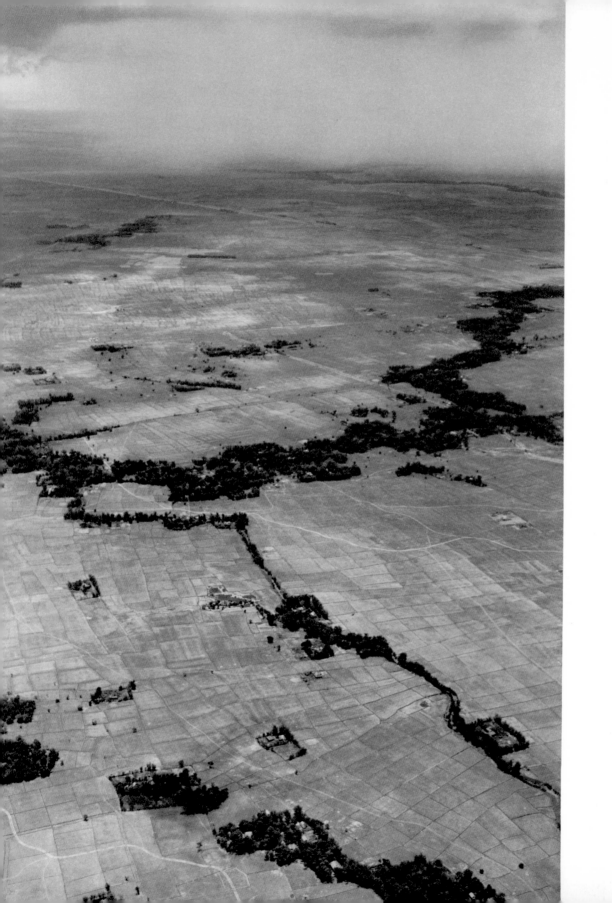

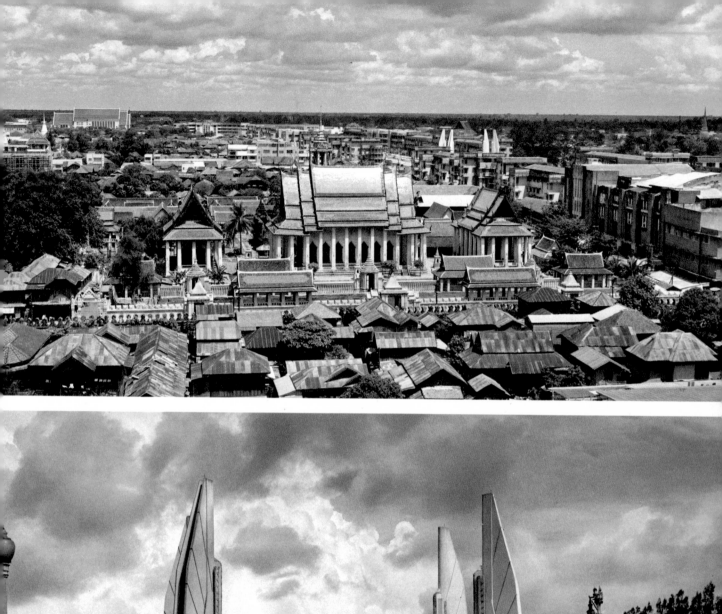
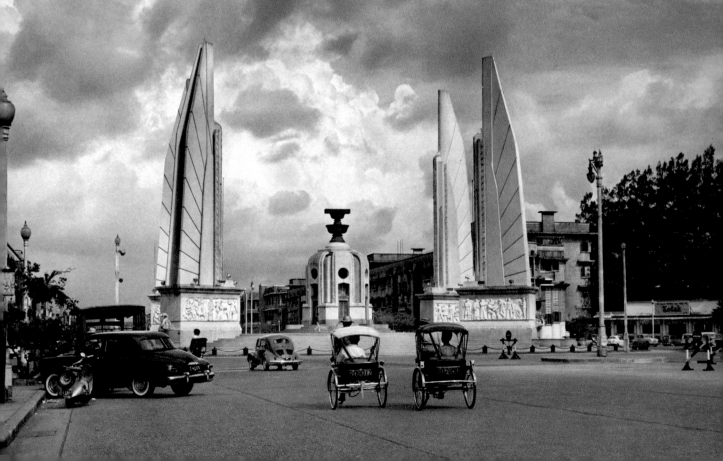

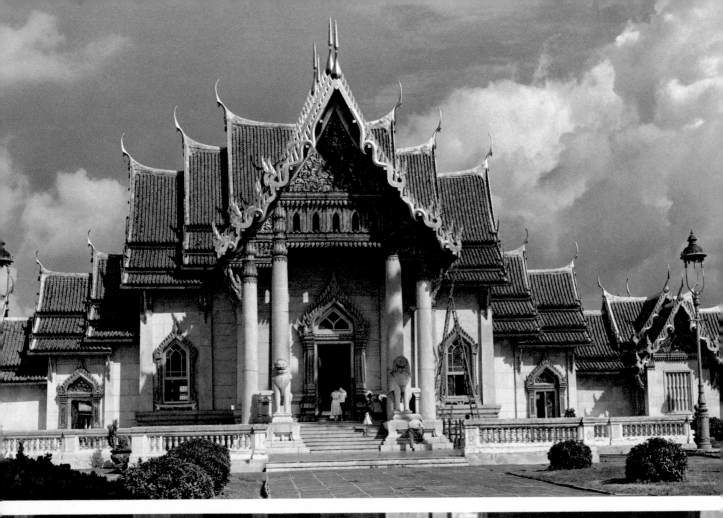

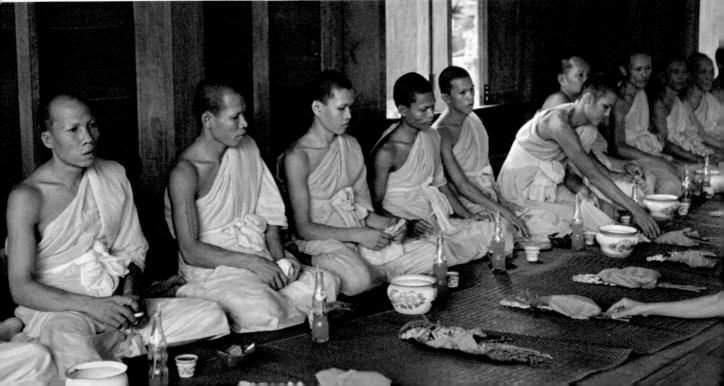

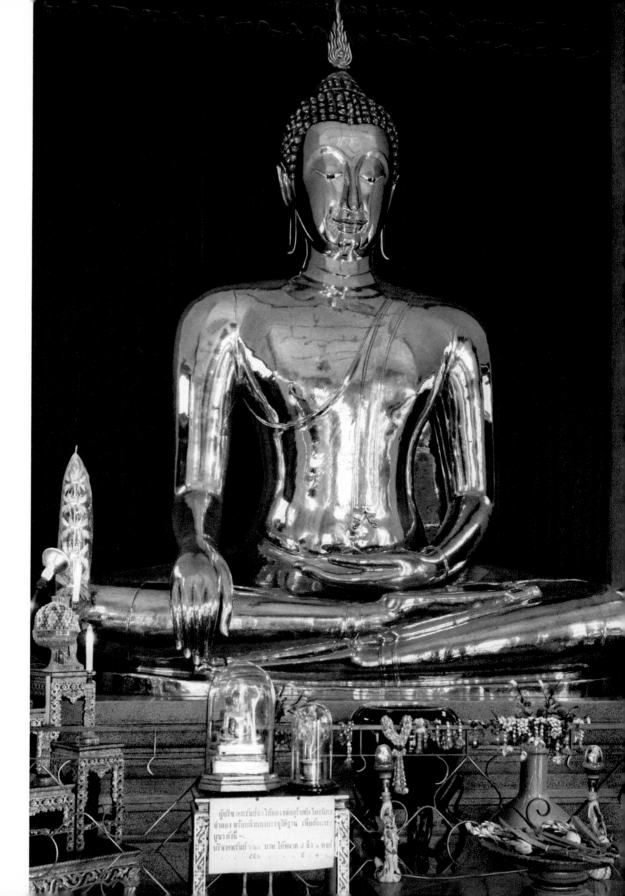

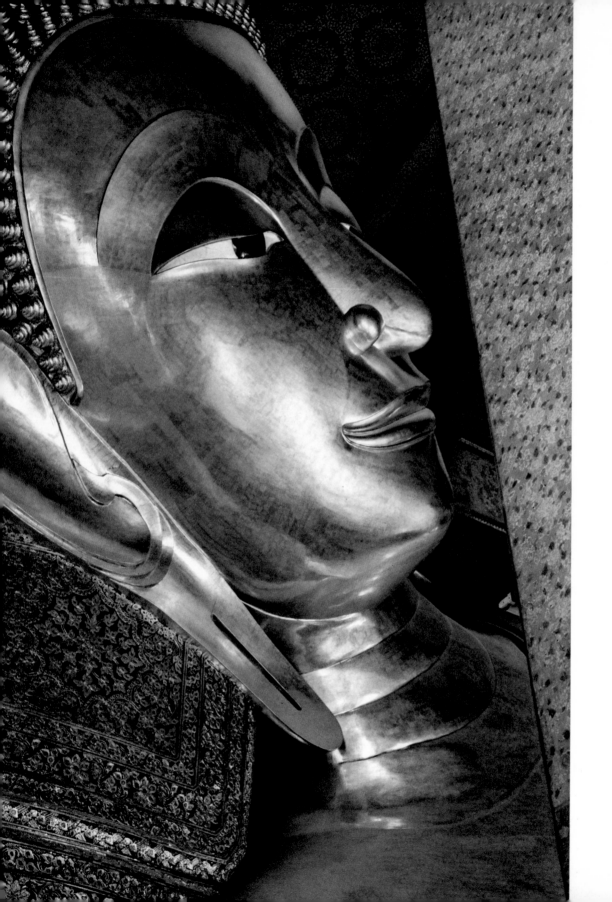

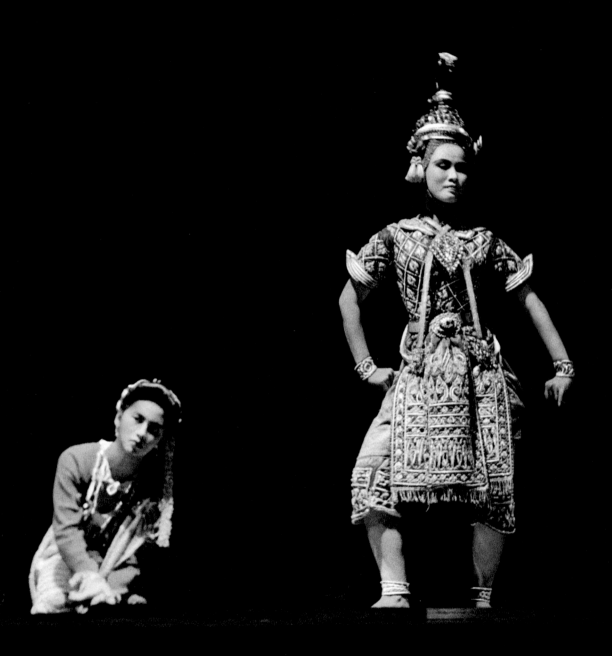

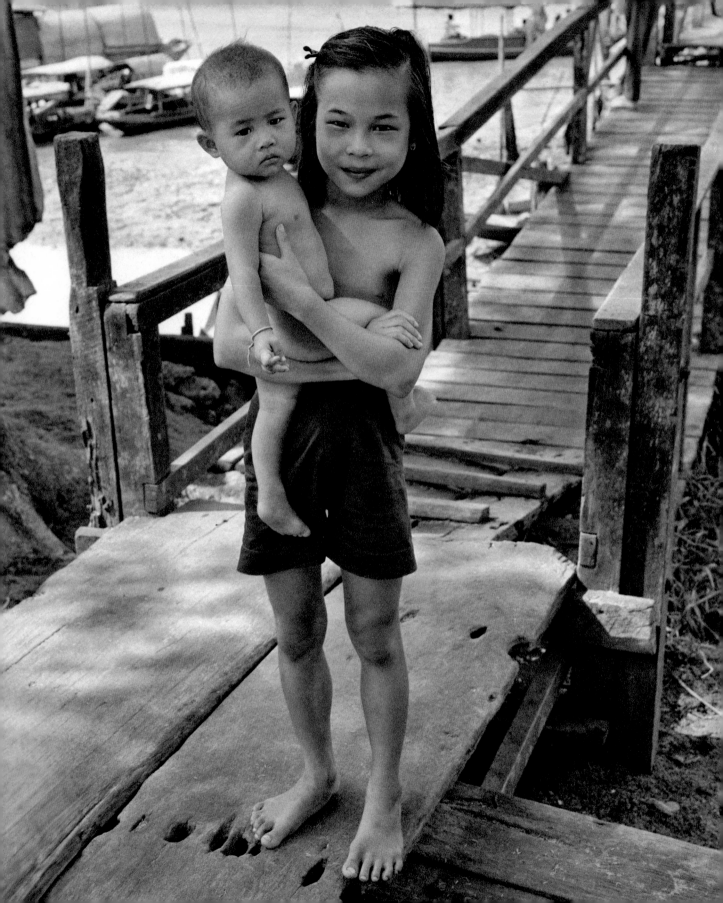

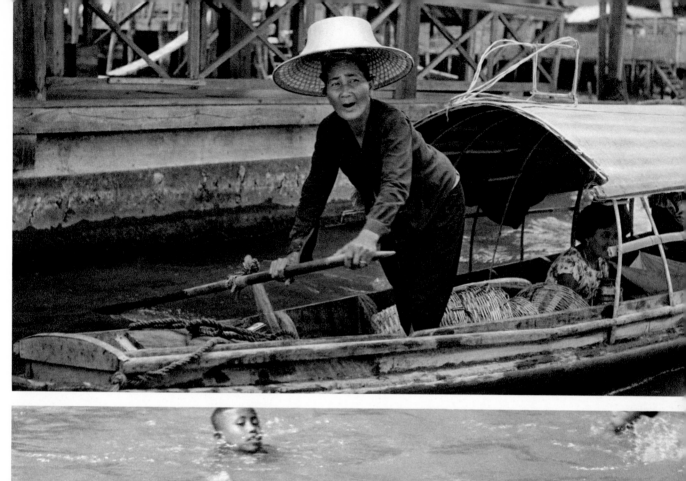

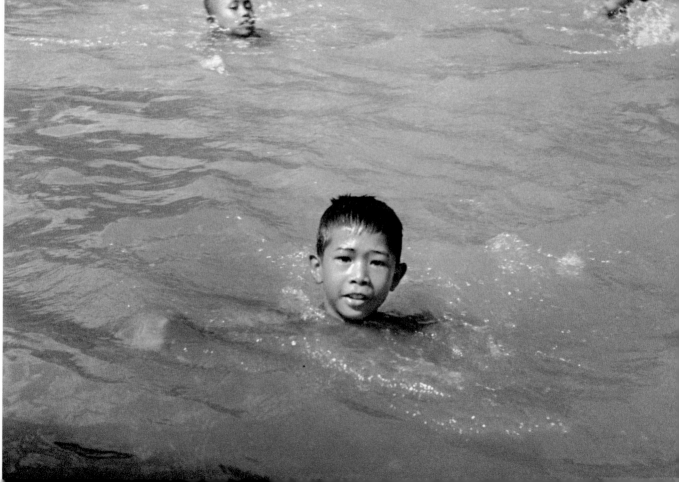

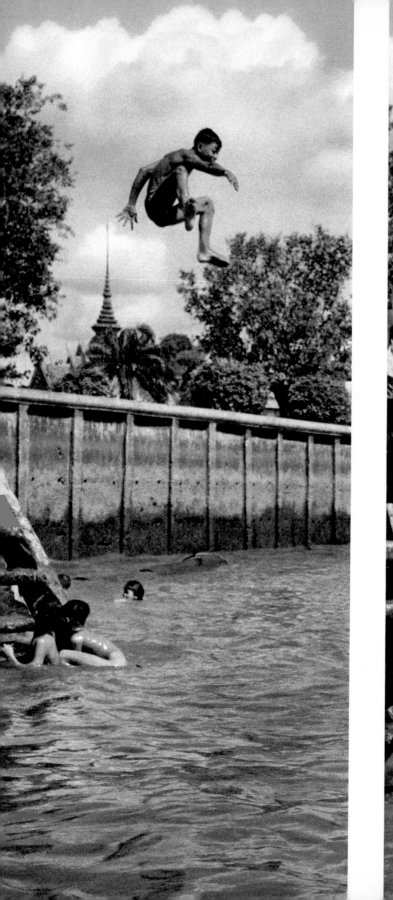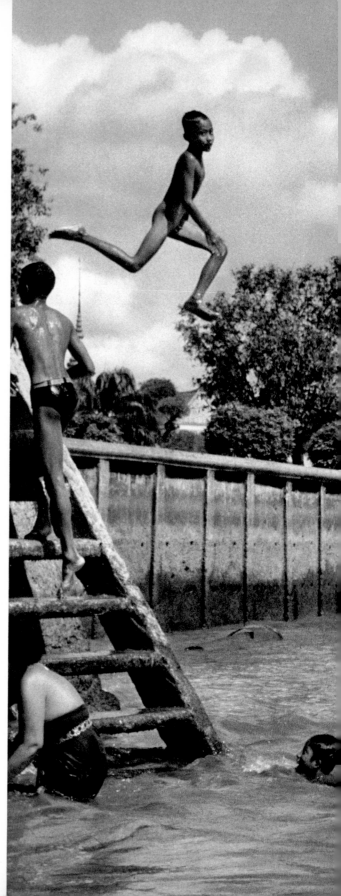

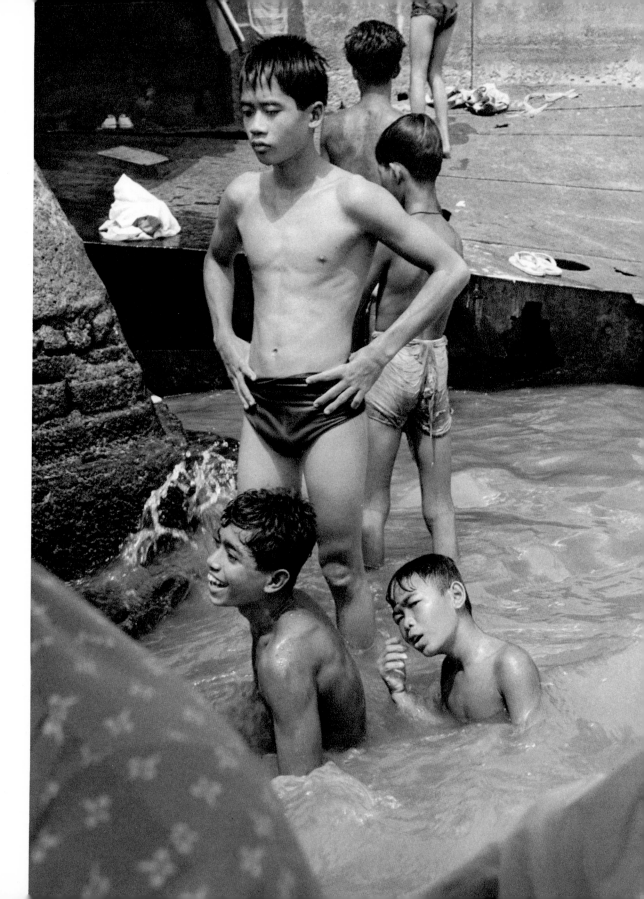

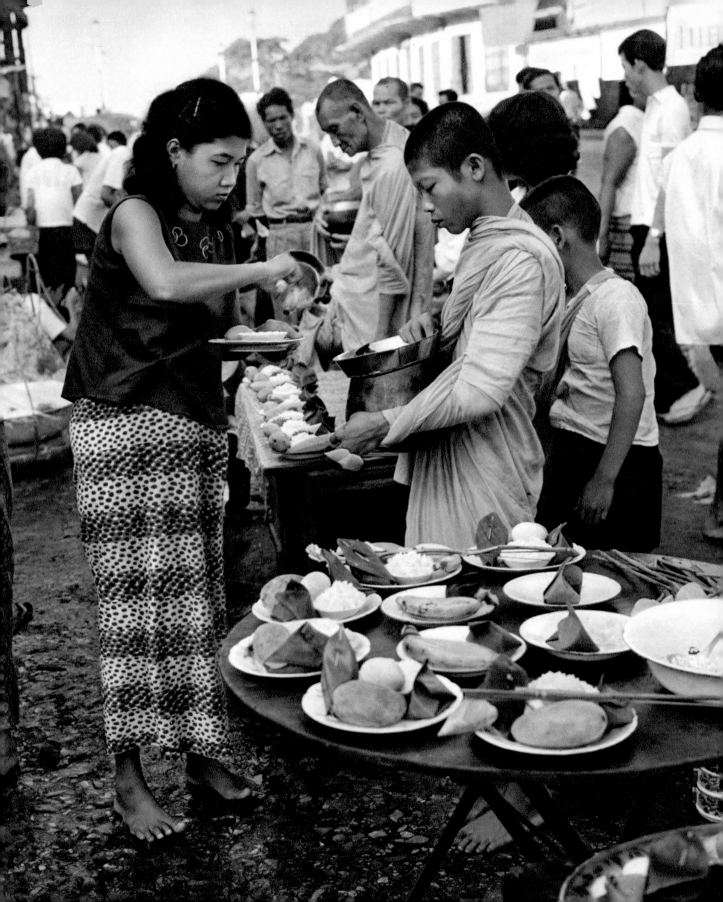

buildings are overwhelming evidence of a tradition kept alive by faith; the best and most beautiful possessions were gathered together here and presented as homage to the great ascetic and conqueror of the world.

There are 300 *wat* (temples) in Bangkok; some of them consisting of a whole collection of buildings; the residence (*kuti*) of the monks may be outside the high wall surrounding the grounds. In the hall of the *Bôt* stood the abbot's throne, decorated with the gilt Buddha statue, in front of the altar—the ceremonial admission of the novice into the holy brotherhood takes place here. Some of the *wihara* (halls of prayer) were as large as the *Bôt*, and had similar high, red, yellow, green, or blue glazed roofs. Covered walks with statues of the Buddha or murals ran round the courtyards; *prangs* (towers) which reminded one of the Angkor model, *prachedis* (relic-memorials), a library, a small stylised garden, palms, and larger-than-life figures as doorkeepers formed part of the richest precincts. The puritanical doctrines of the Hinayana by no means restrained the taste of the patrons or the artists: as well as scenes of the Buddha legend, there were the figures of the Ramayana, the great Indian epic—demons and gods of Hindu mythology; you could see Vishnu with the divine bird Garuda, and Indra riding on the three-headed elephant. Doors and windows were decorated with inlaid mother-of-pearl, the dark timberwork glittered with gay ornaments like precious stones; on the edges of the roofs innumerable bells tinkled gently in the wind. In the dim interior the image of the Enlightened Teacher stood in the place of honour. There were masterpieces among those statues, which were older than their temples; they

Page 318 BANGKOK
The giving of alms is well organised nowadays; in the market merchants prepare gifts for the monks on special tables; but the act of giving has lost none of its simple solemnity; and the youngest generation still wear with undiminished dignity the yellow garments in which they follow the path of the Sakyamuni, the greatest son of India.

were brought here when the capital was moved from Sawankalok or Sukothai to Ayuthia and Bangkok.

One such famous image was transported from one temple to another in 1956 for the 2,500th annual celebration in honour of the Buddha; the larger-than-life statue proved too heavy for a two-ton and even for a five-ton crane; at the next attempt to move it part of the stucco coating splintered off, and then the riddle of its weight, which was excessive even for a bronze figure, was solved: a statue of pure gold was revealed, a masterpiece of the Sukothai period (13th to 14th century). Centuries ago this unprecedentedly valuable treasure had been camouflaged, probably to protect it from enemy looting, and the secret had been forgotten. The shining image was set up in the temporary structure of Wat Traimitr; there it attracted the devotion of the faithful, and donations slowly accumulated which would pay for the construction of a home in keeping with the artistic, material, and religious value of 'Father Traimitr'. Meanwhile, two more gold statues had been found.

One quite small temple, which I found only after a search, deserves special mention; it was called Phra Lak Muang and contained the idol of the god of the city. In the narrow shrine, dimly lit by flickering lights, there was a busy coming and going; the object of worship, decorated with flowers, was in the shape of the linham, the symbol of creation of Shiva. Votive offerings marked the fulfilment of prophecies made here about the finding of a husband, the birth of a child, or a good draw in the lottery. Elsewhere, especially in the country, all kinds of animistic activity went on behind the good Buddha's back.

Beside the colourful magnificence of the temples the sober white memorials of the new secularism thrust themselves forward: the Italian marble splendour of the parliament building, the ministries, hospitals, the four pylons of the 'Monument to Democracy' in Rajademnoen Avenue, new functional structures of the oil magnates, cinemas with screaming posters. But the skyline on the banks of the

Menan was still dominated by the towers and roofs of the old royal palace, of the Wat Po, the Wat Arun, and all the other monastic temples.

The first religious instruction which the Thai receives in his home is: 'I worship the Buddha, the law, and the order.' In contrast to the bewildering diversity of phenomena united within the Buddhist cult in the Mahayana (the Great Vehicle of the northern school), the southern school of the Hinayana, the Lesser Vehicle, which is spread over Ceylon, Burma, Cambodia, and Thailand, observes the teaching of the Gautama in a pure and simple form. You find here nothing of the festive, joyful realism which exists in the Buddhist heaven of the Chinese, nothing of the Lamas' mysticism and belief in spirits, nor the subtle spirituality of the Japanese Zen sect. Five simple commandments accompany the Thai through life: not to kill, not to steal, not to give way to one's desires, not to lie, and to renounce stimulants. For monks there are five further vows: not to eat at forbidden times, not to dance, not to have jewels or perfumes, not to touch money, and to be satisfied with the most simple night's lodging.

The Disciples of Buddha in Our Time

Boys called *Sisya* are among the residents of the 8,000 or so monasteries of Siam as pupils and servants of the monks; they rise to *Nane* or novices, and when, after they have taken the oath, the abbot has given them an alms-bowl, they are finally, as *Phra Song* (venerable monk), full members of the holy community. Anyone who has reached the nine stages of proficiency in the sacred Pali scripts receives the honorary title *Maha Barien*.

Each man has to find the Right Way by meditation, and remain true to it in humility. The rules of the Order are not severe: early in the morning after common prayers the monks set out to receive alms, on their return they breakfast from the gifts received; the rest of the morning is spent in meditation or teaching; at eleven o'clock they assemble for lunch; then they fast for the rest of the day, but they are allowed to drink harmless beverages, chew betel, and smoke. After evening prayers they walk alone or in groups until the bell calls them at nightfall to their simple beds. It is thought becoming for every young Thai, including the king, to come to maturity in the monastery and for some time to make the daily walk with an alms-bowl in the garments of renunciation of the world; the community of monks demands no isolation from life by eternal vows; it stands open for anyone to come and go; it goes on serenely, untouched by time.

Anyone who wanders through the streets early in the morning—whether in the city of Bangkok or in a modest village—meets the monks with their close-cropped heads, clad in yellow robes, and carrying their alms-bowls. They stop in front of the houses or stand motionless at their place in the market, their heads bowed, and wait until a donor hands them his gift. They do not ask, they do not thank. There are some wrinkled faces among them, but most of them are lads scarcely in their twenties. In the towns special market booths have standardised gifts for sale: rice, vegetables and fruits, a flower. A small *Sisya*, who accompanies the *Phra Song*, puts the fruit and flowers, for which there is no room in the rice-bowl, in a bag they have brought with them. It is mostly young girls and women who offer gifts; they kneel with clasped hands before and after offering them, for it is a holy action; everyone is gripped by the devout seriousness of the scene.

The treachery and cunning of our time will surely not stop short of their realm of peace, and the disciples of Buddha may yet have to undergo their sternest test

Pages 323–326 BANGKOK

323 Between an asphalt street and the plain buildings where the police are quartered there was water with a lotus in bloom.

324, 325 In the market early in the morning Buddhist monks stand with their alms-bowls; many young men join them for a year or more. Donors kneel to greet the representatives of the doctrine of compassion and renunciation.

326 Fruits and flowers are especially abundant in the market—in the foreground are baskets of mangosteens.

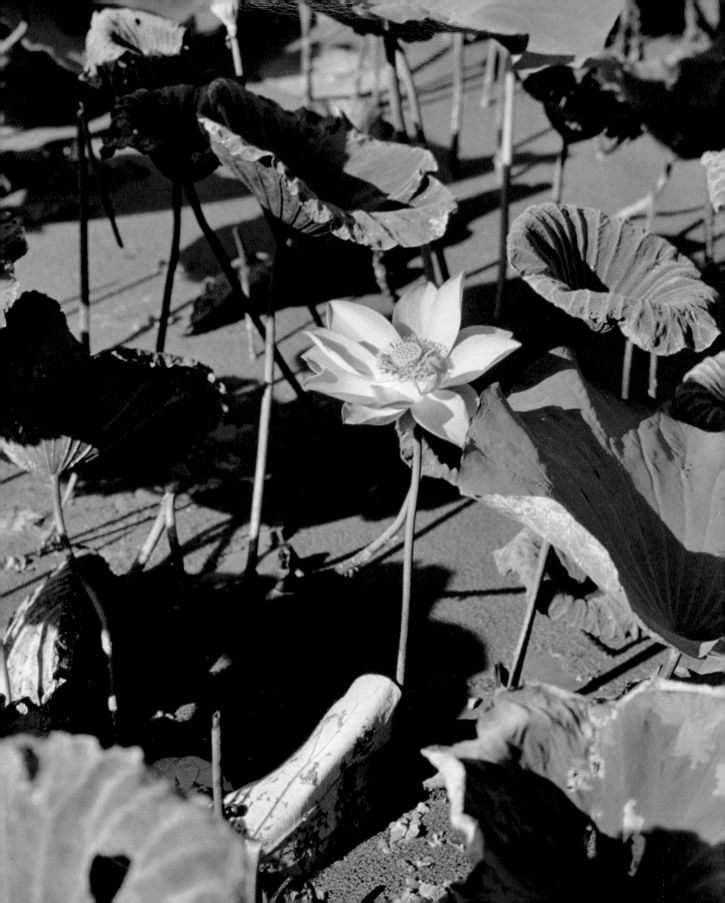

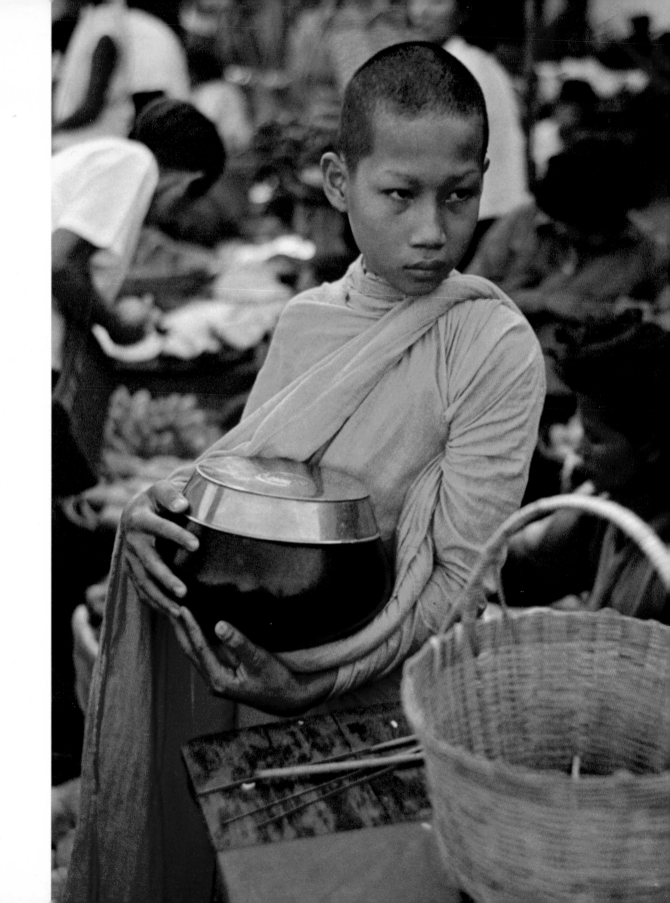

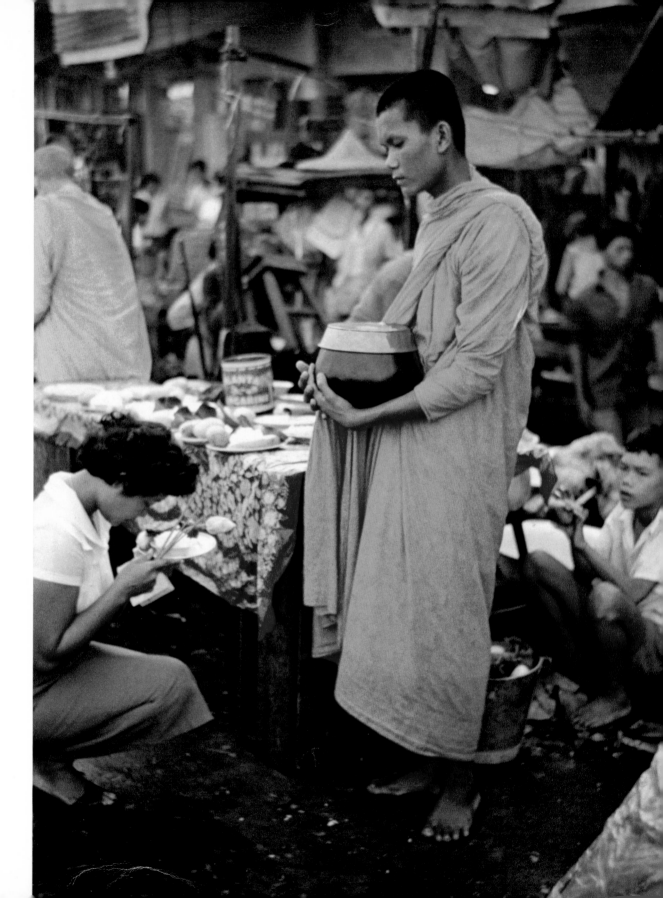

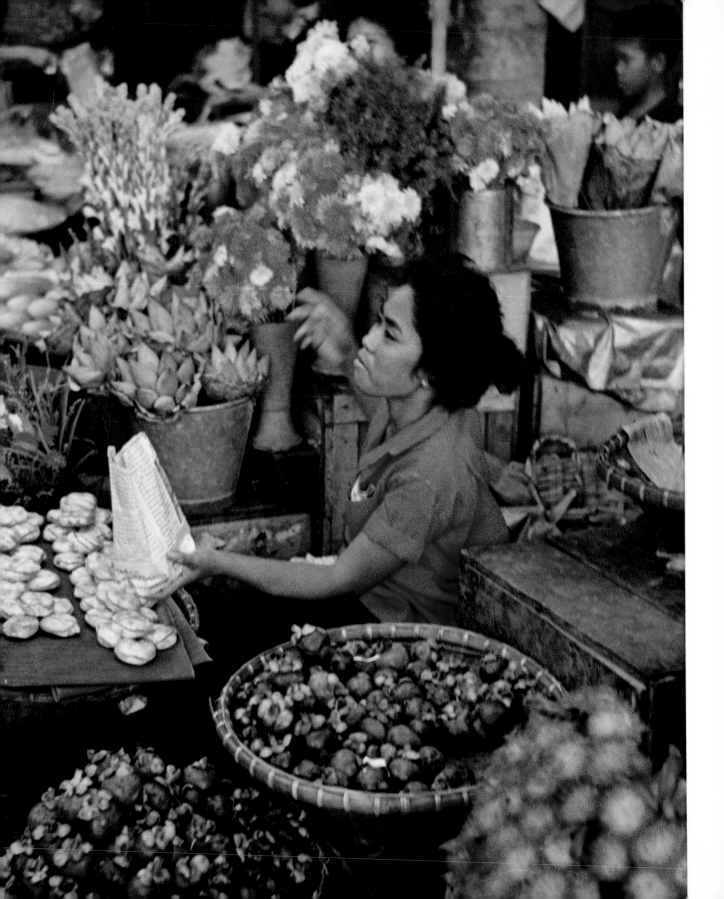

since the Indian sage received his enlightenment under the Bo-tree at Gayà. It is not only the government of the generals, keeping their powerful protecting hand over the kingdom, which is at stake, but rather the anxious question put to me by my visitor in the twilit hotel room at Kowloon, before he said good-bye . . . 'What is the most essential thing today?'

In the fresh early morning air I visited the market near the hotel once more before my departure. Laden rowing-boats were moving along the *klong*; at the edge of the road were mounds of pineapples; small eating-houses were enjoying a lively custom; children on their way to school gathered round the Chinese booths which had sweets for sale; flower-stalls looked inviting with their bright colours. And once again I saw the monks clad in yellow, with heads bowed, and in front of them charming young women knelt and offered rice and lotus-flowers. One man had taken off his shoes in the market throng before presenting his gift; the city street was transformed into a sanctuary.

Departure from Bangkok and the Tropics

I acquired two pounds of mangosteens, whose tender white flesh is hidden under such a hard, dark skin, and stuffed them into one of the bags which are not weighed with one's luggage. In the midday heat I boarded my Swissair machine again.

And now the film was shown in reverse: the Calcutta airport with its shop where you can see the gilt-edged *saris* for the last time; the Karachi reception-building with its night-time activity; at sunrise Arabs in their long garments served coffee at the airport in the desert near Cairo; and at midday we landed in front of the smart reception-buildings at Kloten. On the terrace was a throng of spectators, and among them friends and relatives were waving; the loudspeaker summoned passengers to other flights to London and Athens, Lisbon, Buenos Aires, Belgrade, Stockholm, and New York.

The Flight Home

Asia after Thirty Years of
World History

HOW CAN I sum up my impressions of this journey, and in what way do they differ from my experiences of Asia on previous visits? In the interval of thirty to thirty-five years a great deal has changed in Europe too: the development of technology has entered a new revolutionary phase and changes have occurred in the social system. Asia too has become something different, in itself as well as for us.

In the 1920's the traveller was still greatly impressed by unfamiliar mentalities and cultures: the dominating strength and exclusive art of Islam, the imagery of Hinduism welling up from the depths of the soul, the realm of the Buddha with his transcendental smile, the demons and sages of China, the delicate flowers and bloody swords of the Samurai—all this confronted us as phenomena of world history, beside which the colonial powers exercised the relatively modest function of policemen.

Today the Western type of colonialism is irrevocably past. There is now at last a serious effort to unite the world discovered by the seafarers of the 15th and 16th centuries. Unity is to some extent being enforced by technology; for there are many peoples and cultures, many different images of God, but physics is universal and railways, road surfaces, and sewing-machines are virtually the same everywhere. This technology has been developed almost exclusively in Europe and America, and the political and social ideas which are today absorbing the attention of national leaders in Asia are of the same origin: there is democracy, realised by universal suffrage and various parliamentary systems; there are claims that life should be safeguarded by the State, and there are demands for social justice. Even the ideas that radiate from Moscow go back beyond Catherine and Peter, Marx and Hegel, to the same origins as European enlightenment.

At the end of the First World War, Wilson proclaimed the sovereign rights of the people. The Second World War brought a new message from the United States—the claims of under-developed countries to assistance from highly developed nations. Every politician has to reckon with these claims today; but the nations in whose names they were raised in Asia are mostly quite different from the countries in which the ideas originated. The right to vote is exercised chiefly by illiterates, who have never cared a rap about it and who were given overnight what was in Europe the culmination of a long political development.

The educated classes—and this means here almost exclusively those educated according to the principles of European civilisation—have become a new ruling class of politicians, in whose minds a desire to compensate for the humiliations suffered during their term of apprenticeship and struggle plays its part. With their eagerness to plan, these intellectuals are in constant danger of losing contact with their people, and while they are debating in parliament, a new reformer or saint or demagogue may start the masses off in another direction. Administrative incompetence or corruption are a reason for reviving the old game of power and giving up the appearance of free elections; then the strongest decides what will benefit the people most, what is 'truly' democratic, and what is legal. Since my recent visit three Asiatic countries—Pakistan, Thailand, and Indonesia—have given up the pretence of a parliamentary régime and switched over to a presidential dictatorship. In several cases military leaders have taken over the control of politics, because the army has proved to be the most reliable organisation in the country— it, too, by the way, is a creation of Western instructors.

The bogey of Western imperialism will not last for ever; the young nations must consolidate their position by their own strength; they must justify the freedom which they have achieved in the eyes of their own people and their neighbours;

today they put forward claims as 'under-developed' nations; but tomorrow they will have to honour their obligations to make the most of the money entrusted to them and place their mineral wealth at the disposal of world planning. Their failure to do this will deliver them up to a new kind of colonialism; the new colonial power, however, is already standing at every door, gaining ground at every weak spot; sometimes it comes prepared for a friendly compromise, sometimes with drawn revolver; but it is always aiming inexorably at world domination.

The Population
Problem

Even more urgent and serious than the struggle for supremacy between the two power blocks, in the eyes of many who know Asia well, appears the problem of over-population, which intensifies year by year.

As late as the 18th century, in the old civilised nations of Europe too the birth-rate was high, but every biography of that period reveals a degree of infant mortality which to our minds today is appalling, and only a minority reached old age. With the progress of medicine and hygiene the average expectation of life rose, and the population increase was retarded by the individual making up his mind not to have more children than he was able to support. In the national sphere too there was a new balance of forces: inventions of all kinds created work for the extra population, and made it possible for the general wealth to increase steadily. This much we can recognise today as being the result of a hundred years of development; and even the first pioneers of the development are not conceivable without the two thousand years' history of ideas, without the spirit of research and exploration which ever since the Renaissance has been ever more impetuously pushing towards the limits of the earth; without the individual contribution and vitality of each one of the peoples participating in this evolution.

Among the old civilised nations of Asia only Japan has taken part in this development, or at least, in its latter stages.

Of all the achievements of Western civilisation none has spread so rapidly and generally as the scientific struggle against epidemics and diseases of all kinds. The missionaries were often pioneers of medicine—in Siam the American missionaries were called 'doctors'. Colonial lords as well as native potentates who wished to be able to stand the scrutiny of the world competed in the building of hospitals. Charitable institutions in America supplied vaccines and pharmaceutical products generally. Nations which have gained their independence are meantime redoubling their efforts to train their own people in medicine, and send them out to the farthest villages with their pills and hypodermic syringes. Famines too, which previously used to claim millions among the masses of India and China, can nowadays be tackled much more easily with the aid of mechanical transport.

The ancient balance of birth and death has been disturbed, and births are increasingly in excess from year to year. In the rural districts of Malaya, infant mortality in 1927 was still 263 per 1,000; in 1950 it was 82 and by 1956 it had been reduced to 42. Five years ago the population of India was increasing annually by some 5 million, today it increases by 7 million. At the present moment, it is reckoned that Asia has an excess of births over deaths of 25 million per year, and if this trend continues, the 1,500 million Asians will have increased within a quarter of a century to 3,000 million.

More than half of all humanity lives in Asia, but it has only a seventh of the land surface at its disposal, and an even smaller fraction of the mineral deposits. It has been pointed out that the economic potentialities of some countries are still very far from being fully exploited: in India there are 304 inhabitants per square mile, whereas in Japan there are 505, in England and Wales 770, in the Netherlands as many as 883. But against this it must be said that these are highly industrialised countries which have been most thoroughly cultivated for decades. In India a cow yields scarcely a tenth of the milk of a cow in Switzerland; and an

Indian field produces only a fraction of the crop that can be harvested from the same area in Europe.

All this can be improved by means of artificial fertilisers, sounder methods, properly trained personnel, dams, and above all, money and more money. In this process habits and customs have to be overcome which are centuries old and in some cases even sacred. India is trying to tackle the problem through a system of planning which treats tradition with caution and consideration and leaves a certain margin to individual initiative, whereas China attacks the problem with a ruthless use of the whole of its national labour potential. But both require American or Russian aid over and above what they can achieve themselves.

And each year there are more millions to feed, each year more millions must be found work and a livelihood. To their horror the planners find that all their strenuous efforts are being overtaken by the growth of population, that all their new irrigation systems, agricultural reforms, and newly built factories scarcely suffice to absorb the annual increase, and that the much-hoped-for raising of the standard of living can never be achieved by the present means. As a report by the Ford Foundation has pointed out, by 1965 India will no longer be able to feed a large proportion of its population unless something extremely drastic is to be done. Sir Julian Huxley, the British biologist, on his last journey to Asia, was deeply impressed by this alarming situation, and according to him the fate not only of India, but of the entire world, now hinges on what India can achieve in solving its population problem as related to its economic development.

A few years ago it seemed as though China was about to assume leadership in the campaign for birth-control, but since then nothing further has been heard of this; presumably the leaders in Peking have meanwhile calculated that for the time being they require some further scores of millions for their labour battalions. In Hongkong a 'planned parenthood foundation' has been instituted; in Singapore, a professor has suggested that parents of three children should be given an opportunity to undergo voluntary sterilisation. With the exception of the Roman Catholic Church, which continues to hold strictly to its conception of natural law, Christian Churchmen and representatives of other religions have reluctantly indicated their agreement with, or at least their toleration of, birth-control. Early in 1959, Nehru opened the Sixth International Planned Parenthood Conference, which proceeded to recommend urgent measures for the restriction of births. In this respect the 'enlightened' Asiatic has fewer inhibitions to overcome than the European, who regards the production of a large number of children as something morally desirable, if not indeed as his national duty. But to the Indian or Chinese the ethical problem looks different, a desperate situation is creating new laws and commandments.

The Japanese have progressed farthest: their legislation of 1949 permits abortion and all kinds of prevention of conception, and surgical intervention has since been practiced in more than a million cases each year. While before the war the annual number of births per 1,000 inhabitants was 34, it has dropped to 17; in 1948 the increase in population was 22 per 1,000, in 1957 only 9 per 1,000. It is nowadays considered to be a patriotic duty to limit one's family to three children.

The unity of the world confronts both politician and onlooker with more and more new tasks. Conclusions from analogy—as they present themselves in the study of history—can lead to misjudgments and false decisions. Concepts themselves change with place and time; the elements of situations react in a way contrary to our previous experience. Concepts have probably never before been so confused as they are today, when the old familiar words are applied to a new situation which cannot be understood by any historical comparison. We talk of Red dictatorship, a callous totalitarian régime, Soviet imperialism, but these words are not trump-cards in the struggle for the soul of Asia. Everything would be much simpler if in the Kremlin and the new Forbidden City there was no

Confusion of Concepts

more than the naked pursuit of power, as formerly in the New Chancellery of the Reich. For there is some justification for the socialists even in the most cruel Red terror if, in the last analysis, it makes 'progress' possible; the measures taken by the oppressor do not work to the advantage of a master race as in Fascism, for purges and bitter struggles for control serve the complete realisation of the humanitarian socialist ideology. Hundreds of millions of people used to live a life of privation without anyone doing anything about their material welfare—now an objective is offered to them, a panacea; they have nothing to lose. The free world must make haste; it must play for the highest stakes if it wants to carry over into a new era the heritage of its saints and sages, which has been painfully acquired over the centuries.

The nations of Asia have a huge working potential at their disposal; their talents have been shown in great cultural achievements; mineral resources are waiting to be tapped. But their rhythm of life is different from ours, it is not *their* civilisation; left to themselves they have never hitherto felt the urge to reach the Pole or the highest peaks in the world, to analyse matter to its smallest constituents, or to invent the fastest conveyances. Will they be able to fit in with the course of a world united by technology in good time, so that they can participate not only by means of foreign credit and the results of foreign research but as equal partners in the society of free nations? Or will they still remain dependent on help from the 'developed' countries, tacking between the 'great powers' and playing them off one against the other?

The visitor to Asia is surprised by the almost complete absence of any serious attempt to bring the great national creative achievements into a synthesis with the demands of the machine age. Apart from a few exceptions—such as the followers of Gandhi and the keepers of the Shinto tradition—hardly any start has been made among the leading classes in the East to preserve the heritage of their fathers and to find in it the driving force for a genuine contribution of their own to the further development of mankind. In their struggle against the imperialism of the West politicians in particular make references all the time to the ideas of this same West; there is no question for them of restoring the conditions which existed before the colonial powers took over.

Even the care of ancient monuments was in many cases first suggested by Europeans and Americans like Fenollosa, Fergusson, Havell; these are regarded as museums—Hindus from Delhi no longer think of the magnificent buildings of the Mogul emperors as evidence of a foreign faith and a foreign master, and in Red China the temples of the Lamas, Taoists, and Confucians may be looked on as national show-pieces without any regard for their spiritual significance. Although modern publicity and transport have given new life to the pilgrimages and festivals, divine service itself is in danger of becoming a tourist attraction.

Who can see today what Asia's own creative contribution to the future state of the world will be? What reserves are still slumbering in these peoples who have inherited thriving kingdoms? Will they with their ability and vitality once more become the tool of foreign interests or will they make others conscious of their ascendancy? Only one thing is sure today: they belong to our world; they will also have a voice in our fate.

Index

Numerals in italics refer to plates

Index

Springer
London
Berlin
Heidelberg
New York
Barcelona
Hong Kong
Milan
Paris
Singapore
Tokyo

Miriam Sperber (Ed.)

Radiologic Diagnosis of Chest Disease

Second Edition

With 427 Figures

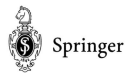

Springer

Miriam Sperber, MD
Department of Diagnostic Imaging, Vall d'Hebron Hospital, Universitat Autonoma,
Barcelona, Spain

Cover illustrations: Insets show conventional chest radiography, MRI and CT, commonly employed in the
diagnosis of chest diseases.

ISBN 1-85233-298-0 2nd edition Springer-Verlag London Berlin Heidelberg

ISBN 0-387-97099-1 1st edition Springer-Verlag New York Berlin Heidelberg
ISBN 3-540-97099-1 1st edition Springer-Verlag Berlin Heidelberg New York

British Library Cataloguing in Publication Data
Radiologic diagnosis of chest disease. – 2nd ed.
    1. Chest – Imaging.   2. Chest – Diseases – Diagnosis
    I. Sperber, Miriam
    617.5'4'0757
ISBN 1852332980

Library of Congress Cataloguing-in-Publication Data
Radiologic diagnosis of chest disease/Miriam Sperber (ed.) – 2nd ed.
    p. ; cm.
    Includes bibliographical references and index.
    ISBN 1-85233-298-0 (alk. paper)
    1. Chest – Imaging.   2. Chest – Radiography.   I. Sperber, Miriam.
    [DNLM: 1. Radiography, Thoracic.   2. Diagnostic Imaging.   3. Thorax – pathology.
4. Thorax – radionuclide imaging.   5. Thorax – ultrasonography. WF 975 R129 2001]
RC941. R26 2001
617.5'40757 – dc21   00-038603

First published 1990
Second edition 2001

Typeset by EXPO Holdings, Malaysia
Printed and bound at the Cromwell Press, Trowbridge, Wiltshire
28/3830-543210 Printed on acid-free paper SPIN 10728391

This book is dedicated with love to my children:
Dr. Steven Sperber, Dr. Galia Angela Sperber and
Alex Sperber, LLB.

Foreword

Prior to the virtual atomic explosion of medical knowledge, at a time when communication was very much slower, a medical book, to be authoritative and believable, had to be written by a very knowledgable, and, per force, usually quite senior person. The choice of texts was limited and tended to be dominated by a few "classic" (a phrase not quite synonymous with dogma). Following the information explosion, the scenario is quite different. Not only is there a geometric progression in the quantity and speed of development of new medical knowledge, but also this development is occurring at very different rates in different countries.

This is particularly true in medical imaging. The result is that it is now virtually impossible to produce a "single author" book that can cover the field or even a subdivision of it. This absolute requirement for multiple authors has in turn created the need for a new type of editor/author who must be multinational in approach, have a uniquely informed appreciation of what is going on in medical imaging research throughout the entire world and possess the depth of personal knowledge and experience to judge correctly what work is the most rigorous and likely to have the greatest impact. This "new-wave" editor must further have the personality and kudos to be able to persuade the chosen few to add still further to their burdens by writing a book chapter!

This book epitomizes what can be achieved by just such an editor, Miriam Sperber, MD. The first edition of this book set a high standard in clarity and concise coverage and the new revised text ensures that even in this fast-moving information era, the book retains its leading position at the cutting edge of medical imaging in pulmonary medicine. Dr. Sperber's eminent team of authors has provided us with a mine of information and I believe that the reader will find that every chapter contains the rarely found gold of new knowledge.

Eric N.C. Milne, MD, FRCR, FRCP (Edin.)

Preface

X-RAYS: Their moral is – that a right way of looking at things will see through almost anything.

Samuel Butler, *Note-Books*, Vol. V

It is always a thrilling experience to prepare a new edition of a textbook, and a daunting one as well. Firstly, there is the natural gratefulness for the gift of life and experience that allows a renewed revision and summary of collected knowledge in a specific area. Then, there is the exciting appreciation of wonderful advances in the studied domain. One worries whether the attempt to bring forward the inspiring progression will be successful, as well as accurately reflect the continuous search for additional answers to existent medical queries.

Thoracic radiology has proven itself to be a fitting component of a new, reinvented and vigorous diagnostic field. To paraphrase Newton, we look back with humility and admiration to the giants that preceded us, and while standing on their shoulders, have the possibility of seeing a bit further. Roentgen's initial vision, courage and determination have been undoubtedly replicated in the works of pioneers of the chest-imaging area, such as Leo Rigler, Felix Fleischner and Benjamin Felson. Their thinking power and dedication serve as an example for an endless line of radiologists working in this field. It is with great sadness that I have to mention here the untimely loss of one of their top representatives, a wonderful friend and supporter, Charles Putman, who was due to contribute a chapter to this volume, and whose professional excellence was matched by extraordinary human qualities. This Preface is dedicated to him.

Nowadays, when reviewing chest radiology, it has become imperative to discuss not only the new and improved diagnostic capabilities resulting from the utilization of advanced techniques, but also the impact that these technologies have on medical therapeutics in general. The high quality and extensive diagnostic details provided by new imaging modalities have ensured that, currently, thoracic radiology occupies a central place in the diagnostic process, as well as in the follow-up of a given patient.

Localization and extension of primary and secondary lesions, early signs and development of diffuse lung disorders, vascular and bony anomalies, and many other pathologic changes, are clearly and reliably identified, due to refinements occurring in recent years in the existent diagnostic techniques. Computed tomography has seen the development of spiral, high resolution and volumetric studies, while Magnetic resonance imaging strives to perfect the use of new imaging materials. Far from being forgotten, conventional radiology is under continuous scrutiny, as the desire exists to improve its capabilities in such vital areas as the intensive care unit or malignancy screening.

Our volume has the goal of faithfully depicting the above, while at the same time underlining the importance of the close cooperation necessary between diagnostic radiologists and their clinical counterparts. We are proud to have been able to include among our eminent authors representatives of both categories, which will certainly enhance the book's ability to correctly reflect the daily diagnostic dilemmas of a medical and radiologic practice. It will also add to its capability of providing necessary and valuable information both to the young trainee and to the experienced specialist.

Moreover, the highly international character of our contributors is of paramount importance in the transmission of the global spirit of modern medical science, and thus will increase the value of the presented material, as a shared experience of experts from important medical centers all over the world.

Our book is being published, appropriately enough, at the dawn of a new millennium. Radiologic sciences can certainly be counted among the greatest discoveries of the last thousand years. It is therefore the time to look forward to many more scientific advancements, with the hope that, in the words of a great luminary of our time, Albert Einstein, "human benefit will remain our main concern, while technology will be a blessing, and not a curse to mankind".

Acknowledgments

Making an orchestra play in unison is never an easy task. My role in this case was immensely facilitated by the quality of the players. I am greatly indebted to all contributors to this volume for agreeing to share their experience and for their exceptional effort in providing material of the highest quality. It was a great pleasure and a privilege to cooperate with them all.

My thanks go also to my dear friends and colleagues, Dragutin Novak, MD, Eric N.C. Milne, MD, and José Cáceres, MD, for their continuous support and encouragement.

My secretaries Nikki Edwards and Gloria Simpson dealt in a splendid manner with often complex organizational jobs.

Last, but not least, my love and thanks go to my family for providing a wonderful and vital foundation for my work. I couldn't do it without them.

Miriam Sperber, MD

Contents

Part 3   Diseases of the Lung and Related Structures

Contributors

J. Andreu
Department of Radiology
Hospital General Vall d'Hebron
Pg de la Vall d'Hebron 119–129
08035 Barcelona
Spain

M.C. Anglade
Hôpital Henri Mondor
Service de Radiologie
Creteil Cedex
France

Y. Berthezene
Department de Radiologie
Hôpital Croix-Rousse
103 Grande rue de la Croix Rousse
69317 Lyon Cedex 04
France

K.A. Buckwalter
Department of Radiology
Indiana University Medical Center
Indianapolis, IN 46204
USA

J. Cáceres
Department of Radiology
Hospital General Vall d'Hebron
Pg de la Vall d'Hebron 119–129
08035 Barcelona
Spain

Roberto Cancellieri
Instituto di Radiologia
Ospedale S. Evgenio
Tor Vergata University
Piazzale dell'Umanesimo 10
00144 Rome
Italy

S.W. Clarke
Royal Free Hospital
Pond Street
London NW3 2QG
England

P.L. Clouet
Department de Radiologie
Hôpital Croix-Rousse
103 Grande rue de la Croix Rousse
69317 Lyon Cedex 04
France

J. Collins
Department of Radiology
University of Wisconsin Hospital and
   Clinics
E3/311 Clinical Science Center
600 Highland Avenue
Madison, WI 53792–3252
USA

D.J. Conces Jr.
Department of Radiology
Indiana University School of Medicine
University Hospital
550 N. University Blvd
Indianapolis, IN 46202–5253
USA

J.-P. Derenne
Service de Pneumologie et Réanimation
Groupe Hospitalier Pitié Salpêtrière AP-
   HP
47–83 Boulevard de l'Hôpital
75651 Paris Cedex 13
France

K.R. Flaherty
Division of Pulmonary and Critical Care
Department of Internal Medicine
University of Michigan Medical Center
Ann Arbor, MI 48109–0360
USA

G.A. Fontana
Department of Critical Care
Section of Respiratory Medicine
University of Florence
Italy

P. Gehr
Institute of Anatomy
University of Berne
Buehlstrasse 26
CH-3000 Berne 9
Switzerland

J.D. Godwin
Department of Radiology
University of Washington Medical Center
Box 357115
Seattle, WA 98195
USA

P.C. Goodman
Radiology Department – Thoracic Imaging
Duke University Medical Center
Durham, NC 27710
USA

N.D. Greyson
Department of Nuclear Medicine
St Michael's Hospital
30 Bond Street
Toronto, Ontario M5B 1W8
Canada

B.H. Gross
Professor and Associate Chairman
Department of Radiology
University of Michigan Hospitals and
  Clinics
Ann Arbor, MI 48109–0030
USA

Harumi Itoh
Department of Radiology
Fukui Medical University
Fukui, 910-1193
Japan

S. Jouveshomme
Service de Pneumologie
Groupe Hospitalier Pitié Salpêtrière AP-HP
47–83 Boulevard de l'Hôpital
75651 Paris Cedex 13
France

E.A. Kazerooni
Division of Chest Radiology
Department of Radiology
University of Michigan Medical Center
Ann Arbor, MI 48109–0326
USA

V. Latrabe
Unite d'Imagerie Thoracique et
  Cardio-vasculaire
Hôpital du Haut-Lévèque
CHU de Bordeaux
Avenue de Magellan
33604 Pessac
France

F. Laurent
Unite d'Imagerie Thoracique et
  Cardio-vasculaire
Hôpital du Haut-Lévèque
CHU de Bordeaux
Avenue de Magellan
33604 Pessac
France

F. Lavorini
Department of Critical Care
Section of Respiratory Medicine
University of Florence
Italy

N. Le Flour
Service de Pneumologie
Groupe Hospitalier Pitié Salpêtrière AP-HP
47–83 Boulevard de l'Hôpital
75651 Paris Cedex 13
France

M. López
Department of Radiology
Hospital General Vall d'Hebron
Pg de la Vall d'Hebron 119–129
08035 Barcelona
Spain

D.A. Lynch
Department of Radiology
Box A030
University of Colorado Medical Center
4200 East Ninth Avenue
Denver, CO 80262
USA

J.P. Lynch III
Division of Pulmonary and Critical Care
  Medicine
University of Michigan Medical Center
Ann Arbor, MI 48109–0360
USA

A. Magalhães
Laboratório de Neuroimgem LIM-21
Hospital das Clinicas
University of São Paolo
av Dr Eneas de Calvalho Aguiar 255
São Paolo 05403–010
Brazil

K. Malagari
2nd Department of Radiology
University of Athens
20 Papadiamaudopoupou Street
11528 Athens
Greece

L. Mancini
Instituto di Radiologia
Ospedale S. Evgenio
Tor Vergata University
Piazzales dell'Umanesimo 10
00144 Rome
Italy

R. Manfredi
Department of Radiology
Università Cattolica del S. Cuore
"A. Gemelli" University Hospital
00168 Rome
Italy

J.R. Manzano
HU Germans Trias
Universitat Autonoma
Barcelona
Spain

P. Marano
Department of Radiology
Unversità Cattolica del S. Cuore
"A. Gemelli" University Hospital
00168 Rome
Italy

B. Marchand
Department de Radiologie
Hôpital Croix-Rousse
103 Grande rue de la Croix Rousse
69317 Lyon Cedex 04
France

E.M. Marom
Department of Radiology – Thoracic
  Imaging
Box 3808
Duke University Medical Center
Durham, NC 27710
USA

F.J. Martinez
Division of Pulmonary and Critical Care
Department of Internal Medicine
University of Michigan Medical Center
Ann Arbor, MI 48109–0360
USA

M. Mascalchi
Department of Clinical Pathophysiology
Section of Radiology
University of Florence
Italy

M. Mata
Department of Radiology
Hospital General Vall d'Hebron
Pg de la Vall d'Hebron, 119–129
Barcelona 08035
Spain

K. McConnochie
Department of Tuberculosis and Chest
  Diseases
Llandough Hospital
Penarth
South Glamorgan CF 64 2XW
Wales

E.N.C. Milne
Department of Radiological Sciences
University of California, Irvine
Medical Center
Orange, CA 92868
USA

M. Montaudon
Unite d'Imagerie Thoracique et Cardio-
  vasculaire
Hôpital du Haut-Lévèque
CHU de Bordeaux
Avenue de Magellan
33604 Pessac
France

J.-F. Mornex
Department de Pneumologie
Hôpital Cardio-vasculaire et
  pneumologique
28 Avenue Doyen Lépine
69500 Bron
France

A. Moscone
Instituto di Radiologia
Ospedale S. Evgenio
Tor Vergata University
Piazzale dell'Umanesimo 10
00144 Rome
Italy

P. Nesme
Department de Pneumologie
Hôpital Croix-Rousse
103 Grande rue de la Croix Rousse
69317 Lyon Cedex 04
France

J. Nishi
Department of Radiology
Kumamoto University
School of Medicine
1-1-1 Honjo
Kumamoto 860-8556
Japan

K. Nishimura
Department of Respiratory Medicine
Graduate School of Medicine
Kyoto University
Sakyo-ku
Kyoto 606-8507
Japan

D. Novak
Institute of Radiology
Adenauerallee 23
53111 Bonn
Germany

S. Oguri
Department of Respiratory Medicine
National Minami-Kyoto Hospital
11 Nakaashihara
Jyouyou-shi
Kyoto 610-0113
Japan

G. Pearson
Section of Chest Radiology
Columbia University College of
  Physicians and Surgeons
630 West 168th Street
New York, NY 10032
USA

T. Pirronti
Department of Radiology
Università Cattolica del S. Cuore
"A. Gemelli" University Hospital
00168 Rome
Italy

M. Pistolesi
Department of Critical Care
Section of Respiratory Medicine
University of Florence
Viale Morgagni 85
50134 Florence
Italy

M. Rebner
Section of Breast Imaging
Department of Diagnostic
  Radiology
Wm. Beaumont Hospital
Royal Oak
MI 48073
USA

P. Reynaud
Service de Chiurgie Thoracique
Hôpital Laennec
Rue de Sevres 42
75007 Paris Cedex 7
France

M. Riquet
Service de Chiurgie Thoracique
Hôpital Laennec
Rue de Sevres 42
75007 Paris Cedex 7
France

Ch. Roussos
University of Athens
Critical Care Department
Evangelismos Hospital
45–57 Hipsilandou Street
Kolonaki
Athens 10671
Greece

M.B. Rubens
Department of Imaging
Royal Brompton Hospital
Sydney Street
London SW3 6NP
England

N.W. Schluger
Department of Medicine
Division of Pulmonary Allergy, and
  Critical Care Medicine
Columbia University College of
  Physicians and Surgeons
630 West 168th Street
New York, NY 10032
USA

G. Sergiacomi
Instituto di Radiologia
Ospedale S. Evgenio
Tor Vergata University
Piazzale dell'Umanesimo 10
00144 Rome
Italy

R. Sheehan
Department of Imaging
Royal Brompton Hospital
Sydney Street
London SW3 6NP
England

T. Similowski
Service de Pneumologie et Réanimation
Groupe Hospitalier Pitié Salpêtrière AP-
    HP
47–83 Boulevard de l'Hôpital
75651 Paris Cedex 13
France

A.K. Simonds
The Royal Free Hospital
Pond Street
London NW3 2QG
England

G. Simonetti
Instituto di Radiologia
Ospedale S. Evgenio
Tor Vergata University
Piazzale dell'Umanesimo 10
00144 Rome
Italy

M. Sperber
Department of Radiology
Hospital Vall d'Hebron
University of Barcelona
Spain

S. Sperber
Department of Medicine
Mount Vernon Hospital
Rickmansworth Road
Northwood
Middlesex MA6 2RN
England

S.G. Spiro
Department of Thoracic Medicine
University College London Hospitals
Middlesex Hospital
Mortimer Street
London W1N 8AA
England

D.L. Spizarny
Department of Diagnostic Radiology
Henry Ford Hospital
Detroit, MI
USA

C. Straus
Service Central d'Explorations
    Functionnelles Respiratoires
Groupe Hospitalier Pitié Salpêtrière,
    AP-HP
47–83, Boulevard de l'Hôpital
75651 Paris Cedex 13
France

J.E. Takasugi
Department of Radiology S-113
Puget Sound VA Health
    Care System
1660 S. Columbian Way
Seattle, WA 98108
USA

M. Takahashi
Department of Radiology
Kumamoto University
1-1-1 Honjo
Kumamoto 860-8556
Japan

R.D. Tarver
Department of Radiology
Indiana University Medical Center
Wishard Memorial Hospital
Indianapolis, IN 46202
USA

S. Tomiguchi
Department of Radiology
Kumamoto University
School of Medicine
1-1-2 Honjo
Kumamoto 860-8556
Japan

N. Vasile
Service d'Imagerie Medicale
Hopital Henri Mondor
51 rue du M.de Lattre de Tassigny
94010 Creteil
France

P. Vock
Department of Radiology
University Hospital Inselspital
3010 Berne
Switzerland

D. Westra
Department of Radiology
Academisch Medisch Centrum
Amsterdam
Holland

M.K. Wood
Department of Thoracic Medicine
University College London Hospitals
Middlesex Hospital
Mortimer Street
London W1N 8AA
England

A.R. Wright
Department of Radiology
St. Mary's Hospital
Praed Street
London W2 1NY
England

M. Zelter
Service Central d'Explorations
    Fonctionnelles Respiratoires
Groupe Hospitalier Pitié Salpêtrière AP-HP
47–83 Boulevard de l'Hôpital
75651 Paris Cedex 13
France

1

Anatomy

1 Normal Anatomy of the Human Lung and Associated Structures

P. Gehr

Introduction to Pulmonary Morphology: An Overview

Functional Morphology

The respiratory tract is part of a system that conducts oxygen from outside air to the mitochondria in the cells throughout the body. It is therefore the most common route of entry for toxic substances from the environment. The same thinness and delicacy of the air–blood barrier in the lung that facilitates the passage of oxygen also reduces its effectiveness as a barrier to toxic substances (Fig. 1.1). As they are transported through the airway system to the gas exchange region, toxic substances may be deposited anywhere on the epithelium, depending on a variety of factors, and enter the tissue.

Variabilities

Apparently there are scarcely any systematic structural variabilities of the human respiratory tract, for example due to body size, growth, age, sex, or ethnic origin, that would fundamentally influence its function. In general there are differences between individuals, mainly genetically based, but they belong to a normal interindividual variability. Differences in organ size are usually proportional to difference in body size. Even the growing human lung, after the age of 2 years, does not seem to deviate principally in its structure from the adult lung (1,2).

However, the effect of body size or growth has been found to be smaller for more distal than for more proximal airways of the conductive zone (trachea, bronchi, and bronchioli). From this it has been predicted that deposition of particulate inhalants would be highest in the newborn and decrease with increasing age to 21 years. This model prediction also indicates that, in general,

smaller individuals will receive greater initial deposition within the conductive zone than will larger individuals, at a given ventilatory state. It is therefore concluded that smaller individuals might be at greater risk from many types of airborne inhalants (3).

At greater age the wall structures of the airways experience some changes, particularly in the connective tissue compartments.

Occasionally the azygos vein is lower in the right upper lobe, causing a fissure. The portion of this lobe on the medial side of the fissure forms the so-called azygos lobe, which is easily detectable on an X-ray by the shadow caused by the four layers of the pleura.

There is very little information about gender-related differences. Up to the age of 14, boys apparently have larger lungs than girls (1). It is controversial whether women's airways are smaller than men's relative to lung size.

Differences between ethnic groups are probably mainly dimensional differences, ie., differences in body size that are reflected in proportional differences in lung size.

There exist considerable morphologic variabilities in the airway system between species. The structure of the wall and the geometry of the conducting airways are very variable. There are also important structural differences at the level of the respiratory bronchioles. In some species they are absent; others, including human, have three to five generations (4,5). These differences are such that they might well influence the deposition and clearance pattern of particulate inhalants. The structure of the gas exchange parenchyma, however, is very similar among mammals, the structural diffusing capacity being directly proportional to body size over six orders of magnitude (6).

Anatomy of the Chest

This section deals with the topography of the chest organs (7–11).

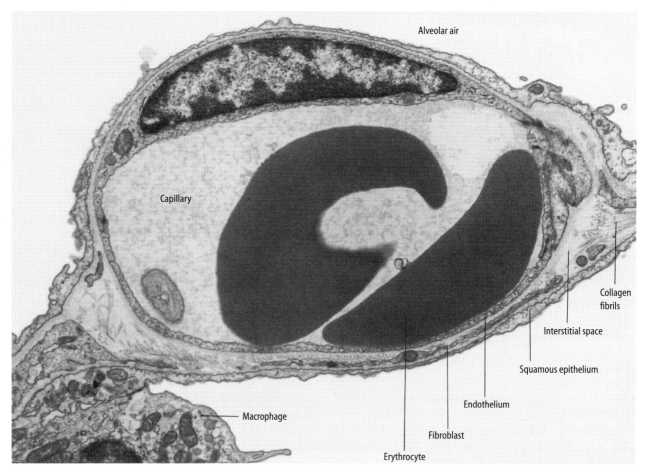

Figure 1.1. Electron micrograph of interalveolar septum demonstrates air–blood barrier, consisting of three layers: endothelium, interstitial space, and epithelium (×14 250)

Chest Wall and Thoracic Cavity

The skeletal boundaries of the *thoracic cavity* are anteriorly the sternum and the rib cartilages, and, laterally and posteriorly, the ribs, the intercostal spaces, and the vertebral column. Cranially an open communication exists to the neck region. Abdominally it is closed by the diaphragm, which bulges deeply into the thoracic cavity; hence the outer borders of the thorax do not coincide with those of the cavity. The diaphragm is flatter at the center than at the periphery, and higher on the right side than on the left. From the highest point on each side the diaphragm slopes suddenly downward to the costal and vertebral attachments; this slope is more marked and longer behind than in front, so that only a narrow space is left between the diaphragm and the posterior wall of the thorax (Figs. 1.2 and 1.3).

The chest capacity does not correspond with the skeletal thorax, because the lower part of the region enclosed by the ribs is encroached upon by the diaphragm and the upper abdominal viscera. The capacity varies with the phase of respiration, which also affects to some extent the positions and relations of the thoracic viscera. Its arbitrary upper limit is usually taken as the plane of the thoracic inlet, but the apices of the lungs extend above this into the neck.

The thoracic cavity is divided by the mediastinum, the region between the lungs that extends from the back of the sternum to the vertebral column and from the thoracic inlet above to the diaphragm below. It contains the heart enclosed within a fibroserous sac, the pericardium, and other organs that are embedded in loose connective tissue. The lungs occupy the right and left parts of the thoracic cavity. Each one is covered with a serous membrane, the pleura, which also lines the walls of the corresponding half of the chest, and forms the lateral boundary of the mediastinum.

The *pleural cavities* are airtight, closed serous spaces that are filled out to a capillary cleft from medial by the lungs. They are lined by the *parietal pleura* (costal, mediastinal, and diaphragmatic portions) on the outer side and by the *visceral pleura* on the inner side.

The costal pleura covers the sternum, the ribs, the constituent parts of the transverse thoracic muscle, and the

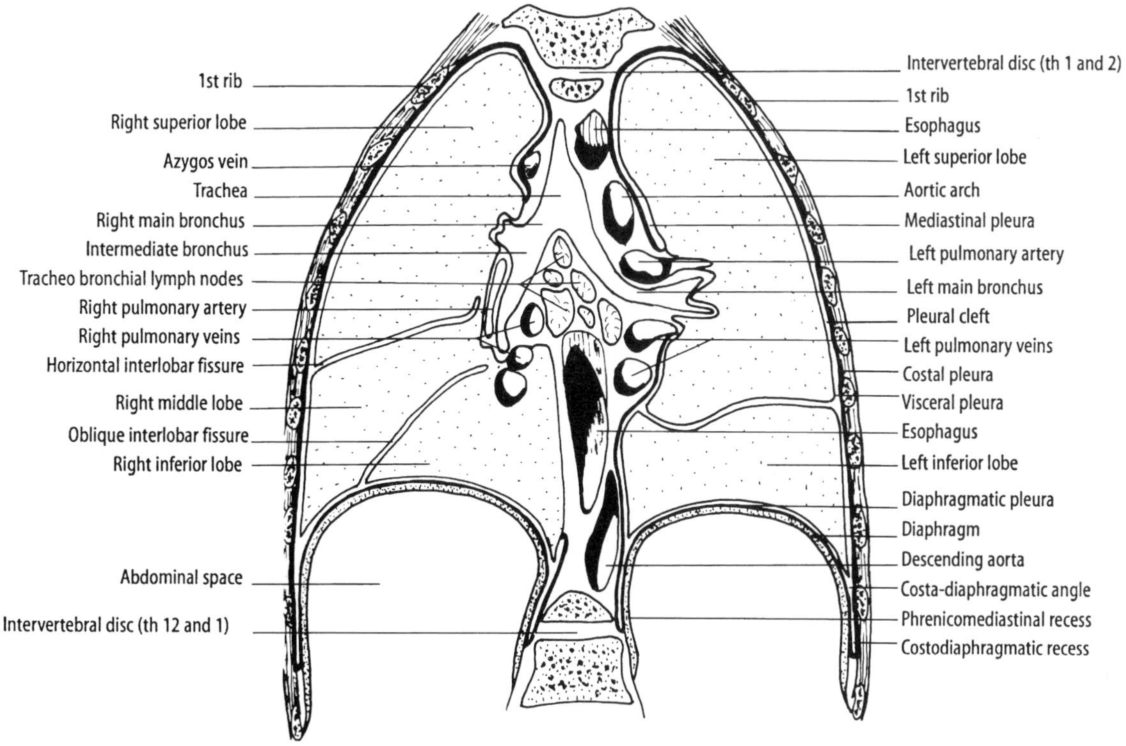
1st rib
Right superior lobe
Azygos vein
Trachea
Right main bronchus
Intermediate bronchus
Tracheo bronchial lymph nodes
Right pulmonary artery
Right pulmonary veins
Horizontal interlobar fissure
Right middle lobe
Oblique interlobar fissure
Right inferior lobe
Abdominal space
Intervertebral disc (th 12 and 1)
Intervertebral disc (th 1 and 2)
1st rib
Esophagus
Left superior lobe
Aortic arch
Mediastinal pleura
Left pulmonary artery
Left main bronchus
Pleural cleft
Left pulmonary veins
Costal pleura
Visceral pleura
Esophagus
Left inferior lobe
Diaphragmatic pleura
Diaphragm
Descending aorta
Costa-diaphragmatic angle
Phrenicomediastinal recess
Costodiaphragmatic recess

Figure 1.2. Frontal section through thorax (redrawn from ref. 9, with permission). Dorsal of midaxillary line.

sides of the bodies of the vertebrae, and forms the dome of the pleura over the apex of the lung. It extends from the internal border of the first rib medially and upward to the apex of the lung, its summit reaching as high as the lower edge of the neck of the first fib; it then descends along the side of the trachea to become continuous with the mediastinal pleura. Owing to the obliquity of the first rib, it extends 3–4 cm above the first costal cartilage, but does not rise above the level of the neck of the first rib. It reaches, like the apices of the lungs, the level of the seventh cervical spine at a distance of 2.5 cm from the median plane. The subclavian artery, directed upward and laterally, occupies a furrow slightly below the summit of the costal pleura.

The mediastinal pleura forms the lateral boundary of the interpleural space or mediastinum. Above the lung it is a continuous sheet between the sternum and the vertebral column. That of the right side is in contact with the right brachiocephalic vein, the upper part of the superior vena cava, the terminal part of the azygos vein, the right phrenic and right vagus nerve, the trachea, and the esophagus. That of the left side is in contact with the arch of the aorta, the left phrenic and left vagus nerves, the left brachiocephalic and superior intercostal veins, the left common carotid and subclavian arteries, and the esophagus. It encloses the structures of the lung root (hilus) and passes into continuity with the visceral pleura. Below the lung root it extends as a double layer, called the pulmonary ligament, from the hilus to the mediastinal surface of the lung, where it is again continuous with the pulmonary pleura. It ends in a free falciform border.

The diaphragmatic pleura covers the upper surface of the corresponding side of the diaphragm. The outer part of its circumference is continuous with the costal pleura; medially it is continuous with the mediastinal pleura along the line attachment of the pericardium to the diaphragm.

The inferior limit of the pleura is on a considerably lower level than the corresponding border of the lung. The costal and diaphragmatic pleurae are here separated only by a narrow slit, the costodiaphragmatic recess (complementary space). In quiet respiration the lower limit of the lung is about 5 cm above the lower limit of the pleura. A similar condition exists behind the sternum and rib cartilages, where the anterior thin margin of the lung falls short of the line of pleural reflection, and where the slit-like cavity between the two layers of pleura forms the costomediastinal recess (complementary space) (Figs. 1.2 and 1.3).

The shape of the thorax is variable, depending on the shape of the vertebral column, the position of the transverse processes, the length, curvature, and direction of the ribs, and the way the ribs are connected to the sternum. According to these anatomic properties two extreme shapes can be distinguished: the short and wide thorax, and the long and narrow thorax. The short and wide thorax is characteristic of infants and, in adults, is found particularly in older people. Shape changes occur during

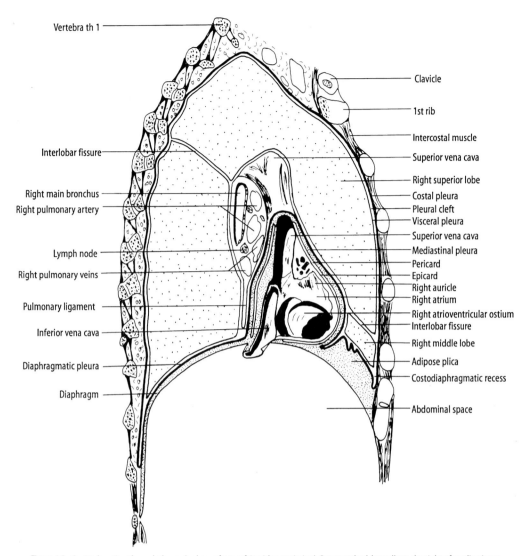

Vertebra th 1

Interlobar fissure

Right main bronchus
Right pulmonary artery

Lymph node

Right pulmonary veins

Pulmonary ligament

Inferior vena cava

Diaphragmatic pleura

Diaphragm

Clavicle

1st rib

Intercostal muscle
Superior vena cava

Right superior lobe
Costal pleura
Pleural cleft
Visceral pleura
Superior vena cava
Mediastinal pleura
Pericard
Epicard
Right auricle
Right atrium
Right atrioventricular ostium
Interlobar fissure

Right middle lobe

Adipose plica
Costodiaphragmatic recess

Abdominal space

Figure 1.3. Sagittal section through thorax (redrawn from ref. 9, with permission). Paravertebral, laterally to the right of mediastinum.

life, depending on the individual's constitution and other factors. In the female the capacity is less, absolutely and proportionately. The sternum is relatively shorter and the thoracic inlet more oblique, the suprasternal notch being level with the third thoracic vertebra rather than the second, as in the male. The upper ribs are also more movable in females, permitting comparatively greater expansion of the upper thorax.

The reniform upper thoracic aperture is bounded dorsally by the first thoracic vertebra, ventrally by the jugular incisure of the sternum and laterally by the first rib. It is ventrally tilted; its anteroposterior diameter is about 5 cm and its transverse about 10 cm. The significantly larger inferior aperture is confined by the 12th thoracic vertebra, the free ends of ribs 10 to 12, and the costal arches, which form the infrasternal arch. On its ventral side it is deeply indented by the epigastric angle (Figs. 1.2 and 1.3).

The *diaphragm*, a musculofibrous dome-shaped sheet, closes the inferior aperture. It is the principal muscle of

inspiration. Its dome presents a concave surface toward the abdomen. The central part of the dome is tendinous, with the pericardium attached to its upper surface and the liver to its lower surface. Its periphery consists of muscular fibers attached to the circumference of the thoracic outlet and converging into the central tendon. The muscle fibers may be grouped into three types: sternal, costal, and lumbar. The diaphragm is pierced for the passage of three larger structures:

1. The aorta, the opening for which is the lowest and most posterior. This opening is at the level of the lower border of the 12th thoracic vertebra, slightly to the left of the median plane. The thoracic duct and occasionally the azygos vein also pass through this opening.

2. The esophageal hiatus, the opening for which is in the muscular part of the diaphragm at the level of the 10th thoracic vertebra. This opening is formed by the splitting of the medial fibers of the right crus, which makes

it elliptical in shape. It is above, in front, and a little to the left of the aortic opening. In addition to the esophagus, the vagus nerve and esophageal branches of the left gastric vessels pass through this opening.

3. The vena caval foramen, the highest of the three large openings. This opening is at about the level of the disc between the eighth and ninth thoracic vertebrae. It is quadrilateral and at the junction of the right leaf with the central area of the tendon so that its margins are aponeurotic. It is traversed by the inferior vena cava and some branches of the right phrenic nerve. Two separate clefts in each crus permit passage of the greater and the lesser splanchnic nerves. The diaphragm is innervated by the phrenic nerve. The phrenic nerves and the lower six or seven intercostal nerves distribute sensory fibers to the peripheral part of the muscle.

The intercostal spaces are limited by the costal sulcus of the upper rib and the upper edge of the lower rib. Their width is variable (i.e., the dorsal lower are narrower than the ventral upper).

Three layers can be distinguished in the *thoracic wall:* (a) the superficial layer, consisting of the skin and the subcutaneous stratum, which contains vessels and nerves embedded in loss connective tissue; (b) the middle layer, consisting of the chest wall muscles and their fasciae (ventral musculi pectorales major, minor, and subclavius; lateral musculus serratus; anterior origin of digitations of the musculus obliquus externus abdominis; dorsal muscles of the shoulder girdle); and (c) the deep layer, consisting of the ribs and the intercostal spaces, which are filled with the musculi intercostales externi, interni, and intimi (from outside). Between the internus and the intimus there are the intercostal vein, the intercostal artery, and the intercostal nerve (from the top).

The subfascial lymph drains into the axillary and infraclavicular lymph nodes. There are four regional groups of lymph nodes: the intercostal, posterior mediastinal, diaphragmatic, and parasternal nodes.

The mammae are an essential part of the plastic formation of the anterior chest wall. They are located in the subcutaneous stratum between the parasternal line and the axillary line between the third and sixth ribs.

Mediastinum

The mediastinum is the partition between the two lungs, and therefore includes the mediastinal pleura of both sides; more generally it is defined as the structure between the two pleural sacs. It can be considered as the continuation of the endothoracic layer of the thoracic wall in the sagittal direction, extending from the sternum in front to the vertebral column behind and from the thoracic inlet

above to the diaphragm below. It may be divided into upper and lower mediastinum, the latter being divided again into anterior, middle, and posterior mediastinum (Figs. 1.2 through 1.4).

The *upper mediastinum* lies between the manubrium sterni in front and the upper four thoracic vertebrae behind. It is bounded below by the plane passing through the sternal angle in front and the lower part of the body of the fourth thoracic vertebra behind; it is bounded above by the plane of the thoracic inlet, and laterally by the mediastinal pleurae. It contains the origins of the sternohyoid and sternothyroid and the lower ends of the longus colli muscles; the aortic arch; the brachiocephalic, left common carotid, and left subclavian arteries; the brachiocephalic veins, the upper half of the superior vena cava and the left superior intercostal vein; the vagus, cardiac branches of the vagus, phrenic, and left recurrent laryngeal nerves; the trachea, esophagus, and thoracic duct; the remains of the thymus; and the paratracheal, brachiocephalic, and some of the tracheobronchial lymph nodes (Fig. 1.4a).

The *anterior lower mediastinum* lies between the body of the sternum in front and the pericardium behind (Fig. 1.4b, c). Above the level of the fourth costal cartilages it is an exceedingly narrow connective tissue cleft, owing to the close approximation of the two pleural sacs. It contains only a few structures such as some lymph nodes and some small branches of the internal thoracic artery.

The *middle lower mediastinum* is the broadest part of the lower mediastinum. Most of its space is taken up by the pericardium with the heart (Figs. 1.3 and 1.4b). In addition it contains the ascending aorta, the lower half of the superior vena cava, the terminal part of the azygos vein, the bifurcation of the trachea, the two main bronchi, the pulmonary arteries, the pulmonary veins, the phrenic nerves, the deep part of the cardiac plexus, and some tracheobronchial lymph nodes.

The *posterior lower mediastinum* is bounded in front by the bifurcation of the trachea, the pulmonary vessels, the pericardium, and the posterior part of the upper surface of the diaphragm; it is bounded behind by the vertebral column from the lower border of the fourth to the 12th thoracic vertebrae, and on each side by the mediastinal pleura (Fig. 1.4b, c). It contains the descending thoracic aorta, the azygos and hemiazygos veins, the vagus and splanchnic nerves, the esophagus, the thoracic duct, and the posterior mediastinal lymph nodes.

Topographically the upper mediastinum shows in ventroposterior direction the remains of the thymus, the left brachiocephalic vein, the brachiocephalic artery, the trachea, the esophagus, and the vertebral column (Fig. 1.4a). From a ventrodorsal radiologic view the main structures, however, lie in the middle lower mediastinum: the heart and the large vessels leading to and from the heart that cause the mediastinal shadows. From above downward, the left border of

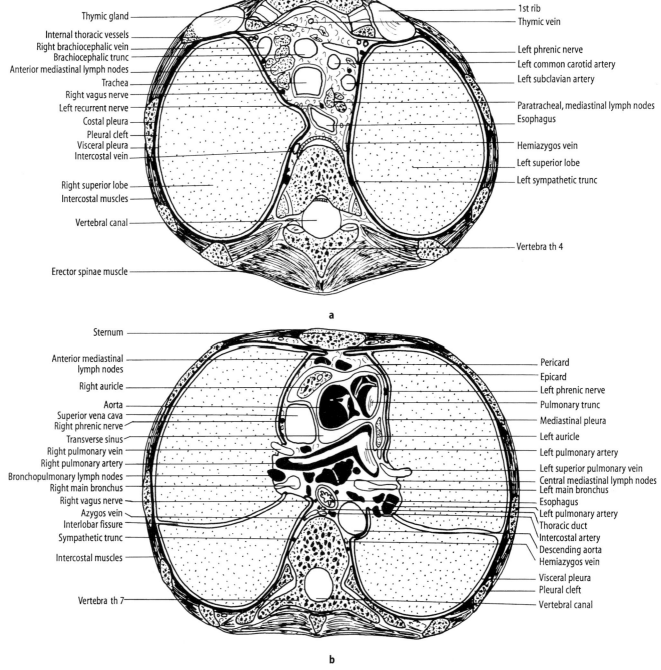

Figure 1.4. Transverse sections through thorax (redrawn from ref. 9, with permission). **a** Section plane on level of fourth thoracic vertebra. **b** Section plane on level of seventh thoracic vertebra.

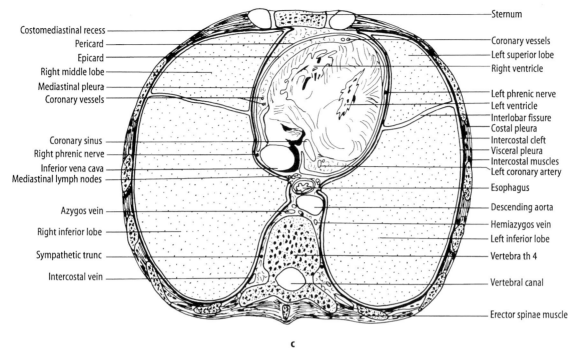

Costomediastinal recess
Pericard
Epicard
Right middle lobe
Mediastinal pleura
Coronary vessels

Coronary sinus
Right phrenic nerve
Inferior vena cava
Mediastinal lymph nodes

Azygos vein

Right inferior lobe

Sympathetic trunc

Intercostal vein

Sternum
Coronary vessels
Left superior lobe
Right ventricle

Left phrenic nerve
Left ventricle
Interlobar fissure
Costal pleura
Intercostal cleft
Visceral pleura
Intercostal muscles
Left coronary artery

Esophagus

Descending aorta
Hemiazygos vein
Left inferior lobe

Vertebra th 4

Vertebral canal

Erector spinae muscle

c

Figure 1.4. c Section plane on level of ninth thoracic vertebra.

this shadow is formed by the left subclavian artery, the arch of the aorta, the left pulmonary artery, the left auricle, and the left ventricle; the right border is formed by the brachiocephalic vein, the superior vena cava, the right atrium, and the thoracic part of the inferior vena cava. On both sides of this mediastinal space the pulmonary vessels entering the lungs constitute the hilar shadows.

Let us follow a few of the main structures that continue through several spaces of the mediastinum. The aorta (ascending) has its origin in the middle lower mediastinum, turns through the upper mediastinum (arch), and continues into the posterior lower mediastinum (descending). The superior vena cava passes from the upper into the middle lower mediastinum. The trachea, located in the upper mediastinum, branches into the right and left main bronchus, located in the middle lower mediastinum. The vagus and the phrenic nerves together enter the upper mediastinum. The vagus nerves pass behind the lung hilus in the posterior lower mediastinum, the right then running on the dorsal side and the left on the ventral side of the esophagus. The right phrenic nerve continues along the upper vena cava and the right contour of the heart, and the left phrenic nerve follows the left contour of the heart in the middle lower mediastinum.

The Extrapulmonary Airways

This section deals mainly with the anatomy and histology of the chest organs (12–17).

The Larynx

The larynx is an organ of phonation, air passage, and sphincteric mechanism (Fig. 1.5). It extends from the oropharynx at the upper border of the epiglottis to the trachea. It projects ventrally between the great vessels of the neck (common carotid artery, internal jugular vein) and the vagus nerve, and is covered anteriorly by the skin, the fasciae, and the depressor muscles of the hyoid bone. Above it opens into the hypopharynx, to which it forms the anterior wall. It is surrounded laterally and anteriorly by the lobes of the thyroid gland. In the adult male it is situated somewhat lower than in the female and the child. Form and size are also different, the length and diameter being larger in men than in women. The average length is 44 mm in males and 36 mm in females; the anteroposterior diameter is 36 mm and 26 mm, respectively.

The skeletal framework of the larynx is formed by the hyoid bone and cartilages (thyroid, cricoid, and arytenoid cartilage; epiglottis), which are connected by ligaments and membranes and are moved by a number of muscles. In effect the larynx itself is suspended from the hyoid bone and slides up and down within a sleeve of connective tissue whenever the hyoid is raised or lowered. The internal lining is a mucous membrane that consists of three pairs of lateral folds, the uppermost aryepiglottic folds, the middle ventricular folds, and the lower vocal folds. They divide the laryngeal cavity into several compartments. The mucosa of the larynx is continuous with that of the pharynx and the trachea and exhibits features of both.

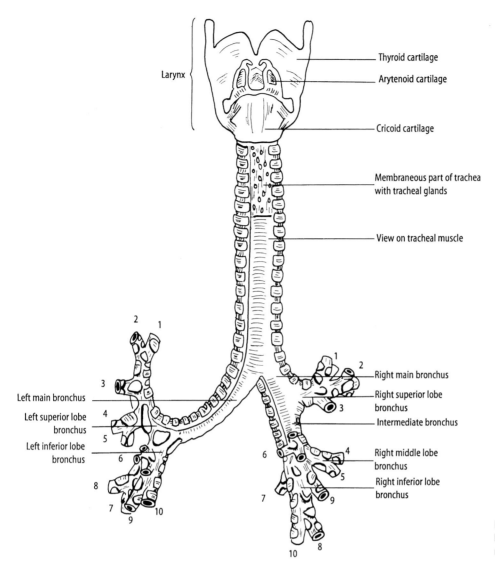

Larynx

Thyroid cartilage

Arytenoid cartilage

Cricoid cartilage

Membraneous part of trachea
with tracheal glands

View on tracheal muscle

Right main bronchus

Right superior lobe
bronchus

Intermediate bronchus

Right middle lobe
bronchus

Right inferior lobe
bronchus

Left main bronchus

Left superior lobe
bronchus

Left inferior lobe
bronchus

Figure 1.5. Airways: larynx to segmental bronchi, segments 1 to 10 (redrawn from ref. 35, with permission). Dorsal view.

Stratified squamous epithelium from above extends partway into the larynx, over the aryepiglottic folds laterally and further ventrally, where it covers the entire lingual side of the epiglottis and the upper half of its laryngeal aspect. It is also present at other points of wear, such as over the vocal folds. Elsewhere it gives way to the typical respiratory pseudostratified, ciliated epithelium, which is coated with a mucus layer. The ciliary beat moves it toward the pharynx. The subepithelial fine connective tissue is rich in elastic fibers. Free cells and also small lymph follicles are abundant here. Underneath, the connective tissue becomes denser and connects the mucosa with the skeletal structures and the cross-striated muscles. Here the laryngeal glands are located.

The chief arteries of the larynx are the laryngeal branches of the superior and inferior thyroid arteries. There are two sets of lymph vessels, a superior group above the vocal folds that drains into the deep cervical lymph nodes situated near the bifurcation of the common carotid artery, and an inferior group below the vocal folds that opens into several lymph node systems, either nodes in front of the cricothyroid ligament, the deep cervical nodes, or nodes alongside the inferior thyroid artery. The nerves are derived from the internal (sensor) and external (motor) branches of the superior laryngeal nerve, the recurrent laryngeal nerve (branches from the vagus nerve), and the sympathetic trunk. Between the vocal folds is the narrow glottal aperture, which is affected by movements of these folds caused by several small, fine, striated muscles. This is the main structural basis for phonation. The closure of the glottal aperture also protects the subsequent airways from penetration of foreign particulate matter. The foreign matter is cleared from the larynx by coughing. With an expiratory effort against the closed glottis for about 0.2 s the pressure in the abdominal, pleural, and alveolar space is raised to 50–100 mmHg or more. Then the glottis is suddenly opened and the air very rapidly forced out (at a rate perhaps exceeding 12 L).

This process blows the foreign matter out (if it is not stuck).

The epiglottis covers the larynx and, hence, protects the lower airways during swallowing. In parallel, the upper airways are covered by the elevation and tension of the soft palate and its firm approximation to the posterior pharyngeal wall by contraction of the muscles of the wall.

The Trachea

The trachea is a hollow cartilaginous and membranous tube, 12 cm long, originating at the base of the larynx and ending below at the carina, where it bifurcates to form the principal bronchus of each lung (Fig. 1.5). It is very mobile and can extend and shorten very rapidly. It is not quite cylindrical, being flattened posteriorly; its external diameter from side to side is about 1.8 cm in the male and a little less in the female. During childhood the diameter in millimeters corresponds approximately with the age in years.

The trachea would collapse during forceful inspiration, or on inspiration against a closed glottis, were it not reinforced by a skeleton of cartilage embedded in its wall. The wall consists of three major layers: a mucosa covering the airspace, a fibrous submucosa containing the cartilage, and an adventitia with which the trachea is embedded in the surrounding tissue.

The tracheal mucosa closely resembles that of the nose and nasopharynx and is virtually identical to that in the lower part of the larynx and in the bronchi. It is lined by a pseudostratified ciliated columnar epithelium, containing many goblet (mucous) cells (Fig. 1.6a, b). It is very sensitive to irritation and responds by increasing in height or even by metaplasia. In addition to ciliated and mucous cells, basal cells stand out because their nuclei form a row close to the basement lamina. These cells do not extend to the free surface and evidently function as a reserve population for the epithelium. There are other types of cells but they have minority representation; they escape notice completely because their distinguishing features are poorly resolved by light microscopy.

The epithelium is covered by a thick mucus lining layer produced by the mucous cells and the tracheal glands. In addition to dead cells, granulocytes, and lymphocytes, it also contains a prominent population of surface macrophages.

The mucus is of a high viscosity and lies above the cilia, which move it oralward by their beat. The cilia are surrounded by a fluid of low viscosity that is produced by the ciliated cells.

Mucus is a protean mixture of molecular species. A main component are the mucins, which, in the respiratory tract, are acid glycoproteins consisting of a polypeptide core and side chains of high molecular weight mucopolysaccharides (proteoglycans), such as sulfated amino sugar or uronic acid (sulfomucins) or sialic acid (sialomucins).

The cilia that move the mucus layer have a diameter of about 0.25 μm and a length of 5–10 μm, the length varying according to location and function (Fig. 1.6a–c). The pattern of movement can be subdivided into two phases, one in which the cilium is extended and moves more quickly and the other in which the cilium is bent and moves more slowly. The first phase produces the main flow of mucus over the cilia; it is therefore referred to as the effective stroke.

The direction of the ciliary beat is always toward the oropharynx, whether in the nasal or in the thoracic parts of the respiratory tract. The beating frequency of tracheal cilia is about 700–1000 at a body temperature of 37 °C. It diminishes toward the periphery. The flow rate of the mucus was found to be about 5–6 mm in the trachea, decreasing to 0.005 mm min^{-1} in the distal bronchioles (18–21). Mucus secretion and ciliary beat are independent, but directional transport of mucus by cilia is an interdependent event.

A variety of different cell types may make up the mature respiratory epithelium (Fig. 1.6a, b). The cellular composition changes, particularly approaching the peripheral airways. There are also interspecies differences as far as the cellular composition is concerned. Among the heterogeneous group of nonciliated epithelial cells, a few are distinguished by the presence of long, straight, and rather thick brush-like microvilli; they are therefore called brush cells and are conspicuous in the trachea of rats, but not easily seen in other species. Other nonciliated cells exhibit an immature character in their structural composition. They are assumed to develop and differentiate into mature epithelial cells of different types and are therefore called indifferent cells. Finally, there is another small basal cell, much less frequently found, characterized by a cytoplasm filled with small dense-core granules, and therefore called small-granule cells (Kulchitsky cells). They constitute a heterogeneous population of neuroendocrine cells generally characterized by the ability to take up amine precursors and store the amines in cytoplasmic granules (amine precursor uptake and decarboxylation; APUD). Occasionally they are found in close association with pulmonary nerves. They are mostly solitary and sparsely distributed along the intrapulmonary and extrapulmonary airways from the trachea to the alveolar ducts. They might, however, occur as clusters in the upper tracheal epithelium, close to the larynx, and are then called neuroepithelial bodies (22). The small-granule cells are difficult to see in routine microscopic slides. Special staining methods may be used to distinguish three different types in the human respiratory tract.

Intraepithelial nerve processes may also be found. Moreover, excretory ducts of the tracheal glands open into

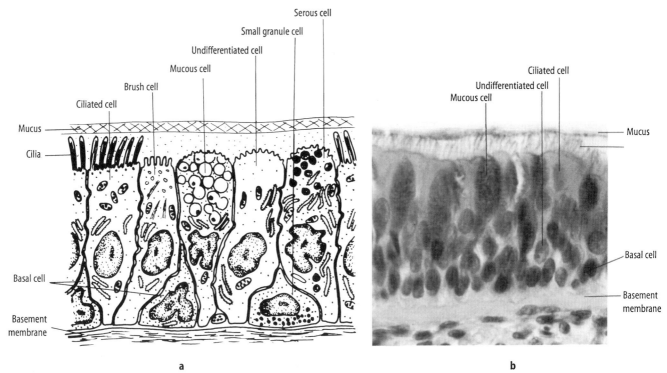

a

b

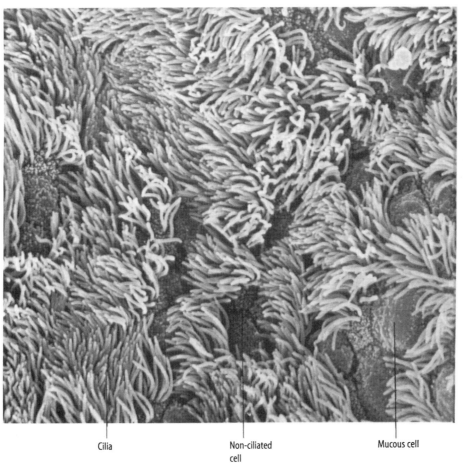

c

Figure 1.6. Histology of tracheal wall. **a** and **b** Epithelium of trachea. Ciliated cells predominate; there are many interspersed goblet mucous (cells). (**a**, redrawn from ref. 10, with permission; **b**, courtesy of ER Weibel, Department of Anatomy, University of Berne, Berne, Switzerland. ×1000.) **c**. Scanning electron micrograph of tracheal epithelium from top (×3100).

the tracheal lumen through the epithelium. In humans these glands are mixed mucous with serous crescents. Around the trachea they generally extend into the submucosa; some secretory portions might even be found in the adventitia. They also be preferentially in the intercartilage compartments.

The fine subepithelial connective tissue (lamina propria) contains interwoven collagenous and particularly abundant elastic fibers, many small blood and lymph vessels, and the usual fixed and free cells of connective tissue. The elastic fibers run in a predominantly longitudinal direction. The submucosa has relatively fewer elastic fibers and more collagen than the propria. It contains the distributing vessels and lymphatics as well as nerves of the tracheal wall. Its connective tissue surrounds the 16 to 20 C-shaped hyaline cartilages that encircle the trachea on its ventral and lateral aspects. The incomplete cartilage rings are separated by interspaces bridged by fibroelastic tissue. The posterior wall, adjacent to the esophagus, is devoid of cartilage. Instead there is a thick layer of smooth muscle bundles that run transversely (Fig. 1.5). They are inserted into the dense fibroelastic connective tissue surrounding the cartilage. The adventitia consists of loose connective tissue containing larger vessels and nerve apposed are lymph nodes.

The arteries for the trachea are mainly from the inferior thyroid. The lymphatics drain into the paratracheal lymph nodes (see Fig. 1.13). The nerves supplying the trachea arise from the recurrent branch of the vagus nerve and from the sympathetic trunk.

The Main Bronchi

The trachea divides into two main extrapulmonar branches called the main (primary, principal) bronch (Fig. 1.5). They are smaller than the trachea, measuring about 1.2 cm in diameter, and also much shorter. The right one is only about 2.5 cm long, whereas the left one is about 5 cm long; the right one is more vertical and the left one more transverse and a little narrower. Their structure is the same as in the trachea. Together with the main pulmonary vessels and nerve they enter the hilum of their respective lungs.

The Lung

Morphologic Overview

The lungs occupy the thoracic cavity, which is smaller on the left than on the right, owing to the position of the heart. Consequently, the right lung is always larger than the left and is subdivided into a greater number of lobes, with three in the right versus two in the left lung. The lobes are separated from each other but confluent at the hilus. They

are covered by the visceral pleura, a connective tissue layer made of collagen and elastic fibers, and lined by a squamous epithelium (mesothelium). Just as the lungs can be subdivided into lobes, the lobes can be subdivided into smaller units, the bronchopulmonary segments, which are incompletely separated from each other by connective tissue sheets originating from the pleura. The right lung is made up of ten such segments, three in the superior lobe, two in the middle, and five in the inferior lobe; the left lung can be subdivided into eight segments, four in the superior and four in the inferior lobe. Deviations from this pattern might occur (occasionally there are five segments in the lower left lobe). Accordingly the main (principal) bronchi give rise to the lobar bronchi, three in the right lung and two in the left lung, which again divide into the segmental bronchi in the same number and distribution as the above-mentioned bronchopulmonary segments. Clinical interest in the branching pattern of the human lungs extends to the level of bronchopulmonary segments. Peripherally the airways continue with this dichotomous branching pattern. Since the two new generations differ in their dimensions (unequal branchings), the branching pattern is called irregular dichotomous. Independent of this pattern there are on the average 10 generations of bronchi whose diameter diminishes from 12.2 to 1.3 mm and whose length diminishes from 47.6 to 4.6 mm from generation 1 to generation 10 (5).

Intrapulmonary Airways

The Conducting System

Structure of Bronchi

As soon as the bronchi enter the lungs (*lobar bronchi*), the cartilage rings disappear and are replaced by irregularly shaped, hyaline cartilage plates that completely surround the bronchi (Figs. 1.5, 1.7). As a result the intrapulmonary airways are cylindrical and not flattened on one side, as are the trachea and the principal (extrapulmonary) bronchi. As one follows the air passages peripherally, the cartilage plates become smaller, elastic, and irregularly distributed around the tube. There is a fourth layer, the smooth muscular layer (tunica muscularis), that completely surrounds the bronchus but does not form a closed ring.

The bronchial lumen is lined by a respiratory mucosa (tunica mucosa) very similar to and continuous with the one in the trachea, consisting of a respiratory epithelium that is covered by a mucus lining layer and of the fine subepithelial connective tissue (lamina propria). The epithelium is set off from the lamina propria by a prominent basement membrane. As a result of contraction of the subsequent smooth muscle layer the mucosa shows a

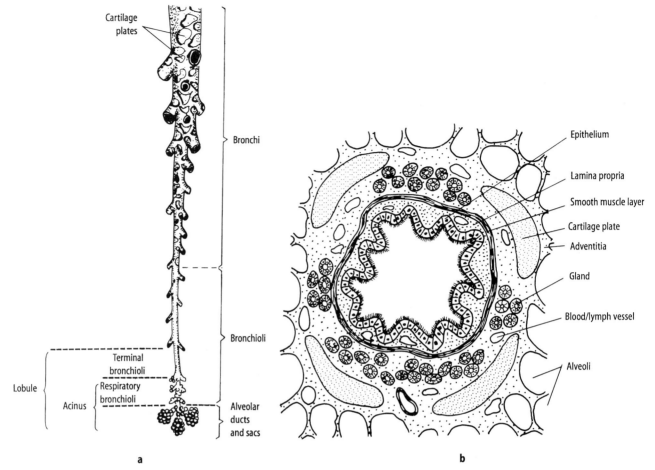

Figure 1.7. Intrapulmonary airways (redrawn from ref. 10, with permission). **a** Subdivision distal of segmental bronchi. **b** Transverse section through a medium-sized bronchus.

marked longitudinal folding on histologic sections. Numerous elastic fibers of the lamina propria are intimately associated with the smooth muscle cells of the muscle layer. Both components play an important part in the changes in lung volume during respiration. The cartilage plates are embedded in a layer of collagenous fibrous connective tissue. Between these plates numerous mucoserous glands are located (Fig. 1.7b).

The outermost tunica adventitia consists of loose connective tissue that contains many elastic fibers. It is continuous with the surrounding pulmonary tissue and accompanies the large vessels. Vessels of the systemic circulation (bronchial arteries), lymphatics, and nerves run in this layer. Diffuse lymphatics tissue occurs regularly in the mucosa and in the adventitia. Lymph nodes can be found in the adventitia of larger bronchi, particularly at bifurcations.

The bronchi are accompanied by the pulmonary arteries (bronchoarterial units). The pulmonary veins (venules) arise from the capillaries of the pleura (systemic, nutritive, bronchial circulation) and of the interalveolar septa and portions of the alveolar duct (pulmonary circulation). They run in the interlobular and intersegmental connec-

tive tissue, independently of the arteries, and join to form the pulmonary veins (Fig. 1.8). In the peribronchial and periarterial connective tissue run the bronchial arteries and veins, the vessels of the systemic circulation (nutrition). Except for the hilar region their blood is brought back by pulmonary veins. There are arterioarterial, bronchopulmonary, and venovenous bronchopulmonary anastomoses. The bronchial vessels do not go beyond the bronchial tree. The bronchial arteries and veins are much smaller than the pulmonary vessels. They arise from the aorta or the intercostal arteries.

There are two main divisions of lymphatics; one set is in the pleura and the other in the pulmonary tissue. They communicate infrequently and drain into the lymph nodes at the hilu. The nerves arise from the pulmonary plexuses at the roof of the lung, which are formed by branches of the vagus nerve and the thoracic sympathetic ganglia.

Structure of Bronchioli

The elastic cartilage plates disappear from the wall when the diameter of the airway approaches 1 mm; the airways

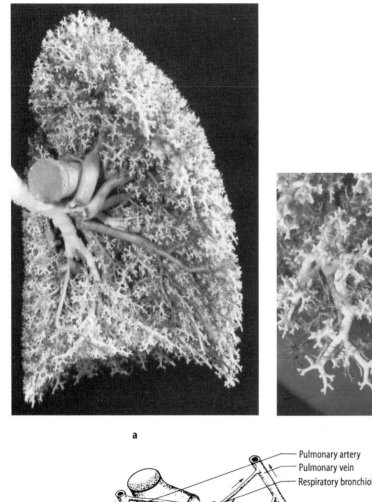

a

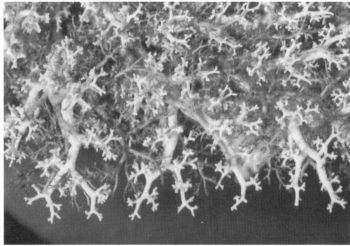

b

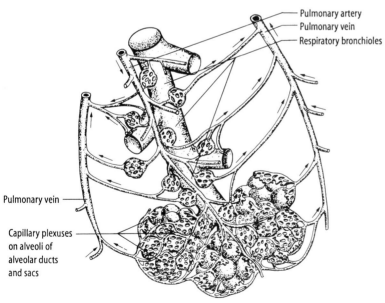

Pulmonary artery
Pulmonary vein
Respiratory bronchioles

Pulmonary vein

Capillary plexuses
on alveoli of
alveolar ducts
and sacs

c

Figure 1.8. Pulmonary blood circulation (the pulmonary system).
a Cast of airway system and pulmonary vascular system. (Courtesy
of W. Weber, Department of Anatomy, University of Berne,
Berne, Switzerland.) **b** Higher magnification of peripheral region
demonstrating the bronchioloarterial units as axial structures of the
lobuli and the interlobular pulmonary veins. **c** Blood circulation of pulmonary lobule (redrawn from ref. 10, with permission).

are now called bronchioles (Fig. 1.9). Gradually other bronchial characteristics are lost and new ones acquired. The bronchioles, generations 11 to 15 (5), are the airways without cartilage, mucoserous glands, and goblet cells. The wall has gradually become thinner. The epithelium is now much lower, columnar to cuboidal, with a unique type of secretory cell (the Clara cell) replacing the mucous cell, and the muscularis is proportionally thicker as compared with that in the bronchi, although not a continuous layer. The subsequent thin connective tissue layer consists of a fine network of interwoven collagenous and elastic fibers that continue into the interalveolar septa; it contains small lymphatics and fine nerves. The bronchioles are accompanied by branches of the pulmonary artery. Two major cell types, ciliated and nonciliated, line the bronchioles. In the larger branches most cells are ciliated, but the nonciliated cells usually dominate the smaller branches. The major nonciliated cell type, the Clara cell, gives the epithelium its special character. It is tall and dome shaped, and protrudes into the bronchiolar lumen to the tips of the cilia. Hence the bronchiolar epithelium has a scalloped contour on sections. There are marked interspecies variations in the structure of Clara cells. The bronchioles comprise on average generations 11 to 16, their diameter diminishing from approximately 1 to 0.6 mm and their length diminishing from approximately 4 to 1.7 mm (5).

The Transitory System

Respiratory Bronchioles

The last generation (no. 6) of the bronchioles are called terminal bronchioles (5). They supply a pulmonary lobule with air (Figs. 1.7, 1.9). The lobules are the structural units of the gas exchange parenchyma and are incompletely separated from each other by the interlobular connective tissue septa. They are about 1 mL in volume. The connective tissue borders of the peripheral (subpleural) lobules reveal a typical texture on the pleural surface (Fig. 1.10). The functional unit is the acinus, which is supplied with air by the two first generations of branches after the terminal bronchioles, the respiratory bronchioles. Hence, one can say that each lobule consists of two acini (Fig. 1.7a).

The respiratory bronchioles are different from the terminal bronchioles in that they have alveoli apposed to their walls – only a few in their first generation (no. 17), but twice as many, on the average, in their last generation (no. 19). These alveoli are the first respiratory structures and therefore have come to give these airway generations the name "respiratory bronchioles" (Figs. 1.7, 1.9). The diameter of one branch does not change much over these three generations, diminishing to a little less than 0.5 mm. The length diminishes still more markedly

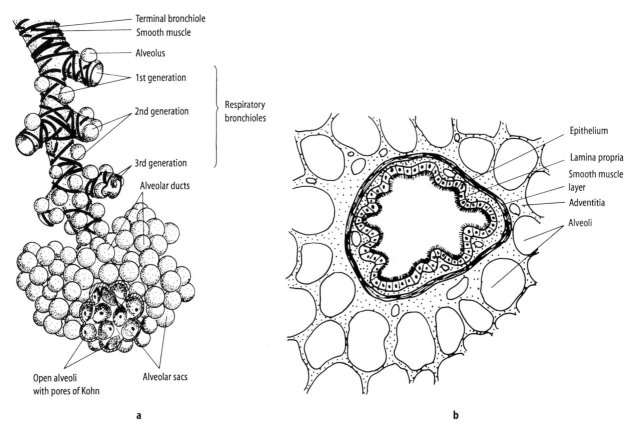

Figure 1.9. The bronchioli (redrawn from ref. 10, with permission). **a** Part of lobule with distal airways. **b** Transverse section through a bronchiole.

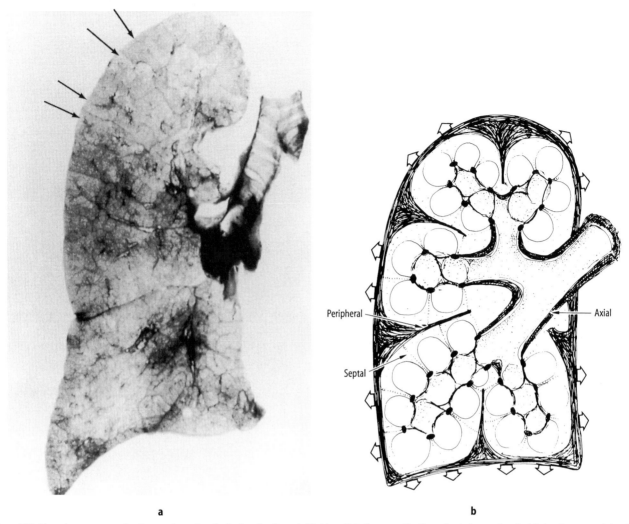

Figure 1.10. The pulmonary connective tissue system. **a** Longitudinal section through dried lung. Note the connective tissue sheets demarcating the lobules; the most peripherally situated lobules reveal the characteristic texture on the pleura (*arrows*). (Courtesy of W. Weber, Department of Anatomy, University of Berne, Berne, Switzerland.) **b** Schematic representation of the fibrous continuum. (From ref. 38, with permission).

from 1.7 to 1 mm. The wall structure is very similar to that of the last generations of bronchioles, except that there are far fewer ciliated cells in the epithelium. At the alveolar rim the epithelium becomes continuous with the thin alveolar lining. Since this portion of the airways is conductive as well as gas exchanging in character, it is called transitory.

Alveolar Ducts

An average of four generations of alveolar ducts, generations 20 to 23 (5), follow the respiratory bronchioles. Their walls are completely covered with alveoli. Each alveolus has an entrance ring, which is a reinforcement of the interalveolar wall by collagenous and elastic fibers and smooth muscle cells. Hence the duct wall in fact consists of alveolar entrance rings (Fig. 1.11). The diameter of the

alveolar ducts also diminishes slightly, the last generation measuring approximately 0.4 mm. The ducts become gradually shorter, with their length diminishing from 1 to 0.6 mm. The last generation (no. 23) ends blindly and is therefore called an alveolar sac. Terminal alveoli cover the peripheral end of the duct. They are the shortest units, being only 0.5 mm long. The diameter stays unchanged. Since this part of the lung consists only of gas exchange units, it is called the gas exchange zone. From the respiratory bronchioles, the pulmonary arteries divide; a branch passes to each alveolar duct and is distributed in a capillary network over all the alveoli that communicate with this duct. The venules arise from these capillaries (Fig. 1.8c). The interstitial fluid is drained along the interalveolar septa into the pleural, interlobular, and peribronchiolar connective tissue, where it is taken up by the lymphatics. No nerves have been observed in interalveolar septa.

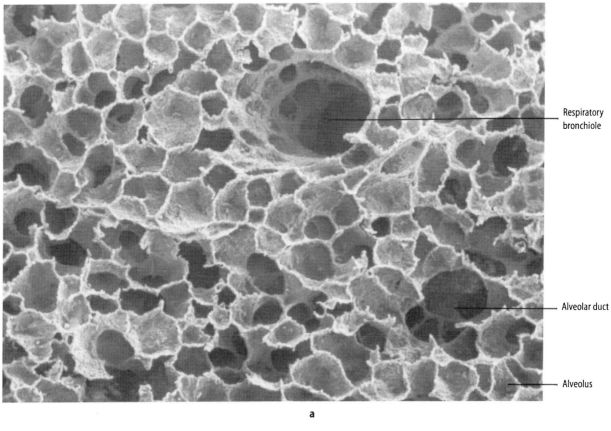

Respiratory
bronchiole

Alveolar duct

Alveolus

a

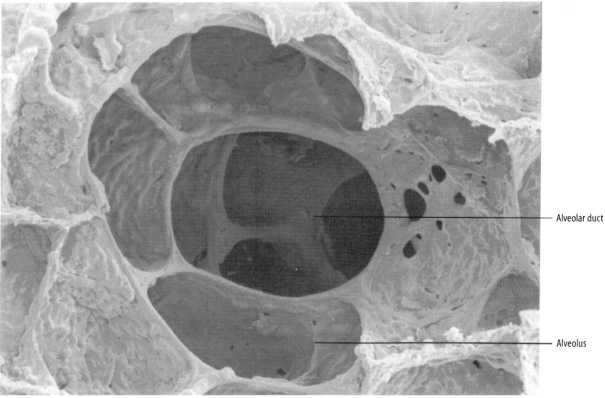

Alveolar duct

Alveolus

b

Figure 1.11. Scanning electron micrographs of gas exchange parenchyma. (From ref. 23, with permission.). **a** Respiratory bronchiole and alveolar duct surrounded by alveoli (×80). **b** Alveolar duct with adjacent alveoli (×240).

The lung is designed to establish optimal conditions for the exchange of oxygen and carbon dioxide between blood and air. In a healthy adult human, over 80% of the lung is gas exchange parenchyma, which consists of 300 million alveoli (5) arranged concentrically around alveolar ducts and sacs (Fig. 1.11). These densely packed alveoli provide a gas exchange surface of 140 m² (23), which is about the size of a tennis court.

The Gas Exchange System

The Gas Exchange Parenchyma

The structural basis for gas exchange is the *alveolar wall*, or, since two adjacent alveoli have a common wall, the interalveolar septum (Figs. 1.1, 1.11). Here air and blood come into close contact and are separated by a barrier as thin as 2 μm, which is only about 1/50 of the thickness of a piece of airmail paper. Nevertheless, this barrier is composed of three layers: the epithelium, interstitium, and endothelium. Oxygen crosses this thin barrier and reaches the erythrocytes, which pass by very closely and frequently touch the endothelium. The capillaries meander around a connective tissue frame, exposing their thin air blood barrier to the alveolar air on either side, and therefore load oxygen from two adjacent alveoli. About 200 mL of blood flow through these capillaries, which is roughly the volume of a red wine glass (23,24).

Crapo et al. (25), by counting pulmonary cells by the mean nuclear caliper diameter method, showed that in the healthy human lung there is on the average a total of 230 × 10⁹ cells. The average includes type I and type II epithelial cells, endothelial cells, interstitial cells (not specified), and macrophages. Type I epithelial cells cover 93% of the alveolar surface; only 7% are covered by the surfactant-producing type II epithelial cells. However, there are twice as many type II as type I epithelial cells. Each type I epithelial cell covers a huge alveolar surface area of 5100 μm². However, there is a large interspecies difference in the number of macrophages. Macrophages (Fig. 1.12) were found to comprise 9% of all cells of the human lung parenchyma (roughly 20 × 10⁹ cells), which is three times as much as in the other species investigated. It is interesting to note that if humans are separated into smokers and non-smokers, the nonsmokers have a percentage of macrophages similar to that found in baboons and rats (approximately 3%), whereas smokers could have six times more.

The Surfactant

The surfactant system is designed to function as a stabilizer of the airspaces; it maintains alveolar stability at end-expiratory volumes and also reduces the work when alveoli are to be opened. The surfactant can be demonstrated in situ by electron microscopy. It consists of the surface active monolayer of phospholipids and an amorphous hypophase that smoothes out the gas exchange surface of the alveoli.

Biochemical analyses revealed that the surfactant material is a complex mixture of phospholipids, neutral lipids, proteins, and carbohydrates. Among the phospholipids, phosphatidylcholine (lecithin) is by far the largest component. The phosphatidylcholine molecules contain two saturated fatty acid constituents. The most frequent fatty acid constituent is palmitic acid; hence the most abundant component of surfactant is dipalmitoyl phosphatidylcholine (DPPC). This is the component that is actually responsible for the surface tension-lowering property.

DPPC is constantly turned over. Therefore its synthesis is a continuous process, for which the type II epithelial cells are responsible. The place of production is the endoplasmic reticulum; the phospholipid is then stored in the lamellated bodies, which are characteristic for the type II cells. They develop from multivesicular bodies. The surfactant material is then secreted onto the alveolar surface, from which it may later be removed and broken down by the alveolar macrophages. Deficiency of the surfactant system is at the origin of the respiratory distress syndrome.

The Connective Tissue System

The conducting airways and their accompanying structures (blood vessels, lymphatics, supporting structures such as cartilage, musculature, glands) are surrounded by connective tissue that originates from the hilus and extends into the fibrous network of the alveolar entrance rings in the wall of the alveolar ducts. According to its location it is called the axial connective tissue. Another connective tissue sheet originates from the visceral pleura that covers the lobes and extends into the depth of the lung, surrounding incompletely the lobules (interlobular septa) and the bronchoarterial units. This tissue sheet is connected to the pulmonary veins and lymphatics. It is called the peripheral connective tissue. These two connective tissue systems are connected with each other by the fine three-dimensional fibrous system of the interalveolar septa. The entirety of this spatial fibrous continuum forms the pulmonary connective tissue system (Fig. 1.10). In particular, with all the histiocytes (connective tissue macrophages) and lymphatics located here, this compartment is important with respect to slow clearance and chronic retention.

The interstitial space follows the continuous fiber system. Hence, the interalveolar septal interstitial space

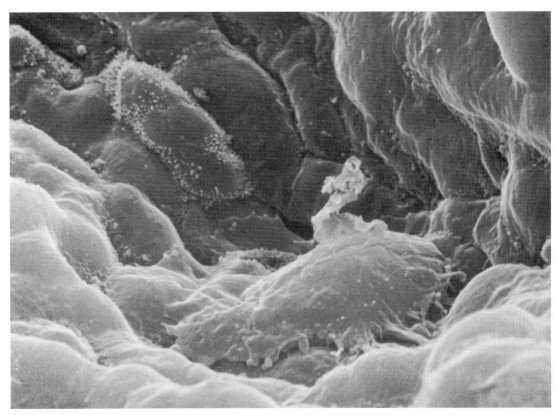

Figure 1.12. Scanning electron micrograph of alveolar macrophage (×2100). (From ref. 23, with permission.)

connects directly with the juxtaalveolar connective tissue sleeves of the airways and blood vessels, and of the interlobular septa, where the lymphatics originate. Although the interalveolar septa do not contain lymphatics, the fiber system establishes a draining pathway from the septa space to the peripheral fluid sumps, where the lymph is removed by lymphatic capillaries.

Inhaled particulate matter may enter the interstitial space freely or engulfed by surface macrophages (26). Free particles may then be phagocytosed by macrophages and retained for a very long time or cleared directly by the draining pathway. This material will continue into the tracheobronchial lymph nodes.

The Glands

The submucosal connective tissue of the nose, pharynx, larynx, trachea, and bronchi houses numerous glands of the branched tubuloacinar type that produce a mixed seromucous secretion. The secretory cells are located at the terminations of the branching ductwork. Up to a dozen such smaller ducts may lead into a collecting duct that can be as long as 1 mm. This duct finally pours its contents into a funnel-like invagination of the airway epithelium, which is covered with ciliated cells (Fig. 1.7).

In cross-section the glands may have a diameter of 0.2 mm, or less than one third of the thickness of the airway wall between the surface and the fibrocartilage layer. The density of the openings in the trachea is of the order of 1 mm^{-2}. The glands become more sparse toward the distal bronchi, paralleling the decreasing amount of cartilage.

The secretion of the glands complements the secretion of the goblet cells of the surface epithelium. Together they make up the mucus layer of these compartments of the respiratory tract, which contains water admixed with some mucins, serum proteins filtered from the blood, secretory immunoglobulin, some immunoglobulin M, the bacteriostatic protein lactoferrin, and some uncharacterized muco- and glycoproteins derived from serous or seromucous cells also present in the glands. In addition there are secretions added from bronchiolar cells located deeper within the lungs. Serous cells are more confined to the glands, but a few may also occur in the surface epithelium.

The Pulmonary Vasculature

Extrapulmonary Vessels

The *pulmonary trunk* conveys deoxygenated blood from the right ventricle of the heart to the lungs (Fig. 1.8). It is about 5 cm long and 3 cm in diameter, and arises from the base of the right ventricle above and to the left of the supraventricular crest. It runs upward and backward, at first in front of the ascending aorta and then to its left side. In the concavity of the aortic arch it divides, at the level of the fifth thoracic vertebra, into right and left pulmonary arteries that are of slightly different sizes.

The whole of the pulmonary trunk is contained within the pericardium. In front the pulmonary trunk is separated from the sternal end of the left second intercostal space by the pleura, the left lung, and the pericardium. Behind are at first the ascending aorta and the left coronary artery. At a higher level the pulmonary trunk lies in front of the left atrium, and the ascending aorta is on its right side. The auricle of the corresponding atrium and a coronary artery lie on each side of its origin. The superfical part of the cardiac plexus lies between the division of the pulmonary trunk and the arch of the aorta.

The *right pulmonary artery* is slightly longer and larger than the left. It runs horizontally to the right, behind the ascending aorta, superior vena cava, and upper right pulmonary vein, and in front of the esophagus and the right bronchus to the root of the right lung, where it divides into two branches. The lower and larger of these goes to the middle and lower lobes, and the upper and smaller accompanies the upper right lobar bronchus.

The *left pulmonary artery* is a little shorter and smaller than the right. It runs horizontally in front of the descending aorta and left bronchus to the root of the left lung, where it divides into two branches, one for each lobe. Above, it is connected to the concavity of the aortic arch by the ligamentum arteriosum, on the left of which is the left recurrent laryngeal nerve and on the right the superficial part of the cardiac plexus.

Before it reaches the hilus, the right pulmonary artery gives off a superior branch to the upper lobe, which at first lies in front of the superior lobe bronchus but soon comes to lie posterolateral to it. The main stem of the right pulmonary artery passes laterally between the superior lobe bronchus and the continuation of the principal bronchus and then lies posterolateral to the latter in the oblique fissure of the lung, supplying branches to the middle and lower lobes. The superior branch of the right pulmonary artery gives off the following branches: apical, anterior descending, anterior ascending, posterior descending, and posterior ascending. The branch to the middle lobe arises from the stem of the right pulmonary artery close to the origin of the superior branch to the lower lobe, and it divides into lateral and medial branches that supply the corresponding segments of the middle lobe. The stem supplies the following branches to the corresponding segments of

the lower lobe: superior, subsuperior, medial basal, anterior basal, lateral basal, and posterior basal.

The left pulmonary artery, having crossed in front of the left principal bronchus to gain its posterolateral aspect in the hilus, gives off the following branches to the upper lobe segments: apical, posterior, anterior descending, anterior ascending, and lingular. Thereafter the artery may supply the following branches to the lower lobe: superior, subsuperior, medial basal, anterior basal, lateral basal, and posterior basal.

The *pulmonary veins* return the oxygenated blood from the lungs to the left atrium of the heart. They are four in number, two from each lung, and are destitute of valves. They commence in the capillary network in the walls of the alveoli, and, joining together, form a single trunk from each lobe, three from the right lung and two from the left. The vein from the middle lobe of the right lung generally unites with that from the upper lobe, so that ultimately two veins, a superior and an inferior, leave each lung. They perforate the fibrous layer of the pericardium and open separately into the upper and posterior part of the left atrium.

In the root of the lung the superior pulmonary vein lies in front of and a little below the pulmonary artery; the inferior is situated at the lowest part of the hilus and on a plane posterior to that of the superior vein. The principal bronchus is behind the pulmonary artery. On the right side the superior pulmonary vein passes behind the superior vena cava, and the lower veins pass in front of the descending thoracic aorta. Within the pericardium, their anterior surfaces are invested by the serous layer of this membrane. Between the veins of the right and left side is the oblique sinus of the pericardium.

The *bronchial arteries* vary in number, size, and origin. There is as a rule a right bronchial artery, which arises from the third posterior intercostal artery or from the upper left bronchial artery. It runs on the posterior surface of the right bronchus, dividing and subdividing along the bronchial tubes, supplying them, the areolar tissue of the lung, and the bronchopulmonary lymph nodes. The left bronchial arteries, usually two in number, arise from the thoracic aorta, the upper opposite the fifth thoracic vertebra and the lower just below the left bronchus. They run on the posterior surface of the left bronchus and have a distribution similar to that of the right bronchial artery.

The *bronchial veins*, usually two on each side, return blood from the larger bronchi, and from the structures at the roots of the lungs. The bronchial veins of the right side open into the terminal part of the azygos vein, and those of the left side into the left superior intercostal or the hemiazygos vein. Some of the blood carried to the lungs through the bronchial arteries returns to the heart through the pulmonary veins.

Intrapulmonary Blood Circulation

The Pulmonary Vessels

The *pulmonary arteries* convey the deoxygenated blood to the lungs. They divide into branches that accompany the segmental and subsegmental bronchi and lie for the most part on their dorsolateral aspects. They continue into the depth of the lung as bronchoarterial units, ending in a dense capillary network in the walls of the air saccules and alveoli (Fig. 1.8). The arteries of neighboring segments are independent of one another. Evidence has been recorded to show that there is a fairly constant relationship between the luminal and mural dimensions of branches of the pulmonary arteries. The pulmonary capillaries in the interalveolar septa form a single layer, the meshes of which are smaller than the vessels themselves.

Arteriovenous shunts have been demonstrated in relation to terminal bronchioles.

The *pulmonary veins* arise from the pulmonary capillaries, the radicles coalescing into larger branches that run through the lung parenchyma, mostly independently of the bronchoarterial units. After communicating freely with other branches they form large vessels, which ultimately come into relation with larger arteries and bronchi, and accompany them to the hilus, the artery usually being dorsolateral and the vein ventromedial to the bronchus.

Whereas in the region of the hilus the pulmonary arteries and veins closely accompany the main divisions of the airways, when traced peripherally the arteries and veins assume different relationships to the bronchopulmonary segments. In general, the centrally placed bronchus and its branches supplying a bronchopulmonary segment are accompanied by branches of the pulmonary arteries, whereas many tributaries of the pulmonary veins run between bronchopulmonary segments, so that each venous tributary drains adjacent segments and each segment is drained by more than one vein (Fig. 1.8). Within a segment the veins collect the blood from the pulmonary capillaries and subsequently run in the interlobular connective tissue septa.

Some of the veins also lie beneath the visceral pleura, including that in the interlobar fissures. Thus a bronchopulmonary segment is not a bronchovascular unit in the sense of possessing its individual bronchus, artery, and vein. There is considerable variation in the above pattern of the airways, arteries, and veins, the veins being more variable than the arteries and the arteries more variable than the bronchi.

The Bronchial Vessels

The *bronchial arteries* supply the blood for the nutrition of the lung. Those supplying the bronchial tubes form in the muscular coat, a capillary plexus from which branches are given off to form a second plexus in the mucus coat. This plexus communicates with branches of the pulmonary arteries, and empties into the pulmonary veins. Others are distributed in the interlobular areolar tissue, and end partly in the deep and partly in the superficial bronchial veins. Finally, some ramify upon the surface of the lung, beneath the pleura, where they form a capillary network. The bronchial arteries supply the walls of the air passages only as far as the respiratory bronchioles. They anastomose with branches of the pulmonary arteries in the walls of the smaller bronchi and in the visceral pleura. In addition to the main bronchial arteries, smaller branches arise from the descending thoracic aorta; one of these may pass in the pulmonary ligament and cause bleeding during surgical removal of the lower lobe.

The *bronchial veins* form two distinct systems. The deep bronchial veins commence as a network in the intrapulmonary bronchioles and communicate freely with the pulmonary veins. They eventually join to form a single trunk that ends in a main pulmonary vein or in the left atrium. The superficial bronchial veins drain the extrapulmonary bronchi, the visceral pleura, and the hilar lymph nodes. They also communicate with the pulmonary veins. The bronchial veins do not receive all the blood conveyed to the lungs by the bronchial arteries, because some enters the pulmonary veins.

The Pulmonary Clearance System

The Lymphatics

The *lymph vessels* of the lung originate in superficial (pleural) and deep (bronchi, pulmonary arteries, and veins) plexuses. In the large bronchi the plexus consists of two networks, a submucosal and a peribronchial (adventitial), whereas in the small bronchi there is only a single plexus that extends as far as the bronchioles but fails to reach the alveoli; there are no lymphatic vessels beyond the alveolar ducts.

The superficial lymph vessels run around the borders of the lungs and the margins of their fissures, and converge to end in the bronchopulmonary lymph nodes. The deep lymph vessels are conducted to the hilus along the pulmonary vessels and bronchi, and end, for the most part, in the same nodes. Anastomoses between the two systems are exceptional.

The tracheobronchial lymph nodes can be classified into five main groups and include some of the largest nodes in the body (Fig. 1.13): (a) paratracheal, at the sides of the thoracic part of the trachea; (b) superior tracheobronchial, in the angles between the lower part of the trachea and bronchi; (c) inferior tracheobronchial, in the

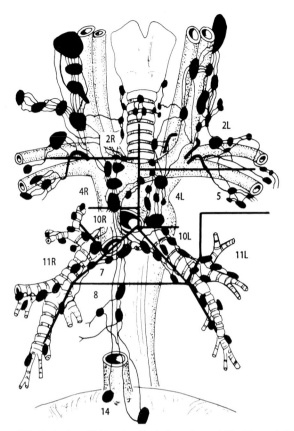

Figure 1.13. Tracheobronchial lymph nodes (redrawn from ref. 36, with permission). American Thoracic Society (27) lymph node mapping is superimposed. *2R/2L*, right/left upper paratracheal nodes; *4R/4L*, right/left lower paratracheal nodes; *5*, aortopulmonary nodes; *7*, subcarinal nodes; *8*, paraesophageal nodes; *10R/10L*, right/left tracheobronchial nodes; *11R/11L*, right/left intrapulmonary nodes; *14*, superior diaphragmatic nodes.

angle between the two bronchi; (d) bronchopulmonary, in the hilus of each lung; and (e) pulmonary, in the lung substance, on the larger branches of the bronchi. These groups are not sharply demarcated. The pulmonary lymph nodes become continuous with the bronchopulmonary nodes at the hilus, and they, in turn, are continuous with the inferior and superior tracheobronchial nodes, while the latter are continuous with the paratracheal group. The American Thoracic Society (ATS) has developed a classification of the mediastinal lymph nodes that attempts to define specific nodal stations in terms of well-recognized anatomic landmarks (27) and to which an additional group of nodes, the superior diaphragmatic lymph nodes, has been added (28) (Fig. 1.13).

The lymph of the upper airways is mostly drained into the upper deep cervical nodes; that from the anterior part of the nasal cavity passes superficially to join that from the skin. Eventually the lymphatics drain into the deep cervical nodes. The deep cervical nodes lie along the carotid sheath and may be subdivided into superior and inferior groups. The efferents of the superior nodes pass to the inferior nodes. The efferents of the deep cervical

lymph nodes then form the jugular trunk, which, on the right side, may end in the junction of the internal jugular and subclavian veins or may join the right lymphatic duct; on the left side, it usually enters the thoracic duct, although it may join either the internal jugular or the subclavian vein. The lymph of the mouth drains into the same system.

The lymph passes through several lymph nodes from the periphery to its entry into the venous blood at the junction of the jugular and subclavian vein in the base of the neck. At the entry a bicuspid valve faces into the vein to prevent reflux of blood into the duct.

Lymphatic vessels generally originate in connective tissue space as anastomosing capillaries. The capillaries flow into larger collecting vessels. Like blood vessels, lymphatic vessels are an arborized system of endothelial-lined tubes. Unlike blood vessels, they do not form a circular system but carry their contents, called lymph, in only one direction, toward the base of the neck. Lymphatic vessels recover (drain) fluids that escape into the connective tissue spaces from blood capillaries and venules and return them to the blood.

Lymphatic capillaries may reach 100 μm in diameter. Their walls are made of flattened endothelium that in some cases may have small apertures. The basement lamina is poorly developed. Collecting vessels are structurally similar to veins but without definite layers.

The lymph consists of interstitial fluid. It carries away proteins and other molecules. Its average protein content is 2 g%, but this shows considerable regional differences. The lymph vessels are, furthermore, the main channels for the clearance of material absorbed by the digestive tract, particularly for the transport of fat. The lymph also contains corpuscular matter such as cell debris and coal particles and cells such as lymphocytes, granulocytes, and macrophages. Under normal conditions in the resting state the amount of lymph produced is about 2 L 24^{-1} (16). Probably 95% comes from the liver and intestine; most of the protein originates in the liver. The flow of lymph is promoted by remitting compression of lymphatic vessels by surrounding structures (muscles, pulsating blood vessels), respiratory movements, force of gravity, and the like. The direction of flow is controlled by valves.

Dense, encapsulated collections of lymphocytes, called lymph nodes, lie across collecting lymphatic vessels; lymph percolates through them. The lymph nodes filter lymph and serve as stations for traffic of T- and B-lymphocytes and their immunological activities. They range from a few millimeters to more than a centimeter in their largest dimension.

The *lymph node* consists of a capsule that encloses lymphocytes and other free cells, which are arranged in a reticulum and supplied by blood and lymphatic vessels and nerves. Its outer surface is convex but contains an indentation, the hilus, through which the efferent lymph vessel leaves the node and blood vessels and nerves enter. Afferent vessels pierce the convex surface and empty into the sinuses of the node. Between the sinuses and partly going through them is a reticulum, a delicate meshwork of reticular fibers and reticular cells. Numerous lymphocytes are dispersed within this reticulum. In the periphery they are closely packed, forming a layer called the cortex. Within the cortex groups of these cells form ovoid lymphatic nodules (follicles) that are the location of B-lymphocytes. T-lymphocytes are located diffusely but densely in the perifollicular zone. Central to the cortex and extending to the hilus lies the medulla. Macrophages are distributed throughout the node. The lymph node is the location where, after an antigen has entered, an immune reaction takes place.

Antibodies are produced by plasma cells in the medulla. They leave the node by the efferent lymphatics. Macrophages that have phagocytosed particulate matter may enter the lymphatics and are then transported into lymph nodes, where they can stay for longer periods of time (26).

The respiratory tract lymph, which originates from the interalveolar septa, flows through lymphatic vessels in the axial and peripheral connective tissue into the lymph nodes associated with the respiratory tract. These are the deep cervical nodes, collecting the lymph of the upper airways, and the tracheobronchial nodes, collecting the lymph of the lower airways and the lungs. The lymph nodes play a major role as far as slow clearance is concerned. The lymph may pass a first set of lymph nodes and continue to second-order lymph nodes, and eventually clear into the blood circulation at the venous angle. The respiratory tract is therefore provided with a unidirectional drainage system with which not only fluid but also free particles and macrophages containing particles are cleared. Most of these particles will actually be retained in the lymph nodes, which act as a filter system for the lymph flowing through them.

Clearance Mechanisms

There are several possibilities for particles to be cleared from the respiratory tract, depending on where they are deposited. Principally, however, there are two main structural pathways: the air passage and the lymph passage.

The Air Passage

Initially, particles that are deposited in airways are swept upward by mucociliary movements. Most of the other particles will be ingested by airway or alveolar macrophages (29), depending on whether they had been deposited in the airways or penetrated into the alveoli; some may enter the epithelium freely. Particle-laden alveolar macrophages first gradually migrate toward ciliated bronchiolar surfaces, from where they will be transported upward by the mucociliary escalator, like particle-laden macrophages of the airways (29–32).

The Lymph Passage

As has been reported, apparently particle-laden alveolar macrophages can also migrate into the interalveolar interstitial space, from where they are transported via interstitial fluid and lymph vessels into the thoracic lymph nodes (26). Free particles entering the interstitial space will be phagocytsed by histiocytes (connective tissue macrophages) and subsequently experience the same fate as the alveolar macrophages. Whether this is a common clearance route, however, is still debated.

Pigmentation of the Lung

At birth the lungs are rose-pink in color; in adult life the color is a dark slate grey, mottled in patches, and as age advances this maculation assumes a black color. The coloring matter consists of granules of inhaled carbonaceous particles contained in histiocytes that are deposited in the areolar tissue near the surface of the lung (in the pleura), but also along the airways in the outer connective tissue sheet (anthracotic pigment). This deposited material increases in quantity as age advances, and is more abundant in men than in women. As a rule, the posterior border of the lung is darker than the anterior. On the upper, less movable parts of the lungs, the surface pigmentation tends to lie opposite the intercostal spaces.

Some macrophages may be retained in the pulmonary connective tissue for long periods of time (years), but their ingested particles will be slowly dissolved.

Pulmonary Innervation

The respiratory tract is mainly innervated by the *autonomic nervous system*. The fibers involved are autonomic afferent, sympathetic efferent, and parasympathetic efferent fibers. Afferent fibers come from stretch receptors in the alveoli and from irritant receptors in the bronchi and bronchioli. They travel via the pulmonary plexus, which is located around the tracheal bifurcation, to the parasympathetic vagus nerve. Irritant receptors in the trachea and cough receptors in the larynx reach the central nervous system via the vagus nerve. Other afferent fibers come from the chemoreceptors in the carotid and aortic bodies and pressor receptors in the carotid sinus and aortic arch; they travel via the glossopharyngeal nerve. Receptors in the nose and the paranasal sinuses give rise to afferent fibers that form part of the trigeminal and glossopharyngeal nerve.

All parasympathetic preganglionic efferent fibers to the tracheobronchial airways are contained in the vagus nerve. The fibers relay with short postganglionic fibers in the vicinity or within the walls, of these airways. They carry motor impulses to the smooth muscle and glands, and produce muscle contraction, gland secretion, and vasodilatation.

The preganglionic efferent fibers emerge from the spinal cord and pass to the sympathetic trunks. Long postganglionic fibers carry impulses to the larynx and upper trachea. Other postganglionic fibers pass to the lower trachea, bronchi, and bronchioli, largely via the pulmonary plexus. Their stimuli relax bronchial and bronchiolar smooth muscle, inhibit glandular secretion, and cause vasoconstriction.

As a whole the intrapulmonary nerve network resembles the airway–arterial system in its pattern of branching. It mainly follows the airway tree, but also accompanies the bronchial (nutritive) vessels. Some fibers run superficially in the connective tissue of the adventitia, and others run more deeply, inside the cartilage. After the cartilage disappears, the two bundles come together to form a single plexus in the adventitia. Ganglion cells are associated with this system. The extent and character of the innervation beyond the respiratory bronchioli still remains controversial. Intraepithelial nerve endings have been found in the trachea as well as in intrapulmonary airways. The visceral pleura receives fibers that come directly from the hilus.

Structure–Function Correlation

The structural diffusing capacity is an estimate of the inner size of the lung (33). The relationship between the gas exchange and the pulmonary structure is given by the diffusing capacity $D_{L_{O_2}}$, which, together with the alveolar–capillary partial pressure difference ($P_{A_{O_2}} - P_{B_{O_2}}$, determines the oxygen uptake of the lung ($\dot{V}_{O_2}$), according to Bohr's (1909) equation:

$$\dot{V}_{O_2} = (\bar{P}_{A_{O_2}} - P_{B_{O_2}}) D_{L_{O_2}}$$

The partial pressure difference can be considered as a functional variable, whereas the diffusing capacity is mainly determined by structural properties; a sufficiently large volume of blood has to be exposed to the air over a sufficiently large surface area and across a sufficiently thin tissue barrier. The morphometric investigation of the human lung has shown that 200 mL of blood are homogeneously distributed over a surface area

of 140 m^2, and are separated from the air by a tissue barrier of less than (1/1000 mm (23). According to the model of Weibel (33) (Fig. 1.14), this reveals a structural diffusing capacity of 2.4 mL O$_2$ s^{-1} mbar^{-1} (300 mL O$_2$ min^{-1} mmHg^{-1}).

In order to find out whether the oxygen uptake during heavy physical work would be limited by this diffusing capacity, experiments have been performed with different groups of animals. Smaller representatives of relatively active versus relatively inactive species, such as dogs versus goats, have been compared with larger representatives of relatively active versus relatively inactive species, such as ponies versus cattle, by estimating oxygen consumption and structural diffusing capacity in the same animal (34). It was found that maximal oxygen consumption was 2.5-fold higher in the more active animals, and that $D_{L_{O_2}}$ and P_{O_2} differences would contribute in equal parts, namely 1.6-fold, to this 2.5-fold higher oxygen consumption. In other words, the 2.5-fold increased capacity of the respiratory system to take up, transport, and deliver oxygen is achieved by increasing the lung's size by 1.6-fold and the blood oxygen capacity by 1.6-fold. Interestingly, it has been found that the increased oxygen capacity of the blood was caused mainly by a larger volume of erythrocytes, and, therefore, that this had to be considered as a structural adaptation as well. Gas exchange structure and blood therefore have been sharing the adaptive effort. The same may be said of the heart and the microcirculation in the muscles.

By integration of the Bohr equation, it was also found that the less active species, at maximal oxygen consumption, used only one quarter to one third of their pulmonary diffusing capacity, whereas the more active species used one half to three quarters. The more inactive animals thus have a rather large surplus of diffusing capacity that can be considered as a "safety factor." With this "safety factor" these animals will be capable of making up for a reduced alveolar P_{O_2} or $D_{L_{O_2}}$ that might be caused by sickness. In the more active animals this surplus is less apparent, and it seems that these animals' maximal oxygen consumption could be limited by their diffusing capacity.

Acknowledgments

The author would like to thank very much Dr. Susan Kayar, Dr. Vinzenz Im Hof, Dr. Peter Vock, and Dr. Eugen van der Zypen for reading the manuscript and for their very helpful advice. The author especially thanks Mr. Karl Babl for the elegant anatomical illustrations. Furthermore, the technical assistance received from Ms. Rosmarie Fankhauser, Ms. Barbara Krieger, and Ms. Renate Luder is gratefully acknowledged.

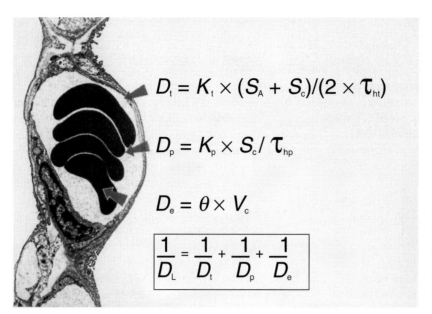

$$D_t = K_t \times (S_A + S_c)/(2 \times \tau_{ht})$$

$$D_p = K_p \times S_c / \tau_{hp}$$

$$D_e = \theta \times V_c$$

$$\frac{1}{D_L} = \frac{1}{D_t} + \frac{1}{D_p} + \frac{1}{D_e}$$

Figure 1.14. Pulmonary diffusing capacity; model of Weibel (33). D_t, D_p, D_e diffusing capacity of tissue, plasma, erythrocytes; D_L total diffusing capacity of the lung for oxygen; S_A, S_C, alveolar, capillary surface area; V_C capillary volume; τht, τhp harmonic mean thickness of tissue, plasma; K_t, K_p, permeation coefficient for oxygen in tissue, plasma; rate of oxygen uptake by whole blood. (Courtesy of ER Weibel, Department of Anatomy, University of Berne, Berne, Switzerland.)

References

1. Thurlbeck WM (1982) Postnatal human lung growth. Thorax 37:564–571.
2. Zeltner TB, Caduff JH, Gehr P, et al. (1987) The postnatal development and growth of the human lung. I. Morphometry. Respir Physiol 67:247–267.
3. Phalen RF, Oldham MJ, Beaucage CB et al. (1985) Postnatal enlargement of the human tracheobronchial airways and implications for particle deposition. Anat Rec 212:368–380.
4. Phalen RF, Oldham MJ (1983) Tracheobronchial airway structures as revealed by casting techniques. Am Rev Respir Dis 128:S1–S4.
5. Weibel ER (1963) Morphometry of the human lung. Academic Press, New York.
6. Gehr P, Mwangi DK, Ammann A, et al. (1981) Design of the mammalian respiratory system. V. Scaling morphometric pulmonary diffusing capacity to body mass: Wild and domestic mammals. Respir Physiol 44:61–86.
7. Schiebler TH, Schmidt W (eds) (1987) Anatomie. Springer-Verlag, Berlin.
8. Toendury G (1981) Angewandte und topographische Anatomie. Georg Thieme Verlag, Stuttgart.
9. Pernkopf E (1980) Atlas der topographischen und angewandten Anatomie des Menschen, Ferner H (ed). Urban und Schwarzenberg, Munich.
10. Netter FH (1979) The Ciba collection of medical illustrations. Vol 7. Respiratory system; Divertie MB, Brass A (vol eds). Ciba Pharmaceuticals, Summit, NJ.
11. Gray H (1973) Gray's anatomy, Warwick R, Williams PL (eds). Longman, Norwich, CT.
12. Fawcett DW (1986) A textbook of histology. WB Saunders, Philadelphia.
13. Weiss L (ed) (1983) Histology. Cell and Tissue biology. Elsevier Biomedical, New York.
14. Ham AW, Cormack DH (1979) Histology. JB Lippincott Company, Philadelphia.
15. Robbins SL, Cotran RS (1979) Pathologic basis of disease. WB Saunders, Philadelphia.
16. Schmidt RF, Thews G (1977) Physiologie des Menschen. Springer-Verlag, Berline.
17. von Mayersbach H, Reale E (1976) Grundriss der Histologie des Menschen. Bd 2. Spezielle Histologie. Gustav Fischer Verlag, Stuttgart.
18. Lee P, Gerrity RT, Hass FJ, et al. (1979) A model for tracheobronchial clearance of inhaled particles in man and a comparison with data. IEEE Trans Biomed Eng BME-26:625–630.
19. Foster WM, Langenback E, Bergofsky EH (1980) Measurement of tracheal and bronchial mucus velocities in man: Relation to lung clearance. J Appl Physiol 48:965–971.
20. Yeates DB, Pitt BR, Spektor DM, et al. (1981) Coordination of mucociliary transport in human trachea and intrapulmonary airways. J Appl Physiol 51:1057.
21. Zwas ST, Katz I, Belfer B, et al. (1987) Scintigraphic monitoring of mucociliary tracheo-bronchial clearnace of technetium-99m macroaggregated albumin aerosol. J Nucl Med 28:161–167.
22. Sorokin SP, Hoyt RF Jr, Pearsall AD (1985) Comparative biology of small granule cells and neuroepithelial bodies in the respiratory system. Am Rev Respir Dis 128:S26–S31.
23. Gehr P, Bachofen M, Weibel ER (1978) The normal human lung: Ultrastructure and morphometric estimation of diffusion capacity. Respir Physiol 32:121–140.
24. Weibel ER, Gil J (1977) Structure function relationship of the alveolar level. Vol 3 Lenfant C (ed) Lung biology in health and disease. Marcel Dekker, New York.
25. Crapo JD, Barry BE, Gehr P, et al. (1982) Cell number and cell characteristics of the normal human lung. Am Rev Respir Dis 125:332–337.
26. Harmsen AG, Muggenburg BA, Snipes MB (1985) The role of macrophages in particle translocation from lungs to lymph nodes. Science 230:1277–1280.
27. American Thoracic Society (ATS) (1983) Clinical staging of primary lung cancer. Am Rev Resp Dis 127:659–664.
28. Glazer HS, Aronberg DJ, Sagel SS, et al (1985) CT demonstration of calcified mediastinal lymph nodes: A guide to the new ATS classification. Am J Radiol 147:17–25.
29. Gehr P, Im Hof V, Geiser M (1988). Reinigungsmechanismen der Luftwege. Therapeutische Umschau 45:287–295.
30. Brain JD (1985) Macrophages in the respiratory tract, Geiger SR (exec ed): Handbook of physiology. Section 3: Fishman AP (s ed). The respiratory system. Vol. 1 Fishman AP, Fisher AB (eds).

Circulation and nonrespiratory Functions; American Physiological Society, Bethesda, MD, pp 447–471.

31. Sorokin SP, Brain JD (1975) Pathways of clearance in mouse lungs exposed to iron oxide aerosols. Anat Rec 181:581–626.

32. Brain JD, Proctor DF, Reid LM (eds) (1977) Respiratory defense mechanisms. Part 1. Lung biology in health and disease; Lenfant C (exec ed). Marcel Dekker, New York, vol 5.

33. Weibel ER (1970/1971) Morphometric estimation of pulmonary diffusion capacity. II. Model and method. Respir Physiol 11:54–75.

34. Weibel ER, Marques LB, Constantinopol M et al (1987) Adaptive variation in the mammalian respiratory system in relation to energetic demand. The pulmonary gas exchanger. Respir Physiol 69:81–100.

35. Sobotta J (1982) Atlas der Anatomie des Menschen. Ferner H, Staubesand J (eds). Urban und Schwarzenberg, Munich, Band 2.

36. Sinelnikov RD (1963) Atlas der Anatomie des Menschen. Ed. 2. Straatlicher Verlag für Medizin, Mosceiv.

37. von Mayersbach H, Reale E (1976) Gmndnss de Histologie des Menscken. Bd 2. Spezielle Histologic. Gustav Fischer Varlag, Stuttgart.

38. Weibel ER, Gil J (1977) Structure–function relationship of the alveolar level. Vol. 3 Lenfant (ed) Lung biology in health and disease. Marcel Dekker, New York.

2

Imaging of the Human Chest

2 Clinical History and Physical Examination

A. Simonds, S. Sperber, and S.W. Clarke

Present and Past Clinical History

Diagnostic skill rests firmly on the ability to elicit a clinical history and physical signs. Details of the duration and mode of onset of the presenting illness should be obtained with special reference to the cardinal respiratory symptoms – cough, sputum, hemoptysis, chest pain, dyspnea, and wheeze. These symptoms must be placed in the context of the patient's past health, previous treatment, family and occupational history, and social background. It is notable that, although radiologic investigation forms an integral part of the assessment of the respiratory system, the majority of cases can be diagnosed accurately on the basis of history alone (1). In other cases, sensible interpretation of history and physical signs will aid the selection of the most appropriate investigative procedures.

A past history of intermittent wheeze in an atopic individual is suggestive of asthma, and recurrent winter chest infections in a smoker may indicate chronic obstructive pulmonary disease (COPD). A previous history of pulmonary tuberculosis and its treatment is clearly of importance, and in individuals with bronchiectasis, pneumonia following measles or pertussis in childhood may be significant. Details of previous chest X-rays should be sought as a matter of priority.

Current and past drug therapy must be noted because drugs such as gold, penicillamine, and bleomycin can cause pulmonary fibrosis, and other medications may lead to allergic alveolitis or provoke bronchospasm. Immunosuppressant drugs are now used widely in the treatment of neoplastic and autoimmune disorders, and in these individuals opportunistic pulmonary infection assumes increasing importance. Family history may suggest hereditary conditions such as cystic fibrosis, atopy, emphysema associated with $\alpha 1$-antitrypsin deficiency, and congenital immunodeficiency states. Other diseases, such as pulmonary tuberculosis and familial mediterranean fever, occur more frequently in certain ethnic groups, and

the geographic location of the patient and a history of foreign travel will raise further possibilities (e.g., an increased incidence of acquired granulomatous lung disease due to coccidia in North and South America, and endemic paragonimiasis in Southeast Asia).

Cigarette smoking is the single most important risk factor in the development of COPD and carcinoma of the bronchus (2). Cessation of smoking or less lifetime smoking exposure affects the distribution of some histologic subtypes of lung cancer and may postpone the age at which lung cancer occurs (3). It is helpful to quantify past smoking history in terms of cigarette pack years. High-risk sexual practices, intravenous drug abuse, and transfusion of blood or blood products are factors that are strongly implicated in the transmission of human immunodeficiency virus (HIV). In patients in whom HIV-associated disease is suspected, close attention should be paid to these aspects of the history and the patient counselled appropriately.

Occupational exposure to nonorganic dusts may lead to various forms of pneumoconiosis. Similarly, inhalation of molds and fungal spores may cause extrinsic alveolitis such as farmer's lung, and exposure to isocyanates and organic dusts can cause occupational asthma. Details of hobbies and pets may yield further clues.

Cough and Sputum Production

Cough is a reflex response to mechanical or chemical irritation of receptors in the larynx, trachea, or major bronchi. The cough mechanism comprises a deep inspiratory effort, followed transiently by forced expiration against a closed glottis. Subsequently, as the glottis opens, air is expelled, carrying with it secretions and particulate matter. This is an effective mechanism for clearing secretions from the major airways, but below subsegmental level the principle method of clearance is via the mucociliary escalator because pressure changes cause small airways to close during coughing.

Cough may be a short-lived accompaniment to upper respiratory tract infections, but can be defined as chronic when it is present for more than 2 weeks. A dry cough occurs in inflammatory conditions such as tracheitis and lymphangitis carcinomatosa, and patients with pulmonary edema may present with a troublesome nonproductive cough. Lesions of the recurrent laryngeal nerve results in abductor paralysis of the vocal cords, producing a weak, prolonged cough described as bovine in character. In some individuals cough becomes habitual following a trivial cause, and occasionally may be perpetuated for psychological reasons.

Normally, sputum production does not exceed 10 mL day^{-1}, and this is usually swallowed. Regular expectoration of sputum is therefore pathologic, and the volume and characteristics of the secretions should be noted. Large volumes of purulent sputum are produced on a daily basis in bronchiectasis. Regular production of mucopurulent sputum is a feature of chronic bronchitis, whereas excessive production of mucoid secretions can occur in asthma, left ventricular failure, and, rarely, in alveolar cell carcinoma. In an acute asthmatic attack precipitated by allergen exposure, the sputum may appear purulent because of the presence of large numbers of eosinophils. Rusty-colored sputum is characteristic of lobar pneumonia, but is now rarely seen.

Hemoptysis

Hemoptysis can be defined as expectoration of blood or blood-stained sputum that is not due to bleeding from the upper respiratory tract or the aspiration of blood from a gastrointestinal lesion. The presence of purulent sputum indicates active infection, and a past history of pulmonary tuberculosis is of obvious relevance. Careful questioning and examination will suggest a primary cardiac cause such as pulmonary hypertension due to mitral valve disease. Profuse bleeding may occur in bronchiectasis, and in patients with mycetoma. Causes such as bronchial carcinoma, tuberculosis, and pulmonary infarction should be considered, but full examination and investigation, including chest X-ray, sputum analysis for malignant cells and acid-fast bacilli, and fiberoptic bronchoscopy, demonstrates no serious pathology in 40–50% of patients with hemoptysis.

Breathlessness (Dyspnea)

Breathlessness is a subjective sensation resulting from a failure to match ventilatory ability and demand. It may be due to a respiratory disease, cardiac pathology, anemia, metabolic derangement (e.g., diabetic ketoacidosis), or psychogenic causes. The degree of breathlessness can be quantified according to the New York Heart Association grading:

Grade I: No dyspnea with ordinary physical activities

Grade II: Dyspnea with moderately severe exertion

Grade III: Dyspnea with slight exertion

Grade IV: Dyspnea at rest

More detailed assessment can be carried out using a visual analog scale or questionnaire to establish the patient's ability to carry out activities of daily living. Of crucial diagnostic importance is the speed of onset of breathlessness, which can be classified as in Table 2.1.

Wheeze

Wheeze is generated by the oscillation of airways and its presence implies airway obstruction due to an intraluminal cause (mucus plug, foreign body, or tumor), bronchoconstriction, or extrinsic compression. Many asthmatics complain of chest tightness or wheeze that may become more prominent at night or on exertion. Nocturnal wheeze may accompany left ventricular failure, and in this respect sometimes can prove difficult to differentiate from asthma.

Chest Pain

As with other forms of pain, chest pain can be elucidated by identifying its character, site and radiation, rate of

Table 2.1. Diagnosis of breathlessness by rate of onset

Rapid onset over minutes
Pneumothorax
Pulmonary embolism
Pulmonary edema
Anaphylactic reaction provoking bronchospasm
Onset over hours
Asthma
Pneumonia
Allergic alveolitis
Pulmonary edema
Onset over months or years
Lung tumor
Interstitial lung disease
COPD
Intermittent onset
Asthma
Left ventricular failure
COPD, chronic obstructive pulmonary disease.

onset, and modifying factors. In respiratory disease, pain originates from the trachea, pleura, chest wall, or mediastinal structures, the lungs themselves being poorly innervated. Pleuritic chest pain is sharp, stabbing, and exacerbated by inspiration. It is usually localized, although referred pain may occur – for example, referral of diaphragmatic pleuritic pain to the shoulder tip or upper abdomen. Pleuritic-type pain is common in pneumonia, pneumothorax, and pulmonary infarction. Pain derived from the trachea is often perceived as a central raw sensation, whereas that experienced as a result of tumor invasion of mediastinal structures or chest wall may be described as a poorly localized, dull ache.

Systemic Symptoms

Weight loss and malaise are features of a wide variety of respiratory disorders. Sweats occur in patients with pneumonia, tuberculosis, lung abcess, HIV-related disease, and lymphoma. It is important to carry out a review of all systems because primary lung disease may present with symptoms outside the respiratory system, and in multisystem disorders the lungs may be only one of the target organs.

Physical Examination

Initial observation will reveal how unwell the patient is and the degree of respiratory distress. This dictates the tenor of the subsequent examination. The patient should be placed in a position of comfort, with the head of the bed raised at 45° (or higher if orthopnea is marked). It is kinder and less tiring for the patient to have the front of the chest examined entirely before progressing to the back. A detailed clinical assessment is carried out by inspection, then palpation and auscultation of the thorax, followed by a general physical examination.

Inspection

Cyanosis, characterized by a blue tinge to the mucous membranes, lips, and nail beds, indicates a significant level of desaturated hemoglobin. The often-quoted figure of 5 g dL^{-1} reduced hemoglobin required to produce cyanosis is an overestimate because concentrations of 1.5 g dL^{-1} are clinically detectable (4), although there is wide interobserver variation in the ability to detect this sign. It follows, however, that cyanosis is more obvious in polycythemic individuals and less easily visible in the anemic patient. Peripheral cyanosis is seen when the

distal circulation stagnates, as in low cardiac output states, or on exposure to the cold. The causes of central cyanosis are given in Table 2.2.

The hands should be carefully examined for the presence of clubbing, tremor, flap, and nicotine staining. Clubbing of the fingers is demonstrated by the loss of the angle between the nail and the nail bed. There is increased curvature of the nail longitudinally and laterally, and in advanced cases swelling of the terminal phalanges, which gives the fingers a drumstick-like appearance. Conditions associated with clubbing are listed in Table 2.3. In hypertrophic pulmonary osteoarthropathy clubbing is accompanied by pain and swelling of the wrists and ankles. This

Table 2.2. Causes of central cyanosis

Respiratory	Cardiac	Others
COPD	Fallot's tetralogy	Methemoglobinemia
Severe asthma	Transposition of aorta and pulmonary artery	Sulphemoglobinemia
Fibrosing alveolitis	Atrial and ventricular septal defect with reversed shunt	
Pulmonary embolism		
Hypoventilation		
Lobar pneumonia with shunt		

COPD, chronic obstructive pulmonary disease.
Modified from ref. 7, with permission.

Table 2.3. Causes of finger clubbing

1. Thoracic tumors
   Carcinoma of lung
   Mesothelioma of pleura
   Thymoma
   Lymphoma
2. Diffuse pulmonary fibrosis
   Fibrosing alveolitis
   Asbestosis
3. Chronic pulmonary infection
   Bronchiectasis
   Abcess
   Empyema
   Cystic fibrosis
4. Cardiac
   Cyanotic heart disease
   Bacterial endocarditis
   Atrial myxoma
   Arteriovenous aneurysm of lung
5. Hepatic cirrhosis
6. Chronic bowel disease
   Ulcerative colitis
   Crohn's disease
   Celiac disease
7. Familial

Modified from ref. 7, with permission.

symptom complex occurs in patients with bronchogenic carcinoma or suppurative lung disease. Roentgenologic examination of affected joints shows subperiosteal new bone formation.

The coarse flap of carbon dioxide retention is often associated with warm, vasodilatated peripheries and a bounding radial pulse. Patients receiving β2 agonist bronchodilator agents commonly have a fine tremor that is similar to that of thyrotoxicosis.

Inspection of the neck may reveal the presence of lymphadenopathy secondary to intrathoracic carcinoma, lymphoma, pulmonary tuberculosis, or HIV-associated disease. The jugular veins are distended in cor pulmonale and in superior vena cava obstruction. In the latter condition, the jugular distension is fixed and accompanied by dilatated venous anastomoses over the upper chest wall, and in some cases swelling of the ipsilateral arm and face. In patients with severe airflow limitation, jugular distension is prominent during expiration as high intrathoracic pressures are generated to overcome the airway obstruction.

Abnormalities of chest wall configuration are of importance because, if severe, they compromise ventilatory mechanics. An increase in anteroposterior thoracic diameter creating a barrel-shaped chest is seen in patients with hyperinflation due to COPD. Developmental abnormalities of the sternum can produce the deformities of pigeon chest (pectus carinatum) and funnel chest (pectus excavatum). Scoliosis, if present, can lead to cardiorespiratory failure if the curvature develops before lung growth is complete, or is associated with respiratory muscle weakness. Iatrogenic chest wall deformity caused by rib resection is found in patients who have undergone thoracoplasty for pulmonary tuberculosis.

Diminished movement of one side of the chest always indicates underlying pathology, such as consolidation, collapse, fibrosis, pleural effusion, or pneumothorax. Flattening of the chest wall apically accompanied by reduced movement and tracheal deviation to the affected side is suggestive of longstanding apical fibrosis.

The rate and pattern of respiration should be noted. A rate above 12 to 16 breaths min^{-1} in adults is seen in anxiety, pneumonia, interstitial fibrosis, emphysema, and cardiac failure. A pattern of apneic episodes followed by a series of crescendo and then decrescendo respiratory efforts characterizes Cheyne–Stokes breathing, which occurs in patients with severe cerebrovascular disease as well as low output cardiac failure, but may be a normal feature of sleep in the elderly.

Pulmonary Signs in Lung Disease

The physical signs found in typical pulmonary conditions are shown in Table 2.4.

Palpation of the Chest

Confirmation of the impression of reduced chest wall excursion can be obtained by clasping the chest wall symmetrically with the fingers, allowing the thumbs to rest lightly on the skin in the midline and part on inspiration (mensuration). This maneuver should be carried out in the upper and lower chest anteriorly and posteriorly, but is unlikely to reveal any chest wall abnormality that has not been identified previously by inspection.

The position of the upper mediastinum is determined by palpating the trachea in the suprasternal notch and assessing any deviation from the midline. The length of the trachea outside the chest is measured by the distance between the cricoid cartilage and the suprasternal notch (cricosternal distance). The average length of three to four fingerbreadths is reduced when the chest is hyperinflated significantly by airway obstruction or emphesema. The position of the apex beat, normally found in the left fifth intercostal space in the midclavicular line, serves to indicate the position of the lower mediastinum. Clearly the apex beat may also be situated laterally to this in primary cardiac disease. Mediastinal shift toward the affected lung occurs following lobar collapse and fibrosis, whereas large space-occupying lesions such as a pleural effusion or a pneumothorax will displace the mediastinum away from the lesion.

Palpation of voice sounds (tactile vocal fremitus) is best achieved by placing the ulnar border of the hand on the chest wall in the upper, middle, and lower zones. Conventionally, the patient is asked to repeat the words "ninety-nine" or "one, one, one". Conduction of these sounds is enhanced when there is underlying consolidation, reduced over areas of collapse and fibrosis, and absent in the presence of a pleural effusion. Thus one may (with vocal resonance) discriminate between consolidation and collapse, fibrosis or effusion – though not to a high degree.

Percussion

Percussive technique is important. The palpating or pleximeter finger should be firmly applied to the chest wall parallel to the ribs and the terminal phalange struck with the middle finger of the opposite hand using a flexion motion at the wrist. The percussion note should be compared on both sides of the chest, starting with direct percussion over the clavicles. The normal chest is resonant anteriorly to the level of the sixth rib (with the exception of an area of cardiac dullness), and posteriorly to the level of the tenth rib. The right hemidiaphragm is approximately 2 cm higher than the left because of the position of the liver. If the liver edge is palpated below the costal margin, percussion over the lower right lung and liver will

Table 2.4. Physical signs of common pulmonary conditions

Disease	Chest movement	Mediastinal shift	Percussion note	Breath sounds	Voice sounds	Added sounds
COPD/ emphesema	Reduced barrel shaped	0	Hyperresonant	Vesicular, prolonged expiration	Reduced	Wheezes
Asthma	Variable, depending on severity	0	Hyperresonant	Vesicular prolonged expiration	Reduced	Wheezes
Pneumonic consolidation	Reduced locally	0	Dull	Bronchial	Increased; whispering pectoriloquy, egophony	Crackles
Collapse	Reduced locally	Toward side	Dull	Vesicular, reduced or absent	Reduced	0
Pleural effusion	Reduced locally	Toward opposite side	Stony dull	Reduced or absent	Reduced or absent;	None or pleural rub
Fibrosis	Reduced	Toward side	Dull	Bronchial	Increased	Crackles
Pneumothorax	Reduced	Toward opposite side	Hyperresonant	Vesicular, reduced or absent	Reduced	0

COPD, chronic obstructive pulmonary disease.
Modified from ref 7, with permission.

establish whether the liver is enlarged or displaced downward by a hyperinflated lung.

Auscultation

Auscultation of the chest will reveal the character of the breath sounds, the presence of added sounds such as crackles and wheeze, and the quality of transmitted voice sounds. Normal breath sounds are inaudible without a stethoscope, although some adventitious sounds can be heard from the end of the bed. Stridor is a harsh inspiratory sound caused by turbulence in the upper airway. It indicates major airway narrowing at the level of the larynx, trachea, or main bronchi.

Using the diaphragm of the stethoscope, the chest should be examined systematically. Care should be taken not to overlook the axillary regions. Normal (vesicular) breath sounds are soft and low pitched and extend through inspiration into expiration. In contrast, bronchial breath sounds are higher pitched, with a blowing quality, and a definite pause can be detected between inspiration and expiration. Bronchial breathing is a reliable sign of pneumonic consolidation, but may be heard over a collapsed lung, over the right upper zone anteromedially by direct transmission of sounds from the trachea (student's pneumonia), and over the trachea proper, which is useful for practice.

Added breath sounds can be divided simply into wheeze, crackles, and pleural rub. *Wheeze* is generated in the large airways by air flowing at high linear velocity

through a stenosis. This explains the occasional finding of a silent chest in severe asthma, when airflow is insufficient to generate wheeze. The pitch of the wheeze depends on the mass and elasticity of the conducting tubing and is unrelated to the length of the airway. Widespread polyphonic wheeze is characteristic of COPD and asthma, whereas a unilateral monophonic wheeze is suggestive of discrete bronchial narrowing by foreign body, tumor, or extrinsic compression. Occasionally, wheeze may be accompanied by an inspiratory "squawk", suggesting fibrosing alveolitis or extrinsic allergic alveolitis (5).

Crackles are sharp, discontinuous popping sounds caused primarily by the abrupt opening of small airways as pressure becomes equalized along their lengths. Persistent late inspiratory crackles are heard in interstitial lung disorders such as fibrosing alveolitis. Fine crackles may be present over areas of consolidation. In severe airflow obstruction early inspiratory crackles can be detected at the mouth. Basal crackles are heard in pulmonary edema and coarse crackles are a prominent feature of bronchiectasis. In the latter situation air bubbling through excessive secretions in the large airways generates moist crackles.

A *pleural rub* is best described as a localized crunching or creaking sound created by friction between inflamed parietal and visceral pleural surfaces in areas adjacent to pulmonary consolidation or infarction. The sound is heard on both inspiration and expiration and can be difficult to distinguish from lung crackles at times.

Egophony is a bleating sound heard occasionally over the surface of a pleural effusion. *Bronchophony* is a term used to describe the enhanced transmission of voice sounds through lung consolidation or cavitation and can be confirmed by the ready transmission of a whispered sound (whispering pectoriloquy).

Extrapulmonary Signs in Lung Disease

A diligent general examination completes the patient's physical assessment. This may reveal extrapulmonary complications of respiratory disease, or highlight a systemic disorder of which the pulmonary disease is only a component. In addition to cyanosis and clubbing, the extrapulmonary manifestations of lung disease include characteristic cutaneous lesions in sarcoidosis, Wegener granulomatosis, and collagen vascular disorders. Carcinoma of the bronchus may be accompanied by a plethora of metastatic and parametastatic phenomena, including peripheral neuropathy, myopathy, dermatomyositis, cerebellar degeneration, and syndromes associated with ectopic hormone release. Patients with hypercapnic respiratory failure may exhibit neuromuscular hyperactivity, drowsiness, and papilledema.

Multisystem disorders that affect the lung include rheumatoid arthritis, the collagen vascular disorders, histiocytosis X, neurofibromatosis, and tuberous sclerosis.

Reliability of Physical Signs

Although the ability to elicit physical signs depends on clinical experience, some signs are more reliable indicators of underlying pathology than others. One study found good agreement between observers in diagnosing clubbing, wheeze, crackles, decreased percussion note, and vocal resonance. There was little agreement over assessment of cricothyroid distance and the presence of cyanosis, tachypnea, tracheal deviation, and whispering pectoriloquy (6).

Radiologic Correlates of Physical Signs

There is a strong correlation between the presence of physical signs and the extent of radiologic shadowing in cryptogenic fibrosing alveolitis, pulmonary edema, lobar pneumonia, and pleural effusion. However, the chest X-ray may prove unhelpful in assessing the severity of the underlying disease in acute asthma, exacerbations of COPD, pulmonary sarcoidosis, pulmonary hypertension, and neuromuscular disorders affecting the respiratory muscles or control of breathing. In all these conditions the chest X-ray may be normal or only mildly abnormal in the face of severe respiratory insufficiency.

Conversely, the chest X-ray is invaluable in diagnosing some conditions that are asymptomatic and associated with few or no physical signs. Solitary pulmonary nodules and brochogenic cysts are classical examples of this category.

References

1. Hampton JR, Harrison MJC, Mitchell JRA, et al. (1975) Relative contributions of history-taking, physical examination and laboratory investigations to diagnosis and management of medical outpatients. Br Med J 2:592.
2. Muscat JE, Stellman SD, Zhang ZF, et al. (1997) Cigarette smoking and large cell carcinomas of the lung. Cancer Epidemiol Biomarkers Prev 6:477–480.
3. Tong L, Spitz MR, Fueger JJ, et al. (1996) Lung carcinoma in former smokers. Cancer, 78:1004–10.
4. Goss GA, Hayes JA, Burdon IGW (1988) Deoxyhemoglobin concentrations in the detection of central cyanosis. Thorax 43:212–213.
5. Earis JE, Marsh K, Pearson MG et al. (1982) The inspiratory 'squawk' in extrinsic allergic alveolitis and other pulmonary fibroses. Thorax 37:923–927.
6. Spiteri MA, Cook DG, Clarke SW (1988) Reliability in eliciting physical signs in examination of the chest. Lancet 1:873–875.
7. Clarke S, Bouchier I, Morris J (1982) Clinical skills, WB Saunders, Philadephia.

3 Conventional Chest Radiography

D. Westra and M. Sperber

Technical Aspects

Posteroanterior and Lateral Chest Radiographs

Plain radiographs of the chest are obtained routinely with the patient in an erect position, with fully suspended respiration, preferentially at total lung capacity (1). The focal point–film distance should be at least 1.80 m. A high kilovoltage (kVp) technique should in general be applied, at least 120 kVp (2,3), preferably with an additional 0.3 to 0.5 mm copper filter (4) and including the use of a grid or air gap between the patient and the film (5). A high kilovoltage technique enhances the visibility of the lungs by reducing the contrast of the bony thorax and also has the advantage of better penetration of the mediastinum (4,6). For proper visualization of the mediastinum an additional penetrated film is often required (Fig. 3.1).

In recent years various techniques have been proposed in order to improve the diagnostic capabilities of conventional chest radiography. Among them, digital chest images obtained with a selenium detector have been shown to allow radiologists the same degree of performance in detecting pulmonary, mediastinal and pleural abnormalities as conventional chest radiography, when computed tomography (CT) was used as a the reference standard (7). A the same time, it has been found that the choice of X-ray film/screen system basically determines the efficacy of screening, and the contrast characteristics of X-ray films together with noise levels that vary at different optical densities, affect the detectability of nodular shadows. Studies have therefore been dedicated to the identification of the most suitable sensitometric characteristics and the effects of the noise level of the X-ray film/screen system on the imaging capabilities (8).

Other technological improvements proposed include the usage of twin screen–film chest radiography, shown to be cost effective and having good potential for use

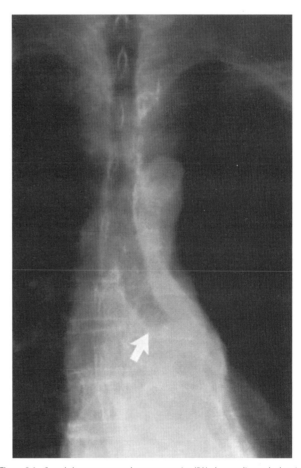

Figure 3.1. Coned-down penetrated posteroanterior (PA) chest radiograph showing obstruction of the left main bronchus by bronchogenic carcinoma (*arrow*). A well-penetrated PA film may adequately show a centrally located bronchial lesion and obviate the need for tomography.

both in standard and portable clinical applications, as they allow improved visualization of radiographic features, especially in the mediastinal and retrocardiac areas (9). Nevertheless, when another technique known as advanced multiple beam equalization radiography (AMBER) has been compared with single or stereoscopic (two films) conventional screen–film radiography, by using receiver operating characteristic (ROC) for statistical analysis, no clinically significant differences were found between the various methods. CT findings were considered as standard, and pathologic conditions studied included infiltrative diseases, emphysema, calcified nodules, and mediastinal and hilar adenopathy (or masses) (10).

The posteroanterior (PA) view is obtained in a symmetric projection. Superposition of the scapulae should be avoided by endorotational position of the arms. The use of wedge filtration to reduce the contrast between the mediastinum and the lungs is recommended for the PA view (5,6,11). Digital radiography of the chest offers specific advantages in this respect (12).

The lateral view should be obtained with uplifted arms and with the left side of the patient turned toward the film. A "right forward" lateral projection has been advocated, in which the right hemithorax is rotated about 10° anterior to the left, for a better demonstration of the hili (13,14). When no abnormalities are expected, chest radiographs should be restricted to only the PA view. The value of routine admission chest radiographs in patient care is still controversial (15). An additional lateral film should be obtained when pathologic lesions are to be expected or when abnormalities are found on the PA film. Other views are occasionally made for special purposes.

Due to the great frequency with which, in most medical centers, CT examinations of the thorax are performed nowadays, it seems that the lateral chest radiograph is relatively rarely employed: this is reflected in the worried title of a recent article "The lateral chest radiograph: is it doomed to extinction?" (16). Still, there are authors who are interested in recapturing the value of the lateral radiographic view of the thorax, emphasizing the fact that, with the advent of the three-dimensional view offered by CT, our understanding and identification of changes from the normal standard are greatly improved, allowing various pathologies such as vascular abnormalities, posteriorly located infiltrates or pericardial effusion to be easily detected (17,18).

In addition to the conventional PA view, an expiration radiograph may provide rough information about respiratory movements (1). The fact that an apparent lack of respiratory movement may be the result of lack of communication between the technician and the patient has also to be taken into consideration. Expiration radiographs are usually employed to demonstrate airtrapping; however, fluoroscopy is a more sensitive method for the discovery of respiratory disturbances.

A low kilovoltage radiograph may be required for the visualization of the skeleton or for demonstrating calcifications (Fig. 3.2). Demonstrating calcified hilar or mediastinal lymph nodes, for example, may be considered a reliable sign of tuberculosis (19).

Lateral Decubitus Chest Radiograph

A radiograph performed with a horizontal X-ray beam in a lateral decubitus position is indicated in addition to the conventional view when free movable fluid is to be demonstrated. Small quantities (less than 100 m) of fluid may be shown when the patient lies in a 20° Trendelenburg position and on the affected side, slightly inclined to the backside and holding the breath in moderate inspiration (1). In the erect patient, a relatively large amount of subpulmonary fluid may remain invisible (20).

For the detection of minimal pleural effusions, a recent study has underlined the value of an expiratory lateral decubitus view. When erect posteroanterior, lateral, and lateral decubitus (in inspiration and expiration) radiographs were performed, in 86% of patients a difference in thickness of the fluid layer found between the expiratory lateral decubitus and the rest of the views (21).

Lordotic View

Apical lesions and middle lobe atelectasis may be better demonstrated on a lordotic view than on a normal PA projection.

Oblique View

Pleural–pulmonary interfaces that differ from the direction of the projecting X-rays in the PA and lateral views are not properly visualized. Oblique views may be needed in such cases (Fig. 3.3). The optimal oblique projection for visualizing the interface in question (tangential view) can be found also by means of fluoroscopy.

The Portable Chest Radiograph

The portable chest radiograph is a valuable aid in the diagnosis and treatment of the intensive care patient. The interpretation of these radiographs should be undertaken with care (22). Some structures, such as the heart, are magnified and the pulmonary blood flow may be redistributed to the apical region as a result of gravity, erroneously suggesting pulmonary vascular congestion (1).

Portable chest radiographs should be marked as such, in order to avoid false-positive readings (22). In a study on the utility and efficacy of portable chest radiographs they were found to have a greater yield of positive findings (45.4%) than is generally considered acceptable, and frequently (37%) demonstrated no change in the patient's clinical status (16).

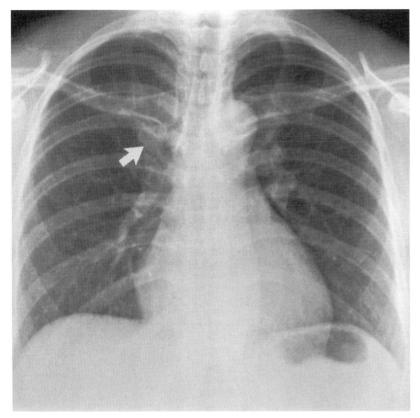

a

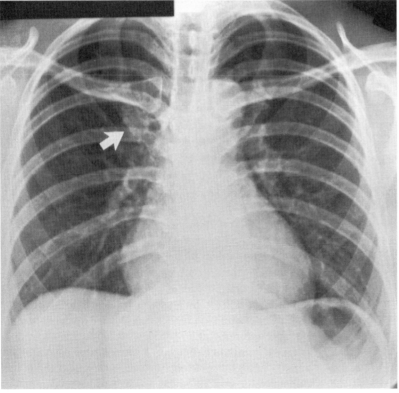

b

Figure 3.2. Calcified first rib cartilage simulating the presence of a pulmonary density (*arrow*). **a** A 120 kVp standard radiograph raising the suspicion of a pulmonary shadow. **b** A 70 kVp PA radiograph. The alleged pulmonary density is obviously caused by a calcified (ossified) first rib cartilage.

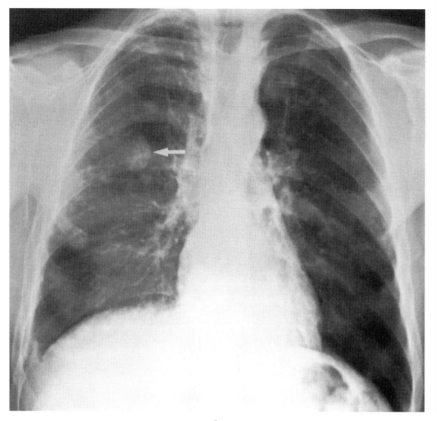

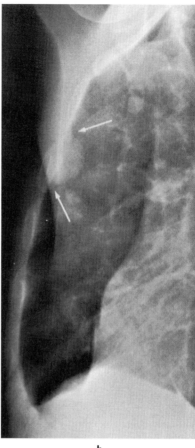

a   b

Figure 3.3. Pleural metastases. **a** Posteroanterior view. The pleural nature of the lesion (*arrow*) can be suspected from the radiological appearance: sharply defined at the inner side and fading away at the periphery. **b** Oblique tangential view showing the exact relation of the mass lesion to the thoracic wall. Obtuse angles (*arrows*) between the lesion and the chest wall suggest the extrapulmonary location.

In the intensive care unit (ICU), despite the development in recent years of new investigative techniques, the portable chest radiograph continues to represent a valuable means of diagnosis. The patient in the ICU is in the majority of cases severely ill and requires the employment of a large number of auxiliary devices such as feeding tubes, chest tubes, intravenous lines, etc., which obviously increases the difficulty of obtaining accurate and clear images. In the performance of a bedside chest radiograph, technical factors are of primordial importance, as is the recognition of false-positive signs resulting from the PA view and the utilization of life support devices. A radiographic examination is mandatory in most medical centers upon the acceptance of a patient to the ICU, as well as a follow-up of treatment and subsequent invasive procedures (23–25).

Stereoscopy

In comparison with the single chest radiograph, a shifted pair of chest films, when viewed either stereoscopically or side by side, may improve the observer's performance (26,27). Repeat chest films are frequently spontaneously shifted in a craniocaudal direction. By binocular viewing of serial chest films according to the shift direction and alternative blinking of the eyes, small changes may be more readily detected (28).

Chest Fluoroscopy

Because the visual perception in fluoroscopy is greatly inferior to that of plain radiographs, chest fluoroscopy should be used only as a supplement to the plain chest radiograph. Chest fluoroscopy may be indicated for making spot films or tangential views, for studying cardiovascular and respiratory movements (such as air-trapping and pneumothorax), for the localization of a pulmonary density, and for guiding purposes (for bronchoscopy, transthoracic puncture, and angio(cardio)graphic procedures). Using fluoroscopy, differentiation is often possible between extrapulmonary lesions fixed to the thoracic wall and more or less mobile intrapulmonary lesions. Also, a pulmonary nodule may be distinguished from a pulmonary vessel visualized end on by rotating the patient during fluoroscopy (20).

Conventional Tomography of the Chest

Conventional tomography of the lungs and mediastinum has largely been replaced by CT. However, there are still indications for this modality.

Conventional tomography can be performed with linear or multidirectional movement of the tomographic system. Tomography with linear movement (linear tomography) has the advantage that relatively short exposure times can be used, which may be required in patients who cannot hold their breath (29). However, the quality of the cross-sectional image in linear tomography is generally reduced in comparison with the multidirectional type because in the first the disturbing shadows are less effectively effaced and the tissue interfaces are less adequately represented (30,31). In linear tomography of the hili, this disadvantage can be more or less compensated for by a 55° oblique tomographic technique (32–34). Nowadays, with most conventional tomographic equipment the patient is examined in a recumbent position. One must be aware of the effect of this position of the patient on the mediastinal structures (22). The use of wedge filtration is strongly recommended while one is performing frontal tomography (29).

Possible indications for conventional tomography:

1. Differentiating normal from pathologic findings, especially in those cases in which benign pathology is suspected (i.e., superposition of shadows, fibrotic changes, or grossly calcified granulomas).
2. In the evaluation of a possibly enlarged hilurn (33,35).
3. As an aid in the interpretation of plain chest radiographs when gross pathology is demonstrated (e.g., prominent mediastinal lymph nodes). The need for CT may then be obviated (36,37) (Fig. 3.4).
4. The examination of the tracheobronchial tree with a view to eventual bronchoscopy (38,39) (Fig. 3.5).
5. The localization of peripheral nodules before bronchoscopy or surgery (40–42) (Fig. 3.6).

Reporting on the Chest Radiograph

Viewing Conditions

A PA chest radiograph is considered to be adequately exposed when the midthoracic vertebral bodies are faintly visible. The lung fields may then be slightly overexposed in some patients, despite the use of high kilovoltage technique and wedge filtration. Proper masking of the film on the viewing box and the use of a spotlight in order to reduce the detrimental effect of ambient light are essential in viewing chest radiographs (40,43). Attention should also be paid to background illumination (44). A white wall behind the observer or the observer's white coat might have a negative effect on the image contrast.

It is recommended, in addition to the normal viewing procedure, that every chest radiograph or chest tomogram be viewed from long distance or through diminishing lenses (1,40,45,46). The contrast in underexposed areas may be enhanced by viewing the film from a position as lateral to the viewing box as possible. There should also be a uniform practice regarding the display of the lateral chest radiograph. The radiograph should routinely be displayed with the patient facing the viewer's left (47).

Several phases are recommended in the study of a chest radiograph (48):

1. *Free search:* the observer scans the radiograph without an orderly pattern.
2. *Direct search:* it is convenient to follow an anatomic pattern, such as bony thorax, extrapleural and extrathoracic soft tissues, diaphragm and pleura, lungs, mediastinum, and heart.
3. Special attention is paid to the clinical problem and search is directed to all possible radiographic abnormalities that may be expected in this connection.

The radiographic report should be built up in two parts, a descriptive part and a conclusive part. Lesions should be depicted in the descriptive part in such a way that the conclusion can be anticipated. In the conclusive part, an attempt should always be made to answer the specific questions that were the reason for performing the radiographic examination.

Pitfalls in Interpretation: Observer Error

Observer error results in false-negative or false-positive readings. In a false-positive reading a detail without pathologic significance is interpreted as a pathologic lesion; in a false-negative reading a pathologic lesion is misinterpreted as nonpathologic. Of positive films 20–30% are called negative and 1–15% of negative films are called positive. Interobserver disagreement in some cases may reach astonishing levels (48–51). Observer error may be reduced by sufficient knowledge and experience, by optimalization of the viewing conditions (see above), by the establishment of quiet surroundings, by frequent rest periods to guard against reader fatigue, and by double readings either by the same observer or by different observers (44,45,52).

A lesion may not be reported because it is too small to be seen. In chest radiographs 0.4 mm is considered to be

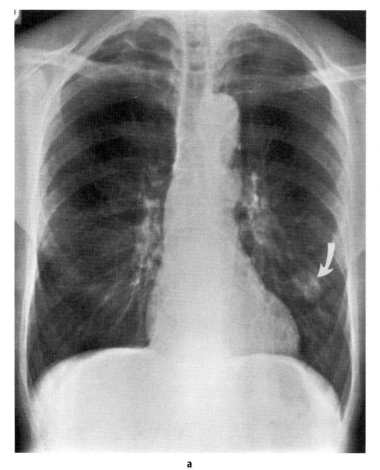

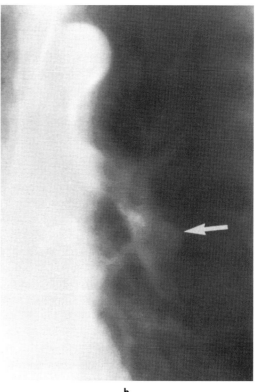

a   b

Figure 3.4. Hilar lymphadenopathy detected by conventional tomography in patient with bronchogenic carcinoma. **a** Posteroanterior view. Peripheral primary tumor in the left lower lobe (*curved arrow*). No definite sign of hilar adenopathy. **b** Frontal tomogram of the left hilus. Enlarged lymph node (*straight arrow*) lateral to the lower lobe artery (*IIa*). The enlarged lymph node was surgically proven to be a metastasis of the primary bronchogenic cancer. Lower lobe bronchus (*IIb*).

the lower limit of visibility for noncalcified intrapulmonary densities (50,53). The chance for such a density to be detected in a PA chest radiograph gradually increases above this size. There is a reasonable expectation (probably about 50%) that a lesion 8–10 mm in size will be visible on the radiograph and perceived by the observer under standard diagnostic conditions (50,54). Pulmonary densities have less chance to be visualized in certain areas, such as the retrocardiac area, the posterior costophrenic sinus, the mediastinal recesses, the pulmonary apices, and areas in close proximity to the pleura and the ribs in general (55). A higher accuracy rate is found for lesions in the upper quadrants compared with lesions in lower quadrants (56). Lesions substantially larger than 10 mm in diameter may be totally obscured in some instances by the superposition of the surrounding images (ribs, pulmonary vessels, etc.) (36,57).

False-positive readings may be caused by technical artefacts, or insufficient knowledge of normal anatomy and its variants. Technical artefacts include those from the developing machine or distortions caused by nonstandard techniques such as portable chest radiographs. Additionally, superposition of extrapulmonary densities over the lung fields on a chest radiograph may simulate an intrapulmonary lesion. Nipples are a common example. The use of nipple markers has therefore been advocated (58). other examples are cutaneous folds, cutaneous papillomas, calcified (ossified) cartilages of the ribs, healed rib fractures, exostoses of the ribs, vertebral exostoses and pleural thickening (59–61). Superposition of normal structures upon each other may also sometime produce "difficult to explain" configurations. Amputation of the female breast or muscular dystrophy may simulate hyperaeration of the lung.

Anatomic variations or anomalies of the vascular structures of the hili or mediastinum may simulate a tumor. Common examples are the confluences of the pulmonary veins, a large azygos or left superior intercostal vein, tortuosity of the thoracic aorta or of the innominate artery, and a right-sided aortic arch (20,62,63).

An unexpected pseudotumor may be caused by mucus plugging. A mucus plug is seldom seen on plain chest

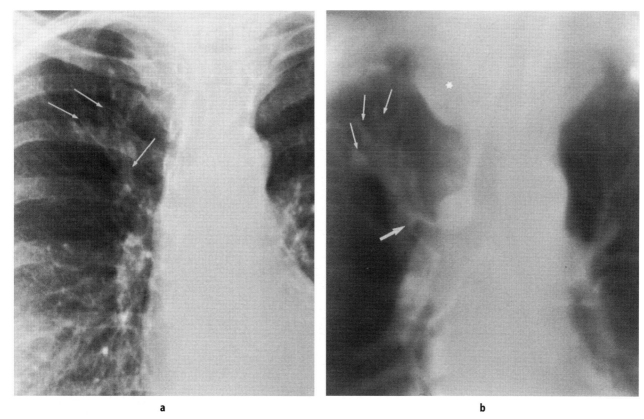

a   b

Figure 3.5. Obstruction of the right upper lobe bronchus demonstrated by conventional tomography. **a** Posteroanterior view. Note the "tramline shadows" (*arrows*) in the right upper lobe indicating the presence of ectatic bronchi with a thickened bronchial wall. **b** Frontal tomogram in recumbent position of the right upper lobe. Obstruction of the right upper lobe bronchus by a bronchial adenoma (*large arrow*) (surgically confirmed). Behind the bronchial obstruction, ectatic bronchi filled with mucus can be seen producing a "gloved hand" configuration (*small arrows*).*, intrathoracic goiter.

radiographs; however, it is not infrequently discovered on conventional tomographs (29,64–66) or CT scans (67). Another well-recognized cause of pseudotumor formation is a localized interlobar effusion in heart failure (68).

Roentgen Anatomy and Image Formation in Conventional Radiography of the Chest

Thoracic Skeleton

In reading the routine high kilovoltage chest radiograph, attention should be paid to the skeleton, despite the fact that the film was not made for that purpose. The first reason for this is to recognize gross deformities that might have important diagnostic or therapeutic consequences for the patient – for example, signs of malignancy, kyphoscoliosis, rib notching or other signs of a systemic disorder (69,70). The second reason is to identify skeletal structures that may mimic pulmonary densities or mediastinal structures, such as old rib fractures, compacta islands, etc. Additional low voltage radiography, bone

scintigraphy, CT or magnetic resonance imaging (MRI) may be indicated for verification.

Techniques used in the precise identification of the ribs are especially useful in the detection of rib abnormalities and localization of lung lesions. The clavicle, the xiphoid process and the sternal angle may be used as anatomic landmarks for rib counting. For rib counting on lateral chest radiographs the sternal angle or the 12th rib may be used. Anatomic rib variants include developmental deformities, cervical rib or short rib detection of thoracic deformities such as funnel chest (pectus excavatum) and barrel-shaped thorax requires an awareness of the strong correlation between the transverse appearance of the thorax and costal shape. Shadows around the rib cage (e.g., rib companion shadows), as mentioned before, may mimic pleural and extrapleural disease on frontal chest radiographs (71).

Extrapleural and Extrathoracic Soft Tissues

Well-known cutaneous shadows usually identified on conventional chest radiographs are the female breasts, the pectoralis muscles and the sternocleidomastoidian

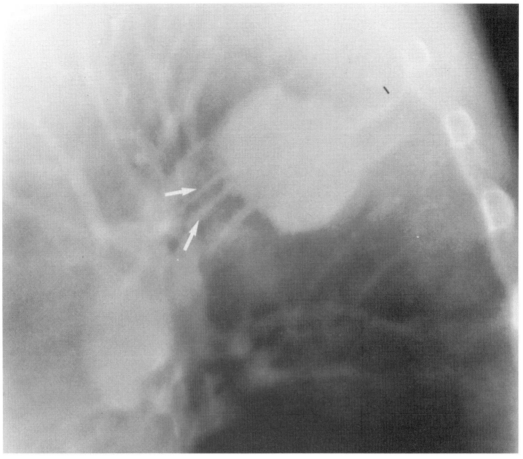

a

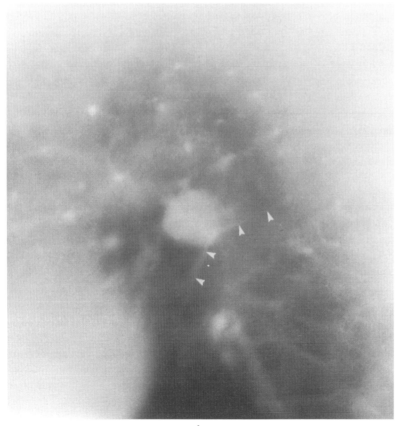

b

Figure 3.6. Tumor localization by conventional tomography. **a** Crosssection through the posterior segmental bronchus of the right upper lobe (*arrows*) clearly identifying the location of the tumor (*t*) in the posterior segment of the upper lobe. *sa*, subsegmental atelectasis behind the tumor with indrawn pleura, often considered erroneously as representing tumor extension. **b** Left lateral tomogram in a different patient with bronchogenic carcinoma. The location of the tumor (*t*) in the left upper lobe is clearly demonstrated by its relation to the oblique fissure (*arrowheads*).

muscles. The nipples are commonly, but not always symmetrically, visualized. In case of an apparent pulmonary nodule that cannot be identified on the lateral radiograph, one should check the patient for the possible existence of a cutaneous lesion. When the latter is not found, fluoroscopy, conventional tomography, and eventually CT must follow, to accurately localize the lesion.

The presence of multiple skin lesions such as in neurofibromatosis may mimic pulmonary metastases when projected over the lung fields. On the other hand, it is easy to overlook a true pulmonary nodule under this conditions (72,73). Muscular dystrophy may also be apparent on the chest radiograph (74), with local muscular distrophy mimicking local hyperlucency of the lung.

Soft tissue calcifications may be difficult to identify on low kilovoltage conventional chest radiographs. When in doubt, CT scans or MRI may be capable of providing an immediate and accurate diagnosis. The abdomen, inasmuch as it is visualized on chest radiographs, is normally underexposed. Nevertheless, abdominal pathology may be unexpectedly discovered. When the basal areas of the lungs are obscured by fluid, the position of the gastric and colonic air bubbles may offer information on the diaphragm's position (Fig. 3.7) (75). Likewise, diaphragmatic rupture may be overlooked when the bowel shadows are mistaken for a pulmonary process or when the herniated stomach resembles an elevated diaphragm. Healed rib fractures in such patients could provide a clue to the real lesion (74).

The Diaphragm

At full inspiration, the level of the right hemidiaphragm is projected in a plane ranging from the anterior end of the fifth rib to the sixth anterior interspace (76). The right hemidiaphragm is usually about half an interspace higher than the left, but appreciable unilateral elevation is not uncommon (77). Diaphragmatic excursions in healthy persons range from about 1 to 8 cm (77).

In a PA view, both domes of the diaphragm can normally be demarcated. In the lateral view, however, the anterior segment of the left hemidiaphragm is commonly obliterated by the heart. When (a part of) the diaphragmatic contour, which is normally visible, is obliterated, an adjacent lesion (i.e., a pulmonary infiltrate) should be suspected at that site. This phenomenon, which can occur everywhere along the pleura, is called the silhouette sign (Fig. 3.8a, b) (78). The interlobar pleura goes into the fissures. A thorough knowledge of the normal position of the pleural fissures is essential for the diagnosis of atelectasis.

When the basilar surface of the lung is elevated, pleural fluid should be differentiated from an elevated diaphragm. On the left side, downward displacement of the gastric bubble may indicate the presence of pleural fluid (79). The value of lateral decubitus views in demonstrating subpleural fluid has already been emphasized. When the diaphragm cannot be located by conventional radiography or ultrasound, CT or hepatic scintigraphy may be necessary to locate it (80,81).

The Pleura

The interface between the pleura and the subpleural aerated lung tissue is visualized as a line only at those places where this interface is struck at a tangent by the X-rays. This is normally the case over the inner surface of the ribs bilaterally in the PA view and anteriorly and posteriorly in the lateral view, along the vertebral column and the mediastinum in the PA view, and over the diaphragmatic cupola in both views. The lines corresponding to these interfaces are sometimes called (pleural) *reflection lines* or extrapleural lines. The pleural interfaces may normally show undulations and impressions caused by ribs and other extrapleural structures of the thoracic wall or by mediastinal structures (82–84). There are essentially two types of pleural reflections: convex and concave toward the lung in the direction of the X-ray beam.

A pleural reflection line corresponding to a pleural surface that is convex toward the aerated lung is accompanied by a dark *Mach's band*. When the pleural surface is concave toward the lung, the line is accompanied by a white Mach's band (Fig. 3.9). The Mach's band phenomenon represents an optical effect (85,86).

In each chest radiograph the pleura should be searched for abnormalities. The normal pleura itself is not separately visualized; however, the distance between a pleural reflection line and the underlying bone structure, such as a rib, represents the pleural thickness plus extrapleural fat. Along the rib this shadow is called the companion shadow of the rib. A broad companion shadow may be found in obese persons and should not be misinterpreted as pathologic pleural thickening (87,88).

Pleural thickening can be diffuse or circumscribed. The image of circumscribed pleural thickening can be caused by extrapleural structures (pleural impression), encapsulated pleural fluid, or thickening of the pleura itself. Also, a subpleural pulmonary density may simulate a pleural process. Diffuse increase of the distance between the reflection line and the underlying bony structure indicates obesity, pleural thickening, or pleural fluid. Pleural thickness can also be estimated or measured at the level of an interlobar fissure, provided this fissure is struck tangentially by the X-rays. The interlobar fissure normally represents the thickness of two (visceral) pleural blades. Subpleural edema may stimulate thickening of the pleural fissures (1,89). A thickened pleura may be calcified. To visualize the calcium to good advantage, a low kilovoltage, somewhat overexposed film is advocated.

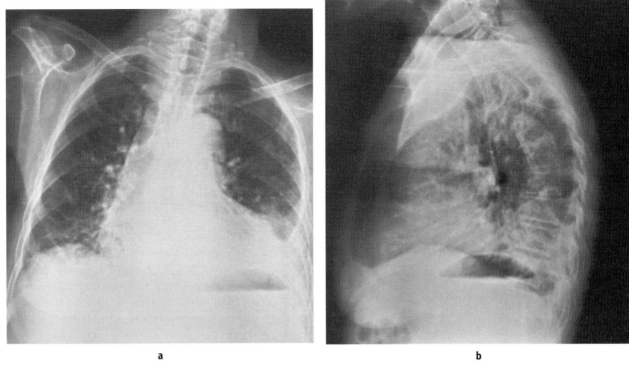

a   b

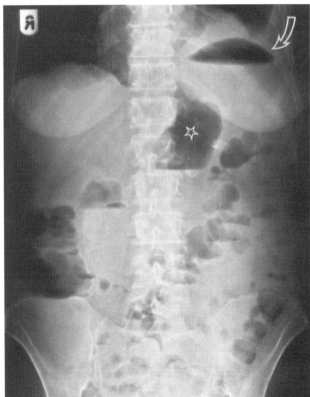

Figure 3.7. Patient with fever. **a** and **b** Posteroanterior (PA) and lateral views. Left costophrenic angle obliterated by the presence of fluid. The diaphragmatic surface of the left lung is invisible on both views because of basal pulmonary infiltration (silhouette sign). **c**. Erect abdominal PA view. The air bubble in the left upper abdomen turns out to be not the gastric bubble, but a subdiaphragmatic abscess (*arrow*). The gastric bubble is displaced downward (*star*).

c

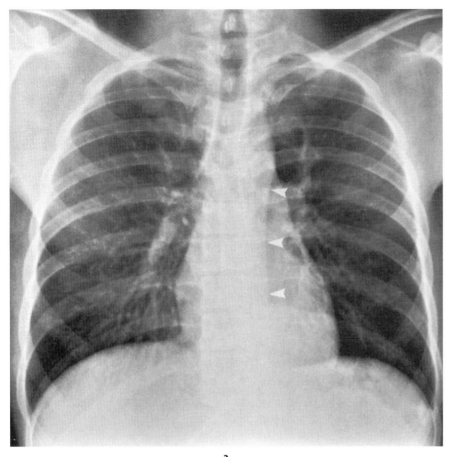

a

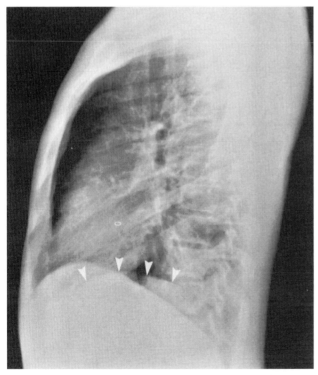

b

Figure 3.8. Silhouette sign in pneumonia. **a** Posteroanterior view. The contour of the lower segment of the descending aorta (*arrowheads*) is not visible because of infiltration of the adjacent lung tissue. The infiltrate is poorly demarcated and can be easily overlooked. **b** Lateral view. The posterior segment of the left diaphragmatic cupola (*arrowheads*) is not visualized because of adjacent pulmonary infiltration.

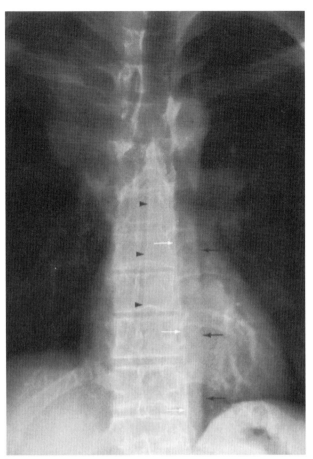

Figure 3.9. Penetrated. coned-down Posteroanterior (PA) chest radiograph Mach's bands in a normal PA view. The contour of the descending aorta is accompanied by a dark Mach's band (*black arrows*). The contour of the left paravertebral line is accompanied by a white Mach's band (*white arrows*). The contour of azygoesophageal recess is identified by *black arrowheads*. *tr.* trachea: *ak.* aortic knob: *rmb.* right main bronchus: *lmb.* left main bronchus.

Extrapulmonary space-occupying lesions should be distinguished from pulmonary processes. When protruding into the lung, extrapulmonary space-occupying lesions in tangential views are characterized by an obtuse angle toward the adjacent pleura, whereas subpleural intrapulmonary processes in most cases show an acute angle (20). However, there are exceptions to this rule (1). If the X-rays are perpendicular to the pleura at the site of the lesion, the contour of the shadow may be very faint because in that direction the attenuation of the X-rays by the thickened pleura is minimal. When a pleural process is projected obliquely, one border may be sharply represented whereas the other border is fading away.

At the apex of the lung, the pleural reflection cannot be exactly related to the ribs on the PA view because the pleural reflection corresponds to a more anterior plane than do the ribs. Therefore apical pleural thickness cannot be measured exactly at that site. Consequently a normal pulmonary apex is sometimes erroneously called an apical cap lesion. The apical pleural reflection line can frequently be traced converging medially and sometimes continuing

into the posterior mediastinal junction line. Frequently, the apical pleural contour has an irregular aspect. This appearance is called an apical cap and is most frequently caused by nonspecific scarring of the subpleural lung parenchyma (90). The apical cap appearance should always be differentiated from the beginning of a tumoral lesion such as the Pancoast tumor. In case of doubt, a CT scan should be performed (91,92).

The lateral or posterior costophrenic sinus may be blunted or obliterated by adhesive processes or by pleural fluid. In the erect patient, pleural fluid of some quantity obliterates the costophrenic sinus with a smoothly ascending border. Sometimes, however, pleural fluid may be accumulated in the infrapulmonary pleural space with or without minimal obliteration of the costophrenic sinus. Frequently, in such cases the lateral segment of the diaphragm may be somewhat elevated (20). On the left side, the presence of infrapulmonary fluid may be suggested by an increased distance between the gastric bubble and the inferior pulmonary border. The fluid can be demonstrated, especially if it is not encapsulated, by decubitus views. For differentiating encapsulated fluid from a solid process, or for differentiating emphysemas and peripheral pulmonary abcesses, ultrasound or CT may be needed (91,93–95).

The Lungs

In searching the lungs for abnormalities it is recommended that the following areas be checked: (a) tracheobronchial tree, (b) pulmonary vessels, (c), hili, and (d) lung parenchyma.

Tracheobronchial Tree

The lumen of the trachea and main bronchi is often visualized on conventional chest radiographs. At those places where the aerated lung abuts the tracheal or bronchial wall, this wall is visualized as a band-like shadow if struck at a tangential plane by the X-rays. At places where the tracheobronchial wall is in contact with other mediastinal structures, only the interface between the wall and the lumen is visualized. The trachea in the PA view shows a slightly S*-shaped curve. After entering the thorax the trachea shows a slight deviation to the right (1). The aortic arch commonly causes a slight tracheal impression on the left.

The trachea in the lateral view is visualized as a column of air that does not normally show an impression (96). The right and left main bronchus more or less overlap each other and constitute the lower section of this air column. The origins of the left and right upper lobe bronchi are often seen superimposed upon the image of the main bronchi as rounded radiolucencies, one above the other (13,96). Narrowing of the air column of the trachea or major bronchi may be caused by an impression by abnormal vessels or space-occupying lesions or by intrinsic processes of the tracheobronchial wall (97–99).

The lateral tracheal band measures I–4 mm at a level 2 cm above the azygos vein (100). A thickened or obscured tracheal band may indicate a mediastinal process such as lymphadenopathy or a pleural or pulmonary process (42,101). Also pleural or subpleural pulmonary processes at that site may enlarge or obscure the band. The lateral tracheal band was visualized in 97% of a series of 100 consecutive patients with no known thoracic disease on high kilovoltage thorax radiographs for which films with a wide exposure latitude were used (102). Consequently, nonvisualization of the tracheal band may not reflect pathology. Actually, the tracheal band may, for example, be obscured by mediastinal lipomatosis (62).

As with the lateral band on the PA view, the posterior wall of the trachea is visualized on the lateral view as a white band, 2–3 mm in width, except in those cases when the esophagus fills the space behind the trachea (62,103,104). On lateral tomograms the posterior tracheal band is interrupted at its lower end by the azygos arch (62). Widening of the posterior tracheal band may be caused by processes that are not visible on the PA view (103). The posterior walls of the right main bronchus and the right intermediate bronchus are most consistently visualized as a continuous band in the lateral view (13,14,62,83). The thickness of the posterior wall of the bronchus intermedius should not normally exceed 3 mm. Thickening of this wall may indicate edema, neoplasm, or enlarged lymph nodes (105).

The following bronchial bands are inconsistently found in the PA view: the left wall of the supraaortic segment of the trachea (102,104), the superior wall of the right main bronchus, the inferior wall of both main bronchi, the medial wall of the intermediate bronchus and the right lower bronchus, and the inferior wall of the lingula bronchus (106,107). Obliteration of only those tracheobronchial bands that are consistently visualized should be considered as a sign of possible lymphadenopathy or other pathologic pulmonary, pleural, or mediastinal processes (97,103,104,108,109). Invisibility of those bands that are inconsistently visualized has limited diagnostic value (102,106).

Intrinsic lesions of the trachea or larger bronchi may be visible on chest radiographs with sufficient penetration and should be searched for, but are often better visualized by conventional tomography or CT.

The smaller bronchi are normally not visualized on plain radiographs. The medium-sized bronchi may be visualized as a double-line shadow (*tramline shadow*) when seen in profile and as a ring-like shadow when seen on end. Prominent tramline shadows may be caused by thickened bronchial walls (e.g., bronchiectasis). The so-called peri-

bronchial cuffing in acute pulmonary edema appears to be caused by edema involving the bronchial wall as well as the peribronchial interstitial space (110). Ectatic bronchi filled with mucus may mimic pulmonary vessels. These various findings may contribute to a general impression of accentuated bronchovascular bundles, producing what is sometimes called a "dirty chest radiograph."

Sometimes ectasis with mucus retention is confined to only one lobar or segmental bronchus and the proximal segments of its ramifications, producing an image of gloved fingers or a gloved hand. This often denotes the presence of a longstanding bronchial obstruction.

Air-containing bronchi standing out in a consolidated segment of lung result in a configuration known as an *air bronchogram* (20). A special example of an air bronchogram is the end-on air bronchogram of the superior segment bronchus of the lower lobe in the PA view, which indicates a consolidative process in this segment and is called the B6 *bronchus sign* (111).

Pulmonary Vessels

In order to distinguish normal from abnormal pulmonary findings on the chest radiograph, it is essential to identify the pulmonary arteries and veins. The normal pulmonary markings, in addition to a limited contribution from the bronchi, consist mainly of the pulmonary arteries and veins. While the pulmonary arteries follow the course of the bronchi, the pulmonary veins are quite variable in their size and course and do not parallel the bronchi. In reporting on the chest radiograph, one should identify the separate vessels and study the vascular pattern as well.

Abnormal pulmonary vascular patterns may reflect heart or lung diseases (112,113). A redistribution of blood flow from one area to another may be the result of impaired perfusion in some areas due to emphysema, tumor, or the like. A redistribution of blood flow in the direction opposite to gravity or general widening of pulmonary veins may reflect pulmonary venous engorgement, but may also result from increased pulmonary blood flow (114). Increased pulmonary blood flow results in a general widening of the pulmonary arteries and veins (113,114). Central widening of all pulmonary arteries with narrowing of the more peripheral arteries may indicate the presence of pulmonary arterial hypertension. Narrowing of peripheral pulmonary arteries combined with hyperaeration may indicate pulmonary emphysema. These different vascular patterns are discussed elsewhere in this volume in connection with specific diseases.

The small pulmonary vessels do not reach the pleura. There is a zone of a few centimeters' width that is recognizable on the chest radiograph where the pulmonary tissue consists only of secondary pulmonary lobules (1). When interlobar fissures are not visualized as a line on conventional radiographs or conventional tomograms, their presence may be indicated by this zone (115–118).

Pulmonary Hili

The complex shadow of the pulmonary hilus is composed mainly of pulmonary arteries and veins, and to a lesser extent bronchi. In addition to the identification of pulmonary vessels and the tracheobronchial system, the hilus should be judged as a whole (119). The hilar shadow may appear enlarged on both the PA and lateral views. When the hilar shadow appears enlarged on the PA view, one should look for abnormalities in the lateral view, because the area beneath the left upper lobe bronchus should be relatively radiolucent on the latter. Enlargement of nodes in the hilar and subcarinal areas increases the opacity in this area (120). As a result, the lateral view can be particularly helpful in analyzing whether a "prominent hilus" is due to enlargement of pulmonary arteries or lymphadenopathy. In order to distinguish a hilar mass from enlarged vessels, or for the visualization of an intraluminal bronchial lesion, conventional tomography or dynamic CT may be required (29,32,121,122).

The Lung Parenchyma

Normally, the lung parenchyma does not produce separate shadows on the chest radiograph. However, when there is loss of lung parenchyma this can be visualized as hyperlucency. On the other hand, increase in water density material exclusively in the lung parenchyma can be visualized as an increase of density. Loss of lung parenchyma is discussed further later in this volume.

Abnormal density material may be situated either in the interstitial compartment of the lung parenchyma or in the alveoli. Depending on its location, the material produces different patterns. Abnormal density material in the interstitial space causes thickening of this space. Only sufficient thickening will be visible on the chest radiograph because the alveolar lumen retains considerable air (123). In a series of 365 patients with histologically proven diffuse infiltrative lung diseases, a normal chest radiograph was found in 9.6% (124).

When the interstitium is sufficiently thickened, a homogeneous veil may be visible, but in most cases a diffuse pattern of discrete densities is produced. Generally speaking, such a pattern is characteristic of interstitial thickening. Interstitial thickening can only be visualized if the adjoining alveoli contain air. The interstitial pattern is superimposed upon the vascular pattern, which remains visible as long as the interstitial pattern is not too dense (125).

When, on the other hand, the alveolar spaces are filled with various materials, especially fluid, a different pattern can be seen. These densities are larger and readily visualized; they are ill defined and tend to coalesce. This pattern is called an "alveolar pattern" or "airspace pattern" (Fig. 3.10) (1,20,125). In the alveolar pattern, the vessels become invisible in the consolidated areas because of the process producing the silhouette sign. For the same reason

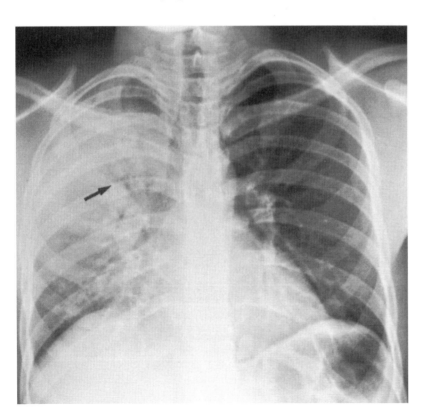

Figure 3.10. Posteroanterior chest radiograph of pneumonia presenting as an airspace consolidation in the major part of the right lung. Note the air bronchogram (*arrow*).

a possible interstitial thickening within an area of alveolar consolidation will not be visualized.

The importance of recognizing abnormal pulmonary patterns is that it may become feasible to refer to a list of diseases that may cause this abnormal pattern. However, there is considerable overlap in alveolar and interstitial patterns. In chronic diffuse infiltrative lung disease, not only the interstitial space but also the alveolar space is more or less involved (124). Alveolar and interstitial patterns may coexist (1). Thus a separate group of combined patterns must be dealt with.

Among these may also be included circumscribed consolidated processes and the sometimes separately described nodular pattern (Fig. 3.11). In all these patterns, the distribution of the lesions throughout the lung may be essential for the diagnosis (1,124,126). The time factor – the rate of progression or regression – can also be very important in the diagnosis of pulmonary parenchymal diseases (51,127).

Mediastinum

The mediastinum is defined best as the extrapleural space within the thorax between the lungs (128). With conventional radiography, including conventional tomography, the interfaces between mediastinum (pleura) and aerated lung are visualized. Within the mediastinum may be visualized air, calcium deposits, or fatty tissue.

Calcium deposits are frequently found in the mediastinum; for example, calcified lymph nodes may be considered a reliable sign of tuberculosis (19). Calcium deposits in the wall of the aorta and large vessels may indicate atherosclerosis; however, the connection between a "calcified aortic knob" and generalized atherosclerosis of the aorta is questionable (129). Another example of calcium deposit in the mediastinum is calcified pericarditis. Fatty tissue of the mediastinum is seldom clearly visualized as such by conventional radiography. However, on the lateral view pericardial fluid may be visualized as a band-like density between the epicardial and pericardial fat (130).

The interface between the mediastinum and the aerated lung is visualized on conventional chest radiographs as the so-called pleural reflection lines or paralines (Fig. 3.12). Such lines should be distinguished from bands or stripes. A pleural reflection line (paraline) represents only one interface, i.e., the border between two areas with different densities. Such a line has no width or density of its own. However, such lines may show the Mach phenomenon (see above). Stripes or bands, in contrast, have a certain width and are white. Bands are

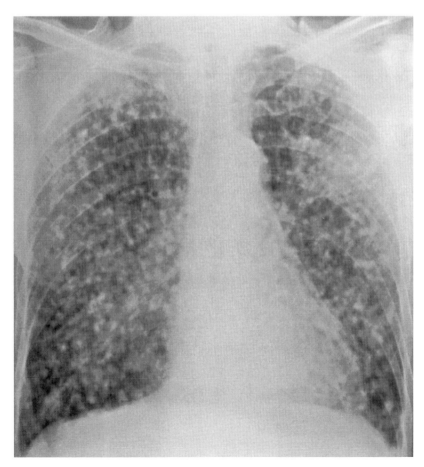

Figure 3.11. Posteroanterior chest radiograph. Nodular pattern in pulmonary metastatses.

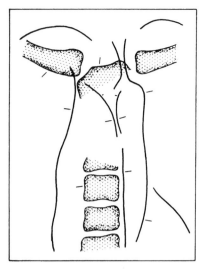 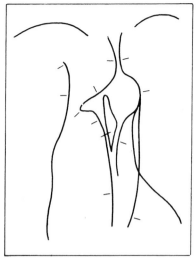 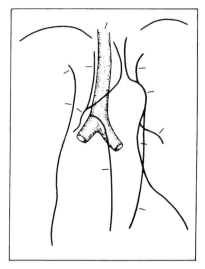

Figure 3.12. Diagram of mediastinal pleural reflection lines. For the sake of clarity the lines are distributed over three figures. (Frequencies of occurrence noted for some lines are taken from ref. 102.)

1. clavicle
2. manubrium sterni
3. spine
4. trachea
5. lateral tracheal band (97%)
6. aortic knob (100%)
7. left subclavian artery (89%)
8. descending aorta
9. reflection A-line
10. reflection B-line
11. vena cava superior (64%)
12. vena anonyma/subclavia
13. azygos arch, paratracheal segment (98%)

14. azygos knob
15. azygoesophageal recess (87%)
16. preaortic recess (7%)
17. subaortic outpouching of esophagus
18. supraazygos (right prevertebral) recess
19. supraaortic (left prevertebral) recess
18/19. posterior superior junction line (32%)
20. right retrosternal recess
21. eft retrosternal recess
20/21. anterior junction line (57%)
22.. anterior mediastinal triangle
23. left paravertebral line (41%)

visualized as such because they are bordered on both sides by air or aerated tissue, so these lines represent two interfaces. When such bands are very thin, they appear as white "lines." Paralines can be used as guidance parameters and play a prominent part in mediastinal diagnosis.

In reporting on the chest radiograph, these pleural lines and bands should be identified and assessed as being normal or abnormal. The following signs may indicate an abnormality: absence of pleural reflection line that is usually visualized, an interrupted segment of the line, a bulging segment in a more or less straight or concave pleural reflection line, or an additonal line not corresponding to a normal anatomic structure. Abnormal pleural reflection lines may reflect a mass lesion within the mediastinum. Mediastinal lipomatosis may affect the pleural reflection lines as well (62).

References

1. Fraser RF, Paré JAP (1977). Diagnosis of diseases of the chest. WB Saunders, Philadelphia.
2. Christensen EE, Dietz GW, Murry RC, et al. (1977) Effect of kilovoltage on detectability of pulmonary nodules in a chest phantom. AJR 128:789–793.
3. Kelsey CA, Moseley RD, Jr, Mettler FA, Jr, et al. (1982) Comparison of nodule detection with 70 kVp chest radiograph. Radiology 143:609–11.
4. Jacobson G, Bohlig H, Kiviluoto R. (1970) Essentials of chest radiography. Radiology 95:445–450.
5. Wilkinson GA, Fraser RG (1975) Roentgenography of the chest. Appl Radiol 4:41.
6. Lynch PA (1985) A different approach to chest roentgenography: Triad technique (high kilovoltage, grid, wedge filter). AJR Radium Ther Nucl Med. 93:965–971.
7. van Heesewijk HP, van der Graaf Y, de Valois JC, et al. (1996) Chest imaging with a selenium detector versus conventional chest radiography: A CT controlled study. Radiology 200:687–690.
8. Maruyama Y (1998) Performance of various x-ray film/screen systems in demonstrating small simulated low-density lung nodules. Nippon Igaku Hoshasen Gakkai Zasshi 58:509–515.
9. McLean D, Gray JE, Swensen SJ, et al. (1998) Clinical evaluation of twin screen–film chest radiography: Cost effective lung and mediastinal imaging. Eur J Radiol 27:61–66.
10. Swensen SJ, Aughenbaugh GL, Brown LR, et al. (1998) Advanced multiple beam equalization radiography: Receiver operating characteristic comparison with screen–film chest radiography. Mayo Clin Proc 73:636–641.

11. Tuengerthal S, Ackermann L, Müller A (1985) Anatomisches geformtes unscharfes bleihaltiges Acrylglasfilter zur Optimierung der Röntgenaufnahme. Röntgen-Bl 38:126–133.

12. Johnson GA, Ravin CE (1983) A survey of digital chest radiography. Symposium on cardiopulmonary imaging. Radiol Clin North Am 21:655–665.

13. Bachman DM, Ellis K, Austin JHM (1978) The effects of minor degrees of obliquity on the lateral chest radiograph. Radiol Clin North Am 16:465–485.

14. Austin JHM (1984) The lateral chest radiograph in the assessment of nonpulmonary health and disease. In Symposyium on nonpulmonary aspects in chest radiology. Radiol Clin North Am 22:687–692.

15. Hubbell FA, Greenfield S, Tyler JL, et al. (1985) The impact of routine admission chest X-ray films on patient care. N Engl J Med 312:209–213.

16. Robinson AE (1998) The lateral chest radiograph: Is it doomed to extinction? Acad Radiol 5:322–323.

17. Giron S, Sans N, Senac JP (1999) Lateral view of the thorax: The profile. J Radiol 80:109–119.

18. Woodring JH (1998) The lateral chest radiograph in the detection of pericardial effusion: A reevaluation. J Ky Med Assoc 96: 218–224.

19. Bismuth V, Coulomb M, Bignon J (1977): Sémiologie radiologique des affections broncho-pulmonaires. In Fischgold H, Doyon D (eds) Traité de radiodiagnostic, Tome IV. Masson, Paris, pp 195–360.

20. Felson B (1973) Chest roentgenology. WB Saunders, Philadelphia.

21. Kocijancic I, Tercelj M, Vidmar K, et al. (1999). The value of inspiratory–expiratory lateral decubitus views in the diagnosis of small pleural effusions. Clin Radiol 54:595–597.

22. Milne ENC (1986). A physiological approach to reading critical care unit films. J Thorac Imaging 1:60–90.

23. Janower ML, Jennas-Nocera Z, Mukai J (1984) Utility and efficacy of portable chest radiograhs. AJR 142:265–267.

23. Swensen SJ, Peters SG, LeRoy AJ, et al. (1991). Radiology in the intensive care unit. Mayo Clin Proc 66:396–410.

24. Fong Y, Whalen GF, Hariri RJ, et al. (1995). Utility of routine chest radiographs in the intensive care unit. A prospective study. Arch Surg 130:764–768.

25. Silverstein DS, Livingston DH, Elcavage J, et al. (1993) The utility of daily chest radiography in the surgical intensive care unit. J Trauma 35:643–646.

26. Brogdon BG, Moseley RD, Kelsey CA, et al. (1978) Perception of simulated lung lesions. Invest Radiol 13:12–15.

27. Kelsey CA, Moseley RD. Mettler FA, Jr (1982) Cost-effectiveness of stereoscopic radiographs in detection of lung nodules. Radiology 142:611–613.

28. Westra D (1972) Binocular differentiation of radiographs (the blinking method). Radiol Clin 41:436–447.

29. Littleton JT (1976) Tomography: Physical principles and clinical applications. Williams & Wilkins, Baltimore, MD.

30. Ziedses des Plantes BG (1971) Body-section radiography. History, image information, various techniques and results. Aust Radiol 15:57.

31. Littleton JT, Durzich ML, Callahan WP (1980) Linear versus pluridirectional tomography of the chest: Correlative radiographic anatomic study. AJR 134:241–248.

32. Favez G, Willa C, Heinzer F (1974) Posterior oblique tomography at an angle of 55 degrees in chest roentgenology. AJR Radium Ther Nucl Med 120:907–915.

33. McLeod RA, Brown LIZ, Miller WE, et al. (1976). Evaluation of the pulmonary hila by tomography. Radiol Clin North Am 14:51–84.

34. Stigsson L, Tyen U (1983). 55 degrees posterior oblique tomograpy in the evaluation of lung tumors. Radiologie 23:224–228.

35. Brown LR, Deremee RA (1976) 55 Oblique hilar tomography. Mayo Clin Proc 51:89–96.

36. Faling LJ, Pugatch RD, Jung-Legg Y, et al. (1981) Computed tomographic scanning of the mediastinum in the staging of bronchogenic carcinoma. Am Rev Respir Dis 124:690–695.

37. Libschitz HI (1983) CT of mediastinal lymph nodes in lung cancer: Is there a "state of the art"? AJR 141:1081–1085.

38. Peace PK, Price JL (1973) Preoperative tomographic assessment of the mediastinum in bronchial carcinoma. Thorax 28:367–370.

39. Lewis, JW, Madrazo BL, Gross SC, et al. (1982) The value of radiographic and computed tomography in the staging of lung carcinoma. Ann Thorac Surg 34:553–557.

40. Brogdon BG, Littleton JT, Durizch ML (1983). Comparison of radiographic imaging techniques in detection of pulmonary nodules. In Littleton JT, Durizch ML (eds) Sectional imaging methods: a comparison. University Park Press, Baltimore, MD, pp 137–153.

41. Chiles C, Ravin CE (1985). Intrathoracic metastasis from an extrathoracic malignancy: A radiologic approach to patient evaluation. Radiol Clin North Am 23:427–438.

42. Schaner EG, Chang AE, Doppman JL et al. (1978): Comparison of computed and conventional whole lung tomography in detecting pulmonary nodules: A prospective radiologic–pathologic study. AJR 131:51–54.

43. Alter AJ, Kargas GA, Kargas SA, et al. (1982). The influence of ambient and viewbox light upon visual detection of low contrast targets in a radiograph. Invest Radiol 17:402–406.

44. Garland LH (1959) Studies on the accuracy of diagnostic procedures. AJR Radium Ther Nucl Med 82:25–38.

45. Tuddenham WJ (1963) Problems of perception in chest roentgenology. Facts and fallacies. Radial Clin North Am 1:277.

46. Westra D (1966) Zonography, the narrow-angle tomography. Excerpta Medica Foundation, Amsterdam.

47. Hall FM (1982) Viewing the lateral radiograph (editorial). AJR 139:1235.

48. Garland LH (1949) On the scientific evaluation of diagnostic procedures. Radiology 52:309–328.

49. Kundel HL (1975) Radiological image perception. Appl Radiol 4:27–96.

50. Brogdon BG, Kelsey CA, Moseley RD (1983) Factors affecting perception of pulmonary lesions. In Pittman CE (guest ed) Symposium in cardiopulmonary imaging. Radiol Clin North Am 21:633–654.

51. Fraser RG, Paré JAP, Paré PD, et al. (1988) Diagnosis of diseases of the chest, 3rd edu. WB Saunders, Philadelphia.

52. Riebel FA (1958) Use of the eyes in x-ray diagnosis. Radiology 70:252.

53. Beckenridge JW, Bird GC (1977) Errors of omission in pulmonary nodule detection. Appl Radiol 6:51–54.

54. Spratt JS, Jr, Ter Pogossian M, Long RTL (1963) The detection and growth of intrathoracic neoplasms: The lower limits of radiographic distinction of the antemortem size, the duration, and the pattern of growth as determined by direct mensuration of tumor diameters from random thoracic roentgenograms. Arch Surg 86:283–288.

55. Greening RR, Pendergrass EP (1954) Postmortem roentgenography with particular emphasis upon the lung. Radiology 62:720–725.

56. Kelsey CA, Moseley RD, Brogdon BG, et al. (1977) Effect of size and position on chest lesion detection. AJR 129:205–208.

57. Capp MP, Gray J, Seeley G, et al. (1974) Psychophysics from a radiologist's point of view. SPIE Proc 46:142–147.

58. Miller WT, Aronchick JM, Epstein DM, et al. (1985). The troublesome nipple shadow. AJR 145:521–523.

59. Bernadac P (1977) Pièges et artefacts de la radiographie pulmonaire standard de face. In Fischgold H, Doyon D (eds): Traité radiodiagnostic, Tome IV. Masson, Paris, pp 125–143.

60. Greene R, McLoud TL, Stark P (1977) Pneumothorax. Semin Roentgenol 12:313–325.

61. King JB (1939) Calcification of the costal cartilages. Br I Radiol 12:2.

62. Heitzman ER (1977) The mediastinum, radiologic correlations with anatomy and pathology. Mosby, St Louis, MD.

63. Westra D (1978) Vascular pseudo-tumours of the mediastinum in asymptomatic patients. A tomographic study. I. Arteries. Radiol Clin 47:100–113.

64. Fischer E. (1963) Durch Schleim vorgetäuschte Wandprozesse der grossen Luftwege. Rofo Fortschr Geb Rontgenstr Neuen Bildgeb Verfahr 98:233-234.

65. Westra D (1975) Der Schleimpfropf, Phantomgeschwulst der grossen Luftwege. Ein tomographisches Bild. Rofo Fortschr Geb Rontgenstr Neuen Bildgeb Verfahr 122:428–434.

66. Karasick D, Karasick S, Lally JF (1979) Mucoid pseudotumors of the tracheobronchial tree in two cases. AJR 132:459–460.

67. Westra D, Verbeeten B, Jr (1985) Some anatomical variants and pitfalls in computed tomography of the trachea and mainstem bronchi. I. Mucoid pseudotumors. Diagn Imaging Med 54:229–239.

68. Millard CF (1971) Vanishing or phantom tumor of the lung: Localized interlobar effusion in congestive heart failure. Chest 59:675–676.

69. Subbarao K, Jacobson HG (1986) Systemic disorders affecting the thoracic cage. In Kattan KR (guest ed) Symposium on nonpulmonary aspects in chest radiology. Radiol Clin North Am 22:497–517.

70. Figley MM (1954) Accessory Roentgen signs of coarctation of the aorta. Radiology 62:671–686.

71. Kurihara Y, Yakushiji YK, Matsumoto J, et al. (1999). The ribs: Anatomic and radiologic considerations. Radiographics 19:105–119.

72. Aughenbaugh GL (1984) Thoracic manifestations of neurocutaneous diseases. In Kattan KR (guest ed) Symposium on nonpulmonary aspects in chest radiology. Radiol Clin North Am 22:741–754.

73. Schabel SI, Schmidt GE, Vujic I (1980) Overlooked pulmonary malignancy in neurofibromatosis. J Can Assoc Radiol 31:135–136.

74. Kattan KR (1984) Some telltales and pitfalls in chest radiology. In Kattan KR (guest ed) Symposium on nonpulmonary aspects in chest radiology. Radiol Clin North Am 22:467–485.

75. Gedgaudas-McClees RK, Torres WE, Colvin RS, et al. (1984) Thoracic findings in gastrointestinal pathology. In Kattan KR (guest ed) Symposium on nonpulmonary aspects in chest radiology. Radiol Clin North Am 22:563–589.

76. Lennon EA, Simon G (1965) The height of the diaphragm in the chest radiograph of normal adults. Br J Radiol 38:937–943.

77. Young DA, Simon G (1972) Certain movements measured on inspiration–expiration chest radiographs correlated with pulmonary function studies. Clin Radiol 23:37–41.

78. Felson B, Felson H (1950) Localization of intrathoracic lesions by means of the postero-anterior roentgenogram: The silhouette sign. Radiology 55:363–374.

79. Mulvey RB (1965) The effect of pleural fluid on the diaphragm. Radiology 84:1080–1086.

80. Trought WS (1981) Ultrasound in the diagnosis of thoracic abnormalities. Pulmonary diagnosis imaging and other techniques. Appleton-Century Crofts, New York.

81. Tarver RD, Godwin JD, Putman CE (1984) The diaphragm. In Kattan KR (guest ed) Symposium on Nonpulmonary Aspects in Chest radiology. Radiol Clin North Am 22:615–631.

82. Whalen JP, Oliphant M, Evans JA (1975) Anterior extrapleural: Superior extension. Radiology 115:525–531.

83. Proto AV, Speckman JM (1979) The left lateral radiograph of the chest. Part I. Med Radiogr Photogr 55:30–74.

84. Proto AV, Speckman JM (1980) The left lateral radiograph of the chest. Part II. Med Radiogr Photogr 56:38–64.

85. Genereux GP (1983) The posterior pleural reflections. AJR 141:141–149.

86. Jaffe CC (1984) Medical imaging, vision, and visual psychophysics. Med Radiogr Photogr 60:1–48.

87. Gluck MC, Twigg HL, Ball MF, et al. (1972) Shadows bordering the lung on radiographs of normal and obese persons. Thorax 27:232–238.

88. Vix VA (1974) Extrapleural costal fat. Radiology 112:563.

89. Grainger RG (1958) Interstitial pulmonary oedema and its radiological diagnosis. A sign of pulmonary venous and capillary hypertension. Br J Radiol 31:201–217.

90. Renner RR, Markarian BP, Pernice NJ, et al. (1974) The apical cap. Radiology 110:569–573.

91. Lackner K, Weiand G, Koster O (1981) Erweiterung der Röntgendiagnostik raumfordernder Prozesse der Thoraxwand durch die Computertomographie. Rofo Fortschr Geb Rontgenstr Neuen Bildgeb Verfahr 134:607–613.

92. Webb WR, Jeffrey RB, Godwin JD (1981) Thoracic computed tomography in superior sulcus tumors. J Comput Assist Tomogr 5:361–365.

93. Stark DD, Federle MP, Goodman PC, et al. (1983). Differentiating lung abscess and empyema: Radiography and computed tomography. AJR 141:163–167.

94. Caron-Poitreau C, Delumeau J, Dabouis G, et al. (1981) Apport de la tomodensitométrie à l'étude des tumeurs primitives de la plèvre. Ann Radiol 24:247–253.

95. Baber CE, Hedlund LW, Oddson TA, et al. (1980) Differentiating empyemas and peripheral pulmonary abcesses. The value of computed tomography. Radiology 135:755–758.

96. Vix VA, Klatte EC (1970) The lateral chest radiograph in the diagnosis of hilar and mediastinal masses. Radiology 96:307–316.

97. Berkmen YM (1984). The trachea: The blind spot in the chest. In Kattan KR (guest ed) Symposium on nonpulmonary aspects in chest radiology. Radiol Clin North Am 22:539–562.

98. Felson B (1983) Neoplasms of the trachea and main stem bronchi. Semin Roentgenol 18:23–37.

99. Muhm JR, Crowe JK (1976) The evaluation of tracheal abnormalities by tomography. Radiol Clin North Am 14:95–104.

100. Savoca CJ, Austin JHM, Goldberg HI (1977) The right paratracheal stripe. Radiology 122:295–301.

101. Kittredge RD (1979) The right posterolateral tracheal band. J Comput Assist Tomogr 3:348–354.

102. Woodring JH, Daniel TL (1986) Mediastinal analysis emphasizing plain radiographs and computed tomograms. Med Radiogr Photogr 62:1–49.

103. Shields JB, Holtz S (1976) The retrotracheal space. Radiology 120:19–23.

104. Bachman AL, Teixidor MD (1975) The posterior tracheal band: A reflector of local superior mediastinal abnormality. Br J Radiol 48:352–359.

105. Schnur MJ, Winkler B, Austin JHM (1981) Thickening of the posterior wall of the bronchus intermedius. A sign of lateral chest radiographs of congestive heart failure, lymph node enlargement and ncoplastic infiltration. Radiology 139:551–559.

106. Rémy J, Lemaître L, Smith M (1981) Die topographischradiologische Anatomie des rechten subkarinaeren und retrobronchialen pulmonalen Recessus. Radiologie 21:324–329.

107. Genereux GP (1983) Conventional tomographic hilar anatomy emphasizing the pulmonary veins. AJR 141:1241–1257.

108. Raider L (1973) The retrotracheal triangle. Chest 63:835-838.

109. Jarlot D, Viallet P, Viallet PF, et al. (1976) Anatomie radiologique du médiastin de profil et applications diagnostiques. J Radiol Electrol 57:916–921.

110. Don C, Johnson R (1977) The nature and significance of peribronchial cuffing in pulmonary edema. Radiology 125:577–582.

111. Friedman PJ (1982) Radiology of the superior segment of the lower lobe. Radiology 144:15–25.

112. Milne ENC (1973) Correlation of physiologic findings and chest roentgenology. Radiol Clin North Am 11:17–48.
113. Kubicka RA (1985) A primer on the pulmonary vasculature. Med Radiogr Photogr 61:14–28.
114. Milne ENC (1978) Some new concepts on pulmonary blood flow and volume. Radiol Clin North Am 16:515–536.
115. Milne ENC, Bass H (1969) The roentgenologic diagnosis of early obstructive pulmonary disease. J Can Assoc Radiol 20:3–15.
116. Frija J, Smith P, Katz M, et al. (1982) Computed tomography of the pulmonary fissures: normal anatomy. J Comput Assist Tomogr 6:1069–1074.
117. Goodman LR, Golkow RS, Steiner RM, et al. (1982) Right mid-lung window: A potential source of error in computed tomography of the lung. Radiology 143:135–138.
118. Milne ENC (1982) Re: the right mid-lung window. Radiology 145:171.
119. Rigler LG, O' Laughlin BJ, Tucker RC (1952) Significance of unilateral enlargement of the hilar shadow in the early diagnosis of the carcinoma of the lung with observation on a method of mensuration. Radiology 59:683–693.
120. Ravin CE (1986) Structures of the hilus and mediastinum. Plain film analysis. 18th International Course, Davos. Thorax.
121. Naidich DP, Zerhouni EA, Siegelman SS (1984) Computed tomography of the thorax. Raven Press, New York.
122. Glazer GM, Francis JR, Gebarski K (1983) Dynamic incremental computed tomography in the study of the pulmonary hili. J Comput Assist Tomogr 7:59–64.
123. Felson B (1966) Disseminated interstitial diseases of the lung. Ann Radiol 9: 325–345.
124. McLoud TC, Carrington CB, Gaensler EA (1983) Diffuse infiltrative lung disease: A new scheme for description. Radiology 149:353–363.
125. Felson B (1978) A new look at pattern recognition of diffuse pulmonary infiltrates. 64th Scientific assembly and annual meeting of the Radiological Society of North America, categorized course in radiology of the chest, 309B.
126. Freundlich IM (1979). Diffuse pulmonary disease. A radiologic approach. WB Saunders, Philadelphia.
127. Felson B (1952) Acute miliary diseases of the lung. AJR Radium Ther Nucl Med 59:32–48.
128. Berne AS, Gerle RD, Mitchell GE (1969) The mediastinum. Normal roentgenanatomy and radiologic techniques. Semin Roentgenol 4:3–21.
129. Dalith F (1961) Calcification of the aortic knob. Its relationship to the fifth and sixth embryonic aortic arches. A radiologic and anatomical study. Radiology 76:213–221.
130. Lane EF, Carsky EW (1968) Epicardial fat. Lateral plain film analysis in normals and in pericardial effusion. Radiology 93:279–284.

Computed Tomography of the Thorax: Lungs and Mediastinum

M. Sperber

Introduction

X-ray cross-sectional images of the human body with computer processing and reconstruction were obtained for the first time in the early 1970s. While leading to a reevaluation of other existing investigative modalities, computed tomography (CT) has since become a well-recognized, valuable diagnostic tool, its use being extended to a large variety of clinical conditions (1–40). CT differs from conventional radiographic techniques, including linear tomography, in its ability to identify abnormalities not only as changes in anatomic form but also as differences in radiographic contrast, therefore enabling a separate visualization of various body tissues.

Depending on the clinical requirements of each examination, the body tissues are studied in the form of reconstructed tomographic slices 1–10 mm thick. Newly developed CT prototypes permit examination of each body slice during a scanning sequence that lasts as little as 2 or even less. "Fast" CT scanning has been demonstrated

to have diagnostic significance, not only by prominently reducing the effects of physiologic motion, but also by allowing the performance of CT angiography (41–43). This modality facilitates the study of the vascularity of a lesion in a short period of time during a contrast bolus injection (successfully used, for example, in the study of thoracic vasculature). The details of the advanced spiral or helical CT technique are discussed at the end of this chapter.

A CT apparatus is basically composed of a scanning gantry with an X-ray source and an array of highly sensitive crystal detectors mounted symmetrically at the extremities of a frame. A centrally collimated fan beam of X-rays is used, and the readings from the detector array are digitized and continuously transferred to a computer during the scanning operation (Fig. 4.1). The accumulated information is registered in the form of picture elements and stored in digital form in the computer's memory.

The obtained image can be displayed in a numerical printout or on a television monitor, with the shade of gray

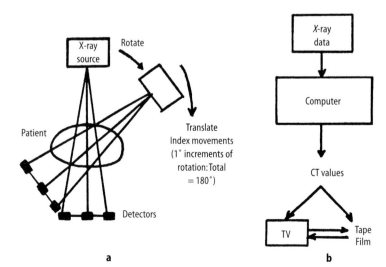

a   b   **Figure 4.1.** Diagram illustrating the principle of a CT apparatus.

corresponding to the calculated absorption coefficients. In computed tomography, the computer uses a sequence of digital numbers to reconstruct the CT image. These CT numbers have been chosen arbitrarily as having water at 0, air at –1000, and bone at +1000. The unit most commonly used to express X-ray attenuation values in a CT representation has been named the Hounsfield unit (HU), to honor the inventor of the CT machine (Fig. 4.2).

The CT numbers obtained have a specific relationship to the brightness level, a relationship that can be represented on a scale having the +1000 limit for white, the –1000 limit for black, and all the values in between represented by various shades of gray. Finding the specific value relating a CT number to a brightness level is called "setting a window" and is a most useful manipulation, allowing the radiologist to recognize fine differences in tissue density by choosing the correct window height and width – in other words, by selecting the desired upper or lower level of contrast between which tissues are imaged.

A certain volume of tissue represented on a CT image is called a voxel. Each voxel is displayed on a cathode ray oscilloscope screen as a picture element, or pixel. A two-dimensional network of pixels forms the matrix; matrices of 256, 320, or 512 elements in diameter are commonly encountered. Several factors influence the Hounsfield value determination, among them the partial volume effect, which means that the pixel delineated in the CT image may include in the volume unit (voxel) tissues of various densities and attenuation qualities, resulting in a Hounsfield number that is the average of the tissues scanned. Recognition of this partial volume effect is a prerequisite for proper diagnosis, especially when specific local measurements are necessary. Other sources for inaccurate Hounsfield values are the alteration of the X-ray radiation used in CT when it passes across materials with a high atomic number, such as bone, iodine, or metallic objects, and patient motion during scanning procedures. This factor reduces the potential precision of the imaging process by producing artefacts.

In the thorax, it is always mandatory to obtain two different images at each thoracic level, because of the variation in attenuation between the mediastinum and the pulmonary parenchyma. Therefore, obtaining a "lung window" means obtaining an image at the widest window width and a window level of about –700, and obtaining a "mediastinal window" means obtaining a narrower window width at a window level of 0. Each CT unit has its own numerical standards, and the particular examination has to be adjusted to them and to the demands of the clinical problems.

In order to accommodate special examinations, a number of technical facilities are usually provided by the CT unit. They include gantry tilt, which permits various changes in the patient's position, and devices that allow magnification of a region of interest or reconstruction of coronal or sagittal images. Reformatted CT images may help the viewer to identify a wide range of abnormalities for which insufficient information is obtained on cross-sectional scans (i.e., determining the real extent of a thoracic aortic aneurysm).

At the present time it is generally acknowledged that CT is a highly sensitive modality for the examination of the thorax. Numerous studies have demonstrated its ability to solve diagnostic problems concerning mediastinal abnormalities, diffuse pulmonary diseases, and pleural pathology as well as its use in pre- and postsurgical and therapeutic evaluation of various lesions. This chapter is designed to review the current diagnostic approach in pulmonary medicine with CT. For more detailed information on this subject, the reader is directed to the chapters that deal with specific diseases, which contain discussions on the place of CT in conjunction with the clinical investigative arsenal, and to other volumes dedicated to this topic (1–3, 44–46).

Thoracic Abnormalities as Viewed by Computed Tomography

Mediastinal and Hilar Pathology

Computed tomography is an ideal modality for the study of the mediastinal and hilar areas because of its ability to

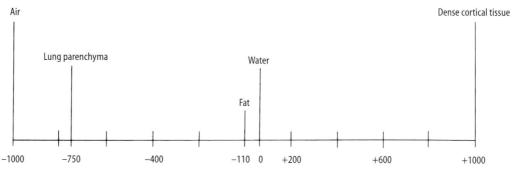

Figure 4.2. CT numbers (Hounsfield units: HU) expressing differences in tissue density.

detect minimal differences in tissue density and provide cross-sectional images of suspected lesions. The differential diagnosis of mediastinal abnormalities is extensive, and often multiple investigative modalities, including conventional tomography and fluoroscopic or barium examinations, are needed in order to arrive to an accurate final diagnosis. Numerous studies have proved the efficacy of CT in the evaluation of mediastinal pathology (10–17, 47–57).

Some of the major indications for the use of CT in the study of the mediastinum are:

1. *Evaluation of mediastinal widening:* CT is able to differentiate between abundant fat deposition, presence of tortuous vessels, primary neoplasms, or enlarged lymph nodes as the major reasons for this abnormality discovered on conventional chest radiographs.

2. *Differentiation of mediastinal lesions based on the attenuation coefficient:* Because of the ability of CT to accurately measure the density of a given mediastinal mass, CT measurements appear to be reliable enough to permit the distinction between solid, cystic, and vascular lesions, as well as helping to identify the presence of minute calcifications or necrotic areas within a mass lesion.

3. *Evaluation of suspected lesions discovered on conventional studies:* On cross-sectional images provided by CT, multiple structures are visible on a single section; therefore, a precise distinction of the suspected abnormality from various mediastinal adjacent structures is possible.

4. *Tumor localization and assessment of metastatic spread:* CT appears to be a most valuable modality in the localization of mediastinal neoplastic lesions, as well as one of the methods of choice in the demonstration of tumor extension to the surrounding mediastinal area, chest wall, and the like. CT has a unique value in the staging of bronchogenic carcinoma; it enables the early discovery of metastatic deposits to the mediastinum and hili from a primary lung tumor.

It has been concluded that an attenuation value around −110 HU can be reliably considered to be a sign of benignity. Less negative coefficients, such as −20 to −40 HU, carry a high probability of malignancy. Benign cystic lesions of the mediastinum present usually as round or oval masses of water density, commonly discovered at the right costophrenic angle (pericardial cysts) or located just inferior to the carina and in the proximity of major bronchi. CT numbers that are higher than those of water can be found in certain areas within the cystic lesion, as a result of their mucoid contents. Generally, the location and density measurements of a mediastinal cyst are characteristic enough to prevent invasive evaluation in an asymptomatic patient, and is reserved for those cases in which the cyst is exerting pressure on adjacent structures.

The extent of a thyroid lesion and its relationship to vital surrounding organs is most accurately established with CT. Scattered calcifications within the tumor, as well as low density cystic portions or areas of necrosis, are easily identified. Characteristically, a thyroid tumor will show prominent enhancement after intravenous administration of contrast material (48,49).

CT is particularly valuable in the study of the thymus gland, which by this method is visualized more clearly than with conventional radiographic techniques, including conventional tomography (50,51). In patients with myasthenia gravis, CT can provide important diagnositic information when one is searching for a possible thymic abnormality. Because in 8–15% of patients with myasthenia gravis a thymoma can be discovered, benign or malignant, and since up to 37% of thymomas are malignant and their resection has a favorable impact on the outcome of the disease in many patients, CT diagnostic information has great clinical value (52,53) (Fig. 4.3). CT is also a reliable modality in the depiction of thymic cysts. Their benignity is usually demonstrated by imaging the homogeneous water-like content and the thin, well-delineated wall. CT-guided needle biopsy may be needed to complete the diagnosis in problematic cases (54,55) (Fig. 4.4).

A teratoma will present calcific deposits or a calcified wall that are clearly identified on CT sections. The extent of other mediastinal tumors, such as seminomas or malignant lymphomas, is also accurately established with CT, a lymphomatous mass often being associated with the presence of enlarged hilar lymph nodes (1,2,11,56).

The discovery of a parathyroid adenoma localized in the upper mediastinum may pose a special diagnostic problem. In such cases, the injection of intravenous con-

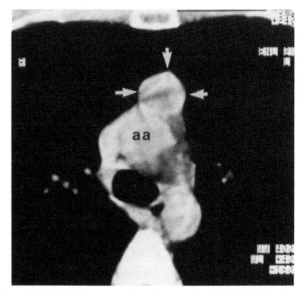

Figure 4.3. Thymoma demonstrated on CT scans as a rounded mediastinal lesion (*arrows*), which should not be misinterpreted as the ascending aorta (*aa*). (Thymoma was surgically confirmed.)

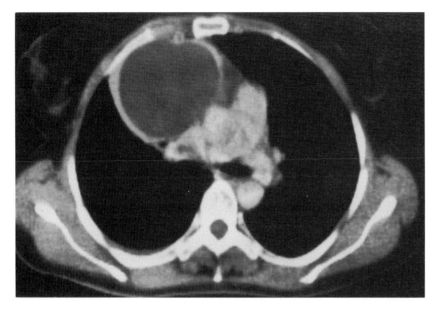

Figure 4.4. Large thymic cyst in the anterior mediastinum exerting pressure on the adjacent structures. The lesion is recognized by its homogeneous content and the well-delineated wall. (Thymic cyst was surgically confirmed.)

trast is advised in order to facilitate the separation of the usually small parathyroid adenoma from the thyroid gland and the surrounding mediastinal vessels (8).

Numerous pathologic processes involve concomitantly the mediastinum and the pulmonary hili. One of the most commonly encountered diagnostic problems in daily practice is the evaluation of an enlarged or questionably prominent hilus and the identification of enlarged hilar lymph nodes, a prominent central pulmonary artery, or a tumoral mass as a reason for this abnormality. Studies have shown that conventional tomography, including the 55*b3 oblique projection, still represents a valuable procedure for the study of the pulmonary hilus (6,16,58). However, the introduction of CT, with its excellent demonstration of the cross-sectional hilar anatomy has added substantial information to the data available from conventional studies. The use of intravenous iodinated contrast material allows accurate differentiation between hilar vasculature and a hilar mass on CT images; obstruction or displacement of the bronchial tree can also be easily identified. A thorough knowledge of mediastinal and hilar anatomy is required in order to diagnose at an early stage abnormalities affecting these areas (4,5,13,14,59–62).

Vascular Anomalies

Congenital and acquired abnormalities of the aortic arch and the great vessels can sometimes be mistaken for mass lesions on plain chest radiographs and CT scans. Generally, whenever the distinction between a mass and a vascular lesion is required on CT examinations of the thorax, intravenous contrast material has to be employed. Using this method, attenuation values of the abnormality in question that are comparable to those of the normal vessels in the area support a vascular etiology. Congenital anomalies of the aortic arch and upper mediastinal vessels are easily identified with CT (18–20). They include an anomalous origin of the right subclavian artery, double or right aortic arch, or a persistent superior vena cava. CT also can be used as a reliable adjuvant to angiography in the confirmation of vascular aberrations typical of coarctation of the aorta and transposition of great vessels, as well as in the search for postsurgical complications that may follow corrections of aortic coarctation, such as dissection, restenosis, or aneurysm formation (21,22).

The value of CT as a radiologic technique has also been demonstrated in the evaluation of thoracic – aortic aneurysm (Figs. 4.5,4.6). The aortic lumen can be precisely measured with CT and is considered to be dilated when it exceeds 4–4.5 cm. The size of the aneurysm and the presence of intramural thrombi and their relationship to the aortic lumen are accurately visualized on CT sections. Arteriosclerotic calcifications, as well as effects of aortic aneurysmal dilatation on adjacent mediastinal structures, are easily demonstrated. If surgical resection of the aneurysm is considered, however, aortography is usually required to supplement the CT findings. CT is also beneficial in the study of the dissection of the thoracic aorta and as an adjuvant to arteriography when the establishment of an immediate diagnosis is of paramount importance in this potentially fatal disorder (23,24,63,64).

Other conditions in which CT seems to add valuable diagnostic information are pulmonary arteriovenous malformations, pulmonary parenchymal varices, abnormal anastomosis secondary to pulmonary inflammation, and pulmonary arterial aneurysm. Although in many cases CT does not eliminate the need for pulmonary arteriography, especially when surgery or embolization are considered as

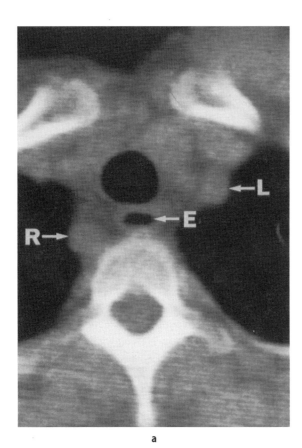
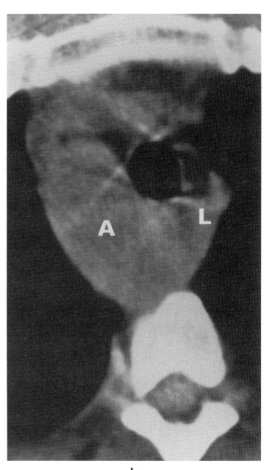

a   b

Figure 4.5. a CT cross-section cephalad to the aortic arch showing an aberrant right subclavian artery (*R*) to the right of the esophagus (*E*). *L* normal left subclavian artery.
b Cross-section of a right aortic arch (*A*) with origin of an aberrant left subclavian artery (*L*). (From ref. 3, with permission.)

therapeutic alternatives, it does provide valuable information concerning the morphology of vascular lesions (65,66).

CT has also been shown to accurately image the characteristic features of pulmonary sequestration, by visualizing the anomalous systemic supply as well as the type of venous drainage (67,68). Pulmonary sequestration is a typical condition in which vascular opacification is best achieved on CT scans by following the rapid sequence (dynamic) injection of contrast material. The useful information obtained with contrast-enhanced CT may obviate the need for arteriographic investigation in selected cases.

Dynamic CT will demonstrate a prominent increase in CT numbers in vascular as opposed to nonvascular lung lesions, based on the supposition that lung lesions that enhance in phase with the pulmonary artery or vein are supplied by the pulmonary circulation, whereas those for which the height of opacification is concomitant with aortic enhancement are probably fed by the systemic circulation. In cases in which a definite diagnosis cannot be established, the suspicion of an aberrant circulation raised

by CT has to be further investigated by an appropriate angiographic examination.

CT has also been shown to be effective in the evaluation of pulmonary thromboembolic phenomena, when central pulmonary emboli have been demonstrated to appear as filling defects in the pulmonary artery after the injection of contrast material (69,70). This pathologic occurrence has been shown to especially benefit from imaging with spiral CT and is mentioned again later.

Solitary Pulmonary Nodules

Computed tomography has been added to the diagnostic modalities used in the evaluation of pulmonary nodules because of its ability to accurately identify calcified tissues and thereby reinforce the diagnosis of a benign process. Possessing a high atomic number, calcium will attenuate the X-ray beam to a greater extent than other elements, and consequently the CT numbers of the tissues containing calcium will be higher than the numbers of other body tissues.

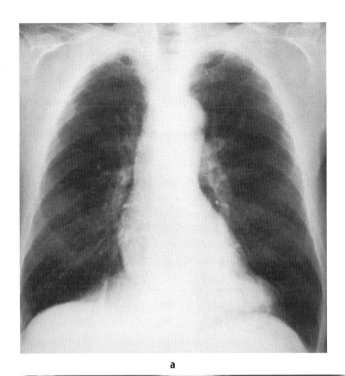

a

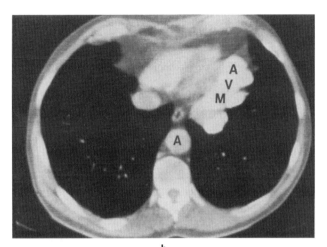

b

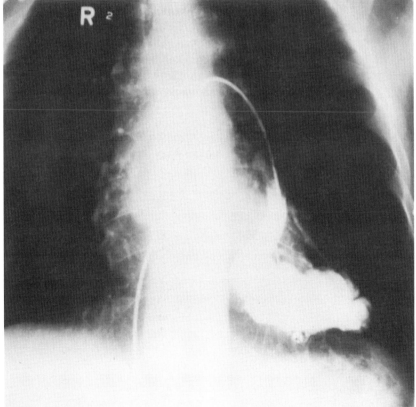

c

Figure 4.6. **a** Posteroanterior chest radiograph showing an irregular lobule visible through the left heart. Its medial margin is not defined. **b** CT scan following the peripheral injection of a bolus of 50 mL of contrast material shows an arteriovenous malformation (*AVM*) that undergoes prominent enhancement, comparable with that seen in the descending aorta (*A*) at the same level. **c** Selective left lower lobe arteriogram confirms the finding of an AVM and its specific blood supply. From ref. 3, with permission.)

Several reports have been dedicated to the subject of quantitatively measuring pulmonary nodules with CT; however, none has yet succeeded in establishing universal values for detection of calcifications in pulmonary nodules. The reason for this difficulty appears to be the fact that more than one element affects the accuracy of the measurements performed by a CT scanner. These factors include the type of CT scanner used in the examination, the partial volume effect, the real slice thickness, and the X-ray beam kilovoltage. Getting small pulmonary nodules to fall into a thinly collimated slice can be a complicated process that requires the performance of a large number of scans. Other technical variants, including the reconstruction algorithm, the type of software and hardware specific for each scanner, and artefacts created by beam hardening or kilovoltage drift, make readings of the same lesion inconsistent, not only from scanner to scanner but also on a single scanner from one examination to the other (25–27).

It has been found that a solid pulmonary nodule has an attenuation value of at least 60 HU. Generally, an attenuation value roughly twice that number or above (more than 140 HU) is a reliable indication of benignity (Fig. 4.7). In most of the series, 15–20% of solitary pulmonary nodules identified as noncalcified on CT sections have been further demonstrated to be benign by operative measures. The remaining cases (around 80% in various reports) are classified as indeterminant and are shown to be benign or malignant almost in equal number (28–32).

Multiple Pulmonary Nodules

Parenchymal pulmonary lesions smaller than 5 mm in diameter will usually not be depicted by conventional chest radiographs. Sometimes the visualization of larger nodules may also be problematic as a result of the density of the pulmonary nodules and their localization. Numerous lesions are overlooked in standard chest radiographs when they do not produce a marked contrast difference with the surrounding lung parenchyma. Also, there is great superposition of bony and soft tissue structures, which often can obscure the presence of a pulmonary nodule.

CT has been demonstrated in numerous studies to represent a major improvement in the evaluation of multiple pulmonary nodules. Its transverse cross-sectional display allows the visualization of such "hidden" anatomic areas as the lung apices, the retrocardiac and retrosternal regions, and the posterior diaphragmatic recesses. Also, CT has superior density contrast when compared with conventional radiography (25,26,71,72).

On CT images, if a nodular density is discovered in the proximity of a vascular structure, the distinction between them may represent a diagnostic problem if the vessel and the nodule are of similar size and density. In such cases, there is need for repeated scanning with the patient in various positions and the pursuit of structures on adjacent sections in order to provide the type of information that will help in the differentiation between the two densities. A pulmonary nodule is usually stable in position, whereas a vessel will change its shape and can be viewed on sequential scans as it connects itself to other vascular structures.

Whole-lung CT has a major clinical impact on patients in whom surgical decisions are made relative to the finding of pulmonary metastasis (e.g., in patients with osteogenic sarcoma). In such patients, as in other patients with a high propensity to metastasis to the lung (e.g., those with breast cancer, malignant melanoma, or testicular carcinoma), CT will provide more information than standard radiographic modalities in the initial

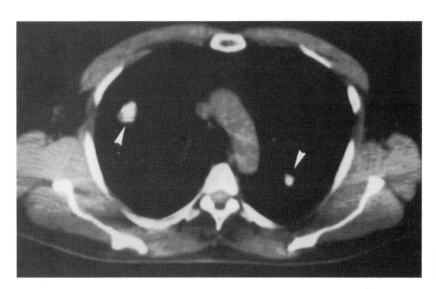

Figure 4.7. Pulmonary nodules (*arrowheads*) demonstrating prominent inner calcifications, a reliable indication of benignity.

screening for metastatic lung disease, as well as in the search for additional lesions when one has already been discovered.

Parenchymal Versus Pleural Disorders

CT, possessing the advantage of cross-sectional imaging, has added a new dimension to the visualization of the pulmonary parenchyma, including its normal components (7–9). Pathologic changes in the pulmonary interstitium, for example, have been shown to be discovered at an earlier stage on CT images than with standard chest radiographs. In such conditions as occupational lung diseases, sarcoidosis, systemic sclerosis, and rheumatoid arthritis, fine interstitial prominence and emphysematous changes are discovered on CT scans at an early stage of the disease. Furthermore, the presence of pulmonary infiltrates (e.g., in malignant lymphoma) is clearly demonstrated by CT. Regression of these infiltrates in response to therapy can also accurately be assessed (73–76).

In sarcoidosis, CT may help in the evaluation of those patients who present with pulmonary parenchymal changes at various stages of their disease. Findings will include ill-defined densities, which are often confluent and may contain an air bronchogram, or more subtle changes such as basal interstitial prominence and irregular peripheral nodules that can be delineated with CT when conventional radiographs are negative or inconclusive (Fig. 4.8). As we will see later on, high resolution CT (HRCT) has been shown to represent a most reliable tool in the identification of the specific parenchymal changes in diffuse lung disorders.

In the search for pulmonary changes resulting from asbestos exposure, CT has been demonstrated to provide valuable information, especially in the initial stages of the disease when the diagnosis of asbestosis can be significantly delayed because of the paucity of symptoms and lack of radiographic signs on conventional chest radiographs (77–81). Abnormalities identified in these patients by CT and not seen on conventional radiographs include pericardial calcifications, posterior diaphragmatic pleural thickening and calcifications, mediastinal pleural thickening, linear parenchymal densities, dilatation of small airways, and small bullae formation. In patients suffering from longstanding asbestosis and presenting with marked alteration in lung functions, CT studies demonstrate progressive increase in radiological abnormalities, including parenchymal fibrosis, emphysematous changes, extensive pleural plaques formation, and calcification (Fig.4.9). In patients in whom the development of a malignant pleural condition is suspected, CT scans have the ability to exclude such a possibility by identifying the areas of localized

pleural thickening ("rounded atelectasis" or "pseudotumor") as benign processes, based on their appearance and behavior on consecutive CT examinations (79,82,83).

The ability of CT to provide diagnostic information additional to that obtained from conventional radiographic studies has also been shown in such pulmonary conditions as tuberculosis, cryptogenic fibrosing alveolitis, pulmonary endometriosis, alveolar proteinosis, and collagen vascular diseases (84–89).

The special area of measurements of lung density in normal physiologic states and in various pathologic conditions has also enjoyed the addition of information received from the CT studies. These studies have been demonstrated to represent a reliable tool for quantitative analysis of lung density, although the method is limited by the presence of artefacts and incomplete inspiration. A histograph, which is an analysis of a frequency distribution, of density values obtained with CT has been shown to be able to differentiate between the various constituents of the lung, which includes separating the parenchymal part of the lung from the vessels. Therefore, its use is advised in the diagnosis of disorders affecting each of these components. Mean lung densities in emphysema, for example, were found to be abnormally low as a result of loss of parenchymal tissue, decrease in intravascular volume, and lung hyperinflation. Measuring lung density with the aid of CT is expected to be particularly valuable in follow-up studies of diffuse pulmonary disease, in which comparable lung levels can be examined, thus permitting the assessment of minimal density variations (90–93).

CT has special value in the study of pleural abnormalities, which have been shown to be discovered by CT at an earlier stage than with conventional radiographic techniques. Calcified and noncalcified pleural plaques are easily identified on CT scans and distinguished from soft tissue shadows. A minimal amount of pleural fluid is also detectable with CT, often when the conventional chest radiograph is negative.

A special diagnostic problem is encountered in those patients in whom a peripheral thoracic cavitary lesion is discovered on conventional studies, often containing an air–fluid level. The diagnostic choice in this case is between a parenchymal or a pleural process. Mainly the possibility of a pulmonary abscess or an empyema is considered. CT scanning is able to help in the differentiation of these two conditions (94,95). Empyema will characteristically have a smooth border and will present a sharp line of separation from the lung parenchyma. Multiple CT positions must be used in this case, because empyema is suspected to change shape with a change in the patient's position. Conversely, a lung abscess will usually present as a thick irregular wall, without being clearly separated from the lung parenchyma. The air–fluid levels within a

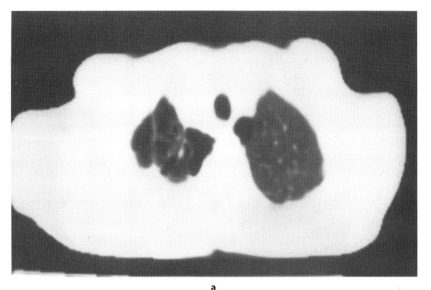

a

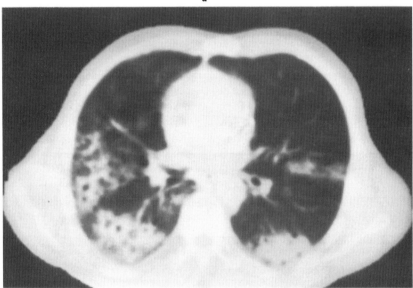

b

Figure 4.8. Apical fibrotic changes (**a**) and multiple pulmonary alveolar densities (**b**) are clearly visualized with CT in a sarcoidosis patient.

pulmonary abscess tend to remain stable when the patient shifts position.

Malignant conditions of the pleura, either primary (malignant mesothelioma of the pleura) or secondary (metastatic deposits to the pleura), are readily identified with CT. Moreover, in conditions such as pleural mesothelioma, CT tends to accurately demonstrate the spread of the tumor to the mediastinum, chest wall, and contralateral hemithorax. Often in such cases conventional chest radiographs underestimate the extent of the disease (96–98) (Fig. 4.10).

Multiple reports have also evaluated and emphasized the role of CT in the recognition of chest wall pathology. CT has been demonstrated to provide more information than conventional techniques when visualizing and accurately localizing chest wall abnormalities such as inflammatory changes secondary to tuberculosis or actinomycosis, posttraumatic changes, or direct tumoral extension (99–102).

Bronchogenic Carcinoma and Posttherapeutic Follow-up of Malignant Tumors

With the advent of CT scanning, the pretreatment period in patients with bronchogenic cancer has been significantly reduced by the ability of this method to localize the primary tumor as well as to discover direct invasion of intrathoracic structures or metastatic spread. Because of the extreme clinical importance of the subject, numerous studies have been dedicated to it, including refinements of regional node localization and identification using CT scanning of the thorax (26,30,71,103–105). CT has the advantage of permitting the visualization of various thoracic components on the same plane. Therefore, chest wall involvement and bony destruction are much easier to discover.

Also, extension of tumor into the mediastinum as well as pleural and pericardial effusions are readily identified. In

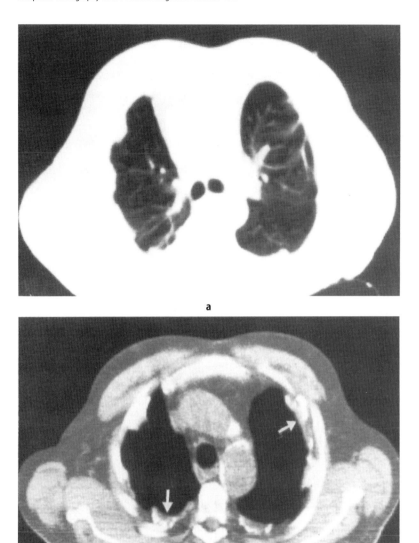

a

b

Figure 4.9. Prominent emphysematous changes (**a**) and extensive pleural thickening and calcification (*arrows*, **b**) demonstrated by CT in an insulation worker exposed to asbestos for 11 years.

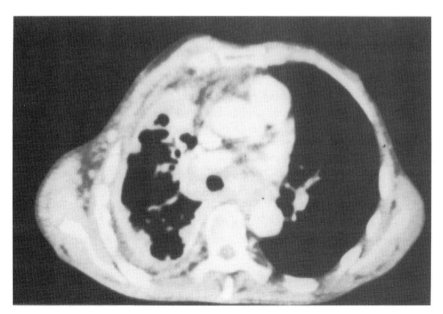

Figure 4.10. Malignant mesothelioma of the pleura developing in the right hemithorax of an asbestosis patient. CT scan clearly demonstrates the extent of the pathologic changes.

many cases such information, which is not obtainable with other preoperative diagnostic modalities, can help to avoid an unnecessary thoracotomy to diagnose an unresectable lesion. CT scanning of the upper abdomen is usually combined with chest CT scanning in order to detect metastatic deposits in the liver and the adrenals, both being common sites for spread of primary lung cancer.

An important fact to mention, however, is that despite the superiority of CT over conventional radiographic techniques, including standard tomography, in the localization of pulmonary lesions, its use as a definitive staging procedure in bronchogenic carcinoma remains controversial (106–109). Some diagnostic difficulties encountered by CT have not been overcome yet. Such difficulties include the inability to differentiate between nodes that are enlarged secondary to inflammatory processes and those that contain a neoplasm, and identification of the presence of microscopic tumor deposits in normal-sized lymph nodes.

In a recent study (110), the ability of chest CT to decrease the use of preoperative bronchoscopy in the evaluation of suspected bronchogenic carcinoma has been questioned. The main focus was on the use of bronchoscopy in the diagnosis and staging of bronchogenic carcinoma presenting as a pulmonary nodule or mass. Selected patients had no typical signs of malignancy such as pulmonary atelectasis, narrowing of the central airways or tumor abutting the central airways. In this study CT failed to detect endobronchial tumor in 11 out of 64 patients (17%), still the authors concluded that CT findings can successfully predict the value of using preoperative bronchoscopy and guide the method of biopsy of a pulmonary mass. In general, by reducing the expenses and risks of either a major operation (exploratory thoracotomy) or minor surgical procedures (mediastinotomy or mediastinoscopy) and by allowing earlier institution of radiation therapy or chemotherapy, CT scanning has become an important, reliable, and cost-effective component of the pretreatment assessment in patients with carcinoma of the lung.

In the postpneumonectomy patient, CT can be used as a reliable tool in the search for immediate postsurgical complications or in the long-term follow-up for tumoral recurrence (111). CT also can be valuable in the preparation for radiotherapy of patients with malignant tumors, resulting in a more accurate delineation of the initial tumor, together with the assessment of any change in the size of the lesion. Radiation-induced changes in the pulmonary parenchyma are identified at an early stage (33,34).

Bronchial Disorders

Aside from bronchogenic carcinoma, a diversity of other neoplasms arise from the bronchial epithelium and bronchial mucosal glands, from cells of neural origin, or from the pulmonary and bronchial mesenchyma. They represent uncommon pulmonary tumors, which, although generally regarded as benign, may include a malignant variety. In addition to invasive methods of investigation such as bronchoscopy with bronchial biopsy, CT can be used as an ancillary diagnostic modality, permitting accurate planning for the biopsy procedures, which is especially valuable because CT is able in most cases to provide information concerning the extraluminal component of bronchial tumors (8,9).

Obstruction of segmental bronchi may cause local atelectasis, which is easily identified on CT sections as a typical triangular density similar to the findings on conventional radiographs. Some specific CT changes have also been described in relation to lobar collapse, occurring in various anatomic locations either secondary to endobronchial obstruction or without it (37,38).

Air bronchograms are often identified on CT sections, confirming the distribution of bronchial segments in consolidated areas. However, patency of various bronchi may be difficult to estimate and their full-length visualization on CT scans may be impossible when they follow a path other than horizontal. By establishing the presence and anatomic extent of bronchial obstruction, CT may accurately delineate recurrence (e.g., occurring often in bronchial adenomas) and in numerous cases may diminish or even obviate the need for frequent bronchoscopic studies.

The diagnosis of bronchiectasis can sometimes be made with CT, in which case thick-walled, dilated bronchi containing air–fluid levels are identified in the lung periphery. Occasionally, findings have to be differentiated from emphysematous changes, which may appear as thick-walled air spaces and may be confused with dilated bronchi. The diferentiation on CT scans can be made by the fact that a bronchus always has accompanying vessels (a pulmonary artery branch) and is arranged in a linear manner, whereas emphysematous blebs have no relation to pulmonary vessels and are most commonly localized in the subpleural region, without any distinguishable pattern of distribution (39,40).

Special attention had been paid to the area of the posterior wall of the left main bronchus, which when thickened, on CT has a reliable pathologic significance. It has been shown that enlargement of lymph glands in the posterior left hilus or subcarinal region in malignant or granulomatous conditions or in cases of inflammatory processes involving the left lower lobe and pleura will produce separation of the lungs, with the air in the bronchial lumen penetrating into the retrobronchial space, and therefore the image of a thickened left retrobronchial stripe will be obtained (89). The present available data thus emphasize the importance of CT in the precise delineation of bronchial anatomy and suggest its complementary use with other investigative modalities in the study of bronchial pathology.

CT-Guided Biopsy

The excellent three-dimensional images provided by CT permit an accurate localization of pulmonary lesions and a precise delineation of their relationships to surrounding structures. Therefore CT also permits correct visualization of the site of penetration of a biopsy needle into a target lesion. A high rate of successful aspiration lung biopsies have been reported (up to 90%) with a considerably low rate of complications such as pneumothorax, transient hypotension, or bacterial contamination.

The need to move the patients back and forth under the CT gantry while the needle is in place and the time required for the various manipulations and CT image formation make CT-guided biopsy a technique somewhat more complicated than percutaneous biopsy under fluoroscopic control. This is particularly true with regard to the evaluation of parenchymal lesions, which can be suitably biopsied under fluoroscopy. However, pleural-based lesions, which are difficult to visualize by conventional radiography, and mediastinal masses, which require contrast enhancement for better delineation, may certainly benefit from CT-directed biopsy (112,113).

High Resolution CT (HRCT)

In the 1980s a big step forward in the diagnostic capabilities of CT was been achieved by the use of thin collimation (114–118). Additionally, high kilovoltage and milliampere settings have been employed with the benefit of limiting the noise on thin section scanning. Other technical adjustments, such as a reduction in the field view or breath-holding methods were also proposed, for the purpose of obtaining images of very high spatial resolution in which superb anatomic and pathologic details are identifiable.

The details of the above technologic improvements are important, as their appropriate usage ensures top quality examinations and the best diagnostic possibilities. Firstly, the thin collimation, one of the most important technical details, has to be kept, as suggested by most of the studies, at an optimum of between 1 and 1.5 mm. A very good visualization of the lung parenchyma is obtained in this manner, with an accurate depiction of small vessels, bronchi and interlobular septae. Owing to the greater contrast between the various elements, changes in lung attenuation are more easily recognized. Moreover, unrelated to the orientation of the scanning plane, the size of the various fissures, vessels and airways is more clearly appreciated with HRCT (119–121).

Basically, thin section imaging permitted a better evaluation of pathologic changes in a large variety of pulmonary disorders. Recent articles have therefore praised this technique for its value in the anatomic localization of multin-

odular disease (121), the study of the pulmonary hilus (42) with the identification of hilar lymph node metastases from lung cancer (122), or the analysis of normal and abnormal changes in the peribronchovascular interstitium (43). The increased degree of visibility brought with it the recognition of various new patterns which various authors attempted to correlate to specific pathologic changes. One of these is the "crazy-paving appearance" corresponding to the presence of a fine reticular pattern superimposed on areas of "ground-glass" opacity. This pattern has been described as being present in exogenous lipoid pneumonia (123), but also in a large variety of other interstitial and airspace lung diseases (124).

The ground-glass opacity, representing volume averaging below the resolution of HRCT, is usually visualized as a hazy increase in lung density, with continuous imaging of pulmonary vessels and bronchi. It is a nonspecific sign; however, it has been shown to have an important diagnostic value suggesting the presence of potentially treatable disorders such as sarcoidosis. Moreover, areas more likely to provide an accurate histologic diagnosis can be identified. A great number of pulmonary diseases have been demonstrated to present, at various stages of their development, areas of ground-glass opacities. Among them are alveolar proteinosis, hypersensitive pneumonitis, *Pneumocystis carinii* pneumonia, pulmonary edema, desquamative pneumonitis, and drug-induced pathologies (125–127). Recently, ground-glass opacities have been described in nodular bronchioloalveolar carcinoma, where it can be the sign of an aggressive biological behavior (128) (Fig. 4.11).

Another valuable feature of HRCT is the capability of retrospective reconstruction. This is based on the utilization of a "high spatial frequency" (bone) algorithm, as opposed to a "low spatial frequency" (soft tissue) algorithm, used in standard CT examinations. The resulting benefit is the creation of images with high diagnostic value owing to enhanced edge detection and the visualization of a sharper lung structure. The reconstruction of scanned data belongs to the all-important part of image processing, during which images are viewed both at lung and at mediastinal settings, including occasional manual adjustments, in order to be able to identify minute pathologic changes (129,130)

A routine HRCT examination of the thorax has to be adjusted to the individual diagnostic needs of a specific patient. Therefore a thicker collimation can be used, for example 3 or 5 mm, and scans can be performed in expiration instead of full inspiration. This procedure has been shown to be beneficial in the identification of typical changes in emphysema, progressive systemic sclerosis, Swyer–James syndrome, tuberous sclerosis and others (120,131,132).

In recent studies, expiratory scans have been employed in chronic airway disease to check the correlation with

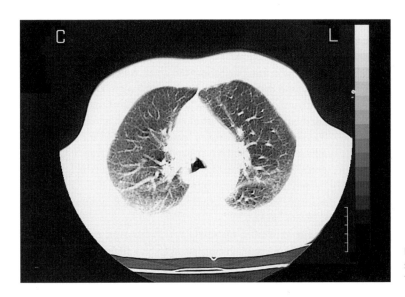

Figure 4.11. HRCT in a patient with extrinsic allergic alveolitis, demonstrating the hazy increase in lung density recognized under the name of "ground-glass opacity".

pulmonary function test results. Their conclusion was that air-trapping may permit detection of airway obstruction in patients with clinically suspected chronic airway disease, even when pulmonary function tests are normal. Moreover, expiratory CT scans allow one to calculate a reduction score for a cross-sectional lung area that appears to be better correlated with the degree of airway obstruction measured on pulmonary function tests (133).

Additionally, scanning performed at end-respiratory volume has been demonstrated to have a special diagnostic value, as it permits the differentiation between areas that have similar appearance, but different etiology, such as crowded pulmonary vessels or atelectasis versus an area of edema (118,134,135). Ultrafast HRCT is another technique that has been employed successfully in the identification of abnormalities at the pulmonary hilus (42) or of air-trapping (136,137). With this method, fast HRCT scans are obtained while the patient exhales. During this time, changes in lung volume and local attenuation are measured, and a diagnosis of air-trapping is made when there is an increase in the pulmonary attenuation following the manoeuver.

Changes in the normal structure of the pulmonary parenchyma such as subpleural lines or dependent density, can also be identified by replacing the standard supine position of the patient in which the examination is performed, with a prone position. In normal patients the observed changes will reverse with a switch in position, but will remain the same in patients with, for example, pulmonary fibrosis (138,139).

While typical parameters for an optimal HRCT examination can be for example 1 s scans, 260 mA and 137 kVp, a reduction in field view can also be of help, as it tends to maximize fine parenchymal details. The amazing capability of HRCT of diagnosing pathologic changes is based primarily on the visualization of an important anatomic

component, the secondary pulmonary lobule, a functional unit never demonstrated as clearly before as with HRCT (127,140–142). Each secondary pulmonary lobule has been found to be approximately 10 mm in diameter, includes three to five terminal bronchioles, and is bordered incompletely by interlobular septae. A terminal bronchiole is located 3–5 mm away from the corresponding lobular border, the pulmonary vein, the pleura and the interlobular septum. It is considered that each secondary lobule contains a variable number of pulmonary acini (10–17,47–53), which are the portions of lung parenchyma participating in gas exchange and located distal to the terminal bronchiole.

Each terminal bronchiole is accompanied by the pulmonary arteriole that distributes blood to the capillaries surrounding the alveoli. The pulmonary venules drain toward the borders of the lobule where they form the pulmonary vein, located within the interlobular septae. These connective tissue septae contain pulmonary lymphatics as well, and are more developed in certain lung areas, such as the anterior and lateral aspects of the upper, middle and lower lung fields, and are not so prominent in the posterior region. This explains why pathologic changes within these septae, such as fluid collection or cell infiltration, are more easily recognized in these areas (140,142–144).

The most important thing is that, on the basis of the above anatomic details, the possibility has been created of describing patterns of abnormality in the secondary lobule, according to their location. Therefore, schematically, diseases affecting the lobule can be classified as centrilobular, bronchovascular, panlobular and perilobular. A centrilobular appearance has been recognized on HRCT in a variety of disorders affecting the central bronchiole, pulmonary artery and lymphatics, and has been shown to take the form of well-delineated or ill-defined single or multiple small opacities. They include bronchopneumonias, occupational lung disorders such as asbestosis and silicosis, perilymphatic diseases such as sarcoidosis, and perivascular conditions such as pulmonary edema, drug reactions and vasculitis (145–147) (Fig. 4.12).

The bronchovascular pattern results from the involvement of the components of the bronchovascular bundle, the interstitial supportive structure, the bronchus, the artery and associated lymphatics. Pathologic signs of conditions that affect the bronchi, such as cystic fibrosis, bronchiectasis or bronchiolitis obliterans include thickening of the bronchial wall and sometimes luminal obstruction with mucus plugs. These and characteristic findings will be well delineated on HRCT scans, eliminating in most of the cases the need for the performance of bronchography.

General interstitial thickening, which can be found in various pulmonary disorders, has been shown by HRCT to have different appearances, according to the specific disease. Therefore, in pulmonary edema, the interstitium will be found to be thickened in rather a "smooth" fashion, while in lymphoma, lymphangitic spread of carcinoma or usual interstitial pneumonia, the interstitium will be thickened in an irregular manner. A nodular form of interstitial thickening can be found in sarcoidosis. It should be remembered that all the above-mentioned diseases, due to the presence of lymphatic channels in the interlobular septae, may present with a combination picture of bronchovascular and perilobular patterns (120,148–154)

When there is a uniform involvement of the secondary lobule by a pathologic process, a panlobular distribution has been described, which preserves central and septal areas. This tendency can be discovered in airspace diseases such as pneumonias or pulmonary hemorrhages, and sometimes even in interstitial conditions such as idiopathic pulmonary fibrosis or the interstitial involvement of sarcoidosis (117,155,156).

Another useful way of classifying pulmonary disorders as visualized on HRCT scans is by their central (parahilar), or peripheral (subpleural) locations. Diseases that have a tendency to be axially located include sarcoidosis, lymphoma, lymphangitic spread of carcinoma and silicosis, while others prefer the periphery of the lung. Examples of the latter are rheumatoid lung disease, scleroderma, asbestosis, desquamative interstitial pneumonia, hypersensitivity pneumonitis, or interstitial lung disease associated with polymyositis–dermatomyositis (139,157–159).

Recognized pathognomonic signs identified on standard CT scans can be discovered on HRCT scans as well. An example of these signs is the air bronchogram, which signifies by its presence the existence of space consolidation. When dealing with cystic lung changes, focal parenchymal abnormalities can be found as a result of parenchymal necrosis and the destruction of the normal supportive lung network. These are in the form of blebs, bullae, and honeycombing. Their origin can be found in such disorders as vascular-embolic phenomena, bronchiectasis, emphysema, infections, and some rarer conditions, including tuberous sclerosis and eosinophilic granuloma (160–162) (Fig. 4.13).

It is to be emphasized that typical findings for interstitial disorders of the lungs, such as micronodules, reticulation, thickening of the septae, ground-glass appearance and, in general, signs of architectural distortion, are all better visualized with HRCT than with standard CT scans. Additionally, lung interfaces separating the pleura from the pulmonary parenchyma and the bronchovascular bundle, when showing irregularities, are better identified with HRCT and at an earlier stage. The obvious result is that the differential diagnosis between a variety of pulmonary abnormalities is much easier to make (121,163–165).

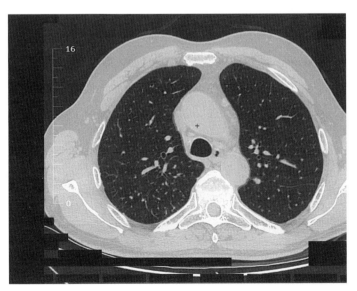

Figure 4.12. Linear and nodular opacities are well-delineated in this patient suffering from sarcoidosis.

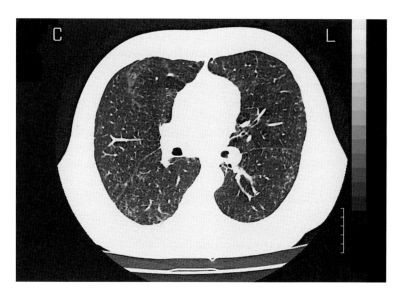

Figure 4.13. Extensive interstitial and emphysematous changes demonstrated by HRCT in a heavy smoker.

When one is overviewing the benefits of HRCT in comparison with conventional CT scanning, some indications become evident and comprise mainly clinical situations in which evaluation of the lung fields is necessary because of a discrepancy between the radiologic and clinical findings, such as absent radiologic findings in a symptomatic patient, or the visualization of abnormalities on conventional chest radiography when the clinical picture is normal. Additional help may arise from the ability of HRCT to discover early and subtle pathologic changes, as well as complications such as superimposed infections or the appearance of fibrocystic changes in patients with diffuse lung disorders. In the event that a transbronchial or open lung biopsy is needed, HRCT can offer a precise localization of the pathologic changes required to be examined.

Nevertheless, although promoting advances, the new modality presents its limitations. The amount of radiation employed to obtain HRCT scans should not be neglected, as it is considerably increased compared with conventional CT examinations. Attempts have been made therefore to propose a low dose technique that, however, has not been shown to have the same satisfactory results, as ground-glass opacities or other subtle findings seemed to be sometimes obscured, and streak artefacts appeared, thus reducing the quality of the images (166–168).

This is the reason that most current protocols include the performance of limited HRCT examinations, i.e., attempting to concentrate on the area where pathology is expected to be found. The resulting danger is to miss some of the existent abnormalities in the nonscanned areas. Other HRCT limitations include the fact that on high resolution scans micronodules are less efficiently visualized than on conventional CT, because on thin scans micronodules may be confused with small vessels on end, or the

confluence of abnormal lines of attenuation. Edge-enhancement properties of HRCT also pose a problem as they makes small nodules appear denser and sometimes may mimic calcifications. In addition, the high resolution and reconstruction algorithms used in HRCT tend to accentuate pleural thickness and increase the difficulty of detecting mediastinal adenopathy.

Despite the above, HRCT became in recent years a valuable tool used in the investigation of diffuse lung disorders, mainly due to its superior ability to imagine the basic anatomic pulmonary unit, the secondary pulmonary lobule. With recognition of anatomy, came the clear identification of pathologic changes such as reticulation, honeycomb cysts, thickened interlobular septae and micronodules. Parenchymal changes due to vascular abnormalities are more difficult to observe. Still, special attention should be paid to changes in vascular diameter, the presence of vascular compression or of an intraluminal filling defect, which are all easily seen with HRCT.

Spiral CT

Described for the first time in 1990 by W.A. Kelender and his colleagues (169), spiral or helical CT of the thorax permits 1 s scans, in a continuous manner and during a single breath-holding episode. The performance of subsecond spiral CT has also been proposed, as it has been found that it results in improved clarity and diminished motion artefacts on mediastinal and pulmonary images when compared with 1 s spiral CT. A narrow collimation (1–3 mm) is of importance with spiral CT, as it is continuous data acquisition and employs data-rendering techniques. The slice thickness chosen is usually 2–10 mm and various reconstruction algorithms and intervals between images are chosen in order to accommodate specific clinical demands (169–173).

When a spiral CT examination of the thorax is being performed, the patient is moved through the gantry and an uninterrupted volume of data is capable of undergoing multiplanar reconstruction and three-dimensional image analysis. Other benefits of this modality include the ability to considerably reduce respiratory artefacts, as well as using contrast material enhancement (169–171,174,175). Vock (174), proposed several protocols of examination, demonstrating the ability to tailor a spiral CT study of the thorax according to the specific area or organ where a pathologic development is suspected (Tables 4.1, 4.2, 4.3).

In the domain of parenchymal lung disease, the remarkable volumetric scanning achieved by spiral CT, together with the highly improved quality of the artefact-free images, has resulted in the capacity to identify mild forms of infiltration, incipient emphysematous changes and peripheral mucus impaction, subtle nodular changes (micronodules) and small bronchiectases. Two methods have been especially emphasized, one which is sliding thin slab maximum intensity projection and the other, sliding thin slab minimum intensity projection. The former has been shown to be of value in the study of micronodular infiltration and bronchiolar abnormalities, due to the ability to retain the

highest attenuated structures within a given slab thickness. The latter is capable of retaining air-filled, low density structures, better than with vascular ones and is especially of interest in the appreciation of mild emphysema (171,176–179).

Other pathologic conditions in which spiral CT has demonstrated its value are those of the pulmonary airways, such as tracheal wall defects, congenital anomalies of the tracheobronchial tree, benign and malignant space-occupying lesions, and postoperative changes, with remarkable facilitation of clinical decisions due to the high morphologic detail offered by this modality, the exploration of a complete volume without gap and excellent multiplanar reformation (180–182).

In the area of pulmonary malignancy, spiral CT has been demonstrated to be able to improve the ability to demonstrate primary thoracic lesions, as well as secondaries from extrathoracic malignancies, clearly identifying the tumor–bronchi relationship or invasion to adjacent structures, and therefore acting as an important tool for planning interventional procedures (183–186). Moreover, studies have shown that spiral CT multiplanar images are superior to conventional axial CT scans in demonstrating neoplastic extension across pulmonary fissures (187).

Volumetric CT and three-dimensional and/or multiplanar reconstruction capabilities have found perhaps

Table 4.1. Spiral CT acquisition protocols of the chest wall and pleura

Acquisition parameter (adult patients)	Region		
	Thoracic inlet	Bone + joints [diaphragm and neighborhood]	Soft tissues, pleura
1. Rotation time	1–2 s	≤2 s, [minimum]	Minimum
2. Scan collimation (slice thickness)	5 mm	2–5 mm (–8 mm)	5–10 mm
3. Table feed per rotation	5 mm	2–8 mm (spine: > 1 segment → 0)[a]	5–16 mm
→ pitch	1	1–1.6	1–1.6
4. kVp	(120–) 140	(120–) 140 [120]	120 (–140)
5. mAs per rotation	200–400	150–400	150–250
6. Gantry angulation	0° (or 10°)	0°, spine ±	0°
7. Scanning direction	si/is	si/is	is/si
8. Scan duration	≤ 30 s	≤ 30s, spine: maximum	≤ 30 s
9. Multiple spiral scans	Usually not	Spine ±	Optional
10. Reconstruction increment	3–5 mm	1–5 (–8) mm	(3–) 5–10 mm
11. Reconstruction center/size (targeting)	As in conventional CT	As in conventional CT	As in conventional CT
12. Reconstruction algorithm	180 (360)° standard	180 (360)° interpolation, high resolution [standard resol.]	180 (360)° standard
13. Patient respiration	Apnea or continuous	(Inspiratory) apnea, (spine: continuous)	(Inspiratory) apnea (+ expir.: pleural shift)
14. Patient position	Supine, arms down	Supine, arms positioned according to indication [elevated]	Supine, arms elevated
15. Contrast	+	–, tumors + [–, +]	Usually +

si, Superoinferior; is, inferosuperior; expir, expiratory; CT, Computed tomography.
[a] With more than one segment of the spinal column, tube heating is usually significant; instead of decreasing the current, many people prefer conventional CT (table feed of 0 per rotation).
From ref. 174, with permission.

Table 4.2. Spiral CT acquisition protocols of the lung

Acquisition parameter (adult patients)	Problem						
	Search for metastases	Cancer staging	Solitary pulmonary nodule	Trauma, intensive care patient	Embolism/ vascular malformation	Bronchial disease (bronchiectasis)	Diffuse infiltrative lung disease
1. Rotation time	Minimum	Minimum	Minimum	Minimum	Minimum	Minimum	Minimum
2. Scan collimation (slice thickness)	4–10 mm –	Hilus 4–5 8–10 mm	1–2 mm	7–10 mm	3–5–7/2–5 mm	1.5–3 mm	1–2 mm = HRCT
3. Table feed per rotation → pitch	4–25 mm 1–2	5–8/8–16 1–1.6	1–3 mm 1–1.5	7–16 mm 1–1.6	(3) 5–7 (10) mm 1–2	0 mm/2–7 mm[a] 1–2	0 mm/2 4 mm[a] 1–2
4. kVp	140 (120)	140 (120)	120	140 (120)	120 (140)	140 (120)	140 (120)
5. mAs per rotation	(50–) 150–250	180–250	150–250	150–250	150–250	150–250	(50–) 150–250
6. Gantry angulation	0°	0°	0°	0°	0°	–20°	0°
7. Scanning direction[b]	is/si	si/is	si/is	si/is	is/si	si/is	is/si
8. Scan duration	≤32 s	≤32 s	≤32 s	≤32 s	≤32 s	≤32 s	≤32 s
9. Multiple spiral scans[c]	(+)	±	–	(+)	–	(+)	(+)
10. Reconstruction increment	(2–) 4–10 mm	(2–) 4–10 mm	1–2 mm	(5–) 10 mm	3–7/2–5 mm	1–2–5 mm (cine)	1–3 mm
11. Reconstruction center/size (targeting)	Lung	Chest (targeting)	Lung area	Entire chest	Central/regional	Central bronchi	Lung (bilateral targeting)
12. Reconstruction algorithm	180 (360)° high	180 (360)° standard + high	180 (360)° standard	180 (360)° standard	180 (360)° standard	180 (360)° high	180 (360)° high
13. Patient respiration	(Inspiratory) apnea	(Inspiratory) apnea	(Inspiratory) apnea	Apnea/shallow respiration	(Inspiratory) apnea	(Inspiratory) apnea (+ expiration)	(Inspiratory) apnea (+ expiration)
14. Patient position	Supine	Supine	Supine	Supine	Supine	Supine	Supine (+ prone)
15. Contrast[c]	–	+	– (+)	+	+/– (+)	–/+	+

HRCT, high resolution computed tomography.

[a] Usually conventional scanning to screen for diffuse disease using 1.5 (1–2) mm slice thickness and 10 mm spacing between slices (less radiation exposure); spiral technique ideal for most suspicious subvolume of lung.

[b] Inferosuperior when scan duration longer than 24 s; is, inferosuperior; si, superoinferior

[c] Not indicated; (+), possibly indicated; +, often indicated.

From ref. 174, with permission.

their best usage in the diagnosis of thoracic vascular abnormalities, including pulmonary embolism. In general, when compared with conventional or digital pulmonary angiography, it becomes evident that spiral CT angiography is a noninvasive modality that requires a small amount of contrast material to be injected, and shows a definite reduction in the procedural complications related to the standard angiographic method, performed often on high risk, seriously ill patients. Additionally, being a three-dimensional procedure with reconstruction capabilities, spiral CT permits images to be viewed after the examination is finished, without the need to excessively irradiate the patient or give more contrast.

More importantly, it has been shown that there is a significant degree of detectability for pathologic changes in pulmonary vessels and the presence of emboli. Studies have nevertheless shown that diagnosis is facilitated when the vessels are central (segmental or larger) and more problematic when subsegmental vessels are involved (188–192). While the use of electron beam scanners has been advised in this condition in order to reduce motion artefacts, visualization of oblique arteries continues to remain difficult, and supports the ongoing discussion about whether spiral CT is capable of replacing pulmonary angiography and ventilation–perfusion scanning as the initial screening tests for pulmonary embolic phenomena (193,194).

Table 4.3. Spiral CT acquisition protocols of the mediastinum

Acquisition parameter (adult patients)	Problem			
	Screening	[Tracheal]/ esophageal disease	Aortic/arterial/venous/ [cardiac] disease	Adenopathy
1. Rotation time	Minimum	Minimum	Minimum	See screening and lung cancer staging
2. Scan collimation = slice thickness	5–10 mm	[3–] 5 (–10)mm	3–5–10 mm	
3. Table feed per rotation	8–20 mm	5–10 mm	5–15 mm	
→ pitch	1–2	1–1.6	1–2	
4. kVp	120	120	120	
5. mAs per rotation	150–250	150–300	180–300	
6. Gantry angulation	0°	0°	0°/[0,–30°]	
7. Scanning direction	is/si	si/is	is (si)	
8. Scan duration	≤40 s	≤32 s	≤ 40 s	
9. Multiple spiral scans	(+)	(+)	–,+/[–]	
10. Reconstruction increment	4–10 mm	[3] 4–10 mm	[3–] 4–10 mm	
11. Reconstruction center/size (targeting)	Mediastinum or entire chest	Mediastinum/(chest)	Mediastinum/chest (collaterals)	
12. Reconstruction algorithm	180 ° (360°) standard	180° (360°) standard		
13. Patient respiration	Inspiratory apnea/ shallow respiration	(Inspiratory) apnea/ [+ expiration]	Inspiratory apnea/ shallow respiration	
14. Patient position	Supine	Supine	Supine	
15. i.v. contrast	+	[–]/+, p.o.	+/[–,+]	

is, Inferosuperior; si, superoinferior; –, not indicated; (+), possibly indicated; +, often indicated; i.v., intravenous, p.o., From ref. 174, with permission.

References

1. Naidich DP, Zerhouni EA, Siegelman SS (1984) Computed tomography of the thorax. Raven Press, New York.
2. Sperber, M (1984) Computed tomography of the lungs: Normal anatomy and most common disorders. Futura Publishing, New York.
3. Senac JP, Giron J (1987) Tomodensitometrie thoracique, 2nd edn. Éditions Axone, Montpellier.
4. Kittredge RD (1981) Computed tomography of the trachea: A preview. J. Comput Tomogr 5:44–49.
5. Naidich DP, Perry PB, Stitic FP et al. (1980) Computed tomography of the bronchi. 1. Normal anatomy. J Comput Assist Tomogr 4:746–753.
6. Webb WR, Ghazer G, Gamsu G (1981) Computed tomography of the normal pulmonary hilum. J Comput Assist Tomogr 5:476–484.
7. Marks BW, Kullus LR (1982) Identification of pleural fissures with computed tomography. Radiology 143:139–141.
8. Goodman LR, Golkow RS, Steiner RM, et al. (1981). The right mid-lung window. Radiology 5:459–467.
9. Speekman JM, Gamsu G, Welob WR (1981) Alterations in CT mediastinal anatomy produced by an azygos lobe. AJR 137:47-50.
10. Crowe JR, Brown LR, Muhn JR (1978) Computed tomography of the mediastinum. Radiology 128:75–87.
11. Moss AA, Gamsu G, Geniant HK (1983) Mediastinum. In Computed tomography of the body. WB Saunders, Philadelphia.
12. Walter VE, Hubener KH (1980) Computer tomographic characteristics of space-occupying processes in the anterior mediastinum and their differential diagnosis. Fortschr Roentgensch 133:391–400.
13. Genereux G, Howie J (1984) Normal mediastinal lymph node size and number. CT and anatomy study. AJR 142:1095–1100.
14. Glazer B, Gross B, Quint L, et al. (1985) Normal mediastinal lymph nodes according to the American Cancer Society mapping. AJR 144: 261–265.
15. McLoud TC, Mayer JF (1982) Mediastinal metastases. Radiol Clin North Am 20:453–468.
16. Webb WR, Gamsu G, Glazer G (1981) Computed tomography of the abnormal pulmonary hilum. J Comput Assist Tomogr 5:476–484.
17. Bein ME, Mancuso AA, Mink JH, et al. (1982). Computed tomography in the evaluation of mediastinal lipomatosis. J Comput Assist Tomogr 2:379–383.
18. Baron RL, Gutierrez FR, Sagel SS, et al. (1981) CT of anomalies of the mediastinal vessels. AJR 137:576.
19. Frija J, Larde D, Katz M, et al. (1982) Le diagnostique tomodensitometrique des anomalies de l'arc aortique chez l'adulte. J Radiol 63:159–165.
20. Webb WR, Gamsu G, Speckman JM, et al. (1982) Computed tomographic demonstration of mediastinal venous anomalies. AJR 139:157–161.
21. Godwin JD, Herfkens RJ, Brundage BH, et al.(1981) Evaluation of coarctation of the aorta with computed tomography. J Comput Assist Tomogr 5:153–156.
22. McLoughlin MJ, Weisbrod J, Wise D, et al. (1981) Computed tomography: congenital anomalies of the aortic arch and the great vessels. Radiology 138: 399–403.
23. Larde D, Belier C, Vasile N, et al. (1980) Computed tomography of aortic dissection. Radiology 136:147–151.
24. Gross SC, Barr L, Eyler WR, et al. (1980) Computed tomography in the dissection of the thoracic aorta. Radiology 136:135–139.

25. Muhm JR, Brown LR, Crowe JL, et al. (1978) Comparison of whole lung tomography with computed tomography in the detection of pulmonary nodules. AJR 131:981–984.

26. Siegelman SS, Zerhouni EA, Leo FP, et al. (1980) CT of the solitary pulmonary nodule. AJR 135:1–14.

27. Gamsu GS, Cann CE, Nicol RF (1981) Calcium quantification in pulmonary nodules using dual-energy CT. Invest Radiol 16:400.

28. Cann CE, Gamsu G, Birenberg FA, et al. (1982) Quantification of calcium in solitary pulmonary nodules using single and dual-energy CT. Radiology 145:493–496.

29. Godwin DJ, Speckman JM, Putman CE, et al. (1982) CT densitometry: Distinguishing benign from malignant pulmonary nodules. Radiology 144:349–351.

30. Levy C, Gray GE, McCollough CE, et al. (1982) The unreliability of CT numbers as absolute values. AJR 139:443–447.

31. Zerhouni EA, Spivey JF, Morgan RH, et al. (1982) Factors influencing quantitative CT measurements of solitary pulmonary nodules. J Comput Assist Tomogr 6:1075–1087.

32. Schaner EG, Chang AE, Doppman JL, et al. (1978) Comparison between conventional and computed tomography of the lungs in detecting pulmonary nodules. A prospective radiologic–pathologic study. AJR 131:51–54.

33. Naidich DP, McCauley D, Khouri NF, et al. (1982) Computed tomography of bronchiectasis. J Comput Assist Tomogr 6:437–444.

34. Fiore D, Biondetti PR, Sartori F, et al. (1982) The role of computed tomography in the evaluation of bullous lung disease. J Comput Assist Tomogr 6:105–108.

35. Webb WR, Gamsu G (1983) Computed tomography of the left retrobronchial stripe. J Comput Assist Tomogr 7:65–69.

36. Gobien RP, Stanley JH, Vujic J (1984) Thoracic CT guidance of thin needle aspiration. Radiology 149:827–830.

37. Bernardino ME (1984) Percutaneous biopsy. AJR 142:41–415.

38. Nakata H, Kimoto T, Nakayama T, et al. (1985). Diffuse peripheral lung disease. Evaluation by high-resolution computed tomography. Radiology 157:181–185.

39. Staples CA, Muller NL, Vedal S, et al. (1987) Usual interstitial pneumonia: Correlation of CT with clinical, functional and radiologic findings. Radiology 162:377–381.

40. Berkmen MY, Davis SD (1990) Radiology of diffuse lung disease. In Radiologic diagnosis of chest disease (Sperber ed.), 1st edn. Springer-Verlag, New York.

41. Shah, RM, Friedman AC. (1998) CT angiogram sign: incidence and significance in lobar consolidations evaluated by contrast-enhanced CT. AJR 170:719–721.

42. Murata K, Takahashi M, Mori M, et al. (1996) CT of pulmonary hilum: Evaluation with thin-section ultrafast CT. Crit Rev Diagn Imaging 37:39–277.

43. Murata K, Takahashi M, Mori M, et al. (1996) Peribronchovascular interstitium of the pulmonary hilum: normal and abnormal findings on thin-section electron-beam CT. AJR 166:309–312.

44. Goldman LW, Fowlkes JB (1995) Medical CT and ultrasound: Current technology and applications. Advanced Medical Publishing, Madison, WI.

45. Lee JKT, Sagel SS, Stanley RJ, et al. (1997) Computed body tomography with MRI correlation, 3rd edn. Lippincot Williams &Wilkins, New York.

46. Naidich DP, Webb WR, Müller NL, et al. (1998) Computed tomography and magnetic resonance of the thorax, 3rd ed. Lippincot Williams & Wilkins, New York.

47. Pugatch RO, Faling LJ, Robbins AH, et al. (1980) CT diagnosis of benign mediastinal abnormalities. AJR 134:685–694.

48. Bashist B, Ellis K, Gold RP (1983) CT of intrathoracic goiters. AJR 140:455–460.

49. Glazer GM, Axel L, Moss AA (1982) CT diagnosis of mediastinal thyroid. AJR 138:495–498.

50. Baron RL, Lee JKT, Sagel SS, et al. (1982). Computed tomography of the normal thymus. Radiology 142:121–125.

51. Dixon AK, Hilton CJ, Williams GT (1981). CT and histological correlation of the thymic remnant. Clin Radiol 32:255–257.

52. Fein GT, Bein ME, Mancuso AA, et al. (1982). Computed tomography of the anterior mediastinum in myasthenia gravis. Radiology 142:135–137.

53. Moore AV, Korobkin M, Powers B (1982) Thymoma detection by mediastinal CT. Patients with myasthenia gravis. AJR 138: 217–222.

54. Goulianos A, Striggaris K, Lolas C, et al. (1982) Thymic cysts. J Comput Assist Tomogr 6:172–175.

55. Lindfors KK, Meyer JE, Dedrick CG, et al. (1987) Thymic cysts in mediastinal Hodgkin's disease. Radiology 136:37–41.

56. Lee J, Sagel ST, Stanley R. (1983). Mediastinum. In Computed body tomography. Raven Press, New York.

57. Krudy AG, Doppman JL, Brennan MF, et al. (1981) the detection of mediastinal parathyroid glands by computed tomography, selective arteriography and venous sampling. Radiology 140:739–744.

58. Glazer GM, Francis IR, Shirazi KK, et al. (1983) Evaluation of the pulmonary hilum: Comparison of conventional radiography, 55 degrees posterior oblique tomography and dynamic computed tomography. J Comput Assist Tomogr 7:983–989.

59. Webb WR, Gamsu G, Glaser G (1981) Computed tomography of the abnormal pulmonary hilum. J Comput Assist Tomogr 5:485-490.

60. Naidich DP, Krouri NF, Stitic FP, et al. (1981). Computed tomography of the pulmonary hila. Abnormal anatomy. J Comput Assist Tomogr 5:468–475.

61. Glazer GM, Francis IR, Gebarski K, et al. (1983) Dynamic incremental computed tomography in the evaluation of pulmonary hila. J Comput Assist Tomogr 7:59–64.

62. Sone S, Higashihara T, Morimoto S, et al. (1983) CT anatomy of hilar lymphadenopathy. AJR 140:887–892.

63. Heiberg E, Wolverson M, Sundaram M, et al. (1981) CT findings in thoracic aortic dissection. AJR 136:13–17.

64. Godwin JD, Webb WR (1981) Dynamic computed tomography in the evaluation of vascular lung lesions. Radiology 138: 629–635.

65. Rankin S, Faling LJ, Pugatch RD (1982) CT diagnosis of arteriovenous malformations. J Comput Assist Tomogr 6:746–749.

66. Miller PA, Williamson BRJ, Minor GR, et al. (1982) Pulmonary sequestration. Visualization of the feeding artery by CT. J Comput Assist Tomogr 6:828–830.

67. Paul DJ, Mueller CF (1982) Pulmonary sequestration (case report). J Comput Assist Tomogr 6:163–165.

68. Godwin JD, Webb RW, Gamsu G, et al. (1980) Computed tomography of pulmonary embolism. AJR 135:691–695.

69. Overfors CO, Godwin JD, Brito BS (1981). Diagnosis of peripheral pulmonary emboli by computed tomography in the living dog. Radiology 141:519–523.

70. Muhm JR, Brown LR, Crowe JL (1977) Computed tomography in the detection of pulmonary nodules. Mayo Clin Proc 52:345–348.

71. Kuhns LR, Borlaza G. (1980) The "twinkling star" sign. An aid in differentiating pulmonary vessels from pulmonary nodules on computed tomography. Radiology 135: 763–764.

72. Putman CE, Rothman SL, Littner MR (1977) Computerized tomography in pulmonary sarcoidosis. Comput Assist Tomogr 1:197–209.

73. Solomon A, Kreel L, McNicol M, et al. (1979) Computed tomography in pulmonary sarcoidosis. J Comput Assist Tomogr 3:754–758.

74. Ellert J, Kreel L (1980) The role of computed tomography in the initial staging and subsequent management of the lymphomas. J Comput Assist Tomogr 9:368–391.

75. Sperber M, Mohan K (1984) Computerized tomography: a reliable diagnostic modality in pulmonary asbestosis. J Comput Assist Tomogr 8:125–132.

76. Katz D, Kreel L (1979). Computed tomography in pulmonary asbestosis. Clin Radiol 30:207–210.

77. Aberle DR, Gamsu G, Ray CS, et al. (1988) Asbestos-related pulmonary and parenchymal fibrosis. Detection with high-resolution CT. Radiology 166:729.

78. McLoud TC (1988) Use of CT in asbestos-exposed persons. Radiology 169:862.

79. Tylen U, Nilsson U (1982) Computed tomography in pulmonary pseudotumors and their relation to asbestos exposure. J Comput Assist Tomogr 6:229–237.

80. Mintzer RA, Gore RM, Vogelzang RL et al. (1981) Rounded atelectasis and its association with asbestos-induced pleural disease. Radiology 139:567–570.

81. Kreel L (1982) Computed tomography of interstitial pulmonary disease. J Comput Assist Tomogr 6:181–198.

82. Warren JB, Kreel L, Johnson L, et al. (1982) Use of computed tomography to demonstrate the extent of tuberculosis. J Comput Assist Tomogr 6:181-198.

83. Hartelius H (1988) Computed tomography in opportunistic lung infections . Acta Radiol 29:171.

84. Hertzanu Y, Heimer D, Hirsch M (1987) Computed tomography of pulmonary endometriosis. Comput Radiol 11:81.

85. Godwin JD, Muller NL, Tagasugi JE (1988) Pulmonary alveolar proteinosis. Radiology 169:609.

86. Rosenblum LJ, Mauceri RA, Wellenstein DE, et al. (1980) Density patterns in the normal lung as determined by computed tomography. Radiology 134:409–416.

87. Hedlund LW, Vock P, Effmannn EL (1983) Evaluating lung density by computed tomography. Semin Respir Med 5(1).

88. Carr DH, Pride ND (1984) Computed tomography in preoperative assessment of bullous emphysema. Clin Radiol 35:43–45.

89. Sperber, M (ed) (1998) Diffuse lung disorders: A comprehensive clinical radiologic overview. Springer-Verlag, Berlin, Heidelberg, New York.

90. Sanders C, Nath PH, Bailey WC (1988) Detection of emphysema with computed tomography. Correlation with pulmonary functions test and chest radiography. Invest Radiol 23:262.

91. Baber CE, Hedlund, Oddson TA (1980) Differentiating empyemas and peripheral pulmonary abscesses. The value of computed tomography. Radiology 135:755–758.

92. Shiu MS, Ho KJ (1983) Computed tomographic characteristics of pleural empyemas. J Comput Assist Tomogr 7:179–182.

93. Alexander E, Clark RA, Colley DP, et al. (1981) CT of malignant pleural mesothelioma. AJR 137:287–291.

94. Mirvis D, Dutcher JP, Haney PJ, et al. (1983) CT of malignant pleural mesothelioma. AJR 140:665–670.

95. Strankinga W, Sperber M., Kaiser M, et al. (1987) The accuracy of diagnostic procedures in the initial evaluation and follow-up of mesothelioma patients. Respiration 51:179–187.

96. Gouliamos AD, Carter BL, Emami B (1980) Computed tomography of the chest wall. Radiology 134:433–436.

97. Leitman BS, Firooznai H, McCauley DI (1983) The use of computed tomography in evaluating chest wall pathology. J Comput Tomogr 7:399–405.

98. Webb WR, Siegel SS (1982) Actinomicosis involving the chest wall: CT findings. AJR 139:1007–1009.

99. Sperber, M, de Verbizier, G, Laurent F, et al. (1990) Bronchogenic carcinoma following thoracic wall actinomicosis. Report on one case with emphasis on CT findings. Comput Med Imaging Graph 14:4.

100. Proto AV, Thomas SR (1985) Pulmonary nodules studied by CT. Radiology 156:149–154.

101. Baron R, Levitt R, Sagel S, White M, et al. (1982) CT in the preoperative evaluation of bronchogenic carcinoma. Radiology 145:727–732.

102. Richey H, Matthews J, Helsel R, et al. (1984) Thoracic CT scanning in the staging of bronchogenic carcinoma. Chest 85:218–221.

103. Webb WR, Gamsu G, Speckman J (1983) CT of the pulmonary hilum in bronchogenic carcinoma. J Comput Assist Tomogr 7:219–225.

104. Brion JP, Depami L, Kuhn G, et al. (1985) Role of computed tomography and mediastinoscopy in preoperative staging of lung carcinoma. J Comput Assist Tomogr 9:480–484.

105. Biondetti PR, Fiore D, Sartori F, et al. (1982) Evaluation of the postpneumonectomy space by computed tomography. J Comput Assist Tomogr 6:238–242.

106. Nabauri P, Mantarardi R, Breyer D, et al. (1980) Computed tomography of radiation-induced lung injuries. J Comput Assist Tomogr 5:568–570.

107. Pagani JJ, Libshitz HI (1982) CT manifestations of radiation-induced change in chest tissue. J Comput Assist Tomogr 6:243–248.

108. Naidich DP, McCauley DI, Siegelman SS (1982) Computed tomography of bronchial adenomas. J Comput Assist Tomogr 6:725–732.

109. Naidich DP, Khouri NF, McCauley D, et al. (1983) Computed tomography of lobar collapse. Part I. Endobronchial obstruction. J Comput Assist Tomogr 7:745–757.

110. Aristizabal JF, Young KR, Nath H (1998) Can chest CT decrease the use of preoperative bronchoscopy in the evaluation of suspected bronchogenic carcinoma.? Chest 113:1244–1249.

111. Naidich DP, Khouri NF, McCauley D, et al. (1983). Computed tomography of lobar collapse. Part II. Collapse in the absence of endobronchial obstruction. J Comput Assist Tomogr 7:758–767.

112. Katzenstein ALA, Fiorelli RF (1994) Non-specific interstitial pneumonia/fibrosis. Histologic features and clinical significance. Am J Surg Pathol 181:136–147.

113. McLoud TC, Carrington CB, Gaensler EA (1983) Diffuse infiltrative lung disease. A new scheme for description. Radiology 149:353–563.

114. Todo G, Itoh H, Nakamo Y, et al. (1982) High resolution CT for the evaluation of pulmonary peripheral disorders. Jpn J Clin Radiol 27:1319–1326.

115. Mayo JR, Webb WR, Gould R et al. (1987). High resolution CT of the lungs: Optimal approach. Radiology 163:507–510.

116. Gamsu G, Klein J (1989) High resolution CT of diffuse lung disease. Clin Radiol 40:554-556.

117. Murata K, Khan A (1989) Pulmonary parenchymal disease: Evaluation with high resolution CT. Radiology 170:629–635.

118. Leung AN, Staples CA, Müller NL, et al. (1991) Chronic diffuse infiltrative lung disease: Comparison of diagnostic accuracy of high resolution and conventional CT. AJR 157:693.

119. Mayo JR (1991) High-resolution computed tomography: Technical aspects. Radiol Clin North Am 29:1043.

120. Grenier P, Cordeau MP, Beigelman C (1993) High resolution computed tomography of the airways. J Thorac Imaging 8:213–229.

121. Swensen SJ, Aughenbaugh GL, Brown LR (1989) High resolution computed tomography of the lung. Mayo Clin Proc 64:1284–1294.

121. Gruden JF, Webb WR, Naidich DP, et al. (1999) Multinodular disease: Anatomic localisation at thin section CT – Multireader evaluation of a simple algorithm. Radiology 210:711–720.

122. Shimoyama K, Murata K, Takahashi M, et al. (1997) Pulmonary hilar lymph node metastases from lung cancer: Evaluation based on morphology at thin-section, incremental, dynamic CT. Radiology 203:187-195.

123. Franquet T, Gimenez A, Bordes R, et al. (1998) The crazy-paving pattern in exogenous lipoid pneumonia: CT–pathological correlation. AJR 170:315–317.

124. Johkoh T, Itoh, H, Müller NL, et al. (1999). Crazy-paving appearance at thin-section CT: Spectrum of disease and pathologic findings. Radiology 211:155-160.

125. Rémy Jardin M, Rémy J, Giraud F, et al. (1993) Computed tomography assessment of ground-glass opacity: Semiology and significance. J Thorac Imaging 8:249–264.

126. Zompatori M, Rimondi MR (1994) Diffuse ground-glass opacity of the lung. A guide to interpreting the high resolution computed tomographic picture (HRCT). Radiol Med 88:576-581.

127. Webb WR, Müller NL, Naidich DP (1996) High-resolution CT of the lung. Lippincott-Raven, New York.

128. Gaeta M, Caruso R, Barone M, et al. (1998) Ground-glass attenuation in nodular bronchioloalveolar carcinoma: CT patterns and prognostic value. J Comput Assist Tomogr 22:215–219.

129. Maguire WM, Herman PG, Khan A, et al. (1993) Comparison of fixed and adjustable window width and level settings in the CT evaluation of diffuse lung disease. J Comput Assist Tomogr 17:847–852.

130. Zwirewich CT, Terriff B, Müller NL (1989) High spatial frequency (bone) algorithm improves quality of standard CT of the thorax. AJR 153:1169–1173.

131. Naidich DP (1991) High-resolution computed tomography of cystic lung disease. Semin Roentgenol 26:151.

132. More ADA, Godwin JD, Dietrich PA, et al. (1992) Swyer–James syndrome: CT findings in eight patients. AJR 158:1211–1215.

133. Lucidarme O, Coche E, Cluzel P, et al. (1998) Expiratory CT scans for chronic airway disease: Correlation with pulmonary function test results. AJR 170:301–307.

134. Noma S, Khan A, Herman PG, et al. (1990) High-resolution computed tomography of the pulmonary parenchyma. Semin Ultrasound CT MR 11:365–379.

135. Mayo JR (1991) High resolution computed tomography: Technical aspects. Radiol Clin North Am 29:1043–1049.

136. Stern EJ, Webb WR (1993) Dynamic imaging of lung morphology with ultrafast high-resolution computed tomography. J Thorac Imaging 8:273–282.

137. Stern EJ, Webb WR, Gamsu G (1994) Dynamic quantitative computed tomography: A predictor of pulmonary function in obstructive lung disease. Invest Radiol 29:564–569.

138. Akira M, Yokoyama K, Yamamoto S, et al. (1991) Early asbestosis: Evaluation with high resolution CT. Radiology 178:409–416.

139. Kim TS, Lee KS, Chung MP, et al. (1998) Nonspecific interstitial pneumonia: High resolution CT and pathologic findings. AJR 171:1645–1650.

140. Bergin C, Roggli V, Coblenz C, et al. (1988) The secondary pulmonary lobule: Normal and abnormal CT appearance. AJR 151:21–25.

141. Heitzman ER, Markarian B, Berger I, et al. (1969) The secondary pulmonary lobule: A practical concept for the interpretation of radiographs. I. Roentgen anatomy of the normal secondary pulmonary lobule. Radiology 93:508–513.

142. Webb WR (1991) High-resolution lung computed tomography: Normal anatomical and pathological findings. Radiol Clin North Am 29:1051.

143. Raskin SP (1982) The pulmonary acinus: Historical notes. Radiology 144:31–34.

144. Müller NL (1991) Clinical value of high-resolution CT in chronic diffuse lung disease. AJR 157:1163.

145. Murata K, Itoh H, Todo G, et al. (1986) Centrilobular lesions of the lung: Demonstration by high-resolution CT and pathologic correlation. Radiology 161: 641–645.

146. Gruden JF, Webb WR, Warnok M (1994) Centrilobular opacities in the lung on high resolution CT: Diagnostic considerations and pathologic correlation. AJR 162:569–574.

147. Bergin CJ, Bell DY, Coblenz CL, et al. (1989) Sarcoidosis: Correlation of pulmonary parenchymal pattern at CT with results of pulmonary function tests. Radiology 171:619–624.

148. Naidich DP (1991) High resolution computed tomography of cystic lung disease. Semin Roentgenol 26:151.

149. Young K, Aspestrand F, Kolbestredt A (1991). High-resolution CT and bronchography in the assessment of bronchiectasis. Acta Radiol 32:439–41.

150. Jonhok T, Ikesoe T, Tomiyama N, et al. (1992) CT findings in lymphangitis carcinomatosis of the lung: Correlation with histologic findings and pulmonary function tests. AJR 158: 1217–1222.

151. Brauner MW, Grenier P, Mompoint D, et al. (1989) Pulmonary sarcoidosis: Evaluation with high-resolution CT. Radiology 172:467–471.

152. Nishimura K, Kitaichi M, Izumi T, et al. (1992) Usual interstitial pneumonia: Histologic correlation with high resolution CT. Radiology 182:337–342.

153. Stein MG, Mayo J, Müller NL, et al. (1987) Pulmonary lymphangitic spread of carcinoma: Appearance on CT scans. Radiology 162:371–375.

154. Johkoh T, Müller NL, Taniguchi H, et al. (1999) Acute interstitial pneumonia: Thin-section CT findings in 36 patients. Radiology 211:859–863.

155. Müller NL (1991) Differential diagnosis of chronic diffuse infiltrative lung disease on high-resolution computed tomography. Semin Roentegenol 26:132.

156. Meziane MA (1992) High-resolution computed tomography scanning in the assessment of interstitial lung disease. J Thorac Imaging 7:3–13.

157. Akira M, Hara H, Sakatani M (1999) Interstitial lung disease in association with polymyositis-dermatomyositis: Long-term follow-up CT evaluation in seven patients. Radiology 210:333–338.

158. Remy-Jardin M, Remy J, Wallaert B, et al. (1993) Pulmonary involvement in progressive systemic sclerosis: Sequential evaluation with CT, pulmonary function tests and bronchoalveolar lavage. Radiology 188:499–506.

159. Hartman PE, Primack SL, Swensen SJ, et al. (1993) Desquamative interstitial pneumonia: Thin-section CT findings in 22 patients. Radiology 187:787–790.

160. Stern E, Webb WR, Golden JA, et al. (1992) Cystic lung disease associated with eosinophilic granuloma and tuberous sclerosis: Air trapping at dynamic ultrafast high-resolution CT. Radiology 182:325–329.

161. Hruban RH, Meziane MA, Zerhouni EA, et al. (1987) High-resolution computed tomography of infiltrative fixed lungs: Pathologic–radiologic correlation of centrilobular emphysema. Am Rev Respir Dis 136:935–940.

162. Santis G, Hodson ME, Strickland B, et al. (1991) High-resolution computed tomography in adult cystic fibrosis patients with mild lung disease. Clin Radiol 44:20.

163. Bessis L, Callard P, Gotheil C, et al. (1992). High-resolution CT of parenchymal lung disease: Precise correlation with histologic findings. Radiographics 12:45–58.

164. Rémy-Jardin M, Rémy J, Deffentaines C, et al. (1991) Assessment of diffuse infiltrative lung disease: Comparison of conventional CT and high-resolution CT. Radiology 181:157–162.

165. Müller NL, Ostrow DN (1991) High-resolution computed tomography of chronic interstitial lung disease. Clin Chest Med 12:97–114.

166. Zwirewich CV, Mayo JR, Müller NL, et al. (1991) Low-dose high-resolution CT of lung parenchyma. Radiology 180:413–417.

167. Naidich DP, Marshall CH, Gribbin C, et al. (1990) Low-dose CT of the lungs: Preliminary observations. Radiology 175:729–731.

168. Soo Lee K, Primack S, Staples C (1994) Chronic infiltrative lung disease: Comparison of diagnostic accuracies of radiography and low- and conventional-dose thin-section CT. Radiology 191:669–673.

169. Kalender WA, Seissler W, Klotz E, et al. (1990) Spiral volumetric CT with single-breath-hold technique, continuous transport, and continuous scanner rotation. Radiology 176:181–183.

170. Costello P (1995) Thoracic imaging with spiral CT. In Fishman EK, Jeffrey RB (eds) Spiral CT: Principles, techniques and clinical applications. Raven Press, New York.

171. Paranjpe DV, Bergin CJ (1994) Spiral CT of the lungs: Optimal technique and resolution compared with conventional CT. AJR 162:561–567.

172. Rubin GD, Leung AN, Robertson VJ, et al. (1998) Thoracic spiral CT: Influence of subsecond gantry rotation on image quality. Radiology 208:771–776.

173. Kalender WA, Polacin A (1991) Physical performance characteristics of spiral CT scanning. Med Phys 18:910–915.

174. Rémy-Jardin, M, Rémy J (ed) (1996) Spiral CT of the chest. Springer, Berlin, Heidelberg, New York.

175. Kalender WA, Polacin A (1991) Physical performance characteristics of spiral CT scanning. Med Phys 18:910–915.

176. Rémy-Jardin M, Rémy J, Artaud D, et al. (1996) Diffuse infiltrative lung disease: Clinical value of sliding-thin-slab maximum intensity projection CT scans in the detection of mild micronodular pattern. Radiology 200:333–339.

177. Engeler CE, Tashjian JH, Engeler CM, et al. (1994) Volumetric high-resolution CT in the diagnosis of interstitial lung disease and bronchiectasis: Diagnostic accuracy and radiation dose. AJR 163:31–315.

178. Toulioupolos P, Costello P (1995) Helical (spiral) CT of the thorax. Radiol Clin North Am 33:843–861.

179. Rémy-Jardin M, Rémy J, Gosselin B, et al. (1996) Sliding-thin-slab, mimimum intensity projection technique in the diagnosis of emphysema: Histopathologic–CT correlation. Radiology 200:665–671.

180. Beigelman C, Howarth NR, Chartrand Lefebre C, et al. (1998) Congenital anomalies of tracheobronchial branching patterns: Spiral CT aspects in adults. Eur Radiol 8:79–85.

181. Quint LE, Whyte RI, Kazerooni EA, et al. (1995) Stenosis of the central airways: Evaluation by using helical CT with multiplanar reconstruction. Radiology 194:871–877.

182. Newmark GM, Conces DJ, Kopecky A (1994) Spiral CT evaluation of the trachea and bronchi. J Comput Assist Tomogr 18:552–554.

183. Costello P, Anderson W, Blume D (1991) Pulmonary nodule: Evaluation with spiral volumetric CT. Radiology 179:875–876

184. Collie DA, Wright AR, Williams JR, et al. (1994) Comparison of spiral-acquisition computed tomography and conventional computed tomography in the assessment of pulmonary metastatic disease. Br J Radiol 67:436–444.

185. Kuriyama K, Tateichi R, Kumatani T, et al. (1994) Pleural invasion by peripheral bronchogenic carcinoma: Assessment with three-dimensional helical CT. Radiology 191:365–369.

186. Kaneko M, Eguchi K, Ohmatsu H, et al. (1996) Peripheral lung cancer: Screening and detection with low-dose spiral CT versus radiography. Radiology 201:798–802.

187. Storto ML, Ciccotosto C, Gudotti A, et al. (1998) Neoplastic extension across pulmonary fissures: Value of spiral computed tomography and multiplanar reformations. J Thorac Imaging 13:204–210.

188. Goodman LR, Curtin JJ, Mewissen MW, et al. (1995) Detection of pulmonary embolism in patients with unresolved clinical and scintigraphic diagnosis: Helical CT versus angiography. AJR 164:1369–1374.

189. Garg K, Sieler H, Welsh CH, et al. (1999) Clinical validity of helical CT being interpreted as negative for pulmonary embolism: Implications for patient treatment. AJR 172:1627–1631.

190. Kim KI, Müller NL, Mayo JR (1999) Clinically suspected pulmonary embolism: Utility of spiral CT. Radiology 210:693–697.

191. Blum AG, Delafau F, Grignon B, et al. (1994) Spiral computed tomography versus pulmonary angiography in the diagnosis of acute massive pulmonary embolism. Am J Cardiol 74:96–98.

192. Kauczor HU, Schwickert HC, Mayer E, et al. (1994) Spiral CT of bronchial arteries in chronic thromboembolism. J Comput Assist Tomogr 1:855–861.

193. Teigen CL, Maus TP, Sheedy PF II, et al. (1995). Pulmonary embolism: Diagnosis with contrast enhanced electron beam CT and comparison with pulmonary angiography. Radiology 194:313–319.

194. Rémy-Jardin M, Rémy J, Petyt L, et al. (1995) Diagnosis of acute pulmonary embolism with spiral CT: Comparison with pulmonary angiography and scintigraphy. Radiology 197(P):303.

5 Magnetic Resonance Imaging of the Thorax

M. Sperber

Technical Considerations

Magnetic resonance imaging (MRI) has revolutionized modem radiology by allowing physicians to obtain images in multiplanar views in a relatively easy manner. This new modality soon became a routine part of the arsenal of diagnostic techniques used in daily practice. However, problems related to its correct integration with other existing methods and to realistic utilization still exist. Basically, in an MRI investigation system, the patient is placed in a strong, uniform magnetic field. This field is produced in most cases by a superconducting magnet that operates at a field strength ranging from 0.5 to 2.0 Tesla. Liquid cryogens are used in connection with this type of magnet, helium for cooling purposes and nitrogen as a thermal cover.

Also on the market are resistive magnets that produce energy at a rate dependent on the current that they carry. They are easily constructed and offer low cost opportunities; however, they provide an unstable magnetic field and therefore their practical use is limited. The other components of an MRI system are the gradient and the radiofrequency coils. The former are used to generate small gradient magnetic fields along the axes of imaging and the latter to transmit and receive radiowaves of preestablished frequencies. Similar to computed tomography (CT), a computer system is required in addition to the above in order to analyze the obtained signals and synthesize information from MR images (Fig. 5.1).

MRI techniques are essentially based on the way the special distribution of hydrogen nuclei (protons) is mapped. When a patient is placed in the magnetic field, the hydrogen nuclei in the body, which are aligned along the axis of the magnetic field, will be deviated because of the short radiowaves transmitted by the radiofrequency coils. The small energy pulses released by this process constitute the basis for the MRI signal.

Tissue parameters have a great impact on MRI, influencing the quality and intensity of images, as well as helping in the characterization of normal and pathologic tissues (1–3). In fact, MRI depends not only on proton density, which is the number of nuclei per volume unit of a specific tissue, but also on several other parameters. Among them the most important are the T_1, and T_2 relaxation times and flow. T_1 *relaxation time* is the time needed for protons that have been rotated 180° away from the plane of the magnetic field to return to their equilibrium plane. The time needed for the signal generated by the protons rotating in the transverse plane to decay and to disappear is called the T_2 *relaxation time.*

Flow effects on MR images are based on the fact that MR signals received from hydrogen nuclei in the blood are dependent on the blood flow velocity. Therefore, compared with stationary blood, flowing blood can produce more or less MR signal as velocity increases. In MRI, contrast injections into the vessels are not required because there is an intrinsic signal intensity difference between flowing blood and the wall of the vessel. The main mediastinal and pulmonary vessels, for example, are demonstrated with great anatomic accuracy (4–6).

In order to understand the way T_1 and T_2 relaxation times of tissue can help to obtain diagnostic MR images, the terms "repetition time" and "time to echo" have to be understood. *Repetition time* (TR) is the interval between the beginning of a pulse sequence and the start of the next pulse sequence. *Time to echo* (TE) is the time between the first 90° pulse and the moment at which a signal is returned from the object under the study and can be read out. By changing the different TR and TE values, one may obtain images that depend on the T_1, and T_2 relaxation times of tissues (T_1- and T_2-weighted images). For example, increased TR values reduce the T_1 characteristics of MR images. While in these cases the scanning time is prolonged, the signal-to-noise ratio is significantly improved. Conversely, shortening the TE values increases the T_1 properties of an image. Long TE values produce more T_2-weighted images.

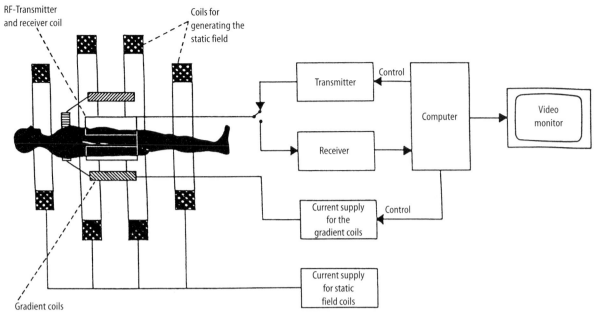

RF-Transmitter
and receiver coil

Coils for
generating the
static field

Gradient coils

Figure 5.1. Diagram representing a basic MRI system.

The choice of pulse parameters appears to be quite important in MRI because a wrong combination of pulses reduces tissue contrast and can mask even large abnormalities. In the study of the mediastinum, for example, the use of T_1-weighted images is recommended because they permit superior differentiation between mediastinal lesions and the bronchovascular system on one side, and between lesions and the mediastinal fat on the other side (Fig. 5.2). In contrast, in the study of lung pathology in general it is important to use T_2-weighted images with long TR values because of the improved signal-to-noise ratio and the relatively increased signal intensity of most masses. T_2-weighted images may also help in the differentiation of high intensity parenchymal consolidation from lower intensity centrally located lesions (7–9).

In an attempt to improve the diagnostic ability of MR examinations, the use of paramagnetic contrast materials has been proposed. Such contrast agents, by shortening proton relaxation times of tissues, permit the use of shorter pulse sequences to obtain high contrast images. Among them, the most representative is gadolinium-diethylenetriamine pentaactetic acid (DTPA), which has been shown to have low toxicity (10,11) and to be able to reduce T_1 and T_2 relaxation times while enhanceing pathologic processes. In the evaluation of thoracic abnormalities by MRI, the use of gadolinium-DTPA has been shown to be beneficial in various conditions, including the demonstration of thoracic masses or as a marker of myocardial necrosis (12–16). Also under study are more sophisticated contrast agents, expected to concentrate specifically in certain organs or pathologic processes.

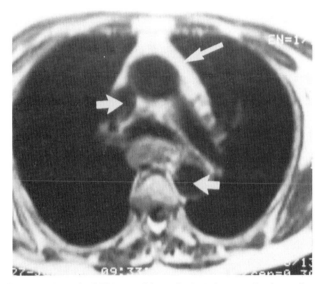

Figure 5.2. T_1-weighted MR image of the mediastinum demonstrating the excellent differentiation of mediastinal structures based on signal intensity (*long arrow*, high signal intensity fat; *short arrows*, low signal intensity vascular system).

Pulse sequences most commonly used in MRI are the *saturation-recovery* (SR), the *inversion-recovery* (IR), and the *spin-echo* (SE) techniques. By far, the SE technique is the most clinically useful type of MRI mode, being sensitive to T_1 and T_2 relaxation times as well as to hydrogen ion density and flow. By this method, changes in TR allow investigators to obtain important differences in contrast between normal and pathologic tissues. SR and IR images have not been shown to offer significant additional information in MRI of the chest (8,17–19), SR because of its low signal capabilities and limitation of multisection views, and IR because of its reduced spatial resolution and long data acquisition times.

Imaging Methodology

MR images can be obtained in a single plane, or by volume data acquisition. There is also the possibility of obtaining single or multiple slices. The *two-dimensional Fourier transformation* (2DFT) has been shown to allow an improved imaging speed and a better image quality (20,21). A three-dimensional technique is also available when data are acquired through a whole volume of tissue and can be reconstructed in various planes. This technique is especially valuable in the imaging of the heart when a process can be visualized during the same phase of the electrocardiogram (ECG) cycle each time.

The availability of a three-dimensional representation of chest pathology by MRI has resulted in a considerable advancement in the diagnosis of thoracic lesions. Coronal and sagittal MR images added to the transverse plane, without the need to move the patient, permit visualization of the entire thorax, as well as of the lower neck and upper abdomen. Extension of disease in areas previously very difficult to image, such as the supraclavicular, subpleural, or subphrenic spaces, is easily demonstrated. Multiplanar imaging has also proven to be an important adjuvant in the performance of fine-needle biopsy or for the planning of transtracheal needle biopsy in cases of subcarinal masses (22–24).

Because MR images may be degraded by artefacts resulting from patient motion, respiration, or cardiovascular movements, gating procedures have been proposed in MRI studies. ECG gating is obtained when the radiofrequency pulses are triggered by the R wave of the ECG. By choosing different time delays, images can be obtained at any period of the cardiac cycle. A 5 ms delay after the peak of the R wave (end-diastole) is commonly used to initiate the imaging sequence. For this reason, cardiac gating is of value in cases in which the heart or the main vascular structures are investigated, and also in the diagnosis of vascular lesions or lung masses situated in the vicinity of the heart. Respiratory gating, on the other hand, has not been shown to be of significant use in MRI of the thorax. The main disadvantage of this technique results from the markedly increased scanning time, which is problematic in patients already suffering from some degree of respiratory distress (25–27).

As mentioned before, it seems that images with relatively short TR intervals (350–500 ms) provide the best spatial resolution and high contrast definition between normal anatomic structures and pathologic tissues. This is especially true in cases of mediastinal lesions, whose commonly intermediate signal intensity can be easily differentiated from the low signal vascular structures and high signal mediastinal fat. However, if the main interest resides in the lungs, it is recommended that more T_2-weighted images be obtained.

Images obtained with long TR intervals produce significant differential change in the signal intensity of various pathologic tissues and are especially valuable in patients in whom the lungs and the pleural space must be investigated simultaneously. Many of the lung masses have prolonged T_2 relaxation times and are seen as areas of increased signal intensity.

In an attempt to reduce prolonged examination times, efforts are being made to develop *fast imaging techniques* that permit examination in patients unable to remain still for prolonged periods of time. In the study of the mediastinum, for example, it seems that images obtained with short TR and TE together with heavy signal averaging succeed in eliminating both cardiac and respiratory motion artefacts. Fast scanning techniques permitting data acquisition for an image in 10–20 s are being introduced. Furthermore, the possibility exists of the development of echo planar pulse sequences (real-time MRI) that allow image acquisition in 50 ms or less (21,28–30). In the study of the heart and related vascular structures, dynamic MRI has a special value when the input and output volumes can be estimated.

At the basis of "ciné-MRI" is a technique named "gradient echo imaging", which visualizes rapidly flowing blood as a bright signal. In this case, a single RF pulse is used to produce an echo signal. A magnetic field gradient is subsequently used to focus the protons and produce an MR (gradient echo) signal. Rapid scanning techniques include as well "GRASS" or "FLASH", which employ low flip angles, gradient refocused echoes, and short TR and TE values to obtain multiple images during a single breath hold. Although selectively used for the moment, "echo planar imaging" (EPI) is a very fast method that provides single images acquired in 40 ms or less, when all the lines of data in the matrix are acquired within the time of a single echo (31–33). For imaging of pulmonary parenchyma perfusion, a technique using pulsed arterial spin labeling (ASL) has been proposed. ASL uses magnetically labeled water as an endogenous, freely diffusible tracer and can be employed in the form of flow sensitive alternating inversion recovery (FAIR) and FAIR with extra radiofrequency pulse (FAIRER) (34).

A recent and exciting development in MRI is the use of hyperpolarized ^3H and ^{129}Xe for the imaging of airspaces and certain tissues. The value of this technique lies in its ability to derive images from the lung parenchyma, which notoriously lacks the sufficient amount of protons to enable a satisfactory MRI visualization. This is the reason behind the current extensive use of CT and especially high resolution CT (HRCT) in the diagnostic work-up of the lung parenchyma. Hyperpolarized gas images strive to reduce the need for the employment of CT, which carries with it patients' exposure to radiation. Mainly, the new technique has the goal to depict and quantify the real-time flow of gases into and out of the lungs.

The nuclear spin polarization of helium and other noble gases is greater than the polarization of water protons and can be enhanced by laser optical pumping. The result is an exceptional gain in polarization that overcomes the loss in signal due to the lower density of the gas. Studies have shown that in this manner a clear demarcation between the lung and surrounding structures can be seen, as the latter give no signal, and in the lungs, well-ventilated areas seem to present a higher signal than the less ventilated ones (e.g., apexes) (35–38). Other attempts have involved the use of inhaled molecular oxygen as a contrast agent to depict directly the transfer of oxygen across the alveolus into the pulmonary vasculature. Molecular oxygen is weakly paramagnetic, but still produces a signal change in the lungs due to their extensive surface area and with this method ventilation disturbances were demonstrated in bullous emphysema and pulmonary embolism (39,40). The search for less expensive contrast agents resulted as well in the trial of fluorinated gases in imaging the lungs, when these agents appeared to be appropriate for the visualization of a steady state rather than transient gas concentrations (41).

Additionally, experimental studies have opened the road to a new approach toward the characterization of pulmonary disorders based on the MR signal received from the lung parenchyma. For example it has been observed that the MR signal obtained from inflated lungs decreases very rapidly as compared with the signal obtained from collapsed lungs. The phenomenon is related to the magnetic field inhomogeneity existing in the air-filled lungs, as air and water have different magnetic susceptibilities. This air–tissue interface effect can be measured by MRI techniques (temporally symmetric and asymmetric SE sequences). When mathematical models were built to explain the internal magnetic field inhomogeneity in aerated normal and diseased lungs, they were found to correspond well with the results of experimental MR measurements in the same cases. The results point toward important clinical applications in the evaluation of various pathologic conditions, mainly acute ones such as pulmonary edema (42).

Magnetic Resonance Spectroscopy

MR spectroscopy was developed initially for analysis of the chemical composition of various substances in the laboratory. Recently, this technique has been applied to the study of compositions of cell cultures and isolated body organs. Moreover, in vivo experiments are increasingly being performed. The most studied paramagnetic ions are ^{31}P, ^{1}H, ^{23}Na, ^{13}C, and ^{19}F. Among them, because of its great metabolic significance, ^{31}P is the one mainly studied in clinical practice. A possible major use of this noninvasive diagnostic modality may be diagnosis and detection of neoplasms and the assessment of their metabolism (43–49). A specific application of spectroscopy in the thorax could be the identification of the relative composition of fluid collections (50,51).

A different technique that makes use of spectroscopic analysis of hydrogen and not phosphorus is chemical shift imaging. The result in this case is not a spectroscopic graph, but an anatomic image. The major use of this method is in the identification of minimal amounts of fat in a given lesion (43). A good example for the clinical utilization of MR spectroscopy is the in vivo localization and identification of molecules with known resonance peaks at specific chemical shifts. By this method, lecithin, one of the markers of fetal lung maturity, can be identified in amniotic fluid by volume-selected proton MR spectroscopy (52).

Clinical Applications

With the development of MRI, a large amount of new diagnostic information has been added to the data available from conventional radiographic studies and CT. In general, diagnostic criteria that have been proposed for the interpretation of MR images are similar to those used in CT. However, it is of paramount importance to understand the major differences between the two modalities, situated mainly in the area of the gray scale ordering of the tissues. In CT, gray scale variations are constant and well established on a range of Hounsfield numbers, whereas in MRI they may vary widely, even for the same tissue. It is essential to clearly comprehend these differences when attempting to interpret MR images.

MR is also able to display anatomy in sagittal and coronal planes supplementary to the transaxial projection, without the need for prolonged reformatting of multiple slices or uncomfortable patient positioning, as in CT.

Because the proton density of the pulmonary parenchyma is very low, one expects to receive minimal signal intensity from it. Centrally located pulmonary vessels and bronchi can be identified on MR images branching from the hilar region into the pulmonary fields. Bronchial and vascular walls produce relatively high signal intensity, whereas their inner content mostly gives a low signal intensity because of the low proton content of air and movement of flowing blood. Coronal and sagittal views are especially useful in the depiction of normal anatomy and pathologic changes in the thorax, because longer sections of bronchi and vessels can be visualized and the continuation of the thoracic structures is preserved (Fig. 5.3).

The value of MRI appears to be mainly in the obviated need for injection of contrast material, without which on CT scans an abnormal mass cannot be differentiated from vascular structures. In this sense, MRI clearly has an

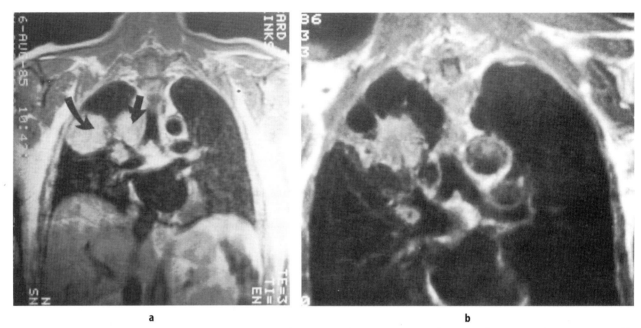

a   b

Figure 5.3. a Coronal MRI view of the thorax clearly facilitates the evaluation of the primary pulmonary masses (*curved arrow*) and their related mediastinal metastases (*short arrow*). **b** Enlarged view.

advantage for defining lesions within or adjacent to the heart and great vessels.

By using ECG-gated imaging, the definition of the mediastinum and pulmonary hili is greatly improved. This imaging technique should be preferred for thoracic evaluation. The most important pulse sequence for evaluating mediastinal and hilar abnormalities is a T_1-weighted SE sequence with short TR and TE, which permits good contrast between lesions and mediastinal fat. Conversely, T_2-weighted images, which have a higher signal-to-noise ratio and a lower contrast-to-noise ratio compared with T_1-weighted images, are more useful for the demonstration of intraparenchymal lesions. Most lung tumors appear to have a high signal intensity on the dark, low intensity background of the lung fields on images obtained with long TR values (e.g., TR 1500/T 30) (Fig. 5.4). However, because SE images obtained with a long TR seem to provide the best spatial resolution and those obtained with short TR the best contrast, in some cases it may be necessary to use pulse sequences with both long and short TR values in order to fulfill these requirements.

Hilar and Bronchial Abnormalities

When it comes to the study of hilar abnormalities, an accurate knowledge of hilar transverse anatomy is required, because walls of vessels and bronchi emit a similar signal. The condition of hilar soft tissues, which give an intermediate signal intensity, is often difficult to diagnose.

Several studies have attempted to compare the value of CT and MRI in the evaluation of the pulmonary hilus. In

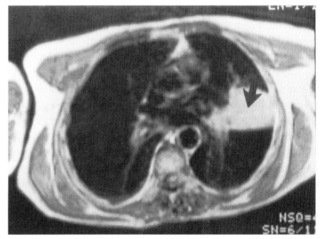

Figure 5.4. Left pulmonary mass with an atelectatic component accurately identified with MRI as an area of increased signal intensity (*arrow*).

general, they have shown the superiority of MRI in diagnosing a hilar mass in cases in which administration of contrast during the CT study was not possible or proved to be inefficient (Fig. 5.5). In addition, small hilar lesions have been mentioned that were not convincingly visualized on CT scans, but were clearly detected on MR images (53–55). Because of the lack of signal from the air in the bronchial tree and flowing blood in pulmonary arteries and veins, MRI, rather than CT, seems to provide more accuracy in the study of the close relationship that exists between visible bronchi, pulmonary artery branches, and hilar lymph nodes.

In fact, on SE images of the thorax, the pulmonary hili are visible as low signal structures composed of vessels, bronchi, and some fat. While MRI seems to be a reliable

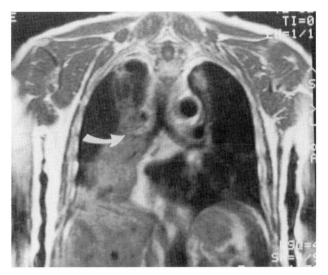

Figure 5.5. Coronal MR T_1-weighted image showing prominent vascular and bronchial obstruction by a right-sided pulmonary tumoral mass (*arrow*).

method of identifying enlarged lymph nodes at various sites in the thorax, easily separating them from the low signal intensity within the vascular lumen, normal-sized lymph glands are seldom identified on SE images. Lymph node calcification, which is commonly encountered in granulomatous disorders of the lungs, in occupational diseases, or in fungus infections, cannot be detected with MRI, since calcium gives no MR signal. Another limitation of MRI in the evaluation of the pulmonary hilus became apparent when patients with bronchogenic carcinoma were examined: the lack of distinction between small adjacent lymph glands, which may appear as single enlarged masses as a result of the limited spatial resolution of MR images.

Studies that have compared MRI, CT, and 55° posterior oblique tomography in the evaluation of patients with lung cancer have demonstrated that pathology is still recognized on the basis of size measurements when enlarged hilar lymph nodes are identified on MR images as regions of increased signal intensity larger than 10 mm in diameter. In general, no significant differences were demonstrated between the three imaging modalities in the overall accuracy of hilar evaluation (55–57).

Calculated MR relaxation times, T_1, and T_2, derived either from spectroscopy data or MR images, failed to allow recognition of specific processes on the basis of these MRI parameters. Comparison of measurements obtained from enlarged lymph nodes present in a large variety of pathologic conditions, including inflammation, tuberculosis, sarcoidosis, and nonspecific enlargement, as well as lymphoma and metastatic carcinoma, showed a clear overlap of T_1, and T_2 values between normal and malignant lymph nodes (54,58).

Some of the suggested reasons for this overlap seem to be related to the great variations in the water content of lymph nodes, a factor on which T_1, and T_2 measurements are mostly dependent (55,58). According to one report

(58), spectroscopic analysis revealed increased T_1, and T_2 values of nodes involved by neoplasm compared with normal specimens and T_2 relaxation times that were greater for acute inflammatory nodes than for nodes involved by granulomatous disease or malignancy. Such findings could not be confirmed by other investigators, and whether T_1, and T_2 relaxation times can provide reliable information for the specific characterization of lymphadenopathy remains uncertain. Measurements with MRI are also seriously impaired by the lower spatial resolution of this modality, due to long scanning times, patient motion, and relatively large slice thickness, which causes volume averaging with the surrounding fat.

Bronchogenic carcinoma presenting as a hilar lesion will usually appear as an irregular, ill-defined mass. The use of sagittal and coronal views in MRI of the chest permits the visualization of longer segments of intrapulmonary bronchi, and therefore bronchial narrowing present in patients with lung cancer is commonly demonstrated with MRI. The primary lung lesion is usually well identified with MRI, as well as its direct or metastatic extension to the mediastinum. The intermediate signal intensity tumor is well separated on MR images from the low signal intensity structures such as the superior vena cava or the pulmonary arteries and the high signal intensity fat (59) (Fig. 5.6).

In a study by Martini et al. (60), mediastinal lymph node dissection or sampling has been performed and correlated with preoperative studies in 34 patients with surgically confirmed carcinoma of the lung. Both CT and MRI have been found to be highly accurate in assessing the presence of mediastinal adenopathy, with a sensitivity rate of 87%. Direct extension into the mediastinum adjacent to a pulmonary mass was easily distinguished from fat with MR when short TR images were used. However, in the above comparative study neither CT nor MRI correlated well with surgical findings, in comparison with which the sensitivity rate for CT was 55% and that for MR 64%.

Bronchogenic carcinoma often presents with distal pulmonary collapse. A study comparing CT and MRI in their ability to identify contour abnormalities secondary to tumor presence, discover bronchial obstruction, and separate proximal tumor from distal collapse has found both methods to be equal in their capacity to visualize a contour abnormality (70% of cases). Because of the poor spatial resolution of MRI, bronchial narrowing could be identified only in 7 patients of 17, whereas CT succeeded in demonstrating bronchial narrowing as a secondary sign of bronchogenic carcinoma in 15 of 16 cases (61).

Another study assessed the accuracy of CT and MRI in staging bronchogenic carcinoma when compared with pathologic and histologic results and found that the sensitivity of CT was 78% and specificity 96%. The values for MRI were 84% and 96%, respectively. MRI seemed to be more accurate than CT in diagnosing mediastinal invasion

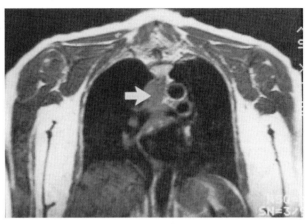

a

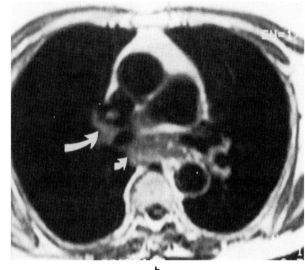

b

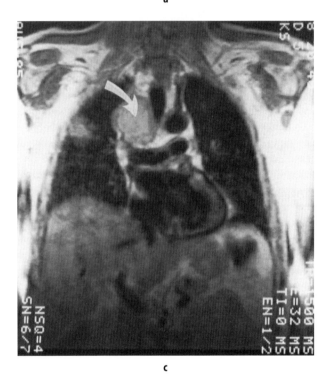

c

Figure 5.6. MR images showing metaslatic deposits at various mediastinal levels (*arrows*). Their relation to normal mediastinal structures is clearly demonstrated. (From ref. 69, with permission.)

and in staging superior sulcus and complex tumors. No great differences have been detected between the two modalities as to the identification of mediastinal node metastases. The sensitivities were CT (82%) and MRI (90%), and specificities CT (88%) and MRI (93%) (62).

In general, it seems that hilar masses or enlarged hilar nodes are more sharply defined and more clearly visualized on MR images when they contrast with the neighboring low signal intensity lung, bronchi, and hilar vessels. In contrast, bronchial abnormalities are better demonstrated on CT, mainly because of the spatial resolution of this modality. Lobar and segmental bronchi are not entirely demonstrated on MR images and one has to be cautious about diagnosing a nonvisualized small bronchus on MR as pathologic.

When separation of a tumoral mass from collapsed lung parenchyma is attempted, a CT examination with bolus injection is usually performed; however, the differentiation remains difficult in most cases. MRI unfortunately does not succeed in adding sufficient information in these pathologies, mainly because of the heterogeneity in the signal intensity of tumors (63) (Fig. 5.7).

An interesting area for comparison between CT and MRI is the detection of pulmonary nodules, single or

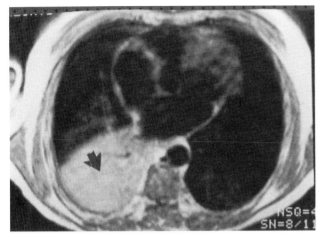

Figure 5.7. MR images of a tumoral process in the right lung, which cannot be differentiated from collapsed parenchyma (*arrow*).

multiple. CT has been demonstrated to be a highly sensitive modality in the diagnosis of pulmonary nodules; however, the distinction between benign and malignant lesions remains difficult in most cases. Additionally, even on CT scans performed with contrast enhancement the discovery of nodules located in the vicinity of vessels may be problematic.

In this sense, on MR images, bright, high signal intensity nodules are clearly separated from the low signal intensity vascular lumen or lung parenchyma. Limitations of MRI of the thorax include its reduced spatial resolution, particularly in the subpleural or diaphragmatic areas where metastatic nodules are often located. Also, because of the low signal-to-noise ratio of the normal lung parenchyma and nonvisualization of most segmental bronchi or normal fissures, it is difficult to establish the exact location of a nodule on MR images. Studies have shown that long repetition times (2.0 s) were beneficial in demonstrating pulmonary nodules, especially those close to blood vessels. CT, with its superior spatial resolution, enabled better detection of nodules close to the diaphragm, the pleura, or each other (64,65).

Additionally, dynamic contrast-enhanced MRI has shown its value in the evaluation of solitary pulmonary nodules. The method has pointed toward significant differences in the degree and kinetics of MR contrast enhancement for specific types of nodules. Malignant lesions seemed to enhance stronger and faster than benign ones. Nevertheless, the strongest contrast enhancement has been found in benign lesions identified histologically as being of the inflammatory-fibrotic type (66). In the case of pulmonary metastases, the use of T_2-weighted turbo-spin-echo (TSE) sequences has been tried and compared with spiral volumetric CT. The conclusion is that, although of limited value in screening, the incidental discovery of a pulmonary lesion on T_2-weighted TSE MR images is highly reliable in representing a pulmonary nodule. However, the malignant nature of such a finding,

on MRI as well as on CT, especially with small nodules, remains uncertain (67).

An interesting diagnostic combination may be obtained from the information offered by dynamic T_1-weighted MRI and positron emission tomography (PET) in patients with lung cancer, when vascular physiology is correlated with glucose metabolism. Parameters of vascular physiology include permeability–surface area (PS) and extracellular contrast agent distribution volume. Experimental results have shown that tumor PS product correlates with glucose metabolism, that chemo- and radiotherapy induce observable and quantifiable changes in these parameters, and that such changes can be measured by in vivo dynamic MRI. Therefore quantitative dynamic T_1-weighted MRI of tumor vascular physiology may have a useful role in the clinical management of lung cancer (68).

Mediastinal Abnormalities

Similarly, to CT, MRI can define the precise location and extent of a mediastinal mass. Additionally, the ability of MRI to provide a three-dimensional representation of pathology greatly facilitates interpretation, widening the range of indications for MRI of the mediastinum. Such indications include evaluation of lesions located in the aortopulmonary window, definition of the relationship to the spinal canal of a mass discovered in the posterior mediastinum, differentiating between solid, vascular, cystic, or lipomatous structures based on signal intensities, and evaluation of pathologic conditions located just above the diaphragm (54,69–74).

Widening of the mediastinum is a commonly encountered clinical problem. It may be the result of a normal variant such as abundant fat deposition or the presence of a tortuous vessel. Pathologic conditions causing mediastinal widening are numerous and include vascular aneurysms, primary tumors, metastatic masses, and enlarged lymph nodes. All these abnormalities have been successfully studied with MRI, which does not require the use of iodinated contrast material and has no ionizing radiation, qualities that make it the method of choice in the investigation of young patients or whenever the amount of irradiation has to be restricted. Additionally, studies have shown that the superior three-dimensional imaging permitted by MRI facilities the diagnosis of vascular abnormalities in the mediastinum, including congenital disorders or acquired conditions such as aneurysms and dissection of the aorta (72–76). In these cases it has been demonstrated that the use of different technical parameters, such as signal intensity variations between the first and second delayed echo, help to differentiate pathologic alterations in blood flow pattern. Morphology, location, and size of aneurysms can be accurately assessed on either short- or long-axis images. Aortic dissection is reliably recognized on MR images, including the identification of the intimal tear in the ascending aorta, the true and false channels, and the eventual involvement of the aortic branches (77–79).

Involvement of the mediastinum in malignant conditions is also a relatively frequent etiology for mediastinal widening. On conventional radiographs metastatic lesions have the tendency to blend in with the surrounding mediastinal components, making their evaluation and accurate localization impossible. CT and MR1 permit a precise separation of the normal mediastinal structures from the suspected abnormality. Studies comparing the utility of these two modalities in the evaluation of questionable lesions discovered on conventional radiographic studies have shown that CT is able to delineate soft tissue abnormalities from vascular structures well, provided contrast injection has been given. MRI is able to offer the same information without requiring intravenous contrast administration. T_1-weighted MR images are most helpful in delineating mediastinal lymph nodes, which are clearly seen as masses of intermediate signal intensity within the high signal intensity of mediastinal fat. Bronchovascular compression or invasion may be confirmed or excluded and the number of invasive procedures, such as mediastinoscopy or exploratory thoracotomy, used for staging purposes can be considerably reduced (54,70,80). The major limitation with MRI remains for the moment the same as that encountered in CT studies – its inability to predict histology by measurements reliable enough to distinguish benign from malignant diseases.

As more clinical experience with MRI has been acquired, several other shortcomings became apparent, such as the relatively poor spatial resolution of MRI compared with CT, as a result of which single mediastinal nodes are difficult to separate from larger groups. Also, volume averaging may result in significant diagnostic problems, especially if only a single pulse sequence study is performed. Reports have shown that volume averaging of mediastinal fat, which has high signal intensity, and low intensity flowing blood may produce a region of intermediate signal intensity that simulates a mediastinal mass or lymphadenopathy (9,81). Imaging with different TR values is therefore strongly advised whenever there is suspicion of a mediastinal mass. Additionally, the presence of calcification in thoracic masses is very difficult to identify with MRI because calcium gives no signal on MR images. This finding, which commonly supports the diagnosis of a benign lesion, cannot be utilized when one is attempting to interpret MR images.

Pleural Abnormalities

Pleural fluid collection is a common finding in patients with bronchogenic carcinoma. With MR, fluid collections are

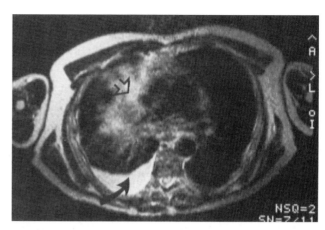

Figure 5.8. T_2-weighted MR image demonstrating a right-sided, high- signal intensity pleural effusion (*long arrow*). Postirradiation mediastinal fibrotic changes are also visible (*short arrow*). (From ref. 69, with permission.)

better visualized on images obtained with long TR and TE values (e.g., 2.0 s (50 ms)$^{-1}$) (Fig. 5.8). Because bronchial carcinoma is often associated with distant metastatic spread, MRI can be used, if there are no time limitations, to accurately locate adrenal or liver metastases. However, MRI is unable to demonstrate bone destruction because of lack of signal from calcified tissues.

With the advent of MRI it was hoped that this modality could provide a reliable tool for the differentiation of inflammatory from noninflammatory effusions. Indeed, initially it seemed that there was a correlation between T_1 and T_2 relaxation times of the effusion and its lipid and/or protein content. Unfortunately, subsequent studies demonstrated a significant overlap of T_1 and T_2 values of various body fluids and only a moderate correlation between protein content and T_1 and T_2 relaxation times (82,83). Typically, blood effusions show a high signal intensity on both T_1- and T_2-weighted images. Similarly, chylous or purulent pleural collections have also a relative high intensity with T_1 and T_2 relaxation times.

In general, pleural abnormalities are easily identified on MR images because of the three-dimensional abilities of this modality. Benign pleural thickening as observed in occupational lung disorders is seen as intermediate signal intensity areas along the thoracic wall. Also of great diagnostic importance is the accurate demonstration of the location and extent of malignant pleural lesions, such as malignant pleural mesothelioma or metastatic deposits. On MR images, malignant mesothelioma appears as a large lobulated mass of high signal intensity on T_2-weighted images (84,85). Compression of the lung parenchyma and mediastinal invasion are clearly demonstrated, as are invasion of the chest wall and soft tissue. Coronal MR images are particularly suited for the visualization of such pathology (Fig. 5.9).

In some cases, primary neoplasms of the chest wall may cause infiltration of the adjacent pleura. Malignant invasion

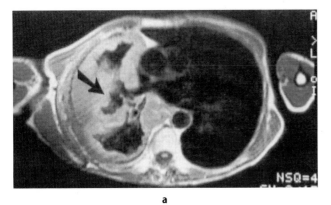
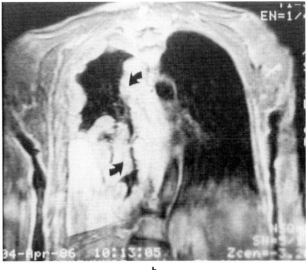

a   b

Figure 5.9. Axial (**a**) and coronal (**b**) MR images demonstrating extensive right pleural and mediastinal involvement by malignant mesothelioma (*arrows*). The lobulated masses appear to be of intermediate signal intensity on T₁-weighted images (**a**) and of high signal intensity on T₂-weighted images (**b**). (From ref 84, with permission.)

is easily recognized as a local change in the signal intensity of the intercostal space and pleural layers when compared with adjacent structures. Tumor and pleural infiltration have the same intermediate signal intensity (84,86).

Other Clinical Applications

An area in which MRI may prove to be a valuable diagnostic technique is the study of the postpneumonectomy thorax. Clinicians are often concerned with immediate and long-term pathologic changes in these cases, especially in patients who undergo pneumonectomy for lung cancer. MR images accurately demonstrate variable degrees of fluid collection, pleural thickening, and mediastinal shift and rotation (Fig. 5.10). They are also expected to reveal the presence of recurrent tumor, shown as an area of high signal intensity. This area is easily differentiated from fibrotic changes, which remain of intermediate signal intensity on both T₁- and T₂-weighted images.

This specific appearance of fibrotic changes on MR images is also useful in the exclusion of malignant changes in patients who received therapy. In this case, intermediate signal intensity areas that do not change their signal intensity from T₁- to T₂-weighted images can reliably be considered as benign fibrotic changes (67,87,88) (Fig. 5.11).

Because a large variety of benign clinical conditions still require an accurate noninvasive mean of diagnosis, attempts have been made to evaluate the potential of MRI in the discovery and determination of extent in such disorders as interstitial diseases, pulmonary embolism, pulmonary airspace disease, and congenital bronchial abnormalities.

Studies have shown that there is a possibility of demonstrating pulmonary emboli with MRI because of the lack of signal from the normal vascular lumen and the intense signal within pulmonary arteries at the level of lodged clots (89–91). Possible difficulties to be taken into consideration are the presence of a slow vascular flow, producing a misleading intraluminal signal, or the concomitant existence of airspace disease or atelectasis, which can give a high signal on MR images covering the existence of small peripheral emboli.

Findings on MR images, when compared with those of CT scans, show that there is a better delineation of the extent of inflammatory changes occurring in intrathoracic abscesses with MRI. Effects on adjacent structures such as vessels, muscles, and bone are clearly demonstrated. Also, there is no need for contrast agent injection for the visualization of the abscess capsule. On CT, if the abscess does not contain gas and does not have a low attenuation number, it is difficult to separate from adjacent structures (92).

In chronic lung disorders, pathogenic changes within the bronchi, such as mucus plugs, have been clearly differentiated on MR images from the pulmonary vessels on the dark background of the pulmonary parenchyma. These findings can underline the value of MRI in the study of children with cystic fibrosis, with the lack of ionizing radiation adding to the utility of MRI in the pediatric age group (93).

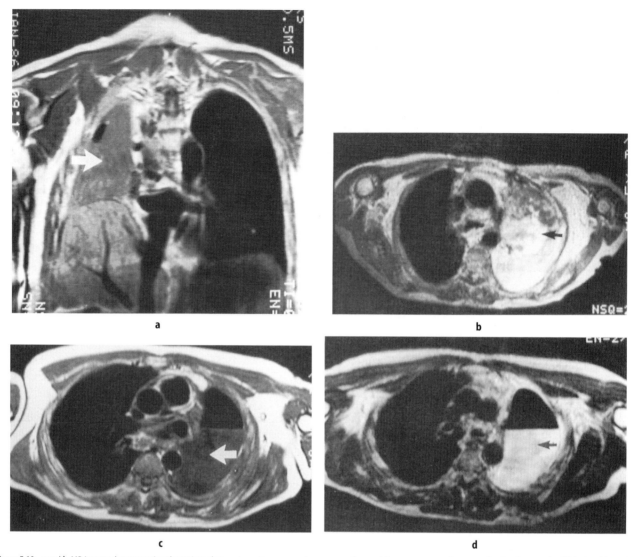

Figure 5.10. a and **b**. MR images demonstrating the various changes in postpneumonectomy spaces (*arrows*). Tumor recurrence is expected to be discovered as high signal intensity areas on T_2-weighted images, in contrast to fibrotic changes, which stay at intermediate signal intensity on both T_1- and T_2-weighted images. Fluid collection is changing its signal intensity from intermediate (with a T_R of 600) **c** to high (with a T_R of 300) (**d**).

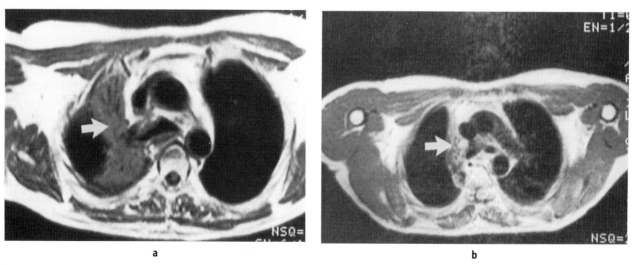

Figure 5.11. Right paramediastinal postirradiation fibrotic changes (*arrows*) appear to be of intermediate signal intensity on T_1-weighted images (**a**). They do not change their signal intensity on T_2-weighted images (**b**).

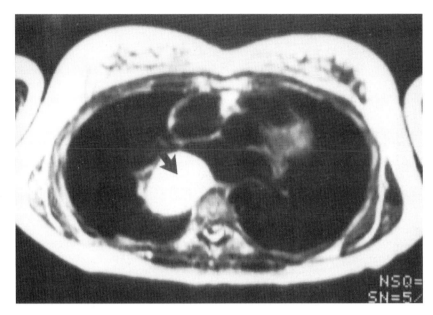

Figure 5.12. MRI performed in a patient with a posterior mediastinal mass demonstrated on SE images a lesion with a very high signal intensity as a result of its fluid viscomucoid content and diagnosed as a bronchogenic cyst (*arrow*). The exact location of the cyst in relation to other mediastinal structures is clearly visualized. (From ref. 69, with permission.)

Fluid-containing congenital abnormalities such as bronchogenic cysts are clearly delineated with MRI. Aside from the clear diagnosis of a cystic lesion permitted by MRI and the visualization of the high intensity fluid content, it is also possible to accurately observe the relationships of the lesion to the mediastinal and pulmonary structures (Fig. 5.12).

Experimental studies have been performed in an attempt to elucidate the value of MRI in the study of diffuse lung disorders (94–96). One of these studies employed a phantom that simulated pulmonary airspace disease with varying degrees of residual aeration. Sixteen patients with a variety of diffuse pulmonary conditions were studied by MRI; mean and standard deviations of T_1 and T_2 measurements were demonstrated on SE images a lesion with a very high signal intensity as a result of its fluid viscomucoid content and diagnosed as a bronchogenic cyst. The exact location of the cyst in relation to other mediastinal structures is clearly visualized, determined for each patient and for each disease process (97) (Fig. 5.12).

Results showed that mean T_1 measurements were similar in patients with pulmonary edema, postobstructive pneumonitis, pulmonary hemorrhage, radiation pneumonitis, and lobar pneumonia. Among the patients with pulmonary edema, the highest T_1 values were found in a patient with acute edema, and the lowest T_1 values in cases in which edema was chronic. Intermediate T_1 values were found in patients with *Pneumocystis carinii* pneumonia, and the lowest T_1 calculated values when compared with all other conditions were found in alveolar proteinosis. Conversely, T_2 measurements were not useful in distinguishing between the various disorders. By using the phantom with its gelatin-foam matrix, the T_1 and T_2 values were plotted against the various combinations of gelatin

and air, and revealed that T_1 and T_2 values remained relatively constant, regardless of the degree of aeration within the tested area.

Still it remains difficult to correlate the above results with in vivo conditions because in disease processes the amount and type of alveolar contents change from one phase of the disease to another. It should probably be considered that these variations result from a combination of water, protein, cells and blood forming the alveolar content, with the possibility of other existing factors to be investigated that contribute to the accuracy of T_1 and T_2 measurements (98–100).

References

1. Wehrli FW, MacFall JR, Newton TH (1983) Parameters determining the appearance of NMR images. In Newton TH, Potts DG (eds) Modern neurology, vol. 2. Clavadel Press, San Anselmo, CA, pp 81–117
2. Ross JS, O'Donovan PB, Novoa R, et al. (1984) Magnetic resonance of the chest: Initial experience with imaging and in-vivo T-1 and T-2 calculations. Radiology 152:95–101.
3. Cohen AM (1984) Magnetic resonance imaging of the thorax. Radiol Clin North Am 22:829–846.
4. Kaufman L, Sheldon P, Norman D, et al. (1984) Nuclear magnetic resonance: Principles of blood flow imaging. AJNR 4:1161-1166.
5. Axel L. (1984) Blood flow effects in magnetic resonance imaging. AJR 143:1157–1166.
6. Bradley WG, Waluch V (1985) Blood flow: Magnetic resonance imaging. Radiology 154:443–450.
7. Young IR, Burl M, Bydder GM (1986) Comparative efficiency of different pulse sequences in MR imaging. J Comput Assisit Tomogr 10:271–286.
8. Gamsu G, Webb WR, Sheldon P, et al. (1983) Nuclear magnetic resonance imaging of the thorax. Radiology 147:478–480.
9. Webb WR, Moore EH (1985) Differentiation of volume averaging and mass on magnetic resonance imaging of the mediastinum. Radiology 155:413–416.

10. Weinmann HJ, Brasch RC, Press WR, et al. (1984) Characteristics of gadolinium–DTPA complex: A potential NMR contrast agent. AJR 142:619–624.

11. Carr DH, Brown J, Bydder GM, et al. (1984) Gadolinium DTPA as a contrast agent in MRI: Initial clinical experience in 20 patients. AJR 143:215–224.

12. McNamara MT, Epstein A, Williams E, et al. (1985) Contrast enhanced MR images of tumors using Gd DTPA (abstract). Radiology 153:145.

13. Tscholokoff D, Higgins CB, McNamara MT, et al. (1986) Early phase myocardiac infarction: Evaluation by MR imaging. Radiology 159:667–672.

14. Fischer M, McNamara MT, Higgins CB (1987) Evaluation of acute myocardial infarction in man with magnetic resonance. Am J Radiol 148:247–251.

15. Crisci R, Di Cesare E, Lupattelli L, et al. (1997) MR study of N2 disease in lung cancer: Contrast-enhanced method using gadolinium DTPA. Eur J Cardiothorac Surg 11:214–217.

16. Yamada K, Jinbo T, Miyahara K, et al. (1996) Contrast-enhanced MRI with gadodiamide injection in rabbit carcinoma models. J Vet Med Sci 58:389–396.

17. Webb WR (1986) Magnetic resonance imaging of the chest. In Kressel HY (ed) Magnetic Resonance Annual 1986. Raven Press, New York, pp 161–176.

18. Webb WR, Gamsu G, Stark D, et al. (1984) Magnetic resonance imaging of the normal and abnormal hila. Radiology 152:89–94.

19. Crooks LE, Ortendahl DA. Kaufman L, et al. (1983) Clinical efficiency of nuclear magnetic resonance imaging. Radiology 146:123.

20. Ortendahl DA, Kaufman L. Crooks LE (1983) A comparison of projection reconstruction and two-dimensional Fourier transformations in NMR imaging. IEEE Trans Nucl Sci NS 30:692.

21. Mansfield P (1984) Real-time echo-planar imaging by NMR. Br Med Bull 40:187–190.

22. O'Donovan PB, Ross JS, Sivak ED, et al. (1984) Magnetic resonance imaging of the thorax: The advantages of coronal and sagittal planes. AJR 143:1183–1188.

23. Webb WR, Jensen BG, Gamsu G, et al. (1984) Coronal magnetic resonance imaging of the chest: Normal and abnormal. Radiology 153:729–735.

24. Webb WR, Jensen BG, Gamsu G, et al. (1985) Sagittal MR imaging of the chest: Normal and abnormal. J Comput Assisit Tomogr 9:471–479.

25. von Schulthess GK, Fisher MR, Higgins CB (1985) Pathologic blood flow in pulmonary vascular disease as shown by gated magnetic resonance imaging. Ann Intern Med 103:317–323.

26. Ehman RL, McNamara MT, Pallack M, et al. (1984) Magnetic resonance imaging with respiratory gating: Techniques and advantages. AJR 143:1175–1182.

27. Tscholakoff D, Higgins CB (1985) Gated magnetic resonance imaging for assessment of cardiac function and myocardial infarction. Radiol Clin North Am 23:449–457.

28. Mezrich RS, Axel L, Dougherty L, et al. (1986) Strip scanning: A method for faster MR imaging. Radiographics 6:833–845.

29. Frahm J, Haase A, Matthaei D (1986) Rapid three-dimensional NMR imaging using the FLASH technique. J Compul Assisit Tomogr 10:363–368.

30. Haacke EM, Bearden FH, Clayton JR, et al. (1986) Reduction of MR imaging time by the hybrid fast scan technique. Radiology 158:521–529.

31. Yokozaki M, Nawano S, Nagai K, et al. (1997) Cine magnetic resonance imaging, computed tomography and ultrasonography in the evaluation of chest wall invasion of lung cancer. Hitoshima J Med Sci, 46:61–66.

32. Sakai S, Murayama S, Murakami J, et al. (1997) Bronchogenic carcinoma invasion of the chest wall:evaluation with dynamic cine MRI during breathing. J Comput Assist Tomogr 21:595–600.

33. Hatabu H, Gaa J, Kim D, et al. (1996) Pulmonary perfusion :qualitative assessment with dynamic contrast-enhanced MRI using ultrashort TE and inversion recovery turbo FLASH. Magn Res Med 36:503–508.

34. Mai VM, Berr SS (1999) MR perfusion imaging of pulmonary parenchyma using pulsed arterial spin labeling techniques: FAIRER and FAIR. J Magn Reson Imaging 9:483–487.

35. Johnson GA, Cates G, Chen XJ, et al. (1997) Dynamics of magnetization in hyperpolarized gas MRI of the lung. Magn Rescon Med 38:66–71.

36. Ebert M, Grossman T, Heil W, et al. (1996) Nuclear magnetic resonance imaging with hyperpolarized helium-3. Lancet 347:9011, 1297–1299.

37. Kauczor HU, Eberyt M, Kreitner KF, et al. (1997) Imaging of the lungs using 3He MRI: Preliminary clinical experience in 18 patients with and without lung disease. J Magn Reson Imaging 7:538–543.

38. Kauczor H, Surkau R, Roberts T. (1998) MRI using hyperpolarized noble gases. Eur Radiol 8:820–827.

39. Edelman RR, Hatabu H, Tadamura E, et al. (1996) Noninvasive assessment of regional ventilation in the human lung using oxygen-enhanced magnetic resonance imaging. Nat Med 2:1236–1239.

40. Chen Q, Jakob PM, Griswold MA, et al. (1998) Oxygen enhanced MR ventilation imaging of the lung. MAGMA 7:153–161.

41. Kuethe DO, Caprihan A, Fukushima E, et al. (1998) Imaging lungs using inert fluorinated gases. Magn Reson Med 39:85-88.

42. Cutillo AG, Ailion DC (1999) Modeling the nuclear magnetic resonance behavior of lung: from electrical engineering to critical care medicine. Bioelectromagnetics 4:110–119.

43. Dixon T (1984) Simple spectroscopic imaging. Radiology 153:189–194.

44. Radda GK (1984) Clinical studies by ^{31}P NMR spectroscopy. Society of Magnetic Resonance in Medicine Scientific Program. Society of Magnetic Resonance, New York.

45. Ra JB, Hilal SK, Cho ZH (1986) A method for in vivo MR imaging of the short T-2 component of sodium-23. Magn Reson Med 3:296–302.

46. Barrett EJ, Alger JR, Zaret BL (1985) Nuclear magnetic resonance spectroscopy: Its evolving role in the study of myocardial metabolism. J Am Coll Cardiol 6:497.

47. Aue WP (1986) Localization methods for in vivo NMR spectroscopy. Magn Reson Med 1:21.

48. Nunnally RL (1983) In vivo monitoring of metabolism with nuclear magnetic resonance spectroscopy. Semin Nucl Med 13:377.

49. Styles P, Blackledge MJ, Oberhaensli R, et al. (1986) Localization techniques for the routine examination of human brain, liver, and heart by 31P NMR spectroscopy. Magn Reson Med 1:1085.

50. Cohen MD, McGuire W, Cory DA, et al. (1986) MR appearance of blood and blood products: An in vivo study. AJR 146:1293–1297.

51. Terrier F, Revel D, Pajannen H, et al. (1986) MR imaging of body fluid collections. J Comput Assist Tomogr 10:953–962.

52. Fenton BW, Lin CS, Seydel P, et al. (1998) Lecithin can be detected by volume-selected proton MR spectroscopy using a 1.5 T whole body scanner: A potentially non-invasive method for the prenatal assessment of fetal lung maturity. Prenat Diagn 18:1263–1266.

53. Cohen AM, Creviston S, Li Puma JP, et al. (1983) NMR evaluation of hilar and mediastinal lymphadenopathy. Radiology 148:739–742.

54. Levitt RG, Glazer HS, Roper CL, et al. (1985) Magnetic resonance imaging of mediastinal and hifar masses: Comparison with CT. AJR 145:9–14.

55. Glazer GM, Gross BH, Aisen AM, et al. (1985) Imaging of the pulmonary hilum: A prospective comparative study in patients with lung cancer. AJR 145:245–248.

56. Dooms G, Hricak H, Crooks LE, et al. (1984) Magnetic resonance imaging of lymph nodes: Comparison with CT. Radiology 153:719–728.

57. Heelan RT, Martini N, Westcott JW, et al. (1985) Carcinomamatous involvement of the hilum and mediastinum: Computed tomographic and magnetic resonance evaluation. Radiology 156:111–115.

58. Dooms GC, Hricak H, Mosley ME, et al. (1985) Characterization of lymphadenopathy by magnetic resonance relaxation times: Preliminary results. Radiology 155:691–697.

59. Webb W (1988) MR imaging in the evaluation and staging of lung cancer. Semin Ultrasound CT MR 9:53.

60. Martini N, Heelan R, Westcott R, et al. (1985) Comparative merits of conventional, computed tomography and magnetic resonance imaging in assessing mediastinal involvement in surgically confirmed lung carcinoma. J Thorac Cardiovasc Surg 90:639–649.

61. Tobler J, Levitt RG, Glazer HS, et al. (1985) Differentiation of proximal bronchogenic carcinoma from distal consolidation or collapse by magnetic resonance imaging. Presentation at the meeting of the Society of Thoracic Radiology, Bal Harbor, FL.

62. Manfredi R, Pirronti T, Bonomo L, et al. (1996) Accuracy of computed tomography and magnetic resonance imaging in staging bronchogenic carcinoma. MAGMA 4:257–262.

63. Shioya S, Haida M, Ono Y, et al. (1988) Lung cancer: Differentiation of tumor, necrosis and atelectasis by means of T_1 and T_2 values measured in vitro. Radiology 167:105.

64. Müller NL, Gamsu G, Webb WR (1985) Pulmonary nodules: Detection using magnetic resonance and computed tomography. Radiology 155:687–690.

65. Webb WR, Jensen BG, Sollitto R, et al. (1985) Bronchogenic carcinoma: Staging with MR compared with staging with CT and surgery. Radiology 156:117–124.

66. Hitmair K, Eckersberger F, Klepetko W, et al. (1995) Evaluation of solitary pulmonary nodules with dynamic contrast-enhanced MR imaging – A promising technique. Magn Reson Imaging 13:923–933.

67. Heelan RT, Panicek DM, Burt ME, et al. (1997) Magnetic resonance imaging of the postpneumonectomy chest: Normal and abnormal findings. J Thorac Imaging 12:200–208.

68. Hunter GJ, Hamberg LM, Choi N, et al. (1998) Dynamic T_1-weighted magnetic resonance imaging and positron emiss-ion tomography in patients with lung cancer: Correlating vascular physiology with glucose metabolism. Clin Cancer Res 4:949–955.

69. Sperber M, Kaiser MC (1987) Mediastinal lesions. In Sperber M, Kaiser MC (eds) Magnetic resonance imaging of the thorax, Warren H. Green Inc., St. Louis, MD.

70. Epstein DM, Kressel H, Gefter H, et al. (1984) MR imaging of the mediastinum: A retrospective comparison with computed tomography. J Comput Assist Tomogr 8:670–676.

71. Sperber M (1984) Mediastinal and hilar abnormalities. In Computerized tomography of the lung – Normal Anatomy and most common disorders, New York, Futura Publishing Co., New York.

72. Struyven J, Grivegnee A, Segebarth C (1987) Cardiovascular system. In Sperber M, Kaiser MC (eds) Magnetic resonance imaging of the thorax. Warren H. Green, Inc., St. Louis, MD.

73. Fletcher BD, Jacobstein MD (1986) MRI of congenital abnormalities of the great arteries. AJR 146:941–948.

74. Dinsmore RE, Liberthon RR, Wismer GL, et al. (1986) Magnetic resonance imaging of thoracic aneurysms: Comparison with other imaging methods. AJR 146:309–314.

75. Boxer RA, LaCork MA, Singh S, et al. (1986) Evaluation of the aorta in the Marfan syndrome by MRI. Am Heart J 111:1001–1002.

76. Naidich DP, Rumancik WM, Ettenger NA (1988) Congenital anomalies of the lungs in adults. MR diagnosis. AJR 151:13.

77. Dinsmore RE, Wedeen VJ, Miller SW, et al. (1986) MRI of dissection of the aorta: Recognition of the intimal tear and differential flow velocities. AJR 146:1286–1288.

78. Amparo EG, Higgins CB, Hricak H, et al. (1985) Aortic dissection: Magnetic resonance imaging. Radiology 155:399.

79. Geisinger MA, Risius B, O'Donnell JA, et al. (1985) Thoracic aortic dissection: Magnetic resonance imaging. Radiology 155:407.

80. Aronberg DJ, Glazer HS, Sagel SS (1985). MRI and CT of the mediastinum: Comparisons, controversies and pitfalls. Radiol Clin North Am 23:439–448.

81. Davies PL, Kaufman L, Crooks LE (1983) Tissue characterization. In Margulis AR, Higgins CB, Kaufman L, Crooks LE (eds) Clinical magnetic resonance imaging. UCSF Radiology Research and Education Foundation, San Francisco.

82. Revel D, Terrier F, Hricak H et al. (1984) Determination of the nature of pleural effusions with MR imaging. RSNA Scientific Program. Radiologic Society of North America, Washington, DC.

83. Brown JJ, van Sonnenberg E, Gerber KH, et al. (1985) Magnetic resonance relaxation times of percutaneously obtained normal and abnormal body fluids. Radiology 154:727–731.

84. Sperber M, Kaiser MC (1987) Pleural and diaphragmatic abnormalities. In Sperber M, Kaiser MC (eds) Magnetic resonance imaging of the thorax. Warren H. Green, Inc., St.Louise, MD.

85. Knuttila A, Halme M, Kivisaari L, et al. (1998) The clinical importance of magnetic resonance imaging versus computed tomography in malignant pleural mesothelioma. Lung Cancer 22:215–225.

86. Haggar AM, Pearlberg JL, Frollick JW, et al. (1987) Chest wall invasions by carcinoma of the lung: Detection by MR imaging. AJR 148:1075–1078.

87. Glazer HS, Lee JKT, Levitt RG, et al. (1985) Radiation fibrosis: Differentiation from recurrent tumor by MR imaging. Radiology 156:721–726.

88. Rholl KS, Levitt RG, Glazer HS (1985) Magnetic resonance imaging of fibrosing mediastinitis. AJR 145:255–259.

89. Thickman D, Kressel HY, Axel L (1984) Demonstration of pulmonary embolism by magnetic resonance imaging. AJR 142:921–922.

90. Moore EH, Gamsu G, Webb WR, et al. (1984) Pulmonary embolus: Detection and follow-up using magnetic resonance. Radiology 153:471–472.

91. Fisher MR, Higgins CB (1986) Central thrombi in pulmonary arterial hypertension detected by MRI imaging. Radiology 158:223–226.

92. Wall SD, Fisher MR, Amparo EG, et al. (1985) Magnetic resonance imaging in the evaluation of abscesses. AJR 144:1217–1221.

93. Brash RC, Gooding CA, Zallemand DP, et al. (1984) Magnetic resonance imaging of the thorax in childhood. Radiology 150:453–463.

94. Cohen MD, Scales RL, Eigen H, et al. (1987) Evaluation of pulmonary parenchymal disease by magnetic resonance imaging. Br J Radiol 60:223.

95. Craig DA, Colletti PM, Ratto D, et al. (1988) MRI findings in pulmonary sarcoidosis. Magn Reson Imaging 6:567.

96. Cutillo AG, Morris AH, Ailion DC, et al. (1988) Quantitative assessment of pulmonary edema by nuclear magnetic resonance methods. J Thorac Imaging 3:51.

97. Moore EH, Webb WR, Müller N, et al. (1986) MRI of pulmonary airspace disease: Experimental model and preliminary clinical results. AJR 146:1123–1128.

98. Skalina S, Kundel HL, Wolf G, et al. (1984) The effect of pulmonary edema on proton nuclear magnetic resonance relaxation times. Invest Radiol 19:7–9.

99. Huber DJ, Kobzik L, Melanson G, et al. (1985) The detection of inflammation in collapsed lung by alternations in proton nuclear magnetic relaxation times. Invest Radial 20:460–464.

100. Schmidt HC, Tsay DG, Higgins CB (1986) Pulmonary edema, an MR study of hydrostatic and permeability types. Radiology 158:297–302.

6 Ultrasound of the Chest

J. Andreu, J. Cáceres, and M. López

Introduction

Ultrasound is a useful imaging technique for evaluating chest diseases. The fact that air and calcium are poor transmitters of sound waves limits the effectiveness of ultrasound when bone structures and pulmonary air are present. However, even with these obstacles, many pleural, mediastinal, and even pulmonary lesions are accessible to sonographic study (1–3).

In the majority of cases, sonographic findings are complementary to other radiologic techniques, such as chest radiography and computed tomography (CT). The advantage of sonography over these methods resides in its capacity to provide information in real time and the fact that it can be performed at the bedside (4). The actual study technique varies and depends on the anatomic area to be examined. The intercostal approach with the patient in a sitting position is the most common, but supine, prone or lateral decubitus positions can also be used. Standard, 3.5 MHz sector or linear-array transducers or high frequency (5, 7 or even 10 MHz) linear transducers that permit more precise spatial resolution (6) are generally employed.

Chest sonography is especially useful for determining the location of lesions in the chest wall, pleura, lung parenchyma, and mediastinum. In some cases, the lesions can be characterized. Since it provides images in real time, ultrasound is also an excellent method for guiding interventional techniques, such as biopsies of masses or drainage of fluid collections (6–8).

Pleura

The pleura are peripheral structures in contact with the chest wall, making them easily accessible to sonographic study. The patient is usually examined by intercostal approach while sitting with his or her back to the radio-

logist. The study begins with standard 3.5 MHz linear or sector transducers to localize the pathologic areas. Further study with 5 or 7 MHz, high frequency transducers provide images of greater clarity. Sonography of the pleural space is useful for studying pleural effusions and masses, for detecting pneumothorax and for guiding interventional techniques.

Pleural Effusion

On ultrasound study, pleural effusion is visualized as a collection (usually anechoic) located between the pleural layers (9–10). Ultrasound has multiple roles for the study of this entity. It can detect small effusions with a sensitivity superior to that of chest radiography, particularly in patients who cannot maintain a lateral decubitus position. It is also a reliable means for differentiating between pleural effusions and other lesions that can simulate pleural effusion on chest radiographs, such as pulmonary consolidations or pleural masses (11). Ultrasound is more reliable than radiography for determining pleural effusion volume (12) and, in some cases, may help to determine the nature of the pleural effusion. Transudates are virtually always anechoic (Fig. 6.1), whereas exudates may be echogenic or show internal septation (Fig. 6.2) (10). The thickness of the pleura can also be evaluated. Pleural thickening associated with effusion is a sign suggesting exudate (10).

When the fluid is echogenic or loculated, it can be mistaken for a pleural mass. Indirect signs of effusion, such as changes in shape with respiration, the presence of septa, and movement of echogenic material within the effusion (swirling) are useful for establishing the correct diagnosis (1). In a small number of cases sonography cannot distinguish between pleural effusion and a mass or pleural thickening (1). Color Doppler can then be used to make the distinction (13).

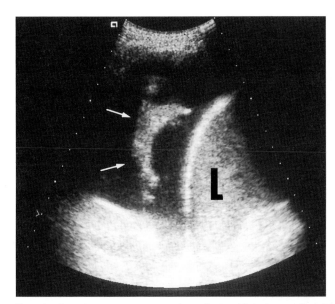

Figure 6.1. Transudate presenting as an anechoic collection. *L*, liver. *Arrows*, collapsed lung.

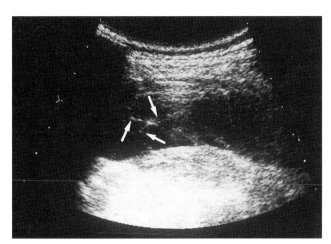

Figure 6.2. Pleural effusion with multiple septa (*arrows*).

Pleural effusion of malignant origin can present any type of echogenicity. The presence of associated pleural nodules is characteristic of malignancy, although it is an infrequent finding (6,10,14). These metastatic implants are best seen in the region of the diaphragmatic pleura and tend to have a nodular shape or present as sheet-like tumor masses (Fig. 6.3). There is no correlation between the histology of the metastasis and the sonographic form of presentation (9,12). In the majority of cases that demonstrate nodules and pleural effusion, cytology of the pleural fluid is positive. When cytology is negative, ultrasound-guided biopsy of the nodules can be performed for definite diagnosis (12).

Tuberculosis is another relatively frequent cause of pleural effusion. Tuberculous pleural effusions are very rich in proteins and tend to present fibrin strands and septa (10,15,16). These features are not, however, exclusively found in tuberculous pleural effusions and can appear in any type of exudate. The septa can be very abundant and lend a lattice-like appearance to the image (16). Pleural effusions of tuberculous origin tend to present with uniform pleural thickening, generally of less than 1 cm (Fig. 6.4). Nodules and micronodules may also be present; this last feature has been described as a characteristic of tuberculous effusions (16).

Pleural Mass

Ultrasound determines the location of masses in the pleura, chest wall and pulmonary parenchyma more precisely than chest radiography (6). Pleural lesions present obtuse angles relative to the chest wall, whereas peripheral pulmonary lesions present acute angles. The presence of rib destruction or muscle infiltration indicates an extrapleural origin of the lesion.

Encapsulated pleural fluid can have a complex, echogenic echostructure. Sonography is used to differentiate encapsulated fluid from a solid mass through secondary findings (e.g., change of shape on breathing) that enable classification of the pleural lesion as fluid (6). The presence of an internal Doppler signal characterizes the lesion as a pleural mass (Fig. 6.5).

Several types of tumor, including fibrous tumor, metastasis and malignant mesothelioma, can present as pleural masses (17). Fibrous pleural tumors appear as homogeneous lesions, with internal vessels in some cases. As mentioned above, pleural metastases are usually associated with pleural effusion. Less commonly, metastases appear as localized, solitary or multiple pleural masses, which are usually hypoechoic. When these masses are large, they can have a heterogeneous echostructure (6). Malignant mesothelioma is usually visualized as pleural thickening, which may or may not be associated with pleural effusion (18). The thickening is usually diffuse, but is sometimes seen as a hypoechoic irregular, lobulated mass in relation to the underlying lung.

Pneumothorax

Ultrasound is a valuable technique for use with intensive care patients, in whom up to 30% of pneumothoraces can be missed (19). It is also useful for identifying pneumothorax when ultrasound-guided interventional techniques of the chest are performed (20). Various studies have demonstrated the high sensitivity and specificity of this technique (21,22). False-positive results are attributed to emphysema, pleural adherences, and pachypleuritis (21).

The examination is performed with the patient in a supine decubitus position, which must be held for at least

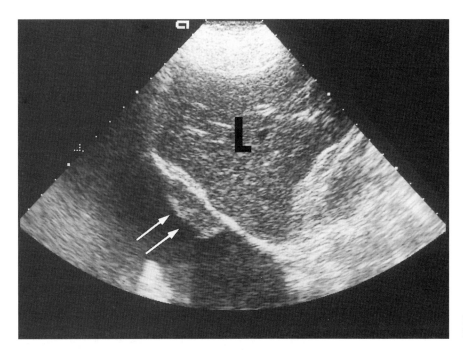

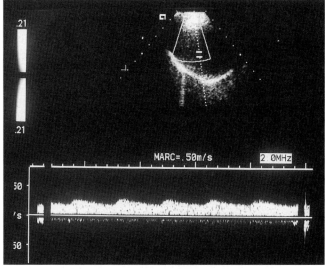

Figure 6.3. Malignant effusion. Note implant (*arrows*) in diaphragmatic pleura. *L*, liver.

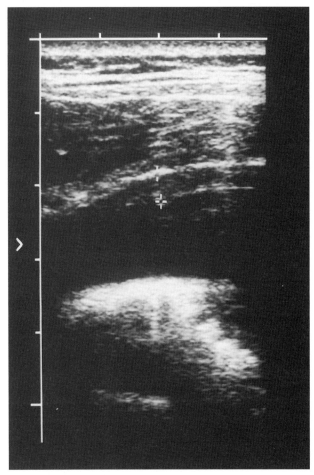

Figure 6.4. Tuberculous effusion. Calipers measure the thickened pleura.

Figure 6.5. Fibrous tumor of the pleura with Doppler signal.

5 min to permit anterior displacement of pleural air. The intercostal approach and high frequency (preferably 7 MHz) linear transducers are used. Studies carried out with 5 MHz transducers have lower sensitivity (21,23).

With high frequency linear transducers, the normal lung appears as a hyperechoic line with posterior reverberation echoes. In real-time studies, this hyperechoic line advances and retreats over the other chest wall structures with the movements of respiration, a feature dubbed "gliding sign" (21,24,25). Focal reverberation echoes in the hyperechoic band, which are characteristic of the normal, properly ventilated lung, are known as "comet tail artefacts" (Fig. 6.6) (21,25).

In pneumothorax, the pleural air is visualized as a hyperechoic line with posterior reverberation echoes, similar to the normal lung. However, neither the gliding sign nor comet-tail artefacts are present (21,25). The absence of these two features establishes the diagnosis of pneumothorax (Fig. 6.7). Another sonographic sign of pneumothorax is the disappearance of a previously visualized lung lesion, which has become hidden by the

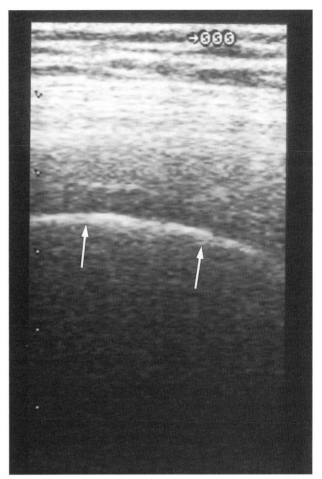

Figure 6.7. Homogeneous hyperechoic line (*arrows*) in pneumothorax.

pleural air (20). This sign is useful in ultrasound-guided interventional procedures. When air and fluid coexist in the pleural space, multiple air fluid levels are evidenced on sonography (24).

For the purpose of diagnosing pneumothorax, ultrasound is indicated for patients in whom upright chest radiograph cannot be performed and in those having an ultrasound-guided interventional technique. One drawback of this method is that the size of the pneumothorax cannot be determined unless there is associated pleural effusion.

Interventional Techniques in the Pleural Space

Ultrasound provides an excellent means for guiding interventional techniques within the pleural space, procedures that are being used with increasing frequency. Ultrasound is used for guiding fine-needle biopsies and it also plays an important role in more sophisticated techniques, such as large-needle biopsy, drainage, and sclerotherapy of the pleural space.

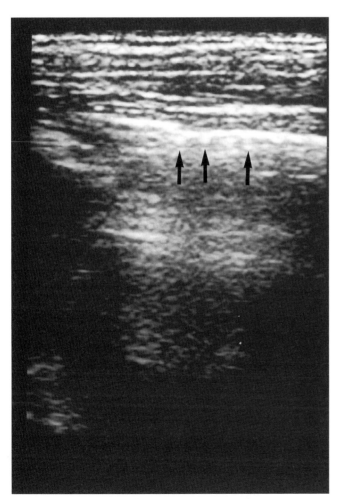

Figure 6.6. Normal lung. Note focal reverberation (*arrows*).

Thoracentesis is required in the majority of pleural effusions (26). This procedure has been guided conventionally by physical examination, based on chest radiograph findings. Nevertheless, in a large number of cases fluid cannot be obtained because the amount of pleural fluid is very small or because the biopsy site is inaccurate. Ultrasound-guided biopsy is of great value in these cases (27).

Thoracentesis is carried out with the patient in an upright sitting position facing away from the radiologist, and using a 20- to 22-gauge needle. The technique is simple and fast, and fluid is obtained in the majority of cases. The incidence of pneumothorax is significantly lower with this technique than with other methods (28,29). Large-needle biopsy is also a common technique for the study of pleural pathology. In patients with nonuniform pleural processes, such as tuberculosis or neoplasm, ultrasound-guided pleural biopsy considerably increases diagnostic effectiveness (30).

Ultrasound has proved to be an ideal technique for biopsy of pleural masses that are not hidden by bone or aerated lung. The results of the ultrasound-guided technique compare well with those obtained by CT (31–32). Fine-needle aspiration can be combined with large-needle biopsy to improve the diagnostic value of the biopsy. This technique provides optimum results for the study of metastatic tumors and mesothelioma (33–35).

Drainage is required in some cases of pleural effusion and ultrasound-guided catheter insertion can be used in selected patients. Another indication for ultrasound guidance is in pleurodesis. As palliative treatment for recurrent malignant pleural effusion, pleurodesis is carried out by introducing a sclerosing agent into the pleural cavity. Ultrasound guidance is a valuable alternative to surgical sclerotherapy (36). The catheters used are smaller and, therefore, less traumatic and better tolerated than those used surgically. The results of ultrasound-guided pleurodesis are good and similar to those obtained in series managed surgically (37,38).

In conclusion, ultrasound is useful for diagnosis of pleural effusion in cases in which chest radiography is inconclusive. In some cases it can help in the etiologic diagnosis of pleural effusion. Ultrasound can differentiate a pleural mass from lung and chest wall masses and a pleural mass from pleural fluid collection. It is valuable for diagnosing pneumothorax and is especially important for intensive care patients. It is also of great value for guiding thoracentesis and for interventional techniques used to study and treat pleural masses and fluid collections.

Lung

The lung is a birefringent structure that blocks acoustic transmission. Ultrasound study is feasible in pulmonary lesions that are in contact with the pleura. The examinations are performed in the supine decubitus position, usually with an intercostal approach. The prone decubitus is used to study the posterior segments. The lower lobes can be studied through the abdomen, with a transhepatic or transsplenic approach. The middle lobe and the lingula are studied with a parasternal approach, using the heart as a window. Finally, the upper lobes are studied by means of the axillary midline in the supraclavicular fossa (39,40).

The pulmonary lesions that can be visualized by ultrasound include consolidations, nodules, and masses. Sonography is useful for determining invasion of the chest wall by lung tumors and can guide interventional procedures for these lesions.

Pulmonary Consolidation

The lung parenchyma can be studied by sonography when the airspace is occupied; at times even deeper associated lesions can be detected (39,41,42). Consolidations are visualized as a triangular or wedge-shaped image, with clearly or poorly defined borders and a hypoechoic or heterogeneous echostructure that moves with respiration (39,41). A bronchogram, a characteristic sign of pulmonary lesions, can be seen within. The presence of a bronchogram excludes lesions of pleural or mediastinal origin.

Two types of bronchograms, air or fluid, can be observed. The air bronchogram is seen as hyperechoic lineal images that bifurcate from the pulmonary hilums and move with respiration (Fig. 6.8) (40). In the proximal bronchi, typical reverberation artefacts produced by air

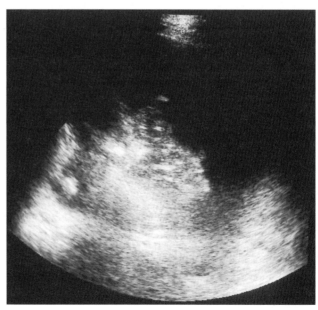

Figure 6.8. Air bronchogram in collapsed lung.

can also appear (40). Fluid bronchograms, appearing less frequently, consist of branching tubular structures with hyperechoic walls and anechoic content (39). These structures must be differentiated from pulmonary vessels, which pulsate and join the pulmonary artery (38,43). In some cases, color Doppler study is required to make this distinction.

The air bronchogram presents in any type of consolidation, whereas the liquid bronchogram is characteristic of obstructive pneumonia. Thus the presence of this sign is suggestive of neoplastic obstruction (39,41). In these cases ultrasound can demonstrate the central tumor, which appears as a homogeneous well-defined lesion within the consolidation, in the hilar area. The echogenicity of the tumor is related to its size: tumors under 5 cm tend to be hypoechoic and larger tumors tend to be heterogeneous, presenting hyperechoic areas that correspond to bleeding or necrosis (39).

Another datum that sonography can provide in the study of consolidations is detection of microabscesses, a characteristic of necrotizing pneumonia. On ultrasound study, microabscesses appear as anechoic or hypoechoic images within the consolidation, of varying size and with poorly defined borders (41,42). Finally, ultrasound enables detection of parapneumonic pleural effusion (41). Thus ultrasound is a useful technique for evaluating pulmonary consolidations and provides data that are difficult to obtain in the chest radiograph, such as presence of parapneumonic effusion, associated masses, and abscesses.

Lung Tumors

To be detected by ultrasound, lung tumors must be peripherally located, be in contact with the pleura, and not be hidden by the bones. Such tumors present as hypoechoic lesions (Fig. 6.9). Lesions over 5 cm in diameter are generally heterogeneous (42). The main task of ultrasound is to determine the location of the lesions and to differentiate them from pleural or chest wall lesions. In a significant number of cases, Doppler signals can be seen within the mass (44). Doppler study is useful for distinguishing benign and malignant lung masses (44–46).

Cavitated lesions (tumors and abscesses) present as hypoechoic lesions with irregular external margins. The cavity area is hyperechoic (47) and, usually, nonhomogeneous. When a sufficient amount of fluid is contained within the lesion, a hyperechoic ring with a hypoechoic centre is seen (42). An air-fluid level may be evidenced if the patient is examined in an upright sitting position (47).

Lung abscesses sometimes affect the visceral pleura. Ultrasound study demonstrates hyperechoic linear images corresponding to adhesions, which limit the respiratory movement.

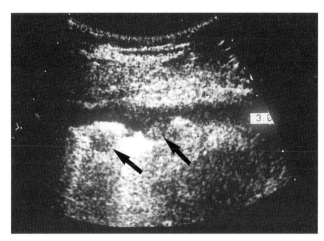

Figure 6.9. Peripheral pulmonary nodules (*arrows*).

Chest wall invasion occurs in a significant number of lung tumors (48). This fact does not contraindicate surgery, but the prognosis and type of surgical treatment varies with chest wall invasion. Such tumor infiltration can be assessed with ultrasound. The relevant sonographic signs include disruption of the pleural line, extension of the tumor to the chest wall, and fixed position of the tumor with respiration. The presence of two of these three signs is sonographically diagnostic of chest wall invasion (49).

Ultrasound has been demonstrated to be a sensitive, specific technique for studying chest wall invasion. CT, the technique of choice for staging lung tumors, has a low sensitivity and specificity for detecting such invasion (50,51). Magnetic resonance imaging (MRI) has shown somewhat better performance than CT (52). However, sonography can be considered a useful, low-cost alternative with high diagnostic value for studying chest wall invasion (51). False positives are rare and usually correspond to pleural adherences or tumors that cannot be properly studied due to their anatomic location (51).

Interventional Techniques in the Lung

Interventional techniques have a great potential value in lung lesions. Cytologic, histologic and microbiologic studies guided by sonography can be used to evaluate these lesions (53,54).

Ultrasound-guided biopsies can be performed in around one-third of tumors. The nodules must be in contact with the pleura. The technique for biopsy is simple and the results are comparable to those obtained by CT (55,56). Potential complications include pneumothorax, and more rarely, hemoptysis or hemothorax (6,55). The incidence of pneumothoraces is clearly lower than in biopsies guided by other techniques (8,55). This lower incidence is attributed to the fact that the needle is introduced through the pleura, which is in contact with the lesion. Thus biopsy of the aerated lung is avoided. Ultrasound is particularly useful for guiding biopsy of apical tumors. Since the brachiocephalic vessels can be seen on sonography, there is much less danger of their being injured (56). It is also useful in small tumors, particularly those adjacent to the diaphragm, where respiratory movement significantly varies their position. Finally, ultrasound-guided biopsy is very useful in peripheral tumors associated with pleural effusion.

In cases of obstructive pneumonitis with negative fibroscopy, sonography can differentiate a proximal mass from collapsed lung and guide the biopsy (39). In cases of pulmonary consolidation that do not respond to standard treatment, biopsy aspiration and ultrasound-guided histologic study can be used to establish the definite diagnosis (41,57,58). Ultrasound is also helpful in abscess biopsy. The microorganism, obtained in the majority of cases, can then be studied to design proper antibiotic treatment (47). The weakness of sonography resides in the fact that the lesion must be in contact with the pleura. Thin-walled cavities are difficult to locate with this technique. Ultrasound is not useful when pneumothorax occurs because the sonographic image of the lung parenchyma becomes hidden by the air (20).

In conclusion, lung lesions in contact with the pleura are accessible to ultrasound study. With use of this method we can determine the location of the lesion in the lung, pleura or chest wall more reliably than with chest radiography. In cases of obstructive pneumonitis, the mass proximal to the pneumonitis can be visualized with a sensitivity similar to CT, but without the need for contrast administration. Invasion of the chest wall by a lung mass can also be determined with ultrasound. Finally, it is a reliable tool for guiding biopsy of selected lung lesions.

Mediastinum

The mediastinum can be easily studied by ultrasound. The patient is usually examined by suprasternal approach in the supine position and by parasternal approach in the lateral decubitus position, with use of 3.5 and 5 MHz transducers. The sonographic study depends on the size and shape of the acoustic window and the distance from the lesion to the transducer.

The mediastinum can be divided sonographically into eight areas (3). The *supraaortic area* is situated above the aortic arch, where the supraaortic trunks and brachiocephalic veins are located. The *right paratracheal area* is located anterior and lateral to the trachea, in the region of the brachiocephalic trunk, the right brachiocephalic vein, the ascending aorta and the right pulmonary vein. The *aortopulmonary window* is situated below the arch and above the pulmonary artery trunk The *prevascular area* is

between the ascending aorta, superior cava and pulmonary trunk, and the sternum. The *subcarinal region* is situated between the carina and the left auricle. The *pericardic area* is situated anterior and lateral to the heart, where the pericardic fat pads are located. The *posterior mediastinal area* is situated between the heart and the trachea and spine. Finally, the *paravertebral area* is located next to the vertebral bodies.

Ultrasound is superior to chest radiography for the study of mediastinal masses. In the supraaortic, pericardic, prevascular and paratracheal areas, it has a sensitivity and specificity similar to CT. In other areas, such as the paravertebral or posterior mediastinal regions, the results are considerably inferior (3). The presence of pulmonary emphysema makes sonographic study difficult (3). Sonography's main tasks regarding the mediastinum include the study of mediastinal masses and guiding interventional procedures.

Mediastinal Masses

The majority of mediastinal masses detected by CT can also be visualized with ultrasound (Fig. 6.10) (3). The fact that some cannot be seen is usually more due to the lack of a suitable window than to poor contrast between the mediastinal connective tissue and the tumor (3). The posterior and paravertebral areas of the mediastinum are more difficult to visualize and only a small number of tumors in these regions can be seen on sonographic study (3).

In the supraaortic and pericardic areas the sensitivity of sonography is similar to that of CT (3). The supraaortic area is ideal, since it is a superficial area with an abundance of vessels, making anatomic orientation

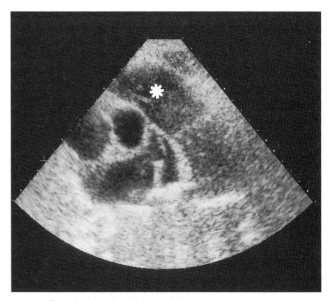

Figure 6.10. Mediastinal mass (*asterisk*) in the prevascular space.

optimum. The sensitivity of sonography is slightly lower than CT in masses located in the prevascular and paratracheal areas (3).

Mediastinal fat presents as a homogeneous, hyperechoic structure around the vascular structures. The majority of mediastinal masses present as hypoechoic lesions. A hypoechoic lesion larger than 1 cm should be considered as abnormal (3). In masses located in deep areas, such as the subcarinal region, the presence of indirect signs of occupation, such as compression of the vascular structures, is useful.

In contrast to CT, normal lymph nodes are not visualized on ultrasound studies with 3.5 MHz, since they have the same echogenicity as mediastinal fat (3,59). Thus all the nodes that are visualized with ultrasound, whether inflammatory or neoplastic, are pathologic. This feature is useful for diagnosis and follow up of Hodgkin lymphomas, whether in adenopathies or in thymic involvement (60,61). Mediastinal nodes often persist after treatment. Nodes visible on CT but not on sonography, correspond to nonviable tumor (3,5). Nodes that are visualized as hypoechoic images on ultrasound study contain viable tumor (61).

Ultrasound has proved to be useful in the follow-up of patients with diseases such as cystic fibrosis, where the presence of adenopathy is a sign indicating the activity of the process (62).

Interventional Techniques in the Mediastinum

The main ultrasound-guided interventional technique for mediastinal pathology is biopsy of mediastinal masses. It is a fast, safe method with a small rate of associated complications (63–67). It is used in masses of unknown origin and when recurrence of mediastinal tumors is suspected. More than half of mediastinal masses are accessible to ultrasound-guided biopsy. Those located in the anterior mediastinum can be most easily biopsied, followed by paratracheal or supraaortic lesions (65). The approach varies according to the location of the lesion. The parasternal approach is preferred, though the suprasternal and supraclavicular approaches can also be used (65).

Depending on the size of the needle, a cytologic or histologic study can be carried out. Initially, two samples with a fine needle are performed. If the amount of material obtained is not sufficient for diagnosis, large needles are used (68). Fine-needle biopsy is effective for establishing diagnosis in the majority of carcinomatous masses. In lymphoma and germ cell tumors, the sensitivity is low. The diagnostic effectiveness increases significantly with use of large-biopsy needles (68).

The biopsy route is an important factor to take into account to avoid complications. Color Doppler study is of great value to avoid injury to vascular structures because of its capacity to visualize vessels that are not seen on gray-scale imaging (69). It is very important to determine the location of the internal mammary artery and vein to avoid serious hematomas (70). Biopsy can be done through the veins when fine needles (22 gauge) are used (66).

Color Doppler is also of value for differentiating between avascular and vascular areas. Avascular areas correspond to areas of necrosis, where cytology tends to be negative (70).

In conclusion, with ultrasound we can evaluate the specific areas of the mediastinum for proper diagnosis and follow up of mediastinal masses. Since radiation is not involved, ultrasound is useful for children and for patients who are allergic to contrast material, in whom CT loses sensitivity. Ultrasound is excellent for guiding biopsy of mediastinal masses. In dyspneic patients biopsies can be carried out in an upright sitting position (69).

Epilogue

Ultrasound is an optimal technique for studying chest pathology. It complements other techniques, such as chest radiography and CT. It is less expensive and more easily accessible than CT and can be performed at bedside, a fact that makes it valuable for intensive care patients. One potential drawback is that ultrasound is operator dependent and proper interpretation requires previous experience. In suitable conditions, it is an excellent technique for guiding interventional procedures. Intracavity sonography (through the esophagus or trachea) is now being developed to study deeper lesions (72,73).

References

1. Lomas DJ, Padley SG, Flower CDR (1993) The sonographic appearance of pleural fluid. Br J Radiol 66:619–624.
2. McLoud TC, Flower CDR (1991) Imaging the pleura: Sonography, CT, and MR imaging. AJR 156:1145–1153.
3. Wernecke K, Vassallo P, Potter R, et al.(1990) Mediastinal Tumors: Sensitivity of detection with sonography compared with CT and radiography. Radiology 175:137–143.
4. Yu C-J, Yang P-C, Chang D-B, et al. (1992) Diagnostic and therapeutic use of chest sonography: value in critically ill patients. AJR 159:695–701.
5. Marglin SI, Laing FC, Castellino RA (1991) Current status of mediastinal sonography in the posttreatment evaluation of patients with lymphoma. AJR 157:469–470.
6. Wernecke K. (1997) Sonographic features of pleural disease. AJR 168:1061–1066.
7. Dodd GD, Esola CC, Memel DS, et al. (1996) Sonography: The undiscovered jewel of interventional radiology radiographics 16:1271–1288.

8. Sheth S, Hamper U, Stanley DB, et al. (1999) US Guidance for thoracic biopsy: A valuable alternative to CT. Radiology 210:721–726.

9. Müller NL (1993) Imaging of the pleura. Radiology 186:297–309.

10. Yang P-C, Luh K-T, Chang D-B, et al. (1992) Value of sonography in determining the nature of pleural effusion: analysis of 320 cases. AJR 159:29–33.

11. Yu C-J, Yang P-C, Wu H-D, et al. (1993) Ultrasound study in unilateral hemithorax opacification. Image Comparison with computed tomography. Am Rev Respir Dis 147:430–434.

12. Eibenberger KL, Dock WI, Amman ME, et al. (1994) Quantification of pleural effusion: Sonography versus radiography. Radiology 191:681–684.

13. Wu R-G, Yuan A, Liaw Y-S, et al. (1994) Image comparison of real-time gray-scale ultrasound and color Doppler ultrasound for use in diagnosis of minimal pleural effusion. Am J Respir Crit Care Med 150:510–514.

14. Goerg C, Schwerk WB, Goerg K, et al. (1991) Pleural effusion: An "acoustic window" for sonography of pleural metastases. J Clin Ultrasound 19:93–97.

15. Martinez OC, Serrano BV, Romero RR (1989) Real-time ultrasound evaluation of tuberculous pleural effusions. J Clin Ultrasound 17:407–410.

16. Akhan O, Demirkazik FG, Ozmen MN, et al. (1992) Tuberculosis pleural effusion: ultrasonic diagnosis. J Clin Ultrasound 20:461–465.

17. Dynes MC, White EM, Fry WA, et al. (1992) Imaging manifestations of pleural tumors. RadioGraphics 12:1191–1201.

18. Miller BH, Rosado-de-Christenson MI, Mason AC, et al. (1996) Malignant pleural mesothelioma: Radiologic–pathologic correlation. RadioGraphics 16:613–644.

19. Tocino IM, Miller MH, Fairfax WR (1985) Distribution of pneumothorax in the supine and semirecumbent critically ill adult. AJR 144:901–905.

20. Targhetta R, Bourgeois J-M, Chavagneux R, et al. (1992) Diagnosis of pneumothorax by ultrasound immediately after ultrasonically guided aspiration biopsy. Chest 101:855–856.

21. Targhetta R, Bourgeois JM, Chavagneux R et al. (1993) Ultrasonic signs of pneumothorax: Preliminary work. J Clin Ultrasound 21:245–250.

22. Lichtenstein DA, Menu Yves (1995) A bedside ultrasound sign ruling out pneumothorax in the critically ill. Lung Sliding. Chest 108:1345–1348.

23. Sistrom CL, Reiheld CT, Gay SB (1996) Detection and estimation of the volume of pneumothorax using real-time sonography: efficacy determined by receiver operating characteristic analysis. AJR 166:317–321.

24. Targhetta R, Bourgeois J-M, Chavagneux R, et al. (1992) Ultrasonographic approach to diagnosing hydropneumothorax. Chest 101:931–934.

25. Wernecke K, Galanski M, Peters PE, et al. (1987) Pneumothorax: Evaluation by ultrasound preliminary results. J Thorac Imaging 2:76–78.

26. Light RW (1997) Diagnostic principles in pleural dizease. Eur Respir J 10:479–481.

27. Weingardt JP, Guico RR, Nemcek AA, et al. (1994) Ultrasound findings following failed, clinically directed thoracenteses. J Clin Ultrasound 22:419–426.

28. Grogan DR, Irwin RS, Channick R, et al. (1990) Complications associated with thoracentesis: A prospective, randomized study comparing three different methods. Arch Intern Med 150:873–877.

29. Raptopouslos V, Davis LM, Umali C, et al. (1991) Factors affecting the development of pneumothorax associated with thoracentesis. AJR 156:917–920.

30. Chang D-B, Yang P-C, Luh K-T, et al. (1991) Ultrasound-guided pleural biopsy with Tru-Cut needle. Chest 100:1328–1333.

31. Scott EM, Marshall TJ, Flower CD, et al. (1995) Diffuse pleural thickening: Percutaneous CT-guiding cutting needle biopsy. Radiology 194:867–870.

32. Metintas M, Ozdemir N, Isiksoy S, et al. (1995) CT-guided pleural biopsy in the diagnosis of malignant mesothelioma. J Comput Assist Tomogr 19:370–374.

33. Hsu W-H, Chiang C-D, Chen C-C, et al. (1997) Value of ultrasonically guided needle biopsy of pleural masses: An under-utilized technique. J Clin Ultrasound 25:119–125.

34. Heilo A. Stenwig AE, Solhein OP (1999). Malignant pleural mesothelioma: US-guided histologic core-needle biopsy. Radiology 211:657–659.

35. Boutin C, Rey F (1993) Thoracoscopy in pleural malignant mesothelioma: A prospective study of 188 consecutive patients. l Diagnosis. Cancer 72:389–393.

36. Morrison Mc, Mueller PR, Lee ML, et al. (1991) Sclerotherapy of malignant pleural effusion through sonographically placed small-bore catheters. AJR 158:41–43.

37. Rashad K, Inui K, Takeuchi Y, et al. (1985). Treatment of malignant pleural effusion. Chest 88:393–397.

38. Hausheer FH, Yarbo JW (1985) Diagnosis and treatment of malignant pleural effusion. Semin Oncol 12:54–75.

39. Yang P-C, Luh K-T, Wu H-D, et al. (1990) Lung Tumors Associated with Obstructive Pneumonitis: US Studies. Radiology 174:717–720.

40. Weinberg B, Diakoumakis EE, Kass EG, et al. (1986) The air bronchogram: Sonographic demostration. AJR 147:593–595.

41. Yang P-C, Luh K-T, Chang D-B, et al. (1992) Ultrasonographic evaluation of pulmonary consolidation. Am Rev Respir Dis 146:757–762.

42. Yang P-C, Luh K-T, Sheu J-C, et al. (1985) Peripheral pulmonary lesion ultrasonography and ultrasonically guided aspiration biopsy. Radiology 155: 451–450.

43. Dorne HI (1986) Differentiation of pulmonary parenchymal consolidation from pleural dizease using the sonographic fluid bronchogram. Radiology 158:41–42.

44. Yuan A, Chang D-B, Yu C-J, et al. (1994) Color Doppler sonography of benign and malignant pulmonary masses. AJR 163:545–549.

45. Hsu W-H, Ikezoe J, Chen C-Y, et al. (1996) Color Doppler ultrasound signals of thoracic lesions. correlation with resected histologic specimens. Am J Respir Crit Care Med 151: 1938–1951.

46. Maldjian PD, Singh-Panghaal S, Wachsberg RH (1997) Use of Doppler sonography to differentiate AIDS-related intrathoracic lymphoma from tuberculosis. J Clin Ultrasound 25: 501–504.

47. Yang P-C, Luh K-T, Lee Y-C, et al. (1991) Lung abscesses: US examination and US-guided transthoracic aspiration. Radiology 180:171–175.

48. Pennes DR, Glazer GM, Wimbish KJ, et al. (1985) Chest wall invasion by lung cancer: Limitations of CT evaluation. AJR 144:507–511.

49. Suzuki N, Saitoh T, Kitamura S (1993) Tumor invasion of the chest wall in lung cancer: Diagnosis with US. Radiology 187:39–42.

50. Glazer HS, Duncan-Meyer J, Aronberg DJ, et al. (1985) Pleural and chest wall invasion in bronchogenic carcinoma: CT evaluation. Radiology 157:191–194.

51. Uhrmeister P, Allmanm K-H, Wertzel H, et al. (1999) Chest wall infiltration by lung cancer: Value of thin-sectional CT with different reconstruction algorithms. Eur Radiol 9:1304–1309.

52. Padovani B, Mouroux J, Seksik, L, et al. (1993) Chest wall invasion by bronchogenic carcinoma: Evaluation with MR imaging. Radiology 187:33–38.

53. Yang P-C, Chang D-B, Yu C-J, et al. (1992) Ultrasound-guided core biopsy of thoracic tumors. Am Rev Respir Dis 146:763–767.

54. Yang P-C (1997) Ultrasound-guided transthoracic biopsy of peripheral lung, pleural, and chest-wall lesions. J Thorac Imaging 12:272–284.

55. Chen C-C, Hsu W-H, Huang C-M, et al. (1995) Ultrasound-guided fine-needle aspiration biopsy of solitary pulmonary nodules. J Clin Ultrasound 23:531–536.

56. Ikezoe J, Sone S, Higashihara T, et al. (1984) Sonographically guided needle biopsy for diagnosis of thoracic lesion AJR 143: 229–242.

57. Yang P-C, Chang D-B, Yu C-J, et al. (1992) Ultrasound guided percutaneous cutting biopsy for the diagnosis of pulmonary consolidations of unknown aetiology. Thorax 47:457–460.

58. Liaw Y-S, Yang P-C, Wu Z-G, et al. (1994) The bacteriology of obstructive pneumonitis. A prospective study using ultrasound-guided needle aspiration. Am J Respir Crit Care Med 149:1648–1653.

59. Wernecke K, Peters PE, Galanski M. (1986) Mediastinal tumors: Evaluation with suprasternal sonography. Radiology 159:405–409.

60. Wernecke K, Vassallo P, Rutsch F, et al. (1991) Thymic involvement in Hodgkin disease: CT and Sonographic Findings. Radiology 181:375–383.

61. Wernecke K, Vassallo P, Hoffmann G, et al. (1991) Value of sonography in monitoring the therapeutic response of mediastinal lymphoma: Comparison with chest radiography and CT. AJR 156:265–272.

62. Dietrich CF, Chichakli M, Bargon J, et al. (1999) Mediastinal lymph nodes demonstrated by mediastinal sonography: Activity marker in patients with cystic fibrosis J Clin Ultrasound 27:9–14.

63. M-Wernecke K, Vassallo P, Peter PE, et al. (1989). Mediastinal tumors: Biopsy under US guidance radiology 172:473–476.

64. Rubens DJ, Strang JG, Fultz PJ, et al. (1997) Sonographic guidance of mediastinal biopsy: An effective alternative to CT guidance. AJR 169:1605–1610.

65. Tikkakoski T, Lohela P, Lappanem M, et al. (1991) Ultrasound-guided aspiration biopsy of anterior mediastinal masses. J Clin Ultrasound 19:209–214.

66. Yang PC, Chang D-B, Lee Y-C, et al. (1992) Mediastinal malignacy: Ultrasound guided biopsy though the supraclavicular approach. Thorax 43:377–380.

67. Gupta S, Gulati M, Rajwanshi A, et al. (1998) Sonographically guided fine-needle aspiration biopsy of superior mediastinal lesion by the suprasternal route. AJR 171:1303–1306.

68. Hsu W-H, Chiang C-D, Hsu J-Y, et al. (1995) Ultrasonically guided needle biopsy of anterior mediastinal masses: Comparison of carcinomatous and non-carcinomatous masses. J Clin Ultrasound 23:349–356.

69. Rubens DJ, Gottlieb RH, Fultz PL (1999) Role of color Doppler imaging in interventional sonography (1999) J Clin Ultrasound 27:259–271.

70. Targhetta R, Bourgeois JM, Dauzat M, et al. (1993) Sonographic guidance in diagnosing anterior mediastinal mass: Importance of visualizing internal mammary vessels. J Clin Ultrasound 21:203–206.

71. Glassberg RM, Sussman SK (1990) Life-threatening hemorrhage due to percutaneous transthoracic intervention: Importance of the internal mammary artery. AJR 154: 1047.

72. Pedersen BH, Vilmann P, Folke K, et al. (1996) Endoscopic ultrasonography and real-time guided fine-needle aspiration biopsy of solid lesions of the mediastinum suspected of malignancy. Chest 110:539–544.

73. Kurimoto N, Marayama M, Yoshioka S, et al. (1999) Assessment of usefulness of endobronchial ultrasonography in determination of depth of tracheobronchial tumor invasion. Chest 115:1500–1506.

7 Conventional and Digital Subtraction Angiography

A. Magalhães

Introduction

Angiography of the thoracic vessels has a key role in the management of pulmonary embolism, hemoptysis, arteriovenous fistula, and aortic aneurysms. In addition to the diagnostic information obtained by this procedure, angiographic catheter techniques are now being used as effective tools in the treatment of pulmonary embolism by intraarterial injections of fibrinolytic drugs (1) and catheter suction embolectomy (2) and in the treatment of hemoptysis (3) and pulmonary arteriovenous fistulae (4) by selective catheter embolization. Angiography is also useful in the planning and follow-up of surgical procedures in conditions such as dissecting aortic aneurysm (5,6) bronchial carcinoma (7), and bullous emphysema (8).

The use of digital subtraction angiography (DSA) has modified to some extent the conventional routine in the investigation of vascular thoracic diseases. Intravenous DSA is performed by introducing a 5F pigtail catheter into the right atrium, usually by percutaneous basilic vein approach. Injection of 40 ml of contrast medium with high iodine concentration 1370 mg results in satisfactory images of the pulmonary artery, the aorta, and their branches. When the study is nondiagnostic as a result of motion artefacts or poor cardiac output, an intraarterial DSA or conventional angiography is usually performed.

Intraarterial DSA has some advantages over conventional angiography because the catheters are smaller, lower doses of contrast media are used, and the examination is quicker and safer. This chapter discusses the angiographic techniques and the specific indications for pulmonary arteriography, bronchial arteriography, thoracic aortography, and superior cavography. Some examples of clinical situations involving the use of DSA or conventional angiography are presented.

Pulmonary Arteriography

Techniques

The first tentative pulmonary artery visualization was performed in 1929 by Forssman, who passed a ureteral catheter into his own heart. The first visualization of pulmonary arteries was achieved by Moniz et al. in 1931 using Forssman's technique and, 1 year later, using intravenous injection (9). Things have improved considerably with the development of the percutaneous route (10) and the use of special catheters (11,12).

Conventional angiography is usually performed with a 6.7F or 8.3F Grollman's catheter introduced by the transfemoral or transcubital approach. Fifty milliliters of contrast media are injected into the main pulmonary artery over 2 s. Selective injection into the right or left pulmonary artery calls for 25 ml over 2 s. In both cases two films per second are obtained during 10 s. DSA is performed with a 5F pigtail catheter inserted into the right basilic vein or cephalic vein and passed into the superior vena cava or the right atrium. When it is necessary, the use of the femoral vein is another alternative. Forty milliliters of contrast media are injected over 2 s. Two images per second are obtained during 20 s. Intraarterial DSA includes the same technique as conventional angiography, except for the use of a small catheter (size 5F) and of contrast that is diluted with an equal amount of normal saline solution and injected in a volume of 30 mL in the main pulmonary artery or 15 mL for the right or left artery. Two images per second are obtained during 15 s.

The Normal Pulmonary Arteriogram

The main pulmonary artery is a broad vessel arising from the pulmonary conus of the right ventricle. It runs upward and posteriorly to its bifurcation into the left and the right pulmonary arteries. The pulmonary artery branches normally follow the segmental bronchi. The right pulmonary artery divides at the right hilus into the ascending branch, which supplies the right upper lobe (apical, posterior, and anterior segmental arteries), and the descending branch, which supplies the middle (middle lobe and superior segmental arteries) and lower (medial, anterior, posterior and lateral basal arteries) lobes. The left pulmonary artery a continuation of the main pulmonary artery divides at the hilus into the ascending branch, which supplies the left upper lobe tapical posterior and anterior segmental arteries) and the descending branch, which supplies the lower lobe (lingular and superior segmental arteries and inferior anteromedial, and lateral basal segmental arteries) (Fig. 7.1).

Congenital Abnormalities

Pulmonary Arteriovenous Fistula

Pulmonary arteriovenous fistula is a congenital lesion. It is often found in the Rendu–Osler–Weber syndrome with telangiectasias of skin and mucous membranes. It is sometimes found as a lesion on the routine chest radiograph. The majority of pulmonary arteriovenous fistulae are multiple and often bilateral in the lower lung fields (13) (Fig. 7.2). Intravenous DSA is the method of choice to establish the diagnosis of an arteriovenous fistula. Intraarterial or conventional angiography is indicated in doubtful cases and when catheter embolization is considered for treatment.

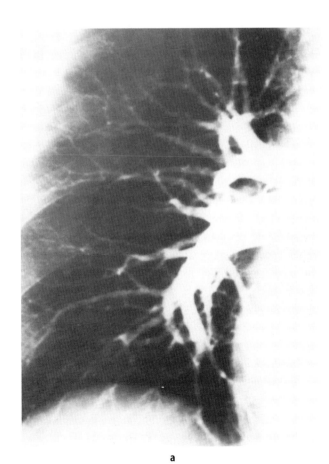

a

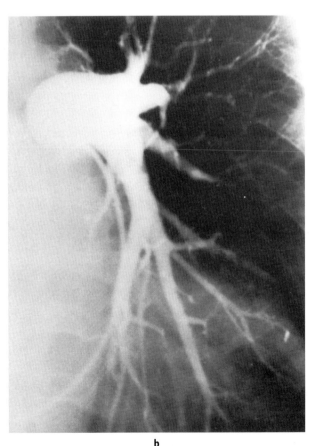

b

Figure 7.1. Normal pulmonary arteriogram. **a** Selective right pulmonary artery and its branches to the right upper, middle, and lower lobes. **b** Selective left pulmonary artery and its branches to the left upper and lower lobes.

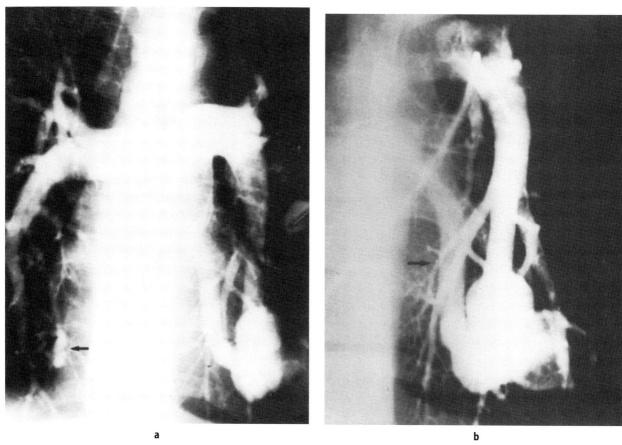

a   b

Figure 7.2. Pulmonary arteriovenous fistulae. Frontal pulmonary angiography demonstrates a large fistula in the left lower lobe (*arrow*) and a small fistula in the right lower lobe (*arrow*).

Stenosis and Hypoplasia of the Pulmonary Artery

These two entities are easily diagnosed by pulmonary angiography. Stenosis of the pulmonary artery can be isolated or may involve multiple sites and can be found in combination with other cardiac defects (Fig. 7.3). The narrowing usually causes a poststenotic dilatation. Hypoplasia or agenesia of the right or the left pulmonary artery is often associated with some type of systemic supply (13).

Acquired Lesions

Pulmonary Embolism

Pulmonary embolism is a very common occurrence (14). Clinical and radiologic signs are usually present but they are nonspecific (15). Nuclear medicine plays an important role in the diagnosis of this condition because a normal perfusion scan usually rules out pulmonary embolism (16.17). When a perfusion scan demonstrates the presence of defects, a ventilation scan should be performed in order to exclude the presence of obstructive pulmonary disease.

When ventilation is intact in an area with a perfusion defect a ventilation-perfusion mismatch is described (see Chapter 11).

Pulmonary angiography should be performed after perfusion – ventilation scanning in ambiguous and mismatch cases (18). It is also indicated when pulmonary embolism is suspected in a patient with chronic obstructive pulmonary disease (18). The angiographic diagnosis of pulmonary embolism is made by the demonstration of intraarterial filling defects (Fig. 7.4). Central occlusions and segmental emboli are easily visualized in the anteroposterior view. Sometimes multiple views are necessary to establish the diagnosis. For suspected subsegmental defects, superselective techniques and magnification should be used (18).

Intravenous DSA is the method of choice in the majority of cases for the identification of pulmonary emboli. When intravenous DSA is doubtful or nondiagnostic as a result of motion artefacts, transcardiac catheterization and an intraarterial DSA or conventional angiography are performed. To avoid the formation of pulmonary emboli in patients with deep vein thrombosis a cava filter is usually placed through the femoral vein or by the jugular route. Severe pulmonary emboli can be treated by direct

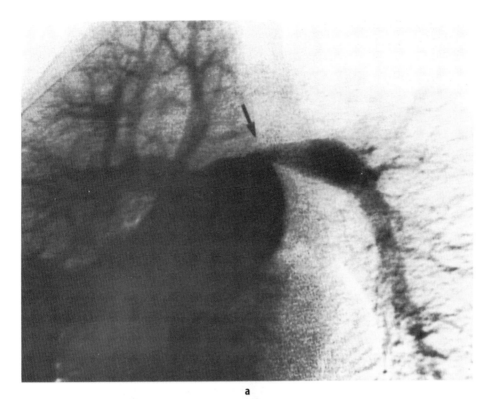

a

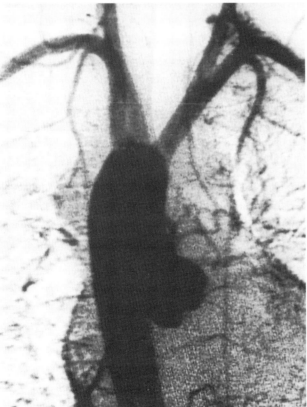

b

Figure 7.3. Pulmonary artery stenosis with dextroposition of the aorta. **a** Left anterior oblique intravenous DSA shows stenosis of the left pulmonary artery (*arrow*). **b** Intraarterial DSA in the same patient demonstrates dextroposition of the aorta and its branches.

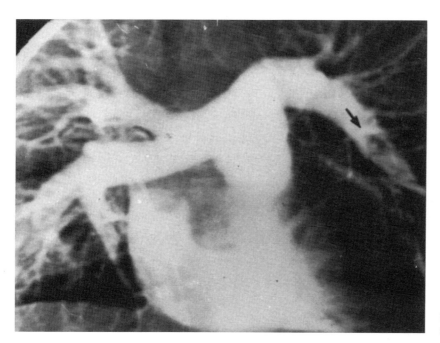

Figure 7.4. Pulmonary embolism. Frontal intravenous DSA shows an embolus in the left lower lobe artery (*arrow*).

pulmonary arterial infusion of streptokinase (1). Pulmonary emboli can also be removed by a transcatheter suction technique (2).

Bullous Emphysema

In bullous emphysema, bullae that are in connection with the bronchial tree tend to increase in size resulting in respiratory insufficiency. Patients with these types of bullae are candidates for surgery (19). Intravenous DSA is able to delineate the bullae and the displacement of adjacent vessels. Angiography therefore provides a means of planning resectional surgery (8).

Bronchial Carcinoma

Occassionally on conventional chest radiograph and tomogram it is difficult to differentiate solid from vascular masses (19). Angiography helps to rule out the presence of vascular lesions such as aneurysms of the aorta and its branches dilatated pulmonary artery and vein, and arteriovenous fistulae. Intravenous DSA easily confirms the nature of the discovered lesion. In the general diagnostic work-up of bronchial carcinoma resectability can be established by performing pulmonary arteriography and cavography (7.20).

Bronchial Arteriography

Techniques

Some of the first radiologic demonstrations of the bronchial pulmonary artery were obtained by Pinet et al. (21) during aortography controlled by hypotension. Viamonte (22) performed the first selective bronchial arteriography. The study of the bronchial arteries should begin with an injection in the thoracic aorta to visualize all arterial pedicles that supply the lungs. The selective opacification of bronchial pedicles could be done with a preshaped catheter for bronchial arteriography and the approach is usually by the transfemoral route (23). Contrast medium is injected by hand (5–10 ml). Seriography is performed at the rate of two films per second during 5–10 s. To obtain better images with DSA, electrocardiographic triggering is recommended (24). In pathologic conditions with systemic hypervascularization of the lungs, opacification of the intercostal arteries, the internal mammary arteries, the branches of the axillary artery, and the inferior diaphragmatic arteries should be obtained (25).

Normal Bronchial Arteriogram

The systemic vasculature of the normal lung is supplied by the bronchial arteries. According to Pinet and Froment (26), the most common patterns of bronchial arteries are:

1. A right intercostobronchial trunk and two left bronchial arteries.
2. A right intercostobronchial trunk and one left bronchial artery.
3. A right intercostobronchial trunk, an inferior left bronchial artery, and a right-left common trunk from which arise an inferior right bronchial artery and a superior left bronchial artery.

The arteries should be searched for at the level of the fifth or sixth thoracic vertebra. They are also projected into the left main bronchus and carina. The origin of the intercostobronchial trunk is posterolateral, and the bronchial arteries that arise directly from the aorta have an anterior origin.

Congenital Abnormalities

Pulmonary Sequestration

A pulmonary sequestration is a mass of lung tissue separated from the rest of the parenchyma and supplied by a systemic artery. The sequestration is commonly found on a routine chest radiograph in a patient with infection of the lungs. A sequestration lesion is usually located in the posterobasal or paramedial part of the lung (26). Intravenous DSA can confirm the diagnosis of a systemic arterial pedicle arising from the lower thoracic aorta or upper segment of the abdominal aorta. Conventional angiography is preferable in case of agenesis of one pulmonary artery. There is a systemic hypervascularization of the entire lung on the side of the agenesis fed by systemic arteries (Fig. 7.5).

Scimitar Syndrome

This syndrome comprises dextrocardiac hypoplasia of the right pulmonary artery; abnormal right pulmonary venous return via the inferior vena cava, or, atypically, via the azygos vein; a characteristic "scimitar" radiographic image; and systemic vascularization of the right lung from the abdominal aorta (26). Intravenous DSA can clearly demonstrate all the abnormalities for this syndrome.

Acquired Lesions

Lesions with Hypervascularization

Acquired lesions of the systemic vasculature of the lungs are characterized by abnormal hypervascularization and the presence of shunts to the pulmonary artery. Bronchial arteries have an increased caliber and become tortuous.

The same alterations are found in other systemic arteries that feed the hypervascularization lesions. If there is a shunt with retrogade opacification of the pulmonary artery, this indicates destruction of the capillary bed in the corresponding territory. Systemic hypervascularization is usually found in tuberculosis, mucoviscidosis, intracavitary aspergillomas, pneumoconiosis, actinomycosis, bronchiectasis, and the sequelae of abcesses (26). These lesions are well demonstrated with selective injection into the bronchial arteries using a DSA technique (24) or by conventional angiography.

Embolization of Systemic Thoracic Arteries

Embolization is indicated in severe hemoptysis (300 ml or more in 24 h), when surgery is contraindicated, and in cases in which the medical treatment fails (26). The main contraindication to therapeutic embolization is the presence of an anterior spinal artery that has a common origin with the systemic arterial pedicle and that, if damaged, can cause paraplegia (3,27). Seriographic verification should be done during the embolization because the spinal artery may become visible only during embolization. The catheter must be well introduced into the pedicles responsible for the hypervascularization. The most commonly used materials for embolization are fragments of Gelfoam and duramater. Minor complications of the procedure are retrosternal and intercostal pain, esophageal burning, and fever. The most common spinal cord complication is spastic paraplegia, which sometimes appears several hours after the performance of the investigation (26).

Thoracic Aortography

Techniques

The first opacification of the thoracic aorta was obtained by Nuvoli in 1936 through direct puncture of the ascending aorta or the left ventricle. Castellanos and Pereiras, in 1939, described a method of countercurrent aortography in infants. Catheter angiography of the thoracic aorta was first obtained through an exposed radial artery by Radner in 1948 and through percutaneous femoral artery catheterization by Pierce in 1951. The refinement of the percutaneous transfemoral technique was made by Odman and Philipson in 1958 (28).

The conventional study of the thoracic aorta is usually performed with a 7F pigtail catheter introduced through the femoral artery by the Seldinger technique. Sometimes the branchial or the axillary approach is used. Contrast material (40–60 ml) is injected into the

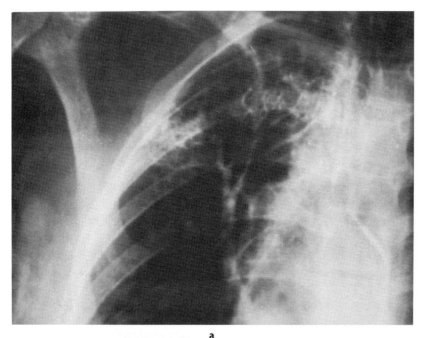

a

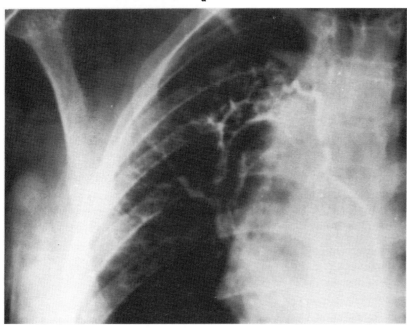

b

Figure 7.5. Pulmonary sequestration in the right lung. a Opacification of one systemic artery in the right upper lobe with its venous return into the pulmonary veins. b Opacification of a second systemic artery with its venous return into the pulmonary veins.

thoracic aorta over 2 or 3 s. Two films per second are obtained during 6 s, in two projections (anteroposterior and left anterior oblique). Intravenous DSA of the thoracic aorta is obtained with a 5F pigtail catheter introduced percutaneously through the antecubital veins into the right atrium or superior vena cava. Forty milliliters of contrast material are injected over 2 s. One image per second is obtained during 25 s in both projections. Intraarterial DSA involves the same technique as the conventional study, except for the use of a small pigtail

catheter (size 4F) and, in general, three times less contrast material.

Normal Thoracic Aortogram

The normal thoracic aorta resembles an inverse and is divided into four segments: the aortic bulb, the ascending aorta, the aortic arch, and the descending aorta. The aortic bulb is formed by the three sinuses of Valsalva,

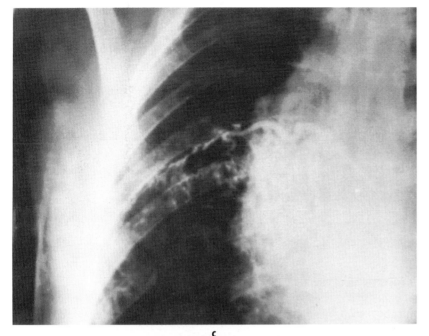

c

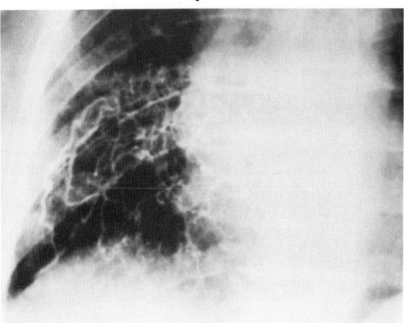

d

Figure 7.5. c and **d** Sequestration of the right lower lobe with two different systemic arteries.

and the coronary arteries originate from it. The ascending aorta is a tube without branches. The aortic arch gives off three large branches: the innominate artery, the left common carotid artery, and the left subclavian artery. Between the arch and the descending aorta there is the isthmus, which is the point where the fourth left brachial arch artery unites with the dorsal aorta in the fetus. In the majority of cases there are no anatomic traces of this segment in adult life, other than the insertion of the ligamentum arteriosum. The descending aorta gives off numerous small branches, the intercostal arteries (29).

Congenital Abnormalities

Patent Ductus Arteriosus

The ductus arteriosus, which connects the pulmonary artery with the descending aorta in fetal life, usually closes after birth and becomes the ligamentum arterio-sum. When the ductus arteriosus remains open, there is a left-to-right shunt with pulmonary plethora, left ventricular enlargement, and congestive heart failure. The angiographic diagnosis is easily obtained by thoracic aortography with opacification of the thoracic aorta, infundibulum of the ductus arteriosus, and pulmonary artery (30). Intravenous DSA demonstrates in this case the opacification of the right chambers, the pulmonary artery, the left chambers, the aorta, the infundibulum of the ductus arteriosus, and then the pulmonary artery again. A patent ductus arteriosus can usually be closed by a catheter (31).

Coarctation of the Aorta

Coarctation of the aorta is a congenital narrowing of the aorta adjacent to the ductus arteriosus. The majority of the patients develop heart failure in infancy with dilatation of the right and left ventricles and pulmonary congestion. In adults, there is the classic finding of rib notching, most prominent at the level of the fourth and fifth ribs. The zone of stenosis is usually localized, however, with preservation of a lumen of variable size; complete interruption of the aortic arch may also be seen (32). Intravenous DSA usually makes the diagnosis of coarctation of the aorta. In doubtful cases intraarterial DSA or conventional aortography is indicated.

Aortic Septal Defects

An aortic septal defect, also called an aortopulmonary window, is a communication between the aorta and the pulmonary artery, located in the ascending aorta. Intraarterial DSA is the method of choice for the diagnosis of this abnormality. Injection of contrast medium into the ascending aorta in this case shows opacification of the pulmonary artery (Fig. 7.6).

Acquired Lesions

Aneurysm of the Thoracic Aorta

A true aneurysm is a dilatation of the vessel wall caused by destruction of the elastic fibers in the media. A false aneurysm results from a traumatic perforation of the wall that is contained by adventitia and perivascular tissue. Arteriosclerosis is the most common cause of thoracic aortic aneurysm. Other causes of aneurysm are syphilis,

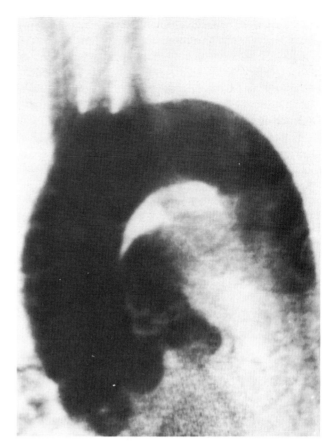

Figure 7.6. Aortic septal defect. Left anterior oblique intraarterial DSA shows opacification of the aorta and its three branches. The pulmonary artery is filled from the ascending aorta through an aortic septal defect.

bacterial infection, and abnormalities. The incidence of traumatic pseudoaneurysms has been increasing with the rise in automobile accidents. An aneurysm of the intra-thoracic branches of the aorta has the same origin as the aorta itself. The innominate and the left subclavian arteries are more frequently involved (33). In atherosclerosis, the association of an aneurysm of the descending thoracic aorta and of the innominate artery can commonly be found. Intravenous DSA makes the diagnosis of a thoracic aortic aneurysm in the majority of cases (34).

Dissecting Aortic Aneurysm

Dissecting aneurysm is produced by separation of the layers of the arterial wall by blood. The most common type begins in the ascending aorta and extends along the arch and descending aorta (type dissection). Type II dissection involves only the ascending aorta and type III dissection begins just beyond the descending aorta. Intravenous DSA can be used to confirm the clinical suspicion of dissecting aortic aneurysm (35), except in patients with congestive heart failure, in whom intraarterial DSA or conventional angiography is preferable. Postsurgery control is successfully achieved with intravenous DSA (6).

Superior Cavography

Techniques

Conventional cavography is usually performed with bilateral 19G needles in each antecubital vein. Fifty milliliters of contrast media are injected simultaneously in both needles over 8 s. One film per second is obtained during 12 s. Sometimes a unilateral needle injection provides the diagnosis. Catheter cavography is used in the presence of collateral channels or partial obstruction close to the superior vena cava (36). DSA uses the same techniques as conventional cavography, except for the contrast material, which is diluted with an equal amount of normal saline solution and injected in an amount of 30 ml in both needles over 5 s, while one image per second is obtained during 20 s.

Normal Superior Cavography and Collateral Pathways

The superior vena cava (SVC) is formed by the junction of the two innominate veins. If there is a low obstruction in the SVC, drainage may be primarily via the azygos and hemiazygos system to the ascending lumbar veins and then to the renal or common iliac veins and the inferior vena cava. If the obstruction is above the azygos vein, drainage may occur retrograde from the innominate veins via three major pathways. One is from the internal thoracic veins to the superior and inferior epigastric veins and then to the superior and veins. Another innominate pathway is from the lateral thoracic veins to the superficial epigastric veins and then to the greater saphenous veins into the common femoral veins and then into the iliac systems. The third pathway is from the highest intercostal and first posterior intercostal veins and then into the azygoshemiazygos system or via the anterior intercostals to the internal thoracic and then to the superior and nferior epigastric veins. Multiple interconnections exist among these collateral channels (Fig. 7.7).

Congenital Abnormalities

A congenital abnormality of the vena cava is a persistent left SVC in conjunction with the right SVC. On plain radiographs, the left SVC may appear as a widening in the area of the aortic arch or the left paramediastinal density (37). Cavography by the left cubital vein makes the diagnosis in these areas.

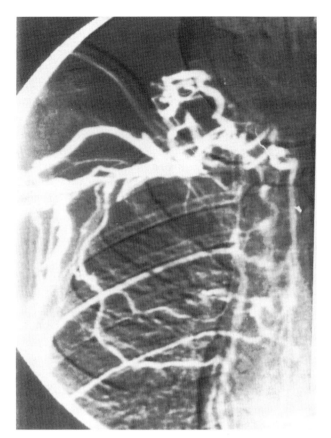

Figure 7.7. Superior vena cava obstruction. Intravenous DSA demonstrates a right innominate vein obstruction with drainage via the intercostal collaterals and the internal thoracic vein.

Acquired Lesions

Lesions of the SVC result in partial or complete obstruction of the vein with the signs and symptoms of the superior vena cava syndrome. The majority of these lesions are mediastinal neoplasms, primary and metastatic lung carcinoma, and lymphoma. Benign lesions causing SVC obstruction are rare, but some causes are known, such as fibrosing mediastinitis, compression by an aortic aneurysm, or compression by huge benign mediastinal tumors (38). Superior cavography is essential in the assessment of SVC-acquired lesions because it demonstrates clearly the obstruction of the vein and the development of collateral pathways.

Interventional Vascular Procedures

Embolization of Bronchial Arteries

Untreated massive hemoptysis has high mortality, and embolization of bronchial arteries is an effective treatment that can obviate major surgical intervention.

Tuberculosis and other inflammatory diseases are the most common causes of massive hemoptysis. Bronchial arteries are variable in size and distribution, but are usually no more than two to each lung, and most arise from the descending thoracic aorta at the level of T5–6. A normal bronchial artery is no larger than 3 mm in diameter. Enlargement can be taken as presumptive evidence of hemorrhagic source, if the origin of bleeding has not been identified bronchoscopically. Peripheral inflammatory lesions can also receive blood from intercostal arteries and chest wall vessels. Innominate, subclavian, and internal thoracic artery injections may be needed for complete evaluation (39).

Pleural thickening should alert one to the presence of such collateral vessels, and embolization of lesions associated with pleural thickening is less likely to result in the long term control of hemoptysis (40). Embolization has stopped pulmonary hemorrhage in 75–90% of patients, but there is a 20% rate of rebleeding within 6 months. The most feared complication of bronchial artery embolization is spinal cord injury (41).

Patients with massive hemoptysis due to pulmonary tuberculosis should be first treated with bronchial artery embolization (42). We present a case of bronchial artery embolization in a patient with massive hemoptysis due to tuberculosis (Fig. 7.8).

New technical developments such coaxial microcatheter systems allow superselective bronchial artery embolization beyond the spinal or mediastinal branches, making superselective embolization safer and more effective than the ordinary method (43).

Embolization of Pulmonary Arteriovenous Malformation

Pulmonary arteriovenous malformation not only can produce problems with blood oxygen desaturation and high output cardiac failure but also are likely to cause cerebral emboli and brain abscess. For the latter reasons, even asymptomatic lesions should be treated by embolotherapy. The great majority of these patients have Rendu–Osler–Weber Syndrome (39) White et al. have had a high degree of success occluding lesions with detachable balloons (44).

A major problem in embolotherapy of pulmonary arteriovenous malformations is recanalization. Sagara et al. found a high incidence of recanalization in pulmonary arteriovenous malformation (PAVMs) embolized with steel coils. Half of the recanalized PAVMs were fed by bronchial artery branches and they conclude that coil embolization should be performed as close as possible to the PAVM to avoid future development of artery-to-pulmonary anastomoses that may cause recanalization (45).

Embolization of Pulmonary Artery Pseudoaneurysm

Pulmonary artery pseudoaneurysm is a rare complication of flow-directed pulmonary artery Swan–Ganz catheterization. The mortality rate associated with pulmonary artery rupture is high and death is due to massive hemoptysis. If the patient survives, a false aneurysm of the pulmonary artery may result from the perforation of the pulmonary artery and may lead to recurrent life-threating hemorrhage (46).

Ferretti et al. described the successful treatment with transcatheter steel-coil embolization of seven false aneurisms in five patients with hemoptysis after the removal of a Swan–Ganz catheter (46).

Multiple pulmonary artery sacular embolization has been described (47).

Removal of Pulmonary Artery Thrombus

Currently available therapeutic options for massive pulmonary embolism include surgical and percutaneous embolectomy and thrombolysis. Limitations of the current treatment options include the need for immediate surgical resources to carry out perative pulmonary embolectomy. Also thrombolysis, although effective in moderate embolic events, may not produce a therapeutic effect quickly in massive embolism. Percutaneous catheter techniques as suction removal or use of catheters for fragmenting and dislodging the pulmonary artery thrombus, although effective in the acute situation, have not found wide acceptance (48).

Mechanical thrombectomy with Amplatz thrombectomy devices were used in five patients with massive pulmonary embolism and provide marked improvement in pulmonary perfusion in three patients at angiography and ventilation–perfusion scanning (49).

The first human experience of removal of thrombus from a patient with acute pulmonary embolism using the hydrolyzer catheter has been described (48).

Pulmonary Artery Stent

Stent insertion into the pulmonary arteries has been reported mainly for periferal stenosis seen in pulmonary transplantation and in congenital cardiac disorders.

Percutaneous stent placement into a severely obstructed right pulmonary artery in a patient with mediastinal tumor mass of unknown etiology with successfull restration of the pulmonary perfusion was reported (50). In patients who present with emergencies such as cor pulmonale or have contraindication to systemic

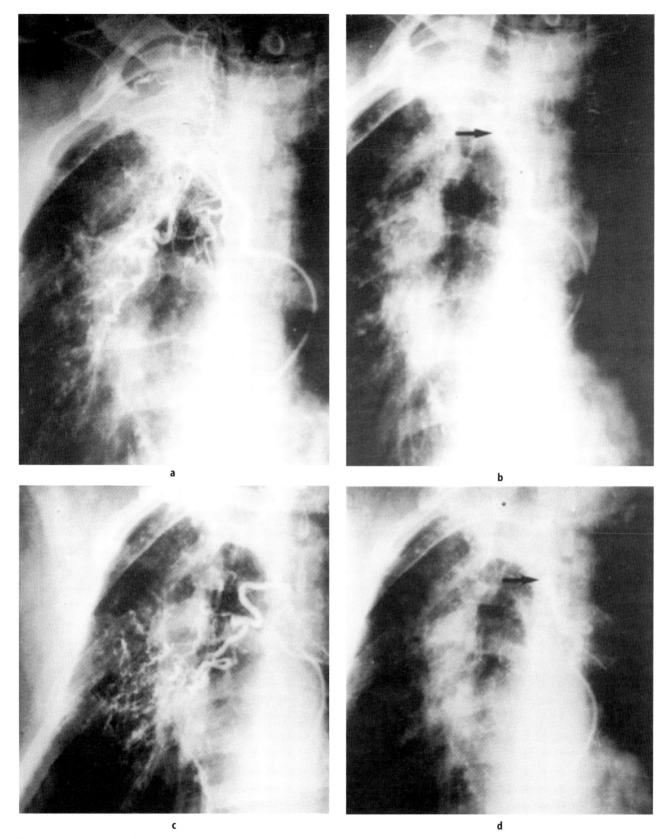

a

b

c

d

Figure 7.8. Bronchial artery embolization. Patient male, 34 years old, with massive hemoptysis due to tuberculosis. **a** Selective arteriography shows a tortuous bronchial artery with multiple ramifications. **b** Postembolization control with liodura fragments shows bronchial artery occlusion (*arrow*). **c** Another bronchial artery was identified more tortuous and well ramified. **d** Postembolization control with liodura fragments shows occlusion of bronchial artery (*arrow*).

thrombolysis, catheter-directed interventions such as intrapulmonary thrombolysis, embolic fragmentation and thrombosuctions are the treatments of choice before surgical embolectomy.

Koizumi et al. (51) reported a patient with pulmonary embolism who developed hypotension and cor pulmonale despite placement of vena cava filter, treatment with thrombolytic agent and failure of percutaneous guidewire fragmentation and thrombosuction. The placement of self-expandable bilateral Z stents into the lower branches through the pulmonary arterial trunks offered immediate relief of cor pulmonale and successful recovery from hypotension (51).

Conclusion

Angiography continues to have great value in the human chest investigation and treatment of vascular congenital abnormalities and vascular acquired lesions of the pulmonary arteries, bronchial arteries, thoracic aorta, and superior vena cava (52,53).

Digital subtraction angiography represents a major technical improvement. Intravenous DSA is the method of choice for the evaluation of most of the vascular disorders in the chest. However, when this study is nondiagnostic as a result of motion artefacts or poor cardiac output, the performance of an intraarterial DSA or conventional angiography is recommended (54).

The advantages of intraarterial DSA over conventional angiography are the use of smaller catheters, lower doses of contrast materials, and quicker and safer examinations.

Angiography catheter techniques are effective tools in the treatment of pulmonary embolism by intraarterial injections of fibrinolytic drugs and catheter suction embolectomy as well as in the treatment of hemoptysis and pulmonary arteriovenous fistulae by selective catheter embolization.

References

1. Resius B, Graor RA (1985) Fibrinolytic therapy in pulmonary tromboembolic disea#atse. Semin Intervent Radiol 2:338–348.
2. Stewart JR, Greenfield LJ (1982) Transvenous vena cava filtration and pulmonary embolectomy. Surg Clin North Am 62:411–430.
3. Rémy J, Arnaud A, Fardon H et al. (1977) Treatment of hemoptysis by embolization of bronchial arteries. Radiology 122:33–37.
4. Castaneda Zuniga WR, Epstein M, Zullikofer C, et al. (1980) Formanek A, Ben-Shachar G, Amplatz K, Embolization of multiple pulmonary artery fistulas. Radiology 134:309–310.
5. Daily PO, Trueblood HW, Stinson EB, et al. (1970) Management of aortic dissections. Ann Thorac Surg 10:237–247.
6. Guthaner DF, Brody WR, Miller DC (1981) Intravenous aortography after aortic dissection repair. AJR 137:1019–1022.
7. Van der Bosch JMM, Gelissen HJ, Wagenaar SS (1983) Exploratory thoracotomy in bronchial carcinoma. J Thorac Cardiovasc Surg 85:733–737.
8. Pearson MG, Ogilvie C (1983) Surgical treatment of emphysematous bullae. Late outcome. Thorax 38:134–137.
9. Dotter CT, Rosch J (1983) Pulmonary arteriography: Technique. In Abrams HL (ed) Abrams angiography. Little, Brown, Boston, MA, pp 707–713.
10. Seldinger SI (1983) Catheter replacement of needle in percutaneous arteriography: A new technique. Acta Radiol 39:368–376.
11. Grollman JH, Gyepes MT, Helmer E (1970) Transfemoral selective bilateral pulmonary arteriography with a pulmonary artery-seeking catheter. Radiology 96:202–204.
12. Grollman JH, Renner JW (1981) Transfemoral pulmonary angiography: Update on technique. AJR 136:624–626.
13. Dotter CT (1983) Congenital abnormalities of the pulmonary arteries. In Abrams HL (ed) Abrams angiography. Little, Brown, Boston, MA, pp 723–741.
14. Rosenow EC, Osmundson PJ, Brown ML (1981) Pulmonary embolism. Mayo Clin Proc 56:161–178.
15. Bell WR, Simon TL, DeMets DK (1977) Clinical features of submassive and massive pulmonary emboli. Am J Med 62:355–360.
16. Gilday MD, Kattidyl PP, Deland FM (1972) Accuracy of detection of pulmonary embolism by lung scanning correlated with pulmonary angiography. AJR 115:732–738.
17. Kelly MJ, Elliot LP (1974) The radiologic evalution of the patient with suspected pulmonary tromboembolic disease. Med Clin North Am 59:3–36.
18. Pond GD (1985) Pulmonary digital subtraction angiography. Radiol Clin North Am 23:243–260.
19. Westermann CJJ (1986) Digital subtraction angiography in pulmonary disease. In Digital subtraction angiography. Philips Medical Systems, Best, Netherlands, pp 143–154.
20. Hoiseth A. Amundsen P (1983) Pulmonary angiography in lung and mediastinal tumors. In Abrams HL (ed) Abrams angiography. Little Brown, Boston, MA, pp 817–843.
21. Pinet F, Gravier J, Pinet A (1959) L'aortographie retrogade sous hipotension controlée. J Radiol Electrol 40:115–126.
22. Viamonte M (1964) Selective bronchial arteriography in man: Preliminary report. Radiology 83:830–839.
23. Viamonte M, Parks RE, Smoak WN (1965) Guided catheterization of the bronchial arteries. Radiology 85:205–230.
24. Ludwig JW, Piers DB (1986) Digital subtraction angiography in bronchial arteriography. In Digital subtraction angiography. Philips Medical System, Best, Netherland, pp 131–141.
25. Remy J, Begnery P, Froment T, Tonnel AB et al. (1975) La vascularization systemique du poumon. Techniques d'exploration et anatomie radiologique apliquées au diagnostique topographique des hemoptises. Ann Radiol 18:47–54.
26. Pinet F, Froment JC (1983) Angiography and embolization of thoracic systemic arteries. In Abrams HL (ed) Abrams angiography. Little, Brown, Boston, MA, pp 845–867.
27. Kardyev V, Symeonov A, Chan Kov I (1974) Etiology, pathogenesis and prevention of spinal cord lesions in selective angiography of the bronchial and intercostal arteries. Radiology 112:81–83.
28. Abrams HL (1983) Technique, indications and hazards. In Abrams HL (ed) Abrams angiography. Little, Brown, Boston, MA, pp 339–352.
29. Abrams HL, Jönsson G (1983) The normal thoracic aorta. In Abrams HL (ed) Abrams angiography, Little, Brown, Boston, MA, pp 353–365.
30. Abrams HL, Jönsson G (1983) Patent ductus arteriosus. In Abrams HL (ed) Abrams angiography. Little, Brown, Boston, MA, pp 367–382.
31. Portsmann W, Wierny L (1983) Nonsurgical closure of patient ductus arteriosus. 14 years experience. In Abrams HL (ed) Abrams angiography. Little, Brown, Boston, MA, pp 2257–2263.

32. Abrams HL, Jönsson G (1983) Coarctation of the aorta. In Abrams HL (ed) Abrams angiography. Little, Brown, Boston, MA, pp 382–412

33. Randal PA, Jarmolowski CR (1983) Aneurysm of the thoracic aorta. In Abrams HL (ed) Abrams angiography. Little, Brown, Boston, MA, pp 417–440.

34. Overtoom TTC (1986) Digital subtraction angiography of the aneurysmatic thoracic and abdominal aorta. In Digital subtraction angiography. Phillips Medical Systems, Best, Nertherlands, pp 73–80.

35. Guthaner DF, Miller DC (1983) Digital subtraction angiography of aortic dissection. AJR 141:157–161.

36. Okay NH, Bryk D (1969) Collateral pathways in occlusion of the superior vena cava and tributaries. Radiology 92:1493–1498.

37. Cha ME, Khoury GH (1972) Persistent left superior vena cava: Radiologic and clinical significance. Radiology 103:375–382.

38. Bettmann MA, Steinberg I (1983) The superior vena cava. In Abrams HL (ed) Abrams angiography. Little Brown Boston, MA, pp 923–938.

39. Wojtowycz M (1995) Handbook of interventional radiology and angiography, 2nd edn. Mosby Year Book, St. Louis, MO.

40. Tamura S, Kodama T, Otsuka N (1993) Embolotherapy for persistent hemoptysis: The significance of pleural thickening. Cardiovasc Interv Radiol 16:85–88.

41. Stoll JF, Bettman MA (1988) Bronchial artery embolization to control hemoptysis: A review. Cardiovasc Interv Radiol 11:263–269.

42. Ramakantan R, Bandekar VG, Gandhi MS, et al. (1996) Massive hemoptysis due to pulmonary tuberculosis: Control with bronchial artery embolization. Radiology 200:691–694.

43. Tanaka N, Yamakado K, Murashima S, et al. (1997) Superselective bronchial artery embolization for hemoptysis with a coaxial microcatheter system. J Vasc Interv Radiol 8:65–70.

44. White RI, Jr, Lynch-Nyhan A, Terry P (1988) Pulmonary arteriovenous malformations: Techniques and long-term outcome of embolotherapy. Radiology 169:663–669.

45. Sagara K, Miyazono N, Inoue H (1998) Recanalization after coil embolotherapy of pulmonary arteriovenous malformations: Study of long term outcome and mechanism for recanalization. AJR 170:727–730.

46. Ferreti GR, Thony F, Link KM (1996) False aneurysm of the pulmonary artery induced by Swan–Ganz catheter: Clinical presentation and radiologic management. AJR 167:941–945.

47. Ghaye B, Trotteur G, Dondelinger RF (1997) Multiple pulmonary artery pseudoaneurysm as: Intrasacular embolization. Eur Radiol 7-2:176–178.

48. Michalis LK, Tsetis DK, Rees MR (1997) Percutaneous removal of pulmonary artery thrombus in a patient with massive pulmonary embolism using the hydrolyser catheter: First human experience. Clin Radiol 52:158–161.

49. Uflaker R, Strange C, Vujic I (1996) Massive pulmonary embolism: preliminary results of treatment with the Amplatz thrombectomy device. J Vasc Interv Radiol 7:519–528.

50. Muller-Hulsbeck S, Bewig B, Schwarzenberg H (1998) Percutaneous placement of a self-expandable stent for treatment of a malignant pulmonary artery stenosis. Br J Radiol 71:785–787.

51. Koizumi J, Kuzano S, Akima T (1998) Emergent Z stent placement for treatment of cor pulmonale due to emboli after failed lytic treatment: Technical considerations. Cardiovasc Interv Radiol 21:254–257.

52. Dieden JD, Friloux LA III, Renner JW (1987) Pulmonary artery false aneurysms secondary to Swan–Ganz pulmonary artery catheters. AJR 149:901–906.

53. Quin MF, Lundell CJ, Klotz TA (1987) Reliability of selective pulmonary arteriography in the diagnosis of pulmonary embolism. AJR 149:469–471.

54. Musset D, Rosso J, Petitpretz P (1988) Acute pulmonary embolism: Diagnostic value of digital subtraction angiography. Radiology 166:455–459.

Pulmonary Function Tests

C. Straus, T. Similowski, J.-P. Derenne, and M. Zelter

Introduction

The lung has two basic simultaneous respiratory functions: the oxygenation of the incoming desaturated venous blood, and the removal of carbon dioxide and consequently of protons (H+) from this incoming blood. To perform this task adequately, both the ventilatory and the circulatory lung systems must be adapted one to another so that the ratio of the distribution of ventilation to perfusion is optimal. Ultimately, this ratio determines the functional quality of gas exchange. Apart from measurement of blood gases, there is no simple test available to give a general assessment of gas exchange in a given patient. Blood gas values, when abnormal, give no clue as to what aspect of lung function is impaired. Furthermore, these values tend to become abnormal only in the late or acute phase of lung diseases, because of the remarkable flexibility of ventilation–perfusion control. The role of pulmonary function testing is to try to sort out precisely what functional part of the ventilatory system is most likely to be related to disease, to identify the type of functional syndrome that affects the patient (obstructive, restrictive or both), and to quantify the impairment in order to allow the follow-up of the disease. Pulmonary function testing cannot identify a specific type of pathology, although these tests tell us whether or not a functional impairment is compatible with a specific type of disease. Because most measurements are done at the mouth, they provide a global evaluation of lung function and do not allow the observer to locate the regional sites of the disease. Correct interpretation of lung testing becomes even more difficult in cases of very heterogeneous lung disease unless the limitations inherent to each type of test are well recognized. For instance, residual lung volume cannot be measured in very heterogeneous obstructive lungs by the helium diffusion technique, even though this technique is reliable in normal and restrictive patients.

Adequate ventilation requires adequate active and passive properties of the ventilatory system and also a normal drive. Ideally, each of these aspects should be tested separately. We should be able to assess separately (a) the active properties of the respiratory muscles, (b) the passive properties of the thoracic wall, and (c) the passive elastic properties of the lung per se (recoil forces). The different lung volumes are determined either by these elastic forces alone (functional residual capacity) or by the interaction of the passive elastic forces and the active action of the muscles (total lung capacity). The conducting airways and their response to various challenges have also to be assessed. In order to proceed, we need to ask the subject to perform so-called forced maneuvers to produce maximum flow. Such maneuvers require full participation of the patient. Correct interpretation relies on a normal thorax configuration and competent muscles. This raises two very important points regarding pulmonary function testing: (a) it is often difficult to discriminate passive from active properties; (b) patient cooperation is critical to obtain correct measurements.

From an engineering viewpoint, most of the pulmonary function tests define the extreme physical properties of the system and bear little relation to normal function, in normal subjects, even during extreme exercise. It is only in pathologic situations that there will be some consistency between the tests and the actual capabilities of the patient, as illustrated by flow–volume curves.

Because of these complex interactions, pulmonary function testing allows logical excercise patterns to be performed and interpreted. There is also a major issue in pulmonary function testing, namely the need for standardization of both the maneuvers and the results. The order in which maneuvers are performed and their temporal sequence may vary the results. Attributing normality or abnormality requires comparison with a carefully designed control population. It is imperative to follow the guidelines issued by leading scientific societies and to refer to their published data.

In the most common usage of the term, pulmonary function tests include spirometry, flow–volume loop, assessment of the mechanical properties of the lung and of the chest wall (the results being influenced by respiratory muscle function and drive), of bronchial reactivity and of carbon monoxide diffusion, and blood gas measurements. Besides these widely available standardized routine tests, more specialized tests evaluate the respiratory muscles and their central control. Assessing respiratory function during exercise is often a mandatory complement of pulmonary function testing.

Ventilatory Flows and Volumes

Oxygen supply and carbon dioxide elimination require continuous alveolar ventilation, and hence cyclic changes in pulmonary volume. In clinical practice, the measurement of ventilatory flows and volumes is the first step in pulmonary function testing. These tests are integrative, depending not only upon the properties of the lungs and the airways but also on those of the chest wall and the respiratory muscles. Muscular activation is necessary for lung inflation and pulmonary emptying, as well as for the performance of maximal respiratory flows. Exact understanding of the physician's commands and adequate execution of breathing by the patient are required. This again underlines the complexing of interpretation of most pulmonary function tests.

The volume of gas contained in the lungs at a specific stage is defined as either a static volume or a capacity (Fig. 8.1), the latter being the sum of two or more static volumes (1). The volume of the lungs in the absence of any respiratory muscle contraction defines the relaxation volume (V_r). V_r corresponds to the equilibrium between the opposite elastic recoils of the lung and chest wall. In normal subjects, V_r is the same as the functional residual capacity (FRC), which corresponds to the end-expiratory volume of tidal ventilation (2). FRC is the sum of the expiratory reserve volume (ERV) and of the residual volume (RV). ERV is the maximal volume that can be expired from FRC. It decreases in the supine position (3). RV is the volume of gas remaining in the lung at the end of a full expiration. Therefore RV cannot be directly measured at the mouth. Since techniques are available to measure FRC, RV is usually calculated by subtracting ERV from FRC (1). The tidal volume (V_T) is the volume of gas inspired or expired during a respiratory cycle. The maximal volume that can be inspired from the mean end-inspiratory level defines the inspiratory reserve volume (IRV). The sum of V_T and IRV is the inspiratory capacity (IC). IC does not change between the sitting position and the reclining position (4). The vital capacity (VC) is the sum of IC and ERV and corresponds to the volume change measured at the mouth between full inspiration and complete expiration. The total lung capacity (TLC) is the total volume of gas in the lungs at the end of a full inspiration. It is usually computed as FRC + IC or FRC + V_T + IRV (1).

Several methods can be used to determine pulmonary volumes and flows. For each individual, the results should be compared with predicted values (1,5,6). When results are compared with imaging data, it is essential to bear in mind the changes in volume induced by changes in posture, because imaging data are generally obtained with the patient supine, and pulmonary function test data in the sitting or standing position.

Measurement Methods

The Spirometer

The spirometer is the oldest method of measuring static lung volumes (7). The classical device consists of an air-filled bell, under which the volume of gas changes with the patient's respiratory movements and which, in response, moves within a water-sealed container (8). The water seal provides good dynamic properties but, recently, dry-type spirometers have been developed as they are easier to decontaminate. The patient wears a nose clip and breaths into the spirometer through a mouthpiece in an unidirectional circuit. The ventilation of the subject induces displacement of the bell in proportion to the mobilized volume. The displacements can be recorded on a paper chart or digitized and computed. To avoid carbon dioxide accumulation due to the closed circuit, a canister filled with soda lime is placed on the expiratory line (Fig. 8.2). A low flow of oxygen is also permitted into the bell to compensate for oxygen consumption. Measurements are

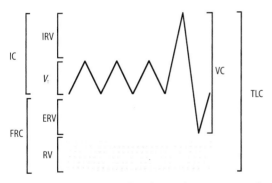

Figure 8.1. Schematic representation of ventilatory volumes, seen on a spirometric tracing. *FRC,* functional residual capacity; *IC,* inspiratory capacity; *V_T,* tidal volume; *IRV,* inspiratory reserve volume; *ERV,* expiratory reserve volume; *VC,* vital capacity; *TLC,* total lung capacity; *RV,* residual volume. *FRC* cannot be directly measured with a spirometer. This requires the use of other techniques such as the multiple-breath helium dilution method, the multiple-breath nitrogen washout method or the plethysmographic technique. From FRC, RV and TLC can be computed as FRC − ERV or FRC + IC, respectively.

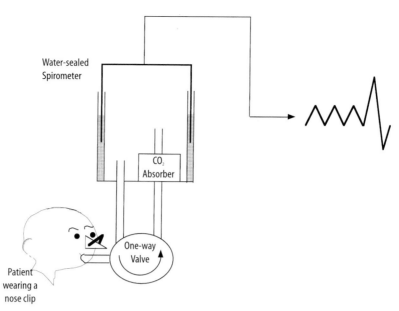

Figure 8.2. Schematic representation of a spirometer.

performed at ambient temperature, pressure and water saturation (ATPS) and therefore must be corrected to allow for the temperature, pressure and water saturation prevailing in the body (BTPS) (1). A spirometer allows measurement of slow and forced VC, V_T, ERV and IRV and, during a forced expiration, the maximal volume expired during the first second (forced expiratory volume in 1 s, FEV_1) (Fig. 8.3). Slow and forced VC should both be measured as they may differ in patients with chronic obstructive pulmonary disease (COPD). It should be stated whether VC or forced VC is used in calculation of the FEV_1/VC ratio.

The Pneumotachometer

The pneumotachometer is a flow-sensing device. The flow signal is integrated to compute volume (1). The pressure differential pneumotachometer consists of a tube contain-

ing a resistive element that causes a pressure drop when gas flows through it. The pressure drop is proportional to the gas flow as long as the latter is laminar. Two types of resistive element are commonly used, either a bundle of capillary tubes (e.g., the Fleisch pneumotachometer) or a grid (e.g., the Lilly pneumotachometer). The hot-wire pneumotachometer is another type of flow sensor, consisting of a heated platinum wire, the temperature of which is maintained constant by an electric current. As the wire is cooled by the gas flow, additional current is needed to maintain the preset temperature of the wire. This current is proportional to the flow. In the turbine-type pneumotachometer, gas flowing through the instrument causes a vane to rotate. It is easy to use at the bedside, but its accuracy is poor. Most of these devices require linearization of the calibration curves to be useful over a reasonable range of flow and must be calibrated regularly to give accurate results.

Pneumotachometers are compact and can be used with an open breathing circuit. Accordingly, they are easier to use and to decontaminate than spirometers.

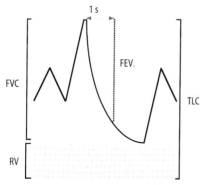

Figure 8.3. Schematic representation of a spirometric tracing obtained during a forced vital capacity (*FVC*) maneuver. *FEV_1* is the maximal volume expired during the first second. *TLC*, total lung capacity; *RV*, residual volume.

The Flow–Volume Curve (Fig. 8.4)

The measurement of flow during a forced inspiration followed by a forced expiration allows one to plot a maximum flow–volume curve with instantaneous flows against volumes (9). Forced expiration is performed from the TLC to the RV. This maneuver defines the forced vital capacity (FVC). A complete flow–volume loop is obtained by performing a maximal inspiration immediately after the forced expiration. The tidal loop must be plotted systematically on the same tracing. The volume is plotted on the x-axis, usually from left to right during the expiration,

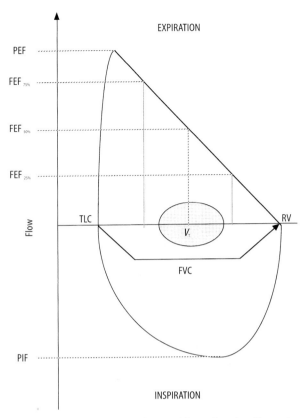

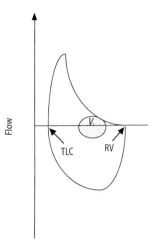

Figure 8.5. Schematic representation of flow–volume loop in an obstructive syndrome. In this example, the forced expiratory flow–volume curve crosses the tidal flow–volume curve, illustrating a flow limitation phenomenon. V_T, tidal volume; *TLC*, total lung capacity; *RV*, residual volume.

Figure 8.4. Schematic representation of a normal flow–volume loop. The *x*-axis corresponds to lung volume and the *y*-axis to flow. V_T, tidal volumes. *TLC*, total lung capacity; *RV*, residual volume; *FVC*, forced vital capacity. *PEF*, peak expiratory flow. *PIF*, peak inspiratory flow. $FEF_{25\%}$, $FEF_{50\%}$, $FEF_{75\%}$, Maximal forced expiratory flows at 25%, 50% and 75% of FVC, respectively.

i.e., from the TLC to the RV contrary to usual practice. The flow is plotted on the *y*-axis, upward for expiration (10).

In addition to FVC, several indices can be derived from flow–volume loops, namely peak inspiratory (PIF) and expiratory (PEF) flows, maximal instantaneous expiratory flow at 25%, 50%, 75% of FVC ($FEF_{25\%}$, $FEF_{50\%}$, $FEF_{75\%}$) and the mean flow between 75% and 25% of FVC (FEF_{25-75}). Below 50% of VC, maximal expiratory flows are no longer dependent upon the expiratory effort of the patient. They reflect only the elastic and resistive properties of the lungs and, in normal subjects, decrease linearly with the pulmonary volume (2,11,12). The computed indexes mentioned above give a quantitative but limited vision of the expiratory data curve, which is still best analysed by eye. Besides numbers, visual inspection of the shape of the flow–volume loop provides important information. For example, a concave shape related to a decrease in $FEF_{25\%}$ and in $FEF_{50\%}$ suggests distal (small) airways obstruction. In severely obstructive patients, the flow–volume loop obtained during tidal breathing can overlap the loop obtained during a forced maneuver, defining flow limitation (Fig. 8.5) (13,14). This paradoxical finding is

due to changes in transmural pressure in flow-limited patients. A flattening of the inspiratory limb of the flow–volume loop suggests extrathoracic obstruction of the airways. A global decrease of the size of the loop, associated to a normal shape, occurs in restrictive diseases.

Measurements of Functional Residual Capacity and Residual Volume

Measurement of FRC by the Multiple-Breath Helium Dilution Method

FRC is the volume of gas remaining in the lungs at the end of a quiet breath. Most commonly, FRC is measured by the multiple-breath helium dilution method (15), as follows. Helium is an inert gas that does not cross the air–blood barrier and therefore equilibrates only in the ventilated compartments of the lungs. To measure FRC, the spirometer is first filled with a known volume of air containing a known amount of helium. Then the patient is connected to the spirometer and breathes quietly from FRC until there is complete equilibration of the gas mixture between the spirometer and the lungs. The concentration of helium is measured inside the spirometer and the lung volume in which helium has been diluted is calculated. If the measurement ends at the end of a tidal expiration, the results correspond to FRC. The limits of this technique are, in addition to the difficulty of decontaminating the closed circuit, its high sensitivity to leaks and the risk of underestimating FRC if there are some slow-filling lung compartments (e.g., severe COPD).

Measurement of FRC by the Multiple-Breath Nitrogen Washout Method

The multiple-breath nitrogen washout method is coupled to the assessment of lung volumes by pneumotachography to provide a measurement of the FRC with an open breathing circuit (16).

The patient breathes through a mouthpiece–valve system. Expired nitrogen is measured "breath by breath" by using a fast responding analyzer. At the end of each expiration, a valve opens and pure oxygen is delivered to the patient during all the inspiratory phase. Thus each breath of pure oxygen washes out some residual nitrogen. The exhaled volume of nitrogen for each breath is calculated from the nitrogen concentration and from the volume of each breath. Values for each breath are summed to provide the total volume of washed out nitrogen. The test is carried out until the nitrogen fraction in the alveolar gas has been reduced to approximately 1% or for a maximum duration of 7 min. FRC is calculated by dividing the total volume of nitrogen washed out by the difference in nitrogen concentration from the beginning to the end of the test. Measurements must be corrected for BTPS conditions and for nitrogen excretion from tissue and blood. The resistance of the valve can prevent some patients from breathing comfortably. Limitations during heterogeneous lung disease with low ventilated area are similar to those of helium dilution.

Plethysmographic Measurement of Thoracic Gas Volume

The plethysmographic technique is the reference method to measure the thoracic gas volume (V_{TG}), most of the time at FRC (8). Indeed, poorly ventilated lung regions may bias the helium dilution and the nitrogen washout methods (17). The plethysmographic technique gives access to the volume of gas in the thorax, be it in communication with the airway or trapped (e.g., bullae). The technique makes use of the Boyle–Mariotte law of pressure–volume changes in a closed container. In order to perform a measurement of the V_{TG}, patients are seated in a body plethysmograph, which consists of a sealed box. They breathe through the mouth in a respiratory circuit, while wearing a nose clip. The circuit includes a pneumotachometer and a pressure transducer for measuring the pressure in the airways. At the end of a normal expiration, the airways are occluded by a shutter. The patient then breathes against the shutter, leading to compression and decompression of a given fixed amount of gas in the chest. The frequency of this "panting" should be 1–2 cycles s^{-1}, the glottis remaining open. The pressure changes in the airway (ΔP) and the volume changes in the body box (ΔV)

during the panting maneuver are recorded and used for the calculation of V_{TG} from the Boyle–Mariotte law (1,18). This law states that the product of pressure and volume for a gas in a chamber is constant under isothermal conditions. Following this law, $V_{TG} = P_{atmospheric} \times (\Delta V/\Delta P)$.

A body plethysmograph equipped with a pneumotachometer allows one to simultaneously assess all ventilatory volumes and flows. The limits of the technique are the impossibility of some patients entering the sealed box (e.g., patients on stretchers, claustrophobic or obese patients) and the relative difficulty of the panting maneuver. In severely obstructive patients, the plethysmographic method can overestimate the V_{TG} if mouth pressure differs from alveolar pressure because of heterogeneous changes in lung elasticity (19). With this proviso, comparison between plethysmographic V_{TG} and FRC measured with the helium dilution method in obstructive patients can provide an evaluation of the volume trapped in the lungs (20). It remains however the reference method.

Measurement of Airway Resistance

In the normal subject, the resistance to the airflow is due mainly to the large bronchi. In obstructive lung disease, resistance of the small airways can become proportionally higher than the resistance of the large airways. Assessing bronchial resistance is particularly relevant to patients having difficulties in performing a reliable forced expiratory maneuver, e.g., children.

Airway resistance is calculated by dividing the difference between alveolar pressure and mouth pressure by the gas flow. Most of the time, in clinical practice, gas flow is measured with a pneumotachometer during a panting maneuver and alveolar pressure is evaluated with a plethysmograph, following principles similar to those used to determine the V_{TG} (21). However, other methods, such as the forced oscillation technique, give access to airway resistance without patient cooperation and permit, at least in theory, partition of proximal and distal resistances (22).

Airway Responsiveness and Pharmacologic Challenges

Bronchial Challenge

Airway hyperresponsiveness denotes an exaggerated response to a bronchoconstricting stimulus. This response is usually assessed by changes in FEV$_1$ but modifications in airway resistance can also be evaluated. From a clinical point of view, the test documents a potential for variable airway obstruction. It is particularly relevant in patients reporting transient symptoms consistent with asthma but whose ventilatory flows and volumes are normal. The high sensitivity and the high negative predictive value of these tests make them particularly suitable for excluding a diagnosis of asthma (23–26). Absolute contraindications to a bronchial challenge are severe baseline airways obstruction ($FEV_1 < 1.2$ L in adults), recent myocardial infarction (< 3 months), arterial aneurysms, and inability to understand the procedures and the implications of the test. Relative contraindications are moderate to severe airways obstruction, recent upper respiratory tract infection (< 2 weeks), exacerbation of asthma, arterial hypertension, pregnancy, and epilepsy requiring drug treatment. Bronchodilator treatments must have been stopped before the test for a period at least equal to the duration of their action. To perform the test, the patient inhales increasing concentrations of a bronchoconstrictor agent. For the assessment of nonspecific bronchial hyperresponsivness, the most commonly used pharmacologic agent is aerosolized methacholine administered with a dosimeter. The maximal cumulative dose is usually 1600 μg. Hyperresponsiveness is defined as a decrease of FEV_1 of more than 20% at a specified dose. The results should be expressed in terms of the cumulative doses of drug that cause a fall of 20% in FEV_1 (PD_{20}). When the fall in FEV_1 exceeds 20%, PD_{20} has to be calculated by interpolation (27). In the case of suspected exercise-induced asthma, nonspecific hyperresponsiveness can also be evaluated by inhalation of dry air during exercise. However, the evaluation of FEV_1 has to be performed after the cessation of the exercise (generally up to 10–15 min) as bronchial response often occurs later. When occupational asthma is suspected, the airway response to a specific agent, for instance flour, can be assessed using quantified aerosols (27). Except in this instance, bronchial challenges are nonspecific tests, since they diagnose a tendency for bronchi to react to a pharmacologic agent but do not provide a formal diagnosis of a specific disease such as asthma. Furthermore a few asthmatic patients fail to respond.

Bronchodilator Studies

Mirroring bronchial challenge, these tests consist of performing spirometry after the administration of a bronchodilator, in order to evaluate the reversibility of airway obstruction. The most frequently used bronchodilators are $\beta2$-agonists, although the effect of either anticholinergic drugs or steroids can also be assessed. Reversibility is defined by an improvement of FEV_1 of at least 12% compared with the predicted value and of at least 200 mL (6). Recent data have shown that bronchodilators can increase inspiratory capacity in obstructive patients showing no improvement in term of FEV_1 (28). Since inspiratory capacity correlates best with dyspnea in obstructive

diseases (29,30), its measurement should probably be systematically associated with FEV_1 in order to assess the effects of a bronchodilator. A bronchodilator study is highly recommended in all obstructive patients. It is of some use in treated asthmatic patients to check indirectly the effectiveness of the treatment.

Functional Ventilatory Semiology

Ventilatory abnormalities can be grouped in syndromes in order to better characterize lung diseases.

Restrictive Syndrome

A restrictive ventilatory syndrome is defined by a decrease in TLC below 80% of the predicted value (1). A reduction in VC alone is never sufficient to characterize a restrictive syndrome because such a decrease may be associated with an increased RV and therefore with a normal or even augmented TLC. This can occur in severe obstructive patients with pulmonary gas-trapping (31). Typically, the flow–volume loop in pulmonary restriction can exhibit a normal shape but a reduced size, because flows are decreased proportionally to volumes (32).

Causes of Restrictive Syndromes (32)

The most typical cause of a restrictive syndrome is a quantitative reduction in lung parenchyma, for example after surgical removal. Typical parenchymal causes are interstitial lung diseases and tuberculosis sequelae. Pulmonary restriction can also be caused by chest wall diseases such as severe kyphoscoliosis or diseases of the pleura. Finally, a restrictive syndrome can be due to neuromuscular disorders. As patients with such diseases may also be smokers an obstructive syndrome can be associated with a restrictive pathology. Careful analysis of the flow–volume loop and of helium and plethysmographic volume measurements have to be performed to identify a real so-called mixed syndrome.

Obstructive Syndrome

The obstructive syndrome is characterized by a disproportionate decrease in FEV_1 compared with the decrease in VC (1). The obstructive syndrome is often defined as a decreased FEV_1/FVC ratio, below 85% of the predicted value. The reduction in FEV_1 is in direct relationship with the severity of the disease. If FEV_1 is superior or equal to 50% of the predicted value, obstruction is defined as mild. FEV_1 between 35% and 49% of the predicted value defines a moderate obstruction. If FEV_1 is inferior or equal to 34% of the predicted value, obstruction is defined as severe (33). The expiratory flow–volume curve is concave (Fig. 8.3) and expiratory flows are reduced at all volumes (14,34). A predominant reduction of flows at low pulmonary volumes (25–50% of VC) suggest a preferential obstruction of the smallest airways. During the evolution of the disease, RV increases; VC can first remain normal and then decreases; TLC increases late in the disease (1). Severe obstructive syndromes are usually associated with hyperinflation, functionally defined as a significant increase in FRC. Hyperinflation seems to be a major cause of dyspnea in obstructive lung diseases (35).

Causes of Obstructive Syndrome

The two most frequent causes of obstructive syndrome are asthma and COPD (1). The variability of airway obstruction characterizes asthma. In many patients, pulmonary function is normal or only slightly altered between intermittent episodes. For example, a persistent obstruction of the small airways can be suggested by a reduction in $FEF_{25\%}$ and $FEF_{50\%}$ or by a concave shape of the flow–volume loop at low volumes. During an asthma attack, however, the FEV_1/FVC ratio clearly decreases. Assessment of nonspecific hyperresponsiveness can help in eliminating the diagnosis of asthma if the symptoms are transient or atypical.

In COPD patients, airway obstruction is usually not reversible with the use of bronchodilators. Nonetheless, reversibility should be assessed systematically. Indeed, some degree of bronchial hyperresponsiveness may be associated with COPD. If positive, the test justifies bronchodilator treatment. Furthermore, bronchodilators can reduce hyperinflation and dyspnea in some COPD patients without necessarily improving FEV_1 (28,30). A decrease in hyperinflation, which can easily be assessed by measuring the inspiratory capacity, should also justify bronchodilator treatment .

Before accepting the association between obstruction and restriction, which characterizes some respiratory diseases (e.g., bronchiectasis, pneumoconiosis, tuberculosis sequelae or sarcoidosis), it is important to eliminate methodological errors. FRC can be underestimated by the helium dilution method in severe obstruction with major air-trapping. The consequence can be an underestimation of TLC that will lead to the erroneous conclusion that both an obstructive and a restrictive syndrome are present. To avoid this pitfall, plethysmographic measurement of the lung volumes should be performed.

Lung Compliance

Definition and Measurement

Lung compliance assesses the elastic properties of the lung, independently of the properties of the chest wall and of muscular effort (36). Lung compliance is defined as the passive volume change per unit of transpulmonary pressure (P_{tp}) change, P_{tp} being the difference between airway pressure (P_{aw}) and pleural pressure (P_{pl}). P_{pl} is evaluated by measuring the esophageal pressure (P_{es}) with an esophageal balloon-catheter inserted through the nose. P_{aw} is recorded at the mouth. Compliance can be measured in quasistatic (36) or static conditions (37,38). The latter is the reference technique. The subject expires passively, starting from TLC, through the mouth, in a respiratory circuit equipped with a shutter that periodically interrupts the expiratory flow. The pressures and the corresponding volume are measured during each flow interruption. Lung compliance is deduced from the relationship between transpulmonary pressure and lung volume.

Significance of Lung Compliance

Reduced lung compliance is a typical feature of pulmonary fibrosis, pulmonary edemas or acute respiratory distress syndrome. Conversely, increased compliance is the hallmark of emphysema, illustrating the decrease of the elastic recoil.

Assessment of Respiratory Muscles

Respiratory muscles are the effectors of the respiratory system. Ventilation depends upon their phasic and continuous contraction in response to neural commands. Failure of this process leads to alveolar hypoventilation and respiratory distress. Virtually, all neuromuscular diseases can affect the respiratory muscles, for example myasthenia gravis, Guillain–Barré syndrome, amyotrophic lateral sclerosis, polymyositis, and others. The involvement of respiratory muscles in steroid-induced myopathy deserves a special mention. Its occurrence has been increasingly recognized in recent years (39). It can explain respiratory manifestations such as exertional dyspnea or restrictive ventilatory defects in patients receiving steroids for nonrespiratory diseases. In patients with primarily chronic respiratory disease such as asthma or COPD, systemic administration of steroids can alter the load-compensating abilities of respiratory muscles and hence worsen the respiratory status.

Static Pressures

The most common way to assess the respiratory muscles is to measure the maximal inspiratory ($P_{i,max}$) or expiratory ($P_{e,max}$) pressure that they can develop (40). The airway pressure is recorded at the mouth during a forceful, briefly sustained respiratory effort, either inspiratory or expiratory, against an occluded valve. A small leak in the valve prevents glottal closure and eliminates pressures generated by the cheek muscles by allowing a small amount of gas to enter and exit the oral cavity. The pressure produced at the mouth by the respiratory muscles indirectly reflects their force.

To account for the force–length relationship of striated muscles, it is essential to know at what volume the static pressures are measured. Inspiratory muscles are at mechanical advantage at low lung volume, hence their maximal pressure generation capability is at RV. Conversely, expiratory muscles are at a mechanical advantage at TLC. It is common practice to measure $P_{i,max}$ and $P_{e,max}$ from FRC. Measuring them at different lung volumes yields more data. In any case, the maximal respiratory pressures should be expressed relative to lung volume. The main limitations of these tests are their strong dependence on the cooperation of the subject and the fact that they assess synergistic muscles without discrimination.

Stimulation

Stimulation techniques alleviate the problem of subject cooperation. They can also isolate one muscle from another. Phrenic nerve stimulation, which allows specific investigation of the diaphragm, is the most established stimulation technique in the field of respiration. It can be performed using either an electric (41) or a magnetic stimulator (42). The electromyographic response of the diaphragm to phrenic nerve stimulation reflects phrenic conduction. Recording a pressure in response to phrenic nerve stimulation permits an evaluation of the contractile properties of the diaphragm. The recorded pressure can be either airway pressure at the mouth (43) or trans-diaphragmatic pressure (41). As with the maximal respiratory pressures, the results for stimulation techniques should be interpreted in relation to lung volume.

Assessment of the Ventilatory Control

The automatic, phasic and continuous contraction of the respiratory muscles is controlled by neural networks located in the brainstem. These networks constitute the ventilatory central pattern generator (CPG) (44). The ventilatory CPG adapts ventilation to the needs of the body in response to numerous afferent inputs. One of the main goals of ventilation is to provide adequate carbon dioxide elimination and oxygen supply. Chemoreceptors continuously monitor the levels of oxygen and carbon dioxide in the blood. As a result, hypercapnia and hypoxemia stimulate the ventilatory CPG and increase the ventilatory drive. In normal subjects, any increase in the respiratory drive leads to an augmentation of ventilation (45). Therefore, the response to hypercapnia is a common way to assess the function of the ventilatory CPG.

Measurement of the Respiratory Drive

The output of the ventilatory CPG is conveyed to the respiratory muscles, which transform the CPG activity into pressure changes that induce lung volume changes. The output of the ventilatory CPG would therefore be assessed ideally by recording the electroneurogram of the phrenic nerve, which conveys the inspiratory signal to the diaphragm. This recording is, however, impossible to perform in clinic. The analysis of ventilatory parameters is the only practical way to assess the CPG output, and analysis of the spirogram can provide information about the respiratory drive (46). However, this implies a fully normal chain of transmission and any abnormality of the bronchi, lung, chest wall, respiratory muscles or nerve conduction may interfere with the evaluation of the respiratory central output from a spirogram.

Occlusion pressure ($P_{0.1}$) has been introduced to circumvent these limits (47–49) as it is measured independently of flow or volume changes. Since $P_{0.1}$ is usually measured at FRC, muscle length and therefore muscle force are standardized. The measurement of $P_{0.1}$ is easy and noninvasive. The subject breathes through a mouthpiece with a one-way valve. During expiration, the inspiratory limb of the apparatus is occluded with a shutter, the subject being unaware of this occlusion. The subsequent inspiration is performed against an infinite resistance and produces a negative pressure in the respiratory circuit. Because a conscious subject does not perceive the occlusion before about 200 ms after the beginning of the effort, the pressure measured in the airway at 100 ms reflects the output of the automatic ventilatory CPG.

Some pitfalls of the $P_{0.1}$ technique should be taken into account when evaluating the ventilatory CPG with this method (49). An increase in FRC, as can occur in emphysema, decreases the force generation ability of the respiratory muscles; hence $P_{0.1}$ may be underestimated. An increased airway time constant can delay the transmission of pleural pressure to the mouth, hence again risking underestimation. Therefore, in patients with COPD, occlusion pressure should not be measured in the airway but with an esophageal balloon-tipped catheter. Paradoxical motion of the rib cage and abdomen may occur during an occluded effort, resulting in marked change in muscle length despite no change in lung volume. As a consequence, inspiratory muscle contraction would no longer be isometric and would depend upon force–length and force–velocity factors. Finally modification of the shape of the pressure wave can also alter the measurement of $P_{0.1}$. For example, positive pressure ventilation can make this wave more convex, which would lead to an overestimation of the pressure value 100 ms after occlusion.

Stimulation of the Ventilatory Central Pattern Generator

Routine assessment of the ventilatory CPG consists in the evaluation of its response to stimulation. Induction of hypercapnia is the most commonly used method. In the open-circuit or steady-state technique (50), the subject breathes various concentrations of carbon dioxide from a reservoir until a steady state is reached. In the rebreathing technique (51), which is the most frequently used, the subject rebreathes from a one-way circuit containing a reservoir of 7% carbon dioxide in oxygen. Because of the closed nature of the circuit, ventilation fails to eliminate carbon dioxide and arterial partial pressure of carbon dioxide (Pa_{CO2}) (estimated from end-tidal P_{CO2}) increases. The subject rebreathes until the concentration of end-tidal P_{CO2} exceeds 9% or until 4 min have elapsed. The response of the ventilatory CPG to hypercapnia is evaluated by measuring the total ventilation and $P_{0.1}$, which normally increase. The normal ventilatory response is linear with a slope between 1.5 and 3 L min^{-1}mmHg^{-1} in 80% of the subjects. This slope characterizes the sensitivity of the response and is similar for the two techniques. The response to hypoxia can also be assessed (52,53). However, this test is more rarely performed because exposure to hypoxia may be hazardous.

Significance of Ventilatory Control Assessment

A decrease in the response to hypercapnia characterizes the hypoventilation syndromes, either congenital or acquired (54).

Investigation of the respiratory drive remains very dependent upon the condition of the respiratory muscles. Interpretation of the results should therefore take into

account their function. For example, in the case of myasthenia gravis, respiratory drive is likely to be normal but muscular function is impaired, leading possibly to a decreased response to hypercapnia (55). In Duchenne and Steinert myopathies, the ventilatory response to hypercapnia is reduced while the augmentation of $P_{0.1}$ with increasing hypercapnia is normal (56).

Assessment of Gas Exchanges

The purpose of ventilation is to provide adequate gas exchanges to the body. The assessment of these exchanges is therefore an important part of pulmonary function testing. The three main methods used to evaluate the gas exchanges are measurement of blood gases at rest, assessment of the diffusing capacity, and the exercise test.

Blood Gases

Specimen Collection and Measurement

Measurement of blood gases is performed on an arterial sample preferably obtained from the radial artery. Arterial specimens may also be drawn from brachial and femoral arteries. Before a radial artery puncture, the adequacy of collateral circulation to the hand via the ulnar artery should be established using the modified Allen's test: both radial and ulnar arteries are occluded by pressing down over the wrist. The subject is instructed to make a fist and then to open and to relax the fingers. At that time, the palm of the hand is pale and bloodless. The ulnar artery is released while the radial remains occluded. If the hand is reperfused in less than 10 s, it is concluded that the ulnar supply is adequate and that the radial artery can be punctured. Blood is collected in a heparinized syringe, which should not contain any air bubbles and should be sealed rapidly from the atmosphere. Analysis of the blood sample must be performed as quickly as possible. Capillary samples are useful when arterial puncture is impractical, especially in children. The ear lobe is often chosen. The region should be heated by warm compresses and lanced.

Commercially available instruments measure the partial oxygen pressure (P_{O2}), the partial carbon dioxide pressure (P_{CO2}) and the pH in arterial blood samples. Bicarbonate concentration and oxygen saturation of hemoglobin (Sa_{O2}) are calculated from these data. Calculated Sa_{O2} is acceptable only if the hemoglobin concentration is normal. Therefore, some devices also measure hemoglobin concentration and Sa_{O2} (57). Most of the time, these instruments provide a measurement of carboxyhemoglobin. This information is required for correct interpretation of the carbon monoxide diffusing capacity (see below).

Pulse oxymetry provides a non-invasive assessment of oxygen saturation (Sp_{O2}). Sp_{O2} estimates Sa_{O2} by analysing absorption of light passing through a capillary bed. The agreement of Sp_{O2} with Sa_{O2} is within 2% from 85% to 100% saturation but decreases below this value. Most pulse oxymeters use a sensor that attaches to the finger or ear lobe (58).

Acid–base Equilibrium (Table 8.1)

The measurement of the arterial pH assesses the acid–base equilibrium. In healthy adults, the pH averages 7.40, ranging from 7.38 to 7.42. Arterial pH below 7.38 defines acidemia. A pH above 7.42 defines alkalemia. Respiratory acid–base disorders are caused by changes in Pa_{CO2}: an increase in Pa_{CO2} induces a respiratory acidosis, a decrease in Pa_{CO2} provokes a respiratory alkalosis. Normal Pa_{CO2} ranges from 35 mmHg to 45 mmHg. Metabolic acid–base disorders are due to changes in bicarbonate concentration. A respiratory acid–base disorder can be compensated for by bicarbonate adaptation, and a metabolic acid–base disorder can be compensated for by ventilatory changes (2).

Hypercapnia and the related respiratory acidosis are the result of alveolar hypoventilation (8). The latter can be due to various neurologic or neuromuscular diseases affecting the respiratory pump. Alveolar hypoventilation can also be caused by an increase in the dead space–tidal volume ratio (V_D/V_T) (54). Conversely, respiratory alkalosis is due to hyperventilation as, for example, in hyperventilation syndrome (59). Metabolic acid–base disorders are beyond the scope of this chapter.

Table 8.1. Blood gas abnormalities

Hypoxemia: Pa_{O2} < 85 mmHg
(Ambient air and sea level conditions)
    Shunt or venous admixture: decreased Pa_{O2} + Pa_{CO2} (<130 mmHg)
    Alveolar hypoventilation: preserved Pa_{O2} + Pa_{CO2} (~130–140 mmHg)

Acidosis: pH < 7.38
    Respiratory: Pa_{CO2} > 45 mmHg (hypercapnia)
    Metabolic: HCO_3 < 25 mmol^{-1}

Alkalosis: pH > 7.42
    Respiratory: Pa_{CO2} < 35 mmHg
    Metabolic: HCO_3 27 mmol/L^{-1}

Hypoxemia (Table 8.1)

The Pa_{O2} of healthy adults at sea level varies from 85 to 100 mmHg. Hypoxemia is defined as a Pa_{O2} less than 85 mmHg (60). Hypoxemia etiologies are numerous. The most frequent mechanism is probably an abnormality of the ventilation–perfusion equilibrium resulting in venous admixture. Other possible causes include alterations of the alveolocapillary diffusing capacity, a right-to-left shunt or alveolar hypoventilation. In the case of pure alveolar hypoventilation, Pa_{O2} + Pa_{CO2} exceeds 130 mmHg (8). A right-to-left shunt can be differentiated from an increased venous admixture by inhalation of pure oxygen for 20 min or longer. If there is no true right-to left shunt, the Pa_{O2} under these conditions exceeds 550 mmHg. In other words, pure oxygen inhalation corrects hypoxemia caused by venous admixture. The blood gases collected in a subject breathing pure oxygen also permit an estimation of the right-to left shunt (2).

Assessment of Diffusing Capacity

Method

An alteration of the capacity of oxygen to diffuse across the alveolocapillary membrane can lead to hypoxemia. The diffusing capacity of the membrane is evaluated by using a small amount of carbon monoxide mixed with inspired air. Carbon monoxide diffuses from the alveoli to the bloodstream and then remains fixed by hemoglobin, hemoglobin's affinity for carbon monoxide being approximately 210 times higher than its affinity for oxygen (61).

The measurement of carbon monoxide diffusion can be performed during steady-state ventilation. However this method is poorly standardized and the results depend upon the ventilation–perfusion ratios. The most commonly used method is the single-breath, or breath-hold technique (61). At the end of a maximal expiration, the subject inspires, up to TLC, a gas mixture containing carbon monoxide in low concentration (0.3%), an inert gas not normally present in the body (for example 10% helium), 21% oxygen, and nitrogen. Then the subject holds her or his breath at TLC for approximately 10 s, during which carbon monoxide diffuses across the alveolocapillary membrane and the inert gas dilutes in the ventilated compartment of the lungs. At the end of this apnea, the expiratory gases are analyzed. The diffusing capacity, also called the transfer factor (T_{LCO}), is calculated from the measurement of the amount of expired carbon monoxide, when the amount of inhaled carbon monoxide is known. The lung volume investigated (V_A) is calculated from the dilution of the inert gas.

In fact this measurement tests the transfer mechanisms from the alveolar space to the complex with hemoglobin, thus including diffusion from the plasma to the red cell cytoplasm and then the kinetics of oxygen fixation by hemoglobin. Many determinants can therefore influence the diffusing capacity: the lung volume, the size of the exchange surface, the alveolocapillary membrane, the capillary volume, the concentration of hemoglobin, the distribution of the ventilation–perfusion ratios and the partial pressure of carbon monoxide in arterial blood (Pa_{CO}) at the beginning of the measurement (61). Tobacco consumption, for instance, can substantially increase Pa_{CO} and should be taken into account when calculating T_{LCO}. An arterial blood sample must be collected and Pa_{CO} measured before the assessment of T_{LCO}. T_{LCO} increases when the subject moves from the upright to the sitting position and from the sitting to the reclining position. Gas diffusion across the alveolocapillary membrane is better assessed by the transfer coefficient K_{CO}, the ratio of T_{LCO} to V_A ($K_{CO} = T_{LCO}/V_A$). K_{CO} is de facto less influenced than T_{LCO} by the exchange surface. The value of T_{LCO} or K_{CO} should also be interpreted according to hemoglobin concentration because anemia decreases T_{LCO} and polyglobulemia increases the diffusing capacity.

Significance of Diffusing Capacity

Measurement of T_{LCO} is an important step in pulmonary function testing. It is usually performed after the assessment of lung volumes in patients with suspected or confirmed disease of the lung parenchyma. The measurement of T_{LCO} is useful for both diagnosis and follow-up purposes. Numerous etiologies and various mechanisms can induce a decrease in T_{LCO} (62). T_{LCO} is reduced in interstitial fibrosis, pneumoconiosis, widespread granulomas, and pulmonary edema. Impairment of the alveolocapillary membrane probably explains the reduction of T_{LCO} in these diseases. Lung resection, for cancer or other reasons, typically results in decreased T_{LCO} but affects K_{CO} much less. T_{LCO} is also reduced in emphysema because of the destruction of the alveolocapillary membrane but in this example, K_{CO} is also decreased. Before CT scans became available, the diagnosis of emphysema relied on the combined poesence of an obstructive syndrome, decreased diffusing capacity, and increased pulmonary compliance (63). A decrease in T_{LCO} can also result from a mismatching of the ventilation–perfusion ratio. T_{LCO} can be diminished in pulmonary vascular disorders, including pulmonary hypertension. The ability of a decrease in T_{LCO} to predict oxygen desaturation during exercise remains controversial (32).

T_{LCO} can be augmented in some circumstances. T_{LCO} can be increased in asthma, in some bronchiectasis and in the very early stages of congestive heart failure. T_{LCO} is also increased in intrapulmonary hemorrhage because carbon monoxide combines with intraalveolar hemoglobin (62).

Exercise Testing

Method

Exercise testing has various purposes: unmasking hypoxemia, quantifying dyspnea, assessing effort limitation factors, either ventilatory, cardiovascular or peripheral (deconditioning), and measuring oxygen consumption and metabolic demand .

During an exercise test, the patient performs a quantified amount of work. This workload is standardized by using a treadmill or a cycle. Blood samples are collected during the test for blood gas determination and the inspiratory and expiratory fractions of oxygen and carbon dioxide can be measured, breathing cycle by breathing cycle, with fast analyzers, although values averaged over several respiratory cycles are quite sufficient in practice. These measurements allow the calculation of oxygen consumption and of carbon dioxide production. Electrocardiogram, blood pressure, and pulse oxymetry must be monitored during the duration of the test.

Major contraindications to exercise testing include: severe hypoxemia in room air, Pa_{CO2} greater than 70 mmHg, FEV_1 less than 30% of predicted, recent (within 4 weeks) myocardial infarction, unstable angina pectoris, second- or third-degree heart block, rapid ventricular or atrial arrhythmia, orthopedic impairment, severe aortic stenosis, congestive heart failure, uncontrolled hypertension, limiting neurologic disorders, dissecting or ventricular aneurysm, severe pulmonary hypertension, thrombophlebitis or intracardiac thrombi, recent systemic or pulmonary embolus, and acute pericarditis (32).

Goals of Exercise Testing

Unmasking hypoxemia is one of the main goals of exercise testing (64). Effort-related desaturation can be due to a decrease in diffusing capacity. It can be observed in emphysema and in interstitial pneumonia and requires further investigation.

Exercise testing also permits assessment of dyspnea. During the test, breathlessness is quantified by using either a visual analog scale or a "Borg-type" scale (65). The test discriminates between respiratory, cardiovascular, and peripheral causes of dyspnea.

Measurement of exhaled gases during exercise allows a noninvasive estimate of the anerobic threshold, also called the ventilatory threshold. The anerobic threshold can be determined by plotting oxygen consumption against carbon dioxide production during exercise of increasing intensity (66). The anerobic threshold is identified by the inflection point of this curve, indicating an abrupt increase in carbon dioxide production. The cardiac frequency corresponding to the anerobic threshold provides the guidance parameter for pulmonary rehabilitation programs. This frequency should be reached but not surpassed during training to ensure that the patient is trained at her or his maximum aerobic level (67).

Conclusion

The information provided by pulmonary function tests should be part of a global strategy of diagnosis, including clinical, radiologic and biologic approaches. The strategy of pulmonary function testing should follow a logical pattern such as that suggested in Figure 8.6. Patient cooperation is required for most of these tests. Because they are mostly noninvasive they can easily be repeated, but many of these tests may prove to be quite exhausting for very sick patients, limiting the feasibility and the reproducibility required for good laboratory practice. Finally interpretation of pulmonary function tests is, needless to say, best performed when both clinical and thorax imaging data are provided to the investigator.

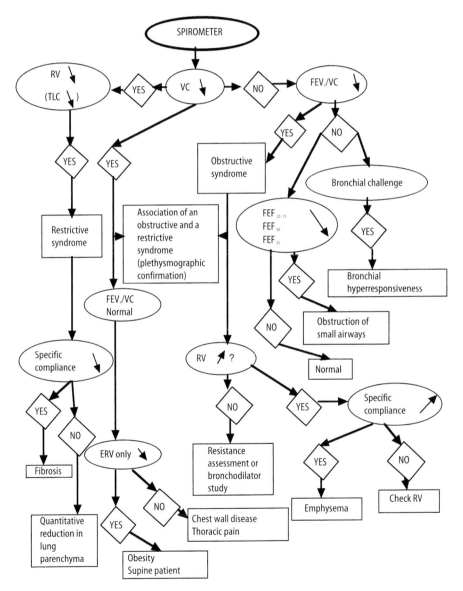

Figure 8.6. Schematic strategy of interpretation of a spirometric investigation. *VC*, vital capacity; *FEV$_1$*, forced expiratory volume in 1s; *RV*, residual volume; *TLC*, total lung capacity; *ERV*, expiratory reserve volume. *FEF$_{25}$* etc., forced expiratory flow at 25% of FVC etc. (from ref. 68, with permission.

References

1. Quanjer PH, Tammeling GJ, Cotes JE, et al. (1993) Lung volumes and forced ventilatory flows. Eur Respir J 6(suppl. 16):15–40.
2. West JB (1990) Respiratory physiology. The essentials, 4th edn. Williams and Wilkins, Baltimore, MD.
3. Becklake MR, Permut S (1979) Evaluation of tests of lung function for "screening" for early detection of chronic obstructive lung disease. In P.T. Macklem and S. Permut (eds) The lung in the transition between health end disease. Marcel Dekker, New York, pp 345–387.
4. Brulot N, Kadas V, Grassino A, et al. (1992) Positional variation in lung volumes in COPD. Am Rev Respir Dis 145:A764.
5. ATS (1995) Standardization of spirometry, 1994 update. Am J Respir Crit Care Med 152:1107–1136.
6. ATS (1991) Lung function testing: Selection of reference values and interpretative strategies. Am Rev Respir Dis 144:1202–1218.
7. Hutchinson J (1846) On the capacity of the lungs, and on the respiratory movements, with the view of establishing a precise and easy method of detecting disease by the spirometer. Lancet i:630–632.
8. Derenne J-P (1981) Physiologie et exploration fonctionnelle respiratoires. In Encyclopédie de Medico-Chirurgicale, Poumon. Elsevier, Paris, pp 6000 A6070–6000 A6090.
9. Hyatt RE, Black LF (1973) The flow–volume curve. A current perspective. Am Rev Respir Dis 107:191–199.
10. Knudson RJ, Slatin RC, Lebowitz MD, et al. (1976) The maximal expiratory flow–volume curve. Normal standards, variability, and effects of age. Am Rev Respir Dis 113:587–600.
11. Leff AR, Schumacker PT (1993) Respiratory physiology. Basics and applications. WB Saunders, Philadelphia.
12. Pride NB, Permut S, Riley RL, et al. (1967) Determinants of maximum expiratory flow from the lungs. J Appl Physiol 23:646–662.
13. Chan ED, Irvin CG (1995) The detection of collapsible airways contributing to airflow limitation. Chest 107:856–859.
14. Bass H (1973) The flow volume loop: Normal standards and abnormalities in chronic obstructive pulmonary disease. Chest 63:171–176.
15. Hathirat S, Renaetti AD, Jr, Mitchell M (1970) Measurement of the total lung capacity by helium dilution in a constant volume system. Am Rev Respir Dis 102:760–770.
16. Darling RC, Cournanad A, Richards DW, Jr (1940) Studies on intrapulmonary mixture of gases. Open circuit methods for measuring residual air. J Clin Invest 19:609–618.
17. DuBois AB, Botelho SY, Bedell GN, et al. (1956) A rapid plethysmographic method for measuring thoracic gas volume. A comparison with a nitrogen wash-out method for measuring functional residual capacity. J Clin Invest 35:322–326.
18. Mead J (1960) Volume displacement body plethysmograph for measurements on human subjects. J Appl Physiol 15:736–740.
19. Rodenstein DO, Stanescu DC, Francis C (1982) Demonstration of failure of body plethysmography in airway obstruction. J Appl Physiol 52:949–954.
20. Rodenstein DO, Stanescu DC (1982) Reassessment of lung volume measurement by helium dilution and by body plethysmography in chronic air-flow obstruction. Am Rev Respir Dis 126:1040–1044.
21. DuBois AB, Botelho SY, Comroe JH, Jr (1956) A new method for measuring airway resistance in a man using a body plethysmograph: Values in normal subjects and in patients with respiratory disease. J Clin Invest 35:327–335.
22. Desager KN, Buhr W, Willemen M, et al. (1991) Measurement of total respiratory impedance in infants by the forced oscillation technique. J Appl Physiol 71:770–776.
23. Cockcroft DW, Hargreave FE (1990) Airway responsiveness. Relevance of random population data to clinical usefulness. Am Rev Respir Dis 142:497–500.
24. Cockcroft DW, Murdock KY, Berscheid BA, et al. (1992) Sensitivity and specificity of histamine PC20 determination in a random selection of young college students. J Allergy Clin Immunol 89:23–30.
25. Britton J (1988) Is hyperreactivity the same as asthma? Eur Respir J 1:478–479.
26. Backer V, Groth S, Dirksen A, et al. (1991) Sensitivity and specificity of the histamine challenge test for the diagnosis of asthma in an unselected sample of children and adolescents. Eur Respir J 4:1093–1100.
27. Sterk PJ, Fabbri LM, Quanjer PH, et al. (1993) Airway responsiveness. Standardized challenge testing with pharmacological, physical and sensitizing stimuli in adults. Eur Respir J 6(suppl. 16):53–83.
28. Tantucci C, Duguet A, Similowski T, et al. (1998) Effect of salbutamol on dynamic hyperinflation in chronic obstructive pulmonary disease patients. Eur Respir J 12:799–804.
29. O'Donnell DE, Lam M, Webb KA (1998) Measurement of symptoms, lung hyperinflation, and endurance during exercise in chronic obstructive pulmonary disease. Am J Respir Crit Care Med 158:1557–1565.
30. O'Donnell DE, Lam M, Webb KA (1999) Spirometric correlates of improvement in exercise performance after anticholinergic therapy in chronic obstructive pulmonary disease. Am J Respir Crit Care Med 160:542–549.
31. Rodarte JR, Hyatt RE, Cortese DA (1975) Influence of expiratory flow on closing capacity at low expiratory flow rates. J Appl Physiol 39:60–65.
32. Ruppel GL (1998) Manual of pulmonary function testing, 7th edn. Mosby, Saint Louis, MO.
33. ATS (1995) Standards for the diagnosis and care of patients with chronic obstructive pulmonary disease. Am J Respir Crit Care Med 152:S77–S121.
34. Ulmer W, Kowalski J, Schmidt EW (1997) The flow–volume curve in patients with obstructive airway diseases. Partial analysis and functional importance. Pneumonol Alergol Pol 65:435–445.
35. O'Donnell DE, Webb KA (1992) Breathlessness in patients with severe chronic airflow limitation. Physiologic correlations. Chest 102:824–831.
36. Yernault JC, Englert M (1974) Static mechanical lung properties in young adults. Bull Eur Physiopathol Respir 10:435–450.
37. Rahn H, Otis AB, Chadwick L, et al. (1946) The pressure–volume diagram of the thorax and lung. Am J Physiol 146:161–178.
38. Turner JM, Mead J, Wohl ME (1968) Elasticty of human lung in relation to age. J Appl Physiol 25:664–671.
39. Dekhuijzen PNR, Decramer M (1992) Steroid-induced myopathy and its significance to respiratory disease: A known disease rediscovered. Eur Respir J 5:997–1003.
40. Agostoni E, Rahn H (1960) Abdominal and thoracic pressures at different lung volumes. J Appl Physiol 15:1087–1092.
41. Similowski T, Yan S, Gauthier AP, et al. (1991) Contractile properties of the human diaphragm during chronic hyperinflation. N Engl J Med 325:917–923.
42. Similowski T, Fleury B, Launois S, et al. (1989) Cervical magnetic stimulation: A new and painless method for bilateral phrenic nerve stimulation in conscious humans. J Appl Physiol 67:1311–1318.
43. Yan S, Gauthier AP, Similowski T, et al. (1992) Evaluation of human diaphragm contractility using mouth pressure twitches. Am Rev Respir Dis 145:1064–1069.
44. Feldman JL, Smith JC (1995) Neural control of respiratory pattern in mammals: An overview. In Dempsey JA and Pack AI (eds) Regulation of breathing. Marcel Dekker, New York, pp 39–70.
45. Fitzgerald RS, Lahiri S (1986) Reflex response to chemoreceptor stimulation. In Geiger SR, Widdicombe JG, Cherniack NS, Fishman AP (eds) Handbook of physiology. Section 3: The respiratory system. American Physiological Society, Bethesda, MD, pp 313–362.
46. Derenne J-P (1977) Méthodes d'investigation clinique des mécanismes régulateurs de la ventilation. Bull Europ Physiopath Resp 13:681–727.

47. Derenne J-P, Couture J, Iscoe S, et al. (1976) Occlusion pressure in man rebreathing CO_2 under methoxyflurane anesthesia. J Appl Physiol 40:805–814.

48. Whitelaw WA, Derenne JP, Milic-Emili J (1976) Occlusion pressure as a measure of respiratory centre output in conscious man. Respir Physiol 23:181–199.

49. Whitelaw WA, Derenne J-P (1993) Airway occlusion pressure. J Appl Physiol 74:1475–1483.

50. Fenn WO, Craig AB (1963) Effect of CO_2 on respiration using a new method of administering CO_2. J Appl Physiol 18:1023–1024.

51. Read DJC (1967) A clinical method for assessing the ventilatory response to carbon dioxide. Austr Ann Med 16:20–32.

52. Dejours P, Labrousse Y, Raynaud J, et al. (1957) Stimulus oxygène chémo-réflexe de la ventiation à basse altitude (50 m) chez l'homme. I. Au repos. J. Physiol. (Paris) 49:115–120.

53. Rebuck AS, Campbell EJM (1973) A clinical method for assessing the ventilatory response to hypoxia. Am Rev Respir Dis 109:345–350.

54. Krachman S, Criner GJ (1998) Hypoventilation syndromes. Clin Chest Med 19:139–155.

55. Spinelli A, Marconi G, Gorini M, et al. (1992) Control of breathing in patients with myasthenia gravis. Am Rev Respir Dis 145:1359–1365.

56. Scano G, Gigliotti F, Duranti R, et al. (1993) Control of breathing in patients with neuromuscular diseases. Monaldi Arch Chest Dis 48:87–91.

57. AARC (1993) In-vitro pH and blood gas analysis and hemoximetry. Respir Care 38:505–510.

58. Severinghaus JW, Kelleher JF (1992) Recent developments in pulse oximetry. Anesthesiology 76:1018–1038.

59. Gardner NG (1996) The pathophysiology of hyperventilation disorders. Chest 109:516–534.

60. Delclaux B, Orcel B, Housset B, et al. (1994) Arterial blood gases in elderly persons with chronic obstructive pulmonary disease (COPD). Eur Respir J 7:856–861.

61. Forster RE (1987) Diffusion of gases across the alveolar membrane. In Fahri LF, Tenney SM (eds) Handbook of physiology: The respiratory system. Section 3: Gas exchange. American Physiological Society, Bethesda, MD, pp 71–88.

62. Cotes JE, Chinn DJ, Quanjer PH, et al. (1993) Standardization of the measurement of transfer factor (diffusing capacity). Eur Respir J 6 (suppl. 16):41–52.

63. Yernault JC, Paiva M (1986) In vivo diagnosis of pulmonary emphysema: An uncompletely resolved issue. Bull Eur Physiopathol Respir 22:95–97.

64. AARC (1992) Clinical practice guideline: Exercise testing for evaluation of hypoxemia and/or desaturation. Respir Care 37:907–912.

65. Hansen JE (1984) Exercise instruments, schemes, and protocols for evaluating the dyspneic patient. Am Rev Respir Dis 129(Suppl):S25–S27.

66. Wasserman K (1984) The anaerobic threshold measurement in exercise testing. Clin Chest Med 5:77–88.

67. ACCP/AACVPR (1997) Pulmonary rehabilitation. Joint ACCP/-AACVPR evidence-based guidelines. Chest 112:1363–1396.

68. Straus C, Zelter M (2000) Sémiologie Fonctionnelle. In Huchon G (ed) Pneumologie pour le practicien. Masson, Paris, in press.

Bronchoscopy and Surgical Procedures for Inspection and Biopsy

M. Riquet and P. Reynaud

Introduction

Histologic or cytologic examinations of representative specimens are necessary for the diagnosis and treatment of many chest diseases. During the 1990s, new procedures and adaptations of already existing techniques emerged that are very important in cases when radiologic diagnosis alone is not sufficient. Some of those new techniques may be performed by qualified radiologists or greatly helped by a participation of radiologists in the procedures.

Bronchoscopy

Rigid Bronchoscopy

Rigid Bronchoscopy is still widely used in the extraction of foreign bodies if they cannot be removed under flexible fiberoptic bronchoscopy. The laser removal of obstructive tracheobronchial tumors, the recalibration of tracheal stenoses, and the placement of tracheobronchial prostheses are also performed with rigid bronchoscopy (1).

Flexible or Fiberoptic Bronchoscopy

Fiberoptic bronchoscopy is used in most diagnostic endoscopic procedures.

Bacterial Infections

To obtain good-quality endobronchial bacteriologic specimens a bronchoscopic protected brush (BPB) doubly protected in two catheters is necessary. The distal end is occluded with a silicone plug. When the end of the catheter is placed in a distal bronchus the brush is pushed forward in the bronchial lumen and then replaced in its sheath, thus avoiding the risk of contamination by the oropharyngeal flora (2).

Histologic Diagnosis

When they are proximal, endobronchial lesions are easily accessible for biopsy, and specimens may be taken with various types of biopsy forceps (simple or window-cupped forceps, serrated jaws). Diagnostic yield depends on the number of biopsies taken (3). In the case of distal lesions that cannot be reached by direct-vision biopsy, washings and brushings may sometimes provide material for a histologic diagnosis.

Transbronchial biopsies (TBB) are required for distal lesions but their diameter must be greater than 2 cm; the biopsy forceps are guided under fluoroscopic control. If the specimens are negative, a transparietal puncture should be made under the control of computed tomography (CT). In lung transplant recipients, an early rejection and the presence of bronchiolitis obliterans can be detected with TBB. This technique is also useful in cases of diffuse disorders, interstitial fibrosis, sarcoidosis, lymphangitis carcinomatosa, and bronchioalveolar carcinoma.

Complications of TBB – the development of a pneumothorax or a severe hemorrhage – are possible.

Bacterial Infections and Histologic Diagnosis

Bronchoalveolar lavage (BAL) may produce some useful findings: inflammatory, immunocompetent or tumoral cells, and mineral particles. This procedure includes the injection of 150–300 mL of sterile saline solution in a segmental bronchus, followed by the collection of residual fluids by careful aspiration. The percentage of recovered fluids is approximately 60–80% of the amount injected. The most appropriate territories are the middle lobe and the lingula (4). The BAL technique permits study of the alveolar cell population. Opportunistic microorganisms, especially *Pneumocystis carinii*, viruses, fungi, atypic mycobacteria, and *Mycobacterium tuberculosis* should be systematically looked for in all immunocompromised patients with pulmonary infection. They may be transplant recipients (5), or patients with acquired immune deficiency syndrome (AIDS) (6,7). This lavage technique helps in the diagnosis of interstitial lung diseases; when associated with multiple biopsies of bronchial segments, with TBB it contributes to the diagnosis of sarcoidosis in approximately 90% of cases. BAL is also used to confirm pulmonary alveolar proteinosis (8).

Rigid and/or Flexible Bronchoscopy Permits Other Procedures

Autofluorescence Endoscopy

This is a technique with which bronchial carcinoma in situ or precancerous lesions may be detected (9). It is reserved to patients at risk, especially heavy smokers. Anomalies are easily visible as areas in which the color of the bronchial mucosa is in contrast with the rest. Directed biopsies give good results in carcinoma in situ, but poor ones in cases of a simple mucosal dysplasia (10).

Photodynamic Therapy

A hematoporphyrin derivative (in most cases, photofrin) preferentially absorbed by cancerous lesions, is injected intravenously the day before the procedure. The area to be treated is illuminated by a dye laser, which induces necrosis of the neoplastic tissues. This technique is reserved for second-line treatment, if a previously treated tumoral lesion has recurred (11).

Cryotherapy (12)

An electrode is placed in contact with an endobronchial tumor. The distal end is cooled down to –180 °C to freeze the tumor in prolonged contact. Cryotherapy may be applied to ambulatory patients and costs less than laser treatment, but this procedure lasts a long time and its response is delayed. Laser therapy is therefore still preferable in cases of very large tumors or very obstructive tracheal lesions.

Brachytherapy

In this technique tumors inaccessible to surgery are irradiated endoluminally by a catheter containing the radioactive source (iridium-192) (13), which is placed in front of the lesion. The doses delivered are greater than those administered externally (14). This technique is more palliative than curative. The association between brachytherapy and chemotherapy is better tolerated than when the chemotherapy is administered at the same time as external radiotherapy (15). In a study of 149 patients treated by brachytherapy, for 73 it was a curative treatment, for 47 a palliative treatment, and 27 also received external radiotherapy. Two months after the end of the treatment, the endoscopic control showed histologic remissions in 64 cases, whilst the symptoms of 79% of the patients were improved (16).

Laser Therapy

Laser, especially neodymium: yttrium-aluminium-garnet (Nd: YAG) has transformed interventional endoscopy. This technique is now quite commonly used to treat endoscopically most tracheal stenoses and nonsurgical tracheal cancers. To avoid a recurrence of the stenosis, however, it is highly recommended to put in place a tracheobronchial prosthesis (17).

Radiofrequency Resection

This technique is used in the excision of endotracheal tumors through coagulation and vaporization of tumoral tissues. In a study of 98 patients, results were deemed satisfactory in 66% of the cases (recalibration >80%), partial in 21.5% (recalibration >50%); failure was observed in 12.5% of these patients (18).

Endobronchial Ultrasound

This modality is presently under evaluation. In this technique an ultrasonography probe is introduced into the operating canal of the endoscope. It permits detection of lymph nodes or other peribronchial masses. Good results may also be obtained from diagnostic punctures made under ultrasonographic control (19).

Video Bronchoscopy

Videoendocopy has been recently introduced into pneumology. Conventional fiberoptics are replaced by a distal camera; digital signals are sent directly to a high definition monitor. The quality of images is higher than that obtained with regular fiberoptic bronchoscopy. The whole investigation and the performed procedures may be recorded and photographs may be taken. This facilitates the discussions between physicians and surgeons, thus allowing the decision-making process to be based on concrete results.

Transesophageal Echography

Transesophageal echocardiography (TEE) or endoscopic ultrasonography of the esophagus appeared in the late 1980s and was widely developed during the 1990s in the field of inspection and biopsy of thoracic diseases: esophageal tumors and compressions, detection of mediastinal and vascular lesions in trauma patients, preoperative staging of nonsmall-cell lung cancers and diagnosis of posterior mediastinal tumors.

TEE employs a modified endoscope with an ultrasound probe at its tip. The instrument is passed through the tumor into the stomach and scanning performed as the probe is withdrawn. Problems occur when the endoscope cannot pass the structure, but the advent of catheter echoprobes that pass down the biopsy channel of a conventional endoscope has helped to solve this problem. It is possible to visualize five to seven alternating hyper- and hypoechoic layers of the esophageal wall (20):

1. The interface between the probe and the mucosa: hyperechoic
2. The mucosa muscularis mucosa: hypoechoic
3. The submucosa: hyperechoic
4. The muscularis propria (circular muscle layer): hypoechoic
5. The connective tissue between the two muscles layers of the muscularis propria: hyperechoic
6. The muscularis propria: hypoechoic (longitudinal muscle layer)
7. The serosa adventitia: hyperechoic

TEE provides an accurate diagnosis for submucosal tumors and enables determin of the layer of origin, the direction of growth, and the consistency of the tumor; TEE can also detect the structure from which an external compression comes (20). Invasion of the esophagus from an adjacent tumor can also be observed.

TEE is useful in the preoperative staging of carcinoma of the esophagus to define extension through the layer of the esophagus, extension to the adjacent organs and involvement of the lymph nodes (21). The sensitivity, specificity, positive predictive value and negative predictive value for the N factor of the TNM classification assessment by TEE approaches 70% (12). Specifically, typical features of malignant lymph nodes include a hypoechoic appearance, which is fairly uniform with smooth borders and a round shape, whereas most of the benign lymph nodes appear either crescent or triangular in shape and not round with homogeneous or centrally echogenic pattern (23). Size alone does not allow differentiation of malignant from benign nodes (24).

The best approach to diagnosing malignancy of the mediastinal nodes was developed in preoperative staging of nonsmall-cell lung cancer by using transesophageal ultrasound-guided fine needle aspiration biopsy (25–27).

Because it gives access to posterior mediastinal or subcarinal lymphnodes, TEE is complementary to mediastinoscopy when staging N in lung cancer and may compete with video-assisted thoracoscopy; both techniques are studied further below. TEE is not only useful in diagnosing with accuracy N status in lung cancer but it also provides indications of the respectability of centrally located tumors invading the esophagus, the aorta, and the heart (28, 29), and enable judging of the effect of treatments at those levels when neoadjuvant therapy has been used.

Owing to the presence of the trachea in the upper part and of the heart in the lower part of the mediastinum, TEE does not permit the exploration of the anterior mediastinum. However, it may be useful as a safe bedside procedure that is excellent for evaluating the superior vena cava and its surrounding structures and in demonstrating the mechanism of superior vena cava syndrome and thus help the physician to choose appropriate management (30). Allowing visualization and biopsy of tumors surrounding the esophagus, TEE is also useful in diagnosing posterior and inferior middle mediastinal masses (31–33), yielding a good sensitivity (89%) and specificity (83%) and presenting as a safe procedure (33).

It is a procedure largely used in cardiology and in cardiac surgery and is very helpful in managing aortic and mediastinal trauma, which is without the scope of this chapter but we will finish this paragraph by stressing it usefulness in assessing vascular anastomoses in lung transplantation (34) and in aiding localization and ensuring complete surgical ligation in arteriovenous malformations (35).

Mediastinoscopy

Cervical mediastinoscopy (CM) was the first surgical procedure (36) for inspection and biopsy in chest disease. CM allows one to obtain tissue material necessary to accurately diagnose the nature of mediastinal lymph nodes whereas CT only suggests malignancy and position emission tomography (PET) permits only confirmation of it without giving further histology. CM is a highly efficient procedure with a global sensitivity of 94%, a global specificity of 100% and an accuracy of 95% when used to diagnose lymphadenopathy (37). Mortality is almost nil and morbidity is low, but the ever-prevent risk of major blood vessel injury dictates that the procedure be performed by a surgical team prepared for the rare necessity of emergency sternotomy.

Recently mediastinoscopy has been incorporated into video surgery and new kind of mediastinocope has been fitted with a video camera (Storz 10970 BV) so as to allow visual documentation for the whole operating team and a more complete and accurate surgical performance (38).

Contrary to what has been widely suggested, CM is a safe and effective technique for establishing histologic diagnosis in superior vena cava obstruction when less invasive techniques have been unsuccessful (39). Cervical arthritis preventing adequate extension of the neck and rendering CM physically impossible remains the only but very rare contraindication. The use of CM remains questionable in cases of tracheostomy.

CM may also be useful in the management of a few tumors of the mediastinum. It permits removal of mediastinal cysts (40) and permits diagnosis and/or removal of tumors located in the anterior mediastinum. In some cases the cervical approach may be replaced by a subxiphoidal approach with good diagnostic access (41).

Nowadays one major indication for mediastinal lymph node biopsy by CM is pretreatment staging of lung cancer specifically targeted to the N factor of the TNM classification (42). Since its introduction as work-up tool in the 60s, CM demonstrating N2 disease has for a long time been interpreted as synonymous of inoperability. However the 5 year survival rate in case of resected N2 disease can approach more than 20%, the prognostic value being influenced only by the number of N2 lymph node anatomic chains involved by the carcinoma (43). It is important to histologically establish pretreatment N2 status before neoadjuvant treatment. Such treatment may be indicated in any respectable N2 lung cancer in order to improve long-term prognosis or may be a solution for unresectable N2 lung cancers in order to try to render some of them respectable, offering then a chance of cure. Unresectability is estimated mainly by CT and any thoracic surgeon with expertise in this field is able to determine the surgical possibilities in consultation with radiologists. Further studies are required to assess the benefits to be obtained by combined medical and surgical treatment in N2 diseases. CM is necessary to be certain of the histologic metastatic status of mediastinal adenopathies and nodes before medical treatment is decided. CM has a few more advantages: it may be used as a routine outpatient procedure (44) and may be repeated with success (45).

A disadvantage of mediastinoscopy is the incompleteness of mediastinal N staging. The only nodes accessible to CM are the paratracheal (levels 2, 3, and 4) and the

subcarinal nodes (level 7) in their anterior part. Further techniques such as extended cervical mediastinoscopy (46) or left parasternal anterior mediastinotomy (47) are required to biopsy nodes located on the left, preaortic (level 6) or aortopulmonary (level 5). Posterior subcarinal nodes (level 7) and esophageal nodes (level 8), as well as pulmonary ligament nodes (level 9), are unreachable. Video-assisted thorascopy, which is considered in the next section is a key for complete staging in such cases.

CM should remain the first mode of mediastinal biopsy before physicians resort to extended techniques.

Thoracoscopy and Video-Assisted Thoracoscopy

Thoracoscopy allows the visualization of the visceral and parietal pleura, the pericardium, the diaphragm and the superior sulcus. It allows deep pleural biopsies and pleurodesis. This procedure has been known since the beginning of the nineteenth century. During the 1990s, video-assisted thoracoscopy (VAT) was developed and this thoracoscopic approach is now employed for inspection and biopsy. VAT requires general anesthesia and one-lung ventilation, and the ability to perform a thoracotomy at any time if needed.

In cases that are not suitable for such a surgical approach, thoracoscopy, i.e., nonVAT, is still an important procedure in pleural pathology (48) and permits many therapeutic applications (49).

VAT compares with nonvideo-assisted thoracoscopy as regards the pleura but permits numerous surgical procedures in respect of the lungs: we now survey the most frequent ones.

In the diagnosis of interstitial lung disease, video-thoracoscopic lung biopsy is a safe and efficient procedure (50,51). Such a diagnostic procedure may be used to intervene only when bronchoscopy, transbronchial biopsies, BAL and CT have failed to yield a diagnosis. Percutaneous cutting-needle biopsy is not recommended in diffuse infiltrative lung disease because of its reported high morbidity relative to its low diagnostic yield (52). The advantage of VAT over open lung biopsy by standard thoracotomy is to offer the possibility of choosing the biopsy sites after careful inspection of the lung surface and, when intraoperative findings are lacking, to target biopsies on chest CT scan abnormalities. However, techniques of cutting-needle biopsy are evolving and will perhaps offer a relatively safe alternative to thoracoscopic lung biopsy in carefully selected patients (52).

In the diagnosis of both benign and malignant peripheral nodules, VAT permits the resection of the lesion and, if benign, its treatment by removal. It competes with percutaneous transthoracic needle aspiration and seems more efficient in cases of benign disease. However, the accuracy and safety of peripheral nodule biopsy have increased owing to improvement in imaging techniques, the use of smaller needles and progress in cytopathologic and histologic interpretation of the obtained material (53). The use of new instruments and methods has improved the quality of the results obtained (53,54). VAT is theorically advised for patients with solitary pulmonary nodules and adequate physiologic reserve (55), but it should also be considered in patients with severe emphysema (56). It is always preferable, to reduce risks, to perform VAT in a thoracic surgery unit. When lung nodules are too small or too deeply located beneath the visceral pleura, it may be helpful to localize them before VAT by CT-guided percutaneous placement of spring hookwires (57). The need for such localization is questionable and denied by some authors (58,59). Indications for preoperative marking should be considered when the distance to the nearest pleural surface is >5 mm in the case of lung nodules <10 mm in size (60). In the diagnosis and staging of lung cancer, VAT is indicated for nodal or tumoral lesions that are not within the reach of the mediastinoscope or when multiple biopsy specimens are necessary (61,62), as we have already mentioned. It is useful to determinate with more accuracy stage IIIA (N2 disease: levels 5, 6, 4L, 7 posterior, 8, and 9) but also stage IIIB (63). VAT will prove unavoidable in the future prior to neoadjuvant treatment when managing lung cancer, for accurate histologic diagnosis and staging.

Finally, VAT is an effective and reliable method of obtaining a diagnosis not only of adenopathy but also of solitary mediastinal lesions not within reach of the mediastinoscope (64). In some cases it allows the complete excision of the mass (65) and such excision is all the more easy when the mass is of moderate size (66) and cystic in nature.

References

1. Colt HG, Dumon JF (1991) Lasers and endoprosthesis in bronchopneumology. Rev Pneumol Clin 47(2):65–73.
2. Pollock HM, Hawkins EL, Bonner JR, et al. (1983) Diagnosis of bacterial pulmonary infections with quantitative protected catheter cultures obtained during bronchoscopy. J Clin Microbiol 17:255–259.
3. Popovich J, Kvake P, Eichenhorn M, et al. (1982) Diagnostic accuracy of multiple biopsies from flexible fiberoptic bronchoscopy. Am Rev Respir Dis 125:521–523.
4. European Society of Pneumology Task Group on BAL (1989) Technical recommendations and guidelines for bronchoalveolar lavage. Report. Eur Respir J 2:561–585.
5. Tiroke AH, Bewing B, Haverich A (1999) Bronchoalveolar lavage in lung transplantation. State of the art. Clin Transplant 13:131–157.
6. Raoof S, Rosen MJ, Khan FA (1999) Role of bronchoscopy in AIDS. Clin Chest Med 20:63–76.
7. Mylonakis E, Barlam TF, Flanigan T, et al. (1999) Pulmonary aspergillosis and invasive disease in AIDS: Review of 342 cases. Chest 114:251–262.
8. Martin J, Coalson JJ, Rogers RM (1980) Pulmonary alveolar proteinosis: The diagnosis by segmental lavage. Am Rev Respir Dis 121:819.
9. Lam S, Kenedy T, Unger M, et al. (1998) Localisation of bronchial intraepithelial neoplastic lesions by fluorescence bronchoscopy. Chest 113:696–702.
10. Masatoshi K, Kim Kyong IL, Tetsuya O, et al. (1999) Early detection of bronchial lesions using system of autofluorescence endoscopy. Diagn Therapeut Endosc 5:99–104.
11. Dougherty TJ, Gomer CJ, Henderson BW, et al. (1998) Photodynamic therapy. J Natl Cancer Inst 90:889–905.
12. Maiwand MO, Homasson JP (1995) Cryotherapy for tracheobronchial disorders. Clin Chest Med 16:427–443.
13. Macha HN, Freitag L (1996) The role of brachytherapy in the treatment and control of central bronchial carcinoma. Monaldi Arch Chest Dis 51:325–328.
14. Hillerdal G (1997) Photodynamic therapy, laser therapy, brachytherapy, stents. Local control of lung cancer. Lakarttidningen 94:2377–2379.
15. Hilaris BS, Mastoras DA (1998) Contemporary brachytherapy approaches in non-small-cell lung cancer. J Surg Oncol 69:258–264.
16. Tredaniel J, Hennequin C, Zalcman G, et al. (1997) Intrabronchial curietherapy. Experience at Hôpital Saint-Louis after the treatment of 149 patients. Rev Mal Respir 14:465–472.
17. Schmidt B, Witt C (1998) Endoscopic interventions in the tracheobronchial system. Zentralbl Chir 123:1134–1139.
18. Marasso A, Bernardi V, Gai R, et al. (1998) Radiofrequency resection of bronchial tumours in combination with cryotherapy: Evaluation of a new technique. Thorax 53:106–109.
19. John J, Shannon RO, Bude JB, et al. (1996) Endobronchial ultrasound-guided needle aspiration of mediastinal adenopathy. Am J Respir Crit Care Med 153:1424–1430.
20. Silva SA, Kouzu T, Ogino Y, et al. (1988) Endoscopic ultrasonography of esophageal tumors and compressions. J Clin Ultrasound 16:149–157.
21. Vilgrain V, Mompoint D, Palazzo L, et al. (1990) Staging of esophageal carcinoma: Comparison of results with endoscopic sonography and CT. AJR 155:277–281.
22. Rice TW, Boyce GA, Sivak MV, et al. (1991) Esophageal ultrasound and the preoperative staging of carcinoma of the esophagus. J Thorac. Cardiovasc. Surg 101:536–544.
23. Wiersema MJ, Hassing WM, Hawes RH, et al. (1993) Mediastinal lymph node detection with endosonography. Gastrointest Endosc 39:788–793.
24. Arita J, Matsumoto T, Kuramitsu I, et al. (1996) Is it possible to differentiate malignant mediastinal nodes from benign nodes by size? Reevaluation by CT, transesophageal echocardiophy and nodal specimen. Chest 110:1004–1008.
25. Wiersema MJ, Kochman ML, Cramer HM, et al. (1994) Preoperative staging of non-small cell lung cancer: Transesophageal US-guided fine-needle aspiration biopsy of mediastinal lymph nodes. Radiology 190:239–242.
26. Silvestri GA, Hoffman BJ, Bhutani MS, et al. (1996) Endoscopic ultrasound with fine-needle aspiration in the diagnosis and staging of lung cancer. Ann Thorac Surg 61:1441–1446.
27. Gress FG, Savides TJ, Sandler A, et al. (1997) Endoscopic ultrasonography, fine-needle aspiration biopsy guided by endoscopic ultrasonography, and computed tomography in the preoperative staging of non small cell lung cancer: A comparison study. Ann. Intern Med 127:604–612.
28. Riquet M, Palazzo L, Saab M, et al. (1992) Bilan d'opérabilité du cancer du poumon: Intérêt de l'échoendoscopie. Presse Med 21:1774–1775.
29. Heslin MJ, Casper ES, Boland P, et al. (1998) Preoperative identification and operative management of intra-atrial extension of lung tumors. Ann Thorac Surg 65:544–546.

30. Ayala K, Chandrasekaran K, Karalis DG, et al. (1992) Diagnosis of superior vena caval obstruction by transesophageal echocardiography. Chest 101:874–876.

31. Rex DK, Tarver RD, Wiersema M, et al. (1991) Endoscopic transoesophageal fine needle aspiration of mediastinal masses. Gastrointest. Endosc; 37:465–468.

32. Pedersen BH, Vilmann P, Folke K, et al. (1996) Endoscopic ultrasonography and real-time guided fine-needle aspiration biopsy of solid lesions of the mediastinum suspected of malignancy. Chest; 110:539–544.

33. Hünerbein M, Ghadimi BM, Haensch W, et al. (1998) Transesophageal biopsy of mediastinal and pulmonary tumors by means of endoscopic ultrasound guidance. J Thorac Cardiovasc Surg 116:554–559.

34. Michel-Cherqui M, Brusset A, Liu N, et al. (1997) Intraoperative transesophageal echocardiographic assessment of vascular anastomoses in lung transplantation. A report on 18 cases. Chest; 111:1229–1235.

35. Almeida AA, Thomson HL, Burstow DJ, et al. (1998) Transesophageal echocardiography in an operation for pulmonary arteriovenous malformation. Ann Thorac Surg 65:267–268.

36. Carlens E. (1959) Mediastinoscopy: A method for inspection and tissue biopsy in the superior mediastinum. Dis Chest 36:343–349.

37. Porte H, Roumilhac D, Eraldi L, et al. (1998) J Cardio Thoracic Surg; 13:196–199.

38. Azorin J, Francisci MP, Tremblay B, et al. (1996) Closure of a postpneumonectomy main bronchus fistula using video-assisted mediastinal surgery. Chest 109:1097–1098.

39. Jahangiri M, Goldstraw P (1995) The role of mediastinoscopy in superior vena caval obstruction. Ann Thorac Surg 59:453–455.

40. Smythe WR, Bavaria JE, Kaiser LR (1998) Mediastinoscopy subtotal removal of mediastinal cysts. Chest 114:614–617.

41. Hutter J, Junger W, Miller K, et al. (1998) Subxiphoidal videomediastinoscope for diagnostic access to the anterior mediastinum. Ann Thorac Surg 66:1427–1428.

42. Moutain CF, Dresler CM (1997) Regional lymph node classification for lung cancer staging. Chest 111:1718–1723.

43. Riquet M, Manac'h D, Dupont P, et al. (1994) Anatomic basis of lymphatic spread of lung carcinoma to the mediastinum: Anatomoclinical correlations. Surg Radiol Anat 16:229–238.

44. Cybulsky IJ, Bennett WF (1994) Mediastinoscopy as a routine outpatient procedure. Ann Thorac Surg 58:176–178.

45. Meerschant D, Vermassen F, Brutel de la Rivière A, et al. (1992) Repeat mediastinoscopy in the assessment of new and recurrent Lung Neoplasm. Ann Thorac Surg 53:120–122.

46. López L, Varela A, Frexinet J, et al. (1994) Extended cervical mediastinoscopy: Prospective study of fifty cases. Ann Thorac Surg; 57:555–558.

47. Jiao X, Magistrelli P, Goldstraw P (1997) The value of cervical mediastinoscopy combined with anterior mediastinotomy in the peroperative evaluation of bronchogenic carcinoma of the left upper lobe. Eur J Cardiothoracic Surg 11:450–454.

48. Urschel JD (1997) Current applications of non videothoracoscopy Int Surg 82:131–133.

49. Weissberg D, Refaely Y (1996) Pleuroscopy: Therapeutic applications. Scand J Thor Cardiovasc Surg 30:1–10.

50. Mouroux J, Clary-Meinesz C, Padovani B, et al. (1997) Efficacy and safety of videothoracoscopie lung biopsy in the diagnosis of interstitial lung disease. Eur J Cardiothoracic Surg 11:22–26.

51. Zegdi R, Azorin J, Tremblay B, et al. (1998) Videothoracoscopic lung biopsy in diffuse infiltrative lung diseases: a 5-year surgical experience. Ann Thorac Surg 66:1170–1173.

52. Niden AH, Salem F (1997) A safe high-yield technique for cutting needle biopsy of the lung in patients with diffuse lung disease. Chest; 111:1615–1621.

53. Noppen MMP, De Mey J, Meysman M, et al. (1995) Percutaneous needle biopsy of localized pulmonary, mediastinal, and pleural diseased tissue with an automatic disposable guillotine soft-tissue needle. Preliminary results. Chest 107:1615–1620.

54. Santambrogio L, Nosotti M, Bellaviti N, et al. (1997) CT-guided fine needle aspiration cytology of solitary pulmonary nodules. A prospective, randomized study of immediate cytologic evaluation. Chest 112:423–425.

55. Mitruka S, Landreneau RJ, Mack MJ, et al. (1995) Diagnosing the indeterminate pulmonary nodule: percutaneous biopsy versus thoracoscopy. Surgery 1118:676–684.

56. Kazerooni EA, Harteken FW, Whyte RI, et al. (1996) Transthoracic needle aspiration in patients with severe emphysema. A study of lung transplant candidates. Chest 109:616–620.

57. Shah RM, Spirn PW, Salazar AM, et al. (1993) Localization of peripheral pulmonary nodule for thoracoscopic excision: Value of CT-guided wire placement. AJR 161:279–283.

58. Yim AP, Ho JK (1995) Digital Localization of peripheral lung nodules with video-assisted thoracic surgery. Chest 107:886–887.

59. Debrosse D, Riquet M, Deslandes P, et al. (1995) Videothoracoscopie des nodules pulmonaires. Peut-on se passer d'un repérage préopératoire? Rev Mal Resp 12:459–464.

60. Suzuki K, Nagai K, Yoshida J, et al. (1999) Video-assisted thoracoscopic surgery for small indeterminate pulmonary nodules. Indication for preoperative marking. Chest 115:563–568.

61. Walle D, Clark S, Tsang G, et al. (1997) Is there a role for video-assisted thoracoscopy in the staging of non-small cell lung cancer? Eur J Cardiothoracic Surg 12:214–217.

62. Mentzer SJ, Swangson SJ, DeCamp MM, et al. (1997) Mediastinoscopy, thoracoscopy, and videoassisted thoracic surgery in the diagnosis and staging of lung cancer. Chest 112:239S–241S.

63. De Giacomo T, Rendina EA, Venuta F, et al. (1997) Thoracoscopic staging of IIIB non-small cell lung cancer before neoadjuvant therapy. Ann Thorac Surg 64:1409–1411.

64. Solaini L, Bagioni P, Campanini A, et al. (1998) Diagnostic role of videothoracoscopy in mediastinal diseases. Eur J Cardio Thorac Surg 13:491–493.

65. Demmy TL, Krasna MJ, Detterbeck FC, et al. (1998) Multicenter VATS experience with mediastinal tumors. Ann Thorac Surg 66:187–192.

66. Riquet M, Mouroux J, Pons F, et al. (1995) Videothoracoscopy excision of thoracic neurogenic tumors. Ann Thorac Surg 60:943–946.

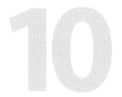

Bronchoalveolar and Serum Markers of Lung Disease

N. Le Flour, S. Jouveshomme and J.-P. Derenne

Introduction

Bronchoalveolar lavage (BAL) allows recovery of both cellular and noncellular components from the epithelial surface of the lower respiratory tract that are thought to be representative of the inflammatory and immune system of the entire lower respiratory tract. Initially developed as a research tool for investigation of the immunopathogenesis of interstitial disorders, BAL is now a standard procedure for diagnostic approach in all kinds of diffuse lung diseases. Appropriate clinical and technical guidelines have been given by European (1,2) and American scientific societies (3).

Bronchoalveolar Lavage

Technique

BAL is performed as part of routine bronchoscopy, after general inspection of the bronchial tree and before biopsy is performed or when brushing in order to avoid excess blood in the recovered fluid, which would alter the concentration of cellular and noncellular components. The bronchoscope is passed into a subsegmental bronchus; 0.9% sterile saline is infused using a syringe through the suction port of the bronchoscope and is retrieved into specimens traps with gentle suction.

At least 100 mL of fluid should be instilled at each pulmonary site (4), and most centres instill 300–400 mL at a single site (1,5). Larger volumes are associated with increased complications (6). Some centres lavage up to three separate sites using 100 mL at each site (5). Prewarming the lavage fluid to 37 °C may prevent coughing and bronchospasm (6,7). Usually, lavage with 100 mL saline yields 40–60 mL of fluid for analysis. The best yield is obtained when lavage is performed in the right middle lobe or in the lingula, but other lobes may be lavaged depending on the location of the radiographic abnormalities. It has been estimated that 100 mL lavage of a bronchial subsegment represents the sampling of about 10^6 alveoli (8).

Contraindications

Although there is no absolute contraindication, performing BAL in some relatively high risk situations should be avoided (3,9): uncooperative patients, patients with a forced expiratory volume in 1 s that is less than 1000 mL. Moderate to severe asthma, hypercapnia, severe hypoxemia with an oxygen saturation less than 90% despite oxygen supplementation, serious cardiac dysrythmia, myocardial infarction within 6 weeks, uncorrected bleeding diathesis, and hemodynamic instability are other classical contraindications.

Safety and Complications

Lavage is a relatively safe procedure. The overall complication rate is less than 3% (10). The most frequent side-effects are cough during lavage and transitory pyrexis for a few hours after the procedure. The latter does not mean pulmonary infection but reflects transient inflammation induced by lavage fluid left in the alveoli (11,12). Lavage may also cause a drop of Pa_{O2}. The extent of the desaturation depends on the volume of fluid instilled and on the underlying lung disease (13). Bleeding and bronchospasm (in normoreactive patients) are rare events (0.7%) (10) and the latter can be prevented by bronchodilator premedication (1,14).

Radiologic alveolar opacities that may appear in the lavaged areas are usually cleared within 24 h (15).

Routine Processing of Bal and Normal Values

Once lavage fluid is obtained it should be processed in a standardized manner in order to allow correct interpretations.

The macroscopic aspect should be noted. It may be: clear in nonsmokers; light brown in smokers or in those professionally exposed to mineral particles; milky in patients with alveolar proteinosis; hemorrhagic in patients with alveolar hemorrhage or after trauma; and yellowish in icteric patients.

Differential cell counts should be performed with a hemocytometer. Several methods have been used to prepare specimens for cytological analysis. Technical recommendations have been given by the European Society of Pneumology Task Group (1) and will be not be developed here. The first aliquots are usually contaminated with proximal airways material. As a result, only the subsequent aliquots, which are relatively enriched for more distal and alveolar contents, should be used for differential cell count.

Each cell type should be expressed either as a percentage of total cells (with exclusion of red blood cells and epithelial cells) or as the total number per unit volume of fluid recovered. In normal nonsmokers, the total number of cells recovered on BAL varies from 4×10^6 to 23×10^6 mL^{-1}. Alveolar macrophages represent the majority of recovered cells, followed by lymphocytes, neutrophils and eosinophils (Table 10.1). There are fewer than 1% basophils and mast cells. Cellular formulae can be established by different methods that influence the results to varying extents, especially for lymphocytes. The differential count is commonly made on cytocentrifuged preparations. Smoking is the major factor that affects BAL fluid cell populations. In smokers, the total cell count and the percentage of macrophages and neutrophils may be three to four times that of nonsmokers. The after smoking cessation increase in neutrophil count may persist for more than 10 years (16).

The diagnosis of *alveolar hemorrhage* may be established by two methods with a good correlation (a) the Golde score, which is based on the hemosiderin content of alveolar macrophages stained with Prussian Blue. One hundred cells are examined and each cell is ranked for hemosiderin content using a scale from 1 to 4. Alveolar hemorrhage is defined by a Golde score of >100 (17). (b) The percentage of siderophages among the alveolar macrophages is counted: alveolar hemorrhage is defined by the presence of 20% or more siderophages (18,19).

Depending on the clinical setting, specific investigations may be performed on the BAL fluid.

Phenotypic analysis: Lymphocytic subpopulations and some malignant cells may be identified by monoclonal antibodies directed against surface antigens. In normal subjects the differential count of BAL lymphocyte subtypes is similar to that of blood lymphocytes (Table 10.2).

Colorations: There is periodic acid–Schiff (PAS) coloration when alveolar proteinosis is suspected, black Soudan in thesaurismosis.

Chemical analysis The supernatant of BAL fluid is composed of three different elements: (a) secretions from the respiratory membrane (surfactant and distal bronchial mucous membrane secretions); (b) products of transmembranous transsudation and exsudation from circulatory blood and interstitial fluids; (c) secretion or degradation products from alveolar cellular components. Several components of the supernatant can be titrated: albumin, immunoglobulins, hyaluronique acid, collagenase, elastase, procollagen, prostaglandins.

Microbiologic and mineralogic analysis. Methods and indications are developed in other chapters.

The different elements of orientation for diagnosis of respiratory diseases are summarized in Table 10.3

BAL in the Diagnosis and Management of Respiratory Diseases

Interstitial Lung Diseases

This is a group of more than 100 different disorders, characterized by an increased number of inflammatory

Table 10.1. Differential cell count in normal nonsmoker BAL

Number of cells (10^3 mL^{-1})	109–149
Macrophages (10^3 mL^{-1})	91–107
%	84–99
Lymphocytes (10^3 mL^{-1})	13–17
%	0.7–14.4
Neutrophils (10^3 mL^{-1})	1
%	<2
Eosinophils (10^3 mL^{-1})	0.2
%	0.2
From ref. 3, with permission.	

Table 10.2. Lymphocytic subpopulations in normal nonsmoker subjects BAL

Cellular type	Phenotype	%
T	CD3	75 (63–88)
T-helper	CD4	53 (36–70)
T-cytotoxic	CD8	28 (15–40)
B	CD19	5 (0–12)
NK	CD57	7 (1–14)
Langherans'	CD1	0–3
From ref. 98, with permission. NK, natural killer.		

Table 10.3. Analysis of alveolitis: an element for diagnosis

Lymphocytic	Neutrophilic	Eosinophilic	Macrophagic	Mixed
Sarcoidosis	Idiopathic pulmonary fibrosis (IPF)	Eosinophilic pneumonia	Pneumoconiosis	Tuberculosis
Extrinsic Allergic Alveolitis (EAA)	Early phase of EAA	Langherans' cell granulomatosis	Langherans' cell granulomatosis	Langherans' cell granulomatosis
Radiation pneumonitis	Collagen vascular diseases	Loeffler syndrome		Drug-induced pneumonia
Sjögren syndrome; rheumatoid arthritis, lupus	Sarcoidosis fibrosis	Churg– Strauss disease		
Silicosis	Asbestosis	Drug-induced pneumonia		
Carcinomatous lymphangitis	Bacterial pneumonia	IPF		
Lymphoma	Drug-induced pneumonia	Sclerodermia		
AIDS Lymphoid pneumonia		Bronchiolitis obliterans and organizing pneumonia		
Tuberculous miliary				
Drug-induced pneumonia				

From ref. 99 with permission. IPF, idiopathic pulmonary fibrosis.

and immune effector cells within the lung parenchyma. It is believed that alveolitis may precede and modulate the derangement of alveolar structures, including thickening and fibrosis, which may eventually lead to sufficient damage of the alveolar capillary membrane to interfere with gas exchange. Assessing the presence and intensity of alveolitis is important in the staging of alveolar diseases and may be of benefit in planning and evaluating therapeutic strategies.

In most situations, BAL does not provide information sufficient to make specific diagnosis but it has an important diagnostic value when considered in conjunction with other information. An abnormal BAL analysis may facilitate the decision to proceed with open lung biopsy.

Sarcoidosis

Sarcoidosis is a multisystem granulomatous disease of unknown origin. Although the clinical course of most sarcoid patients is relatively benign, 20–25% may suffer permanent lung function loss, and in 1–5% of patients the disease may be fatal (20). Pulmonary involvement is present in almost all patients with sarcoidosis and an abnormal chest X-ray is found in 90% of the cases in the course of illness (20). Light microscopy studies have demonstrated that the earliest pathologic pulmonary change in sarcoidosis is lymphocyte accumulation in the alveolar septa, followed by blood monocyte accumulation and formation of noncaseating granuloma (NCG) (21). A tissue diagnosis is desirable to exclude other conditions that may mimic sarcoidosis, such as tuberculosis or lymphomas. The diagnosis is usually confirmed by the presence of noncaseating granulomas on bronchial or transbronchial lung biopsy or on biopsy of other tissues (accessory salivary glands, skin, lymph nodes, conjunctiva, liver).

In 1990 the European Respiratory Society Task Group on BAL stated that the combination of an elevated alveolar lymphocytosis with a T-helper/suppressor (CD4/CD8) ratio >3.5:1 in BAL is consistent with sarcoidosis in an appropriate clinical setting (2), and indeed, the predictive positive value (PPV) of BAL has been shown to be as high as 94% in distinguishing sarcoidosis from other diseases with mediastinal or pulmonary involvement (22–24). However, up to 15% of patients with pulmonary sarcoidosis have a normal BAL lymphocyte count and about 3% have a BAL lymphocyte CD4/CD8 ratio <1 (25).

In patients with proven extrapulmonary sarcoidosis and normal chest X-ray, alveolar lymphocytosis or NCG in transbronchial lung biopsy (TBLB) specimens has been demonstrated in up to 50% of the cases (26–28) and several authors have suggested that BAL could be an important additive investigation in patients with suspected extrapulmonary sarcoidosis and normal chest X-ray (28,29). However, the clinical utility of BAL in diagnosing sarcoidosis in patients with normal chest X-ray is not established (32).

Although the presence of lymphocytic alveolitis is of no prognostic value, an increase in neutrophils or mast cells in the BAL fluid may be indicative of a fibrotic process.

BAL findings in sarcoidosis do not seem to correlate with disease duration and do not predict when therapy may be safely tapered or discontinued. In fact, the correlation between chest X-ray changes, clinical features and lavage lymphocytes counts is poor (30).

In summary, BAL is an important diagnostic tool for sarcoidosis in an appropriate clinical setting, but, at the current time, no cellular or noncellular BAL parameter has been shown to definitively predict the prognosis or to be useful in making therapeutic decisions for individual patients with sarcoidosis.

Idiopathic Pulmonary Fibrosis

Idiopathic pulmonary fibrosis (IPF) is one of the most serious interstitial lung diseases. The prognosis is poor, with a mean survival of 3–6 years, but progression is variable in individual patients. Objective response to corticosteroids is achieved in only 20% of cases and is associated with a better survival (31).

Diagnostic value of BAL: There are no specific diagnostic BAL features in IPF. Neutrophils are the main lavage cell type increased in IPF and are believed, with the eosinophils, to be involved in the inflammatory process that contributes to lung injury and the development of fibrosis (33,34). A combination of increased neutrophils (>4%) and eosinophils (>3%) is observed in about two thirds of the patients with IPF (36).

Prognostic value of BAL: A minority of patients with IPF have slight to moderate increases in lymphocytes in addition to neutrophils and are believed to respond better to corticosteroids, whereas patients with high BAL neutrophil counts, especially when associated with high eosinophil counts, are at increased risk of failing to respond to steroids (34–36). Since the efficacy of corticosteroids in IPF is not yet established, BAL findings may reflect different patterns of progression of the disease (31).

Value of BAL in monitoring and surveillance of therapy: There are few data on serial lavage studies in patients with IPF. One important study, in which 32 patients were followed for a mean of 4 years, showed a significant decrease in all BAL inflammatory cell types, especially neutrophils in responders to corticosteroids, while BAL neutrophil counts remained elevated or increased in non-responders (37).

In conclusion, BAL is an important tool in the understanding of the pathophysiology of IPF. It has only a poor diagnostic value in IPF but may provide some useful prognostic indications that may aid therapeutic decisions (2).

Connective Vascular Diseases

Several connective vascular diseases (CVDs) result in interstitial lung disease similar to IPF, with similar BAL findings (Table 10.4). In addition, inflammatory alveolitis may also be present in a high proportion of patients with CVD without clinical or radiologic evidence of pulmonary involvement (38). The distribution of BAL cell types varies according to the type of CVD and to the presence of ILD as shown in Table 10.4 (39,40).

Diagnostic Value of BAL

Since alveolar inflammation is frequently observed in CVD patients with or without associated ILD, BAL

Table 10.4. Abnormal BAL cell profile in connective tissue diseases

Disease	With ILD	Without ILD
Primary Sjögren syndrome	Neutrophils, lymphocytes (CD8+)	Lymphocytes (CD4+)
Secondary Sjögren syndrome	Neutrophils, lymphocytes (CD8+)	Lymphocytes (CD8+)
Systemic sclerosis	Neutrophils ± eosinophils ± lymphocytes	Neutrophils ± eosinophils ± lymphocytes
Rheumatoid arthritis	Neutrophils ± eosinophils ± lymphocytes (↓ CD4/CD8)	Lymphocytes (CD4+)
Systemic lupus erythematosus	Neutrophils, lymphocytes	Lymphocytes
Mixed connective tissue disease	Neutrophils	Neutrophils
Polymyositis/ dermatopolymyositis	Neutrophils	Neutrophils ± lymphocytes
Ankylosing spondylitis	?	Lymphocytes ± neutrophils
Wegener granulomatosis	Neutrophils ± eosinophils	Neutrophils ± eosinophils
Mixed cryoglobulinemia	?	Lymphocytes
Churg–Strauss syndrome	Eosinophils	Eosinophils

ILD, interstitial lung disease.

cytology is by no means a reliable argument for the diagnosis of ILD. BAL may be useful for the diagnosis of associated lung diseases (infection, pulmonary hemorrage, alveolar proteinosis) or of drug-induced lung disorders.

Interestingly, in Wegener granulomatosis, the antineutrophil cytoplasmic antibody (ANCA) is present in lavage fluid in patients with active disease. Serum ANCA reactivity and the titers of ANCA in BAL fluid both correlate with the presence or absence of active disease (41), suggesting that ANCA are produced by the pulmonary lymphoid tissue.

Prognostic Value of BAL

Early detection of alveolitis in patients with normal chest X-ray provides an accurate prediction of which patients will deteriorate (38). In general, when an increased number of lymphocytes is present in BAL fluid, lung disease is associated with a relatively good prognosis, whereas the presence of a predominantly neutrophilic or eosinophilic alveolitis is associated with a higher risk of functional and radiographic deterioration (42–46). It appears, especially for systemic sclerosis and rheumatoid arthritis, that one of the factors predictive of a significant improvement is the initiation of treatment early in the course of the disease (40).

Extrinsic Allergic Alveolitis

Extrinsic allergic alveolitis (EAA) or hypersensitivity pneumonitis is an interstitial lung disease that results from repeated exposure to a wide range of inhaled organic dusts and related occupational allergens, especially bird and fungal proteins. The presentation of EAA varies from patient to patient and is related mainly to the frequency and intensity of exposure to the causative antigens. Acute, subacute and chronic phases should be distinguished.

In the early phase of the disease, there is a substantial activation of macrophages and an increase of neutrophils and mast cells (46). In a few days, lymphocytes are increased and are the most striking finding during the entire follow-up of the disease process. In a majority of cases, CD8+ lymphocytes are the predominant cells in the BAL and the CD4/CD8 ratio is low. The presence of a marked lymphocytosis (often above 60%) characterized by the CD3+/CD8+/CD57+/CD56+/CD16- (NK marker) phenotype is highly suggestive of EAA (47). The number of cells bearing the proliferation associated markers (CD25 and CD71 antigens) is quite low (48–51).

This phenotype has not been observed in other conditions (47). No cases of EAA have been reported with normal BAL cell count (2).

In the patients who continue to be exposed to antigens, a decrease of BAL lymphocyte count and the recovery of a normal CD4/CD8 ratio may be observed. Increased BAL neutrophil, eosinophil or mast cell counts are associated with an increased risk of developing fibrotic lung disease (52).

In patients who recover and become asymptomatic after removal of the antigen, persistantly increased counts of total BAL lymphocytes may obtain. However, the significance of this alveolitis, its relationship with disease activity, and its prognostic value remain unclear (52).

Pneumoconiosis

Interstitial lung diseases may be associated with occupational or environmental exposure to inorganic dusts and minerals. BAL is performed to provide evidence of mineral dust exposure and the presence of an associated alveolitis. Usually, the intensity of the alveolitis is mild, except in chronic beryllium disease. Most patients have a normal BAL cell profile.

Asbestos

The assessment of asbestos exposure is often difficult because of the large number of occupations in which patients may be exposed to asbestos and because of the long latency between exposure and the development of the disease. In patients with known exposure to asbestos, but without radiographic or functional signs of interstitial lung diseases, the most frequent finding is lymphocytic alveolitis (17–30% of BAL lymphocytes). In patients with asbestosis, there is also an increase in BAL neutrophils with or without an increased number of eosinophils. Neutrophil count correlates positively with the duration of the disease and higher percentages seem to be associated with more severe lung function loss (53). The quantification of asbestos bodies (AB) is done by counting their number. It correlates closely with AB concentration in lung tissue obtained by biopsy or at autopsy. A BAL count >1 AB mL^{-1} is highly indicative of a lung concentration exceeding 1000 AB (g dry tissue)$^{-1}$. Parenchymal concentration of more than 1000 AB (g dry lung tissue)$^{-1}$ is generally associated with past exposure to asbestos.

Silicosis

In coal workers' pneumoconiosis a normal percentage of lymphocytes and a mild increase of neutrophils has been reported in BAL. In other forms of silica exposure, a moderate increase of lymphocytes and sometime of neutrophils has been described (54,55).

Hard Metal Lung Disease

BAL lymphocytes may be mildly increased. An increase of neutrophils or eosinophils has been discribed. There is an increased number of giant cells in BAL fluid (56).

Chronic Beryllium Disease (57,58)

Beryllium has found widespread application in modern industry because of its physical properties and it is used in the manufactures of thermal nuclear reactors, rocket heat shields, and brakes. Inhaled beryllium dusts, oxide or salts can cause acute or chronic lung disease. The acute form has largely been eliminated by control of environmental exposure. The chronic form develops over 1–20 years in 1–3% of exposed persons and is a granulomatous disorder histologically and clinically similar to sarcoidosis. BAL cytology shows the same profile as active sarcoidosis. The antigen has been identified and can be used for a specific diagnosis in vitro. There is a positive proliferative response of CD4+ T-lymphocyte to beryllium salts with a sensitivity and a specificity approaching 100% (58).

Detection and Quantification of Dust Particles and Fibers

The formation of ferruginous bodies occurs after inhalation of dusts of various kinds. When dusts are regularly shaped, true asbestos bodies with a fine central fiber almost invisible with the light microscope are found. Other fibers that are thicker or irregularly shaped lead to the formation of pseudoferruginous bodies, including talc, glass fibers and coal dust particles. The presence of dust particles in the cytoplasm of alveolar macrophages may suggest exposure to crystalline and metallic particles including silica, coal dust, hard metal, antimony, aluminium, iron-rich particles and alloys. The exact analysis of the chemical composition of the particles can be done by electron microscopy making use of energy-dispersive X-ray analysis. Another method is neutron activation analysis, which is useful for the detection of trace metals in cell-free BAL fluid, showing high concentrations of tungsten, tantalium, cobalt and hard metal.

Value of BAL for Clinical Diagnosis and Management (2)

The demonstration of dust in BAL fluid is indicative of exposure but is no evidence of disease. On the other hand, a minority of patients with definite asbestos exposure may have no detectable AB in BAL fluid. The absence of AB in BAL does not exclude asbestos-related pleural disease. In the presence of interstitial lung disease without identified exposure to asbestos, the finding of numerous AB in BAL tilts the balance of probabilities toward a diagnosis of asbestosis because AB are not usually found in patients with other interstitial lung disease . In silicosis, BAL documents silica exposure by detecting birefringent particles in alveolar macrophages with polarized microscopy. About 90% of alveolar macrophages may contain these particles in occupationally exposed workers, while fewer than 5% of macrophages contain such particles in persons with environmental exposure (55). However, detection of dust particles and fibers in BAL is not performed routinely because it does not usually interfere with management decisions.

Histiocytosis X (HX) or Langherans' Cell Granulomatosis (2)

This is a rare chronic granulomatous disorder involving cells of the monophagocytic system. It is characterized by the interstitial accumulation of atypical histiocytes similar to Langerhans' cells (LC). Electron microscopy reveals an indented nucleus and small elongated bodies scattered throughout the cytoplasm, termed "X-bodies". Instead of this ultrastuctural analysis, a more rapid and sensitive technique has been developed to identify the X-bodies, using monoclonal antibodies directed against the antigen surface marker CD1 (OKT6) and PS 100 of the LC. BAL in HX patients usually shows a normal cell count in non-smokers. The differential cell count shows a high percentage of alveolar macrophages, and a slight increase of neutrophils and eosinophils. LC are normally present in the lower respiratory tract and in lung parenchyma of normal subjects, particularly smokers. Therefore, since the presence of LC in BAL is not pathognomonic of HX, at least 5% of CD1-labeled alveolar cells are required to confirm the diagnosis (61). However, false-negative results can be related to patchy distribution or to the advanced stage of the disease.

Eosinophilic Lung Diseases

A great variety of disorders may lead to eosinophilic infiltrates such as asthma, eosinophilic pneumonia, Loeffler syndrome, allergic bronchopulmonary aspergillosis, and Churg–Strauss vasculitis. In these disorders, BAL has an important diagnostic yield when showing an eosinophic alveolitis in an appropriate clinical setting. BAL and blood analysis should be performed in parallel. Eosinopholic pneumonia displays the highest eosinophilic count, which may represent up to 90% of total cells. Eosinophilic lung diseases are usually reversible after initiation of corticosteroid therapy and BAL is helpful for the follow-up of treated patients (2).

Pulmonary Alveolar Proteinosis (2,60,61)

Pulmonary alveolar proteinosis (PAP) is a rare disorder characterized by accumulation of PAS-positive phospholipidic material in the alveolar spaces. PAP can be idiopathic or secondary to infections of the lung (*Nocardia, Mycobacterium tuberculosis, Mycobacterium avium-intracellulare, Pneumocystis carinii*), hematologic malignancies and other conditions altering immune status (Human immunodeficiency virus (HIV) infection), or to exposure to inhaled chemicals and minerals (silica, aluminium dust, insecticides, titanium). The pathogenesis is believed to involve excessive secretion and/or disrupted surfactant clearance. Pathophysiology involves alveolar macrophages that may be defective in the processing and clearing of surfactant.

Segmental BAL appears to be essential in the management of this disease for diagnosis, follow-up and treatment. On gross examination, BAL fluid has a milky appearance. On cytocentrifuged slides stained by MGG, the striking feature is the variable amount of basophilic extracellular deposit mixed with enlarged foamy alveolar macrophages, crystal clefts and cellular debris. This extracellular material as well as the cytoplasmic content of the alveolar macrophages show a pink PAS-positive diastase-resistant staining. On electron microscopy, the ultrastructural appearance is characteristic, with small lamellar bodies of wavy or regular periodicity, tubular myelin structures and myelin-like multilamellated structures with an electron-dense central region, similar to condensed surfactant. Added to this extracellular material, ghost cells, alveolar macrophages, and type 2 pneumocytes are filled with intracellular bodies and empty vacuoles or gray lipid droplets (62).

Biochemical analysis of lavage fluid has shown a preponderance of phospholipids and proteins, consistent with large amounts of pulmonary surfactant within the alveoli. Immunologic studies performed on the lavage fluid show a marked elevation in levels of lung surfactant proteins (SP-A and SP-D). A significant difference in the quantity and repartition of the staining primary and secondary forms of alveolar proteinosis has been suggested, high levels of SP-D in BAL fluid being specific for PAP (60).

The differential cell count does not appear to be helpful in making the diagnosis of PAP. Increases in both lymphocytes and macrophages have been reported (60).

Moderate increases in serum lactate dehydrogenase (LDH) are frequently observed (approximately 25% above normal). Serum levels of lung surfactant proteins A and D are markedly elevated in patients with PAP as compared with healthy volunteers (60).

The value of BAL in the follow-up and treatment of PAP is reported in the section dealing with therapeutic applications, below.

Fat Embolism

In patients with recent trauma, the identification of neutral fat droplets by staining with oil red O within cells recovered by BAL is a rapid and specific method for establishing the diagnosis of fat embolism (63).

Alveolar Hemorrhage (2)

Many disorders are associated with diffuse pulmonary hemorrhage (Table 10.5). The triad hemoptysis, infiltrates on chest X-ray, and anemia is present in most cases. Rapid diagnosis is necessary and BAL appears to be a method of choice. On gross examination, BAL fluid has a bloody or orange-pink color, yet it can be of normal translucent appearance. Total cellular count is increased. Free red blood cells, red blood cells in alveolar macrophages and hemosiderin-laden alveolar macrophages can be observed. The importance of hemosiderin content can be evaluated by the Golde's score (see Chapter 9). An interval of at least 48 h between the episode of acute pulmonary hemorrhage and the performance of BAL is necessary to recover alveolar macrophages with increased amounts of hemosiderin.

Table 10.5. Principal disorders associated with alveolar hemorrhage

Cardiac diseases, intrapulmonary vascular lesions or malformations	Chronic left or right-sided heart failure Pulmonary hypertension Pulmonary venoocclusive disease Pulmonary lymphangiomyomatosis Arteriovenous fistula or other congenital malformations Vascular thrombosis with infarction
Pulmonary hemosiderosis and glomerulonephritis	With anti-basement membrane antibody (ABMA) disease (Goodpasture syndrome)
Coeliac disease	
Idiopathic pulmonary hemosiderosis	
Vasculitis and collagen vascular diseases	Systemic lupus erythematosus Wegener granulomatosis Mixed connective tissue disease Idiopathic thrombocytopenic purpura
Miscellaneous disorders	Diffuse necrotizing infections (leptospirosis, infections in immunocompromised patients) Severe coagulopathy Malignant diseases (leukemia) Bone marrow transplantation
Drugs and toxics	D-penicillamine Amphotericin B Chemotherapy drugs for cancer Isocyanates Cocaine

From ref. 2 with permission.

Drug-induced pneumonitis (2)

The list of drugs that may adversely affect the lung grows longer every day. The goal is to have reliable criteria by which to suspect and recognize iatrogenic lung diseases early enough to prevent the development of irreversible injury. BAL is a useful tool in the diagnostic approach that provides arguments for differentiating iatrogenic causes, and distinguishing them from infectious or malignant etiologies.

BAL can show different profiles. In rare cases, such as exogenous lipoid pneumonia, BAL can be sufficient to confirm a diagnosis. In this disorder, induced by mineral oil, taken as nose drops or laxatives, alveolar macrophages contain large empty vacuoles representing fatty material strongly stained by red oil O (64). Exceptionally, BAL can make the diagnosis of drug-induced pneumonia when showing aurosomes, talc or silicone. In some cases of direct toxicity due to drugs such as bleomycin, nitrofurantoin, cyclophosphamide, eosinophilic pneumonia or secondary alveolar proteinosis can be observed (65).

The most frequent BAL feature observed is an alveolitis characterized by an increase in total recovered cells, among which one particular cell type can be markedly predominant. Hyperlymphocytosis associated with a decrease in the CD4/CD8 ratio is usually observed (66). In methotrexate- or nitrofurantoin-induced pneumonitis, a predominance of CD4 cells has been described (67). Drugs such as amiodarone or amphiphilic molecules can lead to thesaurismosis (68). Ultrastructural studies of BAL show an accumulation of numerous large lamellar inclusions, phospholipidic in nature, mainly in alveolar macrophages, but also in the other cells. These features have been observed in treated patients whether or not they have developed a pneumonitis. In contrast, hyperlymphocytosis associated with thesaurismosis has been observed only in treated patients with pneumonitis. The absence of thesaurismosis makes the diagnosis of amiodarone pulmonary toxicity unlikely (69).

BAL as a Diagnostic Tool in Interstitial Lung Disease

To summarize, BAL remains a powerful investigative tool for diagnosis in some pulmonary diseases: beryllium disease, alveolar proteinosis and Langherans' cell granulomatosis may be diagnosed with certainty, and BAL may provide strong positive predictive value for the diagnosis of sarcoidosis and EAA in an appropriate clinical setting. In asbestosis and silicosis, detection of dust particles and fibers in BAL fluid is indicative of past exposure. For all other interstitial diseases, BAL has been widely used as a research tool and has helped in the understanding of their pathogenesis. However, at present, its clinical utility is limited mainly to the exclusion of other diseases, particularly pulmonary infections.

Pulmonary Infections

The use of BAL as a diagnostic procedure of pulmonary infections has increased dramatically with the epidemic acquired immunodeficiency syndrome (AIDS) and the expanding number of patients receiving organ transplants. Until recently, the use of BAL was limited to the study of interstitial lung diseases and the diagnosis of lung infections by opportunistic microorganisms in severely immunocompromised patients. Over the past decade, the use of BAL has been expanded to include the diagnosis of bacterial pneumonia in nonimmunocompromised patients.

Clinical Utility of BAL in Immunocompromised Hosts

HIV-Positive Patients

Pulmonary complications are common in AIDS patients and are responsible for a significant mortality and morbidity. BAL is the preferred method for obtaining specimens from lower airways in immunocompromised patients with pulmonary infiltrates because of its safety and its high sensitivity for detection of parasites, viruses, fungi, and bacteria (Table 10.6) (70).

Table 10.6. BAL microbiologic diagnosis

Microorganism	Technique, stain	Other techniques
Pneumocystis carinii	Wright–Giemsa (Diff–Quick) Gram–Weigert Toluidine Blue Gomori–Grocott (silver stain)	Monoclonal antibodies Immunofluorescence
CMV, herpes simplex	Virus cell-inclusions (Wright-Giemsa, Papanicolaou)	Monoclonal antibodies pp65 antigenemia (indirect immunofluorescence) Culture DNA probe analysis
Mycobacteria	Ziehl–Neelsen Auramin–Rhodamin	Culture DNA probe analysis
Fungi	Gram–Weigert PAS Gomori–Grocott (silverstain)	Monoclonal antibodies Culture
Bacteria	Gram	Monoclonal antibodies Semiquantitative culture (counting of CFU)
Legionella	Direct immunofluorescence	Culture

CMV, cytomegalovirus; PAS, periodic acid–Schiff; CFU, cell-forming units.

Despite the widespread use of chemoprophylaxis, *Pneumocystis carinii* pneumonia (PCP) remains an important cause of pulmonary disease in HIV-positive patients. Both sensitivity and specificity of BAL for detection of PCP approaches 100% (71). BAL is of no value for monitoring the treatment since *P. carinii* may be found several weeks after initiation of the treatment whatever the clinical outcome (72).

Cytomegalovirus (CMV) is often detected in AIDS patients but is not predictive of active pulmonary disease. Because CMV may be detected in asymptomatic patients as well as in patients with pulmonary disease due to other pathogens, histologic evidence is mandatory for the diagnosis of CMV pneumonitis. Waxman et al. (73) have proposed three diagnostic criteria for CMV pneumonia; (a) positive CMV culture from both BAL and transbronchial biopsy specimens; (b) characteristic cytomegalic inclusion bodies from both BAL and transbronchial biopsy specimens; (c) absence of any other pulmonary pathogen identified by bacterial, fungal, viral, or acid-fast stains or culture.

Pulmonary tuberculosis and *Mycobacterium avium* complex pneumonia are commonly found in HIV-infected patients. BAL is more sensitive than sputum analysis in providing both an immediate diagnosis and a positive culture (74).

HIV-Negative Patients

Pulmonary involvement, both infectious and noninfectious, remains a significant problem in bone marrow transplants (BMT) patients and in patients receiving immunosuppressive drugs for malignant, rheumatologic or dermatologic diseases. BAL is useful for distinguishing drug-induced pneumonia from infectious diseases. Pulmonary complications in BMT occur in 40–60% of patients (74). It is estimated that more than 30% of BMT-related deaths are caused by respiratory complications (75,76). BAL is the method of choice for investigating pulmonary infiltrates in a BMT recipient, because it is relatively safe and easily performed as compared with other invasive diagnostic tools (77). BMT patients are often severely thrombocytopenic but BAL does not induce any serious bleeding complication (78). The major aim of BAL is to pinpoint a treaTable infection, mostly bacterial (Gram-positive), fungal, PCP and CMV (79,80).

The reliability of the detection of CMV in BAL as an indicator of active disease is less controversial than in HIV-positive patients. Actually, 50% of asymptomatic patients with CMV in BAL eventually develop CMV pneumonia, suggesting that detection of CMV in BAL defines a population at risk for the development of CMV pneumonia (79).

BAL may be useful in the diagnosis of alveolar proteinosis and diffuse alveolar haemorrage syndrome. The latter develops about 14 days after BMT, and may be responsive to high doses of corticosteroids (81). Sensitivity of BAL for the diagnosis of PCP in HIV-negative patients is less than in HIV-positive patients (82).

BAL as a Diagnostic Tool in Bacterial Pneumonia in Immunocompetent Patients

The protected specimen brush of Wimberly is the gold standard for the diagnosis of bacterial infection (83). However, several studies investigating the usefulness of BAL in diagnosing bacterial pneumonia in mechanically ventilated patients have been carried out (84). Because the contamination of the BAL fluid by oropharynx bacteria considerably alters its diagnostic yield, a protected BAL technique, with a double lumen distally sealed catheter has been developed (85). Using qualitative bacterial cultures, the sensitivity of BAL in this setting was 80% and the specificity 66%. Since then, the development of culture quantification techniques has improved the specificity of BAL in the diagnosis of bacterial lung infections (16) leading to the formation of guidelines recommending routine use of quantitative cultures of BAL specimens for the diagnosis of bacterial pneumonia in mechanically ventilated patients (86) with a cutoff point of $10^4 \, mL^{-1}$.

Pulmonary Malignancies

The major diagnostic tools for obtaining a diagnosis of cancer remain direct biopsy of bronchoscopically visible tumors and transbronchial biopsy of more distant lesions, with a significantly lower diagnostic yield in the latter. In peripheral lesions, the diagnostic yield of bronchoscopy may be increased by the cytologic analysis of brush or BAL specimens (1).

The criteria for the cytologic diagnosis of lung neoplasms are well established (87), but the exact place of BAL among the diagnostic tools remains poorly defined. The diagnostic yield of BAL varies from 14% to 69% (88). It may be higher in bronchoalveolar cell carcinoma and lymphangitic carcinoma than in other types of primary pulmonary malignancies. BAL may be useful in diagnosing hematologic malignancies affecting the lungs, e.g., like leukemia and pulmonary lymphoma. Hodgkin disease can be diagnosed by the identification of Sternberg cells in BAL cytology specimens (89).

Cytologic analysis must be performed by trained cytologists. A second limitation is that the cytologic diagnosis of malignancy does not always meet with the histopathologic pattern. In one series, cytology agreed with biopsy in only 80% of cases (90). Moreover, severe dysplasy that may develop in airway epithelial cells in clinical circumstances such as pneumonia, viral infection and following chemotherapy can be difficult to distinguish from malignant changes (2).

BAL and Therapy (91,92)

BAL has been used for therapeutic purposes prior to its use as a diagnostic procedure. At present, alveolar proteinosis remains the only definite indication of this procedure.

When the diagnosis of alveolar proteinosis is established, the decision to perform a therapeutic bronchopulmonary lavage should be based upon the patient's tolerance to exercise and on symptomatology, since a spontaneous remission is always possible. Although the technique has not been standardized, the common principles can be outlined as follows. Therapeutic whole-lung lavage is performed under general anesthesia, using a double-lumen endotracheal tube. Both lungs are ventilated with 100% oxygen for 10–15 min. One lung is then excluded from the ventilatory circuit and lavaged with isotonic saline at 37 °C, coming out of a container usually suspended 150 cm above the carena. The usual filling volume is 500–1000 mL. The same volume is then allowed to drain by gravity, with the assistance of mechanical chest percussion. The first recovered aliquots have a milky aspect, which gradually clarifies during the lavage. The filling and draining procedures are then repeated until the effluent is completely clear, which may need 10–40 l. Symptomatic improvement generally takes place within 24–48 h. The other lung is lavaged 3–7 days later. Complications are rare and include hydropneumothorax, bronchospasm and pneumonia. Most patients require repeated whole-lung lavage every 6–12 months. Some authors have shown a significant improvement of alveolar macrophage function after therapeutic whole-lung lavage and a reduction of the rate of secondary infections (93).

Serum Markers in Lung Diseases

In sarcoidosis, *serum angiotensin conversion enzyme* (ACE) concentration is currently measured. Serum enzyme activity may be increased in other conditions and is not specific for sarcoidosis (94). Yet, its positive predictive value is evaluated to 90% in this disease, although normal enzyme activity does not exclude the diagnosis and abnormal levels may persist even in the presence of normal radiograph (30). An increase in ACE has a diagnostic value in an evocative context but serum enzyme activity has no value for prognosis and management of therapy.

Tumor markers: In small cell lung cancer, neuron-specific enolase (NSE) has a sensitivity for diagnosing of 65% and a specificity of 95% for values greater than 25 ng mL^{-1} (95). During treatment, NSE concentration usually decreases but is not a reference method for evaluating the outcome. A rise in NSE may precede recurrence of the disease (95). In nonsmall-cell lung cancer, several other markers have been measured (96). None of them appears sufficiently sensitive or specific and their routine measurement in the screening, staging or evaluation of disease progession is not recommended (97).

In conclusion, serum markers are not reliable diagnostic tools in lung diseases.

Conclusion

In the diagnosis of lung diseases, we employ different tools such as chest X-ray, tomodensitometry, bronchoscopy and serum markers. The last of those have almost no utility. The others are complementary. BAL performed during bronchoscopy may help diagnosis in some diseases.

References

1. European Society of Pneumology Task Group on BAL (1989) Technical recommendations and guidelines for bronchoalveolar lavage (BAL). *Eur Respir J*, 2:561–585.
2. European Society of Pneumology Task Group on BAL (1990) Clinical guidelines and indications for bronchoalveolar lavage (BAL). *Eur Respir J*, 3:937–974.
3. Official ATS Statement (1990) Clinical, role of bronchoalveolar lavage in adults with pulmonary disease. *Am Rev Respir Dis* 142:481–486.
4. Helmers RA, Dayton CS, Floerchunger C, et al. (1989) Bronchoalveolar lavage in interstitial lung disease: Effect of volume of fluid infused. *J Appl Physiol* 67:1443–1446.
5. Rennard SI, Aalbers R, Bleecker et al. (1998) Bronchoalveolar lavage: Performance, sampling procedure, processing and assessment. *Eur Respir J*, 11 (Suppl 26): 13S–15S.
6. Burns DM, Shure D, Francoz RKM, et al. (1983) The physiological consequences of saline lobar lavage in healthy human adults. *Am Rev Respir Dis* 127:695–701.
7. Pingleton SK, Harrison GF, Stechschulte DJ, et al. (1983) Effect of location, pH, and temperature of instillate in bronchoalveolar lavage in normal volunteers. *Am Rev Respir Dis* 128:1035–1037.
8. Helmers RA, Galvin J, Dayton CS, *Dis*, (1989) Small volume bronchoalveolar lavage (BAL) uniformly perfuses the lung segment in interstitial lung disease as assessed by magnetic resonnance imaging (MRI). *Am Rev Respir Dis* 139:A472.
9. Djukanovic R, Dahl R, Jarjour N, et al. (1998) Safety of biopsies and bronchoalveolar lavage. *Eur Respir J* 11 (Suppl. 26): 39S–4!S.
10. Strumpf IJ Feld MK, Cornelius MJ et al. (1981) Safety of fiberoptic bronchoalveolar lavage in evaluation of interstitial lung disease. *Chest* 80:268–271.
11. Standiford TJ Kunkel SL, Strieter RM (1991) Elevated serum levels of tumor necrosis factor-α after bronchoscopy and bronchoalveolar lavage. *Chest* 99:1529–1530.

12. Von Essen SG, Robbins RA, Spurzem JR, et al. (1991) Bronchoscopy with bronchoalveolar lavage causes neutrophil recruitment to the lower respiratory tract. *Am Rev Respir Dis* 144:848–854.

13. Pirozynski M, Sliwinski P, Zielinski J (1988) Effect of different volumes of BAL fluid on arterial oxygen saturation. *Eur Respir J* 1:943–947.

14. NHLBI Workshop Summaries (1985) Summary and recommendations of a workshop on the investigative use of fiberoptic bronchoscopy and bronchoalvolar lavage in asthmatics. *Am Rev Respir Dis* 132:180–182.

15. Gurney JW, Harrison WC, Sears K, et al. (1987) Bronchoalveolar lavage: Radiographic manifestations. *Radiology*, 163:71–74.

16. The BAL Cooperative Group Steering Committe (1990) Bronchoalveolar lavage constituents in healthy individuals, idiopathic pulmonary fibrosis, and selected comparison groups. *Am Rev Respir Dis* 141(5): part 2.

17. Golde DW, Drew WL, Klein HZ, Finley TN, Cline MJ (1975) Occult pulmonary hemorrhage in leukemia. *Br Med J* 2:166–168.

18. De Lassence A, Fleury-Fieth J Escudier E, et al. (1995) Alveolar hemorrhage Diagnostic criteria and results in 194 immunocompromised hosts. *Am J Respir Crit Care Med*, 151:157–163.

19. Cordier JF (1997) Syndromes hémorragiques alvéolaires. In Encyclopédie de Médiciti el Chirurgie, Pneumologie. Elsevier, Paris, pp6–024-D–40, 6 p.

20. American Thoracic Society (1999) Statement on sarcoidosis. *Am J Respir Crit Care Med* 160:736–755.

21. Rosen W, Athanassiades TJ Moon S, et al. (1978) Non-granulomatous interstitial pneumonitis in sarcoidosis: Relationship to the development of epithelialoid granulomas. *Chest* 74:122–125.

22. Winterbauer RH, Lammert J Selland M, et al. (1993) Bronchoalveolar lavage cell populations in the diagnosis of sarcoidosis. *Chest* 104:352–361.

23. Costabel U (1997) CD4/CD8 ratios in bronchoalveolar lavage fluid: Of value for diagnosing sarcoidosis? *Eur Respir J* 10:2699–2700.

24. Drent M, Wagenaar SS, Mulder PHG, et al. (1994) Bronchoalveolar lavage fluid profiles in sarcoidosis, tuberculosis, and non-Hodgkin's and Hodgkin's disease. *Chest* 105:514–519.

25. Kantrow S.P, Meyer K.C, Kidd P, et al. (1997) The CD4/CD8 ratio in BAL fluid is highly variable in sarcoidosis. *Eur Respir J* 10:2716–2721.

26. Wallaert B, Ramon P, Fournier E et al. (1986) Activated alveolar macrophages and lymphocyte alveolitis in extrathoracic sarcoidosis without radiological medistinopulmonary involvement. *Ann NY Acad Sci* 465:201–210.

27. Ohara K, Okubo A, Kamata K, et al. (1993) Transbronchial lung biopsies in the diagnosis of suspected ocular sarcoidosis. *Arch Ophtalmol* 111:642–644.

28. Hoogsteden H, van Dongen J Adriaansen H, et al. (1988) Bronchoalveolar lavage in extrapulmonary sarcoidosis. *Chest* 94:115–118.

29. Sugimoto M, Nakashima H, Ando M, et al. (1989) Bronchoalveolar lavage studies in uveitis patients without radiological intrathoracic involvement of sarcoidosis. *Jpn J Med* 28:50–54.

30. Turner-Warwick M, McAllister W, Lawrence R, et al. (1986) Corticosteroid treatment in pulmonary sarcoidosis: Do serial lavage lymphocyte counts, serum angiotensin converting enzyme measurements, and gallium–67 scans help management? *Thorax* 41:903–913.

31. Turner-Warwick M, Burrows B, Jonhson A (1980) Cryptogenic fibrosing alveolitis: Response to corticosteroid treatment and its effect on survival. *Thorax* 35:593–599.

32. Fujimoto K, Kubo K, Yamaguchi S, et al. (1995) Eosinophil activation in patients with pulmonary fibrosis. *Chest* 108:48–54.

33. Hällgren R, Bjermer L, Lundgren R, et al. (1989) The eosinophil component of the alveolitis in idiopathic fibrosis. *Am Rev Respir Dis* 139:373–377.

34. Haslam PL, Turton CWG, Lukoszek A, et al. (1980) Bronchoalveolar lavage fluid cell counts in cryptogenic fibrosing alveolitis and their relation to therapy. *Thorax* 35:328–339.

35. Watters LC, Schwarz MI, Cherniack RM, et al. (1987) Idiopathic pulmonary fibrosis: Pretreatment bronchoalveolar lavage cellular constituents and their relationships with lung histopathology and clinical response to therapy. *Am Rev Respir Dis* 135:696–704.

36. Peterson MW, Monick M, Hunninghake GW (1987) Prognostic role of eosinophils in pulmonary fibrosis. *Chest* 92:51–56.

37. Turner-Warwick M, Haslam PL (1987) The value of serial bronchoalveolar lavages in assessing the clinical progress of patients with cryptogenic fibrosing alveolitis. *Am Rev Respir Dis* 135:26–34.

38. Wallaert B, Hatron P-Y, Grosbois J-M, et al. (1986) Subclinical pulmonary involvement in collagen-vascular diseases assessed by bronchoalveolar lavage. *Am Rev Respir Dis* 133:574–580.

39. Manganelli P, Salaffi F, Pesci A (1997) Clinical and subclinical alveolitis in connective tissue diseases assessed by bronchoalveolar lavage. *Semin Arthritis Rheum* 26:740–754.

40. Spertini F, Aubert J-D, Leimgruber A (1996) The potential of bronchoalveolar lavage in the prognosis and treatment of connective–vascular diseases. *Clin Exp Rheumatol* 14:681–688.

41. Hoffman GS, Sechler JMG, Gallin JI, et al. (1991) Bronchoalveolar lavage analysis in Wegener's granulomatosis. *Am Rev Respir Dis* 143:401–407.

42. Garcia JGN, Parhami N, Killam D, et al. (1986) Bronchoalveolar lavage fluid evaluation in rheumatoid arthritis. *Am Rev Respir Dis* 133:450–454.

43. Silver RM, Metcalf JF, Stanley JH, et al. (1984) Interstitial lung disease in scleroderma-analysis by bronchoalveolar lavage. *Arthritis Rheum* 27:1254–1262.

44. Kallenberg CGM, Jansen HM, Elema JD, et al. (1984) Steroid-responsive interstitial pulmonary disease in systemic sclerosis – Monitoring by bronchoalveolar lavage. *Chest* 86:489–491.

45. Greene NB, Solinger AM, Baughman RP (1987) Patients with collagen-vascular disease and dyspnea: The value of gallium scanning and bronchoalveolar lavage in predicting response to steroid therapy and clinical outcome. *Chest* 91:698–703.

46. Denis M, Bedard M, Laviolette M, et al. (1993) A study of monokine release and natural killer activity in the bronchoalveolar lavage of subjects with farmer's lung. *Am Rev Respir Dis* 147:934–939.

47. Semenzato G, Agostini C (1989) Editorial. Human retroviruses and lung involvement. *Am Rev Respir Dis* 139:1317–1322.

48. Costabel U, Bross KJ Marxen J, et al. (1984) T lymphocytosis in bronchoalveolar lavage fluid of hypersensitivity pneumonitis. *Chest* 85:514–518.

49. Semenzato G, Agostini C, Zambello R, et al. (1986) Lung T cells in hypersensitivity pneumonitis: Phenotypic and functional analyses. *J Immunol* 137:1164–1172.

50. Semenzato G, Trentin L, Zambello R, et al. (1988) Different types of cytotoxic lymphocytes are involved in the cytolytic mechanisms taking place in the lung of patients with hypersensitivity pneumonitis. *Am Rev Respir Dis* 137:70–74.

51. Haslam P, Dewar A, Butchers P, et al. (1987) Mast cells, atypical lymphocytes, and neutrophils in bronchoalveolar lavage in extrinsic allergic alveolitis. *Am Rev Respir Dis* 135:35–47.

52. Cormier Y, Belandger J Laviollette M (1987) Prognostic significance of bronchoalveolar lymphocytosis in farmer's lung. *Am Rev Respir Dis* 135:692–695.

53. Gellert AR, Macey MG, Uthayakumar S, et al. (1985) Lymphocyte subpopulations in bronchoalveolar lavage fluid in asbestos workers. *Am Rev Respir Dis* 132:824–828.

54. Rom W.N, Bitterman P.B, Rennard S.I, et al. (1987) Characterization of the lower respiratory tract inflammation of nonsmoking individuals with interstitial lung disease associated with chronic inhalation of inorganic dusts. *Am Rev Respir Dis* 136:1429–1434.

55. Costabel U, Teschler H (1989) Inflammation and immune reactions in interstitial lung disease (ILD) associated with inorganic dust exposure. *Eur Respir J* 190:363–364.

56. Davison AG, Haslam PL, Corrin B, et al. (1983) Interstitial lung disease and asthma in hard metal workers: Bronchoalveolar lavage, ultrastructural and analytical findings and results of bronchial provocation tests. *Thorax* 38:119–128.

57. Epstein PE, Dauber JH, Rossman MD, et al. (1982) Bronchoalveolar lavage in a patient with chronic berylliosis: Evidence for hypersensitivity pneumonitis. *Ann Intern Med* 97:213–216.

58. Rossman MD, Kern JA, Elias JA, et al. (1988) Proliferative response of bronchoalveolar lymphocytes to beryllium. *Ann Intern Med* 108: 687–693.

59. Chollet S, Soler P, Dournoro P, et al. (1984) Diagnosis of pulmonary histicytosis X by immunodetection of Langerhans' cells in bronchoalveolar lavage fluid. *Am J Pathol* 115:225–232.

60. Bennet MW, Stern EJ Schmidt RA, et al. (1997) Diagnosing pulmonary alveolar proteinosis. *Chest* 111:460–466.

61. Goldstein LS, Kavuru MS, Curtis-McCarthy P, et al. (1998) Pulmonary alveolar proteinosis. *Chest* 114:1357–1362.

62. Costello JF, Moriarty DC, Branthwaite MA, et al. (1975) Diagnosis and management of alveolar proteinosis: The role of electron microscopy. *Thorax* 30:121–132.

63. Chastre J Fagon J-Y, Soler P, et al. (1990) Bronchoalveolar lavage for rapid diagnosis of the fat embolism syndrome in trauma patients. *Ann Intern Med* 113:583–588.

64. Dougay G, Levade T, Caratero A, et al. (1985) Paraffinose alvéolaire: étude cytologique et biochimique du liquide de lavage bronchoalvéolaire. *Rev Mal Respir* 2:231–237 .

65. Cooper JAD, White DA, Matthay RA (1986) State of the art. Drug-induced pulmonary disease. *Am Rev Respir Dis* 133:321–340.

66. Akoun G, Mayaud C, Milleron B, et al. (1984) Drug related pneumonitis and drug induced hypersensibility pneumonitis. *Lancet,* 1:1362.

67. Akoun G, Mayaud C, Toubol Y, et al. (1987) Use of bronchoalveolar lavage in the evaluation of methotrexate lung disease. *Thorax* 42L:652–655.

68. Israël-Biet D, Venet A, Caubarrere I, et al. (1987) Bronchoalveolar lavage in amiodarone pneumonitis. Cellular abnormalities and their relevance to pathogenesis. *Chest* 91:214–221.

69. Danel C, Israël-Biet D, Venet A, et al. (1988) Ultrastructural comparison of bronchoalveolar lavage (BAL) in patients under amiodarone with or without pulmonary symptoms. *Eur Respir J* 1(Suppl 2): 254S.

70. Weldon-Linne CM, Rhone DP, Bourassa R (1990) Bronchoscopy specimens in adults with AIDS: Comparative yields of cytology, histology and culture for diagnosis of infectious agents. *Chest* 98:24–28.

71. Broaddus C, Dake MD, Stubarg MS, et al. (1985) Bronchoalveolar lavage and transbronchial lung biopsy for the diagnosis of pulmonary infections in the acquired immunodeficiency syndrome. *Ann Intern Med* 102:747–752.

72. Waxman AB, Goldie SJ Brett-Smith H, et al. (1997) Cytomegalovirus as a primary pulmonary pathogen in AIDS. *Chest* 111:128–134.

73. Salzman S.H, Schindel M.L, Aranda C.P, et al. (1992) The role of bronchoscopy in the diagnosis of pulmonary tuberculosis in patients at risk for HIV infection. *Chest* 102:143–146.

74. Dunagan D.P, Baker A.M, Hurd D.D, et al. (1997) Bronchoscopic evaluation of pulmonary infiltrates following bone marrow transplantation. *Chest* 111:135–141.

75. Breuer R, Lossos IS, Berkman N, et al. (1993) Pulmonary complications of bone marrow transplant. *Respir Med* 87:571–579.

76. Krowka MJ Rosenow EC, Hoagland HC (1985) Pulmonary complications of bone marrow transplant. *Chest* 87:237–246.

77. Rennard S.I (1990) Role of bronchoalveolar lavage in the assessment of pulmonary complications following bone marrow and organ transplantation. *Eur Respir J* 3:373–375.

78. Drew WL, Finley TN, Golde DW (1977) Diagnostic lavage and occult pulmonary hemorhage in thrombocytopenic immunocompromised patients. *Am Rev Respir Dis* 166:215–221.

79. Soubani AO, Miller KB, Hassoun PM (1996) Pulmonary complications of bone marrow transplantation. *Chest* 109:1066–1077.

80. Kruger W, Russman B, Kroger N, et al. (1999) Early infections in patients undergoing bone marrow or blood stem cell tranplantation —- A 7 year single centre investigation of 409 cases. *Bone Marrow Transplant* 23:589–597.

81. Chao NJ Duncan SR, Long GD, et al. (1991) Corticosteroids therapy for diffuse alveolar hemorrhage in autologous bone marrow recipients. *Ann Intern Med* 114:145–146.

82. Limper AH, Offord KP, Smith TF, et al. (1989) Pneumocystis carinii pneumonia: Differences in lung parasite number and inflammation in patients with and without AIDS. *Am Rev Respir Dis* 140:1204–1209.

83. Wimberly N, Bass JB Jr, Boyd BW, et al. (1982) Use of a bronchoscopic protected brush for the diagnosis of pulmonary infections. *Chest* 81:556–562.

84. Nieto JMS, Alcaraz AC (1995) The role of bronchoalveolar lavage in the diagnosis of bacterial pneumonia. *Eur J Clin Microbiol Infect Dis* 14:839–850.

85. Rouby JJ Rossignon MD, Nicolas MH, et al. (1989) A prospective study of protected bronchoalveolar lavage in the diagnosis of nosocomial pneumonia. *Anesthesiology* 71:679–685.

86. Meduri GU, Chastre J (1992) The standardization of bronchoscopic techniques for ventilator-associated pneumonia. *Chest* 102:557–564.

87. Johnson WW, Frable WJ (1976) The cytopathology of the respiratory tract: A review. *Am J Pathol* 84:372–424.

88. Bellmunt J DeGracia J Morales S, et al. (1990) Cytologic diagnosis in bronchoalveolar lavage specimens. *Chest* 98:513–514.

89. Morales FM, Matthews JI (1987) Diagnosis of parenchymal Hodgkin's disease using bronchoalveolar lavage. *Chest* 91:785–787.

90. Linder J Radio SJ Robbins RA, et al. (1987) Bronchoalveolar lavage in the cytologic diagnosis of carcinoma of the lung. *Acta Cytol* 31:796–801.

91. Ramirez RJ Schultz RB, Dutton RE (1963) Pulmonary alveolar proteinosis. A new technique and rationale for treatment. *Arch Intern Med* 112:419–431.

92. Danel C, Israël-Biet D, Costabel U, et al. (1992) Therapeutic applications of bronchoalveolar lavage. *Eur Respir J* 5:1173–1175.

93. Claypool WD, Rogers RM, Matuschack GM (1984) Update on the clinical diagnosis, management and pathogenesis of pulmonary alveolar proteinosis (phopholipidosis). *Chest* 85:550–558.

94. Studdy PR, Lapworth R, Bird R (1983) Angiotensin-converting enzyme and its clinical significance -- A review. *J Clin Pathol* 36:938–947 .

95. Pujol J-L (1998) Marqueurs tumoraux sériques. In Arnette Initiatives Santé, *Cancers broncho-pulmonaires,* pp 223–236.

96. Ferrigno D, Buccheri G (1995) Clinical applications of serum markers for lung cancer. *Respir Med* 89:587–597.

97. Official Statement of the ATS and the ERS (1997) Pretreatment evaluation of non-small-cell lung cancer. *Am J Respir Crit Care Med* 156:320–332.

98. Israël-Biet D, Gillet-Juvin K, Taravella O, et al. (1999) Lavage bronchoalvéolaire d'exploration. In Encyclopédie de Nédecin et Chirurge, Pneumologie. 6–000-M–50, 10p.

99. Wallaert B, De Vuyst P, Israël-Biet (1992) Le lavage bronchoalvéolairei Des aspects techniques aux règles d'interprétation. *Rev Mal Respir* 9:39–56.

11   Radionuclide Studies of the Lung

N.D. Greyson

Introduction

Nuclear medicine studies provide unique functional information based on the localizing properties of specific radiotracers in normal or pathologic processes. These images are complementary to conventional X-ray, computed tomography (CT), magnetic resonance imaging (MRI), and angiography, which offer highly detailed anatomy-based images of the lungs, pleura, and mediastinum. Radionuclide studies are noninvasive, widely available, and quantitative. These tests may obviate the need for interventional techniques such as angiography, biopsy, and bronchial alveolar lavage. They may be used in the detection and staging of malignancy, determining the activity of inflammatory processes, and in monitoring the response to therapy or progression of the disease, in a cost-effective, patient-tolerated manner.

Imaging Principles

Radiopharmaceuticals are molecules or compounds that contain a radioactive tracer. The distribution of the pharmaceutical in the body depends on its interaction with normal or pathologic tissues. Many different products are available for assessment of the respiratory system, including those that demonstrate regional ventilation, pulmonary artery perfusion, inflammation and sepsis, primary and secondary tumors, thrombus labeling, and alveolar–capillary permeability. Frequently, multiple studies, each reflecting different functional information, are used in combination.

The radioactive label permits external detection of the distribution of the pharmaceutical. Diagnostically useful radioisotopes are those whose unstable atom results in the emission of a gamma ray, or positron (positively charged electron). The site of this event can be detected using a gamma (or positron) camera, which maps out the distribution of radioactive emissions. The events are recorded and displayed, in planar, tomographic or three-dimensional format. Nuclear images that have relatively low spatial resolution, are "physiologic maps" rather than anatomic displays. They may be visually correlated or electronically merged with radiographs, for precise localization. Diagnosis is made by comparing the patient's results with the known normal localization of that radiopharmaceutical. The regional distribution of the tracer, and its changes over time may be quantified using computer analysis of regions of interest.

Techniques

Ventilation Imaging

Assessment of the patency of the airways is made using radiotracers that follow the ventilation pathways of least resistance to the level of the terminal bronchioles or alveoli. Xenon-133(^{133}Xe), an inert radioactive gas has been used, but it is now largely supplanted by aerosolized Technetium-99m labeled products.

Radioactive xenon ventilation studies are performed using a closed gas distribution system, charged with oxygen. The study is performed in three phases: an initial breath-hold following maximum inhalation of undiluted xenon gas; a 3–5 min equilibration achieved by rebreathing xenon mixed with oxygen; and a washout phase by breathing in room air, and breathing out xenon into a collecting reservoir for disposal. While this approach provides the most physiologic demonstration of airways patency, redistribution, and air-trapping, xenon gas is relatively expensive, and its long half-life produces significant radiation housekeeping difficulties. The dose of xenon gas must be purchased weekly in anticipation of the numbers of expected ventilation studies. This could result in wastage or insufficiency of supplies.

A radioactive aerosol is produced using an oxygen-driven nebulizing system containing a ^{99m}Tc-labeled product. Commonly ^{99m}Tc-diethylene triamine pentaacetic acid (DTPA) or ^{99m}Tc-sulphur colloid are used, but virtually any radiopharmaceutical may be nebulized for ventilation studies. This means that a cheap readily available product is always on hand. Aerosol ventilation may be carried out at normal tidal volume, without breath-holding, even on mechanically ventilated patients.

Aerosol particles less than 1.0 μm in diameter simulate a gas, passing through the airways of least resistance by laminar flow to the terminal bronchiole level. Normally there is very little adhesion of the particles to the mucosa of the proximal tracheobronchial tree, but in the terminal bronchioles and alveoli they stick to the cell surfaces. The activity remains in the lung for up to about 2 hrs, permitting imaging in multiple views. This offers an advantage over xenon studies, which are restricted to a single, usually posterior, set of images. Clearance of the aerosolized tracer is by mucocilliary action, absorption through the alveolar – capillary membrane, and by radioactive decay. The clearance time of soluble materials, such as ^{99m}Tc-DTPA is a measure of membrane permeability, and has been used as an indicator of alveolitis. The distribution of the aerosol also demonstrates the effectiveness of the delivery of aerosolized medication such as pentamidine.

The normal ventilation image (Fig. 11.1, upper row) shows symmetric activity in both lungs, with sharply defined pleural margins, costophrenic angles, diaphragmatic surfaces, cardiac silhouette and great vessels that match the usual contours seen on a chest radiograph. The scan usually demonstrates a normal gradient of ventilation, greater in the bases than in the apices.

In the presence of airways obstruction, or airspace disease, there is interference with the peripheral penetration of aerosol to the pleural surfaces. This results in inhomogeneous ventilation, with defects corresponding to the areas of hypoventilation (Fig. 11.2). With increased airways resistance, normal laminar flow is replaced by turbulence, causing the aerosol particles to stick to the

airways walls at the site of obstruction. The resultant image shows "hot spots" at the level of obstruction (Fig. 11.3).

Perfusion Scanning

^{99m}Tc-labeled macroaggregates of human serum albumin (MAA), 10–60 μm in diameter, are larger than the pulmonary capillaries. When injected intravenously, they flow with the circulation through the right ventricle and pulmonary arteries, and into the pulmonary capillary bed. This results in their transient embolization in the pulmonary bed. To provide a wide margin of safety, approximately 300 000 particles are used in the injection, causing embolization of less than 0.1% of the precapillary arteriole bed (1). The albumin particles are metabolized and pass out of the capillary bed, with a clearance half time of less than 2 h. Although there are theoretical safety issues related to embolization of a compromised circulation such as in pulmonary hypertension or severe emphysema, possible right to left shunting causing microembolization of the systemic circulation, and protein allergy, in reality, significant side-effects are virtually never encountered.

A normal perfusion scan, performed in multiple views has features identical to the normal ventilation image (Fig. 11.1, lower row). Single or multiple areas of decreased perfusion may result from intraluminal obstruction (thrombus or other emboli, pulmonary artery stenosis, vasculitis), extrinsic compression (tumor, mediastinitis), destruction of the vascular bed (emphysema, bullae or abscess), vasospasm secondary to hypercapnea (associated with airspace consolidation, or bronchial obstruction), or vascular diversions (pulmonary arteriovenous malformation, right to left intrapulmonary or intracardiac shunts, postoperative pulmonary-to-systemic vascular anastomoses).

Perfusion abnormalities are characterized by their shape. "Vascular segment" perfusion defects are caused

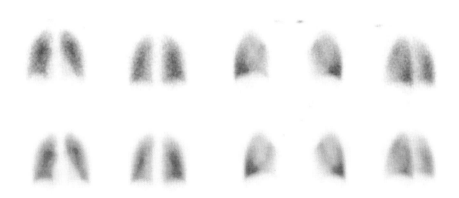

Figure 11.1. Normal ventilation (*upper row*) and perfusion (*lower row*) images. Of the 8 views normally obtained, anterior, posterior, right and left laterals, and the left posterior oblique views are shown. Ventilation and perfusion images match identically. Note the symmetry and homogeneity of activity, with a gradient of ventilation and perfusion favoring the lower lobes. The normal pleura, diaphragm, and cardiac outlines are well defined.

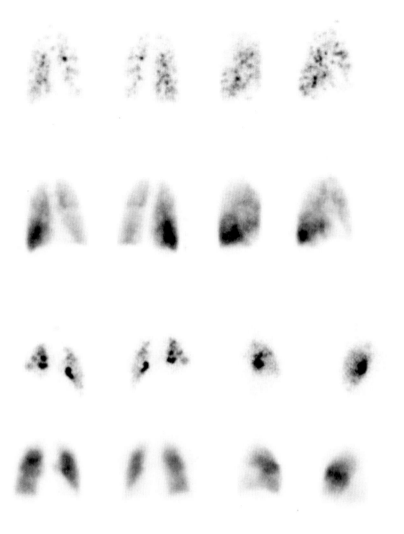

Figure 11.2. Emphysema. The ventilation images (*upper row*) show irregular patchy distribution of aerosol, with poor penetration to the periphery. The perfusion images (*lower row*) show nonsegmental, ill-defined defects. The ventilation pattern is worse than perfusion. There are no "vascular segment defects". This scan is a low probability for PE.

Figure 11.3. Obstructive lung disease. The ventilation images (*upper row*, anterior, posterior, right and left laterals), show very poor ventilation of the bases. The central "hot spots" indicate foci of local airways resistance, with partial obstruction and turbulent flow depositing the aerosol centrally. The perfusion images (*lower row*) show matched, but less severe, lower lobe defects. There are no "vascular segment defects". In conjunction with a clinical low pretest probability, and a normal venous Doppler, this patient has a low probability for PE. With higher probability clinical indications, this would be considered as an intermediate probability for PE, requiring further investigation.

by occlusion of a vessel, cutting off the blood supply to all distal branches. These defects are pleural-based, conical in three dimensions or triangular in two dimensions, usually with the apex directed toward the hilum. (Fig. 11.4). Recent vascular defects are usually so well defined that they can be named according to the lung segment involved. Vascular perfusion defects may be characterized by size (whole lung, lobar, segmental, or subsegmental).

"Nonsegmental" perfusion defects are usually less discrete, may cross segmental or pleural margins, and may not reach the pleural surface ("the peripheral stripe sign"). They may be explained by anatomic structures such as cardiomegaly, or a tortuous aorta, or by radiographic pathology such as pleural effusions ("the fissure sign"), consolidation, atelectasis, or obstructive lung disease (Figs. 11.2, 11.3). Vascular redistribution to the upper zones in congestive heart failure reverses the normal gradient which favors the lower lobes.

The ventilation scan is performed first, followed by the injection of MAA for the perfusion scan. A larger dose of activity bound to MAA is administered compared with the inhaled aerosol. Thus the perfusion pattern is not affected by the activity of the preceding ventilation phase. Gamma camera imaging of both studies is performed in the same positions, so that any perfusion defects may be compared with the ventilation of the same anatomic segment.

Gallium Scanning for Sepsis and Tumor

Gallium-67 citrate (^{67}Ga) is an analog of the ferric ion. Thus it binds preferentially to transferrin, ferritin, and lactoferrin, as well as less avid binding to albumin and other proteins. Gallium also reacts with phosphate, resulting in mild bone localization. A normal gallium scan demonstrates the distribution of iron and albumin stores, with preference to those organs high in lactoferrin, as well

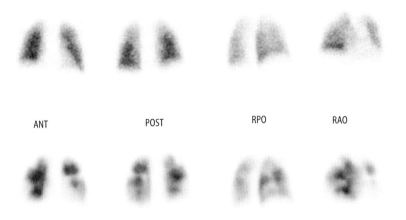

ANT   POST   RPO   RAO

Figure 11.4. Pulmonary emboli. The ventilation images (*upper row*) are normal. The perfusion images (*lower row*) show multiple matched, moderate-sized, bilateral vascular segment shaped perfusion defects. This patient has a high probability for PE, regardless of the clinical presentation. Only primary pulmonary hypertension, vasculitis, or old unresolved PE would produce a similar pattern. *ANT,* anterior; *POST,* posterior; *RPO,* right pulmonary obstruction; *RAO,* right aortic obstruction.

as some skeletal uptake (Fig. 11.5). Normally, there is no visible pulmonary or mediastinal uptake.

Septic or aseptic inflammation, and malignancy may have increased vascularity, which enhances the delivery of the gallium to the abnormal area. Increased vascular permeability permits the protein-bound gallium to exit the capillary bed, and bind to abnormal proteins associated with inflammation or tumor. Gallium also binds onto bacterial and white blood cell walls. Phagocytosis results in intracellular accumulation of gallium, which then binds to lysosomes, which are more plentiful in inflammatory or tumor cells.

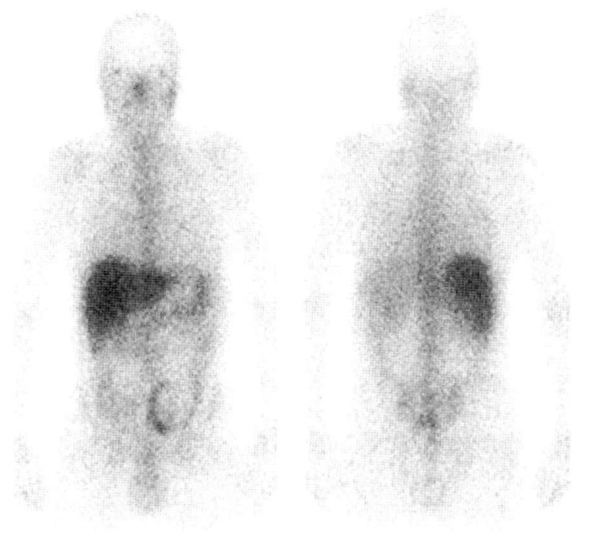

Similar mechanisms occur in both neoplasm and inflammation. Thus a positive scan cannot differentiate between these lesions. Gallium uptake may be considered as a bioassay of the activity of a known inflammatory process (acute versus chronic or quiescent inflammation; response of sepsis to treatment, etc.) (2). Low grade, well-differentiated tumors often have lower gallium affinity ("false negative"), which is a good prognostic sign (3). A good theraputic response will result in lower gallium uptake in tumors inflammation.

Tumour Localization

Fluorine-18 Deoxyglucose (FDG) Imaging by Positron Emission Tomography (PET)

Deyxoglucose labeled with fluorine-18 (^{18}F) is a sensitive detector of cellular metabolism (4). FDG is a glucose analog that follows the phosphorylation pathways, but becomes fixed within the cells prior to ATP production. The degree of accumulation is indicative of the rate of glycolysis or cellular metabolism, and is used in oncology to differentiate benign from malignant lesions, to detect primary tumors and metastases, and to follow response to therapy. Some false-positive results occur in focal inflammatory conditions because of increased local metabolism associated with sepsis and repair.

The detection of FDG requires a special camera, able to image the very high energy pair of photons produced when a positron reacts with an electron. The short half-life of ^{18}F (1.8 h) requires proximity to the cyclotron production facility. It is a relatively expensive product, and not as widely available as gamma-emitting radio-pharmaceuticals.

Figure 11.5. Normal ^{67}Ga-citrate scan. Anterior and posterior views. There is normal activity in the liver, faint bone uptake, some bowel excretion, minimal salivary and lachrymal uptake, and diffuse soft tissue appearance. There is no demonstrable uptake in the lungs, or mediastinum.

Thallium-201 and ^{99m}Tc-labeled Perfusion Agents

Thallium-201 (^{201}Tc) in the form of thallous chloride is a potassium analog. ^{99m}Tc labeled sestamibi (Cardiolite, Dupont Pharmaceuticals Company), and ^{99m}Tc-labeled tetrofosmin (Myoview, Nycomed Amersham) are lipophilic cations. These radiotracers are widely used in assessment of myocardial perfusion however, they have been found to localize in neoplasms. This uptake is proportional to the tumor blood flow, but is also related to the intracellular concentration of mitochondria. The increased negative electrical charge on the mitochondria of neoplastic cells causes the fixation of the positively charged cations.

Monoclonal Antibodies and Peptides

Localization of the radiotracer may be accomplished by the use of specially formulated antibodies directed against specific tumor cells, platelets, or various proteins. Also, tailor-made peptide chains that simulate the binding site of antibodies or hormones may be used to target specific receptors for these agents in tumors or thrombi.

Clinical Applications

Pulmonary Embolism

Ventilation-Perfusion Imaging

Pulmonary embolic disease is a potentially life-threatening occurrence, particularly in immobilized patients, following surgery, or in individuals with deep vein thrombophlebitis. Clinical signs and symptoms are frequently nonspecific (5) and radiographic findings are often absent or nondiagnostic. As pulmonary embolism (PE) is a common comorbid factor, or a direct cause of death, and is a frequent incidental finding at post mortem, it is often misdiagnosed and undertreated. Ventilation – perfusion imaging remains a keystone test in the diagnosis of PE, in conjunction with other noninvasive techniques such as venous Doppler ultrasound, and D-dimer assay. Contrast angiography, either by direct intrapulmonary artery injection (6), or helical CT (7–9) may help to give a more specific diagnosis, particularly in the more proximal branches.

The ventilation–perfusion lung scan is not a "pulmonary embolism scan". It identifies the presence and extent of ventilation and/or perfusion abnormalities, the interpretation of which is used in risk stratification of patients with suspected pulmonary embolism.

Many large clinical trials, such as PIOPED (10–12), and PISA-PED(13), have reviewed the patterns of ventilation–perfusion imaging in patients with suspected PE. The probability of PE was retrospectively based on analysis of these patterns and follow-up of the patients.

PE classically shows-vascular segment-shaped perfusion defects, in areas of normal ventilation (Fig. 11.4) (except when transient bronchospasm is present, or in the presence of consolidation due to infarction, or atelectasis). A normal ventilation – perfusion scan essentially excludes PE, and it is safe to withhold further diagnostic tests, and treatment (14,15). A high probability lung scan (80–95% prevalence of PE) is found in patients with lung scans that show one or more large defects, or multiple medium-sized vascular segment-shaped perfusion defects in areas with normal ventilation and no corresponding radiographic changes. In these patients treatment may be commenced on the base of the scan and a high clinical pretest probability. Absent perfusion of a whole lung may rarely be due to a massive proximal or saddle thrombus, but it is more commonly due to obstruction of the pulmonary artery by malignancy, or intracardiac or intrapulmonary shunts.

"Intermediate probability" scans carry a significant prevalence of emboli (but wide range, from 20% to 80%). These scans show small or moderate-sized perfusion defects with normal ventilation and normal radiographs, or perfusion defects with matched with consolidation, particularly in the lower zones. This category essentially includes any pattern that is not clearly "normal," "high probability," or low probability" for PE (12). To assess the need for treatment in these patients, results must be considered in light of the clinical presentation, the pretest probability of emboli, interpretation of the radiographic findings, venous Doppler, and the D-dimer test.

"Low probability scans" (less than 10% prevalence) demonstrate nonsegmental defects; abnormalities associated with radiographic lesions not suggestive of emboli, or a few very small (less than 25% of a named pulmonary segment) perfusion defects, or perfusion defects smaller than matching radiographic abnormalities, and multiple-mated ventilation and perfusion defects with a normal radiograph (12). Low probability scans exclude significant-sized emboli and have a very low mortality if untreated (16).

"Very low probability" (< 5% prevalence of PE) is associated with very small defects, and a normal radiograph.

The ventilation – perfusion lung scan is a relatively sensitive detector of abnormalities, but it is not specific in the detection of PE. Nevertheless it is still the key diagnostic test to determine the need for immediate treatment, further diagnosis, or dismissal. In the original PIOPED study (10), which relied heavily on the scan pattern, and less on other factors, an abnormal scan was 98% sensitive but only 10% specific for emboli. A high probability scan was 87% specific for PE but occurred in only 40% of PE patients. There was a large number of indeterminate scans, and emboli were present in 14% of low probability studies. Thus, unless the perfusion is absolutely normal, PE cannot be ruled out solely by the scan.

Many modifications to the PIOPED criteria have been proposed (12, 17, 18). The addition of pretest probabilities, and knowledge of specific high risk clinical indicators and ancillary testing, have significantly reduced the number of equivocal reports, with more definitive interpretations that are clinically useful in risk stratification (19). Intermediate or indeterminate categories carry a wide range of probability for PE . In the clinical setting of immobilization, lower extremity trauma, recent surgery, and central venous instrumentation, a defect has a higher likelihood of PE (20). A defect in a patient with known underlying cardiopulmonary disease is less likely to be a PE case (21).

Consistent reporting terminology is necessary to ensure appropriate communication with the referring clinicians (22–25). This facilitates treatment, and avoids expensive, unnecessary or invasive procedures.

Thrombus-Seeking Techniques

The optimistic search for reliable and readily available thrombus-seeking agents, will hopefully convert the diagnosis of pulmonary embolism from the interpretation of a defect to the direct identification of a thrombus (Fig. 11.6). There is an almost unlimited variety of potential thrombus-localizing radiopharmaceuticals. These include radiolabeling the constituents of a thrombus, such as platelets, thrombin, fibrin, or fibrinogen; labeled monoclonal antibodies against various thrombus components; labeled peptide chains to bind onto receptor sites on thrombi or their break-

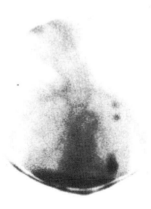

Figure 11.6. Positive identification of PE by ^{99m}Tc-labeled plasmin. Thrombi in the left upper lung, and lingula, adjacent to the left ventricle apex, corresponded to perfusion defects on the lung scan. There was also uptake in several thrombi located in deep venous thrombosis in legs. (Provided courtesy of the Department of Nuclear Medicine, Toronto General Hospital.)

down products; and labeled thrombolytic agents, such as plasmin, urokinase, streptokinase etc. (26–37). However, despite such an extensive potential list, and many decades of research, no one product has emerged as an agent of choice. A completely occluding thromboembolism may not have a sufficiently large surface exposed to the bloodstream to permit interaction of the radiopharmaceutical with the thrombus. False-negative studies may occur in older thrombi that have lost their active thrombogenic characteristics. Some agents are sensitive but not specific, giving false-positive localization in inflammatory sites.

Inflammatory Conditions

Gallium Scanning in Pneumonitis

The lung is susceptible to numerous infectious and non-infectious inflammatory processes, most with conspicuous changes on radiographs or lung CT. Active infections are usually recognizable by clinical signs and symptoms, but radiographic abnormalities often persist even after the acute process has subsided, leaving fibrosis, chronic infiltrates, or granulomas. Many aseptic inflammatory conditions such as fibrosing alveolitis, sarcoidosis, allergic pneumonitis, pneumoconioses, and drug toxicity reactions may undergo a chronic and relapsing sequence, and tuberculosis may recur in previously scarred areas. Conventional radiography and CT may have difficulty in identifying the active component.

The most common radionuclide test for evaluation of the activity of an inflammatory process is the use of ^{67}Ga-citrate. Areas of both septic and aseptic inflammation will show increased localization of gallium in active sites. Areas of fibrosis do not accumulate gallium, whereas areas of active alveolitis, active tuberculosis, sarcoidosis, or *Pneumocystis carinii* pneumonia (PCP) indicate the activity of the disease, and its distribution, but not its cause. Sequential studies will show progression or response to treatment (38).

The intensity of gallium uptake may be semiquantitatively assessed by comparing the intensity of lung uptake with that of neighboring organs. The normal gallium appearance, shows no significant pulmonary uptake (Fig. 11.5). In early inflammation (grade 1), the heart is a "cold" object relative to mild lung uptake, and the pulmonary activity in the chest is greater than the subdiaphragmatic activity. Lung intensity exceeds the thoracic soft tissues in grade 2, the sternum or other bony structures (grade 3), and, finally, has greater uptake than in the liver (grade 4) (Fig. 11.7). The intensity of gallium uptake correlates well with the cellularity of the aspirate obtained by bronchoalveolar lavage (39), but there is also increased uptake in the acellular supernatant fraction of the BAL in PCP (40).

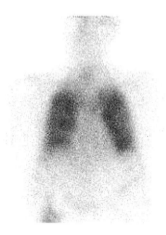
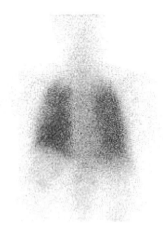

Figure 11.7. Pneumocystis carinii pneumonia. ⁶⁷Ga scan, anterior and posterior views. Diffuse bilateral increased activity. Grade 4 uptake (lung hotter than the liver), in this patient with AIDS.

HIV and AIDS-Related Diseases

Patients who are immunosuppressed due to human immunodeficiency virus (HIV) infection, steroids, post-transplantation, or have marrow replacement diseases are vulnerable to opportunistic infections. Up to 80% of these patients experience PCP, but this complication may be may be radiographically nonspecific, or even occult, in 50% of patients (41). The gallium scan in these patients will show increased lung activity, indicating the active inflammatory process. The usual pattern is diffuse, homogeneous, bilateral, markedly increased uptake. The response to treatment with pentamidine is indicated by normalization of the gallium scan. However, aerosolized pentamidine may not reach some areas as effectively. Some patients on prophylactic pentamidine who develop PCP may have gallium uptake in only part of the lung (42) making the diagnosis less specific (43). Accelerated clearance of ⁹⁹ᵐTc-DTPA aerosol is also demonstrated in the active phase of PCP.

Tuberculosis or atypical tuberculosis causes focal gallium uptake in lymph nodes, or focal distribution within the parenchyma, or other affected sites This appearance is in contrast to the usual diffuse pulmonary uptake pattern of PCP infection.

Kaposi sarcoma may be a complication in one third of acquired minute deficiency syndrome (AIDS) patients. Radiographically, sarcoma in the lungs may not be differentiated from inflammatory infiltrates. It has been shown, however, that Kaposi sarcoma is almost always gallium negative. PCP, tuberculosis or other bacterial pneumonia, and/or Kaposi sarcoma may be present within a nonspecific parenchymal infiltration. On the gallium scan the area of Kaposi sarcoma will be negative, while the other inflammatory processes will be positive. Kaposi sarcoma can be further confirmed by positive uptake within the tumor by thallium or sestamibi scanning, while inflammatory lesions generally have absent uptake by these agents (44,45).

⁶⁷Ga is also a sensitive marker of non-Hodgkin lymphoma. A whole-body scan may be used to stage the distribution of this malignancy.

Sarcoidosis

Gallium is highly sensitive in locating areas of active sarcoidosis. A whole-body gallium scan will reveal the distribution of active intrathoracic and systemic sarcoid lesions. The usual patterns include the pulmonary parenchyma, hilar or peripheral adenopathy, salivary and lachrymal uptake, cutaneous uptake in erythema nodosum, liver and spleen infiltration, and intracranial neural uptake. Intrathoracic uptake of gallium may be diffuse or patchy in the lung parenchyma, or within mediastinal and/or peritracheal lymph nodes, or combined. Regretably, the uptake of gallium is nonspecific and cannot differentiate the hilar adenopathy of sarcoidosis from lymph node involvement by lymphoma. However, in sarcoidosis, the common mediastinal lymph node pattern involves the peritracheal and perihilar lymph nodes in a distribution suggesting the Greek letter lambda (λ). In the presence of the sicca syndrome, or uveoparotitis, the salivary and lachrymal uptake produce an appearance reminiscent of the face of a panda. The combination of the "lambda" and "panda" signs (Fig. 11.8) is virtually exclusive to sarcoidosis, and not seen in lymphoma (46,47). In lymphoma, peripheral lymph node involvement is more common (48).

Cancer Detection and Staging

The principle means of detection of lung malignancies is by plain film or chest CT. However, it may not be possible to differentiate a benign from malignant process within a pulmonary nodule or an enlarged lymph node. Metastases

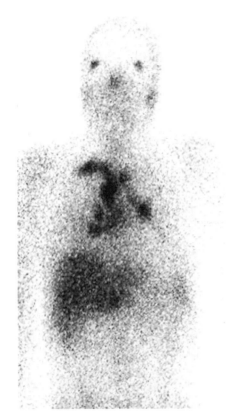

Figure 11.8. Sarcoidosis. Anterior gallium scan shows the classic "lambda sign" (λ) of perihilar and peritracheal lymph node uptake of [67]Ga. This patient also shows the "panda sign" of increased lachrymal and salivary gland uptake. The sign is actually misnamed, as a panda has black ears, not black cheeks.

all nodules are, amenable to intervention. The use of tumor-seeking radiotracers, particularly ^{18}F-FDG, is now becoming widely used for improved detection of primary and metastatic malignant lesions, and for localization of a site for biopsy (49,50). The therapeutic regimen depends on tumor staging. The positive FDG scan helps to select patients for surgery, radiation or chemotherapy (51–53). Detection of tumor spread usually directs the patient away from further surgical intervention (54). Follow-up FDG PET scans may demonstrate response to treatment, or progression of disease.

FDG is expensive, requires special imaging detectors, and the 1.8 h half-life may make it logistically difficult for centers who do not have direct access to a cyclotron. However, the cost efficacy of this technique in preventing unnecessary thoracotomies is now well established (55). Gamma cameras are now available, which may be used for both routine gamma ray nuclear medicine studies, as well as positron detection by dual head coincidence imaging, in those institutions that do not require a dedicated positron camera.

[67]Ga, which is much cheaper and readily available, has been used for lung cancer detection (56,57). However, it may not be able to resolve lesions less than 2 cm in diameter (versus 0.5 cm for PET imaging), and has variable uptake in many tumor cell types. It is still useful in staging of lymphoma (Fig. 11.9).

Thallium, sestamibi and tetrofosmin localize in a variety of tumors (58–61). The uptake of sestamibi and tetrofosmin involves similar pathways of intracellular penetration as various chemotheraputic agents. Lack of uptake of these tracers by malignant tumors correlates with the presence of P-glycoprotein, a factor in multidrug resistance (MDR) to various chemotherapeutic agents. These radiopharmaceuticals may demonstrate the presence of MDR, and predict the possible failure of certain therapeutic regimens (62–64).

and tumor invasion may be difficult to differentiate from nonmalignant granulomas, postsurgical scarring, or post-radiation fibrosis, or they may be obscured by normal mediastinal structures (Fig. 11.9). Histologic sampling may produce specific diagnoses, but not all patients, nor

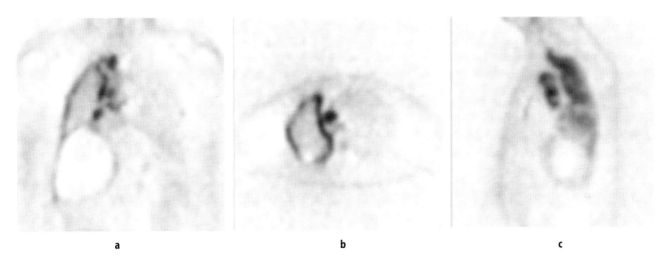

a   b   c

Figure 11.9. [18]F FDG PET in malignant mesothelioma. Coronal (**a**), transaxial (**b**), and sagittal (**c**) tomographic images show marked uptake around the right lung, and in several metastatic foci in right hilar nodes. (Courtesy of the Department of Nuclear Medicine, McMaster University Medical Centre, Hamilton, Canada.)

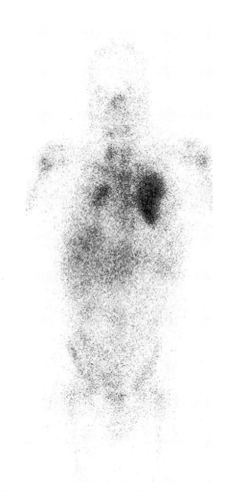

Figure 11.10. Non-Hodgkin lymphoma. Anterior ^{67}Ga scan showing avid uptake in a left lung pulmonary infiltrate, right hilar node, right supraclavicular node, and tiny foci in the liver.

Aerosol Clearance in Alveolitis

Following the administration of ^{99m}Tc-labeled DTPA by aerosol inhalation, there is gradual resorption of this material through the alveolar capillary membrane, into the blood stream, with a normal clearance half-time of more than 60 min (1% per minute). Healthy smokers have an accelerated clearance (4% per minute). In patients with alveolitis, inhalation or radiation pneumonitis, PCP and other infectious processes, sarcoidosis, vasculitis pneumoconiosis, etc., the clearance half-time is markedly accelerated (up to 8% per minute), due to increased capillary permeability and increased porosity of the alveolar epithelial membrane (65–69). An accelerated clearance, even before radiographic changes, is predictive of the possible future development of adult respiratary distress syndrome (ARDS), prompting early therapy (69). It may be used to monitor the progress, or response to treatment of patients who have alveolitis.

Radiation Safety

The clinically useful radiopharmaceuticals are designed to minimize radiation dose. Short-lived tracers are preferred, and isotopes with alpha or beta particle decay are avoided when possible. The radiation burden to the patient depends on the physical decay rate of the tracer (physical $T_{1/2}$), and the duration of the radiopharmaceutical retained in the body (biologic $T_{1/2}$). Combined, these produce the "effective half-time".

Although ^{133}Xe has a long 5 day physical $T_{1/2}$, it is eliminated from the body within minutes of inhalation. Thus it results in a very minimal radiation dose (70). [67]Ga however, has a 3 day physical $T_{1/2}$, and prolonged binding and storage. The potentially high radiation dose is compensated by using a relatively low administered quantity, compared with ^{99m}Tc, which has a 6h $T_{1/2}$. Nuclear medicine studies have an acceptably low radiation dose, in the order of that used in fluoroscopy, spine radiographs, and CT, which results in an insignificant addition to the naturally occurring cancer rate (70).

Pulmonary embolism may be suspected in some pregnant patients, justifying a ventilation – perfusion lung scan. Some radiation dose to the fetus is inevitable, but for the radiopharmaceuticals used in lung scans, this is less then or equal to to the annual natural background radiation exposure (70). Radiation at such low levels does not produce any measurable increase in the incidence of fetal malformations or other complications of pregnancy, compared with the significant incidence of spontaneous genetic problems and miscarrings (71). The hazards of nondiagnosis of a pulmonary embolism, or the inappropriate use of anticoagulants results in a much higher risk of complications than the theoretical effects of these low levels of radiation (72,73).

However, pregnant patients have concerns, and should be counseled about the relative risks of having, or not having, the test. A signed consent to having the test should be obtained. To further offer psychologic support (but probably negligible additional biologic safety), to the pregnant patient, the attending physicians, and ourselves, we may reduce the dose of administered radiopharmaceutical by as much as 50%, and double the imaging time.

Many radioisotopes are excreted in milk in small amounts (74). If a nuclear scan is required during lactation, the mother should be advised that when short-lived tracers such as ^{99m}Tc are used, nursing should be deferred for 24 h. The breast may be pumped and the milk-discarded. For longer-lived radioisotopes, particularly gallium, which binds to lactoferrin, nursing should probably be discontinued completely, as there will be activity in the milk for 1–2 weeks.

Patients may have some residual radiation in their bodies at the conclusion of the diagnostic test. Natural radiation decay accounts for most of the subsequent loss, and some is eliminated in the urine or stool. While the radiation is measurable by sensitive detectors, patients are not considered to be any hazard to the general public or to their family. As a conservative precaution they may wish to remain apart from small children for a day or so, as if they had a cold or the, flu.

Summary

A wide variety of nuclear medicine techniques are available to diagnose and monitor embolic, inflammatory and neoplastic pulmonary conditions. The specific functional information depends on the type of tracer used. Although nuclear images have low spatial resolution they provide a unique physiologic map of metabolic processes occurring in the body which is complementary to the anatomic structural imaging provided by other modalities. Nuclear medicine images are acquired digitally and are thus intrinsically quantitative. This quantitative evaluation may be useful for sequential assessment.

Reference

1. Davis MA, Taube RA (1978) Pulmonary perfusion imaging: Acute toxicity and safety factors as a function of particle size. J Nucl Med 19:1209–1213.
2. Myslivecek M, Husak V, Kolek V, et al. (1992) Absolute quantification of gallium-67 citrate accumulation in the lungs and its importance for the evaluation of disease activity in pulmonary sarcoidosis. Eur J Nucl Med 19:1016–1022.
3. Lentle BC, Catz Z, Dierich HC, et al. (1987) Gallium-67 scintigraphy and non-small-cell bronchogenic carcinoma: A quantitative in-vivo predictive assay? Can Med Assoc J 137:815–817.
4. Brown RS, Leung JY, Kison PV, et al. (1999) Glucose transporters and FDG uptake in untreated primary human non-small cell lung cancer. J Nucl Med 40:556–565.
5. Kemp PM, Tarver DS, Batty V, et al. (1996) Pulmonary embolism. Is the clinical history a useful adjunct to aid the interpretation of the equivocal scan? Clin Nucl Med 21:203–207.
6. van Beek EJ, Reekers JA, Batchelor DA, et al. (1996) Feasibility, safety and clinical utility of angiography in patients with suspected pulmonary embolism. Eur Radiol 6:415–419.
7. Garg K, Welsh CH, Feyerabend AJ, et al. (1998) Pulmonary embolism: Diagnosis with spiral CT and ventilation–perfusion scanning – correlation with pulmonary angiographic results or clinical outcome. Radiology 208:201–208.
8. Robinson PJ (1996) Ventilation-perfusion lung scanning and spiral computed tomography of the lungs: Competing or complementary modalities? Eur J Nucl Med 23:1547–1553.
9. Goodman LR, Curtin JJ, Mewissen MW, et al. (1995) Detection of pulmonary embolism in patients with unresolved clinical and scintigraphic diagnosis: Helical CT versus angiography. AJR 164:1369–1374.
10. The PIOPED Investigators (1990) Value of the ventilation/perfusion scan in acute pulmonary embolism. Results of the prospective investigation of pulmonary embolism diagnosis (PIOPED). JAMA 263:2753–2759.
11. Gottschalk A, Sostman HD, Coleman RE, et al. (1993) Ventilation–perfusion scintigraphy in the PIOPED study. Part II. Evaluation of the scintigraphic criteria and interpretations. J Nucl Med 34:1119–1126.
12. Worsley DF, Alavi A (1995) Comprehensive analysis of the results of the PIOPED study. J Nucl Med 36:2380–2387.
13. Miniati M, Pistolesi M, Marini C, et al. (1996) Value of perfusion lung scan in the diagnosis of pulmonary embolism: Results of the prospective investigative study of acute pulmonary embolism diagnosis (PISA-PED). Am J Respir Crit Care Med 154:1387–1393.
14. van Beek EJ, Kuyer PM, Schenk BE, et al. (1995) A normal perfusion lung scan in patients with clinically suspected pulmonary embolism. Frequency and clinical validity. Chest 108:170–173.
15. Hull RD, Raskob GE, Coates G, et al. (1990) Clinical validity of a normal perfusion lung scan in patients with suspected pulmonary embolism. Chest 97:23–26.
16. Rajendran JG, Jacobson AF (1999) Review of 6-month mortality following low-probability lung scans. Arch Intern Med 159:349–352.
17. Freitas JE, Sarosi MG, Nagle CC, et al. (1995) Modified PIOPED criteria used in clinical practice. J Nucl Med 36:1573–1578.
18. Stein PD, Relyea B, Gottschalk A (1996) Evaluation of individual criteria for low probability interpretation of ventilation–perfusion lung scans. J Nucl Med 37:577–581.
19. Freeman L (1996) The low probability V/Q lung scan: Can its credibility be enhanced? (Editorial). J Nucl Med 37:582–584.
20. Worsley DF, Palevsky HI, Alavi A (1994) A detailed evaluation of patients with acute pulmonary embolism and low-or very-low-probability lung scan interpretations. Arch Intern Med 154: 2737–2741.
21. Stein PD, Gottschalk A, Henry JW, et al. (1993) Stratification of patients according to prior cardiopulmonary disease and probability assessment based on the number of mismatched segmental equivalent perfusion defects. Approaches to strengthen the diagnostic value of ventilation–perfusion lung scans in acute pulmonary embolism. Chest 104:1461–1467.
22. Gray HW, McKillop JH, Bessent RG (1993) Lung scan reports: Interpretation by clinicians. Nucl Med Commun 14:989–994.
23. Gray HW, McKillop JH, Bessent RG (1993) Lung scan reporting language. What does it mean? Nucl Med Commun 14:1084–1087.
24. Kember PG, Euinton HA, Morcos SK (1997) Clinicians' interpretation of the indeterminate ventilation – perfusion scan report. Br J Radiol 70:1109–1111.
25. Kaboli P, Buscombe JR, Ell PJ (1993) Reporting ventilation –perfusion lung scintigraphy: Impact on subsequent use of anticoagulation therapy. Postgrad Med J 69:851–855.
26. Knight LC (1993) Scintigraphic methods for detecting vascular thrombus. J Nucl Med 34(Suppl3):554–561.
27. Dewanjee MK (1987) Methods of assessment of thrombus in vivo. Ann NY Acad Sci 516:541–571.
28. Som D, Oster ZH (1994) Thrombus-specific imaging: Approaching the elusive goal. J Nucl Med 35:202–203.
29. Higashi S, Kuniyasu Y (1984) An experimental study of deep-vein thrombosis using ^{99m}Tc-fibrinogen. Eur J Nucl Med 9:548–552.
30. Smyth JV, Dodd PD, Walker MG (1995) Indium-111 platelet scintigraphy in vascular disease. Br J Surg 82:588–595.
31. Knight LC (1988) Imaging thrombi with radiolabelled fragment E1. Nucl Med Commun 9:849–857.
32. Lavender JP, Stuttle AW, Peters AM, et al. (1988) In vivo studies with an anti-platelet monoclonal antibody: P256. Nucl Med Commun 9:817–822.
33. Lister-James J, Knight LC, Mamer AH, et al. (1996) Thrombus imaging with a Technetium-99m-labelled activated platelet receptor-binding peptide. J Nucl Med 37:775–781.
34. Ciavolella M, Tavolaro R, Di Loreto M, et al. (1999) Immuno-scintigraphy of venous thrombi: Clinical effectiveness of a new antifibrin D-dimer monoclonal antibody. Angiology 50:103–109.
35. Deacon JM, Ell PJ, Anderson P, et al. (1980) Technetium 99m-plasmin: A new test for the detection of deep vein thrombosis. Br J Radiol 53:673–677.

36. Millar WT, Smith JF (1974) Localization of deep-venous thrombosis using technetium-99m-labelled urokinase. Lancet 2:695–696.

37. Kempi V, Van Der Linden W, Von Scheele C (1974) Diagnosis of deep vein thrombosis with 99mTc-streptokinase: A clinical comparison with phlebography. Br Med J 4:748–749.

38. Kao CH, Lin HT, Yu SL, et al. (1994) Lung inflammation in patients with systemic lupus erythematosus detected by quantitative ^{67}Ga-citrate scanning. Nucl Med Commun 15:928–931.

39. Line BR, Fulmer JD, Reynolds HY, et al. (1978) Gallium-67 citrate scanning in the staging of idiopathic pulmonary fibrosis: Correlation with physiological and morphological features and bronchoalveolar lavage. Am Rev Respir Dis 118:355–365.

40. Smith RL, Berkowitz KA, Lewis ML (1992) Pulmonary disposition of gallium-67 in patients with Pneumocystis pneumonia: An analysis using bronchoalveolar lavage. J Nucl Med 33:512–515.

41. Barron T, Birnbbaum N, Shane L, et al. (1987) Pneumocystis carinii pneumonia studied by gallium-67 scanning. Radiology 164:791–793.

42. Katial R, Honeycutt W, Oswald S (1994) Pneumocystis carinii pneumonia presenting as focal bibasilar uptake on galium scan during aerosolized pentamidine prophylaxis. J Nucl Med 35:1038–1040.

43. Kramer EL (1994) PCP, AIDS and nuclear medicine (Editorial). J Nucl Med 35:1034–1037.

44. Abdel-Dayem H, Bag R, DiFabrizio L, et al. (1996) Evaluation of sequential thallium and gallium scans of the chest in AIDS patients. J Nucl Med 37:1662–1667.

45. Turoglu HT, Akisik MF, Naddaf SY, et al. (1998) Tumor and infection localizaton in AIDS patients: Ga-67 and Tl-201 findings. Clin Nucl Med 23:446–459.

46. Sulavik SB, Spencer RP, Palestro CJ, et al. (1993) Specificity and sensitivity of distinctive chest radiographic and/or ^{67}Ga images in the noninvasive diagnosis of sarcoidosis. Chest 103:403–409.

47. Sulavik SB, Spencer RP, Weed DA, et al. (1990) Recognition of distinctive patterns of gallium-67 distribution in sarcoidosis. J Nucl Med 31:1901–1914.

48. Israel HL, Albertine KH, Park CH, et al. (1991) Whole-body gallium 67 scans. Role in diagnosis of sarcoidosis. Am Rev Respir Dis 144:1182–1186.

49. Chiti A, Schreiner FA, Crippa F, et al. (1999) Nuclear medicine procedures in lung cancer. Eur J Nucl Med 26:533–555.

50. Inoue T, Kim EE, Komaki R, et al. (1995) Detecting recurrent or residual lung cancer with FDG-PET. J Nucl Med 36:788–793.

51. Steinhart HC, Hauser M, Allemann F, et al. (1997) Non-small cell lung cancer: Nodal staging with FDG-PET versus CT with corrrelative lymph node mapping and sampling. Radiology 202:441–446.

52. Scott WJ, Schwabe JC, Gupta NC, et al. (1994) Positron emission tomography of lung tumours and mediastinal lymph nodes using F18-fluorodeoxyglucose. Ann Thorac Surg 58:698–703.

53. Guhlmann A, Storck M, Kotzerke J, et al. (1997) Lymph node staging in non-small cell lung cancer: Evaluation by [^{18}]FDG positron emission tomography (PET). Thorax 52:438–441.

54. Bury T, Dowlati A, Paulus P, et al. (1996) Staging of non-small cell lung cancer by whole-body fluorine-18 deoxyglucose positron emission tomography. Eur J Nucl Med 23:204–206.

55. Gambhir SS, Hoh CK, Phelps ME, et al. (1996) Decision tree sensitivity analysis for cost-effectiveness of FDG-PET in the staging and management of non-small cell lung carcinoma. J Nucl Med 37:1428–1436.

56. Ragheb AM, Elgazzar AH, Ibrahim AK, et al. (1995) A comparative study between planar Ga-67, Tl-201 images, chest x-ray, and x-ray CT in inoperable non-small cell carcinoma of the lung. Clin Nucl Med 20:426–433.

57. Matsuno S, Tanabe M, Kawasaki Y, et al. (1992) Effectiveness of planar images and single photon emission tomography of thallium-201 compared with gallium-67 in patients with primary lung cancer. Eur J Nucl Med 19:86–95.

58. Takekawa H, Takaoka K, Tsukamoto E, et al. (1997) Thallium-201 single photon emission computed tomography as an indicator of prognosis for patients with lung carcinoma. Cancer 80:198–203.

59. Greyson ND, Freeman M (1998) Incidental detection of a malignant thymic tumor by Tc-99m sestamibi cardiac imaging. Clin Nucl Med 23:781–782.

60. Arbab AS, Koizumi K, Toyama K, et al. (1996) Uptake of technetium-99m-tetrofosmin, technetium-99m-MIBI and thallium-201 in tumor cell lines. J Nucl Med 37:1551–1556.

61. Bom HS, Kim YC, Song HC, et al. (1998) Technetium-99m-MIBI uptake in small cell lung cancer. J Nucl Med 39:91–94.

62. Piwnica-Worms D, Chiu ML, Budding M, et al. (1993) Functional imaging of multidrug-resistant P-glycoprotein with an organotechnetium complex. Cancer Res 53:977–984.

63. Ballinger JR, Bannerman J, Boxen I, et al. (1996) Technetium-99m-tetrofosmin as a substrate for P-glycoprotein: In vitro studies in a multidrug-resistant breast tumor cells. J Nucl Med 37:1578–1582.

64. Basoglu T, Bernay I, Coskun C, et al. (1998) Pulmonary Tc-99m tetrofosmin imaging: Clinical experience with detecting malignant lesions and monitoring response to therapy. Clin Nucl Med 23:753–757.

65. Coates G, O'Brodovich (1986) Measurement of pulmonary epithelial permeability with 99mTc-DTPA aerosol. Semin Nucl Med 16:275–284.

66. Susskind H, Weber DA, Lau YH, et al. (1997) Impaired permeability in radiation-induced lung injury detected by technetium-99m-DTPA lung clearance. J Nucl Med 38:966–971.

67. Susskind H. Rom WN (1992) Lung inflammation in coal miners assessed by uptake of ^{67}Ga-citrate and clearance of inhaled ^{99m}Tc-labeled diethylenetriamine pentaacetate aerosol. Am Rev Respir Dis 146:47–52.

68. Jacobs MP, Baughman RP, Hughes J, et al. (1985) Radioaerosol lung clearance in patients with active pulmonary sarcoidosis. Am Rev Respir Dis 131:687–689.

69. Tennenberg SD (1987) The use of ^{99m}Tc-DTPA radioaerosol lung clearance in the assessment of acute lung injury: clinical applicability in the adult respiratory distress syndrome. Respir Care 32:757–772.

70. Committee 3 of the International Commission on Radiation Protection (1993) Summary of the current ICRP principles for protection of the patient in nuclear medicine. Pergamon Press, Oxford.

71. Ritenour ER (1986) Health effects of low level radiation: Carcinogenesis, teratogenesis, and mutagenesis. Semin Nucl Med 16:106–117.

72. Sorenson JA (1986) Perception of radiation hazards. Semin Nucl Med 16:158–170

73. van Beek EJ, Kuijer PM, Buller HR, et al. (1997) The clinical course of patients with suspected pulmonary embolism. Arch Intern Med 157:2593–2598.

74. Ahlgren L, Ivarsson S, Johansson L, et al. (1985) Excretion of radionuclides in human breast milk after the administration of radiopharmaceuticals. J Nucl Med 26:1085–1090.

3

Diseases of the Lung and Related Structures

12 Abnormalities of Pulmonary and Mediastinal Vessels

N. Vasile and M.C. Anglade

Introduction

In this chapter the acquired abnormalities of the pulmonary vessels (including the systemic arteries, which contribute to pulmonary vascularization), the superior vena cava, and the azygos vein are described.

Acquired Abnormalities of the Pulmonary Vessels

Pulmonary Arteries

The most frequent acquired disorders of the pulmonary arteries are thromboembolic phenomena, which are described in Chapter 23.

Aneurysm of the Pulmonary Artery (1–4)

Aneurysms of the pulmonary artery are rare. They can be idiopathic or be part of Marfan syndrome. Acquired aneurysms have various etiologies: they may be mycotic, syphilitic, atheromatous, postembolic, or posttraumatic, or they may follow surgery for persistent ductus arteriosus. Acquired aneurysms can be proximal as well as distal, unlike congenital aneurysms, which are usually proximal. Sometimes, as in Hughes–Stovin syndrome, aneurysms can be bilateral and multiple. Mycotic and posttraumatic aneurysms can also be multiple.

Clinical symptomatology in these cases usually depends on the size, the anatomic location, and the eventual complications of the aneurysms. In most cases, pulmonary artery aneurysms are asymptomatic, but they can sometimes be accompanied by chest pain and dyspnea, and rarely by hemoptysis. Clinical manifestations, if present, should in general suggest an impending complication, such as thromboembolism, fissuration, or rupture into the bronchi or mediastinum.

A pulmonary aneurysm may simulate radiologically the presence of a hilar mass. Occasionally, curvilinear calcifications may be noticed in the wall of the aneurysm. Pulmonary angiography, spiral computed tomography (CT) examination or magnetic resonance imaging (MRI) is required for the diagnosis of a pulmonary aneurysm. These techniques are able to identify an increase in the pulmonary artery diameter with loss of continuity of the vessel edge. In some cases, only a part of the aneurysm may opacify because of clots adhering to the aneurysmal wall. CT with bolus injection of contrast material usually adds valuable diagnostic information concerning the presence of an intraluminal clot or an intimal flap of a dissection, as well as mediastinal or pleural effusion (CT numbers specific for blood may support the diagnosis of a rupture).

Pulmonary Artery Enlargement (5,6)

Enlargement of the pulmonary artery can be differentiated from pulmonary aneurysm by the fact that in enlargement the edges of the vessels remain parallel. Enlargement of the pulmonary artery occurs as a result of hypertension; it is present in diseases that produce an increase in pulmonary flow and/or an increase in pulmonary resistance, or an excentric pulmonary flow, or is idiopathic. Pulmonary artery pressure is considered high if it is greater than 30 mmHg. Clinical manifestations of pulmonary hypertension depend on the etiology (Table 12.1)

Roentgenologic signs can be discovered only if pulmonary arterial pressure reaches 50 mmHg. They vary with the basic disorder; however, some signs are common in all instances:

1. Proximal arteries are dilatated and pulsating and there is narrowing of the distal vessels.

Table 12.1. Main etiologies of pulmonary hypertension (PH)

PH with increased vascular resistance		PH with increased flow	PH with increased flow and increased vascular resistance
Precapillary	Postcapillary		
Thromboembolism	Obstruction/stenosis of the pulmonary vein	Left-to-right intra- or supracardiac shunting	Increase of the postcapillary resistances complicating a left-to-right shunt
Obstructive chronic bronchopneumopathy	Left atrium disease		Pulmonary arteriovenous fistula complicating chronic bronchopneumopathy
Diffuse interstitial lung disease	Mitral stenosis		
Neuromuscular disease	Left ventricular failure		
Thoracic deformation Fibrothorax Obesity	Aortic stenosis, regurgitation		

2. In advanced states, there is hypertrophy of the right ventricle.

3. Dilatation of the right ventricle can also be present, with prominence of the pulmonary artery segment in the midpart of the left border and increased convexity of the lower anterior cardiac border on lateral projection. There is also reduction in the size of the retrosternal space.

Spiral CT or pulmonary angiography confirms in these cases the enlargement of the proximal pulmonary arteries and narrowing of the peripheral vessels. The reduction in the size of the peripheral vessels occurs abruptly, producing stagnation of the contrast material. Selective angiography allows a better analysis of peripheral vessels; however, in severe pulmonary hypertension cases, death subsequent to angiography has been reported.

Spiral CT or MRI examination allows differentiation between enlarged pulmonary vessels and hilar tumors. In some cases, the etiology of pulmonary hypertension can be discovered. Some authors have correlated the size of the intrapericardial portion of the right pulmonary artery measured on CT with the degree of pulmonary hypertension (normal value 13.3 ± 1.5 mm). Others have described a correlation between pulmonary hypertension and the index diameter of the main pulmonary artery added to the corporeal area (Fig. 12.1).

Another index has been proposed that consists in measuring on plain films the distance between the midline and the site of emergence of the first branches of the right and left pulmonary arteries. The normal value of this index is the sum of these two measures, reported as the maximal thoracic transverse diameter, and is less than 38%.

These noninvasive methods may offer an appreciation of the severity of the pulmonary hypertension; however, a precise measurement can be obtained only from pulmonary catherization pressure data.

Stenosis and Obstruction of the Pulmonary Artery (7–10)

Extrinsic Compression

Stenosis of the main pulmonary artery may be secondary to intrapericardial space-occupying lesions such as hematomas, sarcomas, bronchogenic cysts, and aneurysm of the sinus of Valsalva or the initial part of the aorta. Stenosis of the right or left pulmonary arteries may result from aortic aneurysm, hilar masses (malignant or benign), and mediastinal lesions.

Clinical manifestations are variable with the disease, being latent in most cases or revealing themselves by the presence of a systolic murmur. In some cases, the symptomatology may simulate the occurrence of a pulmonary embolism: thoracic pain, dyspnea, hypoxemia, and arterial hypertension.

On plain films when no associated abnormalities are present, there is a localized hypoperfusion of the lung with vascular redistribution in other territories. A CT examination can also permit the visualization of the stenotic area; however, its usefulness remains mainly with the evaluation of the primary lesion. Pulmonary angiography is a valuable modality in the diagnosis of pulmonary artery stenosis. It allows a precise evaluation of the stenosis, its site, and the quality of the distal vascularization.

Intrinsic Lesions

Excluding thromboembolic phenomena (discussed in Chapter 23), we will deal only with tumoral pathology. Primary tumors of the pulmonary arteries are very rare and include mainly fibrosarcomas and leiomyosarcomas. They are usually located in the main pulmonary artery, and less often in the pulmonary branches. They are known

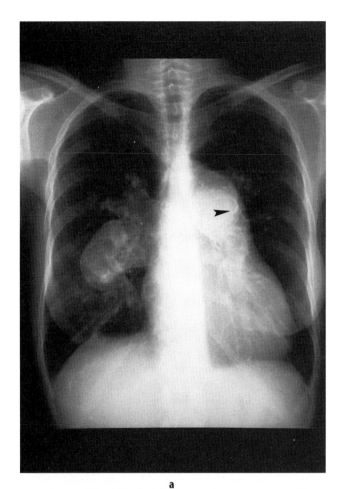

a

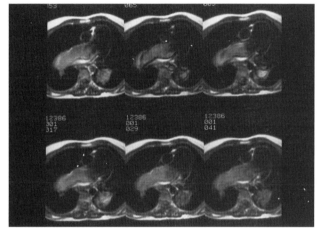

c

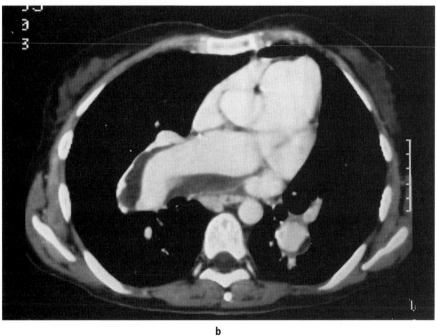

b

Figure 12.1. Female, 32 years old, with 32 years old female, with arterial septal defect. **a** On plain film, dilatation of the proximal pulmonaries arteries with peripheral curvilinear thin calcifications (*arrowhead*); **b** CT and MRI (**c**) scans of the same patient reveal peripheral clots mimicking vessel dissection.

to have hematogenous dissemination and to send metastases to other arterial territories. They can also be the cause of pulmonary infarction. Mediastinal tumors can compress the pulmonary arteries; they can also invade the vessels and lead to an arterial stenosis or obstruction.

Clinical manifestations are commonly discrete and can mimic a pulmonary embolism. When spiral CT is performed, it reveals an arterial obstruction, complete or partial, with the visualization of an irregular growing cast spreading into the secondary branches.

Arteritis (11–17)

Autoimmune diseases of the arteries are of unknown etiology and involve most commonly the aorta and the proximal brachiocephalic arteries, but changes can also occur in other arteries, including the pulmonary arteries.

Takayasu Disease

Takayasu's disease includes destruction of the elastic tissue, intimal proliferation, and adventitial infiltration in the arteries. Pulmonary vessels are involved in 50–80% of cases. In some cases, pulmonary disease precedes the systemic manifestations. The lesions are located mostly in the upper lobes, but complete stenosis of pulmonary arteries can also occur. The disease occurs predominantly in young adult females. While in some cases plain radiographs may appear normal, in others dilatation of the aorta with linear calcification of the aortic arc and pulmonary hypovascularization can be seen.

Imaging reveals the pulmonary artery stenosis. Eventually, the vessels may become completely occluded. Multiple poststenotic dilatations are often present. In cases of complete pulmonary artery obstruction, bronchial collateral circulation can develop. The discovery of pulmonary lesions suggesting Takayasu disease should generally lead to the performance of an aortography to evaluate the systemic extent of the disease.

Behçet disease

Behçet disease has various clinical manifestation. Typically, a mouth ulcer occurring in a young male is associated with rectogenital ulcerations, uveitis, and arthralgia.

Periarterial infiltration with lymphocytes and plasma cells may result in some pathologic changes in the thorax, with areas of diffuse airspace consolidation or peripheral opacities corresponding to pulmonary hemorrhage or pulmonary infarction. In some cases prestenotic dilatations of pulmonary arteries can be observed. Thrombophlebitis is common and may result in superior vena cava

obstruction. CT is the method of choice to evaluate the extent of the thoracic disease.

Hughes–Stovin Syndrome

This rare syndrome, occurring in young males, is characterized by aneurysms of the pulmonary arteries and thrombosis of the peripheral veins. Pulmonary embolism and thrombophlebitis of the vena cava are commonly associated.

Pathology of the Pulmonary Veins (18–20)

Dilatation of the Pulmonary Veins

Juxtaatrial dilatation of the pulmonary veins may be congenital or can occur in acquired mitral valve disease. In the latter condition this is a consequence of an increase in the left auricular pressure. Angiography usually demonstrates the enlarged and tortuous vessels during the stage of pulmonary venous filling. CT examination before contrast injection clearly shows the presence of hilar masses, usually bilaterally. Bolus injection of contrast material demonstrates simultaneous enhancement of these structures and of the left atrium. This differentiates the above pathology from the arteriovenous fistula, which is enhanced earlier, during the stage of right cavities enhancement (Fig. 12.2).

Obstruction of the Pulmonary Veins

Obstruction of the pulmonary veins may occur secondary to various diseases (venous compression by hilar masses, mediastinitis, and extension of left atrial thrombosis) or in the postoperative state after correction of an anomalous venous return. Angiography demonstrates in these cases indirect signs of obstruction: stasis in the pulmonary arterial territory due to pulmonary arterial hypertension with opacification of venous collateral pathways by the parietal or bronchial venous system.

Venoocclusive Disease

This is a rare entity resulting from progressive occlusion of distal pulmonary veins by intimal fibrosis. Fifty percent of cases occur in patients under the age of 16 years. Dyspnea with orthopnea may be present. Hemoptysis is rare. On plain chest radiographs, disseminated interstitial disease of the lungs with Kerley-B lines can be demonstrated. At angiography, the only findings are those of pulmonary hypertension.

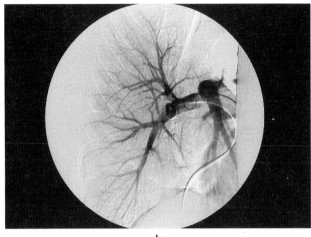

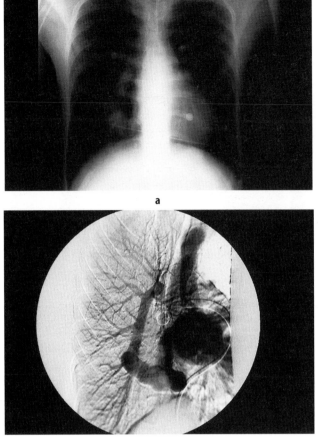

Figure 12.2. Male 18 years old. **a** An episode of chest pain leads to the discovery, on plain film, of a right paracardiac round mass for a vascular connection. **b** The pulmonary angiography performed on the suspicion of a pulmonary arteriovenous fistula shows that the right pulmonary artery is normal but (**c**) the pulmonary vein is unique with juxtaatrial dilatation.

Pulmonary Arteriovenous Fistula

Familial hemorrhagic telangiectasia, or Rendu–Osler–Weber syndrome, is found in 30% of patients with arteriovenous fistulae. Other etiologies for arteriovenous fistula formation are: posttraumatic, metastasis of a primary choriocarcinoma or of a cancer of the thyroid, blood dyscrasias, mitral stenosis, schistosomiasis, and empyema and other conditions associated with pulmonary hypertension. Pulmonary arteriovenous fistulae can be disseminated and multiple, corresponding in 50% of cases to Rendu–Osler–Weber syndrome, or be single and often more prominent in size.

Clinical manifestations are due to the causative disease or to resulting complications. They include hypoxia leading to cyanosis, polycythemia, and clubbing of the fingers. The presence of a right-to-left shunt can lead to a cerebral embolism secondary to thrombosis of the aneurysmal vessel, a brain abscess, or fissuration of the fistulae, with massive hemoptysis.

On plain chest radiographs, lesions appear usually as round or oval densities, single or multiple. On CT scans,

pulmonary nodules of various sizes can be visualized. After bolus injection of contrast, the pulmonary nodules enhance strongly at the time of pulmonary artery enhancement. A dilatated efferent vein can usually also be visualized (Fig. 12.3).

Acquired Disorders of the Bronchial Arteries

Pathologic changes of the bronchial arteries are due to a systemic hypervascularization occurring when pulmonary flow is greatly reduced, such as in congenital heart diseases or in some lung disorders. The systemic collateral pathways are the bronchial arteries, arteries of the triangular ligament, and parietal arteries in the case of pleural adhesions. Two different mechanisms have been described as causing disorders of the bronchial arteries: (a) exclusive systemic vascularization of cicatricial tissue, occurring, for example, in inflammatory lesion or bronchiectasis; and (b) formation of shunts between pulmonary and bronchial circulation by the

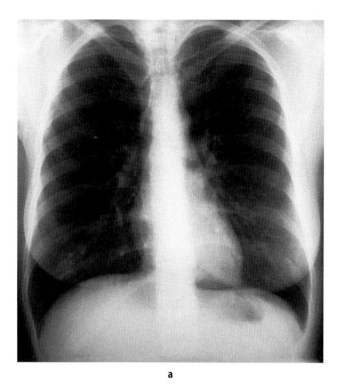

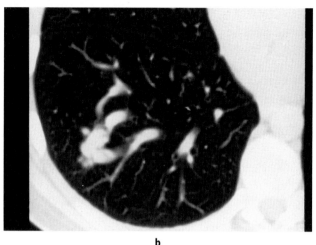

a   b

Figure 12.3. Female, 29 years old, with brain abscess. **a** On plain chest radiograph, there is a round opacity in the right lung. **b** On CT after bolus injection, the node enhances and one efferent vein is seen.

opening of preexisting anastomoses. The main preexisting anastomoses are: precapillary– bronchopulmonary anastomosis, capillary–bronchopulmonary anastomosis, arterioarterial or arteriovenous anastomosis via the vasa vasorum, and transpleural anastomosis between the parietal and pulmonary arteries.

According to the site of the pulmonary lesions and the anastomosis, two types of shunt can be differentiated: anterograde and retrograde. In anterograde shunting a systemic artery revascularizes first a pulmonary arterial branch, then the capillary vessels and the pulmonary veins. This kind of communication occurs in cases of congenital cardiac malformations with an obstruction to the pulmonary outflow tract, or in cases with proximal stenosis of the pulmonary artery with a normal capillary bed. In retrograde shunting a systemic artery vascularizes a pulmonary arterial branch in an upstream direction. This communication occurs whenever the capillary bed is obstructed, as in cases of pleural or parenchymal pulmonary disorders. The above communications may eventually change their direction. An anterograde shunting may, as a result of the high pressure that alters and occludes the capillary bed, become retrograde.

The most common clinical manifestation of bronchial artery disorders, and of all hypervascularization states, is hemoptysis.

Radiological Manifestations

On plain chest radiographs bronchial artery branches may be seen as multiple nodular opacities or tortuous linear shadows within the proximal lung fields. In fact, signs of the basis disorder causing bronchial abnormalities may be the only radiographic finding. In general, one or more systemic arteries (bronchial or parietal) are enlarged and tortuous. The pulmonary artery opacified via the arterial pathway is not always seen, depending on the site of the shunt and the angiographic technique. Distal anastomoses are seldom visualized; however, the draining pulmonary vein is usually opacified. During hemoptysis, bronchial arteriography may reveal the site of the bleeding by blood pooling into the bronchial wall or lumen.

Bronchial Artery Embolization (21–24)

Embolization of the systemic arteries of the lung is an effective treatment for massive hemoptysis and for some cases of bronchial hypervascularization.

Technique

Transcatheter embolization involves the injection of occluding material via the angiographic catheter, a preformed 5F with a distal hole. The catheter is placed under fluoroscopic guidance to monitor the progress of embolization, and frequent injection of contrast material is used.

Embolization materials include resorbable materials, such as Gelfoam, Ivalon (a plastic sponge material that is dry in the compressed state and reexpands when wetted, and nonresorbable materials such as isobutyl 2-cyano-acrylate (IBC), which remains liquid in a nonionized environment but polymerizes when contact with blood occurs. The most frequently used is Gelfoam, Ivalon and IBC being somewhat unreliable in regard to degree of embolization (Fig. 12.4).

Complications

Some slight discomfort is associated with embolization procedures, including chest pain and fever in the 48 h following the examination. Severe complications resulting from the occlusion of spinal arteries (with the possibility of spinal cord injury and paraplegia) and esophageal necrosis have been also described. Therefore, the decision regarding use of embolization and the choice of the most appropriate embolizing material should be in the hands of an experienced vascular radiologist.

Superior Vena Cave Disorders

Aneurysm of the Superior Vena Cava (25)

Aneurysms of the superior vena cava are rare and asymptomatic. They are usually discovered incidentally. The performance of a superior venography will demonstrate in these cases widening of the superior vena cava. CT images

usually show a mass-like structure. These two investigations should also be able to detect thrombosis, which can lead to pulmonary embolism.

Persistent Left Superior Vena Cava (Fig. 12.5) (26–29)

A persistent left superior vena cava results from the absence of involution of the left anterior cardinal vein. This abnormality has no hemodynamic significance and is clinically latent. Its frequency is about 0.3% in the overall population, but it is observed more frequently (4.4%) in association with cardiovascular congenital abnormalities, of which septal defects and anomalous pulmonary veins are the most common.

In most cases, the right superior vena cava is normal, the brachiocephalic vein is small or absent, and the left superior vena cava connects to the coronary sinus and drains into the posteroinferior portion of the right atrium.

CT or MRI features are characteristic. The left vena cava is symmetric with the right one. It is situated anteriorly to the left subclavian artery and exteriorly to the carotid artery. It runs obliquely caudal from left to right, forward to the aortic arch, from the pulmonary hilum toward the coronary sinus.

In some cases, the right vena cava involutes completely, leaving only a left superior vena cava.

Superior Vena Cava Compression (30)

Displacement of the superior vena cava may be caused by mediastinal tumors, aneurysms of the ascending aorta, a right-sided aortic arch, or the absence of the innominate vein. Other reasons for displacement include thoracic

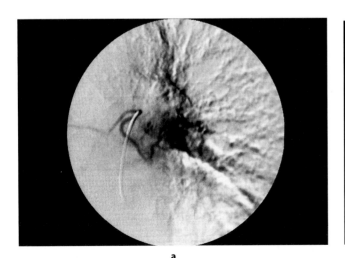

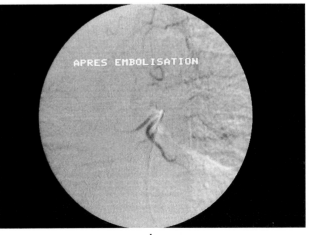

a   b

Figure 12.4. Male, 47 years old, with hemoptysis. Bronchial arteriography shows a localized hypervascularization (**a**) when embolization is performed (**b**).

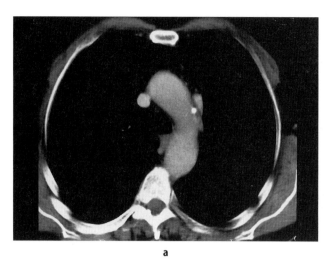
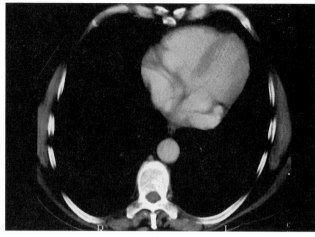

a   b

Figure 12.5. Male, 32 years old. **a** On the CT scan performed for the staging of a non-Hodgkin lymphoma, a persistant left superior vena cava is discovered connecting on the caudal views (**b**) into the coronary sinus.

deformations such as a funnel breast deformity or retractile disease of the left hemithorax.

Compression of the superior vena cava is expressed clinically by the superior vena cava syndrome (dilatation of superficial veins, cyanosis, and superior thoracic edema). CT scanning demonstrates the degree of obstruction and the extent of venous collateral pathways. It permits recognition of the causative pathology.

Superior Vena Cava Obstruction

Compression, thrombosis, and inflammatory or tumoral involvement can all produce obstruction of superior vena cava. CT usually demonstrates the obstruction and the extent of collateral circulation.

Direct signs of obstruction include the findings of an endoluminal filling defect, with possible extension to efferent veins. On CT scan sections before the injection of contrast material, the density varies according to the age of the clot. A fresh thrombus is hyperdense compared with the circulating blood. Later it becomes isodense with the blood, but may also undergo calcification. After contrast injection by bilateral venous injection, the vascular lumen is not opacified and the vessel will present a rim enhancement on CT as a result of enhancement of the vascular wall by the vasa vasorum.

Collateral pathways usually develop in the azygos system. This is the main collateral pathway. Whenever the superior vena cava is occluded below the azygos arch, the azygos vein diverts blood from the obstructed cava toward the lumbar veins and inferior vena cava. With occlusion of the superior vena cava above the azygos vein, there is collateral flow through the intercostal veins into the azygos

vein. When the obstruction involves the arch of the azygos vein, the blood is diverted to the inferior vena cava either by the internal and external mammary veins, which connect the innominate veins, epigastric veins, and inferior caval circulation, or by the vertebral venous plexus, which connects the innominate veins, posterior jugular veins, and vertebral veins to the lumbar veins. All these different collateral pathways may ultimately be connected by intercostal veins.

Abnormalities of the Superior Left Intercostal Vein and of the Internal Mammary Veins

Dilatation of these venous systems has the same causes as azygos vein dilatation, including involvement or obstruction by tumors originating in the lungs or the mediastinum.

The left superior intercostal veins may be enlarged in conditions that produce distension in the hemiazygos and the accessory hemiazygos system (31). It projects over the inferolateral portion of the aortic knob and may be a cause of "aortic nipple" on frontal chest radiographs. (Fig. 12.6).

Abnormalities of the Azygos Vein (31)

The normal azygos vein has a diameter that varies from 5 to 10 mm according to the intrathoracic pressure. The width of the azygos vein is decreased by inspiration and the Valsalva maneuver. Causes for azygos vein dilatation are summarized in Table 12.2. Commonly, radiologic studies are used to distinguish between an enlarged azygos vein and a large lymph node. The diagnosis is

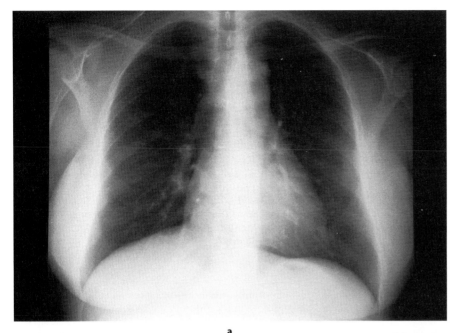

a

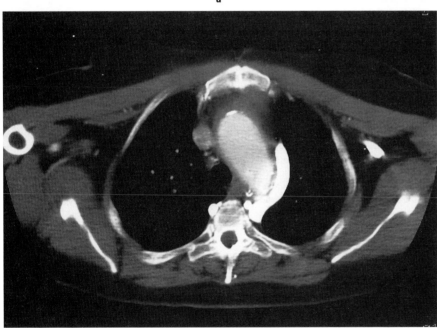

b

Figure 12.6. Female, 65 years old. **a** "Aortic nipple" on frontal chest radiograph. **b** On CT there is lack of enhancement of the superior vena cava. The left superior intercostal vein is enlarged and highly enhanced.

Table 12.2. Main causes of a dilatated azygos vein

Obstruction of superior vena cava
Acquired or congenital obstruction of inferior vena cava
Hypertension in right heart chambers
Obstruction of pulmonary vein
Portal hypertension
Budd–Chiari syndrome
Vertebral arteriovenous fistulae
Pulmonary sequestration
Hypervascularized tumor draining into azygos system
Posttraumatic pseudoaneurysm
Kinking of the aorta
Pregnancy
Idiopathic

usually made on CT scans obtained after injection of contrast material.

One malformation that is often isolated, but is sometimes associated with dextrocardia, partial or total situs inversus, and other congenital malformations, is the infrahepatic interruption of the inferior vena cava with azygos continuation. In this case the azygos vein is widened as a result of failure of development of the suprarenal segment of the inferior vena cava. Through the dilatated azygos vein, blood is carried to the superior vena cava. The diagnosis of this condition, which has a frequency of 0.6–1% in patients with cardiac malformations, can be made by echography, CT and MRI.

References

1. Crivello MS, Hayes C, Thurer RL, et al. (1986) Traumatic pulmonary artery aneurysm: CT evaluation. J Comput Assist Tomogr 10:503–505.
2. Daykin EL, Gal I, Harisson DA (1986) CT demonstration of a traumatic aneurysm of the pulmonary artery. J Comput Assist Tomogr 10:323–324.
3. Ferretti GR, Thony F, Link KM, et al. (1996). False aneurysm of the pulmonary artery induced by a Swan–Ganz catheter: Clinical presentation and radiologic management. AJR 167:941–945.
4. O'Callaghan JP, Heitzman ER, Somogyi JW, et al. (1982) CT evaluation of pulmonary artery size. J Comput Assist Tomogr 6:101–104.
5. Lupi E, Dumont C, Tejada VM, et al. (1975) A radiologic index of pulmonary arterial hypertension. Chest 68:28–31.
6. Charnsangave JC (1979) Occlusion of the right pulmonary artery by acute dissecting aortic aneurysm. AJR 132:274–276.
7. Shield JJ, Cho KJ, Geisinger KR (1980) Pulmonary artery constriction by mediastinal lymphoma simulating pulmonary embolus. AJR 135:14–150.
8. Ilsson HE, Spitzer RM, Erston WF (1976) Primary and secondary pulmonary artery neoplasia mimicking acute pulmonary embolism. Radiology 18:49–53.
9. Kauczor HU, Schwickert HC, Mayer E, et al. (1997) Pulmonary artery sarcoma mimicking chronic thromboembolic disease: Computed tomographic and magnetic resonance imaging findings. Cardiovasc Intervent Radiol 17:185–189.
10. Wieder S, White TJ, Salazar J, et al. (1982) Pulmonary artery occlusion due to histoplasmosis. AJR 138:243–251.
11. Kuniaki H, Masaji N, Naofumi M, et al. (1996) Initial pulmonary artery involvement in Takayasu arteritis. Radiology 159:401–403.
12. Suzuki Y, Konishi K, Hisada K (1973) Radioisotope lung scanning in Takayasu's arteritis. Radiology 109:133–136.
13. Liu YQ, Jin BL, Ling J (1994) Pulmonary artery involvement in aortoarteritis: An angiographic study. Cardiovasc Intervent Radiol 17:2–6.
14. Sharma S, Rajani M, Talwar KK (1992) Angiographic morphology in nonspecific aortoarteritis (Takayasu's arteritis): A study of 126 patients from North India. Cardiovasc Intervent Radiol 15:160–165.
15. Matsunaga N, Hayashi K, Sakamoto I, et al. (1997) Takayasu arteritis: Protean radiologic manifestations and diagnostis. Radiographics 17:579–594.
16. Grenier P, Bletry O, Cornud F, et al. (1984) Pulmonary involvement in Behçet disease. AJR 137:565–569.
17. Teplick JG, Haskin ME, Nedwich A (1984) The Hughes–Stovin syndrome. Radiology 113:607–608.
18. Shackelford GD, Sacks EJ, Mullens JD, et al. (1977) Pulmonary veno-occlusive disease: Case report and review of literature. AJR 128:643–648.
19. Swensen SJ, Tashjian JH, Myers JL, et al. (1996) Pulmonary veno-occlusive disease: CT findings in eight patients. AJR 167:937–940.
20. White CS, Baffa JM, Haney PJ, et al. (1998) Anomalies of pulmonary veins: Usefulness of spin-echo and gradient-echo MR images. AJR 170:1365–1368.
21. Cadotte R, Leger C, Harel C, et al. (1986) Bronchial angiography: Report of 21 patients. J Can Assoc Radiol 37:22.
22. Zhang JS, Cui EP, Wang MQ, et al. (1994) Bronchial areteriography and transcatheter embolization in the management of hemoptysis. Cardiovasc Intervent Radiol 17:276–279.
23. Casteneda-Zuniga WR, Epstein M, Zollikofer CL, et al. (1980) Embolization of multiple pulmonary artery fistulas. Radiology 134:309–310.
24. Haitjema TJ, Overtoom TTC, Westermann CJJ, et al. (1998) Embolisation of pulmonary arteriovenous malformations: Results and follow up in 32 patients. Thorax 50:719–723.
25. Hidvegi RS, Modry DL, Lafleche L (1979) Congenital saccular aneurysm of the superior vena cava: Radiographic features. AJR 133:924–927.
26. Huggins TJ, Lesar ML, Friedman AC, et al. (1981) CT appearance of persistant left superior vena cava. J Comput Assist Tomogr 6:921–924.
27. Baron RL, Guttierrez FR, Sagel SS, et al. (1981) CT of anomalies of the mediastinal vessels. AJR 137:571–576.
28. Webb WR, Gamsu G, Speckman JM, et al. (1982) Pictorial essay: Computed tomographic demonstration of mediastinal venous anomalies. AJR 139:157–161.
29. White CS, Baffa JM, Haney PJ, et al. (1997) MR imaging of congenital anomalies of the thoracic veins. Radiographics 17:595–608.
30. Racke JR, Kaplan H, Conway WA (1980) The significance of superior vena cava syndrome developing in patients with sarcoidosis. Radiology 137:311–312.
31. Hatfield MK, Vyborny CJ, McMahon H, et al. (1987) Congenital absence of the azygos vein: A cause for "aortic nipple" enlargement. AJR 149:273–274.

13 Pneumonias

P.L. Clouet, Y. Berthezene, B. Marchand, P. Nesme, and J.-F. Mornex

Introduction

Pneumonia remains a major cause of death worldwide, accounting for an estimated 5 million deaths per year. In developed countries, the antimicrobial era has brought a 66% reduction in the crude mortality rate associated with the disease, but pneumonia remains the most frequent infectious cause of death and the sixth leading cause overall in the USA (1).

General Clinical and Radiologic Aspects of Pneumonia

Pneumonia presents clinically as an infectious syndrome with symptoms indicating respiratory tract involvement. Physical examination establishes a diagnosis of pneumonia that can be confirmed by radiologic examination.

The posterior–anterior and lateral chest roentgenogram is still the standard in the diagnosis of pneumonia, with good interobserver reliability when infiltrate, multilobar disease, or pleural effusion is present (2). Although computed tomography (CT) has a radiation equivalent of about 100 chest radiographs, it shows findings suggestive of pneumonia approximately 5 days prior to the appearance of an infiltrate on the chest roentgenogram in neutropenic patients with fever of unknown origin (3).

The Infectious Syndrome

The primary symptom is fever; it can vary both in intensity and in chronologic pattern. It may begin abruptly, or, conversely, have a slow and progressive onset; it may be sustained or intermittent in type; it may relapse, and its termination may be marked by remittent episodes or by a rapid and continuous decrease.

The Pulmonary Infectious Syndrome

The principal clinical symptom is coughing, which may initially be dry or productive. Sputum production appears or increases as in patients with chronic bronchitis. Hemoptysis is occasionally seen. The patient typically complains of chest pain when pleural inflammation is present. Dyspnea and cyanosis are less frequent, but may occur in the presence of chronic obstructive lung disease, for example, in patients with chronic bronchitis or asthma.

Pneumonia

The association of alveolitis with consolidation produces a characteristic picture on physical examination, with fine crackles, percussion dullness, increased tactile fremitus, inspiratory rales, and bronchial breath sounds. Pneumonias typically show an alveolar pattern with coalescence of densities to form large homogeneous shadows, and with the presence of an air bronchogram resulting from the air-filled peripheral bronchi being surrounded by airless consolidated tissue. Consolidation may be limited to one lobe or pulmonary segment, or may be more diffusely spread. Lobar pneumonia provides a most characteristic example. Homogeneous confluent densities obliterate the normal vascular pattern throughout the whole lobe, and are bounded by the fissure (Fig. 13.1). The filled airways produce an air bronchogram. In general, lobar pneumonia involves multiple segments. Bronchopneumonia, or lobular pneumonia, presents a more variable picture. The involvement of bronchial and alveolar spaces with peribronchial thickening leads to a fluffy, ill-defined density with or without volume loss. Acute interstitial pneumonia, frequently associated with mycoplasma or viral infections, typically gives a pattern involving finely reticulated densities. Finally, single or multiple

171

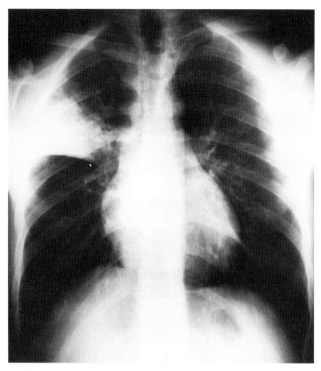

Figure 13.1. Typical upper lobe acute lobar pneumonia in a 24 year old male.

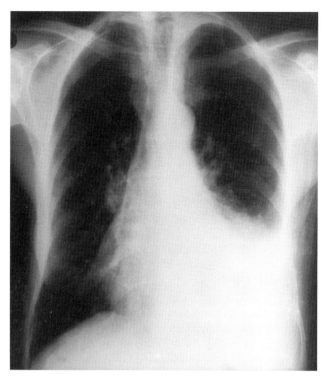

Figure 13.2. Left lower lobe pneumonia with pleural effusion.

nodules may be observed alone, or with any of the above patterns.

Two major types of pneumonia are encountered. In common acute pneumonia there is an abrupt onset with shivering and chills. In typical lobar pneumonia caused by *Streptococcus pneumoniae* findings include a productive cough of pinkish or rusty mucus sputum, a dull percussion tone, and tubular breath sounds with fine rales. Clinical examination may disclose fever blisters (herpes labialis). Severe acute pneumonia is characterized by dyspnea and cyanosis, and may be encountered in specific clinical settings: acute respiratory distress syndrome, chronic respiratory insufficiency, and extensive pneumonias, such as those caused by *Legionella pneumophila*.

Further investigations can be performed in order to gain access to infectious samples for assessment of the agent causing the pneumonia. These investigations include analysis of sputum, transtracheal aspiration, analysis of fiberoptic bronchoscopic aspiration, or bronchoalveolar lavage. A bacterial or a viral isolate from the respiratory tract should be analyzed with caution.

Chest X-rays should be employed in the follow-up of the pneumonia patient, to visualize the progressive clearing of the densities and to detect possible complications (4). The most frequent complications are pleural effusion (Fig. 13.2) and cavitation (Fig. 13.3). These show up as lucent patches in the density and may appear as a single pulmonary abscess (Fig. 13.4) or as multiple centers scattered through the affected region. A delay in the resolution of the chest X-ray of longer than 2 to 3 weeks is quite

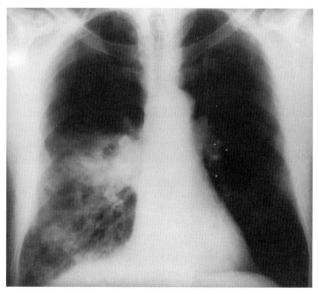

Figure 13.3. Middle lobe pneumonia with cavitation.

frequently associated with certain pathogens, as a result of the anatomic reorganization of the initial inflammatory lesions (so-called chronic pneumonia), or as a result of insufficient treatment schedules.

In older patients with alcoholism or chronic obstructive pulmonary disease, resolution may take as long as 18 weeks. Legionnaires' disease and necrotizing pneumonias may take several months to resolve; bronchoscopy and/or

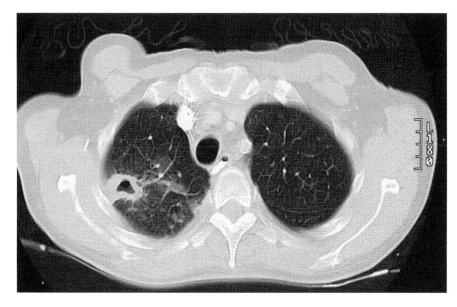

Figure 13.4. CT scan of a right upper lobe pulmonary abscess.

CT are recommended for all chronic nonresolving pneumonias (5). Recurrent pneumonias occur typically in patients with one or more intrathoracic (benign or malignant obstruction, bronchectasis) (Fig. 13.5) or extrathoracic predisposing factors.

Differential Diagnoses

Delayed resolution always requires consideration of possible differential diagnoses, such as pulmonary embolism, bronchial obstruction (benign or malignant), lymphoma and bronchioloalveolar carcinoma (BAC).

BAC radiographic similarity to pneumonia delayed one correct diagnosis by an average of 5 months (6). Many findings reported as key features of BAC (leafless tree bronchogram, cysts or cavities) were present in both BAC and pneumonia. Hence, multifocality indicating tumor spread – peripheral consolidation and nodules – should suggest a diagnosis of BAC (Fig. 13.6).

One other diagnosis is bronchiolitis obliterans with organizing pneumonia where thin-section CT scan through

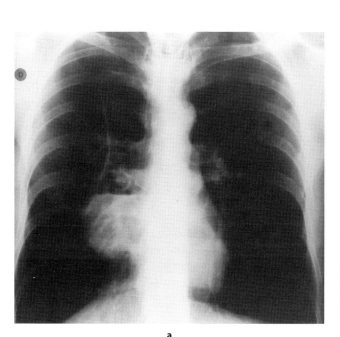

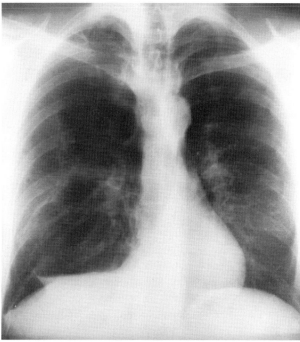

a b

Figure 13.5. **a** Infection of a pulmonary bullon **b** Evolution after 3 weeks of treatment with antibiotics

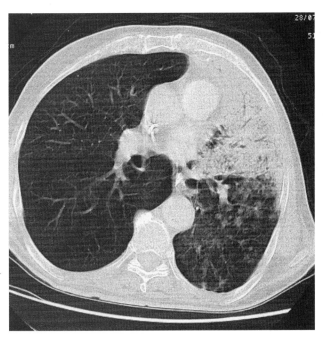

Figure 13.6. Bronchioloalveolar carcinoma in a 62 year old male, demonstrating a left upper lobe consolidation with multiple nodules in the lower lobe.

conditioning system. The isolation and bacteriologic identification of the agent is tedious. The disease has an acute onset with high fever and chills but very few respiratory symptoms (dry cough) or signs pointing to respiratory tract involvement. In contrast extrapulmonary symptoms can be impressive, including confusion, disorientation, hematuria, and renal insufficiency. Chest radiographs show poorly marginated rounded opacities that are patchy and localized at first, but rapidly progress, sometimes within a single day, to involve multiple lobes (Fig. 13.8) and become bilateral. The resulting impairment of pulmonary function may require mechanical ventilation of the patient. The resolution is slow, but pleural effusion and cavitation are rare. Prognosis depends essentially on the rapid identification of the pathogen, which may be obtained from bronchoalveolar lavage samples. A typical radiographic picture shows a dense opacity involving a single lobe or segment, bounded by the pleural fissures.

Staphylococcus aureus can cause unilateral or bilateral pneumonia with formation of pneumoceles. Pleural effusion occurs in up to 50% of patients. The initial radiologic pattern is of multiple bilateral heterogeneous shadows (Fig. 13.9).

Chlamydia psittacis is the causative agent of ornithosis and may infect those exposed to pet birds. The clinical picture is poor as compared with the radiologic examination. Blood-tinged sputum is characteristic, and mediastinal lymph nodes may be found.

Mycoplasma pneumoniae infection generally results in diffuse pneumonia, and may spread epidemically by close contact. The pathologic findings are bronchiolitis and interstitial pneumonia. The radiographic findings are usually less impressive than the physical signs, and may include a unilateral segmental or lobar confluence of patchy consolidation, but bilateral or multiple segment involvement is more typical. Nodular infiltrates may be observed in the lower lobes. Pleural effusion is infrequent. *Mycoplasma pneumoniae* is the causative agent of so-called primary atypical pneumonia, but the more usual manifestations involve the association of a predominant alveolar pattern with an interstitial pattern. Hilar lymphadenopathies are more often seen than in other infections. The pathogen initially induces a peribronchovascular inflammatory process after its fixation to the bronchial epithelium, and both incubation time and resolution of the lesions are long.

Other bacterial diseases can occur. The most usual cause of rickettsial pneumonia is *Coxiella burnetti*, the Q fever agent. The chest radiograph shows patchy areas of consolidation that can be segmental or lobar. The Q fever agent is transmitted by bovine and ovine animals. *Actinomyces israelii* causes an insidious chronic pneumonia that frequently evolves toward a parietal lesion with rib involvement. *Nocardia asteroides* is an uncommon pathogen in normal patients; however, its incidence is

the lung can show bilateral, patchy, rounded opacities in a subpleural location. These opacities have irregular margins and correspond to areas of airspace consolidation.

Clinical and Radiologic Aspects of Causative Agents

Although it is not possible to make a definitive identification of the causative agent on the basis of clinical and radiographic findings, some pathogens are frequently associated with certain signs in a way that can be helpful in making therapeutic decisions.

Bacteria

Typical acute pneumonia is most often caused by *S. pneumoniae*. Pleural effusion, sometimes including empyema, is frequent (50% of cases), and progression, possibly to the other lung, occurs in 40% of patients.

Klebsiella pneumoniae generally causes an acute pneumonia, with dense lobar or segment consolidation and enlargement, generally in elderly patients. The upper lobes are most frequently affected and brick-red. bloody sputum is characteristic. Cavitation, which may evolve to empyema, is a frequent complication (7) (Fig. 13.7).

Pneumonia caused by *L. pneumophila* has a long incubation time (up to 10–15 days), and is associated with exposure to contaminated water, often via an air-

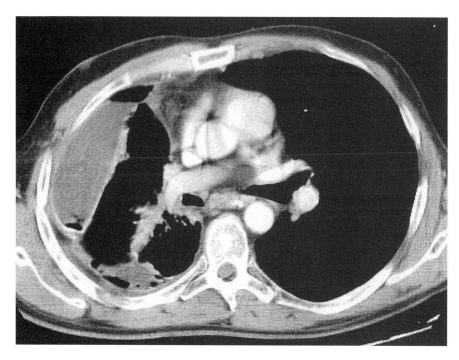

Figure 13.7. CT scan showing a right empyema in a patient with *Klebsiella*

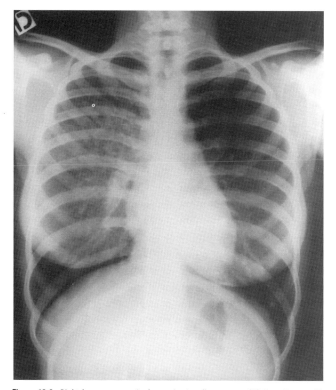

Figure 13.8. Right lung pneumonia due to *Legionella pneumophila* in a 40 year old female showing poorly marginated rounded opacities.

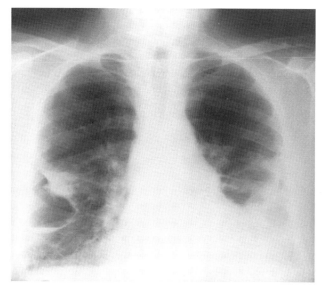

Figure 13.9. *Staphylococcus aureus* bilateral pneumonia in a 60 year old male.

rising in immunocompromised patients. Clinically, the picture is of chronic suppurative pneumonia rather than classic pneumonia.

Other bacteria that rarely cause pneumonia include: *Haemophilus influenzae*, more often responsible for an acute exacerbation of chronic pneumonia; *Pseudomonas aeruginosa*; *Enterobacter*; *Streptococcus pyogenes*; and *Escherichia coli*. Anaerobic bacteria may cause pneumonia, usually associated with cavitation, as do certain unconventional agents such as *Proteus, Serratia, Acineto-*

bacter, Listeria monocytogenes, Brucella melitensis, and *Yersinia pestis*.

Patients infected with human immunodeficiency virus (HIV) need chest roentgenograms for their febrile illnesses. Many of the bacterial infections behave as described above, but atypical presentations are more common. For instance, with salmonella bacteremia, lung involvement was found in up to 35% of patients and cavitary disease was the most common radiologic finding. Suppurative nocardia infections often present with focal consolidation but cavitation and pleural involvement can occur. Patients with HIV are more likely to have multiple nodules or cavitation. The diagnosis of actinomycosis is often delayed if the characteristic cutaneous fistula with yellow granular discharge does not occur, because the radiographic features are not distinctive. Only 15% of the infections involve the thorax, but invasion of the ribs or vertebral bodies can cause a reactive periostitis that can be detected by bone scan. A nonspecific chronic alveolar infiltrate resembling pneumonia, or a mass with or without cavitation and pleural effusion, is common, but hilar lymphadenopathy is rare. Infiltrates have a basilar predominance and tend to involve adjacent lobes via interlobar fissure.

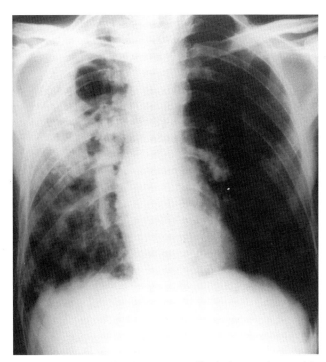

Figure 13.10. Reactivation tuberculosis in a 48 year old male, demonstrating upper lobe consolidation with cavitation.

Mycobacterium Tuberculosis

Primary tuberculosis in the normal host remains dormant. However, radiographic findings in patients with active disease include one or more of the following: parenchymal lower lobe consolidation, hilar and mediastinal lymphadenopathy, and pleural effusion. Loculated pleural effusions may be a source for development of a bronchopleural fistula and active tuberculosis as long as 20–40 years after the initial infection. In patients with acquired immune deficiency syndrome (AIDS), progressive primary tuberculosis is seen as a single focus in one lobe that may progress to extensive involvement of one or both lungs, with cavitation.

Reactivation tuberculosis occurs typically in the first and second year following initial infection. It occurs most frequently in the elderly. A dormant focus becomes active when the immune defense system becomes impaired. The apical and posterior segments of the upper lobe and the superior segment of the lower lobe are most commonly involved (Fig. 13.10). Cavitation and a chronic lesion with calcification may occur. The National Tuberculosis and Respiratory Disease Association requires unchanging radiographs for 6 months for tuberculosis to be labeled as radiographically stable. Endobronchial tuberculosis has been reported in 10–20% of cases and causes airway stenosis and respiratory failure in the acute phase. Patients with active disease showed irregular and thick-walled airways by CT that was reversible. Patients with fibrotic

disease had smooth narrowing of airways and minimal wall thickening that was not reversible. The tuberculoma, a spherical, smooth, sometimes calcified nodule may appear in both primary and reactivation disease. Miliary tuberculosis, described as multiple 1 mm small nodules throughout the lung field, occurs within a few weeks of the initial infection.

Although mediastinal adenopathy or pleural effusion is thought to be typical of recent or primary infection, this classic distinguishing feature is lost in patients with HIV. Recent and remote tuberculosis have similar presentations, and the adenopathy and pleural effusion reflect the status of the ineffective cell-mediated immunity rather than the timing of the disease. The state of HIV infection determines how tuberculosis is manifested radiographically. Initially, in less immunocompromised patients, most infections are the result of reactivation. In later stages, a diffuse symmetric coarse reticular or reticulonodular infiltrate is seen. Cavitation at this stage is rare.

Mycobacteria Other than M. Tuberculosis

All infections of *Mycobacterium kansasii* and *Mycobacterium avium-intracellulare* are primary. *M. kansasii* and *M. avium-intracellulare* have been found to be radiographically indistinguishable from tuberculosis in some studies. Other studies, however, have shown that, unlike in tuberculosis, 50% of patients had a bronchiectatic pattern, solid infiltrates, or nodules in the mid and lower lung field and multiple nodules and infiltrates without upper lobe predominance. Cavities are often thin walled.

In patients with HIV infection, lymphadenopathy with other mycobacterial infection is common, unlike in the normal host. Cavitation is rare. The lung field may be normal or may have patchy infiltrates. Fishman et al. (8) characterized the chest radiographic studies in 96 patients with HIV and *M. kansasii* infections: 75% demonstrated alveolar opacities, 25% had thoracic lymphadenopathy, 19% had cavitation, 12% had pleural effusions, and 6% had interstitial opacities. *Mycobacterium avium-intracellulare* is a common pathogen in end-stage HIV infection. The radiograph can show cavitary upper lobe disease at this point.

Viral Infections

Viral pneumonia accounts for approximately 25% of cases of community-acquired pneumonia. Six radiographic patterns for viral infections have been noted on the chest roentgenogram (2) (a) acute interstitial pneumonia shows thickening of the end-on bronchi and tramlines; a diffuse miliary pattern may also be seen; (b) lobular or sublobular inflammatory reaction reveals patchy airspace filling with diffuse acinar nodular pattern, characteristic of varicella pneumonia; (c) localized hemorrhic pulmonary edema has confluent segmental opacification that is often confused with bacterial lobar pneumonia; (d) generalized hemorrhagic pulmonary edema reveals an acute, disseminated alveolar perihilar pattern, characteristic of influenza virus; (e) pleural exudation; and (f) effusion along with chronic interstitial fibrosis.

Influenza as a result of infection by myxoviruses usually involves the bronchi and produces a clinical picture of bronchial rales with no evidence of parenchymal involvement; however, on some occasions it can produce a typical clinical picture of pneumonia. In these cases the chest X-ray shows typical opacities, but lacks the air bronchogram, giving a diffuse interstitial pattern. After the myxoviruses, adenoviruses are the most frequent causes of viral pneumonia. The radiologic picture is generally that of heterogeneous pneumonia that rarely involves the parenchyma, but that may facilitate the superposition of bacterial pneumonia. In children, respiratory syncytial virus may cause bronchiolitis, giving a picture with haziness at the lung base and a diffuse unilateral or bilateral infiltrate. This is a frequent cause of pneumonia in the young infant with classic sequela such as bronchiectasis.

Cytomegalovirus (CMV) infection occurs in neonatal and immunocompromised patients, for example those who have been diagnosed with HIV and those who have undergone transplantation. Diffuse miliary patterns and bilateral reticulonodular interstitial infiltrates are seen initially. Airspace consolidation progresses to a diffuse hemorrhagic pulmonary edema pattern. Rarely, patchy airspace consolidation with acinar nodules is also seen.

Varicella-zoster pneumonia occurs in approximately 30% of immunocompetent adults with chickenpox during the third to fifth day of the infection. Initially, bronchial wall thickening and peribronchial infiltration with a diffuse miliary or diffuse reticulonodular pattern is seen. Multiple acinar nodules and small pleural effusions may occur. Roentgenographic clearing parallels improvement of the skin rash. Pulmonary nodules may clear over a period of months and some have residual fibrosis and multiple punctate calcification (Fig. 13.11) similar to that seen with residual histoplasmosis.

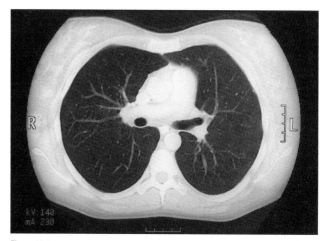

Figure 13.11. Multiple residual micronodules in a 34 year old female with antecedents of varicella pneumonia.

Pulmonary disease due to herpes simplex virus, primarily in immunocompromised patients, develops as an extension of tracheobronchitis or from hematogenous dissemination. Diffuse bronchial wall thickening, extensive peribronchial infiltration, diffuse interstitial or bronchopneumonia patterns are seen (9).

Fungal Infection

Aspergillosis in the normal host or mildly immunocompromised patient is either noninvasive or semiinvasive. A pulmonary mycetoma, a mass of matted hyphae in a ball, is seen initially in the apex, usually in a preexisting cavity (Fig. 13.12). A crescent-shaped air shadow over the mass inside the cavity signifies early mycetoma formation. Extensive pleural thickening at the apex is often a clue to semi-invasive aspergillosis. With a large inoculum, primary invasive aspergillosis may occur in the normal host. Regarding invasive aspergillosis in patients, Tenholder et al. (2) found that 8 out of 10 patients had thick-walled cavities and noncavitating nodules were

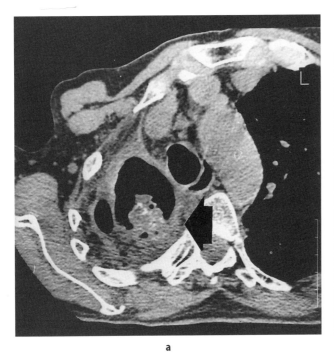

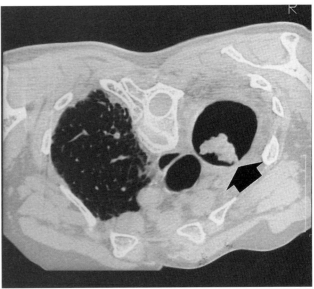

a   b

Figure 13.12. CT scan in a 53 year old male demonstrating a right pulmonary mycetoma (*arrow*) in the dependent portion of the cavity (supine (**a**) and prone (**b**) positions).

found in four out of 10 patients. Lesions were 2–10 cm in diameter and had a wall thickness of 0.4 mm. Invasive aspergillosis in the severely immunocompromised host is variable, with 40% of patients presenting with bilateral multiple nodular infiltrates. Solitary infiltrates, pleural-based nodules, and diffuse alveolar infiltrates have also been reported. Cavitation typically occurs as granulo-cytopenia is improving (Fig. 13.13).

Cryptococcosis is the most commonly encountered deep-seated fungal infection in HIV-infected patients. In the immunocompetent host, 2–10 cm pleural-based alveolar solitary masses, cavitation, lymphadenopathy, and pleural effusion have been reported. In the immunocompromised host, extrapulmonary dissemination is common and diffuse alveolar consolidation or miliary pattern may be seen.

Pulmonary candidiasis in the normal host is quite rare and appears as a consolidated bronchopneumonia. In the immunocompromised host, it is a manifestation of disseminated disease. Candidiasis is radiographically nonspecific, but is usually manifested as bilateral, multiple, patchy infiltrates that do not follow segmental distribution. Cavitation and adenopathy are rare, but pleural effusions occur in up to 25% of patients.

Protozoal Infections

Pneumocystis carinii pneumonia (PCP), the most important protozoal infection, is seen most commonly in

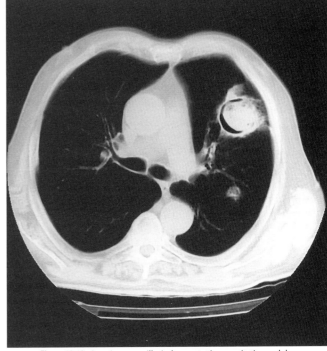

Figure 13.13. Invasive aspergillosis demonstrating a cavitating nodule.

patients with HIV. High resolution CT (HRCT) is more sensitive than the chest radiograph in the detection of PCP in patients with AIDS (Fig. 13.14). Chest radiographic findings have been reported as normal in up to 39% of patients with proven PCP. Patients with normal radio-

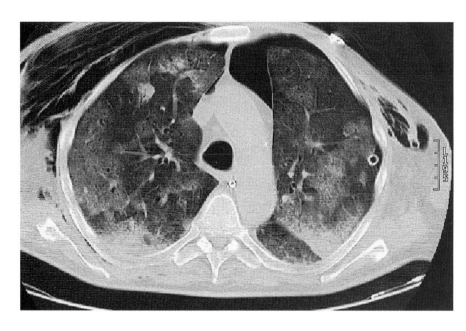

Figure 13.14. *Pneumocystis carinii* pneumonia in a 32 year old male with AIDS, showing multiple patchy ground-glass opacities, bilateral pneumothorax and subcutaneous emphysema.

graphic findings and clinical PCP may especially benefit from indirect testing with HRCT. Patchy ground-glass opacity is the most common abnormality seen on HRCT in PCP, occurring in 92% of patients (with a striking upper lobe predominance). Atypical manifestations seen on HRCT, including miliary or diffuse centrilobular nodules of ground-glass attenuation, have been reported but are unusual (10). Other infections in AIDS patients can also cause a pattern of patchy ground-glass opacity.

When chest CT films of patients with AIDS were compared with those of patients with leukemia and PCP, cystic changes, especially subpleural, were more common in AIDS patients. Lymphadenopathy and pleural effusions are rare.

Toxoplasmosis can present as either heterogeneous or homogeneous consolidation or bilateral interstitial infiltrates. Coarse nodular opacities are also common.

References

1. Farr BM (1997) Prognosis and decisions in pneumonia. N Engl J Med 336:288–289.

2. Tenholder MF, Greene LM, Thomas AM (1998) The role of radiology in pulmonary infectious disease. Curr Opin Pulm Med 4:142–147

3. Heussel CP, Kaukzor HU, Heussel G, et al. (1997) Early detection of pneumonia in febrile neutropenic patients: Use of thin-section CT. AJR 169:1347–1353.

4. Freudlich IM, Bragg DG (1997) A radiologic approach to diseases of the chest. Williams and Wilkins, Baltimore, MD.

5. Donnelly LF, Klosterman LA (1998) The yield of CT of children who have complicated pneumonia and noncontributory chest radiography. AJR 170:1627–1631.

6. Aquino SL, Chiles C, Halford P (1998) Distinction of consolidative bronchioloalveolar carcinoma from pneumonia: Do CT criteria work? AJR 171:359–363.

7. Wescott JL, Volpe JP (1995) Peripheral bronchopleural fistula: CT evaluation in 20 patients with pneumonia, empyema, or postoperative air leak. Radiology 196:175–181.

8. Fishman JE, Schwartz DS, Sais GJ (1997) Mycobacterium kansasii pulmonary infection in patients with AIDS: Spectrum of chest radiographic findings. Radiology 204:171–175.

9. Aquino SL, Dunagan DP, Chiles C et al. (1998) Herpes simplex virus 1 pneumonia: Patterns on CT scans and conventional chest radiographs. J Comput Assist Tomogr 22:795–800.

10. Gruden JF, Huang L, Turner J, et al. (1997) High-resolution CT in the evaluation of clinically suspected Pneumocystis carinii pneumonia in AIDS patients with normal, equivocal, or nonspecific radiographic findings. AJR 169:967–975.

14 Diagnostic Imaging of Pulmonary Tuberculosis

T. Pirronti, R. Manfredi, and P. Marano

Introduction

In recent years, health care workers have shown a growing interest in tuberculosis (TB) and its most frequent location – the lungs. This is a direct result of the increased number of cases, in apparently normal subjects as well as those suffering from acquired immune deficiency syndrome (AIDS) (1–5).

Radiologic examination of the respiratory tract shows, in an increasing number of subjects, signs suggestive of TB in differential diagnosis. This has led radiologists to reconsider the experience of TB in past decades (6–8) from the viewpoint of presently available diagnostic procedures. Among these, computed tomography (CT) undoubtedly supplies the most complete information on the pulmonary system as well as on most other organs. Chest X-ray, however, is still the preliminary modality for obtaining initial diagnostic indications.

The high number of cases diagnosed daily make integration of the radiologic data with the clinical findings essential. Radiologic findings are therefore analyzed in this chapter for the two forms of TB: primary and post-primary.

Primary Tuberculosis

Primary TB is defined as the symptoms and manifestations that accompany the first contact of the host with mycobacteria (6–8). Most patients do not show evident clinical symptoms and contact is confirmed only by a positive tuberculin test. When the host immune system does not respond to the bacterial invasion, symptoms appear that can guide the search for radiologic changes. For years, TB was considered a disease of childhood; in fact its radiologic manifestations were initially described in children (1–9). At present, new cases in adults are markedly increasing; however in most countries the disease is still more common in children. Chest radiography is mandatory in diagnosis: over 60% of pediatric patients present with few or no symptoms at onset, but chest radiographs can also be normal in 15% of patients with primary TB.

Lung contamination is airborne and structures that can be involved, in isolation or in various combinations, are the lymph nodes, parenchyma, trachea, bronchi, and pleura.

Lymph Node Alterations

Nodal involvement is almost constant in primary TB, both in isolated form or associated with parenchymal and/or pleural lesions; over 90% of pediatric forms and about 10% of adult forms at onset show mono- or bilateral hilar and/or mediastinal lymph node enlargement (Fig. 14.1).

This aspect, typical of primary TB, rules out post-primary TB, especially in adults; in fact, nodal enlargement is constant in primary TB of childhood where nodal impairment is often present, with all mediastinal nodes involved. Chest radiography, still the most important means of investigating this disease, often shows mediastinal and mono- or bilateral hilar enlargement.

However, CT can supply additional information on involved lymph nodes and their features. CT (2,3,11,12) has revealed that nodal impairment is much more common than has appeared from chest radiographs in past decades (Fig. 14.2).

Limited adenopathy following caseous inflammation caused by mycobacterium infection appears on CT as isolated nodular formations. After injection of contrast medium, a central hypodense portion can be identified that is indicative of necrosis. Often adenopathy is large, with confluent lymph nodes not recognized as single entities but forming more or less large masses in the entire mediastinum; these masses surround the remaining structures and appear heterogeneous in nature, with hypodense areas due to massive necrosis (Fig. 14.3).

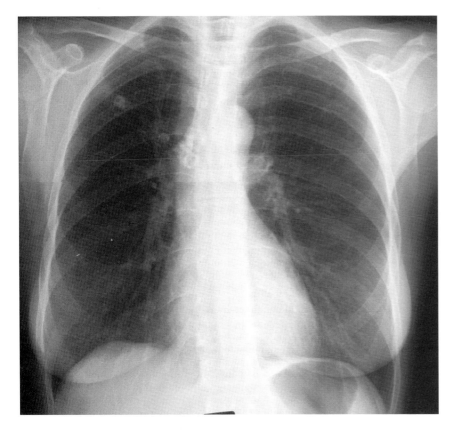

Figure 14.1. Chest radiograph shows primary complex with calcified parenchymal nodule and calcified mediastinal lymph nodes.

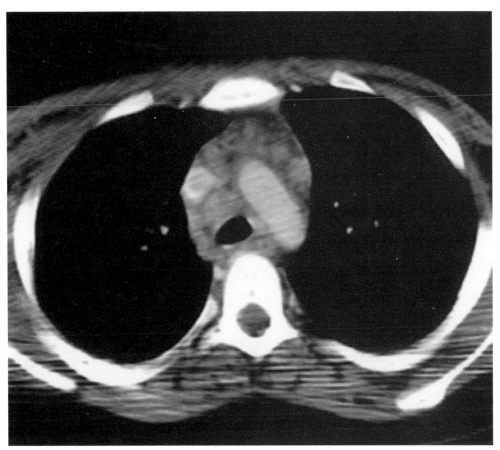

Figure 14.2. Enlarged, partially confluent mediastinal lymph nodes.

These signs apparently suggest a tuberculous etiology, and pose problems of differential diagnosis with lymphomas, especially non-Hodgkin lymphoma, both in adults and children, even when present in the parenchymal or pleural (2,3,6–9,11,12).

In most cases nodal involvement undergoes regression following therapy, with residual fibrosis or nodal calcifications visualized on radiograph or CT scan as minute or gross intranodal calcifications that can readily be differentiated from the egg-shell-shaped calcifications of silicosis and the more rare calcifications of sarcoidosis and treated lymphomas: the latter are both frequently bilateral. Nodal calcification associated with parenchymal nodular calcification represents the Ranke complex. Nodal enlargement, if present, is responsible for more or less marked airway compression, with bronchial narrowing or obstruction and consequent lobar atelectasis, usually of the middle lobe. The oblique orientation of this lobe, its small calibre and close relation to the numerous surrounding hilar and peribronchial lymph nodes cause it to be compressed when enlarged.

Parenchymal Alterations

The typical parenchymal manifestation of primary TB is an ill-defined parenchymal consolidation varying in diameter from 1 to 7 cm (Fig. 14.3); an air bronchogram may be seen at the same time, often progressing to cavitation in adults.

Most parenchymal locations are associated with nodal enlargement, what is sometimes not recognized in the chest radiograph, but can be clearly seen on the CT scan (2,3,5,11–13). On CT, the site of parenchymal consolidation is often accompanied by multiple foci adjacent to the main parenchymal focus as well as in other segments of the same lobe or in segments of other ipsi- or contralateral lobes.

Multiple parenchymal locations appear as blurred lobular, multilobular or subsegmental opacities in close contact with bronchial branches, a condition clearly shown by CT. This is strong evidence for the airborne genesis of the bronchial spread of multiple foci a, differentiated form hematogenous dissemination, which is characterized by small nodules in distal vessels (the "vessel sign"). Hematogenous nodules, when enlarged, are in continuity with bronchial structures, thus making differential diagnosis difficult.

Airborne spread is often concomitant with hematogenous opacities, and signs of both become evident; they are suggested on the chest radiograph, but readily identified on the CT Scan (2,3,11–13) (Fig. 14.4).

Multiple parenchymal opacities may progress to cavitation, with concomitant involvement of several parenchymal foci: this type of spread of pulmonary TB is at present very common both in immunosuppressed and otherwise normal subjects.

The impairment of a whole lobe is not frequent, often being associated with bronchial obstruction and increased lobar volume in the initial exudative phases; the most

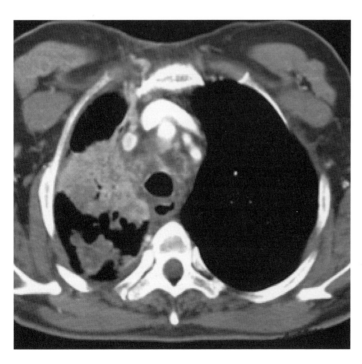

Figure 14.3. Enlarged, partially confluent mediastinal lymph nodes with hypodense center due to necrosis; in the upper right lobe we can also see parenchymal consolidation.

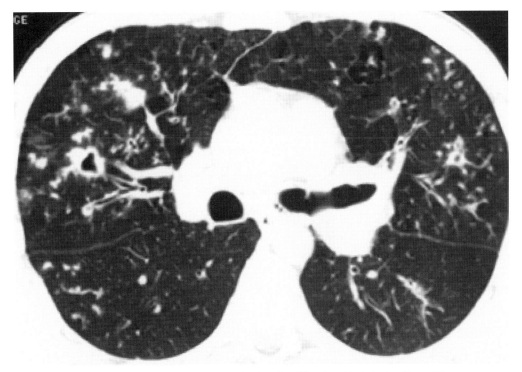

Figure 14.4. Presence of cavitations associated with confluent blurred opacities is clearly evident on CT scans.

typical evolution is that of the middle lobe location, which leads to reduced lobar volume, scissural displacement, and signs of atelectasis.

In about 70% of cases, alterations heal with no sequelae after 6 months to 2 years; in the remaining 30% a radiologically visualized parenchymal scar or Ranke complex may be observed (Fig. 14.3). The American Thoracic Society recommends a control radiograph every 2–3 months after the start of therapy until the resolution or stabilization of alterations (2,3).

A persistent nodular opacity or tuberculoma is not very frequent; most tuberculomas are seen in the upper lobes as nodules (<3 cm) having slow growth and calcification in about 50% of cases (Fig. 14.5). An association with calcified hilar lymph nodes further supports the diagnosis.

An important aspect of parenchymal locations is in miliary TB. In most cases hematogenous dissemination in primary TB has no clinical or radiologic manifestations. Generally, the symptomatic form appears about 6 months after primary infection and the chest radiograph often is without alterations while a nuclear medicine study with ^{67}Ga shows diffuse radionuclide accumulation in the pulmonary parenchyma. Pulmonary change, are seen on radiography and are more precisely defined on high resolution CT, where there are perivascular and periseptal micronodules 1–2 mm in diameter associated with reti-

cular septal thickening similar to that of lymphangitis. Miliary involvement may lead to the formation of larger confluent parenchymal nodules with consequent respiratory insufficiency.

Airway Alterations

Tracheobronchial impairment may be caused by bronchial compression of enlarged confluent lymph nodes, as shown by the effects on pulmonary ventilation (6–8). Compression with calibre reduction may cause areas of reduced ventilation due to subsegmental atelectasis, while complete obstruction causes atelectasis of the middle lobe (Fig. 14.6). When the obstruction is removed, because of reduced nodal volume following antibiotic therapy, the lobe may re-expand or, if the atelectasis was longlasting, it may persist after nodal healing. This is evidenced on CT by the presence of one or more calcifications in the lymph nodes adjacent to the origin of obstructed bronchus (2,3,11,13).

Primary bronchial wall involvement with the diffusion of bronchoscopy is shown to be rather frequent: granulations are observed along the walls of the tracheal and bronchial mucosal surface, and compression of enlarged lymph nodes on bronchial walls is evident. Both bronchoscopy and CT can document the presence of

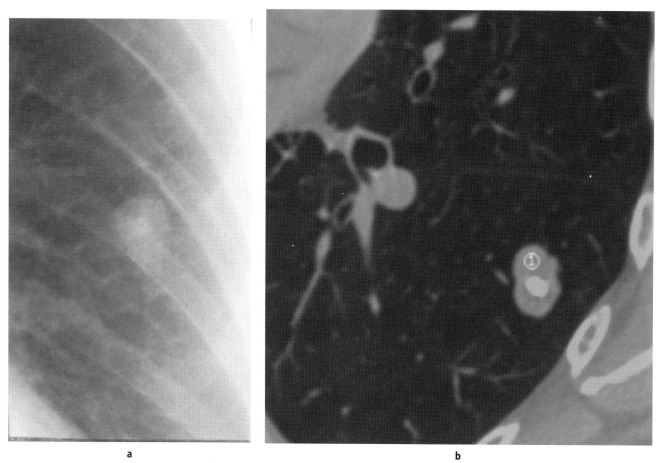

a   b

Figure 14.5. a and **b** The tuberculoma appears as a <3 cm nodule with central calcification.

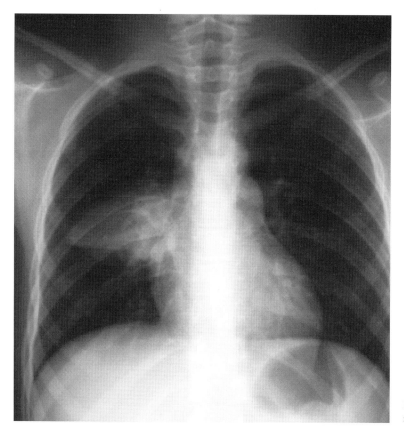

Figure 14.6. Atelectasis of the middle lobe: triangular opacity with scissural displacement.

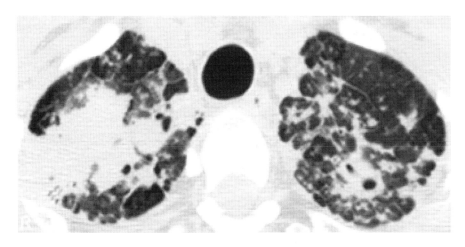

Figure 14.7. CT scan: parenchymal consolidation in the right upper lobe and small cavitated opacities in the left upper lobe.

endobronchial granulation or bronchial wall erosion by nodal calcifications that have entered the bronchial lumen and caused atelectasis or hemoptysis.

Pleural Alterations

The pleural manifestation of primary TB is pleural effusion (2,3,7–9,11–13), considered to be a common late complication of parenchymal alterations. It may be ipsilateral with respect to parenchymal lesions or it may involve both pleurae; in more severe forms pericardial effusion is associated.

Chest radiography, ultrasound and CT are able to show pleural effusion and monitor its evolution; however, none of them is able to identify typical signs of tuberculous effusion. Radiologically, about 50% of patients with primary TB present with isolated pleural effusion, but CT shows the presence of parenchymal lesions and nodal enlargement in most cases.

Postprimary Tuberculosis

Parenchymal Alterations

Postprimary TB has a clinical and radiologic pattern whose pathogenesis is closely related to patient hypersensitivity and acquired immunity status.

Almost all cases of postprimary TB appear in adults as the result of the reactivation of a previous infectious focus. The pathologic features are markedly different from those of primary TB because the body reacts to isolate the bacillus (2,3,6–8). The most frequent sites are the apicodorsal segments of upper lobes and the apical segments of lower lobes, though the other segments are often involved with multiple and bilateral alterations.

The radiologic and pathologic manifestations are closely correlated and may be distinguished in exudative and fibroproductive forms. Circumscribed exudative TB is seen as blurred, acinar, single or multiple opacities lacking defined margins (Fig. 14.7).

Chest radiography documents the site and morphology of these lesions, which tend to cavitation; sometimes striae that connect the opacity to the hilus are observed. Exudative lesions are replaced by irregular, small, better-defined opacities, leaving parenchymal scars.

Detailed assessment of alterations documented on chest radiography is possible on CT scan. The latter shows more lesions and the presence of cavitation, as compared with standard radiography (2,3,11,13–15) (Fig. 14.8).

On CT, the relation of opacities with bronchial branches is revealed, evidencing the airborne spread and its association with hematogenous lesions resulting from bacteremia, which is frequent in these patients.

Cavitation occurs when the caseous material that fills the airspaces undergoes lysis, with outside removal and/or endobronchial diffusion to other segments (Figs 14.9, 14.10,14.11). Excavated opacities are blurred and thick walled; they become gradually smaller, leaving cicatricial striae associated to calcified micronodules or thin-walled cystic formations, the possible sites of mycotic implantation.

The most frequent complication is endobronchial diffusion (2,3,6–8,11,13–16) shown by blurred peribronchial and centrilobular opacities, a few millimeters to some centimeters in diameter, which tend to be confluent. Centrilobular nodules have the "tree-in-bud" appearance, suggestive of airborne activity and diffusion of the disease (Fig. 14.12). A rare complication of tuberculous cavitation is the spontaneous pneumothorax observed in 3–5% of patients with gross cavitations, while in miliary TB hematogenous dissemination is more frequent.

Miliary Tuberculosis

The hematogenous dissemination of tuberculosis bacilli is a frequent, repeated condition during the disease; most bacteremias are not followed by clinical manifestations of the different and multiple locations.

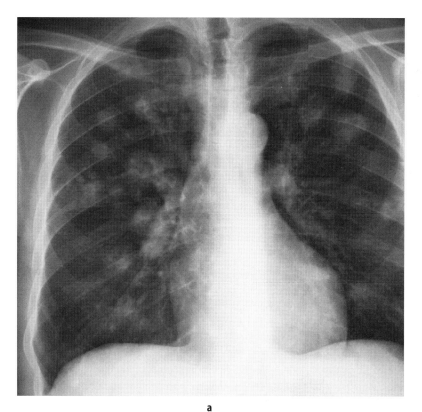

a

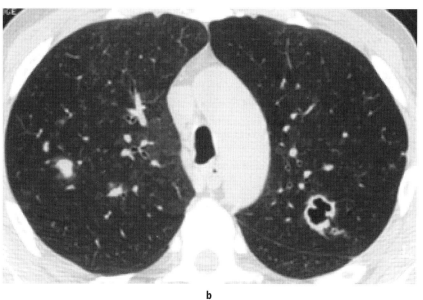

b

Figure 14.8. a Chest radiograph shows multiple opacities of both lungs. **b** Cavitations are better depicted by CT.

When bacteremias are repeated and numerous, with the release of relevant amounts of mycobacteria, the clinical manifestations appear in relation to the affected organs and anatomic structures: meninges, lungs, abdominal organs, etc. (3,6–9,14–16). Pulmonary hematogenous dissemination is shown by the miliary form; radiologically there are numerous micronodular opacities a few millimeters in size and with well-defined margins, distributed bilaterally in both lungs (Fig. 14.13). In about 15% of cases, the distribution may be asymmetric. In childhood,

the association with mediastinal lymphadenopathy, which is also seen occasionally in adults, is more frequent. On CT, the presence of numerous micronodules on all lobes is well documented; even if they are very small in the early phases, their proximity to vessels is often evident, proving their hematogenous spread or periseptal location. Often, diffuse or local thickening of interlobular septa, similar to that of carcinomatous lymphangitis, is observed. In more severe, extensive forms of TB the micronodules may be confluent with blurred bronchial opacities.

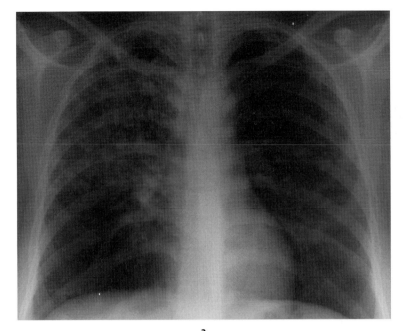

a

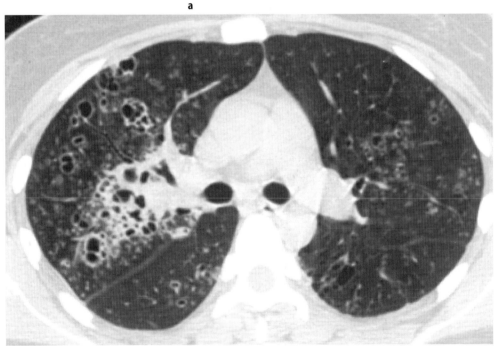

b

Figure 14.9. **a** and **b** Multiple cavitations in the upper lobes, some of them in continuity with the bronchus (**b**).

Airway Alterations

Airway alterations are frequent in postprimary TB (6–8,11,13); bronchial wall involvement by airborne or lymphatic spread may cause more or less marked stenosis, with the formation of areas of expiratory air-trapping or segmental–lobar atelectasis. Sometimes the cause is a nodal calcification, a broncholith with bronchial fistulization and occlusion, the cause of atelectasis. Cylindrical, saccular, segmental, multisegmental or lobar bronchi-

ectasis is frequent, mostly in the upper lobes, or presenting as generally asymptomatic, with abrupt major hemoptysis because of rupture of hypertrophic bronchial arteries (Fig. 14.14).

Pleural Alterations

Pleural effusion is less frequent in postprimary TB, often less marked but commonly associated with parenchymal

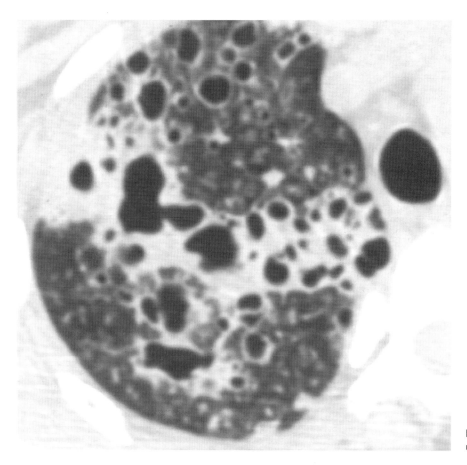

Figure 14.10. Numerous cavitations in the right upper lobe.

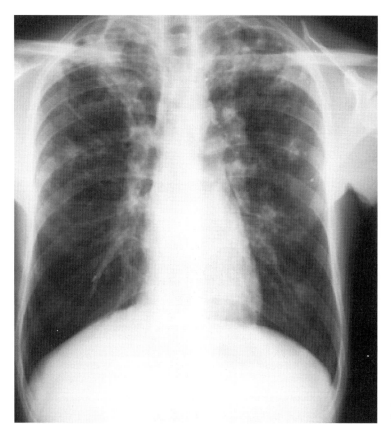

Figure 14.11. Numerous cavitations associated with multiple calcified opacities, predominantly in both upper lobes.

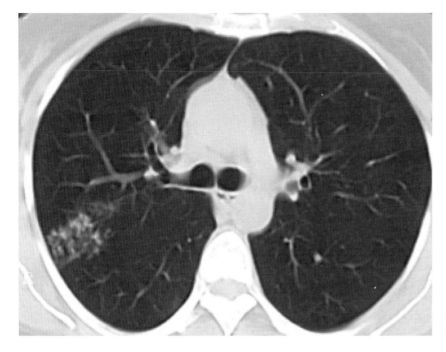

Figure 14.12. "Tree-in-bud" appearance due to small intralobular nodules in the distal bronchioles.

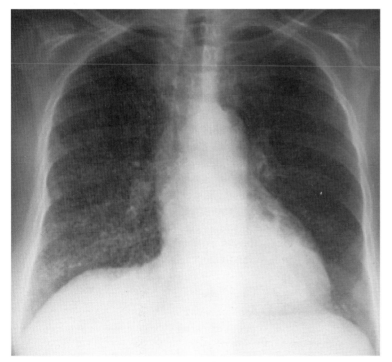

Figure 14.13. Chest radiograph shows numerous bilateral small nodules, predominantly in the right lower lobe and the lingula.

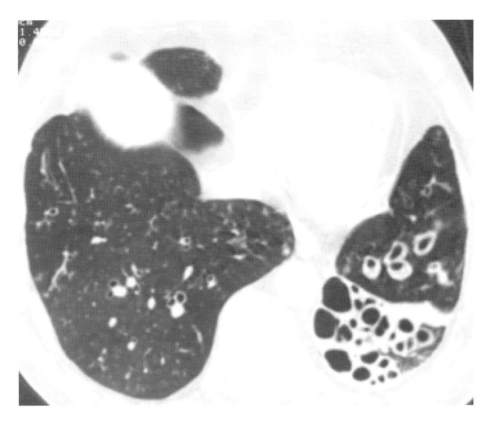

Figure 14.14. Outcome of tuberculous process: saccular bronchiectasis in the left lower lobe.

alterations such as sacculated pleural effusions; broncho-pleural fistulae are possible (17–20).

At present pleural involvement may heal with modest sequelae (Fig. 14.15), but, in the past, calcific pachypleuritis with gross calcified thickening and reduced hemithorax, tracheal attraction and forced contralateral redistribution of pulmonary circulation was frequent. Pleural calcification documented by CT is located at the level of visceral pleura, which accounts for the absence of reduction in parenchymal volume and practically absent compliance.

Tuberculosis and HIV Infection

The human immunodeficiency virus (HIV) is a major factor responsible for the present resurgence in the incidence of TB.

The impaired cell-mediated immunity typical of HIV infection is responsible for the high incidence of TB in patients; in 70% of cases the respiratory tract is involved, with alterations proportional to the severity of immunodeficiency. In patients with CD4 levels equal to or higher than 500 cells mm^{-3}, TB shows clinical and radiologic manifestations similar to those of normal subjects (21–23).

Most frequently, TB is postprimary, with exudative inflammation of the apicodorsal segments of the upper lobes and of apical segments of the lower lobes, which frequently tend to cavitation, associated with pleural effusion (24–26).

Primary TB is also frequent, the outcome being adverse in the presence of severe immunodeficiency. The miliary form becomes manifest when the CD4 title is under 500 mm^{-3} and may be associated with confluent mediastinal lymphadenopathy and areas of colliquation, which are seen as hypodense areas on CT. Pulmonary location in miliary dissemination is frequently associated with the impairment of other organs and structures – peritoneum, meninges, abdominal organs – with complex clinical and radiologic patterns due to the multiorgan involvement.

References

1. Pedicelli G (1993) La tubercolosi polmonare attuale. Problematiche radiologiche. Radiol Med 86:399–417.
2. McAdams HP, Erasmus J, Winter JA (1995) Radiologic manifestations of pulmonary tuberculosis. Radiol Clin North Am 33:655–78.
3. Goodman PC, Jinkis JR (1995) Imaging of tuberculosis and craniospinal tuberculosis. Radiol Clin North Am 20–27.

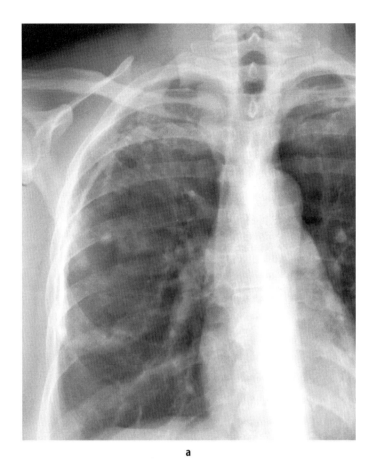

a

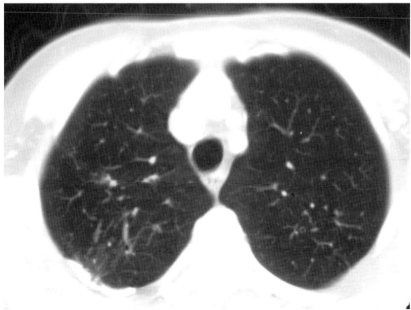

b

Figure 14.15. a Chest radiograph shows outcome of tuberculous process with pleural thickening. **b** Corresponding CT scan.

4. Wilcke JT, Kok Jensen A (1997) Diagnostic strategy for pulmonary tuberculosis in a low-incidence country: Results of chest X-ray and sputum cultured for Mycobacterium tuberculosis. Respir Med 91:281–285.

5. Smuts NA, Beyers N, Gie RP, et al. (1994) Value of lateral chest radiograph in tuberculosis in children. Pediatr Radiol 24:478–480.

6. Fraser RG, Paré JAP (1980) Diagnosi delle malattie toraciche, vol 1. Ambrosiana, Milan.

7. Fraser RG, Paré JAP (1980) Diagnosi delle malattie toraciche, vol 2. Ambrosiana, Milan.

8. Bismuth V, Blery M, Rémy J, et al. (1979) Traité de radiodiagnostic, Tome IV. Masson, Paris.

9. Kim WS, Moon WK, Kim IO, et al. (1997) Pulmonary tuberculosis in children: Evaluation with CT. AJR 168:1005–1009.

10. Ferguson JS, Hornick DB, Dayton CS (1996) Patients with an abnormal chest radiograph and latent tuberculosis. Am Family Physician 54:2495–2500.

11. Naidich DP, Zerhouni EA, Siegelman SS (1991) Computed tomography and magnetic resonance of the thorax. Raven Press, New York.

12. Rotteberg GT, Shaw P (1996) Radiology of pulmonary tuberculosis. Br J Hosp Med 56: 195–199.

13. Reed JC (1997) Chest radiology: Plain film patterns and differential diagnoses. Mosby Year Book, Inc., St. Louis, MO.

14. Jones BE, Ryu R, Yang Z, et al. (1997) Chest radiographic findings in patients with tuberculosis with recent or remote infection. Am J Respir Crit Care Med 156:1270–1273.

15. Nyman RS, Brismar J, Hugosson C, et al. (1996) Imaging of tuberculosis: experience from 503 patients. Tuberculosis of chest. Acta Radiol 37:482–488.

16. Singh SP, Nath H (1994) Early radiology of pulmonary tuberculosis. AJR 162:846.

17. Haramati LB, Jenny Avital ER, et al. (1997) Effect of HIV status on chest radiographic and CT findings in patients with tuberculosis. Clin Radiol 52:31–35.

18. Im JG, Itoh H, Lee KS, et al. (1995) CT pathology correlation of pulmonary tuberculosis. Crit Rev Diagn Imaging 36:227–285.

19. Polverosi R, Zanellato E, Zanlungo P (1995) Pulmonary tuberculosis in non-immunocompromised patients. Current radiologie features. Radiol Med Torino 89:769–775.

20. Nardini S, Schiavon F, Zuin R, et al. (1995) Has the role of radiology changed in the fight against pulmonary tuberculosis? Radiol Med Torino 89:49–56.

21. Greenberg SD, Frager D, Suster B, et al. (1994) Active pulmonary tuberculosis in patients with AIDS: Spectrum of radiographic findings (including a normal appearance). Radiology 193:115–119.

22. Lessnau KD, Gorla M, Talvera W (1994) Radiographic findings in HIV-positive patients with sensitive and resistant tuberculosis. Chest 106:687–689.

23. Small PM, Hopewell PC, Schecter GF, et al. (1994) Evolution of chest radiographs in treated patients with pulmonary tuberculosis and HIV infection. J Thorac Imaging 9:74–77.

24. Sanchez Nistal MA, Gallego Gallego MS, Manfreique Chico J, et al. (1996) Thoracic tuberculosis in adults. A comparative study of radiological findings of HIV seropositive and seronegative patients. Ann Med Internel 13:476–482.

25. Boiselle PM, Tocino I, Hooley RJ, et al. (1997) Chest radiograph interpretation of Pneumocystis carinii pneumonia, bacterial pneumonia, and pulmonary tuberculosis in HIV-positive patients: accuracy, distinguishing features, and mimics. J Thorac Imaging 12:47–53.

26. Daley CL (1995) The typically "atypical" radiographic presentation of tuberculosis in advanced HIV disease. Tuber Lung Dis 76:475–476.

15 Sarcoidosis

J.P. Lynch III and E.A. Kazerooni

Introduction

Sarcoidosis is a poorly understood granulomatous disease that involves the lung and intrathoracic lymph nodes in more than 90% of patients (1–10). However, multisystemic involvement is characteristic and virtually any organ can be affected (3,4,8–10). Skin, eye, and peripheral lymph nodes are each involved in 20–30% of patients (3,7). Clinically significant involvement of spleen, liver, heart, central nervous system, bone, and kidney occurs in 2–7% of patients (3,4,7). Asymptomatic involvement of these organs is far more common (3,4,7). This review focuses on intrathoracic manifestations of sarcoidosis, and only briefly discusses a few specific extrapulmonary manifestations that may be of relevance to radiologists. A comprehensive review of extrapulmonary manifestations of sarcoidosis is presented elsewhere (3).

Epidemiology of Sarcoidosis

Sarcoidosis is worldwide in distribution, but the prevalence varies according to racial and geographic factors. Sarcoidosis is four to eight times more common in blacks than whites (4,11,12). In North America and Northern Europe, the incidence is 6–20 cases per 100 000 (11–14), but in Scandinavia and certain parts of the British Isles, incidence exceeds 80 per 100 000 (13,15). In Spain and Italy, the incidence is much lower 1.36 (16) and 1.2 (17) per 100 000, respectively. Sarcoidosis is recognized in Japan (13,18) but is rarely reported in Central or South America or Africa. Whether this represents lack of recognition or a reduced prevalence of the disease is not clear. More than 70% of patients with sarcoidosis present between age 20 and 45 years (4,10,12). Sarcoidosis is slightly more common in women (1.4/1.0 male to female ratio) (11,12). Some studies cite a higher incidence of sarcoidosis in nonsmokers (19), but this is variable (4). A specific genetic defect has not been identified, but familial cases occur (12). Familial sarcoidosis (defined as having a first- or second-degree relative with sarcoidosis) occurs in 17% of African–American patients with sarcoidosis compared to 6% among Caucasian cases (11). Routine screening of family members of patients with sarcoidosis using chest radiography was studied and is not recommended, as no new cases were detected (20). Certain human leukocyte antigen (HLA) alleles are more common in sarcoidosis (e.g., HLA-B8) (21), but no consistent association exists (4).

Etiology and Immunopathogenesis

Despite exhaustive investigations and a variety of hypotheses regarding causative agents, the etiology of sarcoidosis is enigmatic (22–25). Although the inciting signals evoking the granulomatous response have not been identified, the cells responsible for induction, immunomodulation, and orchestration of the sarcoid granuloma are well characterized (26–28). Interactions between activated mononuclear phagocytes (e.g., macrophages or monocytes) and activated T-helper/inducer (CD4+) lymphocytes are responsible for the induction and evolution of the granulomatous process (27). At sites of active disease, striking increases in CD4+ lymphocytes and increased CD4/CD8 ratios are characteristic (29). Lung T-cells from patients with active pulmonary sarcoidosis release several cytokines that stimulate or amplify immune responses and facilitate T-cell replication and mononuclear phagocyte activation (27,29). Alveolar macrophages from patients with pulmonary sarcoidosis are activated, enhance antigen presentation, express receptors for interleukin-2 (IL-2), and release growth factors that promote fibroblast recruitment and proliferation (27–29). Macrophages play a dual role in orchestrating the granulomatous lesions, by producing monokines that either amplify or downregulate the inflammatory process.

Histopathology

The histological hallmark of sarcoidosis is compact, non-necrotizing (noncaseating) granulomas composed of epithelioid cells and multinucleated giant cells, surrounded by lymphocytes, plasma cells, and fibroblasts in the periphery (4,30) (Fig. 15.1). Macroscopic necrosis suggests an alternative diagnosis (e.g., tuberculosis, fungal infection, vasculitis, etc.). However, foci of micronecrosis may be found (31,32). Since mycobacterial and fungal granulomas can cause nonnecrotizing granulomas, special staining for acid-fast bacilli and fungi should be performed to exclude these infectious etiologies. Basophilic inclusions (Schaumann bodies) or asteroid bodies are occasionally found in giant cells (30). fibrosis is present in varying degrees; hyalinizing, acellular granulomata may coexist (4,30). In the lung, the granulomatous lesions are preferentially distributed along bronchovascular bundles (within the connective tissue sheath of bronchioles) and lymphatics (4,30,33). The predilection for lymphatics differentiates sarcoidosis from other interstitial lung disorders. For example granulomas in hypersensitivity pneumonitis (extrinisic allergic alveolitis) do not follow lymphatics and are distributed randomly (30). In sarcoidosis, mononuclear cell infiltrates (principally lymphocytes and plasma cells) follow the alveolar septae and extend from the granulomata; arteries or veins may be involved (31,32). Other features include small (2–4 mm) or large (>2 cm) parenchymal nodules, which represent coalescent granulomata. Confluent pulmonary mass lesions, with consolidation of lung parenchyma, reflect exuberant granulomatous inflammation (30). The granulomas can either resolve or cause progressive disruption and destruction of the alveolar architecture (4,30).

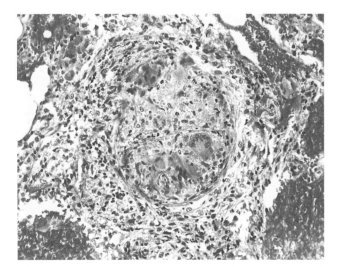

Figure 15.1. Photomicrograph. Transbronchial biopsy demonstrates a sarcoid granuloma with multinucleated giant cells and epithelioid cells. Scattered lymphocytes and fibroblasts are present in the periphery (Hematoxylin-eosin.) (Reproduced from ref. 320, with permission.)

Bronchiectasis, bronchioloectasis, alveolar septal fibrosis, honeycomb cysts, and secondary pulmonary vascular changes reflect end-stage disease (4,30).

Biopsy Procedures

The diagnosis of sarcoidosis can be confirmed (provided the clinical context is appropriate) by biopsies of lung, mediastinal lymph nodes, skin, or other affected sites (4). Fiberoptic bronchoscopy (FB) with transbronchial lung biopsies (TBBs) is the preferred diagnostic procedure in patients with bilateral hilar lymphadenopathy and/or parenchymal infiltrates (1). Surgical (or thoracoscopic) lung biopsies or mediastinoscopic lymph node biopsies have a higher yield, but are expensive and have increased morbidity (34). The characteristic granulomatous lesions are easily assessable to bronchoscopic diagnosis, either by endobronchial or transbronchial lung biopsies (35,36) (Fig. 15.2). The yield of TBBs ranges from 60% to 97%, according to the number of biopsies and radiographic stage (36–41). The yield is higher in radiographic stage II or III disease (40), when biopsies are obtained from sites of greatest radiographic change (37,39), and when multiple biopsies are obtained (37,39). To optimize yield, we obtain 4–6 TBBs (using alligator forceps) from the upper and lower lobes of one lung (total of 8–12 TBBs). Endobronchial biopsies are performed only when gross endoscopic findings are present (e.g., mucosal nodularity, "cobblestoning"; mucosal edema; hypervascularity; bronchostenosis). In this context, the yield of endobronchial biopsies exceeds 85% (35). In contrast, the yield was 37% when the bronchial mucosa was grossly normal. Transbronchial needle aspiration (TBNA) biopsies of mediastinal lymph nodes increases the yield (42–44) but adds a level of complexity, expense, and expertise. Because of the high yield with TBB alone, we do not believe routine use of TBNA is necessary. Bronchoalveolar lavage may suggest the diagnosis, when lymphocytosis or increased CD4/CD8 ratios are found (45,46), but lymphocyte phenotyping is expensive and is not specific (4). Percutaneous needle aspiration biopsies (47), cytologies of sputum (48) or BAL fluid (49,50) may reveal multinucleated giant cells, epithelioid cells, or lymphocytes in patients with sarcoidosis (48,50). In one retrospective study, multinucleated giant cells, epithelioid cells, or increased lymphocytes were identified in BAL fluid in 23 of 26 patients (89%) with pulmonary sarcoidosis (49). However, these findings are nonspecific and may be seen in other granulomatous disorders (including infections) (49). Mediastinoscopic lymph node biopsies or video-assisted thoracoscopic (VAT) lung biopsies are reserved for patients with suspected intrathoracic pathology and nondiagnostic bronchoscopy. Biopsy of extrapulmonary sites is appropriate when specific lesions or abnormalities are identified (e.g., lymphadenopathy, skin lesions, abnormal liver enzymes, etc.) (3).

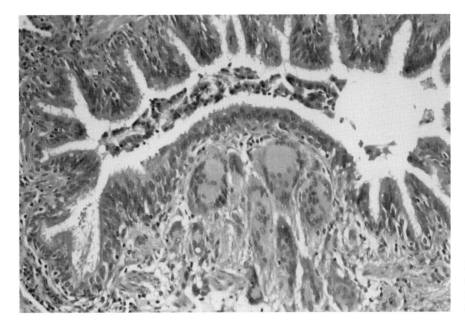

Figure 15.2. Photomicrograph. Endobronchial biopsy demonstrates large multinucleated giant cells in the submucosa underlying a bronchiole. (Hematoxylin-eosin.) (Reproduced from ref. 6, with permission.)

Laboratory Features

Laboratory features are nonspecific. Historically, the Kveim test was used to corroborate the diagnosis of sarcoidosis (25). However, the long delay (4–6 weeks) required for interpretation and the lack of a commercially available antigen rendered this test obsolete. Hypergammaglobulinemia is observed in 30–80% of patients with chronic sarcoidosis (4,51). Hypercalcemia occurs in 2–5% of patients; hypercalciuria, in 15–40% (52,53). These abnormalities of calcium metabolism reflect enhanced sensitivity to vitamin D (53–55). Elevated levels of serum 1,2-dihydroxycalciferol are present in sarcoid patients with hypercalcemia; these aberrations reverse with corticosteroid therapy (56). Elevations in transaminases or alkaline phosphatase are common (5–30%) (3). Leukopenia is present in 5–40% of patients with sarcoidosis; anemia occurs in 4–20% (3,57). Serum angiotensin-converting enzyme (ACE) levels are elevated in 30–80% of patients with sarcoidosis (55,58). Serum ACE levels may reflect total granuloma burden and may parallel disease activity. However, Serum ACE levels do not predict long-term prognosis and normal levels do not exclude active, localized disease (58).

Clinical Features

The clinical spectrum of sarcoidosis is protean, but pulmonary manifestations typically dominate (1). Chest radiographs are abnormal in 90–95% of patients with sarcoidosis (10,51,59,60). Cough or dyspnea may be present in patients with endobronchial or pulmonary involvement

(1,61), but 30–60% of patients with sarcoidosis are asymptomatic, with incidental findings on chest radiographs (10,51,59,62,63). Chronic pulmonary sarcoidosis may cause inexorable loss of lung function and destruction of the alveolar architecture (10,15,51,59,60,64) (Fig. 15.3). Serious extrapulmonary involvement (e.g., heart, nervous system) occurs in 4–7% of patients with sarcoidosis at presentation; the incidence is higher as the disease evolves (3,8,51,59,65). The clinical course and prognosis of sarcoidosis are variable. Spontaneous remissions occur in nearly two thirds of patients but the course is chronic in 10–30% of patients (10,14,15,51,59,60). Fatalities occur in 1–5% of patients, typically due to progressive respiratory failure or central nervous system (CNS) or myocardial involvement (10,14,15,51,59,60,66–70).

Differing mortality rates reflect different genetic and epidemiologic factors and referral bias. Studies in non-referral settings in the USA and Scandinavia comprise predominantly Caucasians, many of whom are asymptomatic (14,15,60,63). In this context, mortality rates are less than 1% and serious morbidity is uncommon. In one study of 775 patients with sarcoidosis in Japan, fewer than one percent died as a direct result of sarcoidosis (71). Huang reported a 2.8% mortality rate among 1090 sarcoid patients in Europe (69). In contrast, published data from referral centers include a disproportionate number of patients with severe or progressive disease, and higher morbidity and mortality (5,8,10,51,59,62,72–74). Ethic or geographic factors also influence clinical expression of disease. Mortality rates are higher in blacks (5,10,51,73,74). In the USA, most deaths are due to pulmonary complications; 13–50% of deaths are attributed to cardiac involvement (68,70,75). In Japan, 77% of deaths have been ascribed to cardiac involvement (76).

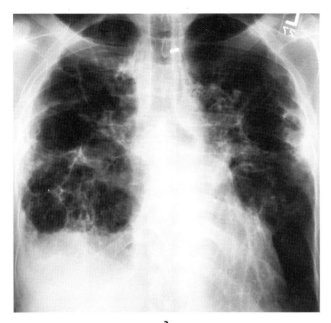

a

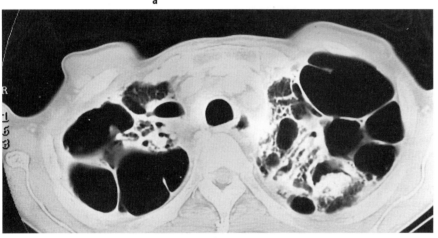

b

Figure 15.3. a Posteroanterior chest radiograph demonstrates severe destruction of both lungs, with severe bullae and cystic radiolucencies secondary to chronic sarcoidosis. **b** CT scan. Severe cystic radiolucencies in upper lung zones. Note the mycetoma in the left lung.

Pulmonary Sarcoidosis

Symptoms of pulmonary parenchymal or endobronchial involvement are nonspecific but include cough (typically nonproductive), dyspnea (1), and, in some cases, bronchial hyperreactivity (61,77). Chest pain is not an uncommon symptom in patients with pulmonary sarcoidosis. However, neither the presence nor degree of enlarged lymph nodes or pleural abnormality correlates with chest pain (78). Physical findings are usually absent. Crackles are present in fewer than 20% of patients with sarcoidosis, even with extensive radiographic involvement (79). Clubbing is rare (79).

Radiographic Features

During the course of the disease, over 90% of patients with sarcoidosis will have or develop abnormal chest radiographs (6,15,59,60,62,66,79–81). The most characteristic finding is

bilateral hilar (often with concomitant right paratracheal) lymph node enlargement, noted in 50–85% of cases (15,51,57,59,60,81,83) (Fig. 15.4). Pulmonary parenchymal infiltrates (with or without hilar lymphadenopathy) are present in 25–50% of patients with sarcoidosis (15,51,57,59, 60,79,81,83). For asymptomatic patients, the suspicion of sarcoidosis is first raised on a chest radiograph obtained for other reasons. This is not surprising given that 30–60% of patients with a new diagnosis of sarcoidosis are asymptomatic, and another 25% of patients present only with extrathoracic symptoms (15,60,79,80).

Chest Radiographic Classification Scheme

The most widely used staging system for sarcoidosis is based on chest radiography. Developed more than four decades ago, this staging scheme pre-dates the introduction of computed tomography (CT) scanners. The published

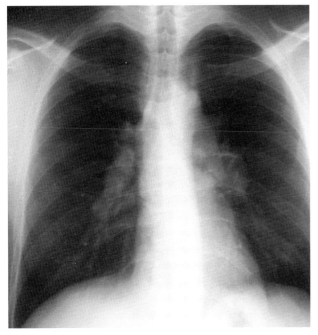

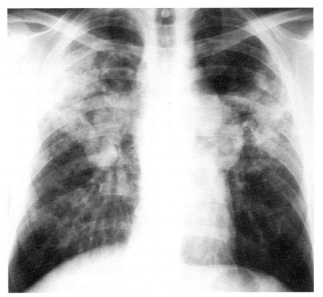

Figure 15.5. Stage II sarcoidosis. Posteroanterior chest radiograph demonstrates nodular infiltrates predominantly involving mid and upper lung zones; massive bilateral hilar lymphadenopathy is present.

Figure 15.4. Stage I sarcoidosis. Chest radiograph from a 35 year old male demonstrating bilateral hilar lymphadenopathy. Lymph nodes in the left paraaortic region and aortopulmonary window are also enlarged.

longitudinal studies of sarcoidosis that evaluated patient prognosis by radiographic stage were based on plain chest radiographs, not on CT (59,62,84). The chest radiograph is normal in stage 0 sarcoidosis; at least 10% of these patients will have biopsy-confirmed intrathoracic sarcoidosis (84). Even if enlarged lymph nodes and/or lung parenchymal abnormalities are found on conventional or high resolution chest CT (HRCT), patients with normal chest radiographs still represent stage 0 disease. Stage I disease is defined when bilateral hilar lymphadenopathy (BHL) is present without lung parenchmal abnormalities. In one HRCT study, all patients with stage I sarcoid on chest radiography had abnormal lung parenchyma on HRCT (85). Stage II disease is defined by the combination of BHL and pulmonary parenchymal abnormalities (Fig. 15.5). In stage III sarcoidosis, pulmonary abnormalities are present without BHL (Fig. 15.6). Stage IV refers to extensive fibrosis with architectural distortion and/or bullae (1,15,79) (Fig. 15.3). In a study of 3676 patients with sarcoidosis from nine countries, 8% presented with stage 0, 51% with stage I, 29% stage II, and 12% with stage III (84). This radiographic classification scheme, despite its simplicity, is prognostically useful, and is discussed in detail later.

Intrathoracic Lymph Node Enlargement

The triad of bilateral hilar and right paratracheal lymph node enlargement (the 1–2–3 sign) is seen in 50–85% of patients with sarcoidosis (15,51,57,59,60,79,81,83). Enlarged lymph nodes in other locations (e.g., aorto-

pulmonary window, subcarinal region, anterior mediastinum, axillae, subphrenic) are less common, but may be evident on CT scans (81,83,86–90). In one study, subcarinal and anterior mediastinal lymph node enlargement was noted in only 12% of patients on conventional chest radiographs, compared with 64% and 48%, by CT (89). Posterior mediastinal or paravertebral lymph node enlargement has been reported in 2–20% of patients with sarcoidosis (91–93). Unilateral hilar enlargement occurs in 3–5% (94,95). Isolated unilateral hilar lymph node enlargement is much more common in tuberculosis and lymphoma than is sarcoidosis; predominant anterior mediastinal lymph node enlargement is more common in lymphoma. Despite the high prevalence of enlarged hilar and mediastinal lymph nodes in sarcoidosis, compression of the airway, pulmonary vasculature, superior vena cava, or innominate veins is rare (96).

Calcification of hilar or mediastinal lymph nodes is noted on chest radiographs in 20% or more of patients with longstanding pulmonary sarcoidosis (>10 years) (81,97–99) (Fig. 15.7). In one study, calcified nodes were identified on CT scans in 20% of patients initially, but in 44% of patients up to 4 years later (100). The distribution and pattern of lymph node calcification in sarcoidosis differs from tuberculosis (101). In one study, CT scans were performed in 28 patients with tuberculosis and 49 patients with sarcoidosis (duration 0–32 years) (101). Calcifications were identified in 53% and 46% of patients with sarcoidosis and tuberculosis, respectively; the lymph nodes in sarcoidosis were larger than in tuberculosis (mean diameter 12 mm versus 7 mm), more often focal (sarcoidosis 58%, tuberculosis 23%) and less likely to be completely calcified (sarcoidosis 27%, tuberculosis 62%).

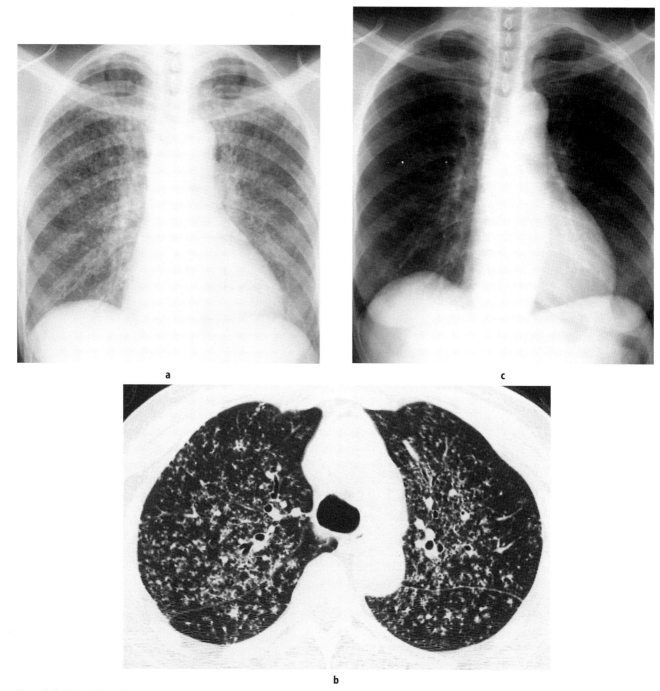

Figure 15.6. a Stage III sarcoidosis. Posteroanterior chest radiograph demonstrates widespread reticulonodular and miliary infiltrates in a 62 year old female with sarcoidosis and severe dyspnea, cough, and weight loss. **b** HRCT scan from the same patient demonstrated widespread nodular and miliary opacities. Transbronchial lung biopsies demonstrated numerous noncaseating granulomas. Special stains and cultures for acid-fast bacilli and fungi were negative. **c** Posteroanterior chest radiograph from the same patient 4 months after corticosteroid therapy demonstrates complete resolution of infiltrates.

Lymph node calcification was bilateral in 65% of patients with sarcoidosis but in only 8% of patients with tuberculosis. Egg-shell calcification of lymph nodes on CT was observed in only 9% of patients with sarcoidosis (101). However, sarcoidosis is the most common cause of this pattern in patients without exposure to silica (96,102).

Lung Parenchymal Abnormalities

Pulmonary parenchymal abnormalities, with or without hilar lymph node enlargement, occurs in 50–60% of patients with sarcoidosis over the course of the disease (15,51,57,59,60,79,81,83). CT is more sensitive than chest

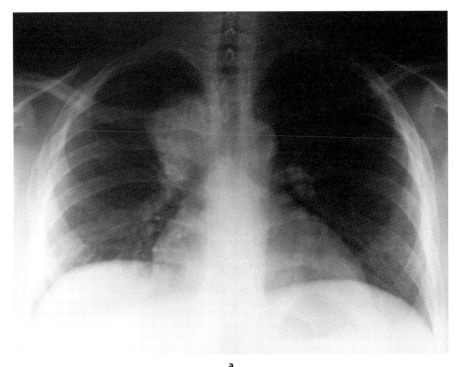

a

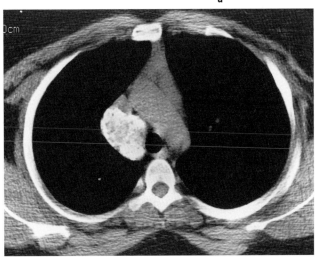

b

Figure 15.7. a Calcified mediastinal (right paratracheal) lymph nodes in a 36 year old women with chronic sarcoidosis and a 3 year history of uveitis. **b** Calcified mediastinal (right paratracheal) mass. CT scan demonstrates dense calcified mass.

radiograph. In one series, HRCT revealed parenchymal lesions in 5 of 27 patients with normal chest radiographs (87). Lung involvement was confirmed by transbronchial or open lung biopsies even when HRCT scans were normal (103). The lung parenchymal abnormality is usually symmetric, involves the central portion of both lungs, and most commonly affects the upper lobes (15,60,79,81). The distribution of sarcoid lesions on CT is consistent with lung biopsy findings; noncaseating granulomas are most commonly found along peribronchovascular sheath lymphatics, and to a lesser extent in subpleural and interlobular septal lymphatics (30,33, 103,104). Sarcoidosis and lymphangitic carcinomatoses

are two disorders with a bronchovascular distribution (33). Asymmetric disease may be seen when the process is developing or resolving (105).

The pattern of lung parenchymal abnormality on chest radiographs is nodular, in 30–60% of patients, reticulonodular in 25–50%, and reticular in 15–20% (81,103, 106–108). Nodules are seen in >90% of patients undergoing HRCT (85,109) (Fig. 15.8). The nodules are usually less than 3 mm, but may exceed 2 cm in diameter (85,103, 106,109). These nodules represent conglomerate granulomas along interlobular septae, centrilobular and subpleural regions (103,104). Thickening of inter- and intralobular septa are seen in 20–90% and 20–70% of

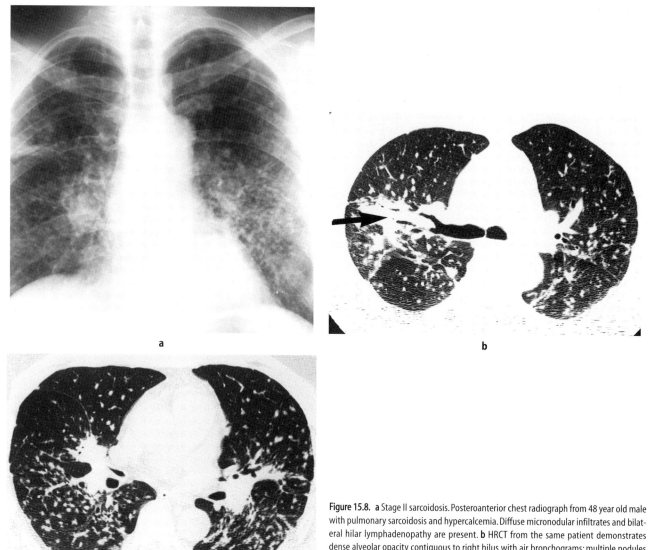

Figure 15.8. a Stage II sarcoidosis. Posteroanterior chest radiograph from 48 year old male with pulmonary sarcoidosis and hypercalcemia. Diffuse micronodular infiltrates and bilateral hilar lymphadenopathy are present. **b** HRCT from the same patient demonstrates dense alveolar opacity contiguous to right hilus with air bronchograms; multiple nodules in both lungs. **c** HRCT demonstrates multiple nodules in both lungs; bilateral hilar lymph nodes with infiltrates radiating from both hili.

patients respectively on HRCT (104). Focal or confluent alveolar opacities with consolidation is noted in 10–20% of patients (82,103,108,110) (Fig. 15.9).

A diffuse ground-glass pattern on conventional radiographs is rare in sarcoidosis (Fig. 15.10). In one series of 1600 patients with sarcoidosis, diffuse ground-glass opacities were noted on chest radiographs in 10 patients (0.6%) (111). Ground-glass opacities resolved in all 9 patients treated with corticosteroids. Diffuse miliary nodules as the predominant pattern were seen in 2 of 150 patients in one series (112), and may be seen in unusual clinical settings such as recurrent sarcoidosis after lung transplantation (113) (Fig. 15.6a).

With longstanding sarcoidosis, the lung parenchyma is destroyed, manifesting radiographically as honeycomb

cysts, fibrosis, architectural distortion, and volume loss, with cephalad retraction and posterior rotation of the hili (15,60,81). On HRCT, the fibrosis/cystic changes predominate along the central bronchovascular bundles and upper lobes (104) (Fig. 15.11). Coalesence of granulomas may simulate conglomerate masses of silicosis. Large bullae, cystic bronchiectasis and enlarged pulmonary arteries (due to secondary pulmonary arterial hypertension) may complicate advanced stage III or IV sarcoidosis (81,114, 115). Pleural thickening is uncommon, but may be found in longstanding cases (81). This may represent inward retraction of extrathoracic soft tissues and extrapleural fat, rather than true pleural abnormality.

Primary cavitary sarcoidosis, with central necrosis due to conglomerate granulomas, is rare (116–118), but

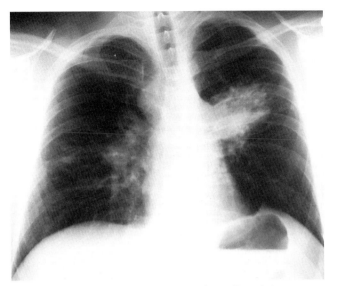

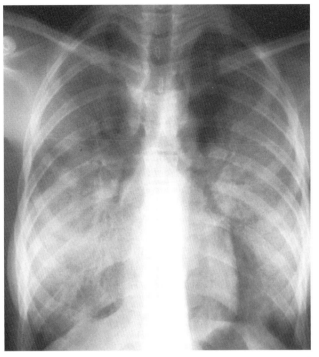

Figure 15.9. Stage III sarcoidosis. Posteroanterior chest radiograph demonstrates mass-like density emenating from left hilum and extending into the lung parenchyma. Bilateral hilar and right paratracheal lymphadenopathy is present.

Figure 15.10. Stage III sarcoidosis. Chest radiograph demonstrates extensive ground-glass, miliary infiltrates throughout both lung fields in a 22 year old black female with a 4 month history of dyspnea. Transbronchial lung biopsies demonstrated confluent non caseating granulomas. Special stains and cultures for acid-fast bacilli and fungi were negative. Corticosteroids (prednisone 40 mg day^{-1}) led to dramatic improvement. (Reproduced from ref. 1, with permission.)

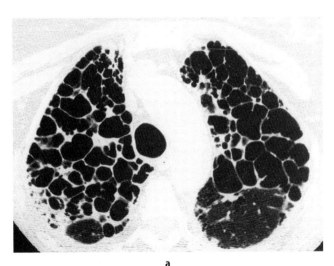

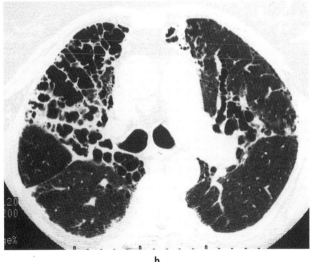

a   b

Figure 15.11. a HRCT scan. End-stage sarcoidosis with virtually complete replacement of upper lobes with cystic radiolucencies. b HRCT scan from the same patient demonstrating patchy involvement with in an axial (perihilar) distribution. End-stage sarcoidosis with cystic radiolucencies is apparent.

has been described in a few patients with acinar or nodular sarcoidosis. In one series of 1254 patients with sarcoidosis, cavitation was evident on chest radiographs in only 8 patients (0.6%) (8). Cavitation is more common on CT, cited in 3 of 159 patients (2%) in one series (106). Cavities usually develop with other lung abnormalities, may resolve spontaneously, or be a site for the development of a fungus ball (mycetoma). Since cavitation is rare, superimposed infection should be considered. This entity is distinct from large bullae or cystic bronchiectasis complicating advanced stage IV, sarcoidosis (81).

Vascular Involvement

Sarcoidosis involving pulmonary arteries or veins is common on open lung biopsies (31,32), but symptoms due to pulmonary vascular involvement, compression, or occlusion are rare. Pulmonary hypertension occurs in 1–4% of patients with sarcoidosis, primarily in patients with severe parenchymal destruction and cor pulmonale (119,120). Pulmonary hypertension without pulmonary parenchymal involvement is rare (121–123). Causes of pulmonary hypertension in sarcoidosis include extrinsic compression from enlarged hilar lymph nodes (96, 124–126), intrinsic involvement of the pulmonary vessels by granulomatous inflammation (119,121,127) and fibrosing mediastinitis (86,128). Sarcoidosis is a rare cause of fibrosing mediastinitis, resulting in stenosis or obstruction of pulmonary arteries (86), innominate veins (129), superior vena cava (130) or bronchi (131). Extensive mediastinal lymphadenopathy from sarcoidosis is a rare cause of superior vena cava syndrome or compression of the innominate veins (1,129,130,132–134). Pulmonary venoocclusive disease is a rare complication of sarcoidosis (135,136).

Pleural Involvement

Clinically significant pleural manifestations (e.g., pleural effusions, pneumothorax, chylothorax) occur in 2–7% of patients with sarcoidosis (81,131,137–139). Conventional chest radiographs demonstrate pleural effusions in only 1–4% of patients with sarcoidosis (81,131,137–139). Pleural effusions and thickening are more common in patients with chronic stage II or III sarcoidosis. The frequency of pleural thickening or small pleural effusions on CT scans is higher (104). Sarcoid pleural effusions are exudative in 70% of patients, with a predominance of lymphocytes (131,140) and elevated CD4/CD8 ratios (131,141). Pleural biopsies may reveal noncaseating granulomas (1). When a pleural effusion develops in a patient with sarcoidosis, other etiologies need to be definitively excluded. Pneumothorax or pleural thickening may be observed in chronic fibrocystic sarcoidosis (1). Ipsilateral pleural thickening is common in patients with mycetomas (142). Spontaneous pneumothoraces, due to rupture of subpleural bullae, occur in 1–3% of patients with fibrotic stage III or IV sarcoidosis (1,131). Pleural calcification was described in a patient with chronic sarcoidosis and a pleural effusion (131). A few cases of chylothorax in patients with sarcoidosis involving mediastinal lymph nodes or the thoracic duct have been reported (143–146).

One patient presenting with focal pleural mass was described (147).

Aspergillomas

Aspergillomas may develop in cystic spaces (typically in the upper lobes) in patients with advanced stage III or IV) sarcoidosis (86,148–153) (Fig. 15.12). Pleural thickening adjacent to a cystic space usually precedes the fungus ball (142). Prevalence of aspergillomas ranges from 1% to 3% in patients with pulmonary sarcoidosis (151,152) but rates are higher with radiographic stage III or IV disease (153).

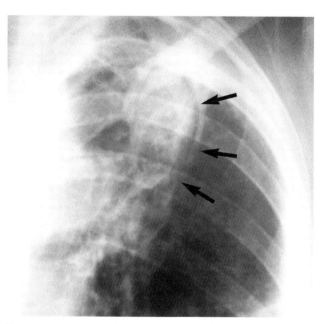

Figure 15.12. Aspergilloma. Posteroanterior chest radiograph: coned down view demonstrates the right upper lobe mass, surrounded by a crescent of air, consistent with a mycetoma.

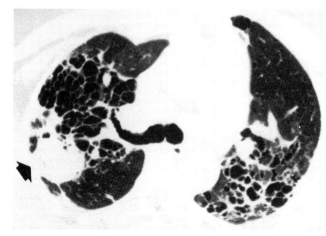

Figure 15.13. HRCT scan. Severe cystic radiolucencies with a proclivity for the bronchovascular bundles; note the mycetoma in the right lung (*arrow*). (Reproduced from ref. 2)

Mycetomas are often asymptomatic but severe, exsanguinating hemorrhage may occur when aspergilli invade vessel walls (96). Prognosis of aspergillomas is poor (fatality rates >50%); most fatalities reflect progression or severity of the underlying pulmonary disease rather than a direct complication of mycetoma (148,151,152).

Surgical resection is advised for localized mycetomas if patients can tolerate surgery and general anesthesia. However, severe respiratory insufficiency or extensive pleural adhesions may preclude surgical resection (148, 154). Systemic antifungal agents are of doubtful value. Other options include intracavitary instillation of amphotericin B (155–157), fluconazole (156), or potassium iodide (154). Bronchial arterial embolization is reserved for severe hemoptysis refractory to medical therapy (152).

Nodular Sarcoidosis and Necrotizing Sarcoid Angiitis and Granulomatosis

Multiple well-circumscribed pulmonary nodules >1 cm in size, known as nummular ("coin-like") or nodular sarcoidosis, occur in 2–4% of patients with sarcoidosis (Fig. 15.14) (86,158–161). Occasionally, nodules exceed 6 cm in size (162). Lung biopsies demonstrate focal nodules composed of coalescent masses of granulomas and hyalinized connective tissue (30). Clinical and radiographic features of "nodular sarcoid" are similar to "necrotizing sarcoid angiitis and granulomatosis (NSG)" (30), an entity characterized by pulmonary vasculitis, granulomas, and pulmonary nodules on chest radiographs (163–170). In NSG, lung biopsies demonstrate a granulomatous vasculitis involving arteries and veins, foci of parenchymal necrosis, and confluent noncaseating granulomata (30,163,166,171). Both nodular sarcoidosis and NSG likely are variants of sarcoidosis. When vasculitis is a prominent feature, the term NSG is applied (30). Most patients with NSG are asymptomatic, but cough, chest pain, or constitutional symptoms may be present (38,166). Chest radiographs reveal multiple, bilateral pulmonary nodules (163,165). Cavitation occurs in a minority of patients (38). Hilar lymphadenopathy is present in 10–60% of cases (163,165,166). Prognosis is excellent. The disease resolves (spontaneously or in response to therapy) in more than 80% of patients (38,163,165).

Bronchostenosis

Bronchostenosis, although uncommon, may develop due to extrinsic airway compression by enlarged lymph nodes or primary airway sarcoidosis (81,85,86,96,111,115,172, 173). Stenosis or compression of bronchi may reflect granulomatous inflammation of the bronchial wall (61), extrinsic compression from enlarged hilar nodes, or distortion of major bronchi due to lung parenchymal sarcoidosis (35,40,61,174–177). The right middle lobe is most commonly affected, because of the small orifice, sharp angulation from the bronchus intermedius, and large number of local lymph nodes (178,179). Stenosis or narrowing, irregularity, distortion, crowding, and areas of focal bronchiectasis have been noted by bronchography (175) or CT scans (180). Bronchostenosis is an incidental finding in 2–26% of patients with sarcoidosis undergoing

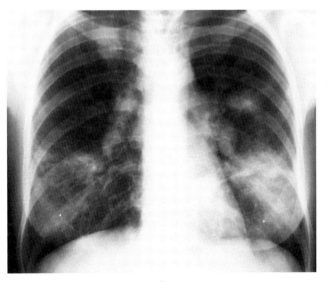
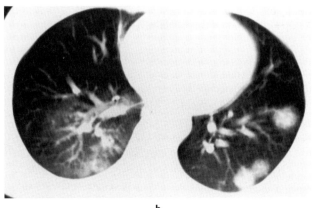

a   b

Figure 15.14. **a** Nodular sarcoidosis. Posteroanterior chest radiograph reveals multiple dense alveolar nodular infiltrates in a 36 year old woman. Bilateral hilar lymphadenopathy is also present. Transbronchial lung biopsies demonstrated multiple, confluent noncaseating granulomas consistent with sarcoidosis. The infiltrates resolved following institution of corticosteroid therapy. (Reproduced from ref. 1, with permission.) **b** Nodular sarcoidosis. CT scan from the same patient demonstrates multiple, large well-dermarcated alveolar nodules in the left lower lobe. Areas of ill-defined alveolar consolidation with small nodules are also noted in the right lower lobe. (Reproduced from ref. 1, with permission.)

bronchoscopy (35,175), but severe, symptomatic bronchostenosis is rare (175,177,181). Corticosteroids may be tried for severe or chronic bronchostenosis, but are usually ineffectual (177). Balloon dilatation of localized stenoses has been successful in anecdotal cases (182).

Computed Tomography

Computed tomographic (CT) scans are more sensitive than plain chest radiographs in delineating lung parenchymal, mediastinal and hilar structures and provide greater anatomic lung detail (85–87,104). Enlarged lymph nodes are often seen on CT in the paratracheal, pretracheal, paraaortic, internal mammary, subcarinal, anterior mediastinal or axillary regions that are not evident on plain chest radiographs (81,83,86,87,89). In a study of 175 patients with chronic infiltrative lung disease who had chest CT, enlarged lymph nodes were detected in 84% of patients with sarcoidosis Rates in other diseases were: idiopathic pulmonary fibrosis, 67%; hypersensitivity pneumonia, 53%; bronchiolitis obliterans organizing pneumonia (BOOP), 36%; age-matched controls, 5% (183). The mean number of enlarged lymph nodes was higher for sarcoidosis (3.2) compared with other infiltrative lung diseases (1.2). However, this additional information is rarely of clinical value. Routine chest CT is expensive and is not necessary to evaluate patients with obvious BHL on chest radiographs (88,184). CT may be helpful in patients with atypical manifestations or with normal chest radiographs when disease is suspected clinically (86). In patients with uveitis and normal chest radiographs, conventional CT may identify lymph node enlargement and raise the suspicion of sarcoidosis as the cause of uveitis (185).

Clinical Significance of Bilateral Hilar Lymph Node Enlargement

The differential diagnosis for BHL includes infection (particularly fungal and mycobacterial organisms) and malignancy (particularly lymphoma). In the absence of specific signs or symptoms, BHL is rarely a presenting feature of malignancy. In one review, BHL was a presenting feature in only 3.8% (8 of 212) of lymphomas, 0.8% (4 of 500) of bronchogenic carcinomas, and 0.2% (2 of 1201) of primary extrathoracic malignancies (57). In a study of 100 consecutive patients with BHL by chest radiography, sarcoidosis was the final diagnosis in 74% of patients (57). Although malignancy was the cause of BHL in 11 patients, all 11 with malignancy were symptomatic and 9 of 11 had palpable extrapulmonary masses on physical examination. Among 52 patients with BHL and a normal physical examination, 50 (96%) had sarcoidosis. Further, all 47 patients who were asymptomatic or exhibited only acute inflammatory features (e.g., uveitis, polyarthritis, or erythema nodosum) had sarcoidosis. Anemia was present in only one of the 74 patients with sarcoidosis, but was common in malignancy. The risk of malignancy is low along patients presenting with BHL and no prior history of malignancy, provided physical examination and routine blood tests are normal (57,186). Histologic confirmation of sarcoidosis is not necessary in asymptomatic patients with symmetric BHL, normal complete blood counts, normal physical examination and no prior history of malignancy. In such patients, follow-up chest radiography should be performed at 3 and 6 months. Biopsy is required only if chest radiographs worsen or specific signs or symptoms develop (186).

High Resolution Thin Section CT Scanning

HRCT using thin collimation (1–1.5 mm) and an edge-enhancing algorithm is superior to conventional CT (using 10 mm collimation and a soft tissue reconstruction algorithm) for evaluating fine parenchymal details and discriminating alveolitis from fibrosis (33,83,100,103,104, 184,187). HRCT scans are particularly useful for detecting subpleural nodules, thick interlobular septa and faint ground-glass attenuation (103). Conventional CT may be superior for detecting miliary and peribronchovascular nodules (103,188). Characteristic features of sarcoidosis on CT include: nodular opacities and micronodules (<3 mm in diameter) along bronchovascular bundles; involvement of the axial interstitium (Fig. 15.15); central bronchovascular thickening and nodularity; confluent

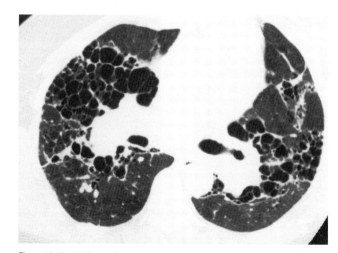

Figure 15.15. HRCT scan from a 58 year old woman with severe sarcoidosis. Severe cystic radiolucencies with a proclivity for the bronchovascular bundles; both hilae are enlarged.

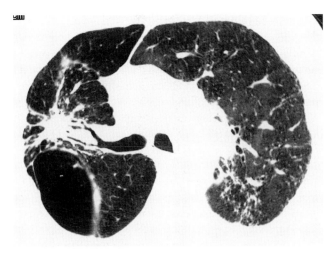

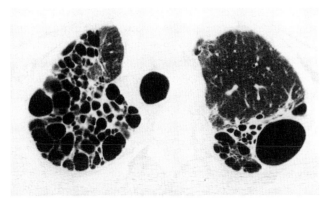

Figure 15.17. HRCT scan from a 42 year old man with sarcoidosis. Severe cystic radiolucencies in the upper lobes, with distortion and destruction of lung parenchyma; the anterior portions of the left lung are relatively preserved.

Figure 15.16. HRCT scan from a 55 year old black male with sarcoidosis demonstrates a focal alveolar opacity distal to right hilum; note the prominent air bronchograms leading to the nodular opacity. A focal cystic radiolucency, representing destroyed lung parenchyma, is present inferior to the nodular mass.

nodular opacities with air bronchograms (Fig. 15.16); ground-glass opacities; crowding and central retraction of bronchi and vessels near the hili; and pleural or subpleural nodules (33,85,103). Progression of the sarcoid lung lesion may form conglomerate masses and distort and destroy lung architecture (85,104). Nonspecific features include irregular interfaces, thickened interlobular septae or pleural surfaces, traction bronchiectasis, distortion or displacement of vessels, bronchi, or interlobar fissures, honeycomb cysts, and bullae (33,81,83,85,104). Miliary nodules are common on CT scans in sarcoidosis, but rarely present in the absence of the other findings (111). The distribution of sarcoid lesions on CT is consistent with lung biopsy findings; granulomas are most commonly found along peribronchovascular sheath lymphatics, and to a lesser extent in subpleural and interlobular septal lymphatics (30,33,103). The parenchymal abnormalities have a predilection for the upper lobes (81,85) (Fig. 15.17, 15.18). Sarcoidosis and lymphangitic carcinomatosis are two disorders with a bronchovascular distribution (33). In contrast, idiopathic pulmonary fibrosis (IPF) is characterized by peripheral and lower lobe predominant interlobular septal thickening and honeycombing; nodules and central bronchovascular thickening are rare in IPF (30).

Lesion Reversibility and CT

Specific CT features have prognostic significance. Honeycomb cysts, bullae, coarse broad bands, distortion of alveolar architecture, or traction bronchiectasis indicate fibrosis and poor responsiveness to therapy (33,100,184). In contrast, ground-glass opacities often represent alveoli-

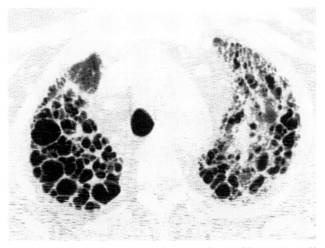

Figure 15.18. HRCT scan. Severe cystic radiolucencies in the upper lobes in a 58 year old women with severe stage IV sarcoidosis.

tis, which may be amenable to therapy (33,100,184). Nodules, alveolar consolidation, and septal thickening may represent either granulomatous inflammation or fibrosis (or a combination) and are potentially reversible following corticosteroid therapy (33,83,100,189). In one series of 20 patients, nodules and alveolar abnormalities always improved or cleared on follow-up CT scans (83). One study analyzed serial HRCT scans and pulmonary function tests in 66 patients with pulmonary sarcoidosis (184). Reversible CT changes included nodular high attenuation lesions, consolidation, ground-glass opacities, and septal lines. By contrast, honeycombing, nonseptal lines, and distortion never improved and sometimes worsened. Ground-glass opacities improved in two patients with disease of recent onset, but in only 2 of 14 with disease of greater than 2 years' duration. Thus CT was no more valuable as a prognostic guide than the combination of information gleaned from conventional chest radiographs and duration of disease. While the value of HRCT has yet to be elucidated, we reserve HRCT for selected patients with stage II or III sarcoidosis in whom the "activity" of the disease is indeterminate. In such cases, the extent and pattern of abnormalities on HRCT may guide therapy. Extensive ground-glass opacities on HRCT favors aggressive therapy whereas extensive honeycomb cysts, distorted alveolar architecture, and traction bronchiectasis support a more conservative approach.

Pulmonary Function Tests

Pulmonary function tests (PFTs), are abnormal in only 20% of patients with stage I sarcoidosis but in 40–70% of patients with radiographic stage II, III, or IV (1,15,51,60, 66,190). Reductions in lung volumes vital capacity (VC) and total lung capacity (TLC) are characteristic (79,191, 192). One third or more of patients with pulmonary parenchymal involvement manifest an obstructive component (with reductions in forced expiratory volume in 1 s (FEV_1),/FVC (forced vital capacity) ratio and expiratory flow rates (79,193–196). Increased airway hyperreactivity following methacholine challenge is common (77), and may reflect granulomatous inflammation within airways or distortion from destroyed bronchioles or lung parenchyma (30,61). The diffusing capacity for carbon monoxide ($D_{L_{CO}}$) may be reduced, but less so than patients with idiopathic pulmonary fibrosis (191–193). Hypoxemia is rare, except in patients with advanced fibrocystic sarcoidosis (190,193).

PFTs correlate only roughly with the severity or extent of disease on chest radiographs (190–192,197) and cannot discriminate alveolitis from irreversible fibrosis (79,190, 198). With severe stage III or IV disease, reductions in FEV, $D_{L_{CO}}$, and lung volumes are prominent (197). Similarly, the extent or pattern of CT aberrations correlate imprecisely with the severity of pulmonary functional aberrations (87).

Although the predictive value of PFTs at a single point in time is limited, serial PFTs are useful to follow the course of the disease in individual patients (79,190). Increases in VC correlate best with symptomatic and radiographic improvement in patients with stage II or III sarcoidosis (1,190). Changes in TLC correlate with VC, and are of marginal incremental value (190). $D_{L_{CO}}$ is less reproducible as a measure of response to therapy. Measurement of oxygen saturation at rest or during exercise was no more sensitive than VC or $D_{L_{CO}}$ (190). Given the complexity and high cost of measuring lung volumes or $D_{L_{CO}}$, spirometry and flow volume loops are the most cost-effective and useful functional tests to assess the course of sarcoidosis. Measurement of $D_{L_{CO}}$, TLC, or gas exchange is appropriate in selected patients. Severe derangements or deteriorating pulmonary function over time warrant a trial of corticosteroid therapy.

Exercise Testing in Sarcoidosis

Exercise testing is a sensitive but nonspecific measure of functional disease in sarcoidosis. Aberrations in cardiopulmonary exercise tests (principally ventilatory limitation and increased dead space to tidal volume ratio (V_D/V_T) with exercise occur in up to 50% of sarcoid patients with normal spirometry and $D_{L_{CO}}$ (192). A widened alveolar – arterial gradient is seen predominantly in patients with reduced $D_{L_{CO}}$ (192). Static PFTs and other indices at rest are not adequate predictors of work capacity (191). Exercise testing may detect functional limitation in patients with normal PFTs, but cardiopulmonary exercise testing has limited practical utility. Neither static PFTs nor exercise tests discriminate alveolitis from fibrosis. Spirometry and oximetry are the most cost-effective measures to follow the course of sarcoidosis longitudinally. In selected patients, a noninvasive 6 min walk test (with oximetry) provides useful adjunctive data.

Radiology and Pulmonary Function

The severity of disease on chest radiographs correlates imprecisely with clinical symptoms or functional impairment (103,190–192,197). With severe stage III or IV disease, reductions in FEV_1, $D_{L_{CO}}$, and lung volumes are prominent (197), but substantial variability exists. Semiquantitative schema based on a modification of the ILO/UC Classification for Pneumoconioses correlate modestly with PFTs, but have marginal prognostic value in individual patients (196,199). Neither chest radiographs nor PFTs discriminate alveolitis from irreversible fibrosis (79,190,198). Similarly, the extent or pattern of CT aberrations do not predict the severity of pulmonary functional aberrations (85,87,103,184). However, in one study of conventional CT scans in 27 patients with sarcoidosis, nodular opacities correlated with less severe dyspnea and larger lung volumes compared with predominantly irregular opacities ($p < 0.05$) (200). Standard CT provided a superior pictorial display compared to chest radiographs, but CT was no better than chest radiographs in estimating functional or clinical impairment (estimation of disease extent to nearest 5%) (200). Brauner and colleagues found moderate to poor correlations between either HRCT or chest radiographs and PFTs (85). Other investigators found low correlations between the extent of abnormality on CT and pulmonary functional impairment (184). In contrast, Bergin et al using a semiquantitative standard CT grade, cited good correlation with pulmonary function FEV_1 % predicted, $r = 0.81$; FVC % predicted, $r = 0.81$; SVC % predicted, $r = 0.67$ (87).

Natural History and Prognosis of Sarcoidosis

The clinical course and prognosis of sarcoidosis is influenced by ethnic and genetic factors (5,7,73,74,201). Black race is associated with a higher rate of extrapulmonary involvement, chronic progressive disease, worse long-term prognosis, and higher rate of relapses (5,7,51,73,74,201). The influence of HLA markers and prognosis and site(s) of organ involvement is controversial (7,21,202). HLA-B8 is associated with acute inflammatory features and a favorable prognosis whereas HLA-B13 is often associated with a progressive and protracted course (203). Some HLA patterns are associated with a good prognosis in Japanese but a poor prognosis in Italians (202,204). In the USA, fewer data are available regarding HLA (4,205).

Certain clinical syndromes have prognostic value. For example, erythema nodosum, BHL, and fever or polyarthritis (Lofgren syndrome) portends an excellent prognosis (21,186,206,207). The constellation of these features is associated with a high rate (>80%) of spontaneous remissions (21,186,206,207). Lofgren syndrome occurs in 30% of Caucasians with sarcoidosis, in 10% of Orientals, but is rare in blacks (51,72,73). In contrast, several clinical features predict a chronic or progressive course. Adverse prognostic factors include: lupus pernio (51); chronic uveitis (51); age at onset greater than 40 years (60); nephrocalcinosis (51); progressive pulmonary sarcoidosis (206,208); involvement of nasal mucosa (51) or central nervous system (209); and cystic bone lesions (51,210).

Influence of Chest Radiographic Stage

Numerous studies affirm the prognostic value of the chest radiographic classification scheme espoused more than four decades ago (10,14,15,51,59,60,63). Although exceptions exist, prognosis is best with stage I and worst with stage II, III or IV disease. Spontaneous remissions occur in 60–90% of patients with stage I disease, in 40–70% with stage II, and 10–20% with stage III (1,10,15,59,60,62,79). By definition, stage IV indicates irreversibility. In a sentinel study by Scadding, 31 of 32 patients (97%) with stage I disease were asymptomatic at 5 years (59). In contrast, only 58% of stage II and 25% of stage III were asymptomatic. Similar findings were echoed in the USA (62). In a long-term follow-up study of 244 patients with pulmonary sarcoidosis (both treated and untreated), chest radiographs normalized in 54% of patients with stage I sarcoidosis but in only 31% with stage II and 10% with stage III (62). More importantly, none of 110 patients with stage II died. In contrast, mortality rates among stage II and III were 11% and 18%, respectively. British investigators noted higher rates of radiographic resolution with stage I (59%) compared to stage II (39%) or stage III (38%) sarcoidosis (51). Swedish investigators followed 505 patients with sarcoidosis (both treated and untreated) for up to 15 years (15). Among 308 patients with stage I disease, 29 (9%) progressed to stage II and only 5 (1.6%) progressed to stage III or IV. Among 128 patients with stage II sarcoid, chest radiographs normalized in 22% after 1 year; 7 patients (5.5%) progressed to stage IV. At 5 year follow-up, chest radiographs had normalized in 82% of patients with stage I sarcoidosis 68% with stage II and 37% with stage III. It is important to emphasize that persistence of BHL does not imply ongoing active disease or the need for therapeutic intervention. Serious morbidity or late sequelae are rare with stage I sarcoidosis. In contrast, morbidity and mortality are appreciable in patients with persistent parenchymal infiltrates (radiographic stages II, III, or IV). We agree with other investigators (66,211,212) that therapy is rarely required for stage I but is often necessary to prevent devastating sequelae in patients with stage II or III disease. But when should intervention be contemplated?

The course of sarcoidosis is usually defined within the 2 years after diagnosis. Danish investigators found that 85% of all remissions occurred within 2 years of initial presentation; chest radiographs normalized in only 12% of patients who remained in stage II after 2 years (60). Only 1 of the 63 patients (1.6%) who presented in stage I progressed after the second year. Other studies have documented that spontaneous remissions occur in 16–39% of patients within 6–12 months from the onset of symptoms (73,213–215). Further, among patients who spontaneously remit, late relapses are uncommon (2–8%) (60,73,213, 214). In contrast, failure to improve within 2 years predicts a chronic or persistent course (51,60,73). A recent multicenter study under the auspices of the British Thoracic Society analyzed 149 patients with stage II or III sarcoidosis (214). Within the first 6 months of observation, chest radiographs improved spontaneously in 58 (39%); 33 (22%) required corticosteroids for persistent or progressive symptoms. The remaining 58 patients with persistent infiltrates at 6 months were randomized to long-term corticosteroids (for 18 months) or no treatment unless symptoms mandated corticosteroid therapy. At long-term follow-up, chest radiographs and PFTs were significantly better in the corticosteroid-treated cohort.

These various studies suggest that therapy is rarely required for stage I sarcoidosis, but is often necessary to prevent devastating sequelae in patients with stage II or III disease. We believe the decision to treat (or withhold treatment) should be made within the first 12 months of onset of symptoms. Delaying therapy beyond this point in patients with persistent radiographic infiltrates or functional deficits may result in irreversible fibrocystic changes.

Ancillary Studies

Bronchoalveolar lavage (BAL) cell profiles (particularly CD4+ helper/inducer cells), serum ACE (4,215) or ^{67}Ga citrate scanning (216) have been used as surrogate measures of alveolitis in sarcoidosis or as a measure of granuloma burden. However, these parameters do not reliably reflect "activity" of disease or predict long-term prognosis.

Radionuclide Scanning

Increased intrapulmonary uptake of ^{67}Ga-citrate is noted in 61–94% of patients with pulmonary sarcoidosis but does not predict prognosis or responsiveness to therapy (79,216,217). Specific patterns of uptake (e.g., uptake in hilar lymph nodes, parotid, salivary, and lacrimal glands) (216) are characteristic of sarcoidosis, and suggest the diagnosis in atypical cases (4). Because of its expense, inconvenience (scanning follows the injection by 48 h), lack of a reproducible gold standard, and exposure to radioisotopes, we see no role for ^{67}Ga scans in either the initial staging or follow-up evaluation of pulmonary sarcoidosis.

Bronchoalveolar Lavage

BAL in patients with active pulmonary sarcoidosis demonstrates increased numbers of lymphocytes, T-helper lymphocytes (CD4+) increased CD4/CD8 ratios, activated alveolar macrophages, diverse lymphokines, monokines, and biochemical markers (28,207, 215,218–222). However, increased CD4/CD8 ratios or biochemical markers cannot distinguish sarcoidosis from other interstitial lung diseases (45,46). BAL provides invaluable insights into the pathogenesis of sarcoidosis, but has marginal clinical or prognostic value (1,207,221–223). BAL cell profiles do not predict prognosis or responsiveness to corticosteroids (1,207) (223). Increased numbers of BAL mast cells (46,224), or neutrophils (46), were associated with a worse prognosis in some studies, but significant variability exists. Despite initial enthusiasm for the predictive utility of CD4/CD8 ratios (55), most studies found no correlation between initial BAL CD4/CD8 ratios and subsequent outcome or responsiveness to corticosteroid therapy (207,223,225). BAL is expensive and invasive, and we do not believe that BAL has a clinical role in determining need for therapeutic intervention.

Extrapulmonary Involvement (Selected Sites)

Lofgren Syndrome

The association of erythema nodosum and BHL (Lofgren syndrome) is an acute form of sarcoidosis that typically has a benign course and excellent long-term prognosis (even without treatment) (51,66,186,206–208). Fever, acute polyarthritis (particularly involving the ankles), and uveitis are common accompanying features (51,186,207). This syndrome is more common in Caucasians (15,186), and is self-limited in more than 85% of patients (51,186, 207). Corticosteroid treatment is reserved for patients with significant arthritis refractory to nonsteroidal anti-inflammatory agents.

Bone Involvement

Osseous involvement has been cited in 1–14% of patients with sarcoidosis (3,8–10,210, 226,227). Virtually any bone can be involved, but the small bones of the hands or feet (typically distal and middle phalanges) are most commonly affected (3,210,226,227). Involvement of long bones, calvarium, skull, orbital bones, vertebrae, ribs or pelvis is rare (210,226,227). Osseous sarcoidosis is more common in blacks and in females, and is associated with chronic multisystemic involvement (3,210,226). The radiographic spectrum is variable. Small, "punched out" lytic cortical lesions (2–4 mm in size) are characteristic; larger cysts involving cortex and medulla may cause pathologic fractures (3,210,226,227). Other radiographic features include osteopenia, "stippled" rarefaction, diffuse latticework or honeycomb pattern, and coarse or fine reticular permeative lesions (3, 210,226,227). Osteosclerotic lesions are rare (3,210,226–228). Radioisotope (^{99m}Tc phosphate) bone scans are superior to conventional radiographs (210,228). Treatment of osseous sarcoidosis is often unsatisfactory. Corticosteroids often fail, and may exacerbate bone loss (210,226). Anecdotal responses have been cited with hydroxychloroquine (229) or chloroquine (227,230).

Cardiac Involvement

Clinical involvement of the heart is recognized in only 2–5% of patients with sarcoidosis (231,232) but much higher rates (20–47%) were cited in necropsy studies (9,68,70,76,233,234). Cardiac involvement may occur at any point in the course of sarcoidosis, and may be the presenting and sole feature (68,70,76,231–234). Sarcoidosis can involve any part of the pericardium, myocardium, or endocardium (231–233). Manifestations include sudden death, arrythmias, intractable heart failure, pericardial effusions, papillary muscle dysfunction and ventricular aneurysms (68,231–233). Diagnosis of cardiac sarcoidosis is difficult. Because of potential morbidity, cardiac biopsies are infrequently performed, even when a diagnosis of myocardial sarcoidosis is suspected. In young patients presenting with cardiac manifestations and no prior history of sarcoidosis, the presence of noncaseating granulomata on endomyocardial biopsies may confirm the diagnosis. However, due to the patchy nature of the disease, endomyocardial biopsies are normal in most patients with myocardial sarcoidosis (231,233,235,236). Among patients with known sarcoidosis, the diagnosis of myocardial sarcoidosis is usually assumed when imaging studies are abnormal and coronary arteriograms are normal. Electrocardiograms (ECGs) or Holter monitors should be performed in patients with suspected cardiac involvement, but are neither sensitive nor specific (3,237, 238). Two-dimensional echocardiograms are useful in detecting right heart failure in patients with severe parenchymal pulmonary sarcoidosis, the role of echo-cardiography with primary cardiac involvement is less clear (237–239). Macroscopic areas of fibrosis or granulo-matous inflammation appear as bright echoes; other abnormalities include focal dyskinesia or hypokinesia, reduced contractility, ventricular or atrial enlargement, and incompetent valves (232,237). Although data are limited, ^{201}Tl imaging may be superior to two-dimensional echocardiography to image cardiac sarcoidosis. Segmental areas of decreased ^{201}Tl uptake correspond to areas of fibrosis or granulomatous replacement (19,232). With exercise or infusion of adenosine or dipyridamole, per-fusion defects noted at rest improve (19,232). Because cardiac sarcoidosis may be lethal, aggressive and prompt therapy with high dose corticosteroids or immuno-suppressive agents is mandatory (3,232,236). Patients with complete heart block or serious arrythmias should receive a permanent endocardial pacemaker – defibrillator (69, 240). Cardiac transplantation has been successful in patients with intractable heart failure refractory to medical therapy (3).

Central Nervous System Involvement

Clinically significant involvement of the central nervous system (CNS) occurs in 2–7% of patients with sarcoido-sis) (67,209,241–243). Manifestations of neurosarcoidosis include cranial nerve palsies (particularly Bell's palsy), meningitis, hypothalamic and pituitary lesions, masses, communicating or obstructive hydrocephalus, peripheral neuropathy, spinal cord involvement, dementia, seizures, narcolepsy, and psychiatric manifestations) (67,209, 241–244). Paresis of the seventh cranial nerve (Bell's palsy) is the most common feature, affecting 49–67% of patients with neurosarcoidosis (67,209,241–244). Facial nerve paresis typically occurs early in the course of sarcoidosis; erythema nodosum, uveitis, polyarthritis, fever, and BHL are frequent concomitant features (209,242–244). CNS sarcoidosis has a predilection for the optic chiasm, hypothalamus, and pituitary gland; visual field deficits, diabetes insipidus, and hypopituitarism may result (67,209,241–244). Virtually any part of the

central or peripheral nervous system can be involved, often with devastating consequences. Because of the inaccessibility of CNS lesions, histologic confirmation is rarely accomplished. Cerebrospinal fluid (CSF) reveals lymphocyte pleocytosis, elevated protein, or decreased glucose in 70–80% of patients with neurosarcoidosis (67,241,242, 244), but these findings are nonspecific. CSF is often normal when involvement is limited to the cranial nerves (67,241, 242,244). Radiographic imaging procedures are essential to establish the diagnosis of neurosarcoidosis, and monitor response to therapy (245–249). Contrast-enhanced CT scans may detect meningeal sarcoidosis, focal or parenchymal mass lesions, periventricular white matter lesions, or obstruc-tive or communicating hydrocephalus, but gadolinium-enhanced magnetic resonance imaging (MRI) is superior (67,245,246). Multiple, well-defined, hyperdense enhanc-ing lesions with surrounding edema are characteristic on contrast-enhanced CT (250). However, CT scans are normal in up to one third of patients with CNS sarcoido-sis, especially when lesions are confined to the cranial nerves or brainstem (250). Gadopentate dimeglumine (gadolinium)-enhanced MRI is the best test to diagnose and follow sarcoidosis involving the brain and spinal cord (246, 249) (Fig. 15.19). Multifocal periventricular and subcortical white matter abnormalities and regions of meningeal enhancement are characteristic of neu-rosarcoidosis (245,246,249). However, as with CT scans, MRI scans can be normal in patients with neurosar-coidosis, particularly when only cranial nerves are involved (245,250). The diagnosis of neurosarcoidosis is presumed in patients with a known history of sarcoido-sis at other sites, and a compatible MRI scan (246–249). Serial MRI scans are the preferred means of monitoring response to therapy (246,249). Corticosteroids are the mainstay of therapy for neurosarcoidosis but 10–50% of cases fail therapy (67,75,241). Other treatment options include: cyclosporine A (241,242), azathioprine (3,209,241, 242), methotrexate (3,241,242), antimalarials (67), and intravenous pulse cyclophosphamide (75). Radiation therapy is reserved for severe neurologic sarcoidosis refractory to pharmacologic therapy (3,209,248,251).

Hepatic Involvement

Asymptomatic granulomas are detected in 21–79% of patients with sarcoidosis, even when signs of liver disease are absent (3,252–254). Hepatomegaly has been noted on physical examination in 2–21% of patients with sarcoido-sis (3,8,9,253,254). Asymptomatic elevations in liver func-tion tests (particularly alkaline phosphatase) are common (3). Despite the high frequency of occult hepatic involve-ment, clinically significant liver disease has been cited in

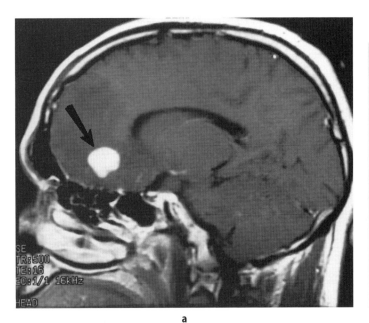
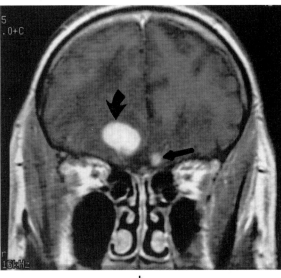

a   **b**

Figure 15.19. a Sarcoidosis involving the brain. MRI scan from the same patient. *Arrow* depicts a large mass lesion in the medial aspect of the right frontal lobe that enhances with gadolinium. Considerable edema in the frontal lobe surrounds the mass lesion. Although no biopsy was obtained, a presumptive diagnosis of central nervous system sarcoidosis was made and prednisone (60 mg per alternate day) was initiated. (Reproduced from ref. 3, with permission.) **b** Sarcoidosis involving the brain. MRI scan from the same patient taken before corticosteroid therapy. *Curved arrow* depicts the large enhanced lesion in right frontal lobe. With prednisone therapy, his lesions regressed substantially and his symptoms resolved. *Straight arrow* depicts an enhancing lesion in the left frontal lobe. (Reproduced from ref. 3, with permission.)

fewer than 5% of patients with sarcoidosis (3). However, serious, even fatal, liver dysfunction can occur (253,255). CT or MRI scans demonstrate nonspecific hepatomegaly or multiple, low attenuation nodules (256–258). One study evaluated consecutive patients with sarcoidosis who were referred for abdominal CT scans (259). Abnormal findings included, hepatomegaly (8%) and low attenuation nodules in liver (6%) or spleen (14%). The presence of hepatic nodular lesions was associated with abdominal symptoms or abdominal lymphadenopathy in more than two thirds of patients (257).

Muscle Involvement

Asymptomatic involvement of muscle occurs in 20–75% of patients with sarcoidosis, but symptomatic muscle involvement is noted in fewer than 0.5% of patients (3,260). Manifestations of primary muscle involvement include acute or subacute myopathy (261), chronic myopathy (262), and granulomatous nodules or mass lesions (260). MRI imaging (263,264), CT scans (264), and ^{67}Ga scintigraphy (263,265) may discern focal granulomatous masses in patients with sarcoidosis involving muscle. MRI scans reveal star-shaped areas of low signal intensity surrounded by areas of high signal intensity (263–265). CT is less sensitive than MRI in evaluating nodular sarcoid myopathy (263–265). Ultrasonography reveals central zones of increased echogenicity and a peripheral area of decreased echogenicity (263).

Splenic Involvement

Asymptomatic involvement of the spleen is common, occurring in 38–77% of patients with sarcoidosis in necropsy series (9,10,266). Splenic granulomas were noted in 24–59% of unselected patients with sarcoidosis undergoing fine-needle biopsy (267–270). However, symptomatic splenic involvement occurs in only 1–3% of patients with sarcoidosis (3,9,10,267). Massive splenomegaly can give rise to abdominal pain, splenic rupture, portal hypertension, refractory leukopenia or pancytopenia (271–274). Constitutional symptoms may be prominent (3,257). Concomitant enlargement of liver and intraabdominal lymph nodes (e.g., portahepatic, paraaortic, celiac) is common (257,259). Granulomatous infiltration of spleen or liver typically appears as diffuse, homogeneous organomegaly on abdominal CT scans (257) (Fig. 15.20). In a minority of cases, multiple, low attenuation nodules (ranging in size from 5 to 20 mm) are found (257,259, 273,274). MRI may also define sarcoid lesions in spleen or liver (258,275). Symptomatic or massive splenomegaly warrants treatment with corticosteroids to avert splenic rupture or other potential complications (257,276). Immunosuppressive or cytotoxic agents or antimalarials may be used in patients refractory to or experiencing adverse effects from corticosteroids (3). Splenectomy may be required for patients with symptomatic, massive splenomegaly refractory to medical therapy (271,277).

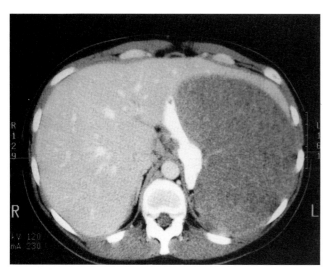

Figure 15.20. Sarcoidosis involving the spleen. CT scan shows massive splenomegaly and diffuse hypoattenuation throughout the spleen. Because of severe abdominal pain, she was treated with corticosteroids (40 mg prednisone daily for 1 month, tapered to 40 mg every other day). Improvement was dramatic. (Reproduced from ref. 3, with permission.)

Therapy of Sarcoidosis

Although indications for treatment are controversial, corticosteroids are the mainstay of therapy for persistent or progressive sarcoidosis (pulmonary or extrapulmonary) (4,66,212). Optimal dose and duration of corticosteroids have not been studied in prospective, randomized trials. Interpretation of efficacy of therapy is confounded by several factors including: high rate of spontaneous remissions; heterogeneous patient populations, dosages, and duration of therapy; inability to discriminate effects of corticosteroids from the natural history of the disease; and lack of validated gold standards for assessment of disease activity (i.e., extent of inflammatory versus fibrotic components). Several prospective studies failed to show long-term benefit with early (routine) use of corticosteroids (278–283). One conclusion that should be drawn from these studies is that "routine" treatment with corticosteroids in all patients with sarcoidosis is inappropriate. Indications for treatment should be focused and circumscribed, since most patients improve without therapeutic intervention. However, several of these placebo-controlled randomized studies enrolled patients with normal or near normal PFTs and no symptoms (280–283). In clinical practice, treatment would not be indicated in such patients. Conversely, patients with more severe disease were excluded from the prospective study designs and often were treated with corticosteroids. Thus these studies do not address the issue of what to do with symptomatic patients with severe or deteriorating disease. Extensive clinical experience supports treating patients with severe or deteriorating pulmonary or extrapulmonary sarcoidosis (5,66,212,213). After an initial

6 months of observation a recent multicenter trial randomized patients with stage II or III sarcoidosis and persistent radiographic infiltrates to receive either corticosteroids or placebo for at least another 18 months (214). Long-term pulmonary function was significantly improved in the patients receiving corticosteroids compared to placebo (214). This supports our view that an empirical trial of corticosteroids should be tried in patients with progressive or persistent pulmonary infiltrates and significant physiologic derangements. It should be emphasized that treatment is not required for stage I disease unless additional features develop. Routine corticosteroids for asymptomatic or minimally symptomatic patients with normal pulmonary function should be discouraged. However, patients may underestimate functional limitations, particularly those with a sedentary life style. Baseline PFTs are required to identify patients who may be candidates for therapy. We treat symptomatic patients (or those with significant pulmonary dysfunction) for the following indications: a deteriorating course, persistent or progressive parenchymal infiltrates on chest radiographs, and moderate or severe pulmonary dysfunction. Early institution of corticosteroids is warranted among patients with radiographic infiltrates and severe pulmonary functional impairment or symptoms. In contrast, the decision to treat can be delayed for up to 12 months in patients with stage II or III sarcoidosis with mild or moderate symptoms, since potential for spontaneous resolution exists. Patients with chronic symptoms lasting more than 1 year should generally be treated, as spontaneous remissions are unlikely to occur in this context. Therapy is rarely efficacious in patients with far-advanced fibrosis, honeycombing, or bullae (radiographic stage IV) (212). In this context, overaggressive treatment leads to excessive toxicities (including opportunistic infections) (284). Treatment of stage IV disease should be limited to patients with a progressive course or ancillary evidence for active alveolitis.

Corticosteroids can be dramatically effective in reversing alveolitis and improving symptoms, chest radiographs, and pulmonary function. In uncontrolled studies, more than 70% of patients with symptomatic pulmonary sarcoidosis responded favorably to corticosteroids (10,15,60, 63,64,66,212,213). Long-term efficacy is less clear, as relapses occur in 16–50% following discontinuation or taper of corticosteroids (1,10,15,60,63,212,213). The appropriate dose and duration of corticosteroid therapy have not been evaluated in controlled, randomized trials. High daily doses of corticosteroids (e.g., prednisone 1 mg kg^{-1} day^{-1} or equivalent) have been used for pulmonary sarcoidosis (213), but lower doses (e.g., prednisone 40 mg daily for 4 weeks, tapered to 40 mg per alternate day by 3 months) are less toxic and are usually effective (1,66). For some patients, initial treatment with alternate day corticosteroids is adequate (e.g., prednisone 40 mg per alternate day for a 3 months trial) (285,286). Higher doses (e.g., prednisone 1 mg kg^{-1} day^{-1}) may be necessary for myocardial or central nervous system disease, or selected patients with severe pulmonary involvement. Responses to corticosteroids are evident within 4–12 weeks. Patients who fail to respond after a 3 month trial are unlikely to respond to a more prolonged course of therapy. Failures to respond to corticosteroids may reflect: the presence of irreversible, fibrotic or cystic disease; inadequate dose or duration of therapy; noncompliance; or intrinsic corticosteroid resistance. Among corticosteroid responders, the dose is gradually tapered (e.g., to 30 mg per alternate day within 6 months and to 20 mg per alternate day within 9 months). The rate of taper needs to be individualized according to clinical responses and adverse effects. Relapses usually respond to reinstitution of daily corticosteroid therapy. A minimum of 12 months of therapy is advised. A more protracted course is warranted for patients who relapse each time the dose is tapered. In selected patients, prolonged (sometimes indefinite) therapy with low dose prednisone (10–20 mg per alternate day) may prevent relapses.

Inhaled Corticosteroids

Inhaled corticosteroids suppress endobronchial or alveolar inflammation, and have been used with anecdotal successes in patients with sarcoidosis limited to the lower respiratory tract (287–292). However, two recent randomized, double-blind studies failed to show benefit with inhaled corticosteroids for pulmonary sarcoidosis (293,294). Inhaled corticosteroids may have a limited role in sarcoid patients with cough, endobronchial inflammation, or bronchial hyperreactivity but are not adequate to treat patients with severe pulmonary parenchymal involvement. In this context, systemic corticosteroids are indicated.

Alternatives to Corticosteroids

Immunosuppressive, cytotoxic, and antimalarial agents with immunomodulatory properties have been used to treat sarcoidosis patients failing or experiencing adverse effects from corticosteroids (3,212,213,295). However, experience is largely anecdotal, and controlled, randomized trials are lacking.

Methotrexate

Methotrexate (dose 10–20 mg orally once weekly) may be effective in patients failing or experiencing adverse effects from corticosteroids (58,212,241,252,296–298) Favorable responses have been cited in more than two thirds of

patients treated with methotrexate (MTX), but relapses occurred in >70% following discontinuation of therapy (252,295). Nonetheless, favorable responses are usually achieved with reintroduction of MTX. Toxicities associated with MTX are protean and include: mucosal ulcerations, gastrointestinal symptoms, hepatitis, cirrhosis, skin rash, stomatitis, alopecia, bone marrow suppression, interstitial pneumonitis, teratogenicity, and opportunistic infections (284). Contraindications to MTX include: alcohol abuse, prexisting liver disease, poor bone marrow reserve, renal failure, or unreliable patients (284). An empirical trial of MTX for 4–6 months is reasonable but continuing therapy beyond this point should be reserved for patients manifesting unequivocal objective improvement. Because of potential hepatic toxicity, serial transaminases should be measured every 4–6 weeks while the patient is on therapy, but do not reliably predict late sequelae (284).

Azathioprine

Azathioprine (dose 100 to 200 mg day^{-1}) has a role in patients failing or experiencing adverse effects from corticosteroids (212). Anecdotal successes have been cited (58,114,299,300), but studies comparing azathioprine with other agents are lacking. Toxicities include: bone marrow suppression, gastrointestinal symptoms (e.g., nausea, vomiting, liver toxicity), skin rash, mucosal ulcerations, idiosyncratic reactions (fever, rash, arthralgias), opportunistic infections, and a slightly increased risk of neoplasia (284). Because of potential bone marrow toxicity, complete blood count, differential, and platelet counts should be performed within 2 weeks of initiation of azathioprine, and monthly while the patient on therapy. Leukopenia (< 3500 mm^{-3}) or thrombocytopenia (platelet count < 100 000) mandates dose reduction.

Cytotoxic Agents

Cytotoxic alkylating agents (e.g., cyclophosphamide and chlorambucil) have been used to treat corticosteroid-recalcitrant sarcoidosis, but data are limited (201,276,278, 301,302). Israel and McComb cited favorable responses in 20 of 31 patients (64%) treated with chlorambucil (201). Only five had failed corticosteroids; the remaining patients requiring unacceptably high doses of corticosteroids for control. Data regarding cyclophosphamide are limited to rare case reports (213, 301) and one small series (302). Lower and colleagues cited favorable responses in 8 of 10 patients with neurosarcoidosis treated with intravenous pulse cyclophosphamide (302). All patients failed corticosteroid therapy; 8 failed methotrexate. Side-effects with alkylating agents include: infertility; gastrointestinal, mucosal, and bone marrow toxicities; heightened risk of infections; alopecia; interstitial pneumonitis; and induction of neoplasia (including hematologic malignancies) (284). Hemorrhagic cystitis and bladder carcinoma complicate the use of cyclophosphamide in 27–50% and 5–7%, respectively (284). Because cyclophosphamide and chorambucil are oncogenic, we prefer alternative agents. However, intravenous pulse cyclophosphamide has a role for patients with severe CNS sarcoidosis refractory to corticosteroids and other immunosuppressive agents (e.g., azathioprine, methotrexate, and/or hydroxychloroquine) (302).

Cyclosporine A

Anecdotal successes were noted with cyclosporine A (CsA) (241,299,303), an immunosuppressive agent which inhibits T-cell activation and proliferation (299,303), but experience with this agent is disappointing (212,241,242, 304,305). In a recent, open-label randomized controlled trial, the combination of CsA (5–7 mg kg^{-1} day^{-1}) and prednisone was no more effective than prednisone alone (305). Despite a theoretical basis for the use of CsA, CsA has a best a limited role in sarcoidosis. Further, CsA is exceedingly expensive (>$500 per month) and is nearly invariably toxic (212,284).

Nonsteroidal Anti-inflammatory Agents (NSAIDs)

Nonsteroidal anti-inflammatory agents (e.g., indomethacin, phenylbutazone) may ameliorate acute arthritic manifestations of sarcoidosis (particularly in Lofgroens' syndrome), but have no role in pulmonary sarcoidosis (212).

Antimalarials

Antimalarials (e.g., chloroquine, hydroxychloroquine) inhibit antigen presentation and cytokine release and are effective in selected patients with sarcoidosis (67,212, 229,300,306–310). Antimalarials concentrate in melanin-containing tissues (e.g., skin, liver, spleen, leukocytes), and may be more efficacious in treating sarcoidosis affecting these sites (212). Anecdotal successes were cited with both chloroquine and hydroxychloroquine for treating sarcoid-induced hypercalcemia or hypercalciuria (306,311,312), or sarcoidosis involving skin (including lupus pernio) (307,308), bone (212,229,307), central nervous system (67) and lung (310,313). Because chloroquine can cause serous ocular toxicity, chloroquine is rarely used. Hydroxychloroquine (Plaquenil), is less toxic

than chloroquine, but probably is less effective (67,212). We use hydroxychloroquine (dose 200 mg twice daily) as adjunctive therapy in patients failing or experiencing adverse effects from corticosteroids. A minimum of a 6 month trial is advised, as responses are delayed for up to 3–6 months. Among responders, the dose may be tapered to 200 mg once daily. Hydroxychloroquine is usually well tolerated, but ocular toxicity (e.g., changes in color vision, blurred vision, retinopathy) is a rare complication (212,308). Ophthalmologic examinations should be performed every 6–9 months while on treatment. Retinal toxicity mandates cessation of therapy. Hydroxychloroquine suppresses gluconeogenesis, increases peripheral utilization of glucose, and reduces insulin requirements (314). This property may be beneficial in patients with severe hyperglycemia due to corticosteroids.

Other Agents

Ketoconazole reduces circulating 1,25-hydroxyvitamin D_3 and serum calcium levels in hypercalcemia due to sarcoidosis (315,316). Anecotal responses have been claimed with pentoxifylline (317), thalidomide (318), and melatonin (4), but none of these agents are of proven efficacy.

Lung Transplantation

Lung transplantation has been successfully accomplished in patients with end-stage pulmonary or cardiac disease secondary to sarcoidosis (319). Recurrence of sarcoid granulomas in the lung allografts is common (320,321), but is rarely clinically significant. Since transplant recipients are treated for life with immunosuppressive agents, these may attenuate or limit the severity of granulomatous inflammation.

References

1. Lynch JP, III, Kazerooni EA, Gay SE (1997) Pulmonary sarcoidosis. Clin Chest Med 18:755–85.
2. Lynch JP, III (1997) Pulmonary sarcoidosis: Current concepts and controversies. Comprehen Ther 23:197–210.
3. Lynch JP, II, Baughman RP, Sharma O (1998) Extrapulmonary sarcoidosis. Semin Respir Infect 13:229–254.
4. American Thoracic Society (1999) Statement on sarcoidosis. Am J Respir Crit Care Med 160:736–755.
5. Johns C, Michele T (1999) The clinical management of sarcoidosis. Medicine 78:65–111.
6. Lynch JP, III, Strieter R (1991) Sarcoidosis. In Lynch, JP III, DeRemee R (eds) *Immunologically mediated pulmonary disorders*, JB Lippincott, Philadelphia, pp 189–216.
7. Newman LS, Rose CS, Maier LA (1997) Sarcoidosis. N Engl J Med 336:1224–1234.

8. Mayock RL, Bertrand P, Morrison CE, et al. (1963) Manifestations of sarcoidosis: Analysis of 145 patients, with a review of nine series selected from the literature. Am J Med 35:67–89

9. Longcope WT, Frieman DG (1952) A study of sarcoidosis based on a combined investigation of 160 cases including 30 autopsies from the Johns Hopkins Hospital and Massachusetts General Hospital. Medicine (Baltimore) 31:1–132

10. Siltzbach L, James D, Neville E, et al. (1974) Course and prognosis of sarcoidosis around the world. Am J Med 57:847–852

11. Rybicki BA, Major M, Popovich J Jr, et al. (1997) Racial differences in sarcoidosis incidence: A 5-year study in a health maintenance organization. Am J Epidemiol 145:234–241

12. Rybicki BA, Maliarik MJ, Major M, et al. (1998) Epidemiology, demographics, and genetics of sarcoidosis. Semin Respir Infect 13:166–173

13. Hosoda Y, Yamaguchi M, Hiraga Y (1997) Global epidemiology of sarcoidosis. What story do prevalence and incidence tell us? Clin Chest Med 18:681–694

14. Henke C, Henke G, Elveback L, et al. (1986) The epidemiology of sarcoidosis in Rochester, Minnesota: A population-based study of incidence and survival. Am J Epidemiol 123:840–845

15. Hillerdal G, Nou E, Osterman K, et al. (1984) Sarcoidosis: Epidemiology and prognosis. A 15 year European study. Am Rev Respir Dis 130:29–32

16. Mana J, Badrinas F, Morera J, et al. (1992) Sarcoidosis in Spain. Sarcoidosis 9:118–122

17. Fazzi P, Solfanelli S, Di Pede F, et al. (1992) Sarcoidosis in Tuscany. A preliminary report. Sarcoidosis 9:123–126

18. Yamaguchi M, Hosoda Y, Sasaki R, et al. (1989) Epidemiological study on sarcoidosis in Japan. Recent trends in incidence and prevalence rates and changes in epidemiological features. Sarcoidosis 6:138–146

19. Tellier P, Paycha F, Antony I, et al. (1988) Reversibility by dipyridamole of thallium-201 myocardial scan defects in patients with sarcoidosis. Am J Med 85:189–193

20. Fite E, Mana J, Alsina JM, et al. (1997) Sarcoidosis: The chest radiograph screening of familial contacts. Respiration 63:160–163

21. Martinetti M, Tinelli C, Kolek V, et al. (1995) "The sarcoidosis map": A joint survey of clinical and immunogenetic findings in two European countries. Am J Respir Crit Care Med 152:557–564

22. Newman LS (1998) Metals that cause sarcoidosis. Semin Respir Infect 13:212–220

23. Hance AJ (1998) The role of mycobacteria in the pathogenesis of sarcoidosis. Semin Respir Infect 13:197–205

24. Moller DR (1997) Etiology of sarcoidosis. Clin Chest Med 18:695–706

25. Teirstein AS (1998) Kyeim antigen: What does it tell us about causation of sarcoidosis? Semin Respir Infect 13:206–211

26. Moller DR (1999) Cells and cytokines involved in the pathogenesis of sarcoidosis. Sarcoidosis Vasc Diffuse Lung Dis 16:24–31

27. Agostini S, Semenzato G (1998) Cytokines in sarcoidosis. Semin Respir Infect, 13:184–196

28. Muller-Quernheim J (1998) Serum markers for the staging of disease activity of sarcoidosis and other interstitial lung diseases of unknown etiology. Sarcoidosis Vasc Diffuse Lung Dis 15:22–37

29. Moller DR (1998) Involvment of T cells and alterations of T cell receptors in sarcoidosis. Semin Respir Infect 13:174–183

30. Colby TV, Carrington CB (1995) Infiltrative lung disease. In: Thurlbeck WM (ed) *Pathology of the lung*, 2nd edn. Thieme Medical Publishers, New York, pp 589–738

31. Rosen Y, Moon S, Hyang C, et al. (1977) Granulomatous pulmonary arteritis in sarcoidosis. Arch Pathol Lab Med 101:170–174

32. Carrington C, Gaensler E, Mikus J, et al. (1976) Structure and function in sarcoidosis. Ann NY Acad Sci 278:265–283

33. Nishimura K, Itoh H, Kitaichi M, et al. (1995) CT and pathological correlation of pulmonary sarcoidosis. Semin Ultrasound CT MR 16:361–370

34. Reich JM, Browns MC, O'Connor EA, et al. (1998) Mediastinoscopy in patients with presumptive stage I sarcoidosis. Chest 113:147–153

35. Armstrong J, Radke J, Kvale P, et al. (1981) Endoscopic findings in sarcoidosis. Characteristics and correlation with radiographic staging and bronchial mucosal biopsy yield. Ann Otol 90:339–343

36. Koerner S, Sakowitz A, Appelman R, et al. (1975) Transbronchial lung biopsy for the diagnosis of sarcoidosis. N Engl J Med 293:268–270

37. Gilman M, Wang K (1980) Transbronchial lung biopsy in sarcoidosis: An approach to determine the optimal number of biopsies. Am Rev Respir Dis 122:721–724

38. Koontz C, Joyner L, Nelson R (1976) Transbronchial lung biopsy via the fiberoptic bronchoscope in sarcoidosis. Ann Intern Med 85:64–66

39. Roethe R, Byrd R, Hafermann D (1980) Transbronchoscopic lung biopsy in sarcoidosis: Optimal number and sites for diagnosis. Chest 77:400–402

40. Poe R, Israel R, Utell M, et al. (1979) Probability of a positive transbronchial lung biopsy result in sarcoidosis. Arch Intern Med 139:761–763

41. Mitchell D, Mitchell D, Emerson C (1980) Transbronchial lung biopsy through fiberoptic bronchoscope in diagnosis of sarcoidosis. Br Med J 280:679–681

42. Morales C, Patefield A, Strollo P-J, et al. (1994) Flexible transbronchial needle aspiration in the diagnosis of sarcoidosis. Chest 6:709–711

43. Pauli G, Pelletier A, Bohner C, et al. (1984) Transbronchial needle aspiration in the diagnosis of sarcoidosis. Chest 85:482–484

44. Wang KP, Fuenning C, Johns CJ, et al. (1989) Flexible transbronchial needle aspiration for the diagnosis of sarcoidosis. Ann Otol Rhinol Laryngol 98:298–300

45. Winterbauer R, Lemmert J, Selland M, et al. (1993) Bronchoalveolar lavage cell profiles in the diagnosis of sarcoidosis. Chest 104:352–361

46. Bjermer L, Rosenhall L, Angstrom T, et al. (1988) Predictive value of bronchoalveolar lavage cell analysis in sarcoidosis. Thorax 43:284–288

47. Vernon S (1985) Nodular pulmonary sarcoidosis: Diagnosis with fine needle aspiration biopsy. Acta Cytol 29:473–476

48. Aisner S, Gupta P, Frost J (1977) Sputum cytology in pulmonary sarcoidosis. Acta Cytol 21:394–398

49. Zaman S, Elshami A, Gupta P (1995) Bronchalveolar cytology in pulmonary sarcoidosis. Acta Cytol 39:1117–1123

50. Hendricks MV, Crosby JH, Davis WB (1999) Bronchoalveolar lavage fluid granulomas in a case of severe sarcoidosis. Am J Respir Crit Care Med 160:730–731

51. Neville E, Walker A, James D (1983) Prognostic factors predicting the outcome of sarcoidosis: An analysis of 818 patients. Quart J Med 208:525–533

52. Goldstein RA, Israel HL, Becker KL, et al. (1971) The infrequency of hypercalcemia in sarcoidosis. Am J Med 51:21–30

53. Sharma OP (1996) Vitamin D, calcium, and sarcoidosis. Chest 109:535–539

54. Niimi T, Tomita H, Sato S, et al. (1999) Vitamin D receptor gene polymorphism in patients with sarcoidosis. Am J Respir Crit Care Med 160:1107–1109

55. Costabel U, Teschler H (1997) Biochemical changes in sarcoidosis. Clin Chest Med 18:827–842

56. Meyrier A, Valeyre D, Bouillon R, et al. (1985) Resorptive versus absorptive hypercalciuria in sarcoidosis: Correlations with 25-hydroxy vitamin D_3 and 1,25-dihydroxy vitamin D_3 and parameters of disease activity. Q J Med 54:269–281

57. Winterbauer RH, Belic N, Moores KD (1973) Clinical interpretation of bilateral hilar adenopathy. Ann Intern Med 78:65–71.

58. Baughman R, Lower E, Lynch J III (1994) Treatment modalities for sarcoidosis. Clin Pulm Med 1:223–231.

59. Scadding J (1961) Prognosis of intrathoracic sarcoidosis in England: A review of 136 cases after five years' observation. Br Med J 2:1165–1172.

60. Romer F (1982) Presentation of sarcoidosis and outcome of pulmonary changes. A review of 243 patients followed for up to 10 years. Dan Med Bull 29:27–32.

61. Lavergne F, Clerici C, Sadoun D, et al. (1999) Airway obstruction in bronchial sarcoidosis: Outcome with treatment. Chest 116:1194–1199.

62. Siltzbach L (1967) Sarcoidosis: Clinical features and management. Med Clin North Am 51:483–502.

63. Reich J, Johnson R (1985) Course and prognosis of sarcoidosis in a nonreferral setting: Analysis of 86 patients observed for 10 years. Am J Med 89:61.

64. Thomas P, Hunninghake G (1987) Current concepts of the pathogenesis of sarcoidosis. Am Rev Respir Dis 135:747–760.

65. Takada K, Ina Y, Noda M, et al. (1993) The clinical course and prognosis of patients with severe, moderate, or mild sarcoidosis. J Clin Epidemiol 46:359–366.

66. Sharma O (1993) Pulmonary sarcoidosis and corticosteroids. Am Rev Respir Dis 147:1598–1600.

67. Sharma OP (1997) Neurosarcoidosis: A personal perspective based on the study of 37 patients. Chest 112:220–228.

68. Gideon N, Mannino D (1996) Sarcoidosis mortality in the United States, 1979–1981: An analysis of multiple-cause mortality data. Am J Med 100:423–427.

69. Huang C, Heurich A, Sutton A, Lyons H (1981) Mortality in sarcoidosis: A changing pattern of the causes of death. Eur J Respir Dis 62:231–238.

70. Perry A, Vuitch F (1995) Causes of death in patients with sarcoidosis. A morphologic study of 38 autopsies with clinicopathologic correlations. Arch Pathol Lab Med 119:167–172.

71. Yamamoto M, Kosuda T, Yanagawa H, et al. (1977) Long-term follow-up in sarcoidosis in Japan. Z Erk Atmungsorgane 149:191–196.

72. Israel H, Karlin P, Menduke H, et al. (1986) Factors affecting outcome of sarcoidosis: influence of race extrathoracic involvement, and initial radiologic lung lesions. Ann NY Acad Sci 465:395–406.

73. Gottlieb JE, Israel HL, Steiner RM, et al. (1997) Outcome in sarcoidosis: The relationship of relapse to corticosteroid therapy. Chest 111:623–631.

74. Johns CJ, Schonfeld SA, Scott PP, et al. (1986) Longitudinal study of chronic sarcoidosis with low-dose maintenance corticosteroid therapy: Outcome and complications. Ann NY Acad Sci 465:702–712.

75. Baughman RP, Lower EE (1997) Steroid-sparing alternative treatments for sarcoidosis. Clin Chest Med 18:853–864.

76. Iwai K, Takemura T, Matsui Y, et al. (1993) Pathological studies on sarcoidosis autopy: II. Early change, mode of progression and death pattern. Acta Pathol Jpn 43:377–385.

77. Bechtel J, Starr T, III, Dantzker D, et al. (1981) Airway hyperactivity in patients with sarcoidosis. Am Rev Respir Dis 124:759–761.

78. Highland KB, Retalis P, Coppage L, et al. (1997) Is there anatomic explanation for chest pain in patients with pulmonary sarcoidosis. South Med J 90:911–941.

79. Sharma O, Badr A (1994) Sarcoidosis: Diagnosis, staging, and newer diagnostic modalities. Clin Pulm Med 1:18–26.

80. Scadding J, Mitchell D (1985) Sarcoidosis, 2nd edn. Chapman & Hall, London.

81. Chiles C, Putnam C (1992) Pulmonary sarcoidosis. Semin Respir Med 13:345–357.

82. Kirks D, McCormick V, Greenspan R (1973) Pulmonary sarcoidosis. Roentgenologic analysis of 150 patients. AJR Radium Ther Nucl Med 117:777–786.

83. Brauner M, Lenoir S, Grenier P, et al. (1992) Pulmonary sarcoidosis. CT assessment of reversibility. Radiology 182:349–355.

84. James D, Carstairs L, Trowell J, et al. (1967) Treatment of sarcoidosis: Report of a controlled therapeutic trial. Lancet 2:526–528.

85. Brauner M, Grenier P, Mompoint D, et al. (1989) Pulmonary sarcoidosis: Evaluation with high-resolution CT. Radiology 172:467–471.

86. Hamper U, Fishman E, Khouri N, et al. (1986) Typical and atypical pulmonary sarcoidosis. J Comput Assist Tomogr 10:928–936.

87. Bergin C, Bell D, Coblentz C, et al. (1989) Sarcoidosis: Correlation of pulmonary parenchymal pattern at CT with results of pulmonary function tests. Radiology 171:619–624.

88. Mana J, Tierstein A, Mendelson D, et al. (1995) Excessive thoracic computed tomographic scanning in sarcoidosis. Thorax 50:1264–1266.

89. Sieder L, Horton E (1990) Hilar and mediastinal adenopathy in sarcoidosis as detected by computed tomography. J Thorac Imaging 5:77–80.

90. Kuhlman JE, Fishman EK, Hamper UM, et al. (1989) The computed tomographic spectrum of sarcoidosis. RadioGraphics 9:449–466.

91. Rosseel B, Vierendeells T, Noppen M, et al. (1986) Posterior mediastinal sarcoidosis. Chest 90:462–464.

92. Kutty C, Varkey B (1982) Sarcoidosis presenting with posterior mediastinal lymphadenopathy. Postgrad Med 71:64–66.

93. Schabel S, Foote G, McKee K (1978) Posterior lymphadenopathy in sarcoidosis. Radiology 129:591–593.

94. Kent DC (1965) Recurrent unilateral hilar lymph node enlargement in sarcoidosis. Am Rev Respir Dis 91:272.

95. Spann R, Rosenow E, III, DeRemee R, et al. (1971) Unilateral hilar or paratracheal adenopathy in sarcoidosis: a study of 38 cases. AJR Rad Ther Nuc Med 126:296–299.

96. Rockoff S, Rohatgi P (1985) Unusual manifestations of thoracic sarcoidosis. AJR 144:513–528.

97. Israel H, Sones M, Roy R, et al. (1961) The occurrence of intrathoracic calcification in sarcoidosis. Am Rev Respir Dis 84:1–11.

98. Israel H, Lenchner G, Steiner R (1981) Late development of mediastinal calcification in sarcoidosis. Am Rev Respir Dis 124:302–305.

99. McLoud T, Putnam C, Pascual R (1974) Eggshell calcification with systemic sarcoidosis. Chest 66:515–517.

100. Murdoch J, Müller N (1992) Pulmonary sarcoidosis: changes on follow-up CT examination. AJR 159:473–477.

101. Gawne-Cain ML, Hansell DM (1996) The pattern and distribution of calcified mediastinal lymph nodes in sarcoidosis and tuberculosis. Clinical Radiology 51:263–267.

102. Gross BH, Schneider HJ, Proto AV (1980) Eggshell calcification of lymph nodes: An update. AJR 135:1265–1268.

103. Muller N, Kullnig P, Miller R (1989) The CT findings in pulmonary sarcoidosis: Analysis of 25 patients. AJR 152:1179–1182.

104. Wells A (1998) High resolution computed tomography in sarcoidosis: A clinical perspective. Sarcoidosis Vasc Diffuse Lung Dis 15:140–146.

105. Stone DJ, Schwartz A (1966) A long-term study of sarcoid and its modification by steroid therapy. Lung function and other factors in prognosis. Am J Med 41:528–540.

106. Grenier P, Brauner M, Valeyre D (1999) Computed tomography in the assessment of diffuse lung disease. Sarcoidosis Vasc Diffuse Lung Dis 16:47–56.

107. Traill ZC, Maskell GF, Gleeson FV (1997) High-resolution CT findings of pulmonary sarcoidosis. AJR 168:1557–1560.

108. Battesti J, Saumon G, Valeyre D, et al. (1982) Pulmonary sarcoidosis with an alveolar radiographic pattern. Thorax 37:448–452.

109. Mathieson JR, Mayo JR, Staples CA, et al. (1989) Chronic diffuse infiltrative lung disease: Comparison of diagnostic accuracy of CT and chest radiography. Radiology 171:111–116

110. McLoud T, Epler G, Gaensler E, et al. (1982) A radiographic classification for sarcoidosis: Physiologic correlation. Invest Radiol 17:129–138

111. Tazi A, Desfemmes-Baleyte T, Soler P, et al. (1994) Pulmonary sarcoidosis with a diffuse ground glass pattern on the chest radiograph. Thorax 49:793–797

112. Scadding JG (1970) The late stages of pulmonary sarcoidosis. Postgrad Med J 46:530–536

113. Kazerooni EA, Jackson C, Cascade PN (1994) Sarcoidosis: Recurrence of primary disease in transplanted lungs. Radiology 192:461–464

114. Pacheo Y, Marechal C, Marechal F, et al. (1985) Azathioprine treatment of chronic pulmonary sarcoidosis. Sarcoidosis 2:107–113

115. Zar H, Cole R (1995) Bullous emphysema occurring in pulmonary sarcoidosis. Respiration 62:290–293

116. Ichikawa Y, Fujimoto K, Shiraishi T, et al. (1994) Primary cavitary sarcoidosis: High resolution CT findings. AJR 163:745

117. Rohatgi P, Schwab L (1980) Primary acute pulmonary cavitation in sarcoidosis. AJR 134:1199–1203

118. Biem J, Hoffstein V (1991) Aggressive cavitary pulmonary sarcoidosis. Am Rev Respir Dis 143:428–430

119. Damuth TE, Bower JS, Cho K, et al. (1980) Major pulmonary artery stenosis causing pulmonary hypertension in sarcoidosis. Chest 78:888–891

120. Battesti J, Georges R, Basset F, et al. (1978) Chronic cor pulmonale in sarcoidosis. Thorax 33:76–84

121. Smith L, Lawrence J, Katzenstein A (1982) Vascular sarcoidosis: a rare cause of pulmonary hypertension. Am J Med Sci 285:38–44

122. Levine B, Saldana M, Hutter A (1971) Pulmonary hypertension is sarcoidosis. A case report of a rare but potentially treatable cause. Am Rev Respir Dis 103:413–417

123. Rodman D, Lindenfeld J (1990) Successful treatment of sarcoidosis-associated pulmonary hypertension with corticosteroids. Chest 97:500–502

124. Hietala S, Stinnett R, Faunce M, et al. (1977) Pulmonary artery narrowing in sarcoidosis. JAMA 237:572

125. Westcott J, DeGraff A (1973) Sarcoidosis, hilar adenopathy, and pulmonary artery narrowing. Radiology 108:585

126. Faunce HF, Ramsay GC, Sy W (1976) Protracted yet variable major pulmonary artery compression in sarcoidosis. Radiology 119: 313–314

127. Mangla A, Fisher J, Libby D, et al. (1985) Sarcoidosis: pulmonary hypertension and acquired peripheral pulmonary artery stenosis. Cathet Cardiovasc Diagn 11:69–74

128. Schowengerdt CG, Suyemeto R, Main FB (1960) Granulomatous and fibrosing mediastinitis. J Thorac Cardiovasc Surg 57:365–379

129. Javaheri S, Hales H (1980) Sarcoidosis: A cause of innominate vein obstruction and massive pleural effusion. Lung 157:81–85

130. Gordonson J, Trachtenberg S, Sargent E (1973) Superior vena cava obstruction due to sarcoidosis. Chest 63:292–293

131. Soskel N, Sharma O (1992) Pleural involvement in sarcoidosis: Case presentation and detailed review of the literature. Semin Respir Med 13:492–514

132. Brandstetter, Hansen D, Jarowski C, et al. (1981) Superior vena cava syndrome as the initial clinical manifestation of sarcoidosis. Heart Lung 10:101–104

133. Kinney E, Murthy R, Ascunce G, et al. (1980) Sarcoidosis: Rare case of superior vena caval obstruction. Penn Med 83:31

134. Radke JR, Kaplan H, Conway WA (1980) The significance of superior vena cava syndrome developing in a patient with sarcoidosis. Radiology 134:311–312

135. Schachter EN, Smith GJW, Cohen GS, et al. (1975) Pulmonary granulomas in a patient with pulmonary veno-occlusive disease. Chest 67:487–489

136. Hoffstein V, Ranganathan N, Mullen J (1986) Sarcoidosis simulating pulmonary veno-occlusive disease. Am Rev Respir Dis 134:809–811

137. Sharma O, Gordonson J (1975) Pleural effusion in sarcoidosis: Report of six cases. Thorax 30:95–101

138. Durand D, Dellinger A, Guerin C, et al. (1984) Pleural sarcoidosis: One case presenting with an eosinophilic effusion. Thorax 39:468–469

139. Beekman JF, Zimmet SM, Chun BK, et al. (1976) Spectrum of pleural involvement in sarcoidosis. Arch Intern Med 136:323–330

140. Nicholls A, Friend J, Legge J (1980) Sarcoid pleural effusion: Three cases and review of the literature. Thorax 35:277–281

141. Flammang d'Ortho M, Cadranel J, Milleron B, et al. (1990) Pleural, alveolar and blood T-lymphocyte subsets in pleuropulmonary sarcoidosis. Chest 98:782–783

142. Libshitz HI, Atkinson GW, Israel HL (1974) Pleural thickening as a manifestation of aspergillus superinfection. AJR Radium Ther Nucl Med 120:883–886

143. Aberg H, Bah M, Waters A (1966) Sarcoidosis complicated by chylothorax. Minnesota Med 49:1065–1070

144. Jarman P, Whyte M, Sabroe I, et al. (1995) Sarcoidosis presenting as chylothorax. Thorax 50:1324–1325

145. Cappell M, Friedman D, Mikhail N (1993) Chyloperitoneum associated with chronic severe sarcoidosis. Am J Gastroenterol 88:99–101

146. Haegeli A, Keller R (1981) Chylothorax bei Sarkoidose. Schweiz Med Wechenschr 111:125–128

147. Loughney E, Higgins BG (1997) Pleural sarcoidosis: A rare presentation. Thorax 5:200–201

148. Israel H, Lenchner G, Atkinson G (1982) Sarcoidosis and aspergilloma. The role of surgery. Chest 82:430–432

149. Jewkes J, Kay PH, Paneth M, et al. (1983) Pulmonary aspergilloma: Analysis of prognosis in relation to haemoptysis and survey of treatment. Thorax 38:572–578

150. Johns C (1982) Management of hemoptysis with pulmonary fungus balls in sarcoidosis. Chest 82:400–401

151. Kaplan J, Johns C (1979) Mycetomas in pulmonary sarcoidosis: Non-surgical management. Johns Hopkins Med J 145:157–161

152. Tomlinson J, Sahn S (1987) Aspergilloma in sarcoid and tuberculosis. Chest 92:505–508

153. Wollschlager C, Khan F (1984) Aspergillomas complicating sarcoidosis: A prospective study in 100 patients. Chest 86:585–588

154. Rumbak M, Kohler G, Eastrige C, et al. (1996) Topical treatment of life threatening haemoptysis from aspergillomas. Thorax 51:253–255

155. Hargis JL, Bone RC, Stewart J, et al. (1980) Intracavitary amphotericin B in the treatment of symptomatic pulmonary aspergillomas. Am J Med 68:389–394

156. Yamada H, Kohno S, Koga H, et al. (1993) Topical treatment of pulmonary aspergilloma by antifungals. Relationship between duration of the disease and efficacy of therapy. Chest 103:1421–1425

157. Jackson M, Flower CD, Shneerson JM (1993) Treatment of symptomatic pulmonary aspergillomas with intracavitary instillation of amphotericin B through an indwelling catheter. Thorax 48:928–930

158. Sharma O, Hewlett R, Gordonson J (1973) Nodular sarcoidosis: An unusual radiographic appearance. Chest 64:189–192

159. Rose R, Lee R, Costello P (1985) Solitary nodular sarcoidosis. Clin Radiol 36:589–592

160. Onal E, Lopata M, Lourenco R (1977) Nodular pulmonary sarcoidosis: Clinical, roentgenographic, and physiologic course in five patients. Chest 72:296–300

161. Romer F (1977) Sarcoidosis with large nodular lesions simulating pulmonary metastasis: An analysis of 126 cases of intrathoracic sarcoidosis. Scand J Respir Dis 58:11–16.

162. Kiyosawa K (1998) Sarcoidosis associated with multiple large pulmonary nodules. Respirology 4:372–376.

163. Liebow AA (1973) The J. Burns Amberson lecture – pulmonary angiitis and granulomatosis. Am Rev Respir Dis 108:1–18.

164. Gibbs A, Williams W, Kelland D (1987) Necrotizing sarcoid granulomatosis: A problem of identity. A study of 7 cases. Sarcoidosis 4:94–100.

165. Churg A, Carrington C, Gupta R (1979) Necrotizing sarcoid granulomatosis. Chest 76:406–413.

166. Churg A (1983) Pulmonary angiitis and granulomatosis revisited. Hum Pathol 14:868–883.

167. Saldana M (1978) Necrotizing sarcoid granulomatosis: Clinicopathologic observations in 24 patients. Lab Invest 38:364.

168. Chittock D, Joseph M, Patterson N, et al. (1994) Necrotizing sarcoid granulomatosis with pleural involvement: Clinical and radiographic features. Chest 106:672–676.

169. Niimi H, Hartman T, Müller N (1995) Necrotizing sarcoid granulomatosis: Computed tomography and pathologic findings. J Comput Assist Tomogr 19:920–923.

170. Hammar SP (1995) Granulomatous vasculitis. Semin Respir Infect 10:107–120.

171. Koss M, Hochholzer L, Geiger D, et al. (1980) Necrotizing sarcoid-like granulomatosis. Hum Pathol 11(Suppl):510–519.

172. Demicco W, Fanburg B (1982) Sarcoidosis presenting as a lobar or unilateral lung infiltrate. Clin Radiol 33:663–669.

173. Littner M, Schachter E, Putman C, et al. (1977) The clinical assessment of roentgenographically atypical pulmonary sarcoidosis. Am J Med 62:361–368.

174. Mendelson D, Norton K, Cohen B, et al. (1983) Bronchial compression: An unusual manifestation of sarcoidosis. J Comput Assist Tomogr 7:892–894.

175. Udwadia Z, Pilling J, Henkins P, et al. (1990) Bronchoscopic and bronchographic findings in 12 patients with sarcoidosis and severe or progressive airways obstruction. Thorax 45:272–275.

176. Westcott J, Noehren T (1973) Bronchial stenosis in chronic sarcoidosis. Chest 63:893–897.

177. Olsson T, Bjormtad-Pettersen H, et al. (1979) Bronchostenosis due to sarcoidosis. Chest 75:663–666.

178. DiBenedetto R, Ribaudo C (1966) Bronchopulmonary sarcoidosis. Am Rev Respir Dis 94:952–958.

179. Munt P (1973) Middle lobe atelectasis in sarcoidosis. Am Rev Respir Dis 108:357–360.

180. Lenique F, Brauner M, Grenier P, et al. (1995) CT assessment of bronchi in sarcoidosis: Endoscopic and pathologic correlations. Radiology 194:419–423.

181. Hadfield J, Page R, Flower C, et al. (1982) Localized airway narrowing in sarcoidosis. Thorax 37:443–447.

182. Brown K, Yeoh C, Saddekni S (1988) Balloon dilatation of the left main bronchus in sarcoidosis. AJR 150:553–554.

183. Niimi H, Kang EY, Kwong JS, et al. (1966) CT of chronic infiltrative lung disease: Prevalence of mediastinal lymphadenopathy. J Comput Assist Tomogr 20:305–308.

184. Rémy-Jardin M, Giraud F, Rémy J, et al. (1994) Pulmonary sarcoidosis: Role of CT in the evaluation of disease activity and functional impairment and in prognosis assessment. Radiology 191:675–680.

185. Kosmorsky GS, Meisler DM, Rice TW, et al. (1998) Chest computed tomography and mediastinoscopy in the diagnosis of sarcoidosis-assoicated uveitis. Am J Opthalmol 126:132–136.

186. Mana J, Gomez-Vaquero C, Montero A, et al. (1999) Lofgren's syndrome revisited: A study of 186 patients. Am J Med 107:240–245.

187. Johkoh T, Ikezoe J, Takeuchi N, et al. (1992) CT findings in pseudoalveolar sarcoidosis. J Comput Assist Tomogr 16:904–907.

188. Rémy-Jardin M, Rémy J, Deffontaines C, et al. (1991) Assessment of diffuse infiltrative lung disease: Comparison of conventional CT and high-resolution CT. Radiology 181:157–162.

189. Lynch D, Webb W, Gamsu G, et al. (1989) Computed tomography in pulmonary sarcoidosis. J Comput Assist Tomogr 13:405–410.

190. Winterbauer R, Hutchinson J (1980) Use of pulmonary function tests in the management of sarcoidosis. Chest 78:640–647.

191. Bradvik I, Wollmer P, Blom-Bulow B, et al. (1991) Lung mechanics and gas exchange during exercise in pulmonary sarcoidosis. Chest 99:572–578.

192. Miller A, Brown L, Sloane M, et al. (1995) Cardiorespiratory responses to incremental excercise in sarcoidosis patients with normal spirometry. Chest 107:323–329.

193. Dunn T, Watters L, Hendrix C, et al. (1988) Gas exchange at a given degree of volume restriction is different in sarcoidosis and idiopathic pulmonary fibrosis. Am J Med Z 85:221–224.

194. Harrison B, Shaylor J, Stokes T (1991) Airflow limitation in sarcoidosis: A study of pulmonary function in 107 patients with newly diagnosed disease. Respir Med 85:59–64.

195. Levinson R, Metzger L, Standley N, et al. (1977) Airway function in sarcoidosis. Am J Med 62:215–222.

196. McCann B, Harrison B (1991) Bronchiolar narrowing and occlusion in sarcoidosis – correlation of pathology with physiology. Respir Med 85:65–67.

197. Nugent KM, Peterson MW, Jolles H, et al. (1989) Correlation of chest roentgenograms with pulmonary function and bronchoalveolar lavage in interstitial lung disease. Chest 96:1224–1227.

198. Huang C, Heurich A, Rosen Y, et al. (1979) Pulmonary sarcoidosis: Roentgenographic, functional, and pathological correlation. Respiration 37:337–345.

199. ILO/UC (1972) 1971 International classification of radiographs of the pneumoconioses. Med Radiogr Photogr 48:67–76.

200. Müller N, Mawson J, Mathieson J, et al. (1989) Sarcoidosis: Correlation of extent of disease at CT with clinical, functional and radiographic findings. Radiology 171:613–618.

201. Israel HL, McComb BL (1991) Chlorambucil treatment of sarcoidosis. Sarcoidosis, 8:35–41.

202. Pasturenzi L, Martinetti M, Cuccia M, et al. (1993) HLA class I, II, and III polymorphism in Italian patients with sarcoidosis. The Pavia–Padova Sarcoidosis Study Group. Chest 104:1170–1175.

203. Lenhart K, Kolek V, Bartova A (1990) HLA antigens associated with sarcoidosis. Dis Markers 8:23–29.

204. Ina Y, Takada K, Yamamoto M, et al. (1989) HLA and sarcoidosis in the Japanese. Chest 95:1257–1261.

205. Raphael SA, Blau EB, Zhang WH, et al. (1993) Analysis of a large kindred with Blau syndrome for HLA, autoimmunity, and sarcoidosis. Am J Dis Child 147:842–848.

206. Gran JT, Bohmer E (1996) Acute sarcoid arthritis: A favorable outcome? A retrospective survey of 49 patients with review of the literature. Scand J Rheumatol 25:70–73.

207. Ward K, O'Connor C, Odlum C, et al. (1989) Prognostic value of bronchoalveolar lavage in sarcoidosis: The critical influence of disease presentation. Thorax 44:6–412.

208. Glennas A, Kvien TK, Melby K, et al. (1995) Acute sarcoid arthritis: occurrence, seasonal onset, clinical features and outcome. Br J Rheumatol 34:45–50.

209. Chapelon C, Ziza JM, Piette JC, et al. (1990) Neurosarcoidosis: Signs, course and treatment in 35 confirmed cases. Medicine (Baltimore) 69:261–276.

210. Rohatgi PK (1992) Osseous sarcoidosis. Semin Respir Med 13:468–488.

211. DeRemee R, Offord K (1992) The treatment of pulmonary sarcoidosis: The house revisited. Sarcoidosis 9:17S–29S.

212. Baughman RP, Sharma OP, Lynch JP, III (1998) Sarcoidosis: Is therapy effective? Semin Respir Infect 13:255–273.

213. Hunninghake G, Gilbert S, Pueringer R, et al. (1994) Outcome of the treatment for sarcoidosis. Am J Respir Crit Care Med 149:893–898.

214. Gibson G, Prescott R, Muers M, et al. (1996) The British Thoracic Society Sarcoidosis Study: Effects of long term corticosteroid treatment. Thorax 51:238–247.

215. Ziegenhagen MW, Benner UK, Zissel G, et al. (1997) Sarcoidosis: TNF-alpha release from alveolar macrophages and serum level of sIL-2R are prognostic markers. Am J Respir Crit Care Med 156:1586–1592.

216. Sulavik S, Spencer R, Palestro C, et al. (1993) Specificity and sensitivity of distinctive chest radiographic and/or Ga67 images in the noninvasive diagnosis of sarcoidosis. Chest 103:403–409.

217. Mana JN (1997) Nuclear imaging ^{67}gallium, ^{201}thallium, ^{18}F-labeled fluoro-2-deoxy-D-glucose positron emission tomography. Clin Chest Med 18:799–811.

218. Jones C, Lake R, Wijeyekoon J, et al. (1996) Oligoclonal V gene usage by T lymphocytes in bronchoalveolar lavage fluid from sarcoidosis patients. Am J Respir Cell Mol Biol 14:470–477.

219. Striz I, Zheng L, Wang Y, et al. (1996) Soluble CD14 is increased in bronchoalveolar lavage of active sarcoidosis and correlates with alveolar macrophage membrane-bound CD14. Am J Respir Crit Care Med 153:544–547.

220. Girgis R, Basha M, Maliarik M, et al. (1996) Cytokines in bronchoalveolar lavage fluid of patients with active pulmonary sarcoidosis. Am J Respir Crit Care Med 152:71–75.

221. Laviolette M, LaForge J, Tennina S, et al. (1991) Prognostic value of bronchalveolar lavage lymphocyte count in recently diagnosed pulmonary sarcoidosis. Chest 100:380–384.

222. Verstraeten A, Demedts M, Verwilghen J, et al. (1990) Predictive value of bronchoalveolar lavage in pulmonary sarcoidosis. Chest 98:560–567.

223. Drent M, van Velzen Blad H, Diamant M, et al. (1993) Relationship between presentation of sarcoidosis and T lymphocyte profile. A study in bronchalveolar lavage fluid. Chest 104:795–800.

224. Ohrn M, Skold C, van Hage Hamsten M, et al. (1995) Sarcoidosis patients have bronchial hyperreactivity and signs of mast cell activation in their bronchoalveolar lavage. Respiration 62:136–142.

225. Veleyre D, Saumon G, Georges R, et al. (1984) The relationship between disease duration and non-invasive pulmonary explorations in sarcoidosis with erythema nodosum. Am Rev Respir Dis 129:938–943.

226. Sartois DJ, Resnick D, Resnick C, et al. (1985) Musculoskeletal manifestations of sarcoidosis. Semin Roentgenol 4:376–386.

227. Neville E, Carstairs LS, James DG (1977) Sarcoidosis of bone. Q J Med 46:215–277.

228. Oven TJ, Sones M, Morrissey WL (1986) Lytic lesion of the sternum. Rare manifestations of sarcoidosis. Am J Med 80:285–287.

229. DeSimone DP, Brilliant HL, Basile J, et al. (1989) Granulomatous infiltration of the talus and abnormal vitamin D and calcium metabolism in a patient with sarcoidosis: Successful treatment with hydroxychloroquine. Am J Med 87:694–696.

230. Rahbar M, Sharma OP (1990) Hypertropic osteoarthropathy in sarcoidosis. Sarcoidosis 7:125–127.

231. Roberts WC, McAllister HA Jr, Ferrans VJ (1977) Sarcoidosis of the heart. A clinicopathologic study of 35 necropsy patients (group 1) and review of 78 previously described necropsy patients (group 11). Am J Med 63:86–108.

232. Sharma OP, Maheshwari A, Thaker K (1993) Myocardial sarcoidosis. Chest 103:253–258.

233. Silverman KJ, Hutchins GM, Bulkley BH (1978) Cardiac sarcoid: A clinicopathologic study of 84 unselected patients with systemic sarcoidosis. Circulation 58:1204–1211.

234. Fleming H (1994) Cardiac sarcoidosis. In James D (ed) Sarcoidosis and other granulomatous disorders. Marcel Dekker, New York, pp 323–334.

235. Ratner SJ, Fenoglio JJ, Ursell P (1986) Utility of endomyocardial biopsy in the diagnosis of cardiac sarcoidosis. Chest 90:528–533

236. Shammas RL, Movahed A (1993) Sarcoidosis of the heart. Clin Cardiol 16:462–472.

237. Fahy GJ, Marwick T, McCreery CJ, et al. (1996) Doppler echocardiographic detection of left ventricular diastolic dysfunction in patients with pulmonary sarcoidosis. Chest 109:62–66.

238. Suzuki T, Kanda T, Kubota S, et al. (1994) Holter monitoring as a noninvasive indicator of cardiac involvement in sarcoidosis. Chest 106:1021–1024.

239. Kinney EJ, Caldwell JW (1990) Do thallium myocardial perfusion scans abnormalities predict survival in sarcoid patients without cardiac symptoms? Angiology 41:573–576.

240. Winters SL, Cohen M, Greenberg S, et al. (1991) Sustained ventricular tachycardia associated with sarcoidosis: Assessment of the underlying cardiac anatomy and the prospective utility of programmed ventricular stimulation, drug therapy and an implantable antitachycardia device. J Am Coll Cardiol 18:937–943.

241. Agbogu BN, Stern BJ, Sewell C, et al. (1995) Therapeutic considerations in patients with refractory neurosarcoidosis. Arch Neurol 52:875–879.

242. Stern BJ, Schonfeld SA, Sewell C, et al. (1992) The treatment of neurosarcoidosis with cyclosporine. Arch Neurol 49:1065–1072.

243. Scott TF (1993) Neurosarcoidosis: progress and clinical aspects. Neurology 43:8–12.

244. Delaney P (1977) Neurologic manifestations in sarcoidosis: Review of the literature, with a report of 23 cases. Ann Intern Med 87:336–45.

245. Sherman JL, Stern BJ (1990) Sarcoidosis of the CNS: Comparison of unenhanced and enhanced MR images. AJR 155:1293–1301.

246. Zouaoui A, Maillard JC, Dormont D, et al. (1992) MRI in neurosarcoidosis. J Neuroradiol 19:271–284.

247. Lexa FJ, Grossman RI (1994) MR of sarcoidosis in the head and spine: Spectrum of manifestations and radiographic response to steroid therapy. AJNR 15:973–82.

248. Seltzer S, Mark AS, Atlas SW (1992) CNS sarcoidosis: Evaluation with contrast-enhanced MR imaging. AJNR 12:1227–1233.

249. Handler MS, Johnson LM, Dick AR, et al. (1993) Neurosarcoidosis with unusual MRI findings. Neuroradiology 35:146–148.

250. Oksanen V (1992) Neurosarcoidosis. Semin Respir Med 13:459–467.

251. Rubenstein I, Gray TA, Moldofsky H, et al. (1988) Neurosarcoidosis associated with hypersomnolence treated with corticosteroids and brain irradiation. Chest 94:205–206.

252. Lower E, Baughman R (1995) Prolonged use of methotrexate for sarcoidosis. Arch Intern Med 155:846–851.

253. Maddrey WC, Johns CJ, Boitnott JK, et al. (1970) Sarcoidosis and chronic hepatic disease: a clinical and pathologic study of 20 patients. Medicine (Baltimore) 49:375–395.

254. Devaney K, Goodman ZD, Epstein MS, et al. (1993) Hepatic sarcoidosis. Clinicopathologic features in 100 patients. Am J Surg Pathol 17:1272–1280.

255. Rudzik C, Ishak KG, Zimmerman HJ (1975) Chronic intrahepatic cholestasis of sarcoidosis. Am J Med 59:383–387.

256. Nakata K, Iwata K, Kojima K, et al. (1989) Computed tomography of liver sarcoidosis. J Comput Assist Tomogr 13:707–708.

257. Warshauer DM, Molina PL, Hamman SM, et al. (1995) Nodular sarcoidosis of the liver and spleen: Analysis of 32 cases. Radiology 195:757–762.

258. Kessler A, Mitchell DG, Israel HL, et al. (1993) Hepatic and splenic sarcoidosis: Ultrasound and MR imaging. Abdom Imaging 18:159–163.

259. Warshauer DM, Dumbleton SA, Molina PL, et al. (1994) Abdominal CT findings in sarcoidosis: radiologic and clinical correlation. Radiology 192:93–98.

260. Zisman DA, Biermann JS, Martinez FJ, et al. (1999) Sarcoidosis presenting as a tumorlike muscular lesion. Medicine 78:112–122.

261. Ando DG, Lynch JP, Fantone JC, III (1985) Sarcoid myopathy with elevated creatine phosphokinase. Am Rev Respir Dis 131:298–300.

262. Gardner-Thorpe C (1972) Muscle weakness due to sarcoid myopathy. Six case reports and an evaluation of steroid therapy. Neurology 22:917–928.

263. Otake S (1994) Sarcoidosis involving skeletal muscle: Imaging findings and relative value of imaging procedures. AJR 162: 369–375.

264. Kurashima K, Shimizu H, Ogawa H, et al. (1991) MR and CT in the evaluation of sarcoid myopathy. J. Comp Assist Tomogr 15: 1004–1007.

265. Kobayashi H, Kotoura Y, Sakahara H, et al. (1994) Solitary muscular sarcoidosis. CT, MRI, and scintigraphic charateristics. Skeletal Radiol 23:293–295.

266. Fordice J, Katras T, Jackson RE, et al. (1992) Massive splenomegaly in sarcoidosis. South Med J 85:775–778.

267. Selroos O (1976) Sarcoidosis of the spleen. Acta Med Scand 200:337–340.

268. Selroos O, Koivunen E (1983) Usefulness of fine-needle aspiration biopsy of spleen in diagnosis of sarcoidosis. Chest 83:193–195.

269. Taavitsainen M, Koivuniemi A, Helminen J, et al. (1987) Aspiration biopsy of the spleen in patients with sarcoidosis. Acta Radiol 28:723–725.

270. Neiman RS (1977) Incidence and importance of splenic sarcoid-like granulomas. Arch Pathol Lab Med 101:518–521.

271. Kruithoff KL, Gyetko MR, Scheiman JM (1993) Giant splenomegaly and refractory hypercalcemia due to extrapulmonary sarcoidosis. Successful treatment by splenectomy. Arch Intern Med 153: 2793–2796.

272. Salazar A, Mana J, Sala J, et al. (1994) Combined portal and pulmonary hypertension in sarcoidosis. Respiration 61:117–119.

273. Britt AR, Francis IR, Glazer GM, et al. (1991) Sarcoidosis: Abdominal manifestations at CT. Radiology 178:91–94.

274. Mathieu D, Vanderstigel M, Schaeffer A, et al. (1986) Computed tomography of splenic sarcoidosis. J Comput Assist Tomogr 10:679–680.

275. Warshauer DM, Semelka RC, Ascher SM (1994) Nodular sarcoidosis of the liver and spleen: Appearance on MR images. J Magn Reson Imaging 4:553–557.

276. Kataria Y (1980) Chlorambucil in sarcoidosis. Chest 78:36–43.

277. Minor RL Jr, Helmers RA (1990) Sarcoidosis and giant splenomegaly. Sarcoidosis 7:119–122.

278. Israel H, Fouts D, Beggs R (1973) A controlled trial of prednisone treatment of sarcoidosis. Am Rev Respir Dis 107:609–614.

279. Selroos O, Sellergren T (1979) Corticosteroid therapy of pulmonary sarcoidosis. A prospective evaluation of alternate day and daily dosage in stage II disease. Scand J Respir Dis 60:215–221.

280. Yamamoto M, Saito N, Tachibana T, et al. (1980) Effects of an 18 month corticosteroioid therapy to stage I and stage II sarcoidosis patients (control trial). In Chretien J, Marsac J, Saltiel JC (eds) Sarcoidosis and other granulomatous disorders. Pergamon Press, Paris, pp 470–474.

281. Eule H, Weinecke A, Roth I (1986) The possible influence of corticosteroid therapy on the natural course of pulmonary sarcoidosis. Ann NY Acad Sci 465:695–701.

282. Harkleroad L, Young R, Savage P, et al. (1982) Pulmonary sarcoidosis: Long-term follow-up of the effects of steroid therapy. Chest 82:84–87.

283. Zaki M, Lyons H, Leilop L, et al. (1987) Corticosteroid therapy in sarcoidosis. A five-year, controlled follow-up study. NY State J Med 87:496–499.

284. Lynch J, III, McCune W (1997) Immunosuppressive and cytotoxic pharmacotherapy for pulmonary disorders: State of the art. Am J Respir Crit Care Med 155:395–420.

285. DeRemee J (1977) The present status of treatment of pulmonary sarcoidosis: a house divided. Chest 71:388–393.

286. Spratling L, Tenholder F, Underwood G, et al. (1985) Daily vs alternate day predinose therapy for stage II sarcoidosis. Chest 88:687–690.

287. Alberts C, van der Mark T, Jansen H (1995) Inhaled budesonide in pulmonary sarcoidosis: A double-blind, placebo-controlled study. Dutch Study Group on pulmonary sarcoidosis. Eur Respir J 8:682–688.

288. Selroos O (1986) Use of budesonide in the treatment of pulmonary sarcoidosis. Ann NY Acad Sci 465:713–721.

289. Spiteri M, Newman S, Clarke S, et al. (1989) Inhaled corticosteroids can modulate the immunopathogenesis of pulmonary sarcoidosis. Eur Respir J 2:218–224.

290. Spiteri M, (1991) Inhaled corticosteroids in pulmonary sarcoidosis. Postgrad Med J 67:237–329.

291. Gupta S (1989) Treatment of sarcoidosis by steroid aerosol: A ten-year prospective study from eastern India. Sarcoidosis 6:51–54.

292. Zych D, Pawlicka L, Zielinski J (1993) Inhaled budesonide vs prednisone in the treatment of pulmonary sarcoidosis. Sarcoidosis 10:56–61.

293. du Bois RM, Greenhalgh PM, Southcott AM, et al. (1999) Randomized trial of inhaled fluticasone propionate in chronic stable pulmonary sarcoidosis: a pilot study. Eur Respir J 13: 1345–1350.

294. Pietinalho A, Tukiainen P, Haahtela T, et al. (1999) Oral prednisone followed by inhaled budesonide in newly diagnosed pulmonary sarcoidosis: a double-blind, placebo-controlled multicenter study. Finnish Pulmonary Sarcoidosis Study Group. Chest 116:424–431.

295. Baughman RP, Lower EE (1999) A clinical approach to the use of methotrexate for sarcoidosis. Thorax 54:742–746.

296. Baughman RP, Lower EE (1990) The effect of corticosteroid or methotrexate therapy on lung lymphocytes and macrophages in sarcoidosis. Am Rev Respir Dis 142:1268–1271.

297. Soriano F, Caramelli P, Nitrini R, et al. (1990) Neurosarcoidosis: Therapeutic success with methotrexate. Postgrad Med J 66: 142–143.

298. Webster G, Razsi L, Sanchez M, et al. (1991) Weekly low-dose methotrexate therapy for cutaneous sarcoidosis. J Am Acad Dermatol 24:451–454.

299. Lewis SJ, Ainslie GM, Bateman ED (1999) Efficacy of azathioprine as second-line treatment in pulmonary sarcoidosis. Sarcoidosis Vasc Diffuse Lung Dis 16:87–92.

300. Sharma OP (1972) Cutaneous sarcoidosis: Clinical features and management. Chest 61:320–325.

301. Demeter S (1988) Myocardial sarcoidosis unresponsive to steroids. Treatment with cyclophosphamide. Chest 94:202–203.

302. Lower EE, Broderick JP, Brott TG, et al. (1997) Diagnosis and management of neurological sarcoidosis. Arch Intern Med 157:1864–1868.

303. Hammond JM, Bateman ED (1990) Successful treatment of life-threatening steroid-resistant pulmonary sarcoidosis with cyclosporin in a patient with systemic lupus erythematosus. Respir Med 84:77–79.

304. Martinet Y, Pinkston P, Saltini C, et al. (1988) Evaluation of the in vitro and in vivo effects of cyclosporine on the lung T-lymphocyte alveolitis of active pulmonary sarcoidosis. Am Rev Respir Dis 138:1242–1248.

305. Wyser CP, van Schalkwyk EM, Alheit B, et al. (1997) Treatment of progressive pulmonary sarcoidosis with cyclosporin A.

A randomized controlled trial. Am J Respir Crit Care Med 156:1371–1376.

306. Adams J, Diz M, Sharma O (1989) Effective reduction in the serum 1,25-dihydroxyvitamin D and calcium concentration in sarcoidosis-associated hypercalcemia with short-course chloroquine therapy. Ann Intern Med 111:437–438.

307. Jones E, Cagen J (1990) Hydroxychloroquine is effective therapy for control of cutaneous sarcoidal granulomas. Am Acad Dermatol 23:487–489.

308. Zic JA, Horowitz DH, Arzubiaga C, et al. (1991) Treatment of cutaneous sarcoidosis with chloroquine. Arch Dermatol 127:1034–1040.

309. Siltzbach L, Tierstein A (1964) Chloroquine therapy in 43 patients with intrathoracic and cutaneous sarcoidosis. Acta Med Scand 425:302–308.

310. British Tuberculosis Association (1967) Chloroquine in the treatment of sarcoidosis. Tubercle 48:257–272.

311. O'Leary T, Jones G, Yip A, et al. (1986) The effects of chloroquine on serum 1,25-dihydroxyvitamin D and calcium metabolism in sarcoidosis. N Engl J Med 315:727–730.

312. Barre PE, Gascon-Barre M, Meakins JL, et al. (1987) Hydroxychloroquine treatment of hypercalcemia in a patient with sarcoidosis undergoing hemodialysis. Am J Med 82:1259–1262.

313. Baltzan M, Mehta S, Kirkham TH, et al. (1999) Randomized trial of prolonged chloroquine therapy in advanced pulmonary sarcoidosis. Am J Respir Crit Care Med 160:192–197.

314. Quatraro A, Consoli G, Magno M, et al. (1990) Hydroxychloroquine in decompensated, treatment-refractory noninsulin-dependent diabetes mellitus. A new job for an old drug? Ann Intern Med 112:678–681.

315. Adams JS, Sharma OP, Diz MM, et al. (1990) Ketoconazole decreases the serum, 1,25-dihydroxyvitamin D and calcium concentration in sarcoidosis-associated hypercalcemia. J Clin Endocrinol Metab 70:1090–1095.

316. Ejaz AA, Zabaneh RI, Tiwari P, et al. (1994) Ketoconazole in the treatment of recurrent nephrolithiasis associated with sarcoidosis. Nephrol Dial Transplant 9:1492–1494.

317. Zabel P, Entzian P, Dalhoff K, et al. (1997) Pentoxifylline in treatment of sarcoidosis. Am J Respir Crit Care Med 155:1665–1669.

318. Carlesimo M, Giustini S, Rossi A, et al. (1995) Treatment of cutaneous and pulmonary sarcoidosis with thalidomide. J Am Acad Dermatol 32:866–869.

319. Nunley DR, Hattler B, Keenan RJ, et al. (1999) Lung transplantation for end-stage pulmonary sarcoidosis. Sarcoidosis Vasc Diffuse Lung Dis 16:93–100.

320. Martinez F, Orens J, Deeb M, et al. (1994) Recurrence of sarcooidosis following allogeneic lung transplantation. Chest 106:1597–1599.

321. Johnson B, Duncan S, Ohori N, et al. (1993) Recurrence of sarcoidosis in pulmonary allograft recipients. Am Rev Respir Dis 148:1373–1377.

16 Chronic Obstructive Pulmonary Disease

E.A. Kazerooni, K.R. Flaherty, and F.J. Martinez

Introduction

Chronic obstructive pulmonary disease (COPD) is characterized by the presence of airflow obstruction that does not markedly change over months of observation and is pathologically usually the result of chronic bronchitis or emphysema (1–3). It is estimated that 14–15 million people in the USA have COPD, with approximately 12.5 million having chronic bronchitis and 1.65–2 million emphysema (2). Asthma is highly prevalent, affecting an estimated 11 million people (4). There is evidence that the prevalence of asthma and COPD are increasing (5). Vollmer and colleagues noted an increased, prevalence of asthma and chronic airflow obstruction (CAO) over the period 1967–1987 in all age groups except males aged 65 and older who were enrolled in a large health maintenance organization (6). Every 5 years between 1950 and 1970 the death rate for obstructive respiratory disease doubled in the USA (7,8). COPD is the fourth leading cause of death in the USA, with 85 544 patients dying from COPD in 1991(2). COPD contributes to considerable patient morbidity, mortality and the expenditure of considerable health care dollars, and, in both the USA and United Kingdom, COPD is one of the most important contributors to work incapacity and restricted activity (9,10). To understand the role of imaging in COPD, it is important to understand the definition, pathophysiology, clinical history, and natural course of COPD, as well as the diagnostic value of physiologic studies, which are discussed first.

Definitions

COPD is a commonly used term without a well-accepted definition. It has been used to include patients with asthma, asthmatic bronchitis, chronic bronchitis, chronic obstructive bronchitis, bronchiectasis, cystic fibrosis, and emphysema. One definition of COPD is "persistent, largely irreversible airflow obstruction in which the underlying pathophysiology is not precisely know" (11). However, if this terminology is used, patients with documented emphysema on computed tomography (CT) would be excluded; yet these patients make up a significant percentage of patients labeled as having COPD. Another definition is "a chronic slowly progressive airway obstructive disorder resulting from some combination of emphysema and irreversible reduction in the caliber of small airways in the lung". Use of this definition may exclude patients with small-airway disease manifesting with bronchiectasis (12). Most commonly, asthma, chronic bronchitis and emphysema are included in the definition. A recent National Heart, Lung and Blood Institute Workshop of the subject states that "The term 'COPD' is generally used in clinical discourse to describe individuals diagnosed with one or more of the following conditions in the course of a lifetime: asthmatic bronchitis, chronic bronchitis, chronic obstructive bronchitis and emphysema" (13). The lack of a single precise definition reflects the difficulty in subclassifying patients into one form of disease or another clinically and physiologically, and has led to difficulty in estimating the true incidence of COPD.

Asthma, chronic bronchitis, and emphysema are the three most common forms of chronic airflow obstruction. Asthma is typically characterized by airway inflammation, airway hyperresponsiveness, and airflow obstruction that is reversible (5,14). Excessive mucus production characterizes chronic bronchitis, which is clinically diagnosed by the presence of a chronic productive cough for 3 months or more in each of two successive years in a patient in whom other causes of chronic cough have been excluded (2). Emphysema is defined pathologically as abnormal permanent enlargement of the airspaces distal to the terminal bronchioles, with accompanying destruction of their walls without obvious fibrosis (2). While the definition of these categories appears precise, the clinical distinction in specific patients between asthma, chronic bronchitis, and emphysema is often confusing, with an overlap of clinical and physiologic features in many patients. This has resulted in the use of terms such as asthmatic bronchitis, when patients have features of both asthma and chronic bronchitis.

It is important to recognize that there are patients with asthma that lack complete reversibility of their airway obstruction, particularly patients with longstanding asthma who develop fixed airflow obstruction, simulating COPD [O'Byrne, 1999 no. 246; Elias, 1999 no. 181] (15). Furthermore, many patients with chronic bronchitis and emphysema have a significant component of broncho-reversibility, thereby simulating asthma (16–19). The significant overlap of clinical syndromes can make the differential diagnosis of chronic airflow obstruction challenging for the physician. These concepts are reflected in physicians' perceptions regarding the diagnosis and management of COPD. In a survey of 75 primary care practitioners, Kesten and Chapman asked each to describe their diagnostic and therapeutic approach to two hypothetical 52 year old male smokers with persistent cough (18). The only difference between the two cases was a tentative diagnosis of chronic bronchitis in one case scenario. Although most physicians requested chest radiographs (80%) and sputum cultures (50%), few utilized spirometry (21%) in diagnosis. Furthermore, beta-agonists were considered first-line therapy for both COPD and asthma. It is apparent that a clear understanding of the various entities presenting with chronic airway obstruction is needed to optimally manage these disorders in practice.

Pathophysiology

There are clear similarities and differences in the pathophysiology of asthma and other forms of chronic airflow obstruction. The role of inflammation in asthma has been widely accepted (5). There is collagen deposition beneath the epithelial basement membrane in addition to extensive inflammation in bronchial biopsy specimens of patients with mild asthma, as well as increased numbers of inflammatory cell and eosinophils in the epithelium of asthmatics (20,21). The degree of subepithelial thickening correlates with lower forced expired volume (FEV_1) and greater peak flow variability, when comparing the findings with the patient's response to nebulized water and methacholine (21). This suggests that the clinical severity of asthma is not only associated with the severity of inflammation, but also to the degree of airway remodeling.

Emphysema occurs due to a protease and antiprotease activity imbalance, with resulting destruction of pulmonary connective tissue, particularly elastin. In smoking-related centrilobular emphysema there is too much protease, while in α1-antiprotease deficiency there is insufficient α1-antiprotease. Elastase is a protease found in the neutrophils and macrophages abundant in the lungs of smokers. Release of greater than normal amounts of elastase destroys elastin and induces emphysema. The free radicals and oxidants found in cigarette smoke may inactivate the protective antiprotease that is present (22). Circulating elastase is distributed preferentially to the lower lobes, which receive a greater proportion of pulmonary blood flow than the upper lobes. In patients with α1-antiprotease deficiency, more protease (elastase) that destroys elastin is delivered to the lower lungs than to the upper lungs, a possible explanation for the lower lobe predominance of α1-antiprotease deficiency related emphysema. In centrilobular emphysema secondary to cigarette smoking in which α1-antiproteinase levels are normal, the relatively greater ventilation–perfusion ratio in the upper portion of the lungs compared with the lung bases favors greater deposition of particulate matter in the upper lungs, and therefore greater release of elastase and upper lobe lung destruction (22).

Pathologically, emphysema is characterized by the abnormal, permanent enlargement of the airspaces distal to the terminal bronchioles, accompanied by destruction of their walls. When properly inflated, the cut surface of the lung as viewed with a dissecting microscope shows enlarged airspaces and destruction of alveolar walls. Numerous holes or fenestrations are also present in the alveolar walls. These holes are larger and more irregular than the normal pores of Kohn. Fenestrations are considered to be one of the earliest manifestations of emphysema and can sometimes be observed grossly. The alveolar septa may appear as a network of thin strands. As the remaining strands become involved, the alveoli coalesce into larger and larger spaces. The walls of these lesions also have fenestrations that gradually enlarge and cause formation of even larger spaces. Histologically, isolated fragments of alveolar septa result. In contrast, normal lung contains alveolar septa that are almost always connected at one or both ends to other alveolar septa (22,23).

The pathologic features of COPD include emphysema, small-airway inflammation and fibrosis, and mucous gland hyperplasia (3). Interestingly, corticosteroid reversibility in COPD may be related to features of asthma and perhaps inflammation as supported by work of Chanez and colleagues, who examined the response to corticosteroids in a group of 25 patients with COPD, documenting that responders had a larger number of eosinophils and higher levels of eosinophilic cationic protein in bronchoalveolar lavage fluid as well as a thicker reticular basement membrane (24). There are however, differences in the types of inflammatory cells and the degree of activation that may exist (5). Lacoste and colleagues noted that, although similar numbers of eosinophils were present in the bronchial biopsies from patients with chronic bronchitis, COPD, and asthma, the cells were not degranulated in chronic bronchitis or COPD patients. In addition, bronchoalveolar lavage fluid from patients with chronic bronchitis and COPD exhibited levels of eosinophilic cationic protein similar to those of normal controls (25).

Clinical History

Cough, wheezing and dyspnea are common features of obstructive lung disease, with considerable overlap in symptoms noted between asthma, chronic bronchitis, and emphysema. historical can help in beginning to define a specific type of obstructive lung disease. Patients with chronic bronchitis and emphysema generally have more constant and progressive symptoms, while a history of atopic disease or occupational exposure can suggest a diagnosis of asthma (26). Although asthma can occur at any age, asthma patients tend to be younger, and a history of symptoms beginning in childhood points toward asthma (27). For example, in the study of Burrows et al. the mean age of patients with predominantly asthmatic bronchitis was 29.6 years, compared with 64.6 years for patients with emphysema (28). α1-Antiprotease deficiency is an exception in which emphysema develops prematurely, with dyspnea developing and a mean age of 40 years for smokers with α1-antitrypsin deficiency and 53 years in nonsmokers (2). Patients of less than 50 years of age who develop moderate or severe chronic airflow obstruction, with either emphysema that is more severe in the lower lobes or a strong family history of obstructive disease, should be tested for α1-antitrypsin. There are well-described cases of early-onset severe emphysema with normal α1-antiprotease serum levels. For example, Silverman et al. described 44 such patients with severe COPD, mean FEV_1 16.9% predicted, and a normal serum α1-antitrypsin level (29). A high proportion of these patients were female (76.9%), and current or ex-smoker first-degree relatives of all patients had significantly lower FEV_1 and FEV_1/FVC (forced vital capacity) ratio values compared with control subjects.

As the role of smoking in the development and progression of COPD is unquestioned, a history of smoking can be helpful in the diagnosis of obstructive lung disease (2). Two groups have documented the reasonable sensitivity, but low specificity, of a smoking history in detecting COPD (30,31).

Physical Examination

Although crude and insensitive, wheezing and prolonged expiration suggest a diagnosis of airflow obstruction on physical examination (27,30). Holleman and Simel recently reviewed 44 studies reporting the value of the physical examination in the diagnosis of obstructive airways disease (32). Although no single finding or combination of findings could be used to reliably exclude airflow obstruction, the most useful findings were wheezing, barrel chest deformity, rhonchi, hyperresonance, subxyphoid apical impulse and prolonged expiration. Interestingly, the interobserver agreement among trained observers in the reported studies was generally acceptable, although kappa values varied greatly from 0.23 to 0.93. Other published data suggest that physicians are poor at estimating the severity of obstruction from physical examination (33). These data highlight the difficulty of judging the severity of airflow obstruction on physical examination alone.

Natural Course

Asthma usually presents in childhood, and may persist into adulthood. In a series of 207 young adults diagnosed with asthma in childhood, Martin et al. reported no difference in pulmonary function between patients who had ceased wheezing during adolescence and controls; in contrast, patients who continued to wheeze had significantly greater pulmonary function abnormality (34). However, bronchial hyperresponsiveness with histamine challenge was noted in 60% of patients who stopped wheezing during adolescence. In a separate study of 101 adults with asthma since childhood, Gerretsen et al noted that 43 (43%) of the patients had active symptoms, with 29/43 or 67% of these patients receiving maintenance therapy for asthma (35). The outcome of childhood asthma is related predominantly to the level of initial bronchial obstruction and airway responsiveness. Panhuysen et al recently reported the outcome of asthma in 181 adult patients followed for 25 years (36). Twenty patients (11%) were considered no longer to have asthma, demonstrating no pulmonary symptoms, no bronchial hyperresponsiveness and a FEV_1 >90% predicted. The absence of asthma at follow up was associated with a younger age, less severe airway obstruction when first tested, a higher FEV_1 at follow-up, and a shorter untreated period supporting the hypothesis that milder disease and early intervention are important components in asthma outcome. In a study of 92 lifelong nonsmokers (mean age 37 years) with asthma, all demonstrating bronchoreversibility when evaluated, Ulrik and Backer reported nonreversible airflow obstruction and an FEV_1 <80% predicted at 10 year follow-up in 21 patients (23%) (37). These patients demonstrated greater bronchoreversibility at enrollment and a more rapid deterioration in FEV_1 over time. It is evident that many patients have persistent clinical and physiologic evidence of asthma from childhood into adulthood, and a subset develop irreversible obstruction.

Patients with different forms of COPD have a different clinical course and prognosis, reemphasizing the need for accurate distinction between them. For example, Burrow et al. examined the survival rate and rate of decline in FEV_1 during 10 years of follow-up in white, non-Mexican Americans with CAO (28). Patients with nonatopic, smoking-related obstructive disease had a greater rate of decline in FEV_1 and decreased survival than patients with chronic asthmatic bronchitis. Similarly, patients with a self-reported history of chronic bronchitis had a steeper drop in FEV_1 than did patients with other forms of CAO in the report of pulmonary function from the Tucson epidemiological study of obstructive lung disease (38).

Cigarette smoking accelerates the normal decline in FEV_1 that occurs with age. Normally, the FEV_1 in non-smokers without respiratory disease declines by 25–30 mL each year, beginning at about age 35 (2). In the Lung Health Study of 5887 male and female smokers between the ages of 35 and 60, deemed at high risk for clinically significant COPD on the basis of a decreased ratio of FEV_1 to forced vital capacity (FVC), cigarette smoking was reported to adversely affect the preservation of FEV_1 (39). In the cohort of patients offered an intensive smoking-cessation program, 35% of patients who stopped smoking had an increase in mean postbronchodilator FEV_1 of 57 mL at the end of the first year of follow-up, while patients who had not stopped smoking had a mean decline of 38 mL.

Physiologic Studies

Pulmonary function tests are the most useful laboratory studies for the evaluation of suspected COPD, and are used for diagnosis, assessment of disease severity and monitoring response to treatment (2,40). Peak expiratory flow rate (PEFR), the maximal flow that can be achieved during a maximal expiratory effort, is easily measured with readily available, inexpensive, simple and reliable devices (41). This measurement has been widely accepted and advocated for the monitoring of patients with airflow obstruction, particularly asthmatics (40). Unfortunately, its diagnostic value during the initial evaluation of a patient with suspected airflow obstruction is less certain. Although there is a close relationship between the FEV_1 and PEFR (41), the PEFR is consistently higher than the FEV_1. In addition, PEFR can be decreased in upper airway obstruction, which limits the diagnostic accuracy of decreased maximal flow rates (42). Data confirming the diagnostic value of PEFR in the diagnosis of COPD are scant. Badgett and colleagues described a diagnostic model for COPD based on history (smoking history), physical examination (decreased breath sounds) and pulmonary function (PEFR) (43). The investigators defined COPD using standard spirometry. The best predictive model (sensitivity of 98% and specificity of 46%) included a history of cigarette smoking (≥30 pack-years), decreased

breath sounds and a PEFR of 350 L min^{-1}. If none of these features was present, only 3% of patients had COPD (43).

Spirometry is the optimal initial diagnostic approach as a simple screen, particularly as spirometers are widely available. Simple guidelines from the American Thoracic Society provide a framework for normal standards and interpretation of results (42). A decrease in FEV_1/FVC ratio from the predicted range is diagnostic of airflow obstruction (42,44). In addition, the severity of airflow obstruction can be assessed by the FEV_1 expressed as a percentage of predicted values (44). A graphical representation of peak expiratory and inspiratory flows versus lung volume (the flow–volume loop) should be included to exclude potential upper airway obstruction (42).

The diagnosis of asthma is based on an appropriate clinical history and evidence of reversible airflow obstruction, National Asthma Education Program, April 1997 no. 74). The importance of accurate diagnosis, monitoring of disease severity and treatment response have been heavily emphasized and now are considered the standard of care (40). Recent data have confirmed the marked difficulty in diagnosing asthma on purely clinical grounds (National Asthma Education Program, April 1997; no. 243; (40,45). Disease severity is often grossly understated by both the patient and the physician, in the absence of spirometric or peak flow measurements (40).

The diagnosis of COPD requires the documentation of airflow obstruction. Measurement of spirometric parameters before and after the administration of a short-acting beta-agonist is used to determine whether there is bronchoreversibility (44). Complete reversibility of airflow obstruction makes the diagnosis of asthma likely, and strongly argues against a diagnosis of chronic bronchitis or emphysema (27). Increasing evidence has confirmed that some patients with asthma develop irreversible airflow obstruction (IRAO) (5,37,46–48). Some investigators have suggested that development of IRAO is closely related to the duration and severity of previous asthma; others have not confirmed this (37,46). In a study of 18 nonsmoking patients with incomplete reversibility of airflow obstruction ($FEV_1 < 75\%$ predicted; mean 59%) despite aggressive high doses inhaled and oral steroids and bronchodilator therapy, all patients had typical historical features of asthma and an increase in $FEV_1 > 15\%$ after the administration of a short acting beta-agonist (46). Compared with 18 age-matched control subjects with completely reversible airflow obstruction, the patients with IRAO had a longer duration of asthma (32 versus 18 years) and more symptomatic disease. Greater airflow obstruction and hyperinflation was also noted in patients with IRAO, while a normal diffusing capacity was seen in both groups. The same investigators contrasted 14 patients with IRAO and 13 patients with COPD (47). The baseline FEV_1, FVC and postbronchodilator FEV_1 did not differ between the two.

Clearly, bronchodilator reversibility cannot be used as a sensitive test to differentiate asthma from chronic bronchitis and emphysema. The presence of bronchodilation during spirometric testing is seen in up to 30% of patients with a clinical diagnosis of COPD (16). Kesten and Robuck explored the diagnostic ability of acute bronchodilator response to separate asthma from COPD in 450 consecutive patients (287 with "unequivocal asthma" and 108 with COPD) (19). The mean increase in FEV_1 from baseline after inhaled albuterol was higher in the asthmatic patients (16.5% versus 10.6%), although considerable overlap was present, which limited diagnostic ability. Furthermore, when the authors defined response by various threshold improvements from baseline (10%, 15%, 20%), a 20% increase in FEV_1 demonstrated the best specificity for a diagnosis of asthma (84%), although all thresholds demonstrated poor sensitivity (19).

Although bronchoreversibility cannot be used to distinguish between asthma and COPD, some have suggested that an acute response to inhaled bronchodilators identified patients with improved survival, less loss of lung function over time and a better response to steroid therapy (16). In addition, the postbronchodilator FEV_1 is the single best predictor of survival in patients with COPD. A value below 30% of predicted is associated with a marked worsening in long-term survival (16). As a result, the postbronchodilator FEV_1 has become instrumental in establishing an appropriate time for considering surgical therapy in patients with advanced COPD.

Multiple investigators have examined the diagnostic value of an increase in FEV_1 after the administration of corticosteroids, with a metaanalysis of 33 published studies from 1966 to 1989 reported by Callahan et al. (49). The investigators used a weighted mean effect of 10% among the studies that met quality criteria (50). Many authors have attempted to identify which patients are most likely to respond to an oral steroid trial, with recent investigators suggesting that these individuals have many features in common with asthmatics. For example, Chancz et al. examined 25 patients diagnosed clinically with COPD and no atopy, wheezing or bronchoreversibility during acute bronchodilator challenge before and after 1.5 mg oral prednisone kg^{-1} for 15 days (24). Twelve of the patients experienced a greater than 12% increase in FEV_1 from baseline, with an absolute increase greater than 200 mL. These patients had features suggestive of asthma, including significantly larger numbers of eosinophils and higher levels of eosinophilic cationic protein in their bronchoalveolar lavage fluid. Fujimoto and colleagues treated 24 patients with pulmonary emphysema diagnosed clinically, physiologically, and, most importantly, by computed tomography (CT) scanning with 20 mg prednisolone per day for 2 weeks (51). An improvement in FEV_1 was noted in 50% of the patients. Importantly, these patients had an increased number of eosinophils in the sputum that

decreased with steroid therapy. As such, steroid responsiveness does not appear to provide an accurate physiologic technique to discriminate asthma from COPD.

The measurement of diffusing capacity for carbon monoxide ($D_{L_{CO}}$) should be considered a routine test in the evaluation of CAO, particularly in more advanced disease, as it has been established as a sensitive test in the detection of emphysema (52). Several groups have reported increased $D_{L_{CC}}$ in patients with asthma (53,54). Unfortunately, the specificity of this test is low and its use must complemental a thorough clinical history and physical examination. Although not completely accurate in suggesting the presence of emphysema, a decreased $D_{L_{CO}}$ in the setting of CAO suggests a component of pathologic emphysema (55). In large epidemiologic studies the presence of a normal $D_{L_{CO}}$ has been associated with a clinical syndrome more consistent with asthma (56). In fact, emphysema has been confirmed with thoracic imaging in some patients with breathlessness and an isolated decrease in $D_{L_{CO}}$ (57). On the other hand, $D_{L_{CO}}$ measurement has potential limitation in differentiating asthma from emphysema. Boulet and colleagues reported a $D_{L_{CO}}$ below 80% predicted in four of 14 asthmatics with incompletely reversible airflow obstruction (47). Only two asthmatic patients had evidence of emphysema on high resolution CT (HRCT) in this study, although it is not clear whether these patients had abnormalities of diffusing capacity. Gelb et al compared lung function and HRCT in 56 consecutive patients noting a strong negative correlation between $D_{L_{CO}}$ and CT emphysema score only in those patients with an $FEV_1 \geq 1$ liter (58). hypothesized that emphysema does not appear to be primarily responsible for expiratory limitation in COPD and cautioned against overinterpretation of decreased $D_{L_{CO}}$ in the setting of severe CAO. Subsequently, the same group reported detailed physiologic parameters in 10 patients with severe CAO (mean FEV_1 32% predicted) but little emphysema on HRCT (58). All patients had significant hyperinflation, decreased $D_{L_{CO}}$ and abnormal pressure–volume curves. In the three patients who died there was a close correlation between CT and anatomic scores for emphysema. In addition, the membranous–bronchiole and respiratory-bronchiole scores were markedly abnormal, suggesting that the major abnormality was severe, intrinsic "small-airways disease." These data suggest that a normal $D_{L_{CO}}$ has potential diagnostic value in establishing a diagnosis of asthma in patients with CAO, while a decreased $D_{L_{CO}}$ should be investigated in the setting of an appropriate clinical and potentially radiographic evaluation.

Radiology

Routine posteroanterior and lateral chest radiographs are part of the initial evaluation of suspected airflow obstruction. The chest radiographic features of asthma, chronic bronchitis, and emphysema may overlap in the same patient, similar to the overlap discussed above in clinical and spirometric features. Most of the radiographic signs of obstructive lung disease lack specificity. Similarly, chest radiographs lack sensitivity, particularly for mild disease, and therefore cannot be used to exclude a diagnosis of obstructive lung disease. For these reasons chest radiographs are used predominantly to support a diagnosis of obstructive lung disease, not to exclude a diagnosis of COPD. The CT findings of the different forms of obstructive lung disease are well described, and CT is the best tool to evaluate the severity of emphysema in vivo. However, similar to chest radiography, CT has a limited role in the primary diagnosis of emphysema. In the small subset of patients with an isolated reduction in diffusing capacity, otherwise normal pulmonary function tests and a normal chest radiograph, HRCT is useful for establishing the diagnosis of emphysema (57,59). In these patients the emphysema is usually mild compared with that of patients with pulmonary function tests abnormalities. When bronchiectasis is suspected, HRCT is the technique of choice for detecting, localizing and characterizing bronchiectasis, having replaced the more invasive bronchogram. Additionally, HRCT examinations performed in expiration may demonstrate areas of air-trapping in patients with small-airway disease, including asthma and bronchiolitis obliterans, when the inspiratory HRCT examination is normal or minimally abnormal (60).

Asthma

The chest radiographic features of asthma include pulmonary hyperinflation with increased lung lucency and mild bronchial wall thickening, with or without bronchial dilatation. Mild pulmonary artery enlargement may occur due to transient pulmonary hypertension (61). Indications for chest radiographs in asthma patients include chronic asthma refractory to medical therapy, fever, immunosuppression, evidence of other lung disease or heart disease, seizures, a history of intravenous drug abuse, and previous thoracic surgery (62).

Compared with chest radiographs, the CT scans of patients with asthma patients are more frequently abnormal, with 37.8% of asthmatics in one series having abnormal chest radiographs versus 71.9% with abnormal CT scans (63). In another series of adult patients with asthma, bronchial wall thickening was seen on chest radiographs in 71% of patients and on CT in 92% of patients; bronchial wall thickening was only identified in 17% of control subjects (64). However, like chest radiographs, CT scans may be normal, particularly in cases of mild asthma. Clinical indications for CT include identifying

coexisting emphysema, other forms of airway disease that mimic asthma, such as hypersensitivity pneumonitis or bronchiolitis obliterans, and identifying complications of asthma, such as suspected allergic bronchopulmonary aspergillosis (62).

With longstanding asthma, bronchial dilatation and bronchial wall thickening are seen on CT, and may be irreversible (63,65–67). Reversible findings on CT include mucoid impaction and lobar collapse, seen in 10–20% of asthmatic patients (63,67). Bronchial wall thickening and bronchial dilatation are more common and more severe in asthmatic patients with moderate to severe airflow obstruction and in patients with a prolonged history of asthma, than in patients with mild obstruction or normal airflow (63,68–70). Given the frequency of bronchial wall thickening in normal subjects, it cannot be used to separate normal patients from asthma patients with mild airflow obstruction (70). The reported frequency of bronchial dilatation in asthma ranges from 20 to 36%, compared with 0 to 7% in normal control subjects (67–68). In one study the prevalence of bronchial dilatation was 77% in asthma patients and 59% of normal controls; these higher numbers are probably due to the high altitude of the study location (Denver–Colorado altitude 1600 m) with reflex vasoconstriction of the pulmonary arteries making the bronchi appear relatively larger (64). The frequency of bronchial wall thickening ranges from 82 to 92% of patients (64,67,69). Patients with non allergic asthma have more extensive airway remodeling on CT than patients with allergic asthma, with a higher frequency of bronchial dilatation, bronchial recruitment, and emphysema (71).

Areas of low attenuation representing air-trapping, secondary decrease in perfusion, or both, can be seen on inspiratory HRCT (70). While patients with chronic, stable asthma may develop a reduction in lung attenuation on CT, in nonsmoking asthma patients emphysema is not a feature on CT (72,73). This reduction in lung attenuation may represent nondestructive hyperinflation. Air-trapping can be demonstrated on expiratory HRCT, and may precede the development of airway dilatation and thickening (65).

Recently, helical CT has demonstrated reversibility of these findings in mild asthmatics. After bronchial provocation with methacholine chloride there is a reduction in lung attenuation and reduction in the cross-sectional area of small airways (less than 5 mm^2) compared with baseline, accompanied by a 26–30% decrease in FEV_1. All findings returned to normal after reversal with albuterol (74). In a similar study, the internal airway lumen diameter decreased 17% from baseline after methacholine inhalation in asthmatics, and increased to 18% above baseline after albuterol inhalation (75). Methacholine-induced bronchial constriction occurs in bronchi of all sizes, but is most severe in bronchi 2–4 mm in diameter

(76). While in normal patients a decrease in bronchial wall thickness accompanies bronchoconstriction, bronchial wall thickness does not decrease in asthmatic patients as measured on HRCT (76).

Chronic Bronchitis

The radiographic features of chronic bronchitis are poorly described compared with asthma and emphysema. Furthermore, the overlap in clinical presentation and pulmonary function among the subtypes of COPD makes identification of patients with chronic bronchitis in the absence of asthma or emphysema difficult. Findings at chest radiography include pulmonary hyperinflation, and bronchial wall thickening manifesting as peribronchial thickening or cuffing, and increased "markings" due to superimposition of the thickened bronchial and bronchiolar walls (77). There is very little published data on CT in chronic bronchitis. The most common HRCT finding is bronchial wall thickening (78). Arakawa et al included four patients with chronic bronchitis in a series of 45 patients with air-trapping on expiratory HRCT (60). While all four patients had air-trapping on expiratory HRCT, one patient had a normal inspiratory HRCT. In the remaining three patients the inspiratory HRCT demonstrated bronchial wall thickening, a "tree-in-bud" appearance secondary to mucoid impaction, and ground-glass opacity presumed secondary to concomitant infection. Remy-Jardin et al. have shown that spirometrically triggered quantitative CT scanning performed at 10% and 90% vital capacity (VC) can be used to distinguish normal patients and patients with chronic bronchitis, from patients with emphysema (79). At 90% VC, lung attenuation is significantly lower in patients with emphysema than in normal controls and in patients with chronic bronchitis. At 10% VC, mean lung attenuation is significantly higher in normal patients compared with patients with chronic bronchitis and emphysema, and patients with the latter two conditions could not be distinguished.

Emphysema

The chest radiographic features of emphysema include both primary signs of lung destruction and secondary signs of pulmonary hyperinflation (Fig. 16.1). The primary signs of lung destruction include irregular radiolucency of the lungs, arterial depletion and thin-walled bullae. The secondary signs of pulmonary hyperinflation reflect air-trapping and increased lung compliance. They include a reduction in the upward convexity or even depression of the diaphragm, an enlarged retrosternal clear space, an increase in the anteroposterior chest dimension ("barrel chest" that is equal in anteroposte-

rior and transverse dimensions), increased height of the lungs, and an abnormally low right hemidiaphragm (1,80,81). The shape and position of the diaphragm correlates with the severity of hyperinflation at pulmonary function testing (82). The primary and secondary signs alone or in combination have variable sensitivity for the detection of emphysema, ranging from 40 to 80% (61). In some circumstances lung volume is normal on chest radiographs, including patients with mild emphysema, an alteration in the shape of the thorax, such as scoliosis, or superimposed interstitial lung disease. Other radiographic signs include apparent microcardia, with a decrease in the transverse dimension of the heart, and a saber-sheath trachea that is narrow in transverse dimension and enlarged in anteroposterior dimension below the level of the thoracic inlet (83). A tracheal index of less than 0.67 (ratio of coronal to sagittal diameter) indicates a saber-sheath trachea (84). Additional signs of emphysema that occur with severe disease complicated by pulmonary arterial hypertension and right heart overload include enlargement of the central pulmonary arteries and right heart chambers.

While moderate to severe emphysema is generally detectable radiographically, in mild emphysema the radiograph is often normal. While the signs of hyperinflation on chest radiographs are the most sensitive for detecting emphysema, these signs lack specificity and can be seen with other forms of obstructive lung disease. In one report when the height of the right hemidiaphragm on the lateral chest radiograph is less than or equal to 2.6 cm, chest radiographs were 67.7% sensitive for detecting patients with obstructive spirometry (85). In the same series, a right lung height of 29.9 cm or more on the posteroanterior chest radiograph was 69.8% sensitive. The false-positive rate for both was 5%. By combining signs of both lung destruction and hyperinflation, the specificity of chest radiographs for emphysema improves, but at the expense of sensitivity. Only the presence of bullae is sufficiently specific for the diagnosis of emphysema on chest radiographs. The insensitivity of chest radiographs for detecting mild to moderate emphysema has limited their usefulness as a diagnostic tool (81,86,87). Chest radiographs are predominantly used to support a suspected diagnosis of emphysema, to evaluate for complications of emphysema, such as pneumonia or lung cancer, or to detect other superimposed lung disease, such as bronchiectasis.

CT provides excellent anatomic detail for both detecting and characterizing emphysema, as well as for quantitatively determining the severity of emphysema. Conventional CT is more accurate than chest radiography, and HRCT is more accurate than conventional CT at demonstrating the presence, severity and distribution of emphysema (88,89). Emphysema appears as areas of abnormally low attenuation in the lung, without

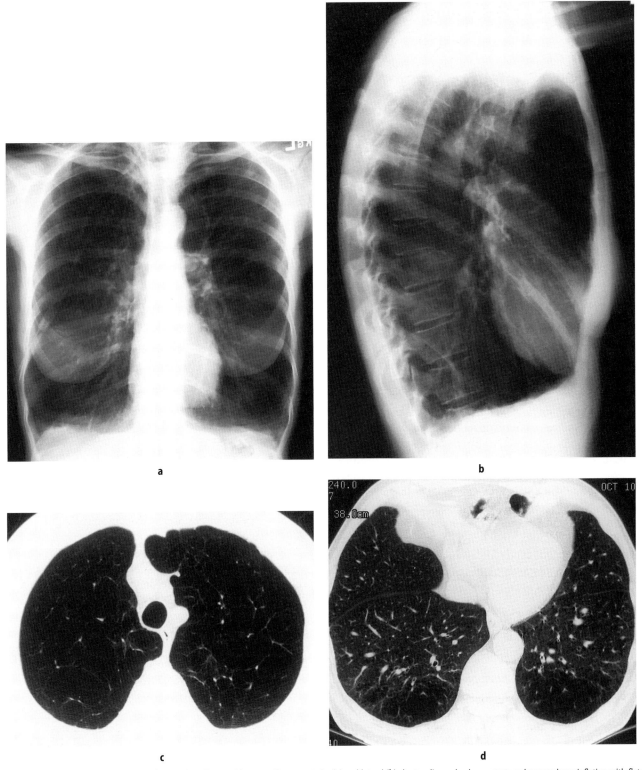

Figure 16.1. Upper lobe predominant emphysema in a 63 year old woman. Posteroanterior (**a**) and lateral (**b**) chest radiographs demonstrate pulmonary hyperinflation with flat hemidiaphragms, increased anteroposterior chest dimension and retrosternal clear space, increased height of the lungs, and a paucity of pulmonary vessels in the upper lobes. Axial HRCT images through the upper lobes (**c**) and lower lungs (**d**) demonstrate more severe anatomic destruction, separation and thinning of pulmonary blood vessels at the lung apices than at the lung bases.

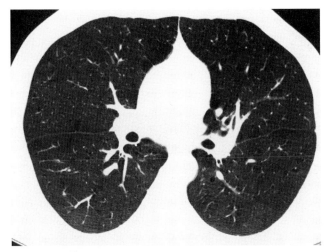

Figure 16.2. Mild centrilobular emphysema: axial 1 mm collimation HRCT image through the mid-thorax demonstrates small focal areas of low attenuation without definable walls, characteristic of mild emphysema.

definable walls (Fig. 16.2). Many investigators have demonstrated excellent correlation of emphysema severity on HRCT and conventional CT with the pathologic severity, using both semiquantitative visual scoring methods or quantitative analysis based on Hounsfield unit (HU) measurements (90–93). In patients with emphysema these methods correlate well with $D_{L_{CO}}$ and pulmonary capillary blood volume in patients, but only moderately with measures of airflow obstruction, such as the FEV_1, FVC and the FEV_1/ FVC ratio. Some authors have therefore speculated that the severity of expiratory airway obstruction in emphysema is not related to the severity of parenchymal destruction (55,96–97). In a study of inspiratory and expiratory CT, the visual emphysema score correlated well with the severity of emphysema, but not with air-trapping. The ratio of the CT attenuation number at expiration to inspiration (E/I ratio) was shown to correlate well with air-trapping, and poorly with the severity of emphysema (98). Haraguchi et al quantified emphysema using regions of interest drawn in the central, intermediate and peripheral lung, as well as in the upper, middle and lower lung. They concluded that central emphysema, not peripheral emphysema, had the greatest correlation with pulmonary function, and furthermore that the more uniform the emphysema between upper and lower lung, or the central and peripheral lung, the more severe the airway obstruction (99).

The quantitative analysis of emphysema severity is referred to as the density mask technique, initially performed on individual axial two-dimensional images (90) (Fig. 16.3.) The density mass can be applied to the entire lung volumes using three-dimensional helical CT to obtain a single volumetric data set acquired during a single inspiration (23,100) (Fig. 16.3d,e). Lung volume,

including total lung capacity (TLC) and residual volume (RV) can also be calculated from inspiratory and expiratory helical CT data with excellent correlation with static lung volumes (101). The thinner the collimation used to acquire the CT images, the better the correlation of CT attenuation-based measurements with the pathologic severity of emphysema (88). CT is the best technique for confirming the presence of emphysema when it is suspected clinically, and for evaluating the severity and distribution of the emphysema, an important selection criterion for lung volume reduction surgery, as patients with focal biapical or bibasilar emphysema have better postoperative outcome than patients with diffuse emphysema (102–106).

Lung perfusion scintigraphy, both planar single photon emission CT (SPECT), provide both qualitative and quantitative assessment of differential pulmonary parenchymal perfusion, locating areas of maximal reduction in blood flow (107). Lung perfusion can be quantified using the count density in different anatomic zones of the lung. However, the distribution of radiotracer indicates relative not absolute perfusion. For example, cold "target" zones of absent perfusion may be seen at the lung apices, with all of the radiotracer depositing at the lung bases (Fig. 16.4). This does not indicate that the lung bases are pathologically normal, but that there is relatively more perfusion and less emphysema in the areas with tracer deposition. Ventilation scintigraphy with[39m] To-DTPA aerosol is of limited value, due to the large amount of central airway distribution that we have experience in nearly half of our patients with emphysema being evaluated for lung volume reduction surgery (108). Ventilation scintigraphy with radiolabeled xenon gas during the washin, equilibrium and washout phases may not have the same limitation, and may demonstrate areas of air-trapping.

Conclusion

Chronic airflow obstruction is a common clinical entity associated with significant morbidity, mortality and the use of extensive health care resources. While there is considerable overlap in the clinical features of the major types of chronic airflow obstruction, pulmonary function and imaging, particularly CT, can assist in identifying the specific or diseases. With the advent of new therapeutic modalities for emphysema, such as lung volume reduction surgery, and with differences in prognosis among the different types of COPD, the importance of making a specific diagnosis is important. Clinical history, physical examination, pulmonary function, and, in selected cases, HRCT scanning, can be used to better define the type of COPD and direct appropriate medical and/or surgical management.

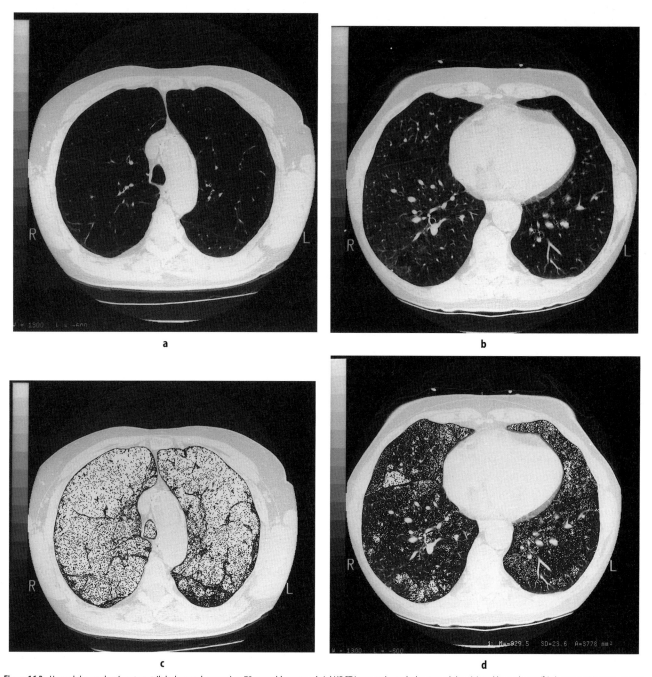

Figure 16.3. Upper lobe predominant centrilobular emphysema in a 72 year old woman. Axial HRCT images through the upper lobes (**a**) and lower lungs (**b**) demonstrate more severe anatomic destruction, separation and thinning of pulmonary blood vessels at the lung apices than the lung bases. Axial density mask (**c** and **d**) through the same level as in **a** and **b**, demonstrating the emphysema as the white areas, again more severe in the upper lungs (all pixels with an attenuation value less than −900 HU). Anterior (*Figure continues.*)

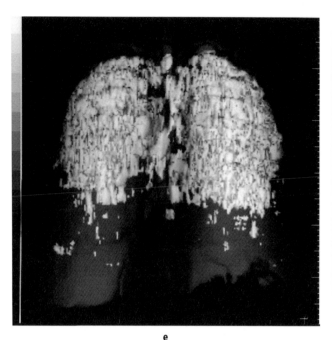
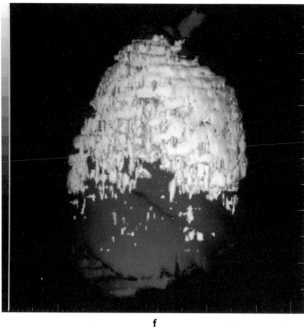

e   f

Figure 16.3. (e) and right lateral (f) projections from three-dimensional shaded surface display reconstructions show the total lung volume in gray and emphysema volume of all pixels less than −900 HU superimposed in white. Dividing the lung in half from apex to base, 71.7% of the upper half of the lungs and 18.8% of the lower half of the lungs represents emphysema, for a CT ratio of 3.8.

References

1. Higgins M (1984) Epidemiology of COPD. State of the art. Chest 85:3S–8S.
2. American Theracic Society (1995) Standards for the diagnosis and care of patients with chronic obstructive pulmonary disease: Definitions, epidemiology, pathophysiology and staging. Am J Respir Crit Care Med 152:578–584.
3. Senior R, Anthonisen N (1998) Chronic obstructive pulmonary disease (COPD). Am J Respir Crit Care Med 157:S139–147.
4. Dykewicz M, Ledford D (1998) Recent findings in asthma likely to impact patient care. Compr Ther 24:187–193.
5. O'Byrne P, Postma D (1999) The many faces of airway inflammation. Asthma and chronic obstructive pulmonary disease. Am J Respir Crit Care Med 159:S41–S66.
6. Vollmer W, Osborne M, Buist A (1998) 20-year trends in the prevalence of asthma and chronic airflow obstruction in an HMO. Am J Respir Crit Care Med 157:1079–1084.
7. Burrow B (1973) Foreward, symposium on chronic respiratory disease. Med Clin North Am 57:545.
8. Burrows B (1990) Airways obstructive diseases: Pathologenetic mechanisms and natural histories of the disorders. Med Clin North Am 74:547–559.
9. Ferris B, Jr (1973) Chronic bronchitis and emphysema. Classification and epidemiology. Med Clin North Am 57:637–649.
10. Murray CJ, L#aaopez AD (1997) Global mortality, disability, and the contribution of risk factors: Global burden of disease study [see comments]. Lancet 349:1436–1442.
11. Fletcher CM, Pride NB (1984) Definitions of emphysema, chronic bronchitis, asthma, and airflow obstruction: 25 years on from the Ciba symposium [editorial]. Thorax 39:81–85.
12. Pride NB, Burrows B (1995) Development of impaired lung function: Natural history and risk factors. In Calverly P, Pride N (eds) Chronic obstructive pulmonary disease. Chapman & Hall, London, pp 69–91.
13. Petty TL, Weinmann GG (1997) Building a national strategy for the prevention and management of and research in chronic obstructive pulmonary disease. National Heart, Lung, and Blood Institute workshop summary, Bethesda, MD 29–31 August 1995 [see comments]. JAMMA 277:246–253.
14. Murray JF, Nadel JA (1994) Textbook of respiratory medicine, vol. 2, 2nd edn. WB Saunders, Philadelphia, p. 2739.
15. Kips J, Pauwels R (1999) Airway wall remodelling: Does it occur and what does it mean? Clin Exp Allergy 29:1457–1466.
16. Anthonisen N (1989) Prognosis in chronic obstructive pulmonary disease: Results from multicenter clinical trials. Am Rev Respir Dis 140:S95–S99.
17. Nisar M, Earis J, Pearson M, et al. (1992) Acute bronchodilator trials in chronic obstructive pulmonary disease. Am Rev Respir Dis 146:555–559.
18. Kesten S, Chapman K (1993) Physician perceptions and management of COPD. Chest 104:254–258.
19. Kesten S, Rebuck A (1994) Is the short-term response to inhaled β-adrenergic agonist sensitive or specific for distinguishing between asthma and COPD? Chest 105:1042–1045.
20. Beasley R, Roche W, Roberts J, (1989) Cellular events in the bronchi in mild asthma and after bronchial provocation. Am Rev Respir Dis 139:806–817.
21. Chetta A, Foresi A, Deldonno M, et al. (1996) Bronchial responsiveness to distilled water and methacholine and its relationship to inflammation and remodeling of the airways in asthma. Am Rev Respir Crit Care Med 153:910–917.

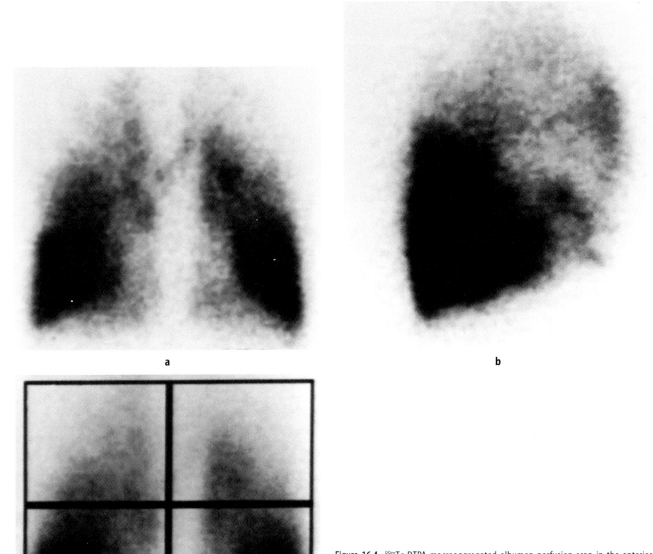

a

b

c

Figure 16.4. ^{99m}Tc-DTPA macroaggregated albumen perfusion scan in the anterior (**a**) and lateral (**b**) projections of a 67 year old man with severe obstructive pulmonary disease secondary to smoking-related centrilobular emphysema. There are focal areas of absent perfusion and in the upper lobes, with most of the perfusion to the lower lungs posteriorly. This corresponded to the severity of emphysema seen on CT. In (**c**) regions of interest can be drawn to quantify the relative distributions of perfusion to different parts of the lungs.

22. Pratt P (1988) Emphysema and chronic airways disease. In, Dail D, Hammar S (eds) Pulmonary pathology. Springer-Verlag, New York, pp 654–659.

23. Kazerooni EA, Whyte RI, Flint A, et al. (1997) Imaging of emphysema and lung volume reduction surgery. Radiogrpahics 17:1023–1036.

24. Chanez P, Vignola A, O'Shaugnessy T, et al. (1997) Corticosteroid reversibility in COPD is related to features of asthma. Am Rev Respir Crit Care Med, 155:1529–1534.

25. Lacoste J, Bousquet J, Chanez P, et al. (1993) Eosinophilic and neutrophilic inflammation in asthma, chronic bronchitis, and chronic obstructive pulmonary disease. J Allergy Clin Immunol 92:537–548.

26. van Scayck C (1996) Diagnosis of asthma and chronic obstructive pulmonary disease in general practice. Br J Gen Pract 46:193–197.

27. McIvor A, Chapman K (1996) Diagnosis of chronic obstructive pulmonary disease and differentiation from asthma. Curr Opin Pulm Med 2:148–154.

28. Burrows B, Bloom JW, Traver GA, et al. (1987) The course and prognosis of different forms of chronic airways obstruction in a sample from the general population. N Engl J Med 317:1309–1314.

29. Silverman E, Chapman H, Drazen J, et al. (1998) Genetic epidemiology of severe, early-onset chronic obstructive pulmonary disease. Risk to relatives for airflow obstruction and chronic bronchitis. Am J Respir Crit Care Med 157:1770–1778.

30. Holleman D, Simel D, Goldberg J (1993) Diagnosis of obstructive airways disease from the clinical examination. J Gen Intern Med 8:63–68.

31. Badgett R, Tanaka D, Hunt D, et al. (1994) The clinical evaluation for diagnosing obstructive airways disease in high-risk patients. Chest 106:1427–1431.

32. Holleman D, Jr, Simel D (1995) Does the clinical examination predict airflow limitation? JAMA 273:313–319.

33. Emerman C, Lukens T, Effron D (1994) Physician estimation of FEV_1 in acute exacerbation of COPD. Chest 105:1709–1712.

34. Martin A, Landau L, Phelan P (1980) Lung function in young adults who had asthma in childhood. Am Rev Respir Dis 122:609–616.

35. Gerritsen J, Koeter G, Postma D, et al. (1989) Prognosis of asthma from childhood to adulthood. Am Rev Respir Dis 140:1325–1330.

36. Panhuysen C, Vonk J, Koeter G, et al. (1997) Adult patients may outgrow their asthma: A 25-year follow-up study. Am J Respir Crit Care Med 155:1267–1272.

37. Ulrik C, Backer V (1999) Nonreversible airflow obstruction in life-long nonsmokers with moderate to severe asthma. Eur Respir J 14:892–896.

38. Postma D, Lebowitz M (1995) Persistence and new onset of asthma and chronic bronchitis evaluated longitudinally in a community population sample of adults. Arch Intern Med 155:1393–1399.

39. Anthonisen N, Connett J, Kiley J, et al. (1994) The effects of smoking intervention and the use of an inhaled anticholinergic bronchodilator on the rate of decline in FEV_1: The lung health study. JAMA 272:1497–1505.

40. National Asthma Education Program NH, Lung and Blood Institute, National Institutes of Health. (1997) Guidelines for the diagnosis and management of asthma. NIH Publications no. 97-4051.

41. Jain P, Kavuru M, Emerman C, et al. (1998) Utility of peak expiratory flow monitoring. Chest 114:861–876.

42. Martinez F (1997) Pulmonary function testing. In Khan M, Lynch J III, (eds) Pulmonary disease. Diagnosis and therapy. A practical approach. Williams & Wilkins, Baltimore, MD, pp 107–141.

43. Badgett RG, Tanaka DJ, Hunt DK (1993) Can moderate chronic pulmonary disease be diagnosed by historical and physical findings alone? Am J Med 94:188–196.

44. American Thoracic Society (1991) Lung function testing: Selection of reference values and interpretative strategies. Am Rev Respir Dis 144:1202–1218.

45. Linden-Smith J, Morrison D, Hernandez P, et al. (1999) Over-diagnosis of asthma? A community survey. Am J Respir Crit Care Med 159 (Suppl 3):A135.

46. Hudon C, Turcotte H, Laviolette M, et al. (1997) Characteristics of bronchial asthma with incomplete reversibility of airflow obstruction. Ann Allergy Asthma Immunol 78:195–202.

47. Boulet L, Turcotte H, Hudon C et al. (1998) Clinical, physiological and radiological features of asthma with incomplete reversibility of airflow obstruction compared with those of COPD. Can Respir J 5:270–277.

48. Brown P, Greville H, Finucane K (1984) Asthma and irreversible airflow obstruction. Thorax 39:131–136.

49. Callahan CM, Dittus RS, Katz BP (1991) Oral corticosteroid therapy for patients with stable chronic obstructive pulmonary disease. A meta-analysis. Ann Intern Med 114:216–223.

50. Callahan C, Dittus R, Katz B (1991) Oral corticosteroid therapy for patients with stable chronic obstructive pulmonary disease. A meta-analysis. Ann Intern Med 114:216–223.

51. Fujimoto K, Kubo K, Yamamoto H, et al. (1999) Eosinophilic inflammation in the airway is related to glucocorticoid reversibility in patients with pulmonary emphysema. Chest 115:697–702.

52. Cotton D, Soparkar G, Graham B (1996) Diffusing capacity in the clinical assessment of chronic airflow obstruction. Med Clin North Am 80:549–564.

53. Collard P, Njinou B, Nejadnik B, et al. (1994) Single breath diffusing capacity for carbon monoxide in stable asthma. Chest 105:1426–1429.

54. Stewart R (1988) Carbon monoxide diffusing capacity in asthmatic patients with mild airflow limitation. Chest 94:332–336.

55. Morrison NJ, Abboud R, Ramadan F, et al. (1989) Comparison of single breath carbon monoxide diffusing capacity and pressure-volume curves in detecting emphysema. Am Rev Respir Dis 139:1179–1187.

56. Knudson R, Kalternborn W, Burrows B (1990) Single breath carbon monoxide transfer factor in different forms of chronic airflow obstruction in a general population sample. Thorax 45:524–529.

57. Klein J, Gamsu G, Webb W, et al. (1992) High-resolution CT diagnosis of emphysema in symptomatic patients with normal chest radiographs and isolated low diffusing capacity. Radiology 182:817–821.

58. Gelb A, Zamel N, Hogg J, et al. (1998) Pseudophysiologic emphysema resulting from severe small-airways disease. Am J Respir Crit Care Med 158:815–819.

59. Chin NK, Lim TK (1998) A 39-year-old smoker with effort dyspnea, normal spirometry results, and low diffusing capacity. Chest 113:231–233.

60. Arakawa H, Webb WR (1998) Air trapping on expiratory high-resolution CT scans in the absence of inspiratory scan abnormalities: Correlation with pulmonary function tests and differential diagnosis. AJR 170:1349–1353.

61. Webb WR (1997) Radiology of obstructive pulmonary disease. AJR 169:637–647.

62. Newell JD, Chan ED, Martin RJ (2000) Imaging of airway disease. In Lynch DA, Newell JD, Lee JS (eds) Imaging of diffuse lung disease. B.C. Decker, Hamilton Ontario, p 173.

63. Paganin F, Trussard V, Seneterre E, et al. (1992) Chest radiography and high resolution computed tomography of the lungs in asthma. Am Rev Respir Dis 146:1084–1087.

64. Lynch DA, Newell JD, Tschomper BA, (1993) Uncomplicated asthma in adults: Comparison of CT appearance of the lungs in asthmatic and healthy subjects. Radiology 188:829–833.

65. Boulet LP, Turcotte H, Hudon C, et al. (1998) Clinical, physiological and radiological features of asthma with incomplete reversibility of airflow obstruction compared with those of COPD. Can Respir J 5:270–277.

66. Carr DH, Hibon S, Rubens M, et al. (1998) Peripheral airways obstruction on high-resolution computed tomography in chronic severe asthma. Respir Med 92:448–453.

67. Grenier P, Mourey-Gerosa I, Benali K, et al. (1996) Abnormalities of the airways and lung parenchyma in asthmatics: CT observations in 50 patients and inter- and intraobserver variability. Eur Radiol 6:199–206.

68. Park JW, Hong YK, Kim CW, et al. (1997) High-resolution computed tomography in patients with bronchial asthma: Correlation with clinical features, pulmonary functions and bronchial hyper-responsiveness. J Invest Allergol Clin Immunol 7:186–192.

69. Park CS, Müller NL, Worthy SA, et al. (1997) Airway obstruction in asthmatic and healthy individuals: Inspiratory and expiratory thin-section CT findings. Radiology 203:361–367.

70. Awadh N, Müller NL, Park CS et al. (1998) Airway wall thickness in patients with near fatal asthma and control groups: Assessment with high resolution computed tomographic scanning. Thorax 53:248–253.

71. Paganin F, Seneterre E, Chanez P, et al. (1996) Computed tomography of the lungs in asthma: Influence of disease severity and etiology. Am J Respir Crit Care Med 153:110–114.

72. Biernacki W, Redpath AT, Best JJ, et al. (1997) Measurement of CT lung density in patients with chronic asthma [see comments]. Eur Respir J 10:2455–2459.

73. Kinsella M, Müller NL, Staples C, et al. (1988) Hyperinflation in asthma and emphysema. Assessment by pulmonary function testing and computed tomography. Chest 94:286–289.

74. Goldin JG, McNitt-Gray MF, Sorenson SM, et al. (1998) Airway hyperreactivity: Assessment with helical thin-section CT. Radiology 208:321–329.

75. Kee ST, Fahy JV, Chen DR (1996) High-resolution computed tomography of airway changes after induced bronchoconstriction and bronchodilation in asthmatic volunteers. Acad Radiol 3:389–394.

76. Okazawa M, Müller N, McNamara AE, et al. (1996) Human airway narrowing measured using high resolution computed tomography. Am J Respir Crit Care Med 154:1557–1562.

77. Takasugi J, Godwin J (1998) Radiology of chronic obstructive pulmonary disease. Radiol Clin North Am 36:29–55.

78. Hartman TE, Tazelaar HD, Swensen SJ, et al. (1997) Cigarette smoking: CT and pathologic findings of associated pulmonary diseases. Radiographics 17:377–390.

79. Remy-Jardin M, Remy J, Boulenguez C, et al. (1993) Morphologic effects of cigarette smoking on airways and pulmonary parenchyma in healthy adult volunteers: CT evaluation and correlation with pulmonary function tests. Radiology 186:107–115.

80. Pratt PC (1987) Radiographic appearance of the chest in emphysema. Invest Radiol 22:927–929.

81. Thurlbeck WM, Simon G (1978) Radiographic appearance of the chest in emphysema. AJR 130:429–440.

82. Pratt PC (1987) Role of conventional chest radiography in diagnosis and exclusion of emphysema. Am J Med 82:998–1006.

83. Greene R (1978) "Saber-sheath" trachea: Relation to chronic obstructive pulmonary disease. AJR 130:441–445.

84. Greene R, Lechner GL (1975) "Saber-sheath" trachea: A clinical and functional study of marked coronal narrowing of the intrathoracic trachea. Radiology 115:265–268.

85. Reich SB, Weinshelbaum A, Yee J (1985) Correlation of radiographic measurements and pulmonary function tests in chronic obstructive pulmonary disease. AJR 144:695–699.

86. Thurlbeck WM, Müller NL (1994) Emphysema: Definition, imaging, and quantification. AJR 163:1017–1025.

87. Nicklaus TM, Stowell DW, Christiansen WR, et al. (1966) The accuracy of the roentgenologic diagnosis of chronic pulmonary emphysema. Am Rev Respir Dis 93:889–899.

88. Miller RR, Müller NL, Vedal S, et al. (1989) Limitations of computed tomography in the assessment of emphysema. Am Rev Respir Dis 139:980–983.

89. Bergin C, Müller N, Nichols DM, et al. (1986) The diagnosis of emphysema. A computed tomographic–pathologic correlation. Am Rev Respir Dis 133:541–546.

90. Müller NL, Staples CA, Miller RR, et al. (1988) "Density mask". An objective method to quantitate emphysema using computed tomography. Chest 94:782–787.

91. Gevenois PA, De Vuyst P, Sy M, et al. (1996) Pulmonary emphysema: Quantitative CT during expiration. Radiology 199:825–829.

92. Gevenois PA, Yernault JC (1995) Can computed tomography quantify pulmonary emphysema? Eur Respir J 8:843–848.

93. Kuwano K, Matsuba K, Ikeda T, et al. (1990) The diagnosis of mild emphysema. Correlation of computed tomography and pathology scores. Am Rev Respir Dis 141:169–178.

94. Müller NL, Thurlbeck WM (1996) Thin-section CT, emphysema, air trapping, and airway obstruction [editorial; comment]. Radiology 199:621–622.

95. Morrison NJ, Abboud RT, Müller NL, et al. (1990) Pulmonary capillary blood volume in emphysema. Am Rev Respir Dis 141:53–61.

96. Gelb A, Schein M, Kuei J, et al. (1993) Limited contribution of emphysema in advanced chronic obstructive pulmonary disease. Am Rev Respir Dis 147:1157–1163.

97. Gelb AF, Hogg JC, Müller NL, et al. (1996) Contribution of emphysema and small airways in COPD. Chest 109:353–359.

98. Eda S, Kubo K, Fujimoto K, et al. (1997) The relations between expiratory chest CT using helical CT and pulmonary function tests in emphysema. Am J Respir Crit Care Med 155:1290–1294.

99. Haraguchi M, Shimura S, Hida W, et al. (1998) Pulmonary function and regional distribution of emphysema as determined by high-resolution computed tomography. Respiration 65:125–129.

100. Kazerooni E, Martinez F, Quint L, et al. (1996) Quantitative helical CT indices of emphysema as predictors of outcome after lung volume reduction surgery. Radiology 201(P):298.

101. Kauczor HU, Heussel CP, Fischer B, et al. (1998) Assessment of lung volumes using helical CT at inspiration and expiration: Comparison with pulmonary function tests. AJR 171:1091–1095.

102. Slone RM, Gierada DS, Yusen RD (1998) Preoperative and postoperative imaging in the surgical management of pulmonary emphysema. Radiol Clin North Am 36:57–89.

103. Slone RM, Pilgram TK, Gierada DS, et al. (1997) Lung volume reduction surgery: Comparison of preoperative radiologic features and clinical outcome [see comments]. Radiology 204:685–693.

104. Kazerooni EA, Curtis JL, Paine R, et al. (1998) Long-term outcome after bilateral apical lung volume reduction surgery (LVRS) via median sternotomy: Predictive value of quantitative helical CT

analysis (QCT) and physiologic severity of hyperinflation. Radiology 209(P):257.

105. Sciurba F (1997) Early and long-term functional outcomes following lung volume reduction surgery. Clin Chest Med 18:259–276.

106. McKenna RJ Jr, Brenner M, Fischel RJ, et al. (1997) Patient selection criteria for lung volume reduction surgery. J Thorac Cardiovasc Surg 114:957–964; discussion 964–957.

107. Mettler FA, Guiberteau MJ (1997) Respiratory system. In Mettler FA, Guiberteau MJ (eds) Essentials of nuclear medicine, 3rd edn. WB Saunders, Philadelphia, pp 167–170.

108. Jamadar DA, Kazerooni EA, Martinez FJ, (1999) Qualitative ventilation–perfusion scintigraphy and SPECT imaging in the evaluation of lung volume reduction surgery candidates: Description and prediction of clinical outcome. Eur J Nucl Med 26:734–42.

17 Pulmonary Disease in the Immunocompromised Host

N.W. Schluger and G. Pearson

Overview

Pulmonary diseases in the immunocompromised host represent an enormous spectrum of illness of growing importance in clinical chest medicine. Because of their continuous exposure to the environment, the lungs are particularly vulnerable to illness if their host defense mechanisms are impaired. The growth of organ transplantation as a clinical endeavor and the attendant use of immunosuppressive therapy to prevent and treat rejection, the emergence of the acquired immune deficiency syndrome (AIDS), and the increasingly aggressive use of anti-inflammatory and immunomodulating therapies to treat collagen-vascular diseases and other inflammatory disorders have all contributed to a greater number of pulmonary complications related to alterations of immune system function. Although the majority of pulmonary complications in the immunocompromised host are infectious in origin, some are drug related, and distinguishing the two is sometimes difficult. Proper diagnosis of lung disease in the immunocompromised host requires knowledge not only of the patient's underlying illness, but also of the treatment for that illness, the interaction between the patient and his or her immediate environment, and the radiographic pattern seen on the plain chest film and computed tomography (CT) scan. Because of the fragile nature of patients with severe immunocompromise, there is often urgency in approaching such cases, and an efficient diagnostic strategy is critical.

In approaching the immunocompromised patient with lung disease it is helpful to review pulmonary host defenses, as different defects in host defense are associated with a propensity for different types of pulmonary complication. A knowledge of the overall organization of pulmonary host defenses can aid in narrowing the differential diagnosis of a compromised host with an abnormal chest radiograph.

Pulmonary Host Defenses

Structural and Physical Components of Host Defense in the Respiratory Tract

Structural or mechanical defenses of the lung offer the initial protection against a wide range of potential respiratory tract pathogens of all types, be they bacterial, fungal, or viral (1). The major components of the physical immune defense system of the lung are airway mucus and the mucociliary escalator. Mucus, composed of a complex mixture of polyanionic proteins, forms a barrier for bacteria that are potential respiratory pathogens. Bacteria are bound by mucus (often through the use of specific types of bacterial adhesin proteins and other molecules), and this binding leads to increased mucous secretion. This increased mucous secretion may make it easier for the mucociliary escalator to remove potential pathogens from the respiratory tract, but it may also occlude small airways and provide an even richer environment in which bacteria can multiply.

Mucus is removed from the airway by two mechanisms: cough and the mucociliary escalator. Ciliated cells are found in the tracheobronchial tree and are composed of a sophisticated system of microtubules arranged in pairs which move (fueled by ATP) in a coordinated fashion ("beating") to remove mucus from the airway. Coughing, which can arise through any one of a complicated set of reflex pathways initiated by stimulation of C-fiber receptors or rapidly adapting receptors, also aids in the expulsion of foreign particles (whether or not they are trapped in the mucus layer) from the lungs.

Examples of impairment in the physical defenses of the lung are abundant and well known, although many patients with such impairment are not usually considered immunocompromised in the usual sense. Patients with cystic fibrosis have an abnormally functioning chloride ion channel and for that reason do not produce normal mucus or normally functioning cilia. This predisposes them to recurrent infections with bacteria such as *Staphylococcus aureus* and *Pseudomonas aeruginosa* (2). As a result of the repeated and constant infection with these and other pathogens, bronchiectasis and chronic inflammation develop, leading to the typical clinical and radiographic changes seen in this disease. Other syndromes associated with ciliary dysfunction and the development of bronchiectasis include Young's syndrome, Kartagener syndrome, immotile cilia syndrome, and yellow nail syndrome. In chronic bronchitis related to cigarette smoking, there is also evidence of ciliary dysfunction. Patients with ciliary dysfunction typically are subject to repeated episodes of infection with organisms such as *Hemophilus influenzae*. The main radiographic features of pulmonary disease in patients with impaired mechanical defenses in the lung are those of bronchiectasis. Computed tomography (CT) of the lung has revolutionized our ability to appreciate bronchiectasis, and has made the performance of bronchography obsolete (3,4). Dilatated airways, i.e., airways seen in the periphery or outer third of the lung (or airways larger than their accompanying blood vessel), are the hallmarks of bronchiectasis. There is often mucus impaction seen in the dilatated or bronchiectatic airway as well. Although in the past bronchiectasis was usually observed as a consequence of repeated bouts of lower respiratory tract infections, such as viral or bacterial pneumonia occurring at an early age, or tuberculosis, these infection syndromes are less common now (at least in countries where medical care is readily available), so that the appearance of bronchiectasis, particularly in a younger patient, should prompt an evaluation for diseases such as those discussed above.

Humoral Immunity in the Lung

Humoral immunity in the lung plays an important role in defense against a large variety of pathogens, particularly bacteria that can cause disease in the lower respiratory tract. Although all immunoglobulin (Ig) isotypes can be found in the lung, the two most important in the host lung are IgA and IgG (5). IgA forms the major component of the mucosal immune system in the lung, and most of the IgA present in the respiratory tract is synthesized locally in the lung, whereas IgG is synthesized locally and transported from the circulation. IgA is important in defense against viral infections and it inhibits growth of microorganisms in the bronchial tree, although it is not a particularly effective molecule in activating complement or enhancing opsonization. Rather, IgA helps to agglutinate microorganisms and enhance their removal by the mucociliary escalator.

In contrast, IgG in the respiratory tree has a significant role in complement activation and opsonization. IgG1, IgG2, and IgG3 are the most efficient activators of complement (via the classical pathway) in the lung.

Deficiencies in immunoglobulin production, either of the IgA isotype or of the IgG isotype (particularly in subclasses IgG_{1-3}) can lead to repeated infections in the respiratory tree (6–11). Selective IgA deficiency is one of the more common immunodeficiencies; it has been reported in 1 in 500 persons in several industrialized nations, and there seems to be a familial occurrence, with autosomal dominant inheritance. Recurrent sinopulmonary infections have been reported in some of these patients, although there is no typical radiographic or clinical pattern to these events.

Common variable immunodeficiency, a disease of differentiation of B-cells, is associated with low levels of both IgG and IgA, but levels of IgM are normal. Patients with common variable immunodeficiency often have recurrent sinopulmonary infections, and they are predisposed to bronchiectasis. Unlike patients with only IgA or IgG deficiency, patients with common variable immunodeficiency may have defects in cell-mediated immunity as well, and they may present with autoimmune disease and granulomatous inflammation of the lungs, spleen, liver, and skin. Treatment is with regular infusions of gammaglobulin which prevents the development of bronchiectasis, which was a common feature of this disease in the past.

Cellular Immunity in the Lung

Cellular immunity plays a major role, if not the major role, in host defense in the lung (12,13). The resident immune cell in the lung is the alveolar macrophage, which is by far the predominant cell in the alveolar space of normal individuals in the resting state. Over 85% of cells recovered by bronchoalveolar lavage (BAL) from healthy nonsmokers are macrophages. These cells are capable of engulfing foreign microbes and inhibiting their growth or killing them directly. In addition, macrophages can send out a variety of signals that will recruit other immune cells to the lung, such as several phenotypes of lymphocytes, which in turn aid the macrophage in its attempt to rid the lung of foreign pathogens. Lymphocytes are generally found in the lung in relatively small numbers and typically comprise 10% of the resident immune cells recovered by BAL from healthy nonsmokers. Lymphocytes found in the lung include both those with helper and cytotoxic phenotypes (CD4 + TH cells, CD8 + cytotoxic T cells, and natural killer (NK) cells). The neutrophil is the third important immune/inflammatory cell type that participates in lung host defense. Neutrophils are recruited to the lungs by a variety of stimuli including cigarette smoke, bacterial products, and chemokines (chemoattractant molecules secreted by macrophages and other cells, which in turn can attract neutrophils to the lung). Neutrophils, probably the cell type most responsible for purulent inflammation such as that seen in bacterial pneumonia, produce hydrogen peroxide and other reactive oxygen species that are directly toxic to invading microbial pathogens.

Specific defects in immune cell function have been described, although in general cellular immune function is most often impaired in the setting of systemic illness or conditions such as AIDS or the postorgan-transplantation state. Diseases such as chronic granulomatous disease, in which macrophages lack the ability to respond to phagocytosis of a pathogen with the typical respiratory burst that produces reactive oxygen species such as superoxide, are rare, but they can result in repeated infections with pathogens such as *S. aureus, S. epidermidis, Serratia marcescens, Salmonella* spp., *Aspergillus* spp. and *Candida* spp. (14). Repeated infections with these pathogens at a young age, in the absence of any other predisposing conditions, should prompt consideration of this syndrome.

Defects in pulmonary host defenses occur only rarely in isolation or on a congenital basis, and the remainder of this chapter focuses largely on the acquired immune deficiency states that are now met increasingly in clinical medicine. These states usually involve impairment in several arms of the lung host defense system and are best considered as syndromes rather than isolated defects in immune function. However, the rare syndromes can serve as paradigms for understanding the immune defenses of the respiratory tract. The more well-defined syndromes, and their clinical sequelae, are listed in Table 17.1.

Major Immunodeficiency Syndromes Affecting the Lungs

The Acquired Immunoe Deficiency Syndrome

Although unknown as a clinical entity prior to the early 1980s, AIDS currently represents the most common acquired immunocompromised state in many parts of the world. Although in urban centers in the industrialized West the major risk factors for acquiring infection with the human immunodeficiency virus (HIV) are intravenous drug use and male homosexual intercourse, heterosexual transmission is probably the major mode of disease transmission in many parts of the world, especially in resource-poor countries. Current estimates by the World Health Organization (WHO) indicate that there are between 30 million 40 million persons around the world infected with HIV, and despite the wider use of potent antiretroviral regimens, it is likely that most of these

people will eventually develop fullblown AIDS (15). Therefore clinicians all over the world will face the daunting challenge of diagnosing and treating pulmonary complications in this patient population for years to come (Table 17.2). As with all immunocompromised hosts, the lungs are a major site of disease and pulmonary infections are a leading cause of morbidity and mortality in patients with HIV. In fact, reports of clusters of cases of *Pneumocystis carinii* pneumonia (PCP) in otherwise apparently healthy homosexual men constituted the first recognition of AIDS (16–19). Early reports on the pulmonary complications of AIDS included, in addition to PCP, cytomagalovirus (CMV) pneumonitis, *Legionella* pneumonia, *Mycobactenum avium* infections, and both lymphocytic interstitial pneumonitis and nonspecific interstitial pneumonitis as common respiratory illnesses (20–22). However, as more careful natural history studies have been done, it is clear that the major pulmonary complications of AIDS are bacterial pneumonia, PCP, and tuberculosis (23,24). Also, in recent years it has been well recognized that airways disease, including bronchiectasis and bronchitis, have become fairly common chronic respiratory illnesses in patients with HIV. It has also been well recognized that some pulmonary complications of HIV infection, such as PCP, occur almost exclusively in persons with CD4 + T-lymphocyte counts below 250 mm^{-3}. In formulating a differential diagnosis, it is important to be aware of the patient's level of immunosuppression as reflected by the T-lymphocyte count.

Bacterial Infections

In patients with HIV infection, even prior to the development of clinical AIDS, there is an excess of cases of bacterial pneumonia compared with age- and sex-matched controls without HIV infection (23). At CD4 + cell counts above 200 mm^{-3}, bacterial pneumonia is probably the most common pulmonary complication of HIV infection, but it is also a very common cause of acute lung disease even in patients with low CD4 + cell counts. The organisms that cause bacterial infections in patients with HIV are both the familiar pathogens causing pneumonia in noncompromised hosts and also organisms more often seen in patients with chronic lung disease. Pathogens commonly recovered from HIV-infected patients with pneumonia include *Streptococcus pneumoniae, Staphylococcus aureus, Hemophilus influenzae, Pseudomonas aeruginosa*, and *Escherichia coli*. Although infections with unusual organisms such as *Rhodococcus equii* (which radiographically can mimic tuberculosis) have occasionally been reported in patients with AIDS, other pathogens often listed as causes of atypical pneumonia, such as *Legionella pneumophila*, and *Mycoplasma pneumoniae*, have not been reported with increased frequency. Similarly, other

Table 17.1. Defects in immune function that can affect the lung

Condition	Type of defect	Mode of acquisition	Clinical syndrome	Typical pathogens
X-linked agammaglobulinemia	Block in early B-cell maturation	X-linked recessive	Paucity of plasma cells, reduced serum immunoglobilins, impaired germinal center formation; presents after the first year of life	Staphylococci, streptococci, *Hemophilus, influenzae*, measles, mumps, varicella
Selective IgA deficiency	Specific immunoglobulin deficiency	Acquired	Recurrent sinopulmonary infections, usually in adulthood	Multiple bacteria
IgG subclass deficiency	Diminished levels of IgG_2, IgG_3, IgG_4	Congenital	Recurrent lower respiratory tract infections, bronchiectasis	Multiple bacteria
Common variable immunodeficiency	Decreased IgA, IgG; increased IgM	Congenital	Recurrent or chronic infections of the lungs and sinuses; bronchiectasis; autoimmunity; granulomatous inflammation	Multiple bacteria
Chronic granulomatous disease	Impaired respiratory burst of macrophages	Congenital	Recurrent and severe lower respiratory tract infections; granulomatous inflammation; usually fatal at an early age	Staphylococci, streptococci, *Klebsiella pneumonia, Eschericha coli, Serratia marcescens, Salmonella* spp., *Aspergillus* spp., *Candida* spp.
Chediak–Higashi syndrome	Defect in granule function	Autosomal recessive	Skin abscesses and progressive pulmonary disease; death by age 10	Multiple pathogens

Ig, immunoglobulin

Table 17.2. Pulmonary complications of HIV infection

Infectious
　Bacterial pneumonias
　　Streptococcus pneumoniae
　　Staphylococcus aureus
　　Klebsiella pneumoniae
　　Hemophilus influenzae
　　Escherichia coli
　　Pseudomonas aeruginosa
　Pneumocystis carinii pneumonia
　Tuberculosis
　CMV pneumonitis
Noninfectious
　Kaposi sarcoma
　Lymphocytic interstitial pneumonitis
　Nonspecific interstitial pneumonitis
　Primary pulmonary lymphoma
　Diseases of the airways
　　Bronchiectasis
　　Chronic bronchitis
CMV, cytomegalovirus.

bacteria such as *Nocardia asteroides*, which have been known to cause pulmonary infections in compromised hosts such as transplant recipients, have not been major pathogens in AIDS.

The radiographic manifestations of bacterial pneumonia in AIDS patients appear similar to those seen in the otherwise healthy host (Fig. 17.1). Typically, localized areas of infiltrates or consolidation suggest a diagnosis of bacterial infection, and in the proper clinical context (e.g., a patient who presents with fever and a productive cough), further diagnostic testing is usually not indicated and the patient can receive an empiric course of antibiotic therapy without undergoing either CT scanning, ^{67}Ga-scanning, or bronchoscopy. As is the case in instances of community-acquired pneumoniain the non-AIDS patient, however, it is well recognized that specific etiologic diagnoses cannot be made with any degree of accuracy for cases of bacterial infections based on chest radiographic findings. Therefore close clinical monitoring is essential for AIDS patients started on antibiotic therapy in order to determine treatment response. A recent study by Boiselle and colleagues addressed the accuracy of chest radiographs in distinguishing bacterial pneumonia from PCP and tuberculosis in patients with HIV and found that in the majority of cases, this could be accomplished accurately (25). However, accuracy in diagnosis of bacterial pneumonia was somewhat lower (64%) than that noted for tuberculosis (84%) or PCP (75%), underscoring the above

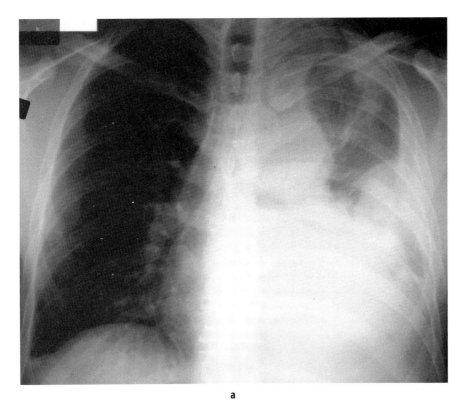

a

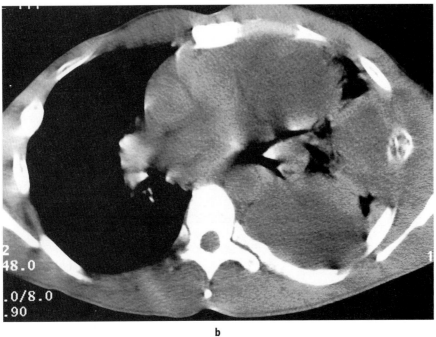

b

Figure 17.1. (a) Chest radiograph and (b) CT scan showing pneumonia and pleural effusion due to *Staphylococcus aureus* in a patient with HIV infection. The CT scan demonstrates extension of the infection into the chest wall, with the pleural fluid collection reaching into the soft tissue of the chest wall (empyema necessitatis).

remarks regarding the need for close clinical follow-up of patients.

Pneumocystis Carinii Pneumonia

AIDS currently represents the setting in which PCP is most commonly seen, although this clinical syndrome was initially described in malnourished children and was later encountered in cancer patients undergoing chemotherapy. In the USA and other industrialized nations, *Pneumocystis carinii* remains the leading opportunistic pathogen causing pneumonia in AIDS patients, although with wider use of highly active antiretroviral therapy for HIV infection itself, PCP seems to be occurring less frequently than before (26,27). Over the last 16 years, the clinical and radiographic findings of PCP in AIDS patients have been very well defined, and the infection is rarely a diagnostic challenge (28,29).

Pneumocystis carinii has recently been reclassified as a fungus, based on DNA sequence analysis. It has long been felt that *P. carinii* is present in the lungs of nearly all healthy persons by the age of 6 or 7, and that most cases of pneumonia are due to reactivation of latent organisms, though direct evidence to support this is lacking (30). Outbreaks of PCP among vulnerable populations have been well described, although respiratory isolation of patients with PCP is not generally recommended.

PCP occurs only rarely in AIDS patients with CD4 + T-cell counts above 200 mm^{-3}. At CD4 + cell counts below 200 mm^{-3}, PCP becomes more common. The clinical syndrome associated with PCP is typically that of gradually increasing dyspnea and/or nonproductive cough, accompanied eventually by fever (31). Physical findings are few but may include dry crackles heard over the lung fields. Laboratory findings almost always include a widened alveolar–arterial oxygen gradient, or oxygen desaturation with exercise, although these are obviously nonspecific findings. The serum lactate dehydrogenase (LDH) concentration is often elevated, although this is a nonspecific finding (32,33).

Chest radiographic examination in PCP usually reveals symmetric, bilateral interstitial infiltrates that may cause a diffuse haziness or ground-glass appearance (29,34). When this pattern is seen in a patient with a low CD4 + cell count and a typical clinical presentation, the diagnosis of PCP can be made with a high degree of confidence. However, other radiographic presentations have been described. Predominantly upper lobe disease has been described in patients receiving aerosolized pentamidine as prophylaxis for PCP (35–38). This mode of prevention, however, is no longer widely used. Pleural effusions have been reported, as have nodular appearing infiltrates, and miliary patterns. Pneumothorax has been frequently noted as a presenting sign in patients with AIDS and PCP, and this finding should suggest the diagnosis (39). In addition, the development of small cystic areas, particularly in the upper lung fields has been noted in patients with PCP, and these lesions are often the precursors to development of pneumothorax (Figs. 17.2, 17.3).

It has been well appreciated that early PCP can present with minimal and nonspecific clinical findings (a dry cough), no physical findings, and a normal arterial blood gas. In these cases, a plain chest radiograph may be normal. Early in the AIDS epidemic, many patients with this clinical presentation underwent ^{67}Ga-scanning in order to make a diagnosis. ^{67}Ga is taken up by activated lung macrophages and will highlight areas of active inflammation. ^{67}Ga-scanning is capable of detecting alveolitis at a low level and is therefore a sensitive indicator of pulmonary inflammation, and useful in detecting or

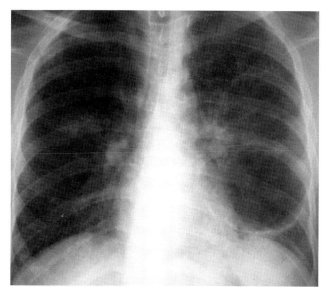

Figure 17.2. Chest radiograph showing typical patchy bilateral infiltrates in an AIDS patient with *Pneumocystis carinii* pneumonia (PCP). There is also a large pneumatocele in the left lower lung field.

suggesting the presence of PCP in many patients (40). However, the test has several limitations. First, it is expensive and may not be widely available. Second, the test is nonspecific. It yields a positive result in any of a large number of diffuse inflammatory disorders of the lungs. Third, the test takes several days to perform: the ^{67}Ga is injected on day 1, and the scan is performed a few days later. In recent years it has been recognized that CT scanning of the chest may provide a better method for detecting PCP in patients with minimal symptoms (41). PCP appears as ground-glass opacity on an high resolution CT (HRCT) scan of the chest, and this finding can be quite specific in the proper clinical context. In addition, HRCT can provide a great deal of information regarding other pulmonary conditions that might be present (42,43). In a study reported by Gruden and colleagues from San Francisco General Hospital, HRCT had a sensitivity of 100% for diagnosis of PCP, a specificity of 80%, and an overall statistical accuracy of 90%. Airways disease was also diagnosed in 23 of 51 patients (41). Hartman and colleagues reported similar advantage for HRCT over ^{67}Ga scanning in the evaluation of AIDS patients with lung disease, as did Kirshenbaum (44,45). Overall, it seems reasonable to replace ^{67}Ga scanning with HRCT for evaluation of clinically equivocal cases of PCP.

Tuberculosis

Tuberculosis remains, even outside the context of HIV infection, a public health catastrophe of almost unimaginable proportions. The WHO estimates that 2 billion

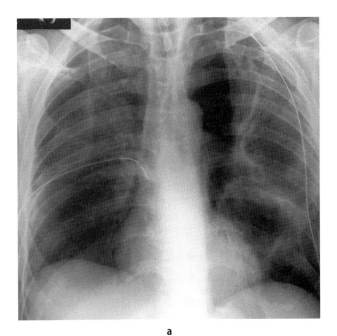

a

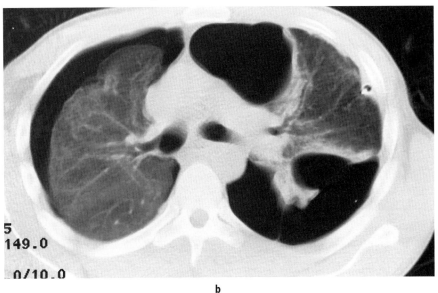

b

Figure 17.3. a Chest radiograph and **b** CT scan showing bilateral pneumothoraces in an AIDS patient with PCP. Bilateral ground-glass opacity is seen in addition to the pneumothoraces.

people, fully one third of the world's population, is infected with *Mycobacterum tuberculosis*, and that there will be nearly 8 million new cases of tuberculosis in the world each year for at least the next years, and 3 million deaths annually (46). At any given time, there are roughly 16 million people with active tuberculosis on the planet, and the vast majority of them live in very poor countries. Coinfection with HIV among tuberculosis patients in many parts of the world, particularly sub-Saharan Africa, is extremely common. The WHO estimates that at least one in three of patients with active tuberculosis in Africa are coinfected with HIV. Further, there is probably a reservoir of at least 10 million HIV-seropositive persons in the world who have latent infection with *M. tuberculosis*. In

parts of Africa, tuberculosis may be the most common pulmonary infection encountered in patients with HIV infection. Such was the case in a recent study from Tanzania (24). The need for rapid and accurate diagnosis of tuberculosis in patients with HIV infection is manifest. Untreated tuberculosis in AIDS patients is associated with substantial morbidity and mortality.

The radiographic findings associated with tuberculosis have been known for nearly a century, and they have been extensively reviewed (47–50). Patients with HIV infection do not present unfamiliar radiographic manifestations of tuberculosis as much as they present a skewed distribution of typical findings, particularly as the CD4 + T-cell count falls. Typical upper lobe disease, often with cavitation, is

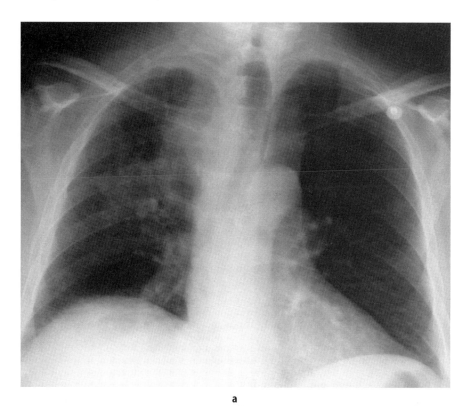

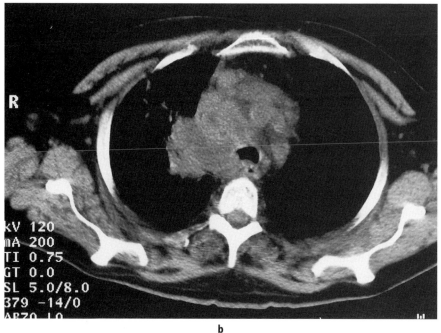

Figure 17.4. Chest radiograph (**a**) and CT scan (**b**) of an AIDS patient with tuberculosis. There is airspace disease in the right upper lobe, as well as significant right paratracheal adenopathy. On the CT scan (**b**), there is clearly necrosis within the paratracheal nodes.

seen in patients with high CD4 + cell counts. However, at lower cell counts, immune function is depressed and patients present with manifestations of tuberculosis more often thought of as reflecting primary tuberculosis. Thus mediastinal or hilar adenopathy with or without parenchymal infiltration strongly hints at a diagnosis of tuberculosis in AIDS patients (Fig. 17.4). Jones and colleagues in Los Angeles found that 34% of AIDS patients

with CD4 + cell counts lesser than 200 mm^{-3} had mediastinal adenopathy, as opposed to only 14% of those with CD4 + cell counts of greater than 200 mm^{-3} (51). Similar findings were reported by Keiper and associates in Philadelphia (52). The differential diagnosis of mediastinal adenopathy in patients with HIV includes tuberculosis, lymphoma, sarcoidosis, and infection with *M. avium* complex organisms. CT scanning can be useful in narrowing

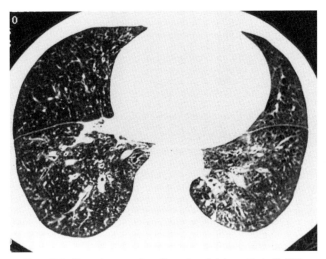

Figure 17.5. CT scan demonstrating miliary tuberculosis in a patient with AIDS.

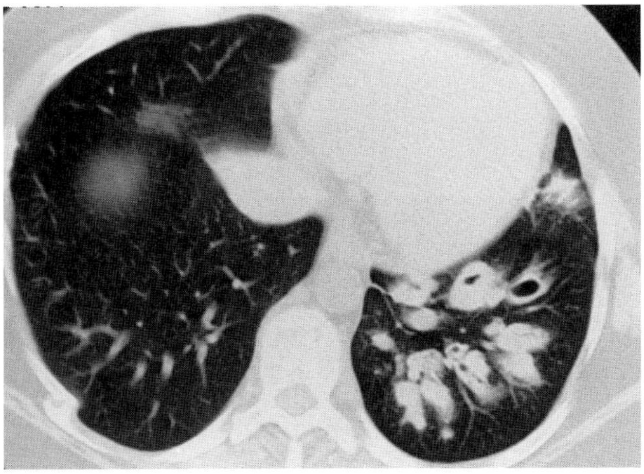

Figure 17.6. CT scan demonstrating multiple focal opacities and dilatated airways in a patient with HIV infection. *Mycobacterium avium* complex was the only pathogen recovered from this patient.

the differential diagnosis of adenopathy in AIDS patient (53). Although the radiographic features of tuberculous mediastinal adenopathy are somewhat nonspecific, the presence of necrosis within the lymph nodes strongly suggests the diagnosis. This finding is uncommon in sarcoidosis or lymphoma. In addition, CT scanning can provide a useful roadmap for transbronchial needle aspiration biopsies of abnormal lymph nodes.

Tuberculous pleurisy is also seen more commonly in patients with HIV infection, although the presence of a pleural effusion in an AIDS patients may also represent pleural involvement with Kaposis' sarcoma, or lymphoma (54). There are no specific radiographic features that allow differentiation between these when they are confined to the pleural space. Although classically tuberculous pleurisy is a manifestation of primary tuberculosis and occurs without parenchymal involvement, effusions have been noted in the presence of lung disease as well. A miliary presentation is more common in patients with HIV infection as well (Fig. 17.5).

Despite the fact that disseminated infection with *M. avium* complex organisms is a well-known complication of advanced AIDS, isolated pulmonary disease caused by this organism is uncommon. When it does occur, it can take the form of isolated mediastinal adenopathy, or as focal infiltrates in the lungs, usually without cavity formation (55) (Fig. 17.6).

Fungal Infections

The occurrence of fungal pneumonias in patients with HIV infection varies widely with geographic distribution. Histoplasmosis (*Histoplasma capsulatum*), coccidioidomycosis (*Coccidioides immitis*), and blastomycosis (*Blastomyces* spp.) have all been reported as complications of HIV infection in areas in which these fungi are endemic (56–58). The most well-described geographic fungal infection in

AIDS patients has been histoplasmosis, which occurs both in the Midwest of the USA and in the Caribbean region. Although in healthy patients histoplasmosis is usually a well-tolerated and relatively mild form of community-acquired pneumonia, in AIDS patients the fungus can disseminate and cause a severe systemic illness (59). The radiographic appearance of histoplasmosis in these cases is that of a miliary pattern, and it can mimic tuberculosis or miliary forms of PCP (Fig. 17.7).

Cryptococcus neoformans (crytpococcosis) is probably the most common form of nongeographic fungus which

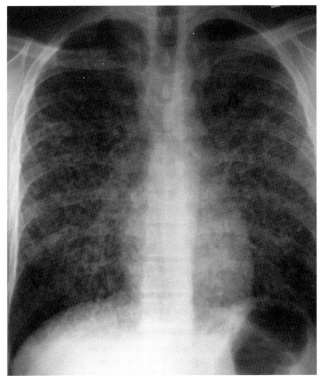

Figure 17.7. Plain chest radiograph demonstrating disseminated histoplasmosis in a patient with HIV infection. There is a typical miliary pattern seen.

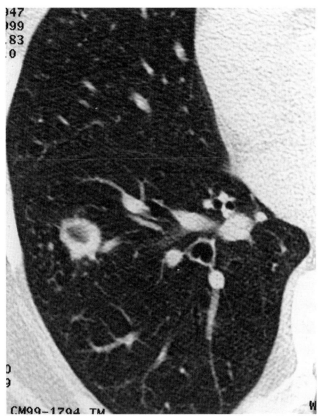

Figure 17.8. Close-up image of a CT scan demonstrating cryptococcus in an AIDS patient. There is a nodular lesion with central necrosis seen.

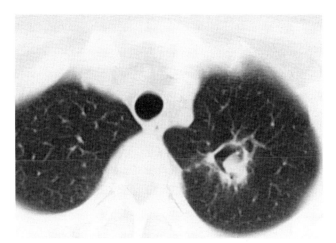

Figure 17.9. CT image of an aspergilloma with some surrounding parenchymal infiltration in the left upper lobe of a patient with AIDS.

occurs in AIDS patients (60,61). In most cases, pulmonary cryptococcosis occurs in the setting of systemic cryptococcal infection or cryptococcal meningitis, although isolated pulmonary cases have been described. Typically, cryptococcal pulmonary disease takes the form of patchy infiltrates, or more typically, nodular densities (Fig. 17.8). These can be relatively stable from a radiographic point of view before enlarging and causing symptomatic illness.

Invasive aspergillosis (*Aspergillus* spp) has been reported in patients with extremely advanced AIDS (CD4 + T-cell count <50 mm^{-3}), usually in the setting of accompanying neutropenia and corticosteroid administration (62). This infection presents radiographically as nodular infiltrates that are usually progressive despite therapy. Invasive aspergillosis is often a postmortem diagnosis in AIDS patients. Aspergillomas have also been reported to occur in patients with HIV (63) (Fig. 17.9).

Viral Infections

CMV, which is known to be a significant cause of morbidity and mortality in other types of compromised host such as bone marrow and solid organ transplant recipients, is frequently recovered from the lungs of AIDS patients. It is usually not found as an isolated pathogen and is generally regarded as a colonizer rather than a cause of disease in patients with HIV (64). However, CMV pneumonitis does occur occasionally, and radiographic findings include ground-glass opacities, consolidation, bronchiectasis, and interstitial thickening without airspace disease (Fig. 17.10). In a report by McGuiness and colleagues from Bellevue Hospital in New York, airspace disease was the predominant finding (65).

Noninfectious Pulmonary Syndromes

Noninfectious pulmonary syndromes in AIDS patients include Kaposi sarcoma, lymphoma, lymphocytic interstitial pneumonitis (LIP), and nonspecific interstitial pneumonitis (NSIP). Of these, only Kaposi sarcoma, which occurs mainly in homosexual men and seems to be declining in incidence, has a typical radiographic presentation (66). On plain films and CT scans, this entity is often manifest as perihilar nodular densities, which in the setting of typical skin findings strongly suggest the diagnosis (Fig. 17.11). Endobronchial Kaposi lesions can also cause blockage of airways and postobstructive pneumonia. Isolated pulmonary lymphoma is an uncommon complication of AIDS. LIP and NSIP present as interstitial processes without unique radiographic features.

Airways diseases, primarily chronic bronchitis and bronchiectasis, are being recognized with increasing frequency in patients with HIV infection. McGuiness and colleagues in New York described findings in patients examined with high resolution CT (HRCT) (3,4). They reported that 8 of their 12 patients had had prior bacterial infections, and that 4 had had opportunistic infections. Although the appearance of bronchiectasis was typical, the rapid pace of development and extent of disease were striking. Associated pneumonitis, often in the form of bronchiolitis appearing as a so-called "tree-in-bud" pattern was also common.

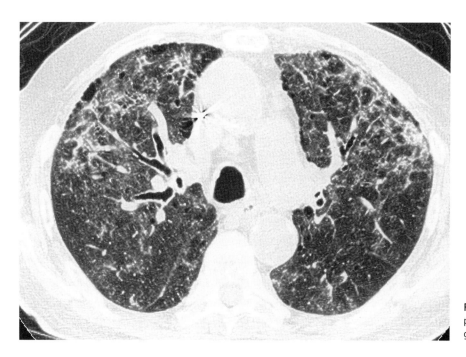

Figure 17.10. CT image of CMV pneumonitis in a patient with AIDS. Bronchiectasis as well as ground-glass opacities are present.

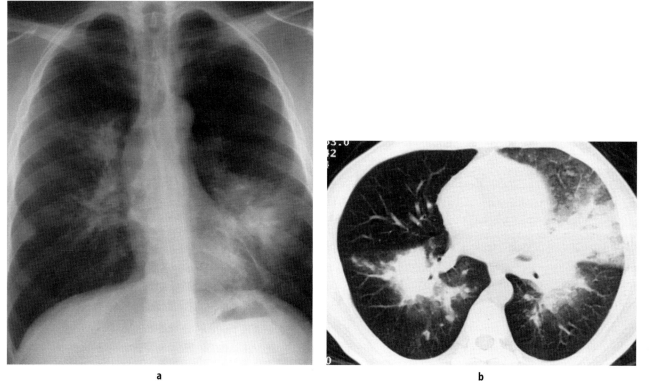

a   b

Figure 17.11. Plain chest radiograph (**a**) and CT scan (**b**) of an AIDS patient with Kaposi sarcoma. Note the typical perihilar location of the densities.

Bone Marrow and Solid Organ Transplantation

Pulmonary complications arising in patients undergoing bone marrow and solid organ transplantation are common, and are usually related to the immunosuppression required to prevent rejection of the allograft (Table 17.3). Although in some countries the number of cadaveric transplants has leveled off or even dropped, wider using of living donors for kidney, liver, and lung transplantation will probably ensure continued growth in the total number of transplants performed in the next several years. Thus familiarity with the pulmonary complications related to these operations will be important for clinicians and radiologists. In fact, there is evidence that demonstrates that prompt diagnosis of pulmonary complications, particularly infections, is associated with a survival benefit (67). There is substantial overlap in the infectious complications related to solid organ transplantation, and the common morbidities associated with these operations will be considered without regard to transplant type (68–76). The complications unique to each of these procedures are discussed separately.

Noninfectious Complications

In the immediate posttransplant period, a large number of noninfectious pulmonary complications may occur (77). Many of these are not related to transplantation per se, but rather are common postoperative findings in patients undergoing major surgery. However, some are tied directly to the specific type of transplant that was performed. Patients undergoing liver transplantation are prone to development of atalectasis and pleural effusions postoperatively in a large number of patients. Most effusions that develop after liver transplantation are right sided, although at times bilateral effusions occur. In a recent series from Spain, Durán and colleagues reported that 70 of 187 patients developed pleural effusion after liver transplant; and the vast majority of these occurred in the first 48 h following surgery (70). Adult respiratory distress syndrome (ARDS) may also occur following solid organ transplantation, and this is often linked to the presence of multiple transfusions, aspiration, sepsis, or acute organ rejection or dysfunction. Pulmonary calcification has been seen following liver and kidney transplantation. The mechanism of this complication is not clear, but it may be related to exogenous calcium administration leading to metastatic deposition of calcium in the soft tissues, including the interstitial space and alveoli. Radiographically, these lesions often present as multiple small nodules, although single, dense, pulmonary lesions have been reported. Pulmonary edema, as part of ARDS or representing fluid overload, is also a common posttransplant finding in solid organ recipients.

Posttransplant proliferative disorder (PTLD) is an immunosuppression related disease that occurs in 1–3% of patients after bone marrow, kidney, and liver transplantation, and in 5–10% of patients after heart, lung, or

Table 17.3. Noninfectious complications of organ transplantation

Complication	Bone marrow transplantation	Kidney transplantation	Liver transplantation	Heart transplantation	Lung and heart–lung transplantation
Alveolar hemorrhage	X				
Aspiration	X				
ARDS	X		X	X	X
Pulmonary edema	X	X		X	X
Thromboembolism	X	X			
Metastatic calcification		X	X		
Bronchiolitis obliterans	X				X
Pleural effusion			X	X	
Acute rejection					X
Airway dehiscence					X
Atalectasis			X	X	
Posttransplant lymphoproliferative disorder	X	X	X	X	X

ARDS, adult respiratory distress syndrome.

heart–lung transplantation (78–83). For reasons that are unclear, PTLD seems to occur earlier in the postoperative period following bone marrow, lung, and heart–lung transplants (first 2–5 months) than after heart, kidney, and liver transplants (23–32 months after surgery). Though pathologically PTLD seems closely related to B-cell lymphoma (and may be causally associated with Epstein–Barr virus infection), reduction in immunosuppression is often the only therapeutic intervention required.

The radiographic appearance of PTLD is usually that of pulmonary nodules which are noncavitary. There is no characteristic distribution for these nodules, and at times there is a small amount of accompanying ground-glass opacity or airspace consolidation.

One of the most important and potentially serious pulmonary complications of transplantation is bronchiolitis obliterans. This lesion is represented pathologically by constrictive bronchiolitis and obliteration of the bronchial lumen by peribronchiolar fibrosis. There may also be granulation tissue within the lumen of the airway. Bronchiolitis obliterans is seen in the context of lung transplantation, heart–lung transplantation, and bone marrow transplantation (84–86). In the context of heart-lung and lung transplantation, this pathologic entity is felt by most to represent chronic rejection, although some linkage to CMV infection has also been proposed. In the context of bone marrow transplantation bronchiolitis obliterans may be a pulmonary manifestation of graft-versus-host disease (GVHD). Whether these lesions occur in the context of lung or bone marrow transplantation, they represent a serious threat to the patient's life. Therefore, early diagnosis and intervention is crucial.

Following lung transplantation, bronchiolitis obliterans (BO) occurs in the majority of patients. In a report from one center in California, the prevalence of this lesion in lung allograft recipients surviving longer than 3 months was 68%, with 28% of patients developing the lesion within the first posttransplant year (87). The eventual risk of developing bronchiolitis obliterans in lung transplant recipients may reach as high as 80%. The timing of development of BO is highly variable. A report from the highly experienced group at the University of Pittsburgh indicated that BO occurs on average 434 ± 422 days following transplantation, though the range of onset was from 60 to 2058 days following surgery (88). Still, most patients who develop BO do so in the first 2 years after undergoing transplantation. The impact of this lesion on survival is striking: in the Pittsburgh series only 40% of those developing BO survived for 4 years, while 4 year survival in the group of patients without BO was 80%.

Radiographic findings in BO following lung or heart-lung transplantation are highly variable. In early BO, the chest radiograph may be normal, and the only symptom of the disease may be a fall in forced expiratory volume in 1 s (FEV_1). However, as the disease progresses and the lesion worsens, radiographic changes begin to appear, although they can be quite nonspecific. Plain films may show volume loss and subsegmental atalectasis, but by the time these findings appear, the disease process may be quite advanced (Fig. 17.12). Recently there has been substantial interest in the use of HRCT for early detection of BO in patients who have undergone lung transplantation. Worthy and colleagues form the University of British Columbia in Vancouver described the findings of BO in 15 patients with biopsy-proven disease (72). Bronchial dilatation was found in 80%, mosaic perfusion (a finding consistent with air-trapping and a radiographic correlate of the physiologic finding of a diminished FEV_1) in 40%, bronchial wall thickening in 27%, and air-trapping on 80%. Bronchial dilatation, mosaic perfusion, and air-trapping were found in 22%, 22%, and 6%, respectively, of control subjects without BO. In another study by Leung and colleagues from Stanford University in California air-trapping was the most sensitive and specific indicator of BO (89). In children, Lau and co-workers from Washington University in St. Louis found essentially similar results (90).

Ikonen and colleagues from Finland have evaluated the use of prospective evaluation with HRCT for early detection of BO (91,92). In a recent study they evaluated 13 consecutive patients with a total of 140 CT scans. Scans were performed monthly for the first 3–6 months following lung transplantation, then every 3 months for the remainder of the first posttransplant year, and every 6 or 12 months thereafter. Additional CT scans were also performed whenever there was suspicion of an intercurrent pulmonary illness. The average number of scans performed per patient was 11 ± 5.7. Ten of the 13 patients studied developed chronic changes seen on CT. These included segmental and subsegmental

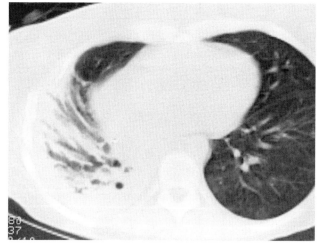

Figure 17.12. CT scan showing advanced bronchiolitis obliterans (BO) in the allograft of a patient who had undergone right lung transplantation. There is extensive consolidation and bronchiectasis.

bronchial dilatation, peripheral bronchial narrowing, diminution of peripheral vascular markings, hyperlucency, mosaic perfusion, peribronchial infiltrates, thickening of septal lines, and both volume contraction and expansion. Eight of the 13 patients in the study developed histologically proven BO. Although the three patients who did not develop BO did not have chronic changes on HRCT, the experience with this technique is too small to recommend routine use of HRCT as a screening tool to detect BO in asymptomatic posttransplant patients.

As noted above, BO also occurs following bone marrow transplantation, where it may be a manifestation of graft versus host disease. Radiographic manifestations of BO following bone marrow transplantation have not, however, been as thoroughly investigated as those seen after lung transplantation. Palmas and colleagues from the Mayo Clinic reported on noninfectious complications following bone marrow transplantation in 179 consecutive patients surviving 3 months after bone marrow transplant (93). The overall incidence of these complications was only 10% (18 patients), much lower than was observed for lung transplant. Of the 18 patients with lung disease, 8 had either bronchiolitis obliterans or bronchiolitis obliterans with organizing pneumonia. In a separate study, Ooi and co-workers from Hong Kong found that findings on HRCT in bone marrow transplant related BO may not be as constant as for the same disease seen after lung transplant (94). In a study of 7 children who have had bone marrow transplant, HRCT findings of BO were similar to those seen following lung transplant and included air-trapping and segmental or subsegmental bronchial dilatation, although bronchial wall thickening was not observed.

Infectious Complications

Infectious complications of most solid organ transplants follow a fairly predictable pattern that was first well described by Rubin in patients undergoing renal transplantation (95). In the first month following transplantation, bacterial infections were more commonly observed that any opportunistic pathogens. These pneumonias have the clinical and radiographic features typical of nosocomial pulmonary infections, and there are no specific radiographic findings that suggest one etiologic organism over another.

Prior to the widespread use of prophylactic therapy with trimethoprim- sulfamethoxazole or other agents, PCP was a significant cause of morbidity and mortality in the early posttransplant period, usually within the first 6 months following surgery (68,69). However, since prophylaxis has become routine, this infection is extremely uncommon. Several studies indicate that when PCP does occur in the non-AIDS setting, the radiographic features

are similar to those seen in HIV-infected individuals, although the clinical course may be somewhat accelerated, and mortality can be high (96).

Fungal infections in organ transplant recipients occur in a manner similar to then occurrence in AIDS patients. In the past few years, a syndrome of *Aspergillus* pseudomembranous tracheobronchitis has been recognized (97,98). This illness can present with signs and symptoms of airway obstruction, and radiographs will show evidence of volume loss, with perhaps an endobronchial lesion seen on HRCT. At bronchoscopy a typical pseudomembrane is seen in the large airways, and biopsies reveal fungal forms. This lesion is typically seen in the same type of patient who develops invasive aspergillosis, namely those with severe neutropenia and steroid use.

Viral pneumonias in organ transplant recipients appear to be a much greater cause of morbidity and mortality than in patients with HIV infection. Important viral pathogens in these patients include the herpesviruses (HSV), respiratory syncytial virus (RSV), and CMV. HSV generally causes mucocutaneous illness in transplant patients, and HSV pneumonia is uncommon. Herpes infections are not seasonal, and their radiographic appearance as pneumonia is that of patchy and diffuse infiltrates, which can show both ground-glass and nodular densities. RSV is seasonal (occurring in the winter and spring) and can cause a devastating illness, particularly in pediatric bone marrow transplant recipients (99,100). The radiographic features of pneumonia caused by RSV are nonspecific, usually presenting as diffuse infiltrates. Early consideration and recognition of this illness is important because specific therapy with antiviral agents such as ribaviran may increase survival , and because there is great potential for transmission to other vulnerable patients if isolation and treatment are not instituted promptly.

CMV is the most significant viral pathogen in transplant patients, especially in bone marrow recipients. In noncompromised hosts, CMV is essentially unknown as a cause of pneumonia, and does not generally cause symptomatic disease of any kind, although serologic evidence demonstrates that a large proportion of the population has had asymptomatic infection. The risk of developing pneumonia (or other illness) due to CMV is directly related to the CMV serostatus of the organ donor and recipient, with the highest risk occurring in situations where a CMV seronegative recipient receives an organ from a CMV seropositive donor (101,102). In these situations, the risk of developing CMV disease is of the order of 70%, whereas, if both donor and recipient are CMV seronegative, disease occurs rarely. In addition, the risk of CMV pneumonia varies with the type of transplant (probably a manifestation of the intensity of immunosuppression needed to prevent rejection of different organs or tissues). Allogeneic bone marrow transplant recipients are at highest risk, followed by those receiving lung, liver, heart, and kidney transplants. Untreated CMV pneumonitis in bone marrow transplant patients has a mortality in excess of 85%, but therapy with gancyclovir and CMV immunoglobulin, if instituted early, can reduce this substantially (103). Prophylactic treatment in high risk patients sharply reduced the incidence of CMV pneumonitis in one study from Australia (104).

In patients who have had bone marrow transplants, CMV pneumonitis generally has onset near the end of the second posttransplant month. In solid organ transplant recipients, the onset may be a month or so later. Radiographic findings in CMV are similar to those seen with other viral infections (105). Abnormalities include reticulonodular opacities, presumably representing interstitial thickening seen in pathology specimens. Airspace consolidation generally does not occur except in cases that have progressed to severe disease, and focal consolidation and nodules are also uncommon. HRCT usually reveals ground-glass opacity in a patchy distribution, with septal thickening (Fig. 17.13).

Other infectious pathogens in organ transplant recipients include *M. tuberculosis*, *Nocardia* spp., and *Legionella* spp. Nocardiosis (Fig. 17.14), which can present as a syndrome of nodular lesions in the lungs and central nervous system, or consolidation with abscess formation in the lung, may be less common since the widespread use of trimethoprim–sulfamethoxazole as prophylactic therapy for PCP (106). The radiographic appearance of tuberculosis or legionellosis is not significantly different from that of AIDS patients and even normal hosts, although as noted above legionellosis is uncommon in patients with HIV infection.

Other Immunocompromised States

The widespread and aggressive use of powerful immunosuppressive agents such as high dose corticosteroids,

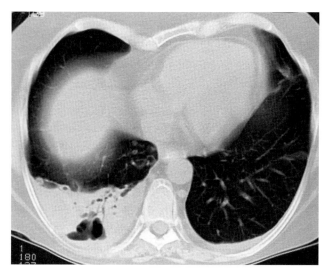

Figure 17.14. CT scan showing focal consolidation and abscess formation due to nocardiosis in a patient who had undergone heart transplantation.

cyclophosphamide, methotrexate and azathioprine in the treatment of collagen-vascular diseases as well as primary lung diseases such as idiopathic pulmonary fibrosis (IPF, cryptogenic fibrosing alveolitis) of the usual interstitial pneumonitis type has greatly enlarged the population of patients at risk for opportunistic infections. In general, the clinical and radiographic appearance of opportunistic pneumonias in these settings is not significantly different from what has been discussed above, but the recognition of them may be more difficult because they can be masked by underlying disease in the lung. This is especially true in the case of patients with IPF or cryptogenic fibrosing alveolitis. In these situations, a heightened clinical suspicion is needed – perhaps more aggressive use of HRCT to look for subtle changes in the lung fields.

Drug-Induced Pulmonary Disease

Many patients with serious underlying disorders such as collagen-vascular illness are treated with drugs that are not only immunosuppressive but can also cause lung disease in and of themselves. For this reason, radiologists and clinicians must have familiarity with the possibility of drug-induced pulmonary disease in these patients. Drug induced reactions to commonly used agents may result in interstitial fibrosis, hypersensitivity pneumonitis, or noncardiogenic pulmonary edema. The list of agents associated with these reactions is long. Commonly used immunosuppressive drugs that cause cytotoxic reactions (most often manifest as pulmonary fibrosis) include azathioprine, cyclophosphamide, and methotrexate. Methotrexate can cause a clinical and radiographic picture consistent with hypersensitivity pneumonitis as well, and cyclophosphamide has

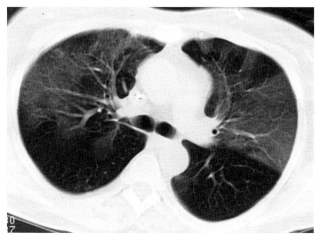

Figure 17.13. CT scan showing typical bilateral ground-glass opacities in the lungs of a patient who had undergone allogeneic bone marrow transplantation for acute leukemia.

been associated with the development of noncardiogenic pulmonary edema, as has the therapeutic pan-T-cell antibody OKT3. In a study by Malik and colleagues from the Mayo Clinic, two major patterns of pulmonary toxicity associated with cyclophosphamide were observed: early-onset and late-onset pneumonitis (107). Early onset pneumonitis (fever, dyspnea, and interstitial infiltrates) responded to corticosteroid administration and prompt cessation of the drug. Late-onset pneumonitis mimicked pulmonary fibrosis and was relentlessly progressive despite withdrawal of the drug. Methotrexate pulmonary toxicity has been described after a review of data from a number of centers treating patients for rheumatoid arthritis (108). Patients with methotrexate pulmonary toxicity presented with dyspnea, cough, and fever, which were present for 2–4 weeks before a diagnosis was made in most cases. No consistent radiographic pattern was identified, but in all cases the chest radiographs and/or CT scans were abnormal.

Conclusion

The spectrum of pulmonary disease in the immunocompromised host is vast, and from a clinical standpoint the magnitude of the challenge is likely to become even greater, as the number of patients undergoing organ transplantation, or who are undergoing treatment with powerful immunosuppressive drugs, or who have HIV infection continues to grow. Very few of the pulmonary complications associated with these disorders have pathognomonic radiographic features, and the key to early diagnosis lies in the recognition of subtle abnormalities on chest radiographs and CT scans in conjunction with a thorough knowledge of the type and timing of respiratory illness associated with various immunocompromised states. Radiologists and clinicians must work side by side in these circumstances in order to lower the substantial morbidity and mortality often accompanying lung disease in these patients with serious underlying diseases.

References

1. Widdicombe J (1997) Physical defenses of the lung. In Stockley RA (ed) Pulmonary defences. John Wiley & Sons, West Sussex, pp 1–16

2. Tummler B, Kiewitz C (1999) Cystic fibrosis: an inherited susceptibility to bacterial respiratory infections. Mol Med Today 5:351–358.

3. McGuinness G, Naidich DP, Leitman BS, et al. (1993) Bronchiectasis: CT evaluation. AJR 160:253–259.

4. McGuinness G, Naidich DP (1995) Bronchiectasis: CT/clinical correlations. Semin Ultrasound CT MR 16:395–419.

5. Jeffries R (1997) Immunoglobulins. In Stockley R (ed) Pulmonary defences. John Wiley & Sons, West Sussex, pp 39–58.

6. Bjorkander J, Bake B, Oxelius VA, et al. (1985) Impaired lung function in patients with IgA deficiency and low levels of IgG2 or IgG3. N Engl J Med 313:720–724.

7. Cantani A, Ferrara M (1988) The lung and primary immunodeficiency. Allergol Immunopathol (Madr) 16:429–437.

8. DeCoteau WE (1974) The role of secretory IgA in defense of the distal lung. Ann NY Acad Sci 221:214–219.

9. Hanson LA, Bjorkander J, Robbins JB (1986) IgG subclass deficiencies. Vox Sang 51(Suppl 2):50–56.

10. Morell A (1994) Clinical relevance of IgG subclass deficiencies. Ann Biol Clin 52:49–52.

11. Rubinstein I, Baum GL (1984) Selective IgA deficiency associated with recurrent sinopulmonary infections in sarcoidosis. Eur J Respir Dis 65:550–552.

12. Pabst R (1997) Localisation and dynamics of lymphoid cells in the different compartments of the lung. In: Stockley R, (ed) Pulmonary defences. John Wiley & Sons, West Sussex, pp 59–76.

13. Poulter L (1997) Pulmonary macrophages. In Stockley R, (ed) Pulmonary defences. John Wiley & Sons, West Sussex, pp 77–92.

14. Meischl C, Roos D (1998) The molecular basis of chronic granulomatous disease. Springer Semin Immunopathol 19:417–434.

15. Nicoll A, Gill ON (1999) The global impact of HIV infection and disease. Commun Dis Public Health 2(2):85–95.

16. Gottlieb MS, Schroff R, Schanker HM et al. (1981) Pneumocystis carinii pneumonia and mucosal candidiasis in previously healthy homosexual men: Evidence of a new acquired cellular immunodeficiency. N Engl J Med 305:1425–1431.

17. Masur H, Michelis MA, Greene JB, et al. (1981) An outbreak of community-acquired Pneumocystis carinii pneumonia: Initial manifestation of cellular immune dysfunction. N Engl J Med 305:1431–1438.

18. Pneumocystis pneumonia – Los Angeles. MMWR Morb Mortal Wkly Rep 30:250–252.

19. Kaposi's sarcoma and Pneumocystis pneumonia among homosexual men – New York City and California. MMWR Morb Mortal Wkly Rep 30:305–308.

20. Murray JF, Mills J (1990) Pulmonary infectious complications of human immunodeficiency virus infection. Part I. Am Rev Respir Dis 141:1356–1372.

21. Murray JF, Mills J (1990) Pulmonary infectious complications of human immunodeficiency virus infection. Part II. Am Rev Respir Dis 141:1582–1598.

22. Murray JF, Felton CP, Garay SM, et al. (1984) Pulmonary complications of the acquired immunodeficiency syndrome. Report of a National Heart, Lung, and Blood Institute workshop. N Engl J Med 310:1682–1688.

23. Hirschtick RE, Glassroth J, Jordan MC, et al. (1995) Bacterial pneumonia in persons infected with the human immunodeficiency virus. Pulmonary complications of HIV Infection Study Group [see comments]. N Engl J Med 333:845–851.

24. Daley CL, Mugusi F, Chen LL, et al. (1996) Pulmonary complications of HIV infection in Dar es Salaam, Tanzania. Role of bronchoscopy and bronchoalveolar lavage. Am J Respir Crit Care Med 154:105–110.

25. Boiselle PM, Tocino I, Hooley RJ, et al. (1997) Chest radiograph interpretation of Pneumocystis carinii pneumonia, bacterial pneumonia, and pulmonary tuberculosis in HIV-positive patients: Accuracy, distinguishing features, and mimics. J Thorac Imaging 12:47–53.

26. Law MG, de Winter L, McDonald A, et al. (1999) AIDS diagnoses at higher CD4 counts in Australia following the introduction of highly active antiretroviral treatment. Aids 13:263–269.

27. Paul S, Gilbert HM, Ziecheck W, et al. (1999) The impact of potent antiretroviral therapy on the characteristics of hospitalized patients with HIV infection. Aids 13:415–418.

28. Crans CA, Jr, Boiselle PM (1999) Imaging features of Pneumocystis carinii pneumonia. Crit Rev Diagn Imaging 40:251–284.

29. Boiselle PM, Crans CA, Jr, Kaplan MA (1999) The changing face of Pneumocystis carinii pneumonia in AIDS patients. AJR 172:1301–1309.

30. Hughes WT (1998) Current issues in the epidemiology, transmission, and reactivation of Pneumocystis carinii. Semin Respir Infect 13:283–288.

31. Elvin K, Lidman C, Tynell E, et al. Natural history of asymptomatic and symptomatic pneumocystis carinii infection in HIV infected patients. Scand J Infect Dis 26:643–651.

32. Garay SM, Greene J (1989) Prognostic indicators in the initial presentation of Pneumocystis carinii pneumonia. Chest 95:769–772.

33. Boldt MJ, Bai TR (1997) Utility of lactate dehydrogenase vs radiographic severity in the differential diagnosis of Pneumocystis carinii pneumonia. Chest 111:1187–1192.

34. Kuhlman JE (1996) Pneumocystic infections: the radiologist's perspective. Radiology 198:623–635.

35. Sanders TG, Northup HM, Wilf LH (1991) Case report: Bilateral upper lobe Pneumocystis carinii pneumonia in a patient receiving aerosolized pentamidine. Clin Radiol 43:356–357.

36. Kennedy CA, Goetz MB (1992) Atypical roentgenographic manifestations of Pneumocystis carinii pneumonia. Arch Intern Med 152:1390–1398.

37. Levine SJ, Kennedy D, Shelhamer JH, et al. (1992) Diagnosis of Pneumocystis carinii pneumonia by multiple lobe, site-directed bronchoalveolar lavage with immunofluorescent monoclonal antibody staining in human immunodeficiency virus-infected patients receiving aerosolized pentamidine chemoprophylaxis. Am Rev Respir Dis 146:838–843.

38. Fahy JV, Chin DP, Schnapp LM, et al. Effect of aerosolized pentamidine prophylaxis on the clinical severity and diagnosis of Pneumocystis carinii pneumonia. Am Rev Respir Dis 146:844–848

39. Sepkowitz KA, Telzak EE, Gold JW, et al. (1991) Pneumothorax in AIDS. Ann Intern Med 114:455–459.

40. Wassie E, Buscombe JR, Miller RF, et al. (1996) ^{67}Ga scintigraphy in HIV antibody positive patients: A review of its clinical usefulness. Br J Radiol 67:349–352.

41. Gruden JF, Huang L, Turner J, et al. (1997) High-resolution CT in the evaluation of clinically suspected Pneumocystis carinii pneumonia in AIDS patients with normal, equivocal, or nonspecific radiographic findings. AJR 169:967–975.

42. Primack SL, Müller NL (1994) High-resolution computed tomography in acute diffuse lung disease in the immunocompromised patient. Radiol Clin North Am 32:731–744.

43. Shah RM, Salazar AM (1998) CT manifestations of human immunodeficiency virus (HIV)-related pulmonary infections. Semin Ultrasound CT MR 19:167–174.

44. Hartman TE, Primack SL, Müller NL, et al. (1994) Diagnosis of thoracic complications in AIDS: Accuracy of CT. AJR 162:547–553.

45. Kirshenbaum KJ, Burke R, Fanapour F, et al. (1998) Pulmonary high-resolution computed tomography versus gallium scintigraphy: Diagnostic utility in the diagnosis of patients with AIDS who have chest symptoms and normal or equivocal chest radiographs. J Thorac Imaging 13:52–57.

46. Dye C, Scheele S, Dolin P, et al. (1999) Consensus statement. Global burden of tuberculosis: Estimated incidence, prevalence, and mortality by country. WHO Global Surveillance and Monitoring Project. JAMA 282:677–686.

47. Washington L, Miller WT, Jr (1998) Mycobacterial infection in immunocompromised patients. J Thorac Imaging 13:271–281.

48. Pirronti T, Cecconi L, Sallustio G, (1998) Diagnostic imaging of pulmonary tuberculosis. Rays 23:93–114.

49. Goodman PC (1990) Pulmonary tuberculosis in patients with acquired immunodeficiency syndrome. J Thorac Imaging 5:38–45.

50. Goodman PC (1995) Tuberculosis and AIDS. Radiol Clin North Am 33:707–717.

51. Jones BE, Young SM, Antoniskis D, et al. (1993) Relationship of the manifestations of tuberculosis to CD4 cell counts in patients with human immunodeficiency virus infection [see comments]. Am Rev Respir Dis 148:1292–1297.

52. Keiper MD, Beumont M, Elshami A, et al. (1995) CD4 T lymphocyte count and the radiographic presentation of pulmonary tuberculosis. A study of the relationship between these factors in patients with human immunodeficiency virus infection. Chest 107:74–80.

53. Harkin TJ, Ciotoli C, Addrizzo-Harris DJ, et al. (1998) Transbronchial needle aspiration (TBNA) in patients infected with HIV. Am J Respir Crit Care Med 157:1913–1918.

54. Frye MD, Pozsik CJ, Sahn SA (1997) Tuberculous pleurisy is more common in AIDS than in non-AIDS patients with tuberculosis. Chest 112:393–397.

55. El-Solh AA, Nopper J, Abdul-Khoudoud MR, et al. (1998) Clinical and radiographic manifestations of uncommon pulmonary nontuberculous mycobacterial disease in AIDS patients. Chest 114:138–145.

56. Conces DJ, Jr (1999) Endemic fungal pneumonia in immunocompromised patients. J Thorac Imaging 14:1–8.

57. Davies SF, Sarosi GA (1997) Epidemiological and clinical features of pulmonary blastomycosis. Semin Respir Infect 12:206–218

58. Bradsher RW (1996) Histoplasmosis and blastomycosis. Clin Infect Dis 22(Suppl 2):S102–S111.

59. Wheat LJ, Connolly-Stringfield PA, Baker RL, et al. (1990) Disseminated histoplasmosis in the acquired immune deficiency syndrome: Clinical findings, diagnosis and treatment, and review of the literature. Medicine (Baltimore) 69:361–374.

60. Cameron ML, Bartlett JA, Gallis HA, (1991) Manifestations of pulmonary cryptococcosis in patients with acquired immunodeficiency syndrome. Rev Infect Dis 13:64–67.

61. Woodring JH, Ciporkin G, Lee C, (1996) Pulmonary cryptococcosis. Semin Roentgenol 31:67–75.

62. Pursell KJ, Telzak EE, Armstrong D (1992) Aspergillus species colonization and invasive disease in patients with AIDS. Clin Infect Dis 14:141–148.

63. Addrizzo-Harris DJ, Harkin TJ, McGuinness G (1997) Pulmonary aspergilloma and AIDS. A comparison of HIV-infected and HIV-negative individuals. Chest 111:612–618.

64. Wallace JM, Hannah J (1987) Cytomegalovirus pneumonitis in patients with AIDS. Findings in an autopsy series. Chest 92:198–203.

65. McGuinness G, Scholes JV, Garay SM (1994) Cytomegalovirus pneumonitis: spectrum of parenchymal CT findings with pathologic correlation in 21 AIDS patients. Radiology 192:451–459.

66. Naidich DP, Tarras M, Garay SM (1989) Kaposi's sarcoma. CT-radiographic correlation. Chest 96:723–728.

67. Johnson PC, Hogg KM, Sarosi GA (1990) The rapid diagnosis of pulmonary infections in solid organ transplant recipients. Semin Respir Infect 5:2–9.

68. Baughman R (1999) The lung in the immunocompromised patient. Respiration 66:95–109.

69. Tamm M (1999) The lung in the immunocompromised patient. Respiration 66:199–207.

70. Durán FG, Piqueras B, Romero M, et al. (1998) Pulmonary complications following orthotopic liver transplant. Transpl Int 11(Suppl 1):S255–S259.

71. Webb WR, Gamsu G, Rohlfing BM, et al. (1978) Pulmonary complications of renal transplantation: a survey of patients treated by low-dose immunosuppression. Radiology 126:1–8.

72. Worthy SA, Flint JD, Müller NL (1997) Pulmonary complications after bone marrow transplantation: high-resolution CT and pathologic findings. Radiographics 17:1359–1371.

73. Edelstein CL, Jacobs JC, Moosa MR (1995) Pulmonary complications in 110 consecutive renal transplant recipients. S Afr Med J 85:160–163.

74. Afessa B, Gay PC, Plevak DJ, et al. (1993) Pulmonary complications of orthotopic liver transplantation. Mayo Clin Proc 68:427–434.

75. Garg K, Zamora MR, Tuder R (1996) Lung transplantation: Indications, donor and recipient selection, and imaging of complications. Radiographics 16:355–367.

76. Soyer P, Devine N, Frachon I, et al. (1997) Computed tomography of complications of lung transplantation. Eur Radiol 7:847–853

77. Conces DJ, Jr (1999) Noninfectious lung disease in immunocompromised patients. J Thorac Imaging 14:9–24.

78. Carignan S, Staples CA, Müller NL (1995) Intrathoracic lymphoproliferative disorders in the immunocompromised patient: CT findings. Radiology 197:53–58.

79. Cleary ML, Warnke R, Sklar J (1984) Monoclonality of lymphoproliferative lesions in cardiac-transplant recipients. Clonal analysis based on immunoglobulin-gene rearrangements. N Engl J Med 310:477–482.

80. Collins J, Müller NL, Leung AN, et al. (1998) Epstein–Barr-virus-associated lymphoproliferative disease of the lung: CT and histologic findings. Radiology 208:749–759.

81. Dodd GDd, Ledesma-Medina J, Baron RL, et al. (1992) Posttransplant lymphoproliferative disorder: Intrathoracic manifestations. Radiology 184:65–69.

82. Rappaport DC, Chamberlain DW, Shepherd FA, et al. (1998) Lymphoproliferative disorders after lung transplantation: imaging features. Radiology 206:519–524.

83. Starzl TE, Nalesnik MA, Porter KA, et al. (1984) Reversibility of lymphomas and lymphoproliferative lesions developing under cyclosporin-steroid therapy. Lancet 1:583–587.

84. Boehler A, Kesten S, Weder W, (1998) Bronchiolitis obliterans after lung transplantation: A review. Chest 114:1411–1426.

85. Schlesinger C, Meyer CA, Veeraraghavan S (1998) Constrictive (obliterative) bronchiolitis: diagnosis, etiology, and a critical review of the literature. Ann Diagn Pathol 2:321–334.

86. Yokoi T, Hirabayashi N, Ito M, et al. (1997) Broncho- bronchiolitis obliterans as a complication of bone marrow transplantation: A clinicopathological study of eight autopsy cases. Nagoya BMT Group. Virchows Arch 431:275–282.

87. Reichenspurner H, Girgis RE, Robbins RC et al. (1996) Stanford experience with obliterative bronchiolitis after lung and heart-lung transplantation. Ann Thorac Surg 62:1467–1472; discussion 1472–1473.

88. Paradis I, Yousem S, Griffith B (1993) Airway obstruction and bronchiolitis obliterans after lung transplantation. Clin Chest Med 14:751–763.

89. Leung AN, Fisher K, Valentine V, et al. (1998) Bronchiolitis obliterans after lung transplantation: Detection using expiratory HRCT. Chest 113:365–370.

90. Lau DM, Siegel MJ, Hildebolt CF, et al. (1998) Bronchiolitis obliterans syndrome: Thin-section CT diagnosis of obstructive changes in infants and young children after lung transplantation. Radiology 208:783–788.

91. Ikonen T, Kivisaari L, Taskinen E, et al. (1997) High-resolution CT in long-term follow-up after lung transplantation. Chest 111:370–376.

92. Ikonen T, Kivisaari L, Harjula AL, et al. (1996) Value of high-resolution computed tomography in routine evaluation of lung transplantation recipients during development of bronchiolitis obliterans syndrome. J Heart Lung Transplant 15:587–595.

93. Palmas A, Tefferi A, Myers JL, et al. (1998) Late-onset noninfectious pulmonary complications after allogeneic bone marrow transplantation. Br J Haematol 100:680–687.

94. Ooi GC, Peh WC, Ip M (1998) High-resolution computed tomography of bronchiolitis obliterans syndrome after bone marrow transplantation. Respiration 65:187–191.

95. Rubin RH, Wolfson JS, Cosimi AB, et al. (1981) Infection in the renal transplant recipient. Am J Med 70:405–411.

96. Kovacs JA, Hiemenz JW, Macher AM, et al. (1984) Pneumocystis carinii pneumonia: A comparison between patients with the acquired immunodeficiency syndrome and patients with other immunodeficiencies. Ann Intern Med 100:663–671.

97. Hummel M, Schuler S, Hempel S, et al. (1993) Obstructive bronchial aspergillosis after heart transplantation. Mycoses 36:425–428.

98. Kramer MR, Denning DW, Marshall SE, et al. (1991) Ulcerative tracheobronchitis after lung transplantation. A new form of invasive aspergillosis. Am Rev Respir Dis 144:552–556.

99. Krinzman S, Basgoz N, Kradin R, et al. (1998) Respiratory syncytial virus-associated infections in adult recipients of solid organ transplants. J Heart Lung Transplant 17:202–210.

100. Fouillard L, Mouthon L, Laporte JP, et al. (1992) Severe respiratory syncytial virus pneumonia after autologous bone marrow transplantation: a report of three cases and review. Bone Marrow Transplant 9:97–100.

101. Meyers JD, Flournoy N, Thomas ED (1986) Risk factors for cytomegalovirus infection after human marrow transplantation. J Infect Dis 153:478–488.

102. Peterson PK, Balfour HH, Jr, Marker SC, et al. (1980) Cytomegalovirus disease in renal allograft recipients: a prospective study of the clinical features, risk factors and impact on renal transplantation. Medicine (Baltimore) 59:283–300.

103. Winston DJ, Ho WG, Bartoni K, et al. (1988) Ganciclovir therapy for cytomegalovirus infections in recipients of bone marrow transplants and other immunosuppressed patients. Rev Infect Dis 10(Suppl 3):S547–S553.

104. Atkinson K, Nivison-Smith I, Dodds A, et al. (1998) A comparison of the pattern of interstitial pneumonitis following allogeneic bone marrow transplantation before and after the introduction of prophylactic ganciclovir therapy in 1989. Bone Marrow Transplant 21:691–695.

105. Kang EY, Patz EF, Jr, Müller NL (1996) Cytomegalovirus pneumonia in transplant patients: CT findings. J Comput Assist Tomogr 20:295–299

106. Chapman SW, Wilson JP (1990) Nocardiosis in transplant recipients. Semin Respir Infect 5:74–79.

107. Malik SW, Myers JL, DeRemee RA, et al. (1996) Lung toxicity associated with cyclophosphamide use. Two distinct patterns. Am J Respir Crit Care Med 154:1851–1856.

108. Kremer JM, Alarcon GS, Weinblatt ME, et al. (1997) Clinical, laboratory, radiographic, and histopathologic features of methotrexate-associated lung injury in patients with rheumatoid arthritis: A multicenter study with literature review. Arthritis Rheum 40:1829–1837.

Radiology of Diffuse Lung Disease

J. Collins

Introduction

The term "diffuse" can be defined as "widely spread or scattered" (1). In the lungs, this can refer to widely scattered disease that is predominantly alveolar, interstitial, a combination of alveolar and interstitial, acute, chronic, symmetric, or asymmetric. Many diseases can present acutely, and become chronic, resulting in overlap between causes of acute and chronic lung disease. A single disease can present in many ways radiologically, sometimes as a focal process, and other times as a diffuse process; sometimes as an interstitial process, and other times as an alveolar process or a combination of interstitial and alveolar. It is therefore important to understand the spectrum of radiologic manifestations for different diseases. This chapter focuses on lung diseases that can present as a diffuse pattern on radiologic imaging, discussing acute and chronic diseases separately.

Acute Diffuse Lung Disease

The term "acute", as regards disease, can be defined as "brief and severe" (2). The term "brief" is nonspecific, but generally means "lasting a short time". "Severe" is also a nonspecific term, generally referring to something that

Table 18.1. Acute diffuse lung disease

Acute alveolitis of fibrosing alveolitis
Extrinsic allergic alveolitis
Drug toxicity
Infectious pneumonitis/bronchitis
Acute radiation pneumonitis
Pulmonary hemorrhage
Pulmonary edema
Alveolar proteinosis

causes distress, or is serious, extreme, intense, or violent. The diseases listed in Table 18.1 are referred to as causes of "acute diffuse lung disease" because of their propensity to present abruptly and resolve in a short period of time, with, and sometimes without, specific treatment.

Acute Alveolitis of Fibrosing Alveolitis

Idiopathic pulmonary fibrosis (IPF), also called usual interstitial pneumonitis, or cryptogenic fibrosing alveolitis, is an inflammatory condition of the lung resulting in endstage fibrosis with honeycombing. The Hamman–Rich syndrome has been used to describe the acute, aggressive form of the disease (3). IPF is a disorder of unknown cause. Most theories concerning pathogenesis implicate injury to alveolar endothelial and epithelial cells by circulating or inhaled agents. An immune response occurs, and activated macrophages secrete factors that activate neutrophils and stimulate fibroblasts to produce collagen. Desquamative interstitial pneumonitis is distinguished from IPF (usual interstitial pneumonitis) by extensive filling of alveoli with macrophages, a uniform histologic appearance, less interstitial component and fibrosis, a younger patient age, and a better prognosis with steroid treatment (Fig. 18.1). Some authors regard desquamative interstitial pneumonitis as an early phase of IPF (4). With disease progression, the active, cellular alveolitis subsides and irreversible fibrosis supervenes.

The distribution of disease in IPF is typically scattered and subpleural. High resolution computed tomography (HRCT) better defines the extent and distribution of disease than does chest radiography. Acute alveolitis can be correctly identified using HRCT by the observation of ground-glass opacity (5). Ground-glass opacity, when not associated with a predominant pattern of honeycombing or traction bronchiectasis, represents an area of reversible disease.

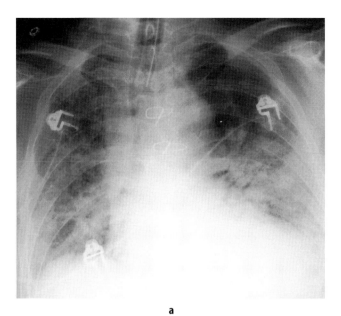
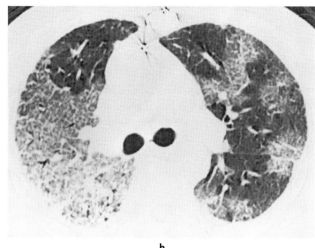

a   b

Figure 18.1. Desquamative interstitial pneumonitis. **a** Anteroposterior supine chest radiograph of a 77 year old man with acute symptoms of cough and shortness of breath shows bilateral diffuse interstitial and airspace disease. **b** HRCT shows bilateral ground-glass opacities and septal thickening, with a peripheral pattern of distribution on the left. Bronchial and vascular markings are still visible.

Extrinsic Allergic Alveolitis

Extrinsic allergic alveolitis (EAA), or hypersensitivity pneumonitis, results from the inhalation of antigenic organic dusts. A large number of causal antigens have been identified, including microorganisms (bacteria, fungi, thermophilic actinomycetes, amebas), animal and plant proteins, drugs, and some low molecular weight chemicals. Histologic changes are classified into acute, subacute, and chronic. The acute illness develops 4–8 h after heavy exposure to the antigen and consists of dry cough, chest tightness, dyspnea, wheeze, fever, chills, malaise, and occasionally hemoptysis. Spontaneous recovery follows separation from the agent, with improvement in 1 or 2 days, and complete recovery in 7–10 days.

The chest radiograph of patients with acute EAA may be normal, or show small pulmonary nodules 1–3 mm in diameter (ranging up to 8 mm), or subtle reticular interstitial opacities (6). These opacities may be so small and profuse that they give a ground-glass appearance. They are almost always bilateral and most commonly found in all lung zones. Patchy areas of consolidation or an interstitial pattern along bronchovascular bundles can develop. HRCT shows diffuse ground-glass opacities and centrilobular nodules (Fig. 18.2) (7).

Drug Toxicity

A number of commonly used drugs have been shown to affect the lungs. Prominent among these are the cytotoxic drugs used in the treatment of cancer and hematologic malignancies. Drugs can affect the lungs by causing hypersensitivity lung disease, diffuse alveolar damage, pulmonary edema, systemic lupus erythematosus, pulmonary vasculitis, and pulmonary hemorrhage. The radiologic abnormalities reflect the type and acuity of the drug reaction.

In the early stages of drug toxicity, the chest radiograph may be normal. When abnormal, the radiograph shows a generalized interstitial, alveolar, or mixed process. Segmental or lobar consolidations are not a feature of diffuse toxic lung damage. On rare occasion, diffuse alveolar damage, caused by cytoxan, bleomycin, and methotrexate, can result in single or multiple pulmonary masses or nodules. Hypersensitivity reactions result in patchy areas of consolidation, often in the periphery of the lung, or a diffuse reticulonodular pattern. Edema resulting from the toxic effect of drugs is indistinguishable from cardiogenic edema. HRCT of patients with acute drug toxicity can show ground-glass opacities when the chest radiograph is normal.

Infectious Pneumonitis/Bronchiolitis

Pneumonias can be classified according to their chest radiographic appearances into bronchopneumonia, lobar pneumonia, spherical (round) pneumonia, and interstitial pneumonia. Although widely used, these terms have limited value because the same organism may produce several patterns and because patterns often overlap in individual patients. Bronchopneumonia is the most

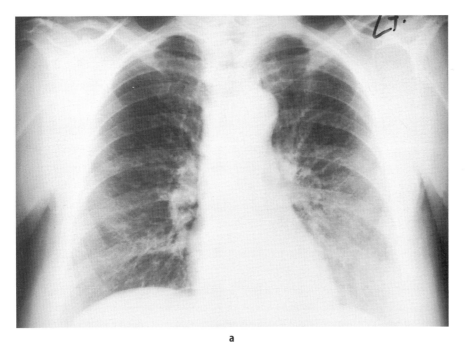

a

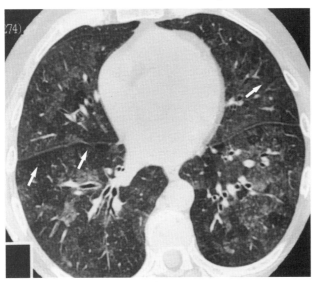

b

Figure 18.2. Extrinsic allergic alveolitis. **a** Posteroanterior chest radiograph of a 59 year old woman with an acute onset of fever, chills, dyspnea on exertion, headache, fatigue, minimal nonproductive cough, and hypoxemia, shows subtle bilateral, diffuse, reticular interstitial opacities. **b** HRCT shows bilateral ground-glass opacities and subtle centrilobular nodules (*arrows*). The patient's symptoms resolved after hospitalization and treatment with antibiotics, but recurred after returning home. She had pet birds and her husband bred pigeons at home. Open-lung biopsy showed noncaseating granulomas and lymphocytes consistent with extrinsic allergic alveolitis from "bird fancier's lung".

common pattern, and is characterized radiologically by patchy consolidation, loss of volume, and absence of air bronchograms. In lobar pneumonia, most commonly bacterial in etiology, the inflammatory exudate begins in the distal airspaces and spreads via the pores of Kohn across segmental boundaries, giving rise to homogeneous nonsegmental consolidation. Initiation of antibiotic therapy usually prevents involvement of a whole lobe. Interstitial pneumonia refers to a radiographic pattern comprising extensive peribronchial thickening, and ill-defined reticulnodular opacities, which may be localized or widespread. The usual causes of interstitial pneumonias are viral and *Mycoplasma pneumoniae* infections. Septic pulmonary

emboli, usually caused by infected venous catheters, result in multiple pulmonary opacities, usually round in shape but sometimes showing the shape of a pulmonary infarct (wedge-shaped opacity based on the pleura and pointing to the hilus), of any size, often cavitating (fig. 18.3), with air bronchograms and a feeding vessel sign (8).

Aspiration pneumonia frequently causes patchy consolidation in the dependent portions of the lungs, usually multilobar and bilateral in distribution. Consolidation with cavitation suggests bacterial or fungal disease rather than viral or *Mycoplasma* infection. Pneumatocele formation can be difficult to distinguish from cavitation. When due to pneumonia, pneumatoceles are usually due to

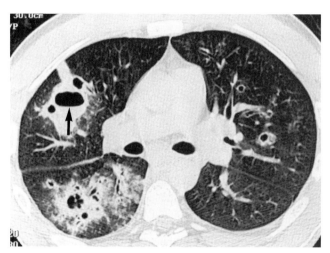

Figure 18.3. Septic emboli. HRCT of a 32 year old man with *S. aureus* septic emboli shows multiple rounded and irregular opacities with cavitation, and occasional air fluid levels (*arrow*).

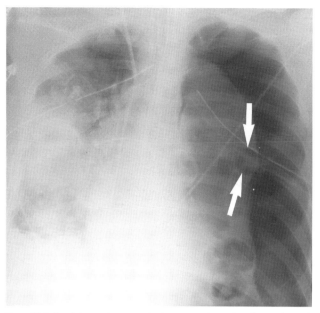

Figure 18.4. Staphylococcal pneumonia. Anteroposterior supine chest radiograph of a 23 year old man with complicated staphylococcal pneumonia shows multiple pneumatoceles (*arrows*) and a large left tension pneumothorax.

infection with *Staphylococcus aureus* (Fig. 18.4). Diffuse miliary nodules are usually due to *Mycobacterium tuberculosis* and various fungi. The nodules are even in size, usually 2–4 mm in diameter, well defined, and uniformly distributed (Fig. 18.5).

Endobronchial spread of infectious organisms can result in centrilobular nodules and linear branching opacities, best seen on HRCT, and is the most common cause of the "tree-in-bud" pattern (9). Bacterial organisms are the most common cause of a bronchiolar pattern of disease on CT, with viral, parasitic, mycobacterial, and fungal organisms less common causes. The term "tree-in-

bud" is commonly associated with endobronchial spread of *M. tuberculosis*, though this pattern is not pathognomonic for tuberculosis. The "tree-in-bud" appearance is characteristic of active and probably contagious tuberculosis, especially when associated with adjacent cavitary nodules in the lungs.

Most pneumonias resolve radiologically within a month, often within 10–21 days, and most of the remainder within

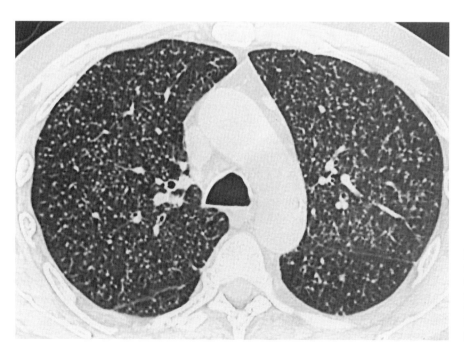

Figure 18.5. Miliary tuberculosis. HRCT of a 53 year old man with a history of alcohol abuse, cigarette smoking, and recent chills and night sweats shows multiple 2–3 mm nodules, randomly distributed throughout both lungs. Sputum culture was positive for acid-fast bacteria, and biopsy showed necrotizing granulomas and "red snappers".

2 months. Beyond 2 months, the most likely reasons for incomplete clearing are that the patient is old or has a systemic disease. However, a predisposing cause such as an obstructing neoplasm should always be considered in adult patients.

Radiation Pneumonitis

If any symptoms related to pulmonary irradiation occur, they are seen during the phase of acute radiation pneumonitis or develop much later as a consequence of fibrosis and lung contraction. The usual symptoms in the acute phase are dyspnea, cough, production of tenacious sputum, and sometimes fever and night sweats. On the chest radiograph, the changes of radiation pneumonitis are generally confined to the field of irradiation. The first change is a diffuse haze in the irradiated region with obscuring of the vascular outlines. Patchy consolidations appear, and these areas may coalesce into a nonanatomic but geometric area of pulmonary opacification. The earliest radiographic changes appear 6–8 weeks after the beginning of radiation therapy. CT is more sensitive than chest radiography in detecting postirradiation changes in the lungs, particularly in showing ground-glass opacities and shrinkage of vessels in the lung peripheral to a central field of irradiation (10).

Pulmonary Hemorrhage

A triad of features suggests diffuse pulmonary hemorrhage (DPH): hemoptysis, anemia, and airspace opacities on the chest radiograph (11). The most common causes of DPH are antibasement membrane antibody disease (Goodpasture syndrome), connective tissue disorders, systemic vasculitides, idiopathic glomerulonephritis, idiopathic pulmonary hemosiderosis, bleeding disorders, drug toxicity, and chemical lung toxicity. Less common causes include mitral stenosis, venoocclusive disease, infectious hemorrhagic necrotizing pneumonia, fat embolism, bone marrow transplantation, and hemorrhagic pulmonary edema of renal failure.

The radiographic changes of acute DPH are the same regardless of etiology and consist of airspace consolidation. When the bleeding is recurrent over a long period of time, interstitial changes may develop, reflecting interstitial fibrosis. The acute consolidation ranges from acinar shadows to patchy airspace consolidation, to widespread confluent consolidation with air bronchograms (12). The consolidation can be widespread or show a perihilar or middle to lower zone predominance and tends to be more pronounced centrally. The consolidation clears within 2–3 days, either completely or partially, leaving a linear or reticular pattern. HRCT shows consolidation or ground-

glass opacity, which can be present when the chest radiograph is normal (13).

Pulmonary Edema

Pulmonary edema is usually due to pulmonary venous hypertension or increased permeability of the alveolar-capillary membrane. Dividing edema into conditions in which the cause is hydrostatic and those in which the cause is capillary damage makes sense, as the treatment is different for each.

Elevated pulmonary venous pressure leads to increased lymphatic drainage. Once the capacity of the pulmonary lymphatics is exceeded, pulmonary edema results. Fluid collects first in the interstitium and then spills into the airspaces. The major causes of hydrostatic edema (also referred to as cardiogenic edema) are cardiac disease, overhydration, and fluid retention as a result of renal failure. The radiographic signs of hydrostatic pulmonary edema include interstitial septal lines, bronchial wall thickening, subpleural pulmonary edema, and airspace opacities, often with air bronchograms. Associated findings include vascular redistribution, enlargement of the cardiac silhouette and vascular pedicle, and pleural effusions. The terms "bat's wing" and "butterfly" patterns have been used to describe the appearance of perihilar airspace disease that is predominantly in the central portion of the lungs, fading out peripherally, leaving an aerated outer "cortex" of lung. A striking feature of hydrostatic edema is rapid change on films taken over short intervals. Rapid clearing is particularly suggestive of the diagnosis.

Adult respiratory distress syndrome (ARDS), a form of noncardiogenic edema, is due to increased pulmonary vascular permeability in response to lung injury. The most common precipitating insults are bacterial sepsis, pneumonia, aspiration of gastric contents, circulatory shock, trauma, burns, and drug overdose. The clinical syndrome is characterized by acute, severe, progressive respiratory distress, diffuse airspace opacities on chest radiography, significant hypoxemia despite high inspired oxygen concentration, and decreased compliance of the lungs.

Radiographic features of ARDS include bilateral, widespread patchy, ill-defined opacities resembling cardiogenic edema, usually without cardiac enlargement, vascular redistribution, or pleural effusions. The opacities progress to produce confluent opacification, usually involving all lung zones both centrally and peripherally, with prominent air bronchograms. CT scans may show that the distribution of the opacities is patchy, with preservation of normal lung regions (14). Patients with abnormal radiographs are all severely hypoxic and require assisted ventilation. During the acute phase,

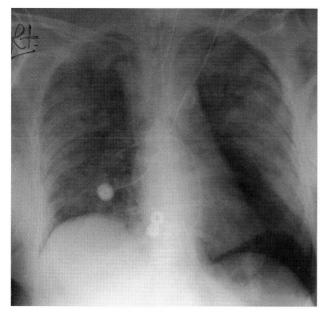

Figure 18.6. Adult respiratory distress syndrome. Anteroposterior supine chest radiograph of a 68 year old woman receiving mechanical ventilation shows bilateral diffuse airspace disease and a large left basilar pneumothorax.

many patients suffer barotrauma caused by positive-pressure ventilation with relatively noncompliant lungs. Pneumothorax, pneumomediastinum, and interstitial emphysema are common, and pneumatoceles may develop within the lungs (Fig. 18.6).

Pulmonary Alveolar Proteinosis

Pulmonary alveolar proteinosis represents a nonspecific response of the type II pneumocyte, the alveolar macrophage, or both, to a variety of injuries (15). Pathologically, there is filling of the alveoli with a lipid-rich, proteinaceous material (positive to periodic acid–Schiff stain), with normal lung interstitium. There is an association between the development of alveolar proteinosis and acute silicosis, exposure to dust or chemicals, hematologic malignancies, and immunologic abnormalities. Patients most commonly present with acute fever, weight loss, and dyspnea, and occasionally with pleuritic chest pain, hemoptysis, and pneumothorax.

The radiographic findings can be striking even when the symptoms and clinical signs are mild. The classic radiographic pattern is bilateral symmetric airspace opacity, particularly in a perihilar or hilar and basal distribution (16). Less commonly, the airspace disease can be asymmetric, unilateral, or lobar. HRCT shows a reticular pattern superimposed on ground-glass opacities, the so-called "crazy paving sign". Resolution of radiologic abnormalities can be spontaneous, but the majority of patients will require treatment with bronchoalveolar lavage.

Chronic Diffuse Lung Disease

A large number of chronic diseases may cause diffuse infiltration of the lungs. Although they are usually referred to as chronic interstitial lung diseases, the majority involve both the interstitium and the airspaces. The preferred term, therefore, is chronic infiltrative lung disease. The clinical and functional features of most of these diseases are similar. The chest radiograph may show patterns suggestive of a particular disease process but rarely allows a confident diagnosis. A number of studies have shown that CT can better assess the type, distribution, and severity of parenchymal abnormalities. Several chronic diffuse lung diseases have been shown to have a characteristic appearance on CT, even when the chest radiograph was normal or showed only nonspecific findings.

A number of signs indicate the presence of chronic infiltrative lung disease on chest radiographs and HRCT. These include abnormal interfaces, irregular linear opacities, thickening of the interlobular septa, nodules, and ground-glass opacities. The differential diagnosis of chronic diffuse infiltrative lung disease is based on the type and distribution of the abnormalities. The most common patterns are summarized in Table 18.2.

Abnormal interfaces between vessels, bronchi, and visceral pleura with the surrounding parenchyma are the most common sign of chronic infiltrative lung disease

Table 18.2. Patterns of chronic infiltrative lung disease

Irregular linear pattern
   Idiopathic pulmonary fibrosis
   Lymphatic spread of tumor
   Asbestosis
   Sarcoidosis

Thickened interlobular septa
   Lymphatic spread of tumor
   Sarcoidosis
   Pulmonary edema
   Idiopathic pulmonary fibrosis

Cystic pattern
   Lymphangioleiomyomatosis
   Langerhan cell histiocytosis
   Idiopathic pulmonary fibrosis

Nodular pattern
   Silicosis and coalworker's pneumoconiosis
   Sarcoidosis
   Langerhan cell histiocytosis
   Extrinsic allergic alveolitis

Ground-glass pattern
   Chronic eosinophilic pneumonia
   Bronchiolitis obliterans organizing pneumonia
   Extrinsic allergic alveolitis
   Idiopathic pulmonary fibrosis

Airspace consolidation
   Bronchiolitis obliterans organizing pneumonia
   Chronic eosinophilic pneumonia
   Bronchioloalveolar cell carcinoma

(17). Irregular linear opacities may be seen in a number of lung diseases, and, in some cases, the pattern and distribution on CT will narrow the range of diagnostic possibilities. For example, IPF is characterized by the presence of reticular opacities and honeycombing in the subpleural and basilar portions of lung. The fibrosis in patients with sarcoidosis is usually more severe centrally along the bronchovascular bundles (18).

Thickening of the interlobular septa is a common finding in chronic infiltrative lung diseases, and, when extensive, is seen on CT as a pattern of multiple polygonal lines. In patients with interstitial fibrosis, the thickening is irregular; in lymphangitic spread of tumor the thickening is nodular; in sarcoidosis the thickening is irregular and often associated with architectural distortion; and in pulmonary edema the thickening is smooth.

Nodules 1–10 mm in diameter can be seen with a number of chronic infiltrative lung diseases. In sarcoidosis, the nodules are usually less than 5 mm in diameter, with smooth or irregular margins, characteristically in a perilymphatic distribution (bronchovascular bundles, subpleural regions, and interlobular septa) (19). In silicosis, the nodules have an upper lung zone distribution.

Ground-glass opacity is defined as hazy increase in lung opacity without obscuration of underlying bronchi or blood vessels, and is commonly seen on CT with a number of acute and chronic diffuse lung diseases. In IPF, areas of ground-glass opacity correlate with active alveolitis (in the absence of extensive honeycombing or traction bronchiectasis).

Lung volumes can also provide a clue as to the etiology of chronic diffuse lung disease. Fibrotic disorders (IPF) are characterized by marked restriction and small lung volumes. On the other hand, Langerhan cell histiocytosis and sarcoidosis, in the early stages, are usually associated with normal lung volumes, but lymphangioleiomyomatosis produces air-trapping with large lung volumes.

Idiopathic Pulmonary Fibrosis

IPF is characterized histologically as alveolitis and mononuclear cell inflammatory changes in the alveolar wall. Eventually, fibrosis develops. This end stage is referred to as honeycomb lung. These changes can be seen with collagen-vascular diseases and in response to certain drugs such as bleomycin, cyclophosphamide, or busulfan.

The characteristic radiographic findings in IPF are diffuse linear and reticular interstitial opacities obliterating normal vessels, in a subpleural and bibasilar distribution. Small, well-formed cystic spaces less than 1 cm in diameter are designated as a "honeycomb" pattern. Identification of honeycombing and severe architectural distortion indicate end-stage disease. HRCT

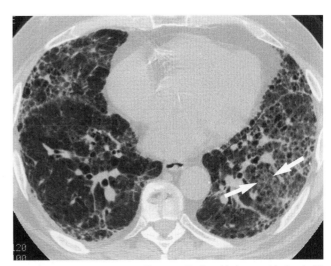

Figure 18.7. Idiopathic pulmonary fibrosis. HRCT of an elderly man with chronic IPF shows extensive honeycomb lung with a subpleural and bibasilar distribution. Areas of ground glass opacity (*arrows*) represent fibrosis beyond the resolution of HRCT, and not reversible lung disease.

shows irregular septal thickening, irregular interfaces between lung and pleura, bronchiolectasis, honeycombing, and traction bronchiectasis, in a subpleural and basilar distribution (fig. 18.7). HRCT gives a better estimate of disease extent and shows more extensive honeycombing than does chest radiography (20).

Pulmonary Lymphatic Carcinomatosis

Pulmonary lymphangitic carcinomatosis refers to tumor growth in the lymphatics of the lung. It is seen most commonly in carcinomas of the breast, lung, stomach, and colon. The radiographic manifestations include reticular opacities, Kerley B lines, and subpleural edema (21). The major lymph vessels are located in the bronchovascular bundles, in the interlobular septa, and in the subpleural regions of the lung. The distribution of tumor cells within these structures results in CT findings of uneven thickening of bronchovascular bundles and of interlobular septa, giving them a beaded chain appearance (fig. 18.8) (22). Nodular thickening of interlobular septa helps to distinguish lymphangitic spread of tumor from pulmonary edema on CT, which causes smooth thickening of the interlobular septa. Tumor spread, however, can also result in smooth septal thickening, and "polygonal lines" on CT.

Asbestosis

Asbestosis is defined as pulmonary interstitial fibrosis caused by asbestos exposure. The chest radiograph has limited sensitivity in detecting subtle changes of asbestosis. Considerable observer error is noted,

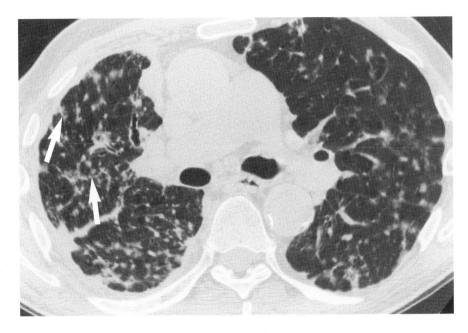

Figure 18.8. Lymphangitic spread of tumor. HRCT of a 76 year old man with adenocarcinoma of the prostate shows "beaded" septal thickening (*arrows*), a typical appearance of lymphangitic tumor spread in the lungs.

particularly in patients with a normal or near-normal chest radiograph (23). When abnormal, chest radiographs show small linear or reticular opacities that predominate in the lung bases. These may progress from a fine reticulation to a coarse linear pattern with honeycombing. The findings are similar to those seen in IPF. The presence of pleural thickening or plaques lends support to the diagnosis of asbestosis, although plaques are not invariably present.

CT is superior in characterizing and quantifying parenchymal abnormalities and in the detection of early asbestosis. Five major parenchymal abnormalities are identifiable on HRCT: (a) curvilinear subpleural lines (linear density of variable length within 1 cm and parallel to the chest wall), (b) thickened interstitial short lines (thickened interlobular septa that consists of lines 1–2 cm in length in the peripheral lung extending to the pleura), (c) subpleural dependent density (a band of increased density 2–20 mm thick bordering the dependent pleura), (d) parenchymal bands (linear densities from 2–5 cm in length coursing through the lung usually in contact with the pleura), and (e) honeycombing (24).

Silicosis and Coal Worker's Pneumoconiosis

Silicosis refers to lung disease caused primarily by inhalation of free silica. Exposed individuals usually work in quarries, drill or tunnel quartz- containing rocks, cut or polish masonry, clean boilers or castings in iron and steel foundries, or are exposed to sandblasting. The chronic form of the disease requires 20 years or more exposure to high dust concentrations before radiographic abnormalities are evident (25). The basic

lesion of silicosis is a hyalinized nodule, containing silica particles.

Early in the course of disease, chest radiographs show 1–3 mm nodules, sometimes calcified, most prominent in the posterior portions of the upper two thirds of the lungs. A reticular interstitial pattern may also be seen. With time, the nodules increase in size and, number, and coalesce to form masses termed "progressive massive fibrosis". As the nodules coalesce, contraction of the upper lobes is observed and bullae form peripheral to the masses. Initially, the masses are seen in the periphery of the lung, and, with time, they migrate towards the hili, leaving emphysematous lung between the fibrotic mass and the chest wall. Similar radiographic findings are seen with coal worker's pneumoconiosis, although the two diseases are pathologically different.

HRCT can detect disease in patients with normal chest radiographs, but may be normal in the presence of pathologically proven infiltrative lung disease (26). CT findings include subpleural micronodules (similar to those seen in sarcoidosis and lymphangitic spread of cancer), diffuse nodules up to 7 mm in diameter, emphysema, progressive massive fibrosis, diffuse interstitial fibrosis leading to honeycombing, and lymph node enlargement and calcification (Fig. 18.9).

Lymphangioleiomyomatosis

Lymphangioleiomyomatosis is a rare disease characterized by progressive proliferation of smooth muscle in the walls of bronchi, bronchioles, alveolar septa, pulmonary vessels, lymphatics, and pleura (27). The process often leads to obstruction of the bronchioles with

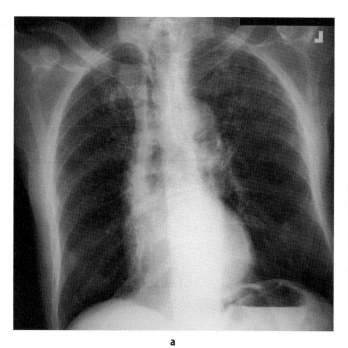

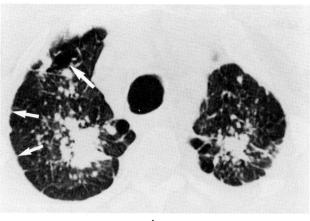

a   b

Figure 18.9. Complicated silicosis. **a** Posteroanterior chest radiograph of a 73 year old man employed as a foundry worker for over 20 years shows small bilateral nodules, involving predominantly the upper lung zones. **b** HRCT shows multiple small nodules, many of which are in a subpleural, lymphatic distribution (*small arrows*), central "progressive massive fibrosis", and adjacent areas of emphysema (*large arrow*).

air-trapping and the development of thin-walled lung cysts that may rupture and cause pneumothorax. Obstruction of the lymphatics can occur, with subsequent development of chylous pleural effusions, and compression of venules may lead to hemoptysis. The disease occurs in women of childbearing age.

Chest radiographs show diffuse reticular interstitial disease that may be associated with cysts. The lung volumes are either normal or increased. Pneumothorax is seen in about 40% of patients and chylous effusions in 60%. HRCT shows thin-walled cysts that may be difficult to recognize on chest radiography. The cysts are distributed diffusely throughout the lungs. The intervening lung parenchyma is normal. Cystic airspaces similar to those seen in lymphangioleiomyomatosis have been described in patients with Langerhan cell histiocytosis; however, in Langerhan cell histiocytosis, a nodular component is also commonly present. Furthermore, Langerhan cell histiocytosis characteristically involves the upper two-thirds of the lungs and spares the costophrenic angles, whereas lymphangioleiomyomatosis involves the lungs diffusely (28). Cystic airspaces are also commonly seen with pulmonary fibrosis, although IPF is characterized by the presence of a reticular pattern and honeycomb spaces with a predominant distribution in the basilar and subpleural regions, unlike the diffuse distribution seen in lymphangioleiomyomatosis. In IPF, the honeycomb cysts are surrounded by

abnormal parenchyma, whereas most of the cysts in lymphangioleiomyomatosis are surrounded by normal lung.

Langerhan Cell Histiocytosis

Langerhans' cell histiocytosis (also referred to as histiocytosis X and eosinophilic granuloma) is an idiopathic disease characterized by benign proliferation of mature histiocytes. Early stages of the disease are characterized by multiple granulomas composed of histiocytes, Langerhan cells, and varying numbers of eosinophils in the alveolar septa, bronchial walls, and perivascular areas. In the later stages, interstitial fibrosis and thin-walled cysts may develop. The disease occurs in young or middle-aged adults. Cigarette smoking is reported in over 90% of patients (29).

Chest radiographs show reticular, nodular, reticulonodular, and cystic abnormalities, often in combination (30). The disease is usually bilateral and diffuse with an upper lung zone predominance. Lung volumes are usually normal or increased. CT is superior to chest radiography in showing the morphology and distribution of lung abnormalities (Fig. 18.10). Many lesions that appear reticular on chest radiographs are shown to represent cysts on CT. CT shows no central or peripheral predominance of lesions, but does show that many small nodules are distributed in the

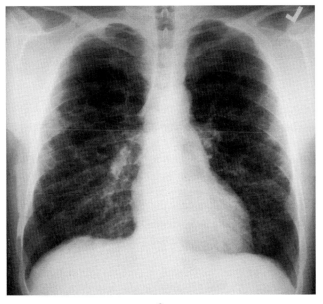
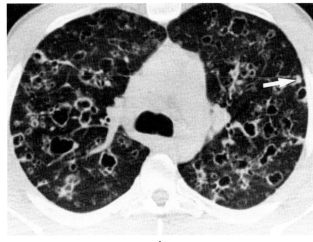

a   b

Figure 18.10. Langerhan cell histiocytosis. **a** Posteroanterior chest radiograph of a 32 year old man with progressive shortness of breath shows large lung volumes, bilateral reticular interstitial opacities, and thin-walled cysts. **b** HRCT better shows the bilateral, diffuse, irregular, thin-walled cysts, and scattered small nodules (*arrow*). The cysts seen in patients with lymphangioleiomyomatosis can look similar, but tend to have a smoother contour, and are not characteristically associated with parenchymal nodules.

centers of secondary pulmonary lobules around small airways. The number of nodules ranges from single to numerous, and are usually solid but can have lucent centers, presumably corresponding to small "cavities". The nodule margins are usually indistinct and often irregular, and the intervening lung parenchyma is normal (28).

Sarcoidosis

Sarcoidosis is a relatively common systemic disorder of unknown cause characterized by noncaseating granulomata, which may resolve spontaneously or progress to fibrosis (31). It most often occurs in young adults, with a greater prevalence in African-Americans. Pulmonary manifestations are present in 90% of patients, 20–25% of whom have permanent functional impairment (32). The diagnosis of sarcoidosis is based on the typical radiographic and clinical presentation supported by histologic evidence of sterile noncaseating granulomata in one or more organs.

The chest radiograph is abnormal in about 90% of patients and is classified according to the presence of enlarged hilar or mediastinal lymph nodes, pulmonary lesions, and fibrosis. About 60–70% of patients with sarcoidosis have a characteristic radiologic appearance consisting of enlarged hilar and paratracheal lymph nodes with or without concomitant parenchymal changes (33). In 5–10% of patients, the radiograph is normal. When present, pulmonary lesions consist of one or a combination of fine

to coarse reticular interstitial markings, small nodules, confluent "alveolar" opacities (although, histologically, only interstitial involvement is seen), honeycombing, bullae, and architectural distortion.

Sarcoid granulomata are distributed mainly along the lymphatics in the bronchovascular sheath, and to a lesser extent, in the interlobular septa and pleura. This distribution is responsible for the high rate of success in diagnosis by bronchial and transbronchial biopsies (31). The smallest lesions often are visible only on CT, with characteristic parenchymal abnormalities consisting of nodular opacities along the bronchovascular bundles, interlobular septa, major fissures, and subpleural regions (34). In the majority of cases, the nodules have irregular margins. Ground-glass opacities are commonly seen on HRCT, and probably represent active alveolitis and interstitial granulomas. CT is superior to chest radiography in demonstrating early fibrosis and distortion of the lung parenchyma. CT may show parenchymal abnormalities in patients with a normal chest radiograph or in patients with only hilar adenopathy apparent on the chest radiograph. CT, however, may be normal in patients with pulmonary involvement proved by transbronchial biopsy. The distribution of sarcoid granulomata along the lymphatics is similar to that seen with pulmonary lymphangitic carcinomatosis. Both may cause a beaded appearance of the bronchovascular bundles and interlobular septa, and the pattern may be identical on CT. In general, however, the septal thickening in sarcoidosis is usually less extensive than that seen in pulmonary lymphangitic carcinomatosis, and often associated with distortion of the lobular architecture.

Extrinsic Allergic Alveolitis

This entity was discussed earlier in this chapter along with other causes of acute diffuse lung disease. EAA, however, can manifest as an acute, subacute, or chronic illness. Acutely, heavy exposure to the inciting antigen causes diffuse airspace consolidation. The consolidation resolves within a few days to reveal a fine nodular or reticulonodular pattern, characteristic of the subacute phase. The chronic stage is characterized by the presence of fibrosis, which may occur months to years after the initial exposure. CT is superior to chest radiography in showing subtle centrilobular nodular opacities. HRCT is superior to conventional CT in showing areas of ground-glass opacity.

Chronic Eosinophilic Pneumonia

The term chronic eosinophilic pneumonia is used when no extrinsic causes, such as fungal hypersensitivity, drug reaction, or helminth infestation, can be identified to explain pulmonary eosinophilia. It is an idiopathic condition characterized by infiltration of the lungs with eosinophils, usually associated with an increased number of eosinophils in the circulating blood. Chest radiographs characteristically show homogeneous peripheral airspace consolidation. The combination of blood eosinophilia, peripheral opacities on the chest radiograph, and rapid response to steroid therapy often obviate the need for lung biopsy (35). In many cases, however, a peripheral predominance of airspace opacities may not be evident on chest

radiography. In many cases, CT shows a peripheral pattern of disease when this pattern is not evident on the chest radiograph. CT, therefore, can be helpful when the clinical findings are suggestive of chronic eosinophilic pneumonia but the radiographic pattern is nonspecific.

Bronchiolitis Obliterans Organizing Pneumonia

Bronchiolitis obliterans organizing pneumonia (BOOP), also referred to as cryptogenic organizing pneumonia, is one of the most common causes of chronic diffuse lung disease, accounting for more than 20–30% of cases (36). The typical presentation is that of a 1–5 month history of low grade fever, malaise, and dry cough. Pathologically, BOOP is characterized by granulation tissue plugs in alveoli, alveolar ducts, and occasionally small airways. Pathologic changes are nonspecific, however, and similar changes are seen in a wide range of disorders. The most commonly identified disorders are infections, connective tissue disorders, and drug toxicity (37).

The chest radiograph shows patchy airspace consolidation that does not respond to broad-spectrum antibiotics. The consolidation on chest radiography often contains air bronchograms, and, in about half of cases, has a predominantly peripheral distribution, although this is often better appreciated on CT. CT typically shows bilateral and asymmetric areas of consolidation with air bronchograms, ranging from about 1.5 cm in diameter to segmental size, often with associated ground-glass opacities (38). A predominantly subpleural distribution of the consolidation is seen in about 50% of cases, and peribronchovascular distribution, similar to a bronchopneumonia, is seen in 30–50% of cases (Fig. 18.11) (39).

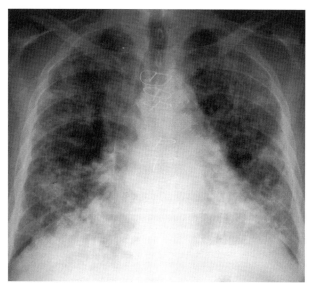

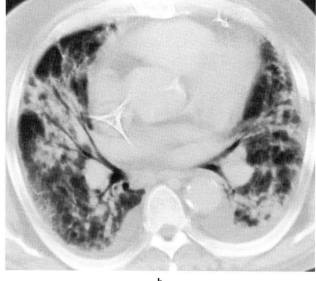

a   b

Figure 18.11. Bronchiolitis obliterans organizing pneumonia. **a** Posteroanterior chest radiograph of a middle-aged man with a recent upper respiratory tract infection, cough, shortness of breath, and hypoxemia shows bilateral patchy airspace opacities. **b** HRCT shows airspace disease in both a peripheral and bronchovascular distribution, characteristic of BOOP.

Bronchioloalveolar Cell Carcinoma

Bronchioloalveolar cell carcinoma is a subtype of adenocarcinoma, and accounts for 2–5% of lung cancers (40). The characteristic pathologic feature is a peripheral neoplasm showing lepidic growth, with the malignant cells growing along the "scaffolding", or alveolar walls, of the lung. The tumor can present as a solitary pulmonary nodule or unifocal or multifocal areas of pulmonary consolidation, with the former having the best prognosis.

Bronchioloalveolar cell carcinoma can be a very slow growing tumor. It occasionally manifests on chest radiography as a slowly progressive airspace process, sometimes present radiographically over several years, (Fig. 18.12). Because it can resemble pneumonia, it is important to document clearing of radiographic abnormalities after treatment for presumptive pneumonia, and exclude alternative diagnoses such as slow-growing bronchioloalveolar cell cancer.

On chest radiography, the tumor appears as a solitary lobulated or spiculated pulmonary nodule, with a propensity for a subpleural location, often with air bronchograms, or as ill-defined or multiple opacities, an ill-defined opacity resembling pneumonia, patchy multifocal areas of consolidation, or multiple ill-defined nodules. CT better shows air bronchograms, and may also show small rounded collections of air within the tumor opacities, referred to as "pseudocavitation". Also described with these tumors is the "CT-angiogram sign", in which the vessels coursing through the tumor stand out clearly against a background of abundant low attenuation mucus within the tumor.

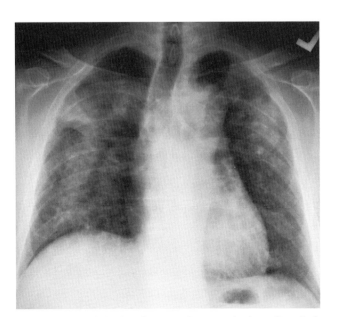

Figure 18.12. Bronchioloalveolar cell carcinoma. Posteroanterior chest radiograph of a middle-aged man shows bilateral diffuse airspace disease. Serial chest radiographs showed that the process was progressing over a 3 year period.

References

1. Steinmetz S (ed) (1993) Random House Webster's dictionary. Ballantine Books, New York, p 182.
2. Steinmetz S (ed) (1993) Random House Webster's dictionary. Ballantine Books, New York, p 8.
3. Hamman L, Rich AR (1944) Acute diffuse interstitial fibrosis of the lung. Bull Johns Hopkins Hosp 74:177–212.
4. Tubbs RR, Benjamin SP, Reich NF, et al. (1977) Desquamative interstitial pneumonitis – cellular phase of fibrosing alveolitis. Chest 72:159–166.
5. Müller NL Staples CA, Miller RR, et al. (1987) Disease activity in idiopathic pulmonary fibrosis: CT and pathologic correlation. Radiology 165:731–734.
6. Mindell HJ (1970) Roentgen findings in farmer's lung. Radiology 97:341–346.
7. Akira M, Kita N, Higashihara T, et al. (1992) Summer-type hypersensitivity pneumonitis: Comparison of high-resolution CT and plain radiographic findings. AJR 158:1223–1228.
8. Kuhlman JE, Fishman EK, Teigen C (1990) Pulmonary septic emboli: Diagnosis with CT. Radiology 174:211–213.
9. Aquino SL, Gamsu G, Webb WR, et al. (1996) Tree-in-bud pattern: frequency and significance on thin section CT. J Comput Assist Tomogr 20:594–599.
10. Libshitz HI, Shuman LS (1984) Radiation-induced pulmonary change: CT findings. J Comput Assist Tomogr 8:15–19.
11. Bradley JD (1982) The pulmonary hemorrhage syndromes. Clin Chest Med 3:593–605.
12. Müller NL, Miller RR (1991) Diffuse pulmonary hemorrhage. Radiol Clin North Am 29:965–971.
13. Cheah FK, Sheppard MN, Hansell DM (1993) Computed tomography of diffuse pulmonary haemorrhage with pathological correlation. Clin Radiol 48:89–93.
14. Maunder RJ, Shuman WP, McHugh JW, et al. (1986) Preservation of normal lung regions in the adult respiratory distress syndrome: Analysis by computed tomography. JAMA 255:2463–2465.
15. Prakash UBS, Barham SS, Carpenter HA, et al. (1987) Pulmonary alveolar phospholipoproteinosis: Experience with 34 cases and a review. Mayo Clin Proc 62:499–518.
16. Davidson JM, McLeod WM (1969) Pulmonary alveolar proteinosis. Br J Dis Chest 63:13–28.
17. Zerhouni EA, Naidich DP, Stitik FP, et al. (1985) Computed tomography of the pulmonary parenchyma. II. Interstitial disease. J Thorac Imaging 1:54–64.
18. Müller NL, Kullnig P, Miller RR (1989) The CT findings of pulmonary sarcoidosis: Analysis of 25 patients. AJR 152:1179–1182.
19. Lynch DA, Webb WR, Gamsu G, et al. (1989) Computed tomography in pulmonary sarcoidosis. J Comput Assist Tomogr 13:405–410.
20. Staples CA, Müller NL, Vedal S, et al. (1987) Usual interstitial pneumonia: Correlation of CT with clinical, functional, and radiologic findings. Radiology 162:377–381.
21. Janower ML, Blennerhaset JB (1971) Lymphangitic spread of metastatic tumor to lung. Radiology 101:267–273.
22. Stein MG, Mayo J, Müller N, et al. (1987) Pulmonary lymphangitic spread of carcinoma: Appearance on CT scans. Radiology 162:371–375.
23. Weill H (1987) Diagnosis of asbestos-related disease. Chest 91:802–803.
24. Aberle DR, Gamsu G, Ray CS, et al. (1988) Asbestos-related pleural and parenchymal fibrosis: Detection with high-resolution CT. Radiology 166:729–734.
25. Ziskind M, Jones RN, Weill H (1976) Silicosis: State of the art. Am Rev Respir Dis 113:647–665.
26. Padley SPG, Hansell DM, Flower CDR, et al. (1991) Comparative accuracy of high resolution, computed tomography in the diagnosis of chronic diffuse infiltrative lung disease. Clin Radiol 44:222–226.

27. Corrin B, Liebow AA, Friedman PJ (1975) Pulmonary lymphangiomyomatosis: A review. Am J Pathol 79:348–382.

28. Moore ADA, Godwin JD, Müller NL, et al. (1989) Pulmonary histiocytosis X: Comparison of radiographic and CT findings. Radiology 172:249–254.

29. Hance AJ, Basset F, Saumon G, et al. (1986) Smoking and interstitial lung disease: The effect of cigarette smoking on the incidence of pulmonary histiocytosis X and sarcoidosis. Ann NY Acad Sci 465:643–656.

30. Lacronique J, Roth C, Battesti JP, et al. (1982) Chest radiological features of pulmonary histiocytosis X: A report based on 50 adult cases. Thorax 37:104–109.

31. Colby TV, Carrington CB (1988) Infiltrative lung disease. In Thurlbeck WM (ed) Pathology of the lung, Thieme Medical Publishers, New York, pp 425–518.

32. Crystal RG, Bitterman PB, Rennard SI, et al. (1984) Interstitial lung diseases of unknown cause: disorders characterized by chronic inflammation of the lower respiratory tract. N Engl J Med 310:154–166.

33. McLoud TC, Epler GR, Gaensler EA, et al. (1982) A radiographic classification of sarcoidosis: Physiologic correlation. Invest Radiol 17:129–138.

34. Brauner MW, Grenier P, Mompoint D, et al. (1989) Pulmonary sarcoidosis: Evaluation with high-resolution CT. Radiology 172:467–471.

35. Dines DE (1978) Chronic eosinophilic pneumonia: A roentgenographic diagnosis. Mayo Clin Proc 53:129–130.

36. Adler BD, Padley SPG, Müller NL (1995) High-resolution CT in the differential diagnosis of chronic infiltrative lung disease. Appl Radiol 45–48.

37. Geddes DM (1991) BOOP & COP. Thorax 46:545–547.

38. Bouchardy LM, Kuhlman JE, Ball WC, et al. (1993) CT findings in bronchiolitis obliterans organizing pneumonia (BOOP) with radiographic, clinical, and histologic correlation. J Comput Assist Tomogr 17:352–357.

39. Müller NL, Staples CA, Miller RR (1990) Bronchiolitis obliterans organizing pneumonia: CT features in 14 patients. AJR 154:983–987.

40. Auerbach O, Garfinkel L (1991) The changing pattern of lung carcinoma. Cancer 68:1973–1977.

19 Cystic and Cavitary Lung Disorders

K. Nishimura, S. Oguri and H. Itoh

Introduction

A "cystic lesion" is a nonspecific term used to describe an area of decreased lung opacity identified radiologically (1–4). These lesions can be focal or multifocal, bilateral or sometimes unilateral. The lesion should be distinguished from air-trapping caused by pathologies of the bronchus or blood vessels, and from a decrease in opacity due to mosaic perfusion. According to the definition by Webb et al., a cystic airspace is a thin-walled (usually < 3 mm), well-circumscribed, air-containing lesion with a diameter of 1 cm or more, and must be visible on high resolution computed tomography (HRCT) (3,4). The definitions with respect to the size and wall thickness are arbitrary, and there has been no consensus on the differentiation of a cystic lesion from other pathologic lesions with decreased lung opacity, such as cavities.

Cystic airspaces are commonly seen in patients with histiocytosis X and lymphangioleiomyomatosis (LAM), but can also be observed in other diseases (4). Honeycombing can also result in cystic airspaces. The term "cyst" is sometimes used to describe the dilatated airways observed in patients with cystic bronchiectasis. However, it is not typically used to refer to low attenuation areas due to emphysema.

Pulmonary Histiocytosis X

Pulmonary histiocytosis X (HX) is also called pulmonary Langerhans' cell histiocytosis or eosinophilic granuloma of the lung. The histologic characteristics of the initial clinical stage are a peribronchial distribution of granulomatous nodules, accompanied by either Langerhans' histiocytes or eosinophilic infiltration, or both (5). At advanced stages, the cellular granulomas may become fibrous or may form cystic lesions of unknown cause (6,7).

Most patients are young or middle-aged adults, and present with nonspecific symptoms of their respiratory tract such as a cough or dyspnea (6–8). Approximately 20% of these patients also have a pneumothorax (9). Male patients are slightly more predominant, and over 90% are smokers, suggesting that smoking may be a cause of this disease (5,10). However, the symptoms usually develop only after several years of smoking, and do not correlate with the cumulative amount of smoking, in contrast to other smoking-related pulmonary disorders such as emphysema or lung cancer. Therefore there is probably an underlying reaction mechanism that causes this disease, and smoking merely triggers this reaction cascade.

Chest radiographs often reveal diffuse and non-specific infiltrates that are reticulonodular, reticular or small nodular. Therefore, HX is often categorized as an interstitial lung disease, but is best distinguished from idiopathic pulmonary fibrosis by its preferential distribution to the upper lung (Fig. 19.1). However, it is usually difficult to identify the cystic airspaces using chest X-rays alone.

Cavitating small nodular opacities and small cystic opacities are distinct features of HX that may be found by CT (Figs 19.1, 19.2) (11–14). In addition, there are small nodular opacities without cavities that tend toward a centrilobular distribution. Moore et al. reported 12 cases of cystic airspaces and 8 cases of small nodular opacities in 17 HX patients (11). Furthermore, Brauner et al. reported that 17 of 18 patients with HX showed thin-walled cysts, and 14 had small nodular opacities that were usually less than 1 cm in diameter (12). According to Grenier et al. in a study of 51 patients with HX, 47% had nodular opacities less than 3 mm in diameter, 45% had opacities ranging from 3 to 10 mm, and only 24% had opacities larger than 10 mm (14). The number of nodular opacities varied from one case to another, and this variability probably reflects the activity of the disease (11,12).

Small cystic opacities have been called thin- or thick-walled cysts, cystic airspaces or cavitated nodules (11,12). Grenier et al. reported that in 51 patients with HX, 88% showed thin-walled cysts (less than 2 mm) whereas 55% showed thick-walled cysts (more than 2 mm) (14). The pres-

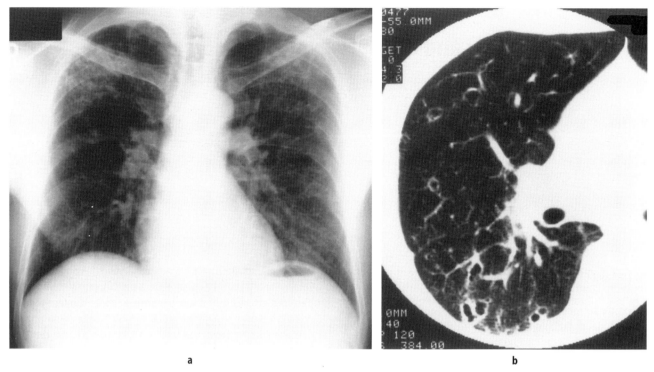

a   b

Figure 19.1. Eosinophilic granuloma of the lung in a 44 year old male. **a** Posteroanterior chest radiograph shows reticulonodular infiltrates predominantly distributed in bilateral upper lungs. **b** CT scan with 5 mm collimation using targeted reconstruction in the same patient as in **a**, obtained at the same time, shows small cystic lesions with oval or lobulated shapes.

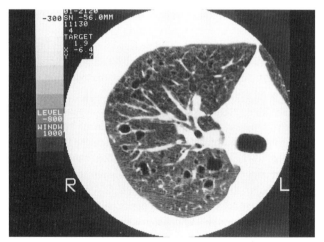

Figure 19.2. A 34 year old man with eosinophilic granuloma of the lung. CT scan with 5 mm collimation scan using targeted reconstruction shows thin-walled cystic airspaces.

ence of a distinct wall surrounding the cyst is useful in distinguishing HX from low attenuation areas due to emphysema. The cyst is usually circular in shape, but may manifest as bizarre shapes such as bilobed, clover-leaf shaped, or branched (11). These unusual shapes are generated by the fusion of several cysts, or occur sometimes because the cyst corresponds to a bronchus with dilatated, thin walls. The cysts tend to distribute preferentially to the upper lung, and the size of the cysts is usually larger in the upper lung as well. Cystic airspaces with these characteristics determined by HRCT strongly support the diagnosis of HX.

In many cases, the lung parenchyma between the cysts or nodules looks normal on CT scans, but irregular interfaces (interface sign), fine reticular opacities and ground-glass opacities may be observed in some cases (4). These appearances are usually indicative of intralobular fibrosis, early cyst formation and a confluence of cysts.

Based on a follow-up investigation using HRCT, these nodular opacities, thick-walled cysts and ground-glass opacities have been reported to regress with time. In contrast, the thin-walled cysts, linear opacities and emphysematous lesions either did not change or even progressed (15).

A comparative study of the CT appearance of these lesions with pulmonary function testing revealed a significant correlation between the diffusion capacity (DL_{co}) and the extent of the lesions. However, the extent of the airflow limitation did not correlate with the CT analysis (16). In addition, even in those cases where no airflow limitation was detected by the pulmonary function tests, an expiratory CT was able to demonstrate the presence of air-trapping and to indicate the presence of local airflow limitation (17).

Lymphangioleiomyomatosis

Lymphangioleiomyomatosis (LAM) is found only in premenopausal women, and can be characterized by the abnormal growth of atypical smooth muscle in the lung parenchyma and in the lymphatic vessels of the thorax and abdomen (18,19). The lung parenchyma develops emphysematous lesions or thin-walled cysts via an unknown mechanism. It has been speculated that the growth of smooth muscle cells along the bronchioles may cause air-trapping. This growth of smooth muscle cells can also be observed in extrapulmonary lymph nodes such as the hilus and mediastinum, and results in an enlargement of the intrapulmonary lymphatics and thoracic duct, followed by chylous pleural effusion. Due to occlusion of the pulmonary vein, pulmonary hemorrhage can also be observed.

For most patients, the initial symptom is a shortness of breath, and 40% of these patients also present with pneumothorax. Chylous pleural effusion is also a common symptom, and hemosputum and hemoptysis are observed in 30–40% of the patients (19–25). LAM is only found in women who have pregnancy potential. Although there have been a few reports of LAM in postmenopausal women, these studies may not be trustworthy. Pregnancy can induce and often worsen LAM.

It appears to share some common features with the pulmonary involvement in patients with tuberous sclerosis. The relation of tuberous sclerosis with LAM has been debated. Renal angiomyolipomas are frequently found in patients with LAM.

The prognosis used to be quite unfavorable, but in recent years it has been reported that the 10 year survival rate was 20–40%, except for one study (20–22,23,26,27). There are

some reports to support the therapeutic benefits of anti-estrogen therapy, including an oophorectomy, but randomized controlled trials have not been performed. Therefore, there are still many questions about the effects of such treatments (23,26). Due to its progression, LAM is one disease in which lung transplantation has been performed.

Chest radiography in patients with LAM often does not show any specific features. There is usually an accompanying volume loss in interstitial lung disorders that are typical of diffuse infiltrative lung diseases. In contrast, LAM patients often develop hyperinflation instead. A complication such as a pneumothorax or chylous pleural effusion is often the key to identifying this disease.

The CT features of patients with LAM are characterized by numerous thin-walled cysts surrounded by a relatively normal lung parenchyma (Fig. 19.3) (28–36). The reported size of these cysts ranges from 2 to 50 mm, and the cysts grow bigger with the progress of the disease. The thickness of the cyst wall also ranges from what is barely detectable by HRCT to about 4 mm, but it tends to be thin. Typically, the cystic lesions are widely distributed throughout the entire lung, and there is no tendency toward a preferential distribution.

The majority of the lung parenchyma between the cysts is normal, but in some cases there may be a thickened interlobular septum, interstitial lesions or ground-glass opacities (4,18). The ground-glass opacity may correspond

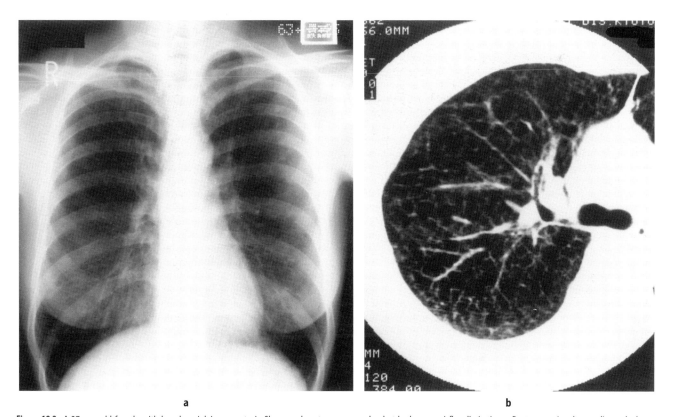

a   b

Figure 19.3. A 37 year old female with lymphangioleiomyomatosis. She was almost a never smoker but had severe airflow limitation. **a** Posteroanterior chest radiograph shows hyperinflation associated with slightly increased vascular markings. **b** Targeted CT image through the right upper lung shows numerous low attenuation areas or small cystic abnormalities with or without thin walls.

to alveolar hemorrhage. On CT scans, there may also be enlargement of the hilar and mediastinal lymph nodes or pleural effusion. The former is believed to be due to the growth of smooth muscle cells in the lymph nodes, whereas the latter is thought to reflect chylous effusion.

A study examining the relationship between pulmonary function testing and the extent of the lesions observed on CT scans revealed that the diffusion capacity and airflow limitation correlated significantly with the extent of the disease observed by CT scans (34). In addition, when the LAM lesions in the lung are quantified using quantitative CT techniques, the CT index correlates significantly with physiologic measurements of the airflow, lung volume, diffusing capacity, and exercise performance, thus indicating the usefulness of a quantitative CT index for the evaluation of the disease severity (35). When examined using inspiratory CT, the size of the cysts was found to decrease upon expiration, indicating a communication between the cysts and the airway (17,36).

It is often an issue as to how to distinguish LAM from HX. Using CT images, the following three points are useful for differentiation: nodular components are often observed in HX, but are rare in LAM; irregularly shaped cysts are common in HX, but are rare in LAM; and HX lesions distribute preferentially to the upper lung and spare the costophrenic angle, whereas LAM lesions usually distribute diffusely over the whole lung.

It has been reported that micronodular pneumocyte hyperplasia is a rare manifestation of tuberous sclerosis or LAM. Although this is a histologic definition of multiple, well-demarcated nodules usually measuring up to 8 mm in size, micronodular pneumocyte hyperplasia should be considered if small nodular opacities are observed in patients with LAM (37).

Bronchiectasis

Reid morphologically classified bronchiectasis into three groups: saccular, varicose, and cylindrical. Reid's classification is the most commonly used, although saccular and varicose bronchiectases are sometimes combined and are termed cystic bronchiectasis. Cystic bronchiectasis ought to be distinguished from other cystic lesions in some cases. In particular, when there is an isolated cystic lesion on a section from CT scans, one must examine the continuity of the lesion to the proximal bronchus, and then judge whether it is bronchiectasis.

It is easy to diagnose cystic bronchiectasis by CT (Figs. 19.4, 19.5). However, for cylindrical bronchiectasis, it is sometimes difficult to determine the presence of dilatation. To diagnose bronchiectasis by CT, it is necessary to identify the bronchial wall because inflammatory thickening of the bronchial wall is an important factor for the diagnosis, along

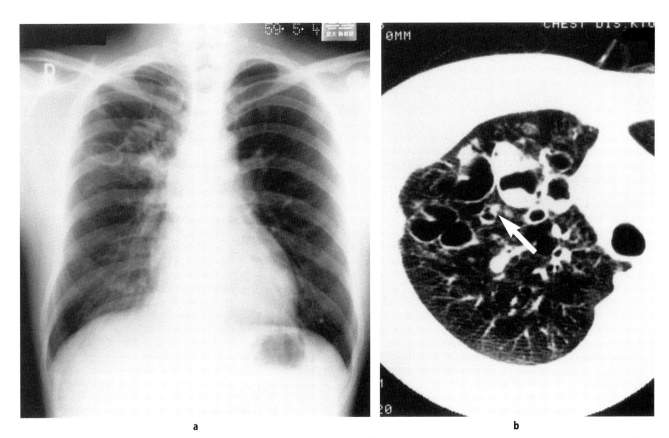

a   b

Figure 19.4. Cystic bronchiectasis with unknown cause localized in right upper lobe in a 38 year old female. **a** Posteroanterior chest radiograph shows reticular or linear opacities in right upper lung. **b** CT scan with 5 mm collimation scan using a high spatial resolution algorithm shows markedly dilatated airways as well as signet-ring sign (*arrow*).

with dilatation of the airway. The "signet-ring sign" is frequently observed on CT scans from patients with bronchiectasis; this is a ring-shaped opacity (representing a dilatated, thick-walled airway) associated with a small, soft tissue opacity corresponding to the adjacent pulmonary artery (4).

Bronchography had been the most reliable method for making the diagnosis of bronchiectasis. In 1984, Müller et al examined 13 lungs and compared the diagnoses obtained by bronchography and CT (38). The CT diagnosis matched the bronchographic diagnosis in only 6 lungs. On the other hand, in 1985, Mootoosamy et al. examined bronchography versus CT in 36 lobes from 15 lungs, and demonstrated the usefulness of CT by matching all 22 positive and 14 negative diagnoses of bronchiectasis between these two techniques (39). In addition, Grenier et al. examined 44 lungs from 36 patients using bronchography and CT scans that were obtained at 1.5 mm collimation (40). They found that both techniques showed the same 25 as positive and the same 15 as negative. Bronchography has therefore been replaced by CT. The diagnostic power of CT compared with bronchography for determining bronchiectasis is approximately 55–100% for sensitivity and 92–100% for specificity (38–49). Therefore, there is a possibility that bronchiectasis may be missed using CT alone. Of course, a clear demonstration of bronchiectasis by CT will leave little need to perform bronchography (41).

Hansell et al. reported that patients with bronchiectasis frequently manifest air-trapping, even in those lobes that show no dilatation. Therefore, they speculated that the airway disease may precede the development of bronchiectasis (50).

Allergic Bronchopulmonary Aspergillosis (ABPA)

This is an allergic asthma caused by the growth of the fungus *Aspergillus* in the airway. The features of ABPA on chest radiographs are recurrent migratory infiltrates and central bronchiectasis. In addition, ABPA may also cause mucus plugging, airspace consolidation, and lobar or segmental collapse. Bronchiectasis is found more often in the proximal than in the distal airways, and consists mostly of a cystic or varicose dilatation. CT may detect the dilatation as an isolated cyst (4,51–54). The presence of central bronchiectasis is included in the secondary diagnostic criteria for ABPA. Expiratory CT scans have been reported to be useful for the detection of early-stage air-trapping, because it can sometimes detect air-trapping that cannot be detected during the inspiratory phase.

Cystic Fibrosis

This is an autosomal recessive genetic disorder found most frequently among Caucasians (55,56). Bronchiectasis and bronchial wall thickening are most frequently observed in patients with cystic fibrosis. These abnormali-

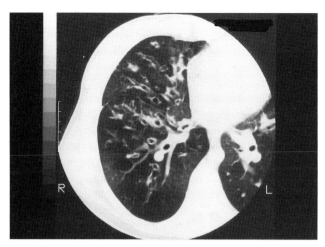

Figure 19.5. Cystic bronchiectasis in a 23 year old female patient with cystic fibrosis. HRCT scan with 2 mm collimation demonstrates cystic and cylindrical dilatation of bronchi and bronchial wall thickening. (Courtesy of Katashi Satoh and Satoko Hojo

ties can be easily detected by chest radiographs (57). The CT features include cystic or cylindrical bronchiectasis, bronchial wall thickening, mucus plugging, and hyperinflation (Fig. 19.5) (4,56–60).

Bronchiolitis Obliterans (BO)

BO is characterized by airflow limitation caused by the inflammation and fibrosis of the bronchioles. It has also been called constrictive bronchiolitis in recent years (61). It can be found with rheumatoid arthritis as well as with polymyositis/dermatomyositis, or it may be idiopathic. BO has also been reported as a manifestation of chronic rejection after lung or bone marrow transplantation (62). Hyperinflation is the most characteristic radiologic feature of BO, whereas the most frequent CT appearance is focal, decreased lung attenuation (4,62). This attenuated area contains pulmonary vessels with a decreased caliber. These changes correspond to the air-trapping or to the decrease in blood flow in the involved area; this is usually termed mosaic perfusion. It may manifest as either proximal or distal bronchiectasis. Expiratory CT has been reported to allow a clear demonstration of mosaic perfusion and air-trapping (36).

Diffuse Panbronchiolitis (DPB)

DPB is a unique disease found mainly in Asian countries (63,64). It is characterized by chronic respiratory tract infections and airflow limitation, and is always complicated by paranasal sinusitis (4,63). The histologic characterization of this disease is an interstitial accumulation of foamy macrophages in the respiratory bronchiolus, frequently accompanied by proximal bronchiectasis (65). The chest radiologic features include diffuse small nodular infiltrates and hyperinflation (63). The main CT features are branching linear opacities and associated small nodular opacities; the latter show a centrilobular distribution (66). Akira et al. categorized the CT appearance of patients with DPB into four types, and type 4 indicates large cystic areas of high attenuation accompanied by dilatated proximal bronchi (67,68). Thus they showed that cystic lesions develop as the DPB progresses, and are an essentially irreversible phenomenon. In addition, although rare, there have been reports of DPB-like bronchiolitis lesions as a human T-cell lymphotrophic virus type 1 (HTLV-1) related bronchopulmonary disease found in carriers of the adult T-cell leukemia virus (69).

Honeycombing

Honeycombing is defined as the macroscopic appearance of bronchiolectasis surrounded by fibrous lesions (70,71). It is generally viewed as the nonspecific, final stage of pulmonary fibrosis, and is therefore sometimes called an "end-stage" lung (72). Honeycomb cystic airspaces range from a few millimeters to several centimeter in diameter, and are characterized by clearly definable walls which can be thick. The cystic airspaces of the honeycomb tend to

share walls. The mechanism and process of chronic honeycombing formation is almost unknown.

Coarse reticular shadows on chest radiographs often correspond to honeycombing (73). The superiority of CT over chest radiography as a detection method for honeycombing is well known. On CT scans, aggregates of cysts that are thick walled, bigger than 2 mm in diameter, and relatively similar in size indicate honeycombing. The spaces between the dilatated bronchioles consist of fibrous lesions instead of air-containing alveoli. Therefore the cysts are in contact with each other through a thick wall. Such aggregates of small cysts are typical, but are difficult to observe even using HRCT when the honeycombing consists of cysts less than 1 mm in diameter. In this case, mildly dilatated airways can be observed in a high-attenuation area (air bronchiologram-like appearance) (70). This latter feature is sometimes difficult to distinguish from lesions with airspace consolidation. The details of diffuse infiltrative lung disorders are discussed in Chapter 19.

Usual interstitial pneumonia (UIP) is the major lung pathology of idiopathic pulmonary fibrosis (IPF) or cryptogenic fibrosing alveolitis (74). It is also the most common pathologic pattern in the pulmonary involvement of various collagen-vascular diseases. The frequency of UIP in the pulmonary involvement of various collagen-vascular diseases depends on the type of disease (75,76).

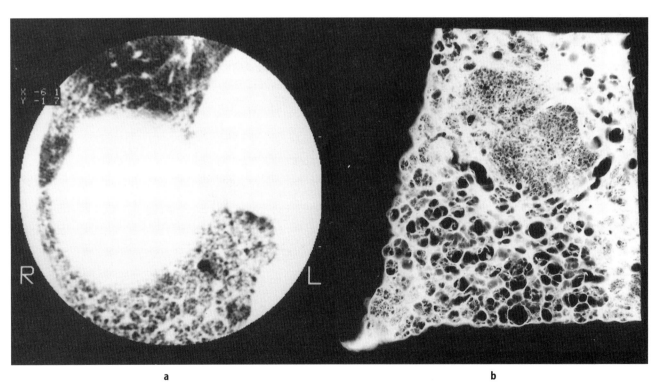

a   b

Figure 19.6. Macroscopic honeycombing in UIP. **a** CT in a 65 year old man, through the right lung base, demonstrates accumulated cystic spaces with thick walls. Since the patient died of exacerbation of idiopathic pulmonary fibrosis an autopsy was performed 36 days after this CT scan was performed. **b** Contact radiograph of the postmortem right lower lung, fixed using Heitzman's solution. The gross honeycombing corresponded to the accumulated cystic spaces with thick walls seen at CT scan. The histologic examination of the postmortem lungs revealed both UIP and diffuse alveolar damage.

For example, the pulmonary involvement of systemic sclerosis is thought to be almost always UIP (76). An important feature for the histologic diagnosis of UIP is that both the normal alveolar areas and the areas of fibrosis are observed in the same tissue specimen (secondary pulmonary lobule), with a patchy distribution (77). The fibrous lesions may begin at the alveolar septum, but there is no clear explanation on how they develop to the final stage of fibrosis and honeycombing. Since there are aggregates of alveoli in the wall of the honeycomb, the regions affected by the honeycombing also show a decrease in volume. Honeycombing is found at a very high frequency in UIP, but such lesions do not have any histologic value for making the diagnosis (Fig. 19.6) (70,78–82).

The various effects of smoking on IPF have been studied (83,84). When smokers develop IPF, any dysfunction that should otherwise be revealed by pulmonary function testing could be masked or modified. Histologically, this modification indicates the copresence of pulmonary emphysema caused by smoking and pulmonary fibrosis. The chest radiologic findings may reveal isolated or interspersed cystic lesions that are not continuous with the honeycombing. Such cysts are often distributed to the upper lungs, and are categorized as emphysema or emphysematous bullae. On CT scans, pulmonary emphysema is described as low attenuation areas without walls. However, because of the fibrous lesions in the surrounding area, pulmonary emphysema may appear like a cyst with a wall.

The long-term prognosis of *pulmonary sarcoidosis* is relatively favorable. Honeycombing is found only in a small proportion of patients with sarcoidosis (85–87). Sarcoidosis is discussed in Chapter 15.

Pulmonary histiocytosis X or *eosinophilic granuloma of the lung* is a disease with a generally favorable prognosis. However, in some cases, the fibrosis worsens and results in death. Since it is a relatively rare disease, the mortality rate of this disease is not known. A centrilobular fibrosis is believed to be important in this case. Since the lesions may distribute over the entire lung at advanced stages, it is often difficult to diagnose this disease even using CT.

The pulmonary lesions of *asbestosis* also show honeycombing, and its CT features are discussed in Chapter 26. In most cases, *desquamative interstitial pneumonia (DIP)* and *lymphocytic interstitial pneumonia (LIP)* do not show any honeycombing upon biopsy. However, honeycombing may develop later and can be detected by CT.

Acute interstitial pneumonia (AIP) is an interstitial pneumonia that shows a relatively acute progression, and has neither any preceding pulmonary lesions nor any obvious extrapulmonary cause (88,89). Clinically, similar histologic features have been recognized as the final state of the lung on the autopsies of patients diagnosed with adult respiratory distress syndrome (ARDS) or other extensive lung diseases; these features are pathologically categorized as those belonging to diffuse alveolar damage (DAD), or acute lung injury (90). Ground-glass opacities accompanied by a volume loss are recognized on chest radiographs of most cases showing histologic lesions characteristic of DAD. The stage showing microscopic honeycomb formation corresponds histologically to organized DAD, and CT scans reveal air bronchiologram-like distal airways inside the high attenuation areas (70). However, this feature on the CT scans is not enough to diagnose the presence of microscopic honeycombing by itself (89). The honeycombing caused by DAD stays at the microscopic level, and usually does not grow to macroscopic honeycombing.

Emphysema

Emphysema is defined histologically as permanent, abnormal enlargement of the airspaces distal to the terminal bronchiole, which is accompanied by the destruction of the walls of the involved alveoli, but is not associated with any obvious fibrosis (91). On the basis of localization of these lesions in the secondary pulmonary lobule, emphysema can be categorized as follows: centrilobular or centriacinar emphysema, panacinar or panlobular emphysema, and paraseptal or distal acinar emphysema. The radiological appearance of emphysema is discussed in Chapter 17.

Centrilobular emphysema is found preferentially in the upper lung, and appears on CT scans as a small, low attenuation area without any obvious walls (92–96). In contrast, low attenuation areas may not been clearly observed in panlobular emphysema even using CT, and thus a mild lesion of this type is more difficult to recognize than centrilobular emphysema (97). Paraseptal emphysema can be recognized as small subpleural cysts or bullae. Some patients with emphysema show multiple bullae on CT scans, and the walls of these cysts may or may not be clearly recognizable, but in either case it is termed bullous emphysema (Fig. 19.7). It is often difficult to determine the relative contribution of the parenchymal emphysema and the bullae to the overall pulmonary dysfunction. It is also often difficult to determine the indications for the surgical resection of the bullae.

Infective Lung Disorders with Cavitary or Cystic Lesions

Pulmonary Tuberculosis

Tuberculosis is one of the most frequent pulmonary infectious diseases that cause cavitating lesions. Pulmonary tuberculosis is usually categorized into either primary pulmonary tuberculosis or reactivation tuberculosis.

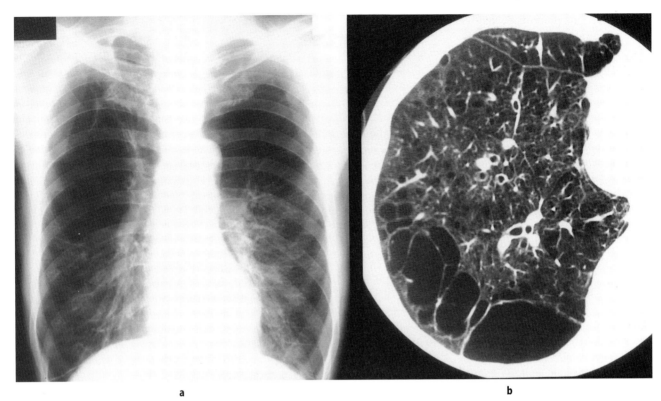

a   b

Figure 19.7. Bullous emphysema in a 67 year old male. He was a former smoker with moderate airflow limitation. Forced expiratory volume in one second (FEV$_1$) was 1.14 L (41% predicted). **a** Posteroanterior chest radiograph shows hyperinflation. **b** Targeted CT image with 2 mm collimation through the right lower lung demonstrates low attenuation areas corresponding to emphysema associated with several cystic airspaces.

Previously, it has been believed that tuberculous pleuritis or miliary tuberculosis follows the primary complex. These concepts ought to be reexamined, since the aged population now often experiences miliary or pleural tuberculosis. The radiological appearance of pulmonary tuberculosis is discussed in Chapter 14.

The radiologic features of primary tuberculosis are airspace consolidation, lobar or segmental collapse, and hilar or mediastinal lymphadenopathy. Cavitation has been reported in 29% of tuberculosis patients (98). Many cases of tuberculosis, which is recognized as a community-acquired disease at many clinics daily, are actually reactivation tuberculosis; its roentgenographic features are summarized by focal consolidation and cavitation observed at the apex or upper lobe. It is most important to suspect tuberculosis based on the chest radiologic features and to look for acid-fast bacilli in the sputum. Of course, it is best to obtain the diagnosis prior to conducting a CT scan. However, in recent years, there have been an increasing number of reports on the CT features of pulmonary tuberculosis (99–107).

Webb et al. summarized the HRCT findings of active tuberculosis as follows: patchy unilateral or bilateral airspace consolidation frequently peribronchial in distribution, thin- or thick-walled cavitation, scattered airspace nodules, and the superimposition of centrilobular branching structures (4). Im and colleagues reported that cavi-

tating nodules were found as a HRCT feature in 69% of 41 patients with active pulmonary tuberculosis (103). Most of these cavities were thick walled, but thin-walled cavities are often seen as well in patients undergoing, and after treatment. In pulmonary tuberculosis, it has been generally thought that there is no special relationship between the CT features of these lesions and their activity. Nevertheless, antituberculous chemotherapy usually helps the cavities to resolve. In addition, CT is useful for the diagnosis of mycetoma (fungus ball), which often complicates the cavitating lesions, especially after treatment for tuberculosis.

Nontuberculous (Atypical) Mycobacterial Infections

Although there are regional differences in the incidence and type of nontuberculous mycobacterial infections, *Mycobacterium avium intracellular complex* (MAC) and *Mycobacterium kansasii* are the two most common pathogens that cause lung lesions (108). There have been several reports on the CT features of in nonimmuno-compromised patients and human immunodeficiency virus (HIV)-infected hosts with MAC-related pulmonary disease (108–115), which manifests radiographic features very similar to those tuberculosis (109,110). However, some authors concluded that there were prominent features indicative of widespread bronchiectasis, particularly if it involves the right middle lobe and lingula (114,115). Cavities, small nodular opacities and airspace consolidation are also frequently observed on CT scans.

Pneumocystis Carinii Pneumonia (PCP)

Immunocompromised patients, especially HIV-infected patients, are highly susceptible to PCP, and the infiltrates often spread to bilateral lungs (116–119). The characteristic CT features of PCP are ground-glass opacities and airspace consolidation that distribute preferentially from the hilus to the internal layers of the lung, with a "patchwork" or "mosaic" pattern (4,117). The "patchwork" distribution pattern of these lesions is unique for this disease, and less involved areas are present between the lesions. Another characteristic is the presence of thick-walled, irregular, and septated cavities or thin-walled cysts (119). There have also been some reports on the relationship between cyst formation and a pneumothorax (120). The fact that the cysts are found preferentially in the upper lobe, together with other reports, indicates that about 35% of PCP cases result in cyst formation. Bronchiectasis is also frequently observed in patients with PCP using CT (121). PCP is further discussed in Chapter 18.

Septic Embolism and Infarction

Septic pulmonary embolisms and infarctions are observed in patients with sepsis or in patients with a intravenous fixed catheter. When there are multiple nodules at varying stages of cavitation, it should be considered as a differential diagnosis. On CT scans, they show nodular or wedge-shaped triangular opacities at the peripheral regions of the lung, especially in the subpleural areas, and these lesions are often accompanied by cavitation with thick walls (122, 123). The nodular lesions may also manifest feeding vessels.

Invasive Pulmonary Aspergillosis

Invasive pulmonary aspergillosis is a pneumonia caused by *Aspergillus*. This pathogen infects only immunocompromised patients, in contrast to the other two pulmonary diseases which are caused by *Aspergillus* and occur in nonimmunocompromised patients, i.e. aspergilloma and allergic bronchopulmonary aspergillosis. It is an opportunistic infection, and those immunocompromised patients who have a hematologic malignancy such as leukemia are the most susceptible.

Aspergillus has a tendency to invade the pulmonary vessels, and therefore frequently causes hemosputum or hemoptysis. Invasive aspergillosis causes diffuse or focal airspace consolidation, nodules, and cavitating lesions (124–127). A relatively characteristic feature of invasive aspergillosis on CT is the halo sign, which is a ground-glass opacity surrounding a nodule (124). Pathologically, this feature corresponds to coagulation necrosis or hemorrhaging in the area surrounding the nodules. It has been reported that thick-walled, cavitating lesions are the most common radiologic manifestation of invasive aspergillosis in acquired immune deficiency syndrome (AIDS) (126).

Pulmonary Cryptococcosis

Pulmonary Cryptococcosis can be categorized into the following two types; a community-acquired disease in nonimmunocompromised patients, and an opportunistic cryptococcus infection in patients with HIV infection or in other immunocompromised hosts (128–130). These fungal infections have great regional variability in the world, and thus one must be aware of the regional frequency and pathology for its differential diagnosis.

Nonimmunocompromised patients with pulmonary cryptococcosis manifest no or only mild symptoms (130). The chest radiographic features include focal or multiple nodular opacities, whereas CT scans reveal nodules with cavities at a higher frequency (Fig. 19.8). These nodules are concentrated in a relatively limited area, but can distribute diffusely to bilateral lungs. They are often found in the subpleural region, may sometimes accompany pleural indentation with irregular edges, and may need to be differentiated from an adenocarcinoma of the lung. Many reports on the CT features of this disease are cases of pulmonary cryptococcosis as a complication of AIDS. About 30% of the pulmonary cryptococcosis cases in AIDS patients manifest nodules that have been observed at an early stage of the HIV infection. Adenopathy or pleural effusion may sometimes be seen as well. Atypical, miliary nodules or ground-glass opacities can also be observed, and in these cases it may be necessary to distinguish it from PCP.

Other Fungal Diseases

Pulmonary nocardiosis is a subacute or chronic lung infection caused by *Nocardia asteroides*. Nocardiosis can be found in nonimmunocompromised hosts, but more often in immunocompromised patients with lymphomas as well as AIDS. In addition, it is known to occur as a complication of pulmonary alveolar proteinosis, pulmonary tuberculosis, and chronic granulomatous diseases. There

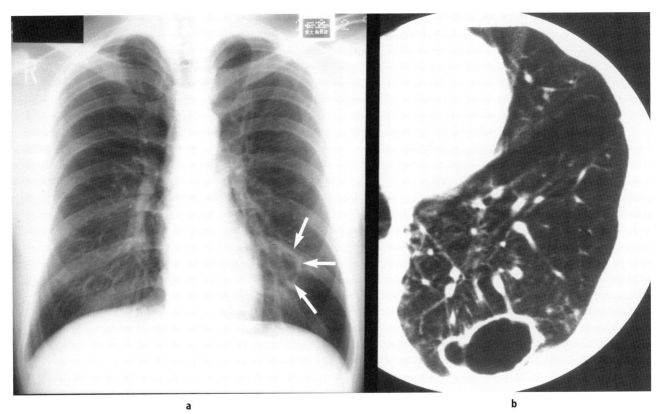

Figure 19.8. Pulmonary cryptoccocosis without evidence of dissemination in a 27 year old asymptomatic nonimmunocompromised male patient. **a** Posteroanterior chest radiograph shows single cystic space (*arrows*) located in the inner zones of the left lower lung. **b** Targeted CT image through the left lower lung demonstrates solitary large cyst with wall thickeness of about 5 mm, located in 10th segment of the left lung.

are only a limited number of reports on its radiologic appearance, but diffuse infiltration and multiple nodules as well as cavitation are commonly observed.

Cavitation is also a common feature of coccidioidomycosis and histoplasmosis, and is occasionally observed in blastomycosis, actinomycosis, and sporotrichosis. Cavitating pneumonia is also seen in immunocompromised patients with invasive candidiasis.

Lung Abscess

The lung abscesses or chronic pneumonia caused by *Staphylococcus, Legionella*, and Gram-negative bacilli including *Klebsiella* occasionally undergo necrosis and cavity formation. Cavitation is also common for hematogenous lung abscesses. The radiologic appearance of lung abscesses is discussed in Chapter 22.

Parasitic Cavity

Hydatid cysts of the lung are occasionally associated with cavitary formation. Multiple small cavities can be seen in

patients with paragonimiasis, and amebic lung abscesses have been reported in patients with hepatic amoebiasis.

Noninfectious Granulomatous Lung Diseases

The chest radiologic features of *Wegener granulomatosis* are parenchymal opacification, nodular opacities, bronchial and pleural abnormalities (131–136). Bilateral or unilateral nodular opacities of various sizes are clearly observed on CT scans, and are accompanied by cavities in about 50% of the cases (131,132). The walls of the cavitating lesions are usually thick. Some nodules demonstrate an angiocentric or bronchocentric distribution on CT scans. Wedge-shaped nodular opacities adjacent to the pleura are a common feature, and pleural effusion is also frequently observed. For laboratory findings, antineutrophil cytoplasmic autoantibody specific for antiproteinase 3 (c-ANCA) is useful for a diagnosis of Wegener granulomatosis.

The pathologic characteristics of *pulmonary sarcoidosis* include a perilymphatic distribution of noncaseating granuloma. The characteristic feature on CT scans is peribronchovascular small nodules (86,87). Airspace consolidation as well as large nodules with diameters greater than 1 cm can also be observed on CT scans. Such large nodules may be cavitated in rare cases (86). Grenier et al. reported that these large cavitated nodules were found in 3% of patients with pulmonary sarcoidosis (14). There are also reports describing cases of pulmonary sarcoidosis which presented as bullous emphysema with severe airflow limitation (137).

Neoplasmatic Cavitation

Lung Cancer and Metastatic Carcinoma

Regardless of the histologic diagnosis, lung cancers can manifest cavity formation, possibly due to necrosis of the central region of the tumor. In squamous cell carcinomas, cavities with thick walls are often formed. In addition, the cancers can grow inside bullae or along the walls, and can show features resembling cavitary formation on chest radiographs and CT. It has been reported that cystic airspaces are observed within lobar or diffuse consolidation on the CT scans of patients with bronchioloalveolar carcinoma (138). There is often cavity or cystic formation inside the multiple nodular opacities caused by metastases from malignant tumors (Fig. 19.9).

Lymphoproliferative or Lymphoinfiltrative Lung Disorders

Lymphoproliferative or lymphoinfiltrative lung disorders include various diseases, from highly malignant ones such as malignant lymphoma to those that are currently considered to be benign. On the basis of several characteristic histologic features, there are a number of terms used to describe diseases with diffuse or local lymphoproliferative or lymphoinfiltrative lung involvement: lymphoid interstitial pneumonia, pseudolymphoma, lymphomatoid granulomatosis, plasma cell granuloma, mucosa-associated lymphoid tissue lymphoma (MALTOMA), and multicentric Castlemann disease. Furthermore, lymphoproliferative or lymphoinfiltrative lung disorders have been reported as the lung manifestation of Sjögren syndrome and AIDS (Fig. 19.10). Gene analysis is currently considered to be a valuable technique in determining whether the lymphoid hyperplasia is related to a tumor.

Cavitation is less common in patients with non-Hodgkin lymphoma than in those with Hodgkin disease. However, the cavitation of pulmonary nodules is rather rare in patients with non-Hodgkin lymphoma (139,140). The lung lesions of multicentric Castlemann disease also manifest cystic formation at high frequency in addition to centrilobular ill-defined nodules, thickening of the bronchovascular bundles and interlobular septal thickening (141). In addition, CT appearance of lymphocytic interstitial pneumonia may show ground-glass attenuation, airspace consolidation, ill-defined nodules and cysts (142).

Pulmonary Sequestration

Pulmonary sequestration is defined as the supply of blood from the systemic circulation to a part of the lung where there is no communication with a normal bronchus. There are two types of pulmonary sequestra-

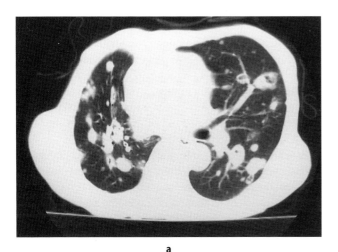

a

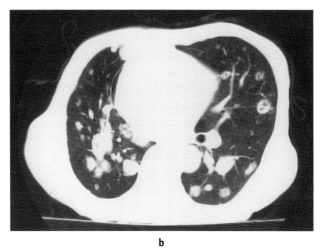

b

Figure 19.9. Postoperative recurrence of adenocarcinoma of lung. Multiple cavitary nodules are demonstrated at CT scans in a 73 year old female who underwent right upper lobectomy 10 years prior to the scan.

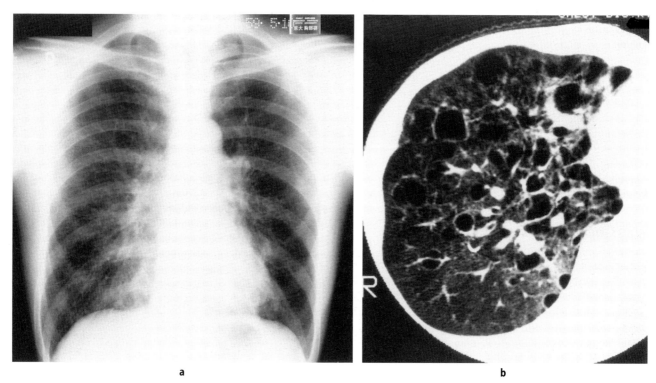

a   b

Figure 19.10. Lymphoproliferative lung disorders associated with Sjögren's syndrome in a 44 year old male. **a** Posteroanterior chest radiograph shows ground-glass opacities predominantly distributed in the inner zones of bilateral lower lungs and mild hyperinflation. **b** Targeted CT image through the right lower lung demonstrates several cystic airspaces with a variety of wall thickness.

tion: intralobar pulmonary sequestration, which shares a pleura with the normal lung; and extralobar pulmonary sequestration, which is enclosed in an independent pleura.

About 75% of pulmonary sequestration is intralobar. Since there is no pleura between the sequestration and the normal lung, it can often result in infection via an acquired communication with the bronchi. Therefore, cystic airspaces are frequently observed in intralobar pulmonary sequestration. The sequestration develops almost exclusively in the posterior basal segment (S10) of the left lower lobe (Fig. 19.11). Blood flows into the sequestration through an artery branching from the aorta, and flows out into the pulmonary veins. On the other hand, extralobar pulmonary sequestration is less prone to infection because it is surrounded by a layer of visceral pleura.

Without infection, the sequestration is seen as a homogeneous tumor adjacent to the left diaphragm. Complications with infection result in the formation of multiple cystic lesions, and sometimes the presence of air–fluid levels. Therefore the formation of multiple cysts is more frequent in intralobar pulmonary sequestration. Thoracic aortography provides the definitive diagnosis, but contrast CT may also reveal abnormal blood vessels branching from the aorta.

Mediastinal Cysts and Other Extrapulmonary Lesions

Most mediastinal cysts are congenital in origin, and these cysts comprise about 9% of the mediastinal mass in an adult. The radiologic appearance of mediastinal tumors and cysts is discussed in Chapter 34.

Bronchogenic cysts are the most common, and appear on CT scans as circular or oval shapes with smooth edges. The walls are too thin to recognize. Bronchogenic cysts can be observed anywhere along the mediastinum, but are often found in the middle to posterior mediastinum.

The CT features of *esophageal duplication cysts* are similar to those of bronchogenic cysts, and therefore these two types of cyst are difficult to distinguish. Sixty percent of esophageal cysts are found in the lower portion of the posterior mediastinum (143).

Pericardial cysts are thin-walled sacs formed during the development of the pericardium. They are connected at the pericardial cavity via the funiculus, but there is no communication. Those cysts that have a communication with the lumen of the pericardial cysts are called pericardial cyst diverticuli. In 90% of these cases, the cysts are in contact with the diaphragm. In 65% and 25% of these cases, they are found at the right and left cardiophrenic angles, respectively.

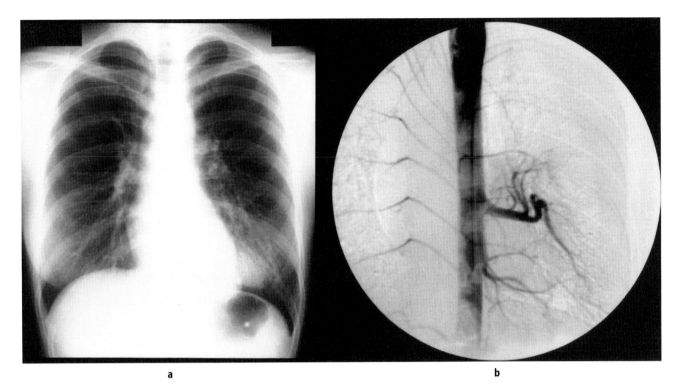

a   b

Figure 19.11. Intralobar pulmonary sequestration in a 23 year old female. **a** Posteroanterior chest radiograph shows mass-like opacity in left lower lung, but cystic abnormality is not evident in this case. **b** Thoracic aortography demonstrates feeding artery originating from descending aorta. Surgical procedure proved her to be having intralobar pulmonary sequestration.

Patients with a *pneumothorax*, a *pneumomediastinum*, or a diaphragmatic hernia show intrathoracic air that can be easily diagnosed by CT scans.

References

1. Tuddenham WJ (1984) Glossary of terms for thoracic radiology: Recommendations of the Nomenclature Committee of the Fleischner Society. AJR 143:509–517.
2. Lillington GA (1987) A diagnostic approach to chest diseses. Differential diagnosis based on roentgenographic patterns, 3rd edn. Williams & Wilkins, Baltimore, MD.
3. Webb WR, Müller NL, Naidich DP (1993) Standardized terms for high-resolution computed tomography of the lung: A proposed glossary. J Thorac Imaging 8:167–175.
4. Webb WR, Müller NL, Naidich DP (1996) High-resolution CT of the lung, 2nd edn. Lippincott-Raven Publishers, Philadelphia.
5. Travis WD, Borok Z, Roum JH, et al. (1993) Pulmonary Langerhans' cell granulomatosis (histiocytosis X). A clinico-pathologic study of 48 cases. Am J Surg Pathol 17:971–986.
6. Colby TV, Lombard C (1983) Histiocytosis X in the lung. Hum Pathol 14:847–856.
7. Marcy TW, Reynolds HY (1985) Pulmonary histiocytosis X. Lung 163:129–150.
8. Schünfeld N, Frank W, Wenig S, et al. (1993) Clinical and radiologic features, lung function and therapeutic results in pulmonary histiocytosis X. Respiration 60:38–40.
9. Lewis JG (1964) Eosinophilic granuloma and its variants with special reference to lung involvemet: A report of 12 patients. Q J Med 33:337–359.
10. Mogulkoc N, Veral A, Bishop PW, et al. (1999) Pulmonary Langerhans' cell histiocytosis. Radiologic resolution following smoking cessation. Chest 115:1452–1455.
11. Moore ADA, Godwin JD, Müller NL, et al. (1989) Pulmonary histiocytosis X: Comparison of radiographic and CT findings. Radiology 172:249–254.
12. Brauner MW, Grenier P, Mouelhi MM, et al. (1989) Pulmonary histiocytosis X: Evaluation with high-resolution CT. Radiology 172:255–258.
13. Kulwiec EL, Lynch DA, Aguayo SM, et al. (1992) Imaging of pulmonary histiocytosis X. Radiographics 12:515–526.
14. Grenier P, Valeyre D, Cluzel P, et al. (1991) Chronic diffuse interstitial lung disease: Diagnostic value of chest radiography and high-resolution CT. Radiology 179:123–132.
15. Brauner MW, Grenier P, Tijani K, et al. (1997) Pulmonary Langerhans' cell histiocytosis: Evolution of lesions on CT scans. Radiology 204:497–502.
16. Kelkel E, Pison C, Brambilla E, et al. (1992) Value of high resolution tomodensitometry in pulmonary histiocytosis X: Radiological, clinical and functional correlations. Rev Mal Respir 9:307–311.
17. Stern EJ, Webb WR, Golden JA, et al. (1992) Cystic lung disease associated with eosinophilic granuloma and tuberous sclerosis: air trapping at dynamic ultrafast high-resolution CT. Radiology 182:325–329.
18. Corrin B, Liebow AA, Friedman PJ (1975) Pulmonary lymphangioleiomyomatosis. A review. Am J Pathol 79:347–382.
19. Carrington CB, Cugell DW, Gaensler EA, et al. (1977) Lymphangioleiomyomatosis: Physiologic–pathologic–radiologic correlations. Am Rev Respir Dis 116:977–995.
20. Taylor JR, Ryu J, Colby TV, et al. (1990) Lymphangioleiomyomatosis. Clinical course in 32 patients. N Engl J Med 323:1254–1260.

21. Kitaichi M, Nishimura K, Itoh H, et al. (1995) Pulmonary lymphangioleiomyomatosis: A report of 46 patients including a clinicopathologic study of prognostic factors. Am J Respir Crit Care Med 151:527–533.

22. Sullivan EJ (1998) Lymphangioleiomyomatosis. A review. Chest 114:1689–1703.

23. Moss J, Ross R, Vaughan M, et al. (1999) Report of workshop on lymphangioleiomyomatosis. Am J Respir Crit Care Med 159:679–683.

24. Oh YM, Mo EK, Jang SH, et al. (1999) Pulmonary lymphangioleiomyomatosis in Korea. Thorax 54:618–621.

25. Chu SC, Horiba K, Usuki J, et al. (1999) Comprehensive evaluation of 35 patients with lymphangioleiomyomatosis. Chest 115: 1041–1052.

26. Krishna G, Berry G, Kao P, et al. (1999) Update on the treatment of lymphangioleiomyomatosis. Clin Pulm Med 6:126–132.

27. Johnson SR, Tattersfield AE (1999) Decline in lung function in lymphangioleiomyomatosis. Relation to menopause and progesterone treatment. Am J Respir Crit Care Med 160:628–633.

28. Merchant RN, Pearson MG, Rankin RN, et al. WKC (1985) Computerized tomography in the diagnosis of lymphangioleiomyomatosis. Am Rev Respir Dis 131:295–297.

29. Rappaport DC, Weisbrod GL, Herman SJ, et al. DW (1989) Pulmonary lymphangioleimyomatosis: High-resolution CT findings in four cases. AJR 152:961–964.

30. Sherrier RH, Chiles C, Roggli V (1989) Pulmonary lymphangioleiomyomatosis: CT findings. AJR 153:937–940.

31. Templeton PA, McLoud TC, Müller NL, et al. (1989) Pulmonary lymphangioleiomyomasosis: CT and pathologic findings. J Comput Assist Tomogr 13:54–57.

32. Lenoir S, Grenier P, Brauner MW, et al. (1990) Pulmonary lymphangiomyomatosis and tuberous sclerosis: Comparison of radiographic and thin-section CT findings. Radiology 175:329–334.

33. Müller NL, Chiles C, Kullnig P (1990) Pulmonary lymphangiomyomatosis: Correlation of CT with radiographic and functional findings. Radiology 175:335–339.

34. Aberle DR, Hansell DM, Brown K, et al. (1990) Lymphangiomyomatosis: CT, chest radiographic, and functional correlations. Radiology 176:381–387.

35. Crausman RS, Lynch DA, Mortenson RL, et al. (1996) Quantitative CT predicts the severity of physiologic dysfunction in patients with lymphangioleiomyomatosis. Chest 109:131–137.

36. Worthy SA, Brown MJ, Müller NL (1998) Technical report: Cystic air spaces in the lung: Change in size on expiratory high-resolution CT in 23 patients. Clin Radiol 53:515–519.

37. Muir TE, Leslie KO, Popper H, et al. (1998) Micronodular pneumocyte hyperplasia. Am J Surg Pathol 22:465–472.

38. Müller NL, Bergin CJ, Ostrow DN, et al. (1984) Role of computed tomography in the recognition of bronchiectasis. AJR 143:971–976.

39. Mootoosamy IM, Reznek RH, Osman J, et al. (1985) Assessment of bronchiectasis by computed tomography. Thorax 40:920–924.

40. Grenier P, Maurice F, Musset D, et al. (1986) Bronchiectasis: Assessment by thin-section CT. Radiology 161:95–99.

41. Pang JA, Hamilton-Wood C, Metreweli C (1989) The value of computed tomography in the diagnosis and management of bronchiectasis. Clin Radiol 40:40–44.

42. Young K, Aspestrand F, Kolbenstvedt A (1991) High resolution CT and bronchography in the assessment of bronchiectasis. Acta Radiologica 32:439–441.

43. Marti-Bonmati L, Catala FJ, Ruiz Perales F (1991) Computed tomography differentiation between cystic bronchiectasis and bullae. J Thorac Imaging 7:83–85.

44. Kang EY, Miller RR, Müller NL (1995) Bronchiectasis: Comparison of preoperative thin-section CT and pathologic findings in resected specimens. Radiology 195:649–654.

45. van der Bruggen-Bogaarts BAHA, van der Bruggen HMJG, van Waes PFGM, et al. (1996) Screening for bronchiectasis. A comparative study between chest radiography and high-resolution CT. Chest 109:608–611.

46. Smith IE, Jurriaans E, Diederich S, et al. (1996) Chronic sputum production: Correlations between clinical features and findings on high resolution computed tomographic scanning of the chest. Thorax 51:914–918.

47. King MA, Stone JA, Diaz PT, et al. (1996) α1-Antitrypsin deficiency: Evaluation of bronchiectasis with CT. Radiology 199:137–141.

48. Lucidarme O, Grenier P, Coche E, et al. (1996) Bronchiectasis: Comparative assessment with thin-section CT and helical CT. Radiology 200:673–679.

49. Miszkiel KA, Wells AU, Rubens MB, et al. (1997) Effects of airway infection by Pseudomonas aeruginosa: A computed tomographic study. Thorax 52:260–264.

50. Hansell DM, Well AU, Rubens MB, et al. (1994) Bronchiectasis: Functional significance of areas of decreased attenuation at expiratory CT. Radiology 193:369–374.

51. Currie DC, Goldman JM, Cole PJ, et al. (1987) Comparison of narrow section computed tomography and plain chest radiography in chronic allergic bronchopulmonary aspergillosis. Clin Radiol 38:593–596.

52. Kullning P, Pongratz M, Kopp W, et al. (1989) Computerized tomography in the diagnosis of allergic bronchopulmonary aspergillosis. Radiology 29:228–231.

53. Neeld DA, Goodman LR, Gurney JW, et al. (1990) Computerized tomography in the evaluation of allergic bronchopulmonary aspergillosis. Am Rev Respir Dis 142:1200–1205.

54. Panchal N, Bhagat R, Pant C, et al. (1997) Allergic bronchopulmonary aspergillosis: The spectrum of computed tomography appearances. Respir Med 91:213–219.

55. Hojo S, Fujita J, Obayashi Y, et al. (1997) Two cases of cystic fibrosis in Japanese/German twins. Jap J Thorac Dis 35:1259–1264.

56. Hojo S, Fujita J, Miyawaki H, et al. (1998) Severe cystic fibrosis associated with ΔF508/R347H+D979A compound heterozygous genotype. Clin Genet 53:50–53.

57. Friedman PJ (1987) Chest radiologic findings in the adult with cystic fibrosis. Semin Roentgenol 22:114–124.

58. Hansell DM, Strickland B (1989) High-resolution computed tomography in pulmonary cystic fibrosis. Br J Radiol 62:1–5.

59. Santis G, Hodson ME, Strickland B (1991) High resolution computed tomography in adult cystic fibrosis patients with mild lung disease. Clin Radiol 44:20–22.

60. Taccone A, Romano L, Marzoli A, et al. (1991) Computerized tomography in pulmonary cystic fibrosis. Radiol Med 82:79–83.

61. Kraft M, Mortenson RL, Colby TV, et al. (1993) Cryptogenic constrictive bronchiolitis. A clinicopathologic study. Am Rev Respir Dis 148:1093–1101.

62. Morrish WF, Herman SJ, Weisbrod GL, et al. (1991) Bronchiolitis obliterans after lung transplantation: findings at chest radiography and high-resolution CT. Radiology 179:487–490.

63. Homma H, Yamanaka A, Tanimoto S, et al. (1983) Diffuse panbronchiolitis. A disease of the transitional zone of the lung. Chest 83:63–69.

64. Randhawa P, Hoagland MH, Yousem SA (1991) Diffuse panbronchiolitis in North America. Report of three cases and review of the literature. Am J Surg Pathol 15:43–47.

65. Kitaichi M, Nishimura K, Izumi T (1991) Diffuse panbronchiolotis. In Sharma OP (ed) Lung diseases in the Tropics. Marcel Dekker, Inc., New York, pp 479–509.

66. Nishimura K, Kitaichi M, Izumi T, et al. (1992) Diffuse panbronchiolitis: Correlation of high-resolution CT and pathologic findings. Radiology 184:779–785.

67. Akira M, Kitatani F, Yong-Sik L, et al. (1988) Diffuse panbronchiolitis: Evaluation with high-resolution CT. Radiology 168:433–438.

68. Akira M, Higashihara T, Sakatani M (1993) Diffuse panbronchiolitis: Follow-up CT examination. Radiology 189:559–562.

69. Sugimoto M, Kitaichi M, Ikeda A, et al. (1998) Chronic bronchiolo-alveolitis associated with human T-cell lymphotrophic virus type 1 infection. Curr Opin Pulm Med 4:98–102.

70. Nishimura K, Kitaichi M, Izumi T, et al. (1992) Usual interstitial pneumonia: Histologic correlation with high-resolution CT. Radiology 182:337–342.

71. Itoh H, Murata K, Konishi J, et al. (1993) Diffuse lung disease: Pathologic basis for the high-resolution computed tomography findings. J Thorac Imaging 8:176–188.

72. Westcott JL, Cole SR (1986) Traction bronchiectasis in end-stage pulmonary fibrosis. Radiology 161:665–669.

73. Heitzman ER (1984) The Lung. Radiologic–pathologic correlations, 2nd edn. Mosby, St. Louis. MO.

74. Crystal RG, Fulmer JD, Roberts WC, et al. (1976) Idiopathic pulmonary fibrosis: Clinical, histologic, radiographic, physiologic, scintigraphic, cytologic, and biochemical, aspects. Ann Intern Med 85:769–788.

75. Yousem SA, Colby TV, Carrington CB (1985) Lung biopsy in rheumatoid arthritis. Am Rev Respir Dis 131:770–777.

76. Chan TYK, Hansell DM, Rubens MB, et al. (1997) Cryptogenic fibrosing alveolitis and the fibrosing alveolitis of systemic sclerosis: Morphological differences on computed tomographic scans. Thorax 52:265–270.

77. Carrington CB, Gaensler EA, Coutu RE, et al. (1978) Natural history and treated course of usual and desquamative interstitial pneumonia. N Engl J Med 298:801–809.

78. Akira M, Sakatani M, Ueda E (1993) Idiopathic pulmonary fibrosis: Progression of honeycombing at thin-section CT. Radiology 189:687–691.

79. Wells AU, Rubens MB, du Bois RM, Hansell DM (1993) Serial CT in fibrosing alveolitis: Prognostic significance of the initial pattern. AJR 161:1159–1165.

80. Mino M, Noma S, Kobashi Y, et al. (1995) Serial changes of cystic air spaces in fibrosing alveolitis: a CT–pathological study. Clin Radiol 50:357–363.

81. Hartman TE, Primack SL, Kang EY, et al. (1996) Disease progression in usual interstitial pneumonia compared with desquamative interstitial pneumonia. Assessment with serial CT. Chest 110:378–382.

82. Lee JS, Gong G, Song KS, et al. (1998) Usual interstitial pneumonia: Relationship between disease activity and the progression of honeycombing at thin-section computed tomography. J Thorac Imaging 13:199–203.

83. Wiggins J, Strickland B, Turner-Warwick M (1990) Combined cryptogenic fibrosing alveolitis and emphysema: The value of high resolution computed tomography in assessment. Respir Med 84:365–369.

84. Hanley ME, King TE, Jr., Schwarz MI, et al. (1991) The impact of smoking on mechanical properties of the lungs in idiopathic pulmonary fibrosis and sarcoidosis. Am Rev Respir Dis 144:1102–1106.

85. Hiraga Y, Yamamoto M, Tachibana T, et al. (1981) Pulmonary fibrosis in severe pulmonary sarcoidosis. In Mikami R, Hosoda Y (eds) Sarcoidosis. University of Tokyo Press, Tokyo, pp 291–300.

86. Nishimura K, Itoh H, Kitaichi M, et al. (1993) Pulmonary sarcoidosis: Correlation of CT and histopathologic findings. Radiology 189:105–109.

87. Nishimura K, Itoh H, Kitaichi M, et al. (1995) CT and pathologic correlation of pulmonary sarcoidosis. Semin Ultrasound, CT MR 16:361–370.

88. Katzenstein ALA, Myers JL, Mazur MT (1986) Acute interstitial pneumonia: A clinicopathologic, ultrastructural and cell kinetic study. Am J Surg Pathol 10:256–267.

89. Primack SL, Hartman TE, Ikezoe J, et al. (1993) Acute interstitial pneumonia: Radiographic and CT findings in nine patients. Radiology 188:817–820.

90. Katenstein AA, Bloor CM, Leibow AA (1976) Diffuse alveolar damage – the role of oxygen, shock, and related factors. A review. Am J Pathol 85:210–228.

91. Snider GL, Kleinerman J, Thurlbeck WM (1985) The definition of emphysema. Report of a National Heart, Lung, and Blood Institute, Division of Lung Diseases Workshop Report. Am Rev Respir Dis 132:182–185.

92. Bergin C, Müller NL, Nichols DM, et al. (1986) The diagnosis of emphysema. A computed tomographic–pathologic correlation. Am Rev Respir Dis 133:541–546.

93. Foster WL, Jr, Pratt PC, Roggli VL, et al. (1986) Centrilobular emphysema: CT-pathologic correlation. Radiology 159:27–32.

94. Hruban RH, Meziane MA, Zerhouni EA, et al. (1987) High resolution computed tomography of inflation-fixed lungs. Pathologic-radiologic correlation of centrilobular emphysema. Am Rev Respir Dis 136:935–940.

95. Miller RR, Müller NL, Vedal S, et al. (1989) Limitations of computed tomography in the assessment of emphysema. Am Rev Respir Dis 139:980–983.

96. Kuwano K, Matsuba K, Ikeda T, et al. (1990) The diagnosis of mild emphysema. Correlation of computed tomography and pathology scores. Am Rev Respir Dis 141:169–178.

97. Spouge D, Mayo JR, Cardoso W, et al. (1993) Panacinar emphysema: CT and pathologic findings. J Comput Assist Tomogr 17:710–713.

98. Woodring JH, Vandiviere HM, Fried AM, et al. (1986) Update: The radiographic features of pulmonary tuberculosis. AJR 146:497–506.

99. Kuhlman JE, Deutsch JH, Fishman EK, et al. (1990) CT features of thoracic mycobacterial disease. Radiographics 10:413–431.

100. Hill AR, Premkumar S, Brustein S, et al. (1991) Disseminated tuberculosis in the acquired immunodeficiency syndrome era. Am Rev Respir Dis 144:1164–1170.

101. Ikezoe J, Takeuchi N, Johkoh T, et al. (1992) CT appearance of pulmonary tuberculosis in diabetic and immunocompromised patients: Comparison with patients who had no underlying disease. AJR 159:1175–1179.

102. Tsao TCY, Juang YC, Tsai YH, et al. (1992) Whole lung tuberculosis. A disease with high mortality which is frequently misdiagnosed. Chest 101:1309–1311.

103. Im JG, Itoh H, Shim YS, et al. (1993) Pulmonary tuberculosis: CT findings – early active disease and sequential change with anti-tuberculous therapy. Radiology 186:653–660.

104. Leung AN, Brauner MW, Gamsu G, et al. (1996) Pulmonary tuberculosis: Comparison of CT findings in HIV-seropositive and HIV-seronegative patients. Radiology 198:687–691.

105. Hatipoglu ON, Osma E, Manisali M, et al. (1996) High resolution computed tomographic findings in pulmonary tuberculosis. Thorax 51:397–402.

106. Lee KS, Hwang JW, Chung MP, et al. (1996) Utility of CT in the evaluation of pulmonary tuberculosis in patients without AIDS. Chest 110:977–984.

107. Poey C, Verhaegen F, Giron J, et al. (1997) High resolution chest CT in tuberculosis: Evolutive patterns and signs of activity. J Comput Assist Tomogr 21:601–607.

108. Miller WT Jr, Miller WT (1993) Pulmonary infections with atypical mycobacteria in the normal host. Semin Roentgenol 28:139–149.

109. Primack SL, Logan PM, Hartman TE, et al. (1995) Pulmonary tuberculosis and Mycobacterium avium-intracellulare: A comparison of CT findings Radiology 194:413–417.

110. Laissy JP, Cadi M, Cinqualbre A, et al. (1997) Mycobacterium tuberculosis versus nontuberculous mycobacterial infection of the

lung in AIDS patients: CT and HRCT patterns. J Comput Assist Tomogr 21:312–317.

111. Hartman TE, Swensen SJ, Williams DE (1993) Mycobacterium avium-intracellulare complex: Evaluation with CT. Radiology 187:23–26.

112. Moore EH (1993) Atypical mycobacterial infection in the lung: CT appearance. Radiology 187:777–782.

113. Swensen SJ, Hartman TE, Williams DE (1994) Computed tomographic diagnosis of Mycobacterium avium-intracellulare complex in patients with bronchiectasis. Chest 105:49–52.

114. Lynch DA, Simone PM, Fox MA, et al. (1995) CT features of pulmonary Mycobacterium avium complex infection. J Comput Assist Tomogr 19:353–360.

115. Obayashi Y, Fujita J, Suemitsu I, et al. (1999) Successive follow-up of chest computed tomography in patients with Mycobacterium avium-intracellulare complex. Respir Med 93:11–15.

116. Hartman TE, Primack SL, Müller NL, et al. (1994) Diagnosis of thoracic complication in AIDS: Accuracy of CT. AJR 162:547–553.

117. Kuhlman JE, Kavuru M, Fishman EK, et al. (1990) Pneumocystis carinii pneumonia: Spectrum of parenchymal CT findings. Radiology 175:711–714.

118. Bergin CJ, Wirth RL, Berry GJ, et al. (1990) Pneumocystis carinii pneumonia: CT and HRCT observations. J Comput Assist Tomogr 14:756–759.

119. Chow C, Templeton PA, White CS (1993) Lung cysts associated with Pneumocystis carinii pneumonia: Radiographic characteristics, natural history, and complications. AJR 161:527–531.

120. Goodman PC, Daley C, Minagi H (1986) Spontaneous pneumothorax in AIDS patients with Pneumocystis carinii pneumonia. AJR 147:29–31.

121. McGuinness G, Naidich DP, Garay SM, et al. (1993) AIDS associated bronchiectasis: CT features. J Comput Assist Tomogr 17:260–266.

122. Kuhlman JE, Fishman EK, Teigen C (1990) Pulmonary septic emboli: Diagnosis with CT. Radiology 174:211–213.

123. Balakrishnan J, Meziane MA, Siegelman SS, et al. (1989) Pulmonary infarction: CT appearance with pathologic correlation. J Comput Assist Tomogr 13:941–945.

124. Hruban RH, Meziance MA, Zerhouni EA, et al. (1987) Radiologic-pathologic correlation of the CT halo sign in invasive pulmonary aspergillosis. J Comput Assist Tomogr 11:534–536.

125. Logan PM, Primack SL, Miller RR, et al. (1994) Invasive aspergillosis of the airways: Radiographic, CT, and pathologic findings. Radiology 193:383–388.

126. Staples CA, Kang EY, Wright JL, et al. (1995) Invasive pulmonary aspergillosis in AIDS: Radiographic, CT, and pathplogic findings. Radiology 196:409–414.

127. Won HJ, Lee KS, Cheon JE, et al. (1998) Invasive pulmonary aspergillosis: prediction at thin-section CT in patients with neutropenia – a prospective study. Radiology 208:777–782.

128. Patz EF Jr, Goodman PC (1992) Pulmonary cryptococcosis. J Thorac Imaging 7:51–55.

129. Lee LN, Yang PC, Kuo SH, et al. (1993) Diagnosis of pulmonary cryptococcosis by ultrasound guided percutaneous aspiration. Thorax 48:75–78.

130. Aberg JA, Mundy LM, Powderly WG (1999) Pulmonary cryptococcosis in patients without HIV infection. Chest 115:734–740.

131. Cordier JF, Valeyre D, Guillevin L, et al. (1990) Pulmonary Wegener's granulomatosis. A clinical and imaging study of 77 cases. Chest 97:906–912.

132. Kuhlman JE, Hruban RH, Fishman EK (1991) Wegener granulomatosis: CT features of parenchymal lung disease. J Compt Assist Tomogr 15:948–952.

133. Weir IH, Müller NL, Chiles C, et al. (1992) Wegener's granulomatosis: findings from computed tomography of the chest in 10 patients. Can Assoc Radiol J 43:31–34.

134. Maskell GF, Lockwood CM, Flower CDR (1993) Computed tomography of the lung in Wegener's granulomatosis. Clin Radiol 48:377–380.

135. Reuter M, Schnabel A, Wesner F, et al. (1998) Pulmonary Wegener's granulomatosis. Correlation between high-resolution CT findings and clinical scoring of disease activity. Chest 114:500–506.

136. Attali P, Begum R, Ban-Romdhane H, et al. (1998) Pulmonary Wegener's granulomatosis: Changes at follow-up CT. Eur Radiol 8:1009–1113.

137. Judson MA, Strange C (1998) Bullous sarcoidosis. A report of three cases. Chest 114:1474–1478.

138. Trigaux JP, Gevenois PA, Goncette L, et al. (1996) Bronchioloalveolar carcinoma: Computed tomography findings. Eur Respir J 9:11–16.

139. Cordier JF, Chailleux E, Lauque D, et al. (1993) Primary pulmonary lymphomas. A clinical study of 70 cases in nonimmunocompromised patients. Chest 103:201–208.

140. Jackson SA, Tung KT, Mead GM (1994) Multiple cavitating pulmonary lesions in non-Hodgkin's lymphoma. Clin Radiol 49:883–885.

141. Johkoh T, Müller NL, Ichikado K, et al. (1998) Intrathoracic multicentric Castleman disease: CT findings in 12 patients. Radiology 209:477–481.

142. Ichikawa Y, Kinoshita M, Koga T, et al. (1994) Lung cyst formation in lymphocytic interstitial pneumonia: CT features. J Comput Assist Tomogr 18:745–748.

143. Macpherson RI (1993) Gastrointestinal tract duplications: Clinical, pathologic, etiologic, and radiologic considerations. Radiographics 13:1063–1080

20 Pulmonary Manifestations of Systemic Diseases

B.H. Gross, K.A. Buckwalter, D.L. Spizarny, M. Rebner, and M. Sperber

The chest may be involved in any of a number of systemic diseases. Because the chest is easily and frequently imaged (via chest radiography, conventional tomography, computed tomography (CT) including high resolution computed tomography (HRCT), ultrasonography, and magnetic resonance imaging (MRI)) such involvement is often manifested radiographically. Indeed, one could probably write an entire textbook on pulmonary involvement in systemic diseases. Instead, this chapter attempts to highlight chest radiographic manifestations of some of the more common systemic diseases that affect the chest, with a few unusual and interesting entities also included.

Metabolic Diseases

Renal Disease

There are a variety of chest radiographic manifestations of renal disease. For the purpose of this chapter, diseases that affect the kidneys and lungs specifically (e.g., Goodpasture syndrome and Wegener granulomatosis) will be covered separately (see below). Apart from these, there are two major categories of renal disease, nephrotic syndrome and renal failure, that have quite different chest manifestations. Nephrotic syndrome affects the chest only when hypoproteinemia leads to anasarca, resulting in pleural effusion. In this setting pleural effusion is usually bilateral.

Renal failure produces many abnormalities in the chest, not all of which involve the lung parenchyma. A common manifestation of renal failure is pericardial effusion (Fig. 20.1) secondary to uremic pericarditis. In many cases echocardiography is necessary for accurate diagnosis. Fluid balance may be difficult to manage in patients with renal failure, and fluid overload may be associated with pleural effusion. Thoracic soft tissues may also be affected by renal failure, with some patients demonstrating metastatic calcification (see below).

Among the most important effects of renal failure are those involving the lung parenchyma. Diffuse bilateral airspace disease is often seen, and the differential diagnosis includes pulmonary edema, hemorrhage, and pneumonia. It is important to emphasize that any patient with chronic renal failure is at risk of developing pulmonary hemorrhage, even in the absence of concurrent pulmonary disease (e.g., Goodpasture syndrome or

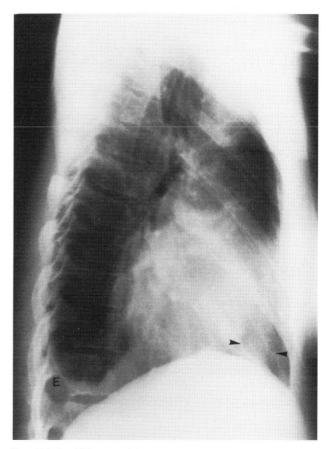

Figure 20.1. Renal failure. Lateral chest radiograph demonstrates pericardial effusion, manifested by separation of epicardial and epipericardial fat planes (*arrowheads*), as well as a small left pleural effusion (*E*).

Wegener granulomatosis) (1). Opportunistic infection can also occur, particularly after renal transplantation, and cytomegalovirus infection is especially frequent in this setting.

Liver Disease

Liver disease rarely causes pulmonary parenchymal abnormalities. In a few cases patients with liver failure may present with pulmonary hemorrhage as a part of a generalized bleeding diathesis. Right lower lobe atelectasis and/or right pleural effusion may result from inflammatory, vascular, or neoplastic abnormalities of the liver (e.g., hepatic infarction). Finally, generalized hepatomegaly may cause elevation of the right hemidiaphragm with compressive right lung atelectasis.

More commonly, liver disease results in pleural effusion, which may be a manifestation of anasarca secondary to hypoproteinemia, in which case it is often bilateral. Alternatively, portal hypertension may result in ascites with transdiaphragmatic migration of fluid, more commonly affecting the right pleural space (Fig. 20.2).

Metastatic Calcifications

Extensive metastatic pulmonary or soft tissue calcifications may occur in patients with chronic hypercal-

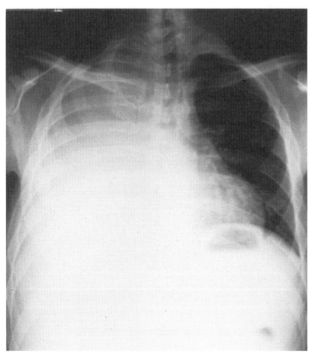

Figure 20.2. Wilson disease. Posteroanterior chest radiograph reveals a massive right pleural effusion.

cemic states (2). These include longstanding renal disease, secondary hyperparathyroidism, multiple myeloma, hypervitaminosis D, milk-alkali syndrome, and sarcoidosis. Abnormal serum calcium and phosphorus levels, alkalinity at the site of calcium deposition, and decreased renal function predispose to these calcifications. In some cases, extensive metastatic calcifications may cause respiratory failure. Bone scanning with technetium methylene diphosphonate can confirm the diagnosis (3).

Hematologic Disorders

Hemophilia

Hemophilia is a bleeding diathesis caused by inherited deficiency of clotting factor VIII. It is the most common inherited coagulation factor disorder, affecting roughly 1 in 10 000 males (4). Because it is a sex-linked recessive disorder it affects men almost exclusively. Women who are heterozygous for the gene are carriers unaffected by the disease. Hemophilia may cause bleeding in any organ or cavity of the body. However, pulmonary, pleural, and pericardial hemorrhage are relatively uncommon. In recent years, CT and MRI have shown their efficacy not only in the demonstration of the common soft tissue and intracranial hemorrhages in hemophiliac patients, but also in the immediate and accurate discovery of pathologic changes such as unsuspected mediastinal hematomas (5).

Hemophilic pulmonary hemorrhage causes acute alveolar disease. In hemophilic patients who have had multiple episodes of pulmonary hemorrhage a pattern of small irregular shadows in the lungs may signal the development of secondary pulmonary hemosiderosis.

An unfortunate complication of hemophilia is acquired immune deficiency syndrome (AIDS), generally secondary to transfusion of infected blood products. In fact, the usual cause of acute alveolar disease in a hemophilic patient is not hemorrhage, but opportunistic infection. Pneumocystis carinii is a common organism in this setting.

Sickle Cell Disease

'Sickle cell disease" is a term referring to any one of several hereditary disorders characterized by the presence of hemoglobin (Hb) S. The most often discussed is sickle cell anemia, in which the major oxygen transport molecule is Hb S-S. The disease is common, occurring in 0.3–1.3% of North American blacks; sickle cell trait (i.e., heterozygous individuals) occurs in approximately 71% of this population. The disease presents only after the first 6 months of life, when fetal hemoglobin, Hb F, is replaced by Hb S. The abnormal hemoglobin is less efficient at oxygen transport, and the presence of Hb S-S results in the characteristic sickle shape of the red blood cells that occurs when the oxygen tension is reduced. This shape increases the viscosity of the blood and causes sludging, often resulting in infarction.

The clinical course is unpredictable, with multiple episodes of sickle cell crisis characterized by bone and joint pain, fevers, and prostration. Affected individuals are particularly susceptible to infection by encapsulated bacteria because of the recurrent splenic infarcts, which eventually result in "autosplenectomy," thus impairing the normal trapping and clearance of these organisms from the systemic circulation. Of particular note is the increased incidence of pneumococcal pneumonia and salmonella osteomyelitis.

Findings on chest radiographs are fairly typical when considered as a group. As expected, the chronic anemia results in moderate cardiomegaly and fullness of the pulmonary vasculature. Multiple pneumonias and/or pulmonary infarcts result in pulmonary parenchymal scarring. An acute crisis episode may cause pleural effusion and focal airspace disease or atelectasis, all nonspecific findings. Gallstones may be visible in the right upper quadrant of the abdomen. Changes in the bony thorax are caused by the chronic anemia and multiple bone infarcts (6). There is diffuse sclerosis of the skeleton and coarsening of the trabecular pattern. Infarcts of the central portion of the vertebral bodies result in the typical H-shaped vertebral body associated with sickle cell disease (Fig. 20.3). Infarcts of the humeral heads result in focal sclerosis of the epiphysis, termed "snow capping" because of the resemblance to a snow-capped mountain (7).

Advanced investigative modalities such as CT and MRI have shown their value in the identification of the large variety of pathologic changes characterizing this disorder (8). Complications such as the development of chronic pulmonary disorders and vasoocclusive phenomena can be clearly identified with thin-section and spiral CT (8,9). In the event of acute chest syndrome in sickle cell disease, CT can show evidence of microvascular occlusion (10).

Intrathoracic Lymphoma and Leukemia

Lymphoma subclassifications change frequently, and although overly simplified, separation into Hodgkin and non-Hodgkin lymphomas is useful when one is discussing radiographic manifestations. In general, intrathoracic lymphoma and leukemia can involve lymph nodes, lung parenchyma, heart and pericardium, and pleura.

Lymphadenopathy

Lymphadenopathy is the most common intrathoracic manifestation of lymphoma. Although frequency of involvement is dependent on the series cited, intrathoracic adenopathy at presentation is more common with Hodgkin lymphoma. Filly et al. (11) found that 67% of Hodgkin lymphoma patients presented with intrathoracic disease (99% of these had adenopathy), whereas 43% of non-Hodgkin lymphoma patients presented with intrathoracic disease (87% of these had adenopathy). They found single intrathoracic nodal group involvement common in non-Hodgkin lymphoma (40%) and uncommon in Hodgkin lymphoma (15%) (12). Although uncommon, bilateral hilar adenopathy without mediastinal adenopathy occurred in both groups (12). Nodal masses can be quite large, especially with Hodgkin disease (Fig. 20.4).

Intrathoracic leukemic adenopathy occurs in 25% of patients (13). It is more frequent with lymphocytic leukemias (13). Because leukemia is systemic, specific nodal site analysis is less important; however, single intrathoracic nodal group involvement has been reported (12).

On chest radiographs, mediastinal and hilar contour deformities are the hallmarks of lymph node detection. Paratracheal stripe widening, lumpy hilar enlargement, aorticopulmonary window convexity, azygoesophageal stripe displacement, paraspinal stripe widening, cardiophrenic angle bulging, and other contour deformities are consistent with specific nodal group enlargement. By directly visualizing the mediastinum, CT has replaced barium swallow and plain film tomography as the second step in intrathoracic lymph node detection. CT detects enlarged lymph nodes and masses missed on chest radiographs (14), and CT can directly affect management in certain lymphoma patients (15). At the same time, subpleural nodular masses are commonly discovered with CT (16).

Pulmonary Lymphoma and Leukemia

Primary lung lymphoma, defined as parenchymal involvement without adenopathy, is rare. When lymphoma involves the lung, lymphadenopathy is almost always present (12). Blank and Castellino (12) found that 11.6% of Hodgkin's lymphoma patients had lung involvement, compared with 3.7% of non-Hodgkin lymphoma patients.

The varied pathologic and radiographic presentations of pulmonary lymphoma are secondary to widespread distribution of pulmonary lymphatic tissue. Lymph nodes occur near vascular and bronchial branches, and peribronchial, perivascular, and intralobular septal lymphatic tissues are joined by a diffuse lymphatic vessel network (17).

B.H. Gross, K.A. Buckwalter, D.L. Spizarny, M. Rebner, and M. Sperber

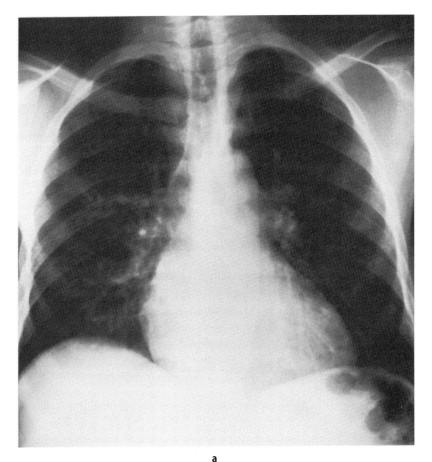

a

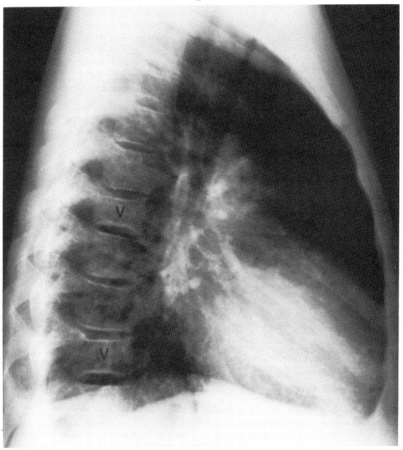

b

Figure 20.3. Sickle cell disease. **a** Posteroanterior chest radiograph reveals cardiomegaly and generalized bony sclerosis. **b** Lateral view shows typical H-shaped vertebrae (*V*).

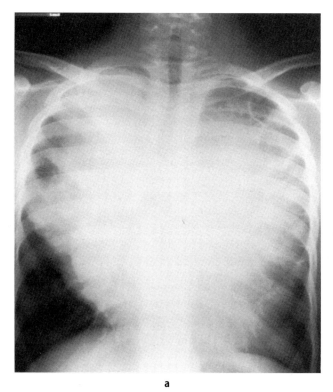

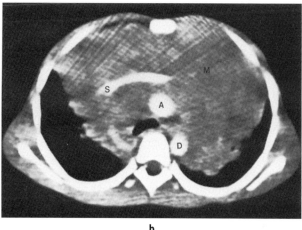

a   b

Figure 20.4. Hodgkin disease. Massive mediastinal lymph node enlargement. **a** Posteroanterior chest radiograph. **b** CT scan at the level of the carina. *M*, mass; *S*, superior vena cava; *A*, ascending aorta; *D*, descending aorta.

Extension of lymphomatous adenopathy into lung causes normally sharp mediastinal–lung and hilar–lung interfaces to become shaggy. Massive peribronchial and perivascular involvement can consolidate the lung, causing very well-defined air bronchograms. Peripheral involvement can cause lymphomatous nodules, which can be well defined or patchy and solid or cavitated. Pulmonary lymphoma may evolve rapidly, with widespread disease developing in days (12).

Lung disease is common in leukemia, and chest radiographic abnormalities are nonspecific. Focal disease usually presents as consolidated or atelectatic lung. Diffuse disease usually causes peribronchial thickening, a diffuse reticular pattern, or diffuse airspace disease. Due to alveolar collapse or alveolar filling with malignant cells an air bronchogram may often be discovered on conventional chest radiographs and CT images. On high resolution CT thickening of the bronchovascular bundle can be seen, together with prominence of the septal lines (18,19).

Tenholder and Hooper (20) reviewed 98 leukemics with lung disease and found that, during treatment, focal disease was 74% infectious (bacterial in 87% and opportunistic in 13%) and diffuse disease was 65% noninfectious. If diffuse disease was infectious, it was almost always (93%) opportunistic (20). Most infectious complications in lymphoma and leukemia include bacteria, among which may appear some of the more unusual ones, such as *Legionella pneumophilia* or *Mycoplasma pneumoniae*, mycobacteria, fungi, *Pneumocystis carinii* and viruses (21–23). CT may be useful in the early discovery of these abnormalities. A good

example is served by invasive pulmonary aspergillosis in which CT findings include the recognition of a nodule with a surrounding area of ground-glass opacification or the so-called "CT halo sign" (24,25). Etiologies of noninfectious diffuse disease included hemorrhage, congestive heart failure, and leukemic infiltration.

Pleural Lymphoma and Leukemia

At initial diagnosis, pleural effusion, especially as the only lymphomatous manifestation, is uncommon in Hodgkin and non-Hodgkin lymphomas (12). When effusion occurs, it may be chylous, can be unilateral or bilateral, and is usually small to moderate in size. Pleural effusion can be secondary to lymphatic obstruction, pulmonary venous obstruction or pleural invasion (12).

Congestive heart failure and infection probably cause most pleural effusions in leukemics. However, leukemic pleural infiltration, lymphatic obstruction by adenopathy, and subpleural infarcts surrounded by leukemic cells are responsible for some leukemic pleural effusions (12).

Cardiac and Pericardial Lymphoma and Leukemia

Lymphoma and leukemia can directly invade myocardium, causing cardiac enlargement. However, roentgenographic cardiac enlargement is more commonly secondary to pericardial effusion (12). Postmortems on leukemics demonstrate small pericardial effusions in 21% and cardiac leukemic infiltration in 18% (13). Apparent cardiac enlargement can also be secondary to mediastinal or pericardial adenopathy.

Amyloidosis and the Plasma Cell Dyscrasia

Amyloidosis is a condition of localized or diffuse deposition of a protein (amyloid) with the identifying characteristic of fibrils arranged in a cross or β-pleated sheet configuration (26). Amyloidosis has traditionally been classified as secondary to a known predisposing cause (e.g., chronic inflammation, multiple myeloma) or else primary. Biochemical analysis has shown that amyloid in primary amyloidosis is identical to that found in multiple myeloma, suggesting that both are plasma cell dyscrasias.

The respiratory tract is involved in about half of patients with amyloidosis, although radiographic abnormalities are much less frequent. Disease confined to the respiratory tract is more common than respiratory involvement as a part of systemic amyloidosis. There are three major forms of involvement: tracheobronchial (reportedly the most common), nodular (more common in our experience), and diffuse parenchymal. Nodular amyloidosis is commonly asymptomatic, but the other forms of amyloidosis generally cause clinical symptoms, especially when there is radiographically demonstrable disease.

As the different forms of involvement would suggest, there are many potential chest radiographic manifestations of amyloidosis. However, several presentations are somewhat suggestive of this condition. When pulmonary nodules are oval, lobular, indolent, and/or calcified, amyloidosis should be considered. Diffuse lung disease in a relatively asymptomatic patient, either in a small, irregular shadow pattern or else with coalescent parenchymal abnormality, suggests amyloidosis. Finally, extensively calcified lymph nodes also raise this possibility (Fig. 20.5). Since special staining of histologic material with Congo red is required to establish the diagnosis, the radiologist can play a key role simply by mentioning that amyloidosis deserves consideration.

Other plasma cell dyscrasias may result in chest radiographic abnormalities, but this is often because there is associated amyloidosis. This is most typical of multiple myeloma, which causes amyloidosis in 10% of patients. However, Waldenström macroglobulinemia, has been reported to cause pulmonary disease in nearly 26 patients (27,28). Common findings to date have included pleural effusion (usually unilateral), parenchymal small irregular opacities, lung nodules, and hilar lymph node enlargement.

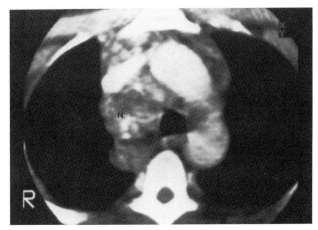

Figure 20.5. Amyloidosis. CT scan reveals a calcified right paratracheal lymph node mass (N).

Collagen Vascular Diseases

Rheumatoid Arthritis

Rheumatoid disease is probably due to altered immunologic mechanisms. The vast majority of patients have elevated titers of rheumatoid factor and some have antinuclear antibodies and positive lupus erythematosus cell preparations. Rheumatoid arthritis is more common in females, but extraarticular manifestations of the disease predominate in males. These extraarticular features include subcutaneous nodules, vasculitis, skin ulceration, adenopathy, neuropathy, splenomegaly, episcleritis, and pericarditis (29). Pleuropulmonary disease may also occur in 5–75% of cases, depending on rheumatoid factor status and the diagnostic criteria utilized.

The pleuropulmonary manifestations may be subdivided into six categories (30):

1. Diffuse interstitial fibrosis
2. Pleural effusion
3. Necrobiotic nodule
4. Caplan syndrome
5. Rheumatoid disease with pulmonary arteritis and hypertension
6. Rheumatoid disease with diffuse patchy bronchiolitis

Diffuse interstitial fibrosis is caused by an early interstitial pneumonia that is replaced by fibrosis and honeycomb lung. Radiographically, initially one sees nodular densities that develop into a reticular pattern, often most prominent at the lung bases.

Basically, the radiographic and histopathologic features of pulmonary rheumatoid arthritis are similar to idiopathic pulmonary fibrosis. HRCT will demonstrate at an early stage the fine interstitial changes.

Pleural abnormality is the most frequent thoracic manifestation of rheumatoid arthritis. The pleural fluid is an exudate with a high protein content and low glucose level. The pleural glucose level does not rise after intravenous glucose infusion, in contradistinction to the low pleural glucose seen in tuberculous pleural effusions. Radiographically, the effusion may persist for months or years, and is most often unilateral.

CT has greatly increased our capability of identifying and quantifying pulmonary fibrosis (31). At the same time specific pathologic changes are illustrated, especially with HRCT, when recent studies have identified bronchiectasis and bronchielectasis, interstitial pneumonitis, pulmonary nodules, ground-glass attenuation, bronchiolitis and honeycombing (32–34).

Necrobiotic nodules are associated with advanced rheumatoid arthritis and subcutaneous nodules. They are often multiple and thick walled. Cavitation is common (Fig. 20.6). If the arthritis wanes, the cavities may disappear.

Caplan syndrome consists of multiple nodules in rheumatoid patients who were or are coalworkers and were hypersensitized to dust particles. The nodules appear similar to the necrobiotic nodules of patients without pneumoconiosis.

Rheumatoid disease with pulmonary arteritis and hypertension may manifest with signs of cor pulmonale.

Ankylosing Spondylitis

Ankylosing spondylitis consists of synovitis, chondritis, and periarticular osteitis of the sacroiliac, apophyseal, and costovertebral articulations. Disease progression is characterized by erosion of subchondral bone, cartilage destruction, and bony fusion. Aortic insufficiency develops in 4–10% of patients.

By fixing the thorax in an inspiratory position, ankylosing spondylitis causes overinflation and restriction of pulmonary function. Rarely, patients may develop bullous changes and pulmonary fibrosis, essentially limited to the upper lobes (Fig. 20.7). These fibrobullous lesions may contain mycetomas and are occasionally secondary to atypical mycobacterial infection (35).

Dermatomyositis

This autoimmune disorder manifests as proximal muscle weakness of the limbs and neck. Approximately half the cases are associated with a violaceous skin rash. The disease occurs twice as often in females as in males. Two age peaks occur, the first during the first decade of life and the second in the fifth and sixth decades. When

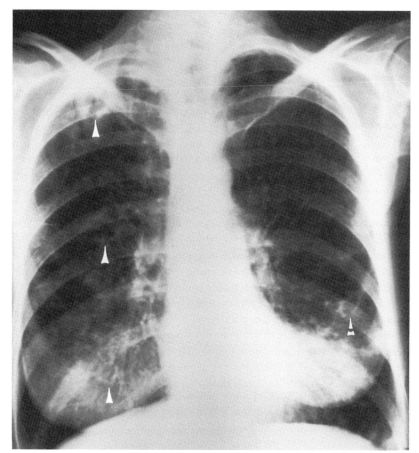

Figure 20.6. Rheumatoid arthritis. Multiple cavitary lung nodules (*arrowheads*).

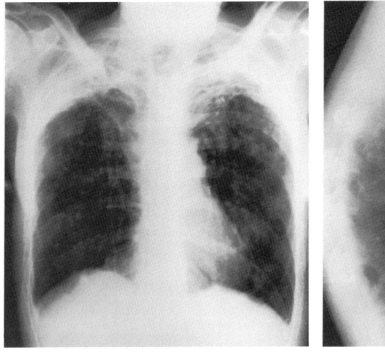 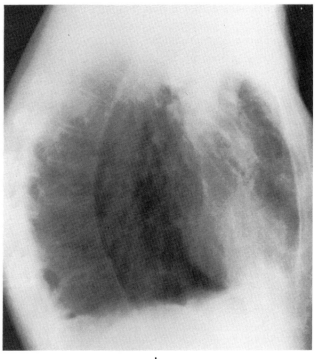

a   b

Figure 20.7. Ankylosing spondylitis. **a** Posteroanterior radiograph shows upper zone honeycomb lung. **b** Lateral radiograph demonstrates a typical "bamboo spine".

muscular weakness affects the thorax, atelectasis and pneumonia may result.

Chest radiographs are often normal. When abnormality occurs there is often a reticulonodular pattern and/or plate-like atelectasis at the lung bases. The esophagus may be abnormally distended, and soft tissue calcifications also occur. Some patients with longstanding disease may develop interstitial fibrosis, again predominantly at the lung bases. An association between dermatomyositis and carcinoma of the stomach, prostate, pancreas, and ovary has been proposed (36).

Scleroderma

Scleroderma, or diffuse systemic sclerosis, is a collagen disease characterized by sclerosis and atrophy of the skin, gastrointestinal tract, musculoskeletal system, heart, and lungs. Affected patients are often 30–50 years old, and the disease affects females approximately three times as often as males.

Ninety percent of scleroderma patients have morphologic and functional signs of pulmonary fibrosis. However, only a minority have abnormal chest radiographs (37). Radiographic changes, when present, usually consist of interstitial disease with a marked basilar predominance (Fig. 20.8). Early on there may be fine reticulation, but, with time, volume loss, coarse reticulation, and eventually fibrosis with honeycombing occur. Pleural involvement is

rare. Aspiration pneumonia may occur secondary to esophageal dysmotility, and as with dermatomyositis, soft tissue calcification is sometimes a prominent feature.

Systemic Lupus Erythematosus

This collagen-vascular disease involves the vascular system, the skin, the serous and synovial membranes, and the connective tissues of almost any viscus. There is a 10:1 female–male predominance. Death rates are three times higher in black than white women in the USA. Clinical manifestations include alopecia, photosensitivity, oral ulcerations, arthritis, pleuritis, pericarditis, and anemia. Hemoptysis is rare but may be massive (38).

Thoracic radiographic abnormalities may be seen in the lungs, pleura, and cardiovascular structures. These include cardiac enlargement, pericardial effusion, pleural effusion, and patchy areas of atelectasis or consolidation usually at the lung bases. Diffuse interstitial lung disease and cavitary nodules are rare in lupus patients. Other pulmonary pathology includes pulmonary hypertension, pulmonary vasculitis, pulmonary embolism (most probably due to circulating anticardiolipin antibodies), alveolar hemorrhage and various pulmonary infections resulting from the use of corticosteroids and immunosuppresive drugs (39–43). Pleural effusions are often bilateral. Cardiac silhouette enlargement generally is due to pericardial effusion, but sometimes may result from lupus cardiomyopathy.

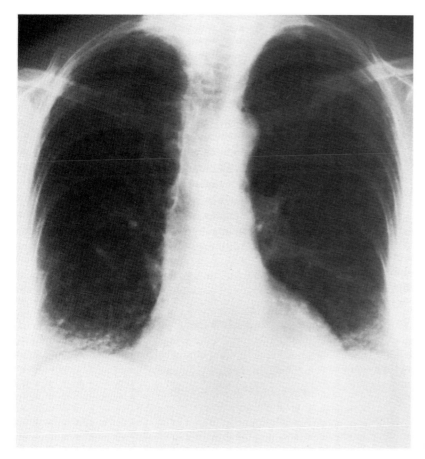

Figure 20.8. Scleroderma. Honeycombing is limited to the lung bases.

Immunological Disorders

A variety of lung and immune system responses to antigenic stimuli lead to pulmonary immunological disorders. Different immunologic responses cause different pathologic presentations. Antigen–antibody complexes deposited in vessel walls trigger vasculitis (44). Activated T-cells and macrophages stimulate granuloma formation (45). Parasites cause inflammation dominated by eosinophilia. These pathologic responses cause characteristic, although often nonspecific, radiographic findings.

Pulmonary Angiitis and Granulomatosis

In 1972, Liebow (46) discussed five distinctive focally destructive infiltrative vascular and granulomatous diseases not associated with infection or rheumatoid arthritis. They are Wegener granulomatosis, limited Wegener granulomatosis, lymphomatoid granulomatosis, necrotizing sarcoidal angiitis and granulomatosis, and bronchocentric granulomatosis. Although precise etiologies remain unknown, increasing evidence suggests immunologic pathogenesis, possibly immune complex deposition (44). In 1951, Churg and Strauss (47) described allergic granulomatosis, a vasculitis associated with eosinophilic pulmonary infiltration.

Wegener Granulomatosis

The classic Wegener granulomatosis triad is upper and lower respiratory tract necrotizing granulomatous vasculitis and glomerulonephritis. Although the etiology remains unknown, evidence suggests that immune complexes, possibly antigenically specific, play a pathogenetic role (44). The often dramatic response to cytotoxic therapy, usually corticosteroids and/or cyclophosphamide, supports an immunologic etiology.

Paranasal sinus mucosal membrane thickening, which can progress to bone and cartilage destruction, characterizes upper respiratory tract pathology (48). Small arterial and venous vasculitis and necrotizing granulomatous inflammation characterize the pulmonary involvement. Glomerulonephritis characterizes the renal disease and includes capillary tuft necrosis and thrombosis and eosinophilic fibrinoid degeneration (48).

Patient presentation is often nonspecific, and usually includes fever, sinusitis, arthralgias, and cough (49). Although a wide age range has been reported, in one series mean age at presentation was 40 years (49). Lungs, paranasal sinuses, and kidneys are the frequently involved organs, but cardiac, central nervous system, and ocular Wegener granulomatosis occurs (49). Wegener granulomatosis occurs in a "limited" form (50). These patients have pulmonary granulomatous vasculitis without renal, paranasal sinus, or other organ involvement.

The classical chest radiograph shows multiple pulmonary nodules; one third of these cavitate. Patchy, often nodular airspace disease is also common (48). However, patients can have solitary masses, pleural effusions (51), or tracheobronchial narrowing (52). Adenopathy is uncommon (48).

The appearance on CT scans of this entity has been reported in several studies. A variety of pulmonary pathologic changes has been reported, including the presence of multiple nodules or masses with distinct feeding vessels, sometimes cavitation or scarring and pleural tags connected to these lesions. Additionally, some patients presented areas of pulmonary consolidation, pleural thickening and pleural effusion. Both CT and MRI have been shown to be beneficial in demonstrating not only the pulmonary abnormalities in this disorders, but the pathologic changes occurring in the paranasal sinuses, orbits and the central nervous system (53–55).

Lymphomatoid Granulomatosis

Histologically midway between pulmonary lymphoma and Wegener granulomatosis is lymphomatoid granulomatosis. Liebow et al. originally described lymphomatoid granulomatosis as "an angiocentric and angiodestructive lymphoreticular proliferative and granulomatous disease involving predominantly the lungs" (56).

Unlike Wegener granulomatosis, lymphomatoid granulomatosis frequently involves the skin and central nervous system and infrequently involves the upper respiratory tract or causes glomerulonephritis (57). Unlike lymphoma, lymphomatoid granulomatosis infrequently involves lymph nodes, spleen, or bone marrow.

Patients present nonspecifically, with weakness, fatigue, weight loss, and fever (44). Because up to 50% of lymphomatoid granulomatosis patients progress to malignant lymphoma, many authors believe lymphomatoid granulomatosis is a primary pulmonary lymphoma that should be treated aggressively (58). The disease is progressive, with a 65–90% mortality incidence (58).

Radiographically, lymphomatoid granulomatosis can present with single or multiple pulmonary nodules or masses that can cavitate, patchy airspace disease, or a reticulonodular pattern. Hilar adenopathy is uncommon. In one study, 21% of 141 patients have been reported as having unilateral lung lesions, the rest presented with bilateral abnormalities (59). Other studies showed that

diffuse lung infiltrates are more common, with localized infiltrates and pulmonary effusion less frequently seen (60,61).

Other Pulmonary Angiitides and Granulomatoses

Originally thought to represent a granulomatous vasculitis, bronchocentric granulomatosis is now believed to be a bronchitis with vascular involvement (44). Not associated with systemic vasculitis, bronchocentric granulomatosis occurs with asthma, eosinophilia, and allergic bronchopulmonary aspergillosis (44). The radiographic findings resemble those of allergic bronchopulmonary aspergillosis. Segmental atelectasis, impacted bronchi, and linear opacities occur more often unilaterally, in the upper lobes (48).

Necrotizing sarcoidal granulomatosis is distinguished from sarcoidosis by the presence of severe arteritis. Involved lung has sarcoid-like noncaseating granulomas and intramural granulomatous arteritis (44). Patients present with fever, malaise, weight loss, cough, and/or chest pain (44). Chest radiographs demonstrate multiple pulmonary nodules, patchy opacities, and occasionally hilar adenopathy (44). Unlike the other granulomatous vasculitides, for necrotizing sarcoidal granulomatosis conservative management using corticosteroids without cytotoxic agents is currently recommended (44).

Allergic Granulomatosis (Churg–Strauss Disease)

Allergic granulomatosis, first described by Churg and Strauss in 1951, has characteristics similar to Wegener granulomatosis and polyarteritis nodosa (47). Unlike Wegener granulomatosis, allergic granulomatosis commonly has cardiac, gastrointestinal, skin, and central nervous system involvement. Patients often have asthma and peripheral and tissue eosinophilia. Unlike polyarteritis nodosa, allergic granulomatosis has universal pulmonary involvement, vascular and extravascular granulomatous lesions, and involvement of capillaries and venules.

Pathologically, necrotizing vasculitis, granuloma formation, and eosinophilic infiltration are characteristic (44). The granulomas may show fibrinoid necrosis rather than coagulative necrosis (48). Pulmonary radiographic manifestations include patchy airspace disease (Fig. 20.9), noncavitary pulmonary nodules, and pleural effusion (44). The pulmonary infiltrates are commonly transient and of even distribution. HRCT has demonstrated that eosinophilic infiltration in vascular and lymphatic walls

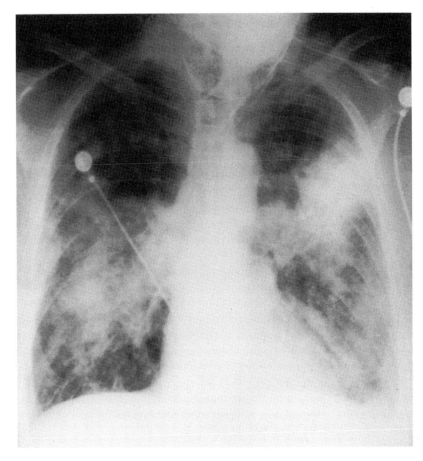

Figure 20.9. Allergic granulomatosis. Patchy bilateral perihilar airspace disease.

results in the appearance of irregular, stellate-shaped arteries on HRCT images (62,63).

Pulmonary Hemorrhage Syndromes

Hemoptysis, anemia, and radiographic airspace disease are the symptom triad of pulmonary hemorrhage syndromes. Several distinct etiologies, clinical presentations, and classifications have been described (2,64).

Goodpasture Syndrome

Antiglomerular basement membrane antibody crossreacting with lung basement membrane, pulmonary hemorrhage, and glomerulonephritis define Goodpasture syndrome. Cytotoxic tissue-specific antibody, usually immunoglobulin (Ig) G, deposits in renal glomeruli and causes linear immunofluorescent staining (2). Goodpasture syndrome occurs predominantly in young males, and presents with hemoptysis and later onset of renal disease (48). Dyspnea, fatigue, weakness, cough, and hematuria can occur. Immunosuppressive agents and plasmapheresis can reverse pulmonary and renal abnormalities (2).

Acute pulmonary hemorrhage causes diffuse, occasionally patchy airspace disease, resembling pulmonary edema, with a perihilar distribution, sparing the costophrenic angles and apices (65). Without further hemorrhage, airspace disease is replaced by a reticular pattern that resolves in less than 2 weeks (48). After repeated episodes, interstitial fibrosis, probably representing hemosiderin deposition within interstitial tissue, causes a permanent reticular pattern (48).

Alveolar Hemorrhage with Rapidly Progressive Glomerulonephritis

Alveolar hemorrhage with rapidly progressive glomerulonephritis can occur with or without basement membrane immune complex deposition (64). Immune complexes usually include IgG and can cause granular immunofluorescence (64). Some authors suggest that immunofluorescent negative alveolar hemorrhage with rapidly progressive glomerulonephritis is actually immune complex disease that has either escaped detection or has undergone granulocytic removal of immune complexes (2). Clinical presentation and radiographic manifestations are similar to Goodpasture syndrome, usually including uremia, hemoptysis, and a chest radiographic pattern of diffuse airspace disease.

Alveolar Hemorrhage with Collagen-Vascular Disease and Systemic Vasculitis

Alveolar hemorrhage may occur with systemic lupus erythematosus, Wegener granulomatosis, and other vasculitides. Immune complex deposition occurs, and renal disease is variable (2). Symptoms relate to the underlying disease, and radiographs resemble those of Goodpasture syndrome.

Idiopathic Pulmonary Hemosiderosis

Hemoptysis, iron deficiency anemia, and fleeting consolidations are the symptom triad of idiopathic pulmonary hemosiderosis. Renal disease does not occur. Children and young adult males are usually affected. Although most patients were reported without immunopathologic data, those subjected to pulmonary immunofluorescence studies have been negative (2). Radiographic abnormalities include alveolar, patchy or diffuse lung infiltrates, with a perihilar or basilar predominance. In young patients hilar or mediastinal adenopathy can be observed.

With time, radiographic opacities may be replaced by a diffuse reticular pattern . If recurrent bleeding occurs the final result will be generalized fibrosis (66,67). Moreover, CT and MRI are capable to show typical changes in the lung parenchyma, the latter images being due to the collected intra-alveolar hemosiderin and its paramagnetic qualities. HRCT images demonstrate in this disorder a characteristic ground-glass appearance during bleeding episodes, and following them, areas of patchy or nodular infiltrates (67,68).

Eosinophilic Lung Disease

This heterogeneous group of disorders is characterized by pulmonary eosinophilic inflammation with or without peripheral blood eosinophilia. Paré and Fraser (48) divided eosinophilic lung disease into three categories: (a) idiopathic, (b) specific etiology, and (c) angiitis and/or granulomatosis.

Acute idiopathic eosinophilic pneumonia (Loffler syndrome) is characterized by blood eosinophilia and acute patchy peripheral transient nonsegmental pulmonary consolidations. Patients are often atopic and asthmatic. Although cough is a common complaint, patients may be asymptomatic (17). Airspace disease may be distinctly peripheral in distribution (the reverse "bat-wing pattern") (Fig. 20.10). Radiographic abnormalities resolve in less than 2 weeks (17).

Patients with chronic eosinophilic pneumonia often have fever, weight loss, dyspnea, and hypoxemia.

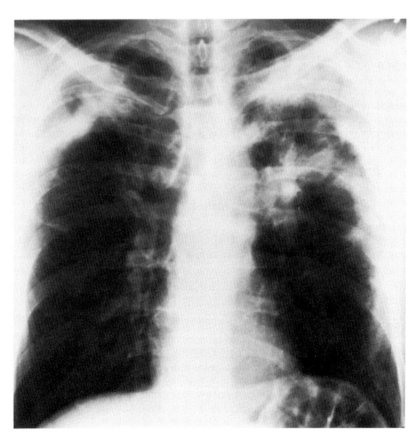

Figure 20.10. Eosinophilic pneumonia. Patchy airspace disease in a distinctively peripheral distribution.

Radiographs resemble those of patients with Lóffler syndrome, but the consolidations persist. Corticosteroids usually cause rapid clearing (48).

Specific etiologies of eosinophilic lung disease include drugs (such as penicillin and nitrofurantoin), parasites, and fungi (such as *Aspergillus fumigatus*). The radiographic findings are diverse and include peripheral consolidations (penicillin and some parasites), basilar small irregular shadows (nitrofurantoin), and mucoid impaction, bronchiectasis, and atelectasis (allergic bronchopulmonary aspergillosis). In general, acute eosinophilic pneumonia is characterized by diffuse patchy infiltrates, while in the chronic form the opacities are usually peripheral. Bronchiectasis may also be a hallmark of the chronic type, excellently demonstrated by CT (69,70).

Wegener granulomatosis, lymphomatoid granulomatosis, allergic granulomatosis, and necrotizing sarcoidal granulomatosis may also show pulmonary and blood eosinophilia. These topics are discussed earlier in this chapter.

Miscellaneous Diseases

Histiocytosis X

Histiocytosis X is a granulomatous disease of unknown etiology. It is subdivided into three separate diseases, primarily distinguished by age and severity. Systemic involvement is associated with considerable morbidity, in contrast to the benign course of a solitary bone lesion. Letterer–Siwe disease occurs in infants and children and is the most severe form of the disease, with widespread systemic involvement and a generally fatal course. Hand–Schuller–Christian disease is a less severe form and occurs in childhood or adolescence. Most patients survive into adult life. Eosinophilic granuloma is a disease of young adults, occurring primarily in young Caucasian males between adolescence and age 30. This is the least severe form of the disease, confined primarily to the lungs and bones. There is some overlap among the three entities.

When it involves the lungs, eosinophilic granuloma produces interstitial disease that often progresses to fibrosis. One third of patients are asymptomatic at the time of diagnosis. Initially, there is a symmetric nodular pattern that spares the lower lungs. The nodules are between 1 and 10 mm in size and represent granulomas. Cavitation of the nodules is uncommon. Alveolar consolidation is rare but can occur early in the disease when the alveoli fill with eosinophils and histiocytes. The disease progresses to a reticulonodular pattern and finally to fibrosis with large cystic spaces and honeycomb lung (Fig. 20.11). Involvement of the ribs results in well-defined, focal osteolytic lesions. The lesions may be expansile, and patho-

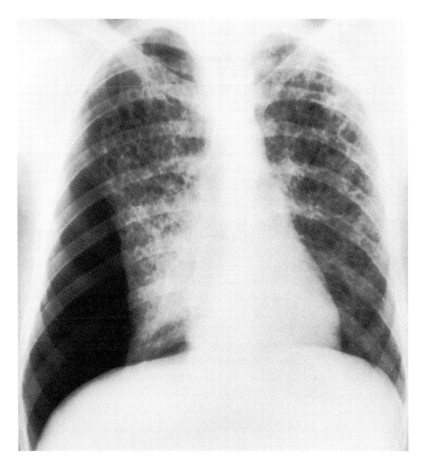

Figure 20.11. Eosinophilic granuloma. Bilateral honeycombing, predominantly in the upper zones, with a large spontaneous right pneumothorax.

logic fractures may occur and may produce extrapleural masses. Involvement of vertebral bodies may cause severe collapse resulting in "vertebra plana".

HRCT provides detailed information on the parenchymal pathologic changes in these conditions. In pulmonary histiocytosis X, this modality succeeds in demonstrating the typical changes of pulmonary nodules and cysts. At the same time, the very accurate depiction of the lung pathologic changes allows an estimation of the extent of the disease, its progression or regression, and has been shown to correlate well with lung diffusing capacity (71,72).

Phakomatoses

Neurofibromatosis

Neurofibromatosis, or von Recklinghausen disease, is an autosomal-dominant disorder involving multiple organ systems. The incidence of the disease is approximately 1 in 3000 births. Spontaneous mutation is responsible for about 50% of all cases. Although it may involve all three germ cell layers, neurofibromatosis affects primarily tissues of ectodermal and mesodermal origin. Café-au-lait spots and cutaneous neurofibromas are frequent presenting signs. Severe disfigurement may occur, with gigantism of a limb, pseudoarthroses, and large lytic bone defects. Patients often have neurofibromas, tumors comprising all elements of the nerve bundles, including Schwann cells, nerve fibers, and fibroblasts. There is also an increased incidence of schwannomas. There is a significantly increased incidence of malignancy, particularly neurofibrosarcomas, which occur in 5% of all patients. These tumors frequently metastasize to the chest. Five to 10 percent will develop central nervous system tumors as well. Pheochromocytomas occur in 1% of patients, sometimes in association with multiple endocrine neoplasia syndrome, type IIB.

The thoracolumbar spine and the thoracic cage are involved in almost half of all cases (73). Approximately 10% of patients will develop a progressive angular scoliosis of the lower thoracic spine. A discrete paravertebral mass in the thorax is more likely to be a lateral meningocele than a tumor; conversely, most cases of lateral meningoceles are associated with neurofibromatosis. Dural ectasia occurs commonly and is more often responsible for posterior scalloping of vertebral bodies than local neurofibromas. Rib notching, both at the superior and inferior margins, and "twisted ribbon" ribs are frequently due to the primary modeling defect, although neurofibromas may cause some of the findings.

Cutaneous neurofibromas may project over the chest and simulate pulmonary nodules. Rarely, a neurofibroma or schwannoma will present as a parenchymal or endobronchial nodule. Extensive, slowly growing, smoothly marginated neurofibromas of the vagus nerve trunks may occur in the middle mediastinum, resulting in widening of the mediastinal silhouette. These tumors are usually asymptomatic. They are generally low attenuation soft tissue masses on contrast-enhanced CT, but they may be as high in attenuation as muscle, depending on their collagen content (74). Schwannomas and neurofibromas cannot reliably be differentiated by CT. Magnetic resonance of neurofibromas shows them to be isointense, with adjacent neural tissue on T_1-weighted images but hyperintense on T_2 weighted images (75).

Interstitial pulmonary fibrosis occurs rarely and results in linear or nodular opacities, generally most pronounced at the lung bases, sometimes progressing to a honeycomb pattern. Apical bullous disease can occur as well (73).

Tuberous Sclerosis

Tuberous sclerosis, or Bourneville disease, is a triad of adenoma sebaceum, of the face, mental retardation, and seizures. Although it is transmitted in an autosomal-dominant fashion, 80% of all cases are sporadic. Death occurs by age 20 in over 75% of patients. Brain neoplasms (principally cerebral and paraventricular hamartomas), renal angiomyolipomas and cysts, cardiac rhabdomyomas, and sclerotic bone lesions are associated with this disease.

Pulmonary involvement is rare, occurring in fewer than 1% of all patients. Exertional dyspnea is the major symptom, and chronic cough and hemoptysis occur frequently. Although the disease has no sex predilection, 84% of patients with pulmonary symptoms in one study were women. Pathologically, there is proliferation of smooth muscle in the walls of blood vessels, bronchioles, lymphatic vessels, and alveolar septa. Because of this, some authors consider a related disease, lymphangiomyomatosis, to be a forme fruste of tuberous sclerosis. This may also explain the increased incidence of pulmonary findings in women. Radiographs show a fine linear pattern in the lung bases that may progress to honeycombing. Signs of cor pulmonale may develop, with enlargement of the central pulmonary arteries and right ventricular enlargement. Spontaneous pneumothorax occurs frequently (73).

Focal or diffuse sclerotic lesions may be present in the skeleton. Small contour defects in the cortex of long bones and ribs are typical. Histologically, the lesions are hamartomas. Sclerotic pedicles and "ivory" vertebrae may occur; rarely, lytic lesions of the clavicles are seen.

Ataxia-Telangiectasia

Ataxia-telangiectasia (Louis–Bar syndrome) is a rare disease characterized by progressive cerebellar ataxia and conjunctival and cutaneous venous telangiectasias. The disease is hereditary, with autosomal-recessive transmission. There is a 10% incidence of cancer, and death before age 20 is common. The most common malignancy is non-Hodgkin lymphoma. Because of an immune deficiency of both T- and B-lymphocytes, recurrent infections (particularly involving the paranasal sinuses and lungs) are common. Most often, *Pseudomonas, Staphylococcus*, and viral pneumonias are encountered (73). There is a notable absence of *P. carinii* infections. Because of the recurrent infections, linear fibrotic changes and bronchiectasis may be present on chest radiographs. Adenopathy is conspicuously absent; its presence may herald the onset of malignancy.

Myositis Ossificans Progressiva

Myositis ossificans progressiva (synonyms include Munchmeyer disease, fibrogenesis ossificans progressiva, and fibrodysplasia ossificans progressiva) is a rare hereditary disease of unknown etiology. Most cases are sporadic, although there is an increased association with advanced paternal age. The disorder affects tissues of mesodermal origin, resulting in progressive ossification of striated muscle, ligaments, and tendons. It occasionally involves the skin, but there is no involvement of smooth muscle. Clinically, the disease presents frequently with torticollis secondary to early involvement of the sternocleidomastoid muscles. Progression occurs erratically, and eventually there is involvement of the shoulder girdles, spine, and pelvis. Fusion of the hips usually occurs in the third decade, resulting in wheelchair confinement. Nearly all of the patients have bilateral microdactyly of the first toes, a key diagnostic sign clinically and radiologically. Conductive hearing loss and mental retardation are common.

Chest radiographs are striking, with columns of solid bone in the soft tissues of the chest wall a characteristic feature (7). Similar-appearing ossified columns occur around the shoulders, sometimes forming pseudoarthroses, and the ossification can also be seen in the soft tissues of the neck. Scoliosis and vertebral body dysplasia are common. The chest wall is usually thin because the patients are often nutritionally deprived secondary to involvement of the masseter muscles. Restrictive lung disease results from the severe deformity of the chest wall; death is commonly due to respiratory failure, frequently with pneumonia.

Osler–Weber–Rendu Disease

Osler–Weber–Rendu disease (hereditary hemorrhagic telangiectasia) is, as the name implies, an inherited disorder that is autosomal dominant in transmission. It is characterized by telangiectasias in the skin, mucous membranes, and various internal organs, with arteriovenous (AV) fistulae in the lungs. In fact, approximately half of patients with pulmonary AV fistulae have Osler–Weber–Rendu disease (30).

Patients with Osler–Weber–Rendu disease may manifest with extrapulmonary bleeding, including epistaxis, hematemesis, and cerebrovascular hemorrhage. Alternatively, pulmonary symptoms may be a prominent feature of disease. Hemoptysis is the most common presenting complaint caused by pulmonary AV fistulae, but dyspnea is also frequently present. Clinical signs such as cyanosis, clubbing, and polycythemia may be present (30). Central nervous system complications are an important by-product of pulmonary AV fistulae. Because the filtering function of the pulmonary capillary bed is bypassed, cerebral abscesses are frequent in this patient population.

Radiographically, Osler–Weber–Rendu disease may demonstrate pulmonary AV fistulae (Fig. 20.12). Fistulae tend to show feeding arteries and draining veins, but in some cases the resemblance to lung nodules is disquieting. The vascular nature of an AV fistula is well shown by CT (76), but pulmonary angiography is usually required if resection of lesions is contemplated because they are often multiple and very small (30).

References

1. Albelda SM, Gefter WB, Epstein DM, et al. (1985) Diffuse pulmonary hemorrhage: A review and classification. Radiology 154:289–297.
2. Sanders C, Frank MS, Rostand SG, et al. (1987) Metastatic calcification of the heart and lungs in end-stage renal disease: Detection and quantification by dual-energy digital chest radiography. AJR 149:881–887.
3. Rosenthal D1, Chandler HL, Azizi F, et al. (1977) Uptake of bone imaging agents by diffuse pulmonary metastatic calcification. AJR 129:871–874.
4. Braunwald E, Isselbacher KJ, Petersdorf RG, et al. (1987) Harrison's principles of internal medicine, 11th edn. McGraw-Hill, New York.

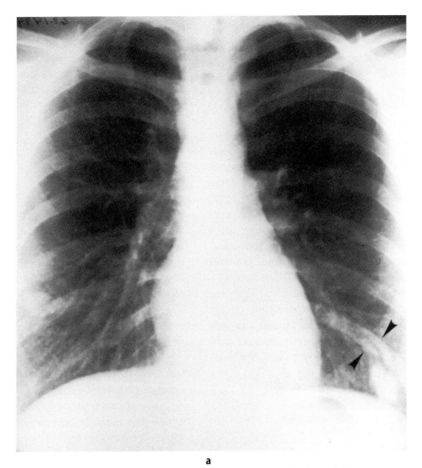

a

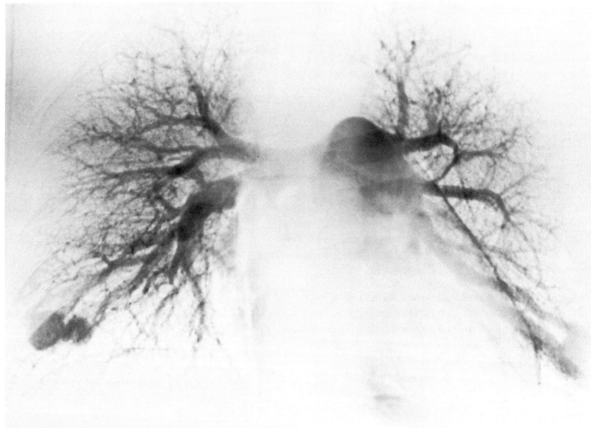

b

Figure 20.12. Osler–Weber–Rendu disease. **a** Posteroanterior radiograph shows bilateral lung nodules, one in the left lower lobe with a visible feeding artery and draining vein (*arrowheads*). **b** Subtraction view from pulmonary angiography reveals the vascular nature of the lung nodules.

5. Siefkin AD, Igarashi P, Allen R, et al. (1984) Unsuspected mediastinal hematoma diagnosed by computed tomography. J Comput Tomogr 8:211–214.

6. Gumbs RV, Higginbotham-Ford EA, Teal JS, et al. (1987) Thoracic extramedullary hematopoiesis in sickle-cell disease. AJR 149:889–893.

7. Resnick D, Niwayama G (1988) Diagnosis of bone and joint disorders, 2nd edn. WB Saunders, Philadelphia.

8. Selvidge SD, Gavant ML (1999) Idiopathic pulmonary vein thrombosis: Detection by CT and MR imaging. AJR 172:1639–1641.

9. Howlett DC, Hatrick AG, Jarosz JM, et al. (1997) The role of CT and MRI in imaging: The complications of sickle cell disease. Clin Radiol 52:821–829.

10. Acquino SL, Gamsu G, Fahy JV, et al. (1994) Chronic pulmonary disorders in sickle cell disease: Findings at thin-section CT. Radiology 193:807–811.

11. Filly R, Blank N, Castellino RA (1976) Radiographic distribution of intrathoracic disease in previously untreated patients with Hodgkin's disease and non-Hodgkin's lymphoma. Radiology 120:277–281.

12. Blank N, Castellino RA (1980) The intrathoracic manifestations of the malignant lymphomas and the leukemias. Semin Roentgenol 15:227–245.

13. Klatte EC, Yardley J, Smith EB, et al. (1963) The pulmonary manifestations and complications of leukemia. AJR 89:598–609.

14. Rebner M, Gross BH, Robertson J, et al. (1987) CT evaluation of mediastinal masses. Comput Radiol 11:103–110.

15. Khoury MB, Godwin JD, Halvorsen R, et al. (1986) Role of chest CT in non-Hodgkin lymphoma. Radiology 158:659–662.

16. Shuman LS, Libshitz HI (1984) Solid pleural manifestations of lymphoma. AJR 142:269.

17. Heitzman RE (1984) The lung: radiologic–pathologic correlations, 2nd edn. Mosby St. Louis, MO.

18. Bragg DG (1987) Radiology of the lymphomas. Curr Probl Diagn Radiol 16:183.

19. Primack SL, Müller NL, (1994) High-resolution computed tomography in acute diffuse lung disease in the immunocompromised patient. Radiol Clin North Am 32:731.

20. Tenholder MMF, Hooper RG (1980) Pulmonary infiltrates in leukemia. Chest 78:468–473.

21. Perez CR, Leigh MW (1991) Mycoplasma pneumoniae as the causative agent for pneumonia in the immunocompromised host. Chest 100:860.

22. Ingram CW, Tanner DC, Durack DT, et al. (1993) Pneumonia caused by rapidly growing mycobacteria in patients with cancer. Chest 87:503.

23. Degregorio MW, Lee WMF, Linker CA, et al. (1982) Fungal infections in patients with acute leukemia. Ann J Med 73:543.

24. Kuhlman JE, Fishman EK, Burch PA, et al. (1987) Invasive pulmonary aspergillosis in acute leukemia: The contribution of CT to early diagnosis and aggressive management. Chest 92:95.

25. Kuhlman JE, Fishman EK, Burch PA, et al. (1988) CT of invasive pulmonary aspergillosis. AJR 150:1015.

26. Glenner GG (1980) Medical progress: Amyloid deposits and amyloidosis – the beta-fibrilloses. N Engl J Med 302:1283–1292, 1333–1343.

27. Gross BH, Felson B, Birnberg FA (1986) The respiratory tract in amyloidosis and the plasma cell dyscrasias. Semin Roentgenol 21:113–127.

28. Winterbauer RH, Riggins RCK, Griesman FA, et al. (1974) Pleuropulmonary manifestations of Waldenström's macroglobulinemia. Chest 66:368–375.

29. Gordon DA, Stein JL, Broder I (1973) The extra-articular features of rheumatoid arthritis. A systematic analysis of 127 cases. Am J Med 54:445–452.

30. Fraser RG, Paré JAP (1978) Diagnosis of diseases of the chest, 2nd edn. WB Saunders Philadelphia.

31. Coxson HO, Hogg JC, Mayo JR, et al. (1997) Quantification of idiopathic pulmonary fibrosis using computed tomography and histology. Am J Respir Crit Care Med 155:1649–1656.

32. Rémy-Jardin M, Rémy J, Cortet B, et al. (1994) Lung changes in rheumatoid arthritis: CT findings. Radiology 193:375–382.

33. Fuji M, Adachi S, Shimizu T (1993) Interstitial lung disease in rheumatoid arthritis: Assessment with high resolution computed tomography. J Thorac Imaging 8:54–62.

34. Gabbay E, Tarala R, Will R, et al. (1997) Interstitial lung disease in recent onset rheumatoid arthritis. Am J Respir Crit Care Med 156:528–535.

35. Jessamine AG (1968) Upper lung lobe fibrosis in ankylosing spondylitis. Can Med Assoc J 98:25–29.

36. Bohan A, Peter JB (1975) Polymyositis and dermatomyositis. N Engl J Med 292:344–347.

37. Bianchi FA, Bistue AR, Wendt VE, et al. (1966) Analysis of 27 cases of progressive systemic sclerosis. J Chron Dis 19:953–977.

38. Hunninghake GW, Fauci AS (1979) Pulmonary involvement in the collagen vascular diseases. Am Rev Respir Dis 119:471–503.

39. Roncoroni AJ, Alvarez C, Molinas F (1992) Plexogenic arteriopathy associated with pulmonary vasculitis in systemic lupus erythematosus. Respiration 59:52–56.

40. Alarcon-Segovia D, Deleze M, Oria CV, et al. (1989) Antiphospholipid antibodies and the antiphospholipid syndrome in systemic lupus erythematosus. A prospective analysis of 500 consecutive patients. Medicine 68:353–365.

41. Zamora MR, Warner ML, Tuder R, et al. (1997) Diffuse alveolar hemorrhage and systemic lupus erythematosus. Medicine 76:192–202.

42. Widemann HP, Matthay RA (1989) Pulmonary manifestations of the collagen vascular diseases. Clin Chest Med 10:677–722.

43. Lynch JP, III, Hunnighake GW (1992) Pulmonary complications of collagen vascular disease. Annu Rev Med 43:17–35.

44. Leavitt RY, Fauci AS (1986) Pulmonary vasculitis. Am Rev Respir Dis 134:149–166.

45. Hunninghake GW, Garrett KC, Richerson HBG, et al. (1984) Pathogenesis of the granulomatous lung diseases. Am Rev Respir Dis 130:476–496.

46. Liebow AA (1973) The J. Burns Amberson Lecture: Pulmonary angiitis and granulomatosis. Am Rev Respir Dis 108:1–18.

47. Churg J, Strauss L (1951) Allergic granulomatosis, allergic angiitis, and periarteritis nodosa. Am J Pathol 27:277–294.

48. Paré JAP, Fraser RG (1983) Synopsis of disease of the chest. WB Saunders Philadelphia.

49. Fauci AS, Haynes BF, Kats P, et al. (1983) Wegener's granulomatosis: Prospective clinical and therapeutic experience with 85 patients for 21 years. Ann Intern Med 98:76–85.

50. Carrington CB, Liebow AA (1966) Limited forms of angiitis and granulomatosis of Wegener's type. Am J Med 41:497–527.

51. Gonzalez L, Van Ordstrand HS (1973) Wegener's granulomatosis. Radiology 107:295–300.

52. Stein MG, Gamsu G, Webb WR, et al. (1986) Computed tomography of diffuse tracheal stenosis in Wegener granulomatosis. J Comput Assist Tomogr 10:868–870.

53. Kuhlman JE, Hruban RH, Fishman EK (1991) Wegener's granulomatosis: CT features of parenchymal lung disease. J Comput Assist Tomogr 15:948–952.

54. Weir IH, Müller NL, Chiles C, et al. (1992) Wegener's granulomatosis: findings from computed tomography of the chest in 10 patients. Can Assoc Radiol J 43:31–34.

55. Provenzale JM, Allen NB (1996) Wegener's granulomatosis: CT and MR findings. Am J Neuroradiol 17:785–792.

56. Liebow AA, Carrington CRB, Friedman PJ (1972) Lymphomatoid granulomatosis. Human Pathol 3:457–558.

57. Dee PM, Arora NS, Innes DJ, Jr (1982) The pulmonary manifestations of lymphomatoid granulomatosis. Radiology 143:613–618.

58. Glickstein M, Komstein MJ, Pietra GG, et al. (1986) Nonlymphomatous lymphoid disorders of the lung. AJR 147:227–237.

59. Katzenstein ALA, Carrington CB, Liebow AA (1979) Lymphomatoid granulomatosis: A clinicopathological study of 152 cases. Cancer 43:360–373.

60. Dee PM, Arora NS, Innes DJ, Jr. (1982) The pulmonary manifestations of lymphomatoid granulomatosis. Radiology 143:613–618.

61. McNiff JM, Cooper D, Howe G, et al. (1996) Lymphomatoid granulomatosis of the skin and lung. An angiocentric T-cell rich B-cell lymphoproliferative disorder. Arch Dermatol 132:1464–1470.

62. Chumbley LC, Harrison EG, Jr, DeRemee RA (1977) Allergic granulomatosis and angiitis (Churg–Strauss syndrome): Report and analysis of 30 cases. Mayo Clin Proc 52:477–484.

63. Buschman DL, Waldron JA, Jr, King TE, Jr. (1990) Churg–Strauss pulmonary vasculitis. High-resolution computed tomography scanning and pathologic findings. Am Rev Respir Dis 142:458–461.

64. Leatherman JW, Davies SF, Hoidal JR (1984) Alveolar hemorrhage syndromes: Diffuse microvascular lung hemorrhage in immune and idiopathic disorders. Medicine 63:343–361.

65. Primack Sl, Miller RR, Müller NL (1995) Diffuse pulmonary hemorrhage: Clinical, pathologic and imaging features. AJR 164:295–300.

66. Akyar S, Ozbek SS (1993) Computed tomography findings in idiopathic pulmonary hemosiderosis. Respiration 60:63–64.

67. Buschman DL, Ballard R (1993) Progressive massive fibrosis associated with idiopathic pulmonary hemosiderosis. Chest 104:293–295.

68. Rubin GD, Edwards DK, Reicher MA, et al. (1989) Diagnosis of pulmonary hemosiderosis by MR imaging. AJR 152:573–574.

69. Mayo FR, Müller NL, Road J, et al. (1982) Chronic eosinophilic pneumonia: CT findings in six cases. AJR 153: 727–730.

70. Needle DA, Goodman LR, Gurney JW, et al. (1990) Computerized tomography in the evaluation of allergic bronchopulmonary aspergillosis. Am Rev Resp Dis 142:1200–1205.

71. Brauner MW, Grenier P, Mouelhi MM, et al. (1989) Pulmonary histiocytosis Evaluation with high-resolution CT. Radiology 172:255–258.

72. Grenier P, Valeyre D, Cluzel P, et al. (1991) Chronic diffuse interstitial lung disease: Diagnostic value of chest radiography and high resolution CT. Radiology 179:123–132.

73. Aughenbaugh GL (1984) Thoracic manifestations of neurocutaneous diseases. Radiol Clin North Am 22:741–756.

74. Bourgouin PM, Shepard JO, Moore EH, et al. (1988) Plexiform neurofibromatosis of the mediastinum: CT appearance. AJR 151:461–463.

75. Higgins CB, Hricak H (1987) Magnetic resonance imaging of the body. Raven Press, New York.

76. Godwin JD, Webb WR (1981) Dynamic computed tomography in the evaluation of vascular lung lesions. Radiology 138:629–635.

21 Pulmonary Abscess and Empyema

G. Simonetti, G. Sergiacomi, A. Moscone, R. Cancellieri, and L. Mancini

Introduction

Pulmonary abscess and empyema have been well known as suppurative diseases since the early history of medicine. Owing to their different locations, evolutions and treatments, we shall consider them here as distinct and separated pathologic entities.

In particular, the usefulness of interventional radiology (IR) procedures is stressed in this chapter. Advanced imaging techniques such as ultrasound (US), computed tomography (CT) and magnetic resonance imaging (MRI) have a distinct role in diagnosis and as guides in IR procedures, even if the plain film roentgenogram is still the first diagnostic step (1–4).

Lung Abscess

At present, because of the use of antimicrobials, pulmonary abscess is a relatively rare condition (10–13 patients per 10 000 hospital admissions) that occurs more frequently in males than in females, roughly in the ratio 3:1 (3,5–7). Lung abscess can be defined as a pus-containing necrotic lesion of the lung parenchyma, often with an air–fluid level inside. (Fig. 21.1). Necrotizing pneumonia is a pathologic process similar to lung abscess, characterized by multiple small cavities less than 2 cm in diameter, as has been described (8).

Both pulmonary abscess and necrotizing pneumonia may be associated with infections caused by pyogenic bacteria, mycobacteria, fungi, and parasites. Pulmonary infarction, primary and metastatic malignancies, and the necrotic conglomerate lesions of silicosis and coal miner's pneumoconiosis can be relatively complicated by lung abscess, which can occur often with infection or sometimes bland.

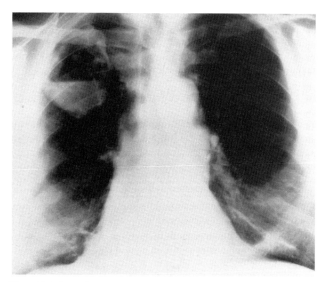

Figure 21.1. Lung abscess in posteroanterior view on chest radiograph showing a round mass with an air fluid level.

Classification of Lung Abscesses

This is based on the differentiation between three physiopathologic entities:

1. Aspiration lung abscess
2. Lung abscess due to preexisting specific pneumonia
3. Lung abscess due to concomitant pulmonary disease or metastatic extrathoracic sites

Aspiration Lung Abscess

Aspiration lung disease is more frequent in hospitalized patients, owing to the more frequent occurrences of nosocomial diseases, particularly in subjects who are unconscious or undergoing anesthesia. Anaerobic bacteria are the most likely pathogens to cause the abscesses encountered today (8). The importance of conditions favoring aspiration in the pathogenesis of lung abscess from anaerobes, especially in the presence of periodontal disease, has already been stressed (9–11). However, reduced or absent cough reflex, seizures, swallowing disorders of neurologic or mechanical origin, and chronic alcoholism also frequently favor the occurrence of lung abscess (12,13). In these cases, saprophytes in the cavity are the most common microbial agents passing through the lower airways and in the lung; in particular anaerobic bacteria in non-hospitalized subjects and both optional anaerobic and aerobic agents in hospitalized patients (14–16).

Klebsiella pneumoniae, *Pseudomonas aeruginosa*, *Staphylococus aureus*, *Nocardia*, and *Actinomyces* species are other bacteria not uncommonly involved in pathogenesis of lung abscess, and cavitation is decidedly rare in the atypical pneumonia syndrome.

Lung Abscess due to Preexisting Specific Pneumonia

The respiratory tract is provided with a vast array of local and systemic defence mechanisms that attempt to maintain sterility of the lung parenchyma and terminal bronchioles. Several types of respiratory tract infection or pathogen may be associated with deficiencies in a specific pulmonary defence mechanism. For instance, excessive aspiration of oropharyngeal secretions into the lower airways is possible, owing to alterations of consciousness, disordered swallowing mechanisms, or improper epiglottic function. Organisms typically found in the oropharynx, such as anaerobes and streptococci, are recovered as pathogens in the lung (17).

Paramyxoviruses, especially influenza viruses, due to their high tropism to bronchial airway wall cells can either infect and destroy ciliated cells or impair bactericidal activity of the phagocytes; this is why postinfluenza pyogenic pneumonia may develop (18,19).

Most of the infections soon in patients with asplenia, hypogammaglobulinemia, or dysglobulinemia seem to be caused by encapsulated bacteria such as *Streptococcus pneumoniae* and *Haemophilus influenzae* (20,21). The recruitment of polymorphonuclear leukocytes could be limited by granulocytopenia resulting from disease, immunosuppressive or antineoplastic therapy, and the development of Gram-negative bacillary pneumonia could be facilitated (22,23).

The kind of pathogen involved in the pathologic process is greatly influenced by environmental factors. In hospitalized patients, 60% of the pneumonias are caused by Gram-negative bacteria (of which 45% are enteric bacteria), 14% are due to staphylococci and 6% to pneumococci. In nonhospitalized patients the organisms are somewhat different, consisting of pneumococci, and to a lesser extent Gram-negative bacteria (7).

The lung necrosis trend of aerobic bacteria is rather low compared to that of anaerobic bacteria, mirroring the lower frequency of aerobic lung abscesses.

Gram-Positive Germs

Streptococcus Pyogenes and Diplococcus Pneumoniae

Streptococcus pyogenes remains the single most frequent cause of community-acquired pneumonia among hospitalized subjects (24–26). The incidence of pneumococcal pneumoniae is approximately 2 cases per 1000 persons yearly (27), the disease occurrence being much higher in elderly and infant patients. Other groups, including human immunodeficiency virus (HIV)-infected individuals, renal or bone marrow-transplanted subjects, and military recruits, are recognized as having higher annual attack rates of pneumonia (28,29).

Pneumococci are found in the oropharynx in 30% of asymptomatic individuals, depending on the season (30). Transmission of the organism is from person to person, although the exact mode is unknown. Aerosolized droplets, expeled by talking, sneezing, or coughing, and also transferred by physical contact, may play a role.

Although actually infrequent, *Streptoccoccus pneumoniae* may represent a complication of infections such as influenza, measles, hooping-cough, and varicella. The tissue necrosis trend in *Diplococcus pneumoniae* infection is low, and, since the introduction of antibiotics, abscess formation has become extremely rare in this condition.

Staphylococcus Aureus

Staphylococcus aureus accounts for fewer than 5% of cases of community-acquired pneumonias (26,31). The disease usually affects newborns, infants and, in particular, individuals requiring hospitalization (7,15,32). Chronic alcoholism, diabetes, underfeeding, and cystic fibrosis represent predisposing conditions to infection. Pneumonia caused by the hematogenous spread of *Staphylococcus* usually occurs in the setting of endocarditis or an infected vascular site, septic pelvic thrombophlebitis, brain abscess, and bone infections (33). Intravenous drug abuse is frequently involved, especially with developing septic pulmonary embolisms.

The occurrence of abscess formation as a complication of staphylococcal pneumonia in the adult is estimated to be 25–75% (34). Pneumatoceles, which may contain air–fluid levels, are observed in between 40% and 60% of subjects affected by staphylococcal pneumonia. These are usually thin walled, but radiographically may be exactly like an abscess formation when trapped within the injured lung (35) (Fig. 21.2).

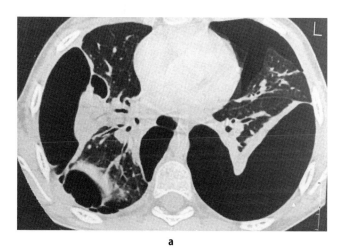

a

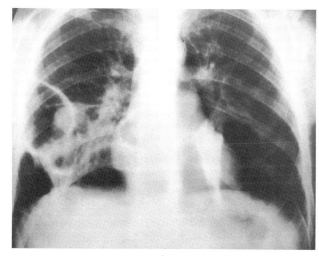

b

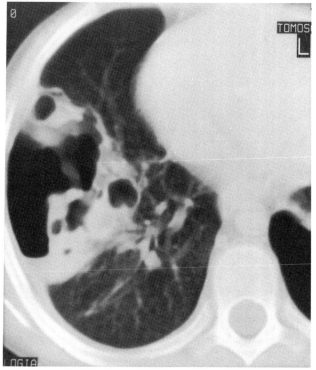

c

Figure 21.2. a Pneumatocele in a child affected by staphylococcal pneumonia in posteroanterior view on chest radiograph. **b** CT scan showing thin-walled multiloculated cysts. **c** CT scan with multiple cystic pattern. Follow-up after 2 months showing partial resolution of the thoracic pattern.

Gram-Negative Germs

Hemophilus Influenzae

Hemophilus influenzae, the major bacterial pathogen of early childhood, has nowadays an important role in adult infections (36,37). The explanation for the apparent increased occurrence of infection is unknown; however, it could be related to the more frequent use of invasive diagnostic measures (such as transtracheal aspiration), declining adult immunity, and the increased numbers of immune-suppressed subjects. The bacterium can be recovered from the rhinopharynx in 90% of 5 year old children (38). whereas, in adults, the most common pre-

disposing conditions to development of *Hemophilus* pneumonia are chronic lung disease, HIV infection, and alcoholism (14,37,39).

Klebsiella Pneumoniae

In early studies, *Klebsiella pneumoniae* was considered to be solely responsible for for 18–64% of community-acquired and 30% of nosocomial Gram-negative pneumonias (40). Most *Klebsiella* lower respiratory tract infections occur in subjects over 40 years old. Alcoholism is a common underlying condition (66%), although diabetes also predisposes to infection (41,42,43). *Klebsiella pneumoniae* pneumonitis is acquired mostly by aspiration and is usually located in the upper lobes, especially the right: the clinical course is often rapid, and extensive tissue necrosis and abscess formation are found in over 50% of cases.

Other Enterobacteriaceae

Among Enterobacteriaceae family, there are other genera as well as *Klebsiella* that may be associated with pneumonia; *Escherichia, Proteus, Morganella, Providencia, Serratia, Salmonella, Citrobacter, Erwinia,* and *Hafnia* have been documented (44–48). These infections usually are community-acquired or nosocomial and tend to involve elderly persons with debilitating underlying disease, alterations of consciousness, renal failure, alcoholism, and diabetes mellitus; immune-suppressed subjects are at greatest risk. The epidemiology and manifestations of pneumonia due to each causative germ are insufficient to distinguish them on a clinical basis alone. These agents may produce abscesses anywhere in the body, in fact 5–15% of subjects with *Escherichia coli* bacteremia could develop metastatic infections in bones, brain, liver, and lung (49,50).

Pseudomonas Aeruginosa

The pathogenesis of nonbacterial infection is much like that of pneumonia due to Enterobacteriaceae; it includes elderly and debilitated individuals, often with complicating chronic pulmonary or cardiac disease (51). *Pseudomonas aeruginosa* secondary infections usually occur in the ear, lung, skin, and urinary tract of subjects whose primary pathogen has been eradicated by antibacterial treatment (52,53).

Bacteremic *Pseudomonas* pneumonia is typically associated with conditions of altered host defences. Even if only 5% of today's general population is affected by *Pseudomonas*, more than 50% of hospitalized patients with malignancy will carry the organism (54).

This disease tends to be bilateral, definitely preferring the lower lobe and with usually multiple abscess formation in 33% of patients (52,53).

Aspergillosis

The *Aspergillus* infection is a mycosis that can be produced by several sources of fungus present in the upper respiratory airways, sometimes as saprophytes. The host's immune status will determine the outcome of the disease (55).

In the primary forms, rare in immunocompromised patients, the radiologic pattern consists of homogeneous

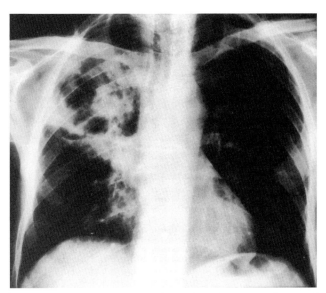

Figure 21.3. Posteroanterior view on chest radiograph showing a "mycetoma" colonizing a preexisting tubercular cavity.

lung consolidations, which can progress into abscesses; in the absence of cavitation, it appears similarly to *Pneumococcus* pneumonia (56). Clinically, low grade fever, productive cough, hemoptysis and chest pain are present.

In secondary forms, radiologic studies show a "mycetoma", fungal hyphae crowding in a pulmonary cavity. In most cases, the fungus is present as a saprophyte in a cavitation produced by other agents, such tuberculosis (TB), as sarcoidosis, histoplasmosis, or bronchiectasies, and the fungus, in micellar form, does not invade the cavity walls. The "mycetoma" is localized more frequently in the upper lung zones, probably due to the frequent presence of tubercular cavitations (Fig. 21.3). Generally the patient is asymptomatic; eventually, the clinical conditions may worsen, probably due to the primary disease responsible of the cavitation process. Productive cough may be present and hemoptysis is seen in 45–70% of patients; when the bleeding is severe, lobectomy is recommended to prevent heavy hemorrhages (14).

Invasive pulmonary aspergillosis is the most frequent and severe manifestation seen in immunocompromised patients, mostly in leukemic subjects, treated with cytostatic myeloinibitor drugs, who show a polymorphonucleocyte level less than 500 mm^{-3} (57). In these subjects the risk of increased virulence of saprophytic respiratory and digestive foci is very high (58). The possible evolution of the above mentioned lesions may be excavation or confluence in larger masses (Fig. 21.4).

Later on, following the normalization of granulocyte level, or after effective therapy, angioinvasive aspergillosis is typically represented by eccentric excavation; it is considered a good prognositic sign, since it indicates an immune response to the infection (55,59).

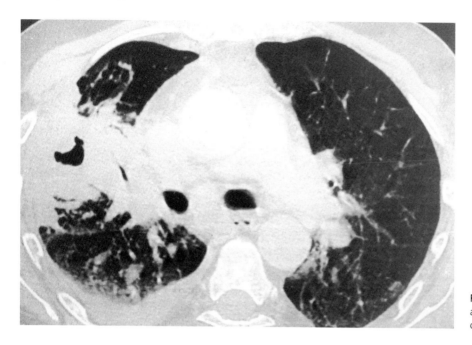

Figure 21.4. CT scan demonstrating an angioinvasive aspergillosis resulting from confluence in a larger mass of singular nodular lesions with an "air crescent sign".

In a few cases, the infection can spread from the nodular lesions toward the airspaces, as in broncho-pneumonic disease (transbronchial invasion) or, hematogenously, evolving into a miliary form. The infection can also invade the mediastinal structures, provoking rare complications such as pneumopericarditis, through a bronchopericardial fistula (60).

Lung Abscess due to Concomitant Pulmonary Disease or Metastatic Extra-thoracic Sites

A secondary lung abscess usually occurs as a complication of a wide variety of underlying pulmonary disorders, bronchial neoplasm seeming to be the most frequent (7,61). An infected, cavitated squamous cell carcinoma may resemble both clinically and radiographically a primary lung abscess and itself may be a relatively frequent complication of a transbronchial biopsy of such a mass lesion (62). Bronchoesophageal fistula, pulmonary sequestration, foreign body inhalation, cystic fibrosis, wrong positioning of a central venous catheter, bronchial anatomic variations, and barium aspiration may be other underlying conditions leading to a secondary lung abscess formation. In fact, each preexisting cavity could be secondarily infected by pyogenic bacterial agents leading to secondary abscess formation (63–66).

Aseptic embolism complicated by bronchogenous origin infection is the most common type of secondary abscess formation in pulmonary embolism. This form is often complicated by septicemia, and the occurrence of hemorrhages has been mentioned (56,67,68).

Cavitation in pulmonary infarction may be completely aseptic. These aseptic cavitating infarcts are either single (75%) or right sided (69%) and usually follow an area of consolidation after a few weeks. The principal localizations of these infarcts are usually the apical or posterior segment of an upper lobe and the apical segment of a lower lobe. The majority (85%) have notched inner margins and well-defined outer margins, with cross-cavity band shadows. Air–fluid levels are common, especially when the primary aseptic cavitation is complicated by infection (69,70).

In the past, septic embolism was almost exclusively a complication of septic pelvic thrombophlebitis due to both septic abortion and postpuerperal uterine infections (71). Today, septic embolism is a frequent condition in drug-addicts, and HIV-positive patients, following repeated injections (72,73). An increasingly common cause is iatrogenic, namely, infections secondary to intravenous catheters inserted for cytotoxic therapy (74–77). Subcutaneous injections can also be responsible for local suppuration, which invades veins.

Another cause of septic embolism is right-sided bacterial endocarditis complicating septic infections (33,34,72,78,79). The pathogens most frequently involved are *Staphylococcus aureus*, and Gram-negative bacteria (80). The cavities are usually thin walled and may simulate pneumatoceles, whereas others may present radiographically as a "target" lesion (81). A coalescence of smaller abscesses can grow to form a giant lung abscess, and complications such as empyema and bronchopleural fistula may occur (82,83). Enlargement of hilar and mediastinal lymph nodes may be a common finding in *S. aureus* septic embolism.

Wegener granulomatosis, multiple excavating metastases, collagen diseases, lymphoma, and occasionally sarcoidosis may simulate the radiographic pattern of septic emboli.

Diagnostic Imaging

Primarily, conventional radiography and CT can be helpful in locating the position of suppurative lesions, since physical examination is not sufficiently specific (3,4). Some 67% and 33% respectively of lung abscesses are represented on conventional chest radiographs as round and ovoid-shaped lesions, the dimensions of which, in both posteroanterior and lateral projections, can be nearly the same (84). The shape of the lesion can also be clearly delineated in oblique and both right and left lateral decubitus views, as well as its relationship to the chest (85). A surrounding pneumatosis usually separates the cavity of the lung abscess from the chest wall without extending to the edge of the lung; however, chest angles are acute (11,86).

The range of variation of the initial cavity size is 1–7 cm; but giant lung abscesses have also been reported (5,6). The radiograph can also be rapidly altered by the state of the cavity as the latter may fill or may empty partially or completely during measurement.

Pleural effusions and transgression of an interlobar fissure are frequent occurrence, the first has been reported in 25% of patients with pulmonary abscesses, and the second is also not unusual (1,7). Rupture in the pleural space, producing pyopneumothorax, is rare in subjects under current therapeutic conditions. Lung abscess is frequently associated with enlargement of hilar and mediastinal lymph nodes (58) (Fig. 21.5).

Differentiation between pleural disease and parenchymal lung disease can be easily depicted by US, with an accuracy of 90% (87). Pleural fluid can be reliably diagnosed as an anechoic image taking up the space delimited by the posterior costophrenic angle and diaphragm (88). Even if US is able to visualize pleural fluid, differentiation between lung abscess and empyema is difficult, moreover correlation radiographs are strictly necessary and may be useful in planning interventional procedures (89).

Because it gives a better demonstration of the three-dimensional shape of thoracic processes and improved visualization of the pleural space and the pleuro-pulmonary interface, CT is the method of choice as conventional radiographic findings cannot completely determine the diagnosis of a lung lesion (84). CT imaging of an abscess is similar to that of conventional radiography. Air, cavity fluid, parenchymal consolidation and partially aerated lung are responsible for the wide range of attenuation values of the tissue mass of the abscess. Localization and behavior of peripheral abscesses is indicated by the acute angle formed with the chest wall, confirming that the lesions are predominantly in the lung parenchyma. (Fig. 21.6) Pleura reactions and thickening are identified as a less well-defined shape which may assume a more obtuse or tapering margin (90) (Fig. 21.7).

The abscess–lung interface can be studied only by viewing CT slices performed with the parenchyma window; the same kind of examination is essential distinguish trapped normal lung surrounded by pneumonia from a cavitating abscess (84). If case the interface the main mass of the lesion and the adjacent lung is infected, as it usually is, it may develop a blurred, indistinct margin. The bronchi and the pulmonary vessels are not distorted or bowed by an abscess, but terminate abruptly at the wall,

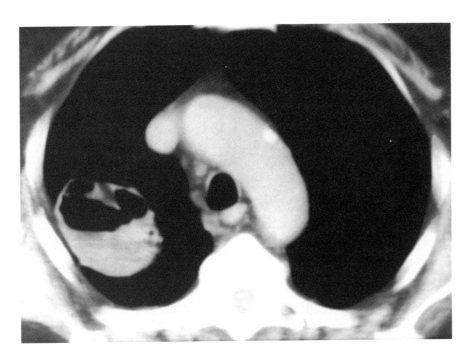

Figure 21.5. CT scan (mediastinal window) of a lung abscess associated with mediastinal adenopathy.

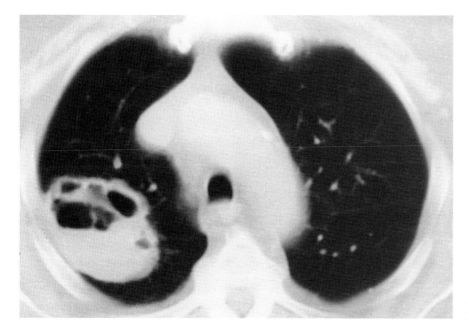

Figure 21.6. CT scan of a lung abscess demonstrating the acute angle formed against the chest wall.

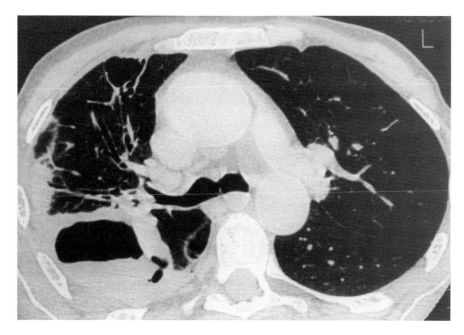

Figure 21.7. CT scan showing a lung abscess associated with pleural reaction, characterized by a more obtuse angle with the chest wall and tapering margins.

since the infection erodes the surrounding lung (1,5,90). (Fig. 21.8).

No correlation between CT findings and the etiologic agent could be demonstrated. MRI is a biologically safe (ie., ionizing radiation free) examination useful in evaluation of abscesses; because of increased spatial resolution it improves soft tissue contrast and is able to visualize a lesion in multiple planes (2,91). Many authors agree that, compared with CT, MRI in this area offers a better appreciation of the inflammatory process and its extension to surrounding structures (muscular bundles, for example are better detected by MRI). (92) (Fig. 21.9).

Empyema

Pulmonary infections are often associated with pleural effusions, which can be characterized as either transudates or exudates (93). Transudates are benign serous collections resulting from oncotic and hydrostatic pressure variations in the pulmonary and systemic circulation, whereas exudates are caused by pleural involvement and inflammation. Empyema may eventuate from most evolution benign parapneumonic exudates, if they go untreated.

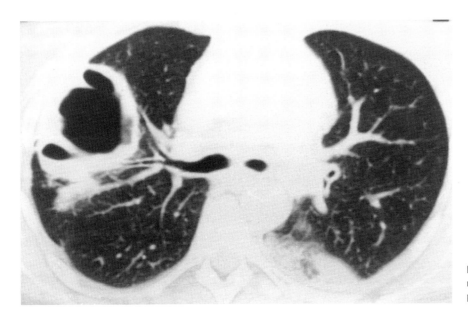

Figure 21.8. CT scan of lung abscess involving the surrounding parenchyma, showing distorted bronchi and pulmonary vessels.

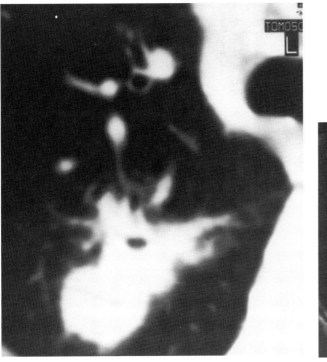

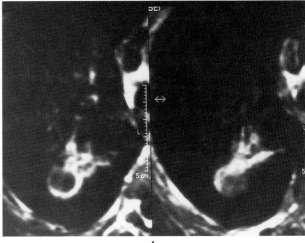

a

b

Figure 21.9. Necrotizing pulmonary carcinoma. Correlation between CT study and MRI findings on Fast Spin Echo T$_1$ (FSE T)-weighted images. **a** CT scan showing an air–fluid level inside the mass. **b** MRI better characterizes the necrotic changes of the lesion as a low signal intensity area.

A definition of empyema could be: "presence of pus in the pleural space; localized or completely involving the pleura." Since the pathology is localized, empyema may occur encapsulated, interlobar, mediastinal, or subpulmonary. The American Thoracic Society classifies empyemas in three stages according to their relationship to the natural history of the disease:

1. Exudative

2. Fibrinopurulent

3. Organized.

In empyema, the pleural space is secondarily invaded by pathogens usually arising from a contiguous site of infection such as lung abscess, pneumonia, TB and fungal infections, mediastinitis, or subphrenic abscess. When a bronchopleural fistula is found, empyema may occur occasionally as a result of a penetrating chest wound or thoracic surgery and as a complication of tumor penetrating the pleura (7). Nowadays empyema is a relatively rare occurrence due to early diagnosis and antibiotic therapy in the treatment of pneumonia; in the past, pneumococci and other streptococci were the most frequent causes of empyema. Currently, most empyemas occur as complications of pneumonia and involve anaerobes (94). Enteric Gram-negative bacteria may be recovered in the case of empyema complicating nosocomial pneumonia, while *Staphylococcus aureus* is the most common causative germ involved in complications following trauma or hemothorax.

Postsurgical empyema can be a complication of lung resections and esophageal surgery. A wide range of microbes, including *S. aureus*, Gram-negative germs and anaerobes may cause these infections. The pleural space may be contaminated intraoperatively, or infected postoperatively by a contiguous focus of infection or by seedings of pleural dead space.

The clinical manifestations of empyema are those of underlying disease. In most cases, an acute empyema is a really serious infection including severe clinical symptoms. Cases of empyema resulting from pneumonia present cough, fever, dyspnea, purulent sputum, and chest pain. Postoperative fever, excessive amounts of pleural fluid due to surgical procedure, and air inside the pleural cavity (probably originating from a bronchopleural fistula) are suggestive of postsurgical empyema diagnosis. The patient may also be seriously toxic or comatose (7).

Diagnostic Imaging

Differential diagnosis between empyema and abscess follows several criteria. Many authors agree the most reliable and consistent of these seems to be the cavity shape, as empyema usually tends to be lenticular and abscesses tend to be round shaped (5).

Several further findings may suggest empyema without being pathognomonic, since they may occur also in the case of lung abscess:

1. Air–fluid level development, increasing within a space where an effusion was noted before.
2. Pleural signs of tapering borders at the edge of an air–fluid cavity.
3. Air–fluid level overtaking a fissure shown on posteroanterior or lateral decubitus views.
4. Enlargement on posteroanterior or/and lateral view of the air–fluid level cavity to the lateral chest wall. Right–left lateral decubitus views could be useful in detecting small fluid volumes (<250 mL).

Empyema diagnosis cannot be excluded by immobile pleural fluid because further stages of the disease may be associated with loculated collection. Lateral decubitus view with decumbent diseased lung, allows a for better appreciation of the underlying pneumonia and detection of loculation (85) (Fig. 21.10).

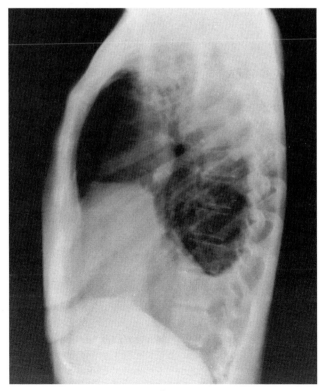
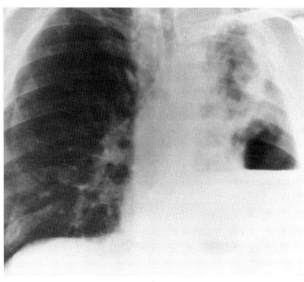

a   b

Figure 21.10. **a** and **b** Posteroanterior and lateral views on chest radiographs showing a pleural purulent fluid collection in the left lung.

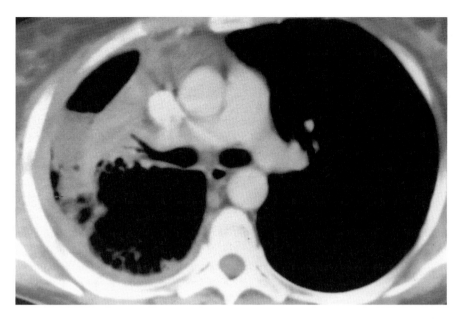

Figure 21.11. CT scan (mediastinal window) viewing a fluid pleural collection associated with and air–fluid level and pleural tapering margin.

Enlargement of the area of empyema usually causes loss of the typical lenticular shape of the lesion, which becomes spherical, and thus similar to the abscess form. Empyema and lung abscess should follow different treatment strategies. Lung abscess needs to be treated by antimicrobial agents, whereas empyema usually requires both antibiotic therapy and drainage.

CT offers a better insightation into the extent of the disease because of thanks to its cross-sectional planes and high contrast resolution. A supine decubitus CT study, performed with serial 10 mm thick sections and intravenous contrast medium administration, is able to characterize and delineate the full extent of most lung abscesses and empyemas (1). Spiral CT examination followed by Three-dimensional reconstruction offers a precise delineation of the pleural collection, allowing a better approach to interventional procedures. Certain CT features are useful in identifying an empyema (95): early in the course of empyema development, the shape of the lesion tends to be ovoidal, conforming to the pleural space. This finding is one of the basic criteria of plain film diagnosis and can be applied to CT. However, the shape may be round in the case of more widespread and loss recent empyemas.

The inside margin of the empyema cavity tends to be smooth, whereas the inner margin of the lung abscess is usually rough (Fig. 21.11). The empyema wall, whenever distinguishable, appears relatively thin and uniformly thick, whereas the lung abscess has an irregular, wider wall. The interface between adjacent lung and both lesions is clearly more defined in empyema than in lung abscess (Fig. 21.12).

Material within an empyema lesion tends to show a restricted range of attenuation values compared to inhomogeneous material inside a lung abscess. The bronchi and pulmonary vessels anatomic configuration seems also to be distorted and bowed where they connect to the bronchial tree. Identification of the limit between parietal and visceral pleura, "split pleura sign," is highly

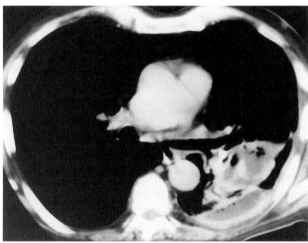

Figure 21.12. CT scan (mediastinal window) of a pulmonary purulent abscess complicated by empyema, showing a sharper interface between empyema and the adjacent lung.

specific for empyema, since it has never been found in lung abscesses. This finding may be seen clearly after administration of intravenous contrast medium, which enhances the appearance of inflamed pleura (96–98).

CT diagnostic accuracy was 100% as against 47% specificity provides significant in plain radiographs (1).

Interventional Radiology

Percutaneous puncture of pulmonary pathology was first performed in 1883 by Leyden to obtain bacterial analysis (99). Various thoracic fluid collections may be treated by interventional radiologic techniques. Percutaneous catheter drainage under local anesthesia, using a combination of US, CT, and fluoroscopic guidance systems, seems to be an effective and safe alternative technique in nonoperative drainage of lung abscesses and thoracic empyemas (100–102).

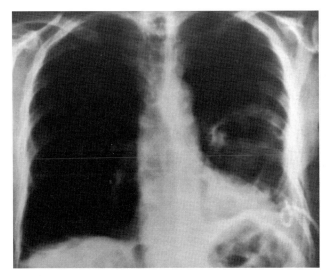

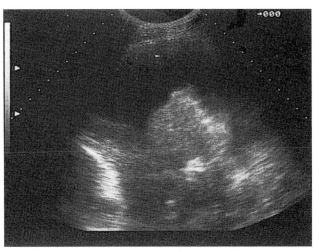

Figure 21.14. US-guided percutaneous drainage of a purulent fluid collection using a 3.5 MHz probe; the white dot inside the fluid collection represents the tip of the needle.

Figure 21.13. Posteroanterior view on chest radiograph showing percutaneous drainage of a pleural fluid collection by means of a pig-tail catheter.

The ongoing sepsis is usually due to suboptimal positioning of the thoracostomy tube, which leaves undrained pus; however, surgical treatment still carries considerable morbidity and mortality in subjects affected by debilitating diseases (103–106). The success rate for drainage of various thoracic collections ranges from 80% to 95%, and depends on the complexity of the collection and the underlying status of the patient (101,107–111). Percutaneous drainage of pleural fluid collections should be considered as first-line therapy in patients with an infected pleural space or pleural effusions, and in those whose fever persists despite adequate antibiotic therapy (112, 113) (Fig. 21.13).

Availability of the modalities, imaging characteristics, location of the collection and operator expertise influence the choice of imaging to guide drainage. US is particularly helpful in identifying laterally loculated collections without exposing the patient and operator to radiation (Fig. 21.14). CT is the preferred modality for medial or fissural collections or for those that are obscured on US due to overlying lung (114) (Fig. 21.15). However, a great disadvantage associated with CT-guided interventions has been the lack of real-time imaging capability. To overcome this limitation, a CT fluoroscopy system was developed, providing real-time imaging reconstruction (115).

The great advantage of fluoroscopic CT versus conventional CT consists in either more accurate positioning of

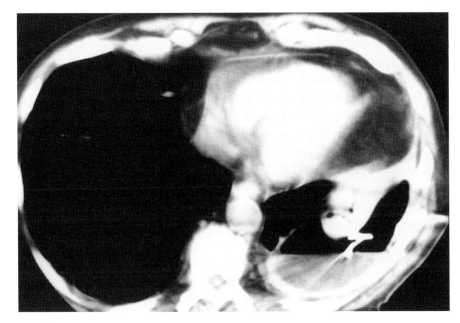

Figure 21.15. CT scan (mediastinal window) showing percutaneous drainage of a pleural empyema.

puncture devices or reduction of examination time (116). Fluoroscopy is used for tube exchanges and to determine cavity communications via the injection of contrast material into the cavity.

MRI currently has no role in the percutaneous drainage of thoracic collections (114).

A stylus is usually used to mark the optimal approach to the skin. The entrance site is prepared using aseptic technique. After local anesthesia a fine 22 gauge needle is introduced. This needle is useful in ascertaining a safe access route and allowing bacteriologic and cytologic studies. The puncture site is located on the upper rib's edge to avoid bleeding and damage of the intercostal nerve. The catheter can be inserted using the Seldinger or Trocar technique; catheter size varies from small 5 French sheath to 30 French catheters. The choice of catheter depends on the viscosity of the fluid collected.

An important philosophy in approaching lung abscess drainage is that "bigger is not better". Small-bore catheters are often the treatment of choice as they are well tolerated; easy to insert, they have response rates similar to those large of bore tubes (117–119) (Fig. 21.16).

Usually single lumen catheters are used in order to reduce the risk of pneumothorax. Once the catheter is placed, the lung abscess or pleural empyema is evacuated as completely as possible and cavity is irrigated with saline solution (114). The catheter is connected to an underwater sealed device employing negative pressure and usually can be removed within 1 week; if residual collection persists, a further catheter can be inserted (102).

Complications can be avoided by meticulous imaging and planning. The complication rate depends on additional pulmonary diseases, such as emphysema or fibrosis, the location of the lesion and the type of needle used. The most frequent complication after these interventional procedures is represented by partial pneumothorax.

Percutaneous treatment of thoracic fluid collections is effective in most cases. The choice of imaging to guide drainage is essential as these collections are often loculated and pose a hazard for delicate structures that are nearby or interposed (114).

References

1. Stark DD, Federle MP, Goodman PC, et al. (1983) Differentiating lung abscess and empyema: Radiography and computed tomography. AJR 141:163–167.
2. Huber DJ, Kobzik L, Melanson G, et al. (1985) Detection of inflammation in collapsed lung by alterations in proton nuclear magnetic relaxation times. Invest Radiol 20:460–464.
3. Thorn GW, et al. (1977) Harrison's principles of internal Medicine, 8th edn. McGraw-Hill New York, vol 1, pp 362–367.
4. Alexander JC, Wolfe WG (1980) Lung abscess and empyema of the thorax. Surg Clin North Am 60:835–849.
5. Baber CE, Hedlund LW, Oddson TA, et al. (1980) Differentiating empyemas and peripheral pulmonary abscess: the value of computed tomography. Radiology 135:755–758.
6. Yellin A, Yellin EO, Lieberman Y (1985) Percutaneous tube drainage: The treatment of choice for refractory lung abscess. Ann Thorac Surg 39:226–270.

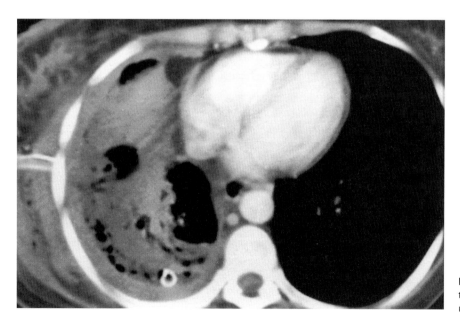

Figure 21.16. CT scan (mediastinal window) of percutaneous drainage of a dense pleural necrotic collection, using a large-bore tube.

7. Le Roux BT, Mohlala ML, Odell JA et al. (1986) Suppurative disease of the lung and pleural space. Part I: Empyema thoracis and lung abscess. Curr Probl Surg 13:1–89.

8. Bartlett J, Gorbach S, Finegold S (1974) Bacteriology and treatment of primary lung abscess. Am Rev Respir Dis 109:510–518.

9. Bertemen YM (1980) Aspiration and inhalation pneumonias. Semin Roentgenol 15:73.

10. Cameron EWJ, Appelbaum PC, et al. (1980) Characteristics and management of chronic destructive pneumonia. Thorax 35:340.

11. Mengoli L (1985) Giant lung abscess treated by tube thoracotomy. J Thorac Cardiovasc Surg 90:186–190.

12. Chidi CC, Mendelsohn HJ (1974) Lung abscess. A study of the results of treatment based on 90 consecutive cases. J Thorac Cardiovasc Surg 68:168–172.

13. Bartlett JG, Gorbach SL, Finegold SM (1974) The bacteriology of aspiration pneumonia. Am J Med 56:103–112.

14. Bartlett JG, Gorbach SL, Tally FP, et al. (1974) Bacteriology and treatment of primary lung abscess. Rev Respir Dis 109:510–518.

15. Brook I, Finegold SM (1979) Bacteriology and therapy of abscess in children. J Pediatry 94:10.

16. Bartlett JG, Finegold SM (1974) Anaerobic infections of the lung and pleural space. Am Rev Respir Dis 110:56–77.

17. Johanson WG, Harris GD (1980) Aspiration pneumonia, anaerobic infections, and lung abscess. Med Clin North Am 64:385–394.

18. Warhauer D, Goldstein E, Akers T (1977) Effects of influenza viral infection on the gestion and killing of bacteria by alveolar macrophages. Am Rev Respir Dis 115:269–277.

19. Douglas RG (1979) Influenza: The disease and its complications. Hosp Pract 11:43–50.

20. Notter DT, Grossman PL, Rosenberg SA, et al. (1980) Infections in patients with Hodgkin's disease: A clinical study of 300 consecutive adult patients. Rev Infect Dis 2:761–800.

21. Siber GR (1980) Bacteremias due to Haemophilus influenzae and Streptococcus pneumoniae: Their occurrence in children with cancer. Am J Dis Child 134:668–672.

22. Valdivieso M, Gil-Extemera B, Zornoza J, et al. (1977) Gram-negative bacillary pneumonia in the compromised host. Medicine 56:241–254.

23. Pierce AK, Edmunson EB, McGree G, et al. (1966) An analysis of factors predisposing to Gram-negative bacillary necrotizing pneumonia. Am Rev Respir Dis 94:309–315.

24. Sullivan RJ, Dowdle WR, Marine WM, et al. (1972) Adult pneumonia in a general hospital. Arch Intern Med 129:935–942.

25. Fang GD, Fine M, Orloff J, et al. (1990) New and emerging etiologies for community-acquired pneumonia with implications for therapy. A prospective multicenter study of 359 cases. Medicine 69:307–316.

26. Mufson MA, Chang V, Gill V, et al. (1967) The role of viruses, mycoplasmas and bacteria in acute pneumonia in civilian adults. Am J Epidemiol 86:526–544.

27. Farr B, Mandel GL (1983) Gram-positive pneumonia. In Pennington JE (ed) Respiratory infections: diagnosis and management. Raven Press, New York, pp 217–226.

28. Mufson MA (1990) Streptococcus pneumoniae. In Mandel GL, Douglas RG, Bennet JE (eds) Principles and practice of infectious diseases, 3rd edn. John Wiley & Sons, New York, pp 1539–1550.

29. Winston DJ, Schiffman G, Wang DC, et al. (1979) Pneumococcal infections after human bone marrow transplantation. Ann Intern Med 91:835–841.

30. Gerber CJ, Farmer WC, Fulkerson LL (1978) Beta-hemolytic streptococcal pneumonia following influenza. JAMA 240:242–246.

31. Bentley DW (1980) Staphylococcal pneumonia: Coping with a medical emergency. J Respir Dis 1:23–4.

32. Mark PH, Turner JAP (1968) Lung abscess in childhood. Thorax 23:216–220.

33. Olsson RA, Romansky MJ (1962) Staphylococcal tricuspid endocarditis in heroin addicts. Ann Intern Med 57:755–762.

34. Fischer AM, Trever RW, Curtin JA, et al. (1958) Staphylococcal pneumonia: A review of 21 cases in adults. N Engl J Med 258:919.

35. Fraser RG, ParÈ JAP (1978) Diagnosis of diseases of chest, 2nd edn. WB Saunders, Philadelphia.

36. Everett ED, Rahm AE, Adaniya R, et al. (1977) Haemophilus influenzae pneumonia in adults. JAMA 238:319–321.

37. Wallace RJ, Musher DM, Martin R (1978) Haemophilus influenzae pneumonia in adults. Am J Med 64:87–93.

38. Smith AL, Pappas P, Plorde J (1983) Haemophilus influenzae pneumonia. In Pennington JE (ed) Respiratory infections: diagnosis and management, Raven Press, New York, pp 269–281.

39. Levin DC, Schwartz MI, Matthay RA, et al. (1977) Bacteremic Haemophilus influenzae pneumonia in adults: A report of 24 cases and a review of the literature. Am J Med 62:219–224.

40. Crane LR, Lerner AM (1983) Gram-negative bacillary pneumonias. In Pennington JE (ed) Respiratory infections: diagnosis and management. Raven Press, New York, pp 227–250.

41. Pierce AK, Sanford JP (1974) Aerobic gram-negative bacillary pneumonias. Am Rev Respir Dis 110:647–658.

42. Edmondson EG, Sanford J (1967) The Klebsiella–Enterobacter–Serratia group. Medicine 46:323.

43. Manfredi F, Daly WJ, Behnke RH (1963) Clinical observation of acute Friedlander pneumonia. Ann Intern Med 58:642.

44. Mertz JJ, Scharer L, McClement JH (1967) A hospital outbreak of Klebsiella pneumonia from inhalation therapy with contaminated aerosol solutions. Am Rev Respir Dis 95:454–460.

45. Tillotson JR, Lerner AM: Characteristics of pneumonias caused by Escherichia coli. N Engl J Med 177:115–122.

46. Berk SL, Neuman P, Holtsclaw S, et al. (1982) Escherichia coli pneumonia in the elderly with reference to the role of E. coli K1 capsular polysaccharide antigen. Am J Med 72:899–902.

47. Yu VL (1979) Serratia marcescens. Hospital perspective and clinical review. N Engl J Med 300:887–893.

48. Pierce AK, Edmunson EB, McGee G, et al. (1966) An analysis of factors predisposing to Gram-negative bacillary necrotizing pneumonia. Am Rev Respir Dis 94:309–315.

49. Fields BN, Uwaydah MM, Kunz LJ, et al. (1967) The so-called "Paracolon" bacteria: A bacteriologic and clinical reappraisal. Am J Med 42:89–106.

50. Tillotson JR, Lerner AM (1967) Characteristics of pneumonia caused by Escherichia coli. N Engl J Med 277:115.

51. Rose HD, Hechman MG, Unger JD (1973) Pseudomonas aeruginosa pneumonia in adults. Am Rev Respir Dis 107:416–422.

52. Unger JD, Rose HD, Unger GF (1973) Gram negative pneumonia. Radiology 107:283.

53. Renner RR, Coccaro AP, Heitzman ER, et al. (1972) Pseudomonas pneumonia: A prototype of hospital-based infection. Radiology 105:555.

54. Schimpff SC, Young VM, Greene WH, et al. (1972) Origin of infection in acute nonlymphocytic leukemia: Significance of hospital acquisition of potential pathogens. Ann Intern Med 77:707–714.

55. Russel W, Gilmore FR (1951) Solitary pulmonary necrosis comparison of neoplastic and inflammatory condition. Radiology 56:708–716.

56. Cole LR, Dundee JC (1955) Cavitation in bland infarcts of the lung. Can Med Assoc J 72:907–910.

57. Putman CE, Godwin JD, Silverman PM, et al. (1984) CT of localized lucent lung lesions. Semin Roentgenol 19:173–18.

58. Rohlfing BM, White EA, Webb WR, et al. (1978) Hilar and mediastinal adenopathy caused by bacteria abscess of the lung. Radiology 128:289–293.

59. Brock RC (1947) Aetiology of lung abscess. In Studies in lung abscess. Guy's Hosp Rep 96:141.

60. Jaffe RB, Koschmann EB (1970) Septic pulmonary emboli. Radiology 96:527–532.

61. Wallace RJ, Cohen A, Awe RJ, et al. (1979) Carcinomatous lung abscess. JAMA 242:521–522.

62. Hsu JT, Barrett CR (1982) Lung abscess complicating transbronchial biopsy of a mass. Chest 80:230–232.

63. Canny GJ, Marcotte JE, Levison H (1986) Lung abscess in cystic fibrosis. Thorax 41:221–222.

64. Norman WJ, Moule NJ, Walrond ER (1974) Lung abscess: A complication of malposition of a central venous catheter. Br J Radiol 47:498–50.

65. Johnston RF, Flegal EE (1969) Displaced bronchus, lung abscess, and retrograde perfusion. Dis Chest 55:69–72.

66. Master KM (1978) Diffuse metallic nodular densities and lung abscess. Chest 74:657–658.

67. Chester EM, Krause GR (1972) Lung abscess secondary aseptic pulmonary infarction. Radiology 39:647–654.

68. Vidal R, Leveen HH, Yarnoz M, et al. (1971) Lung abscess secondary to pulmonary infarction. Ann Thorac Surg 11:557–564.

69. Libshitz HI, Pagani JJ (1981) Aspergillosis and mucormycosis: Types of opportunistic fungal pneumonia. Radiology 140:301–306.

70. Wilson AG, Joseph AEA, Butland RJA (1986) The radiology of aseptic cavitation in pulmonary infarction. Clin Radiol 37:327–333.

71. Jaffe RB, Kochmann EB (1970) Intravenous drug abuse: pulmonary, cardiac and vascular complications. Am J Radiol 109:107–114.

72. Julander I (1983) Staphylococcal septicaemia and endocarditis in 80 drug addicts. Scand J Infect Dis 41:49–54.

73. Leung AN, Brauner MV, Gamsu G et al. (1996) Pulmonary tuberculosis: comparison of CT findings in HIV seropositive and HIV seronegative patients. Radiology 198:687–691.

74. Levy JA (ed) (1994) HIV and the pathogenesis in AIDS. ASM Press, Washington DC.

75. Hershey CO, Tomford JW, McLaren CE et al. (1984) The natural history of intravenous catheter-associated phlebitis. Arch Intern Med 144:1373–1375.

76. Kuhlman JE, Fishman EK, Teigen C (1990) Pulmonary septic emboli: diagnosis with CT. Radiology 174:211–213.

77. Collins CG (1951) Suppurative pelvic thrombophlebitis. II. Symptomatology and diagnosis. Surgery 30:311–327.

78. Cherubin CE, Baden M, Kavaler F (1968) Infective endocarditis in narcotic addicts. Ann Intern Med 69:1091–1098.

79. Sapira JD (1968) The narcotic addict as a medical patient. Am J Med 45:555–588.

80. Gumbs YV, McCauley DI (1982) Hilar and mediastinal adenopathy in pulmonary embolic disease. Radiology 142:313–315.

81. Gross BH, Spitz HB, Felson B (1982) The mural nodule in cavitary pulmonary aspergillosis. Radiology 143:619–622.

82. Briggs JH, McKerron CG, Souhami RL (1967) Severe systemic infections complicating "mainline" heroin addiction. Lancet 2:1227–1231.

83. Husseay HH, Katz S (1945) Septic pulmonary infarction: Report of 8 cases. Ann Intern Med 22:526–542.

84. Williford ME, Godwin JR (1983) Computed tomography of lung abscess and empyema. Radiol Clin North Am 21:575–583.

85. Schachter EN, Kreisman H, Putman C (1976) Diagnosis of problems in suppurative lung disease. Arch Intern Med 136:167–17.

86. Weis W (1973) Cavity behavior in acute, primary, nonspecific lung abscess. Am Rev Respir Dis 108:1273–1284.

87. Doust BD, Baum JK, Maklad NF, et al. (1975) Ultrasonic evaluation of pleural opacities. Radiology 114:132–140.

88. Landay MJ, Conrad MR (1979) Lung abscess mimicking empyema on ultrasonography. AJR 133:731–734.

89. Lang FC, Filly RA (1974) Problems in the application of ultrasonography. AJR 133:731–734.

90. Williford ME, Hidalgo H, Putman CE, et al. (1983) Computed tomography of pleural disease. AJR 140:909–914.

91. Wall SD, Fisher MR, Amparo EG, et al. (1985) Magnetic resonance imaging in the evaluation of abscesses. AJR 144:1217–1221.

92. Barkhausen J, Stoblen F, Dominguez-Fernandez E, et al. (1999) Impact of CT in patients with sepsis of unknown origin. Acta Radiol 40:552–55.

93. Light W, MacGregor I, Luchsinger PC, et al. (1972) Pleural effusions: The diagnostic separation of transudates and exudates. Ann Intern Med 77:507–513.

94. Bartlett JG, Gorbach SL, Thadepalli H, et al. (1974) Bacteriology of empyema. Lancet 1:338–340.

95. Shin MS, Ho K (1983) Computed tomographic characteristics of pleural empyema. JCAT 7:179–183.

96. Bressler EL, Francis IR, Glazer GM, et al. (1987) Bolus contrast medium enhancement for distinguishing pleural from parenchymal lung disease: CT features. JCAT 11:436–440.

97. Waite RJ, Carbonneau RJ, Balikian JP, et al. (1990) Parietal pleural changes in empyema: Appearances on CT. Radiology 175:145–150.

98. Williford ME, Godwin JD (1983) Computed tomography of lung abscess and empyema. Radiol Clin North Am 21:575–581.

99. Leyden OO (1983) Über infektiose pneumonie. Dtsch Med Weschenschr 9:52.

100. van Sonnenberg E, Nakamoto SK, Mueller PR, et al. (1984) CT and ultrasound-guided catheter drainage of empyemas after chest-tube failure. Radiology 151:349–353.

101. van Sonnenberg E, Ferruci JT, Mueller PR, et al. (1982) Percutaneous drainage of abscesses and fluid collections. Technique, results and applications. Radiology 142:1–10.

102. Westcott JL (1985) Percutaneous catheter drainage of pleural effusion and empyema. AJR 144:1189–1193.

103. Davis WC, Johnson LF (1978) Adult thoracic empyema revisited. Am Surg 44:362–368.

104. Cameron EWJ, Whitton JD (1977) Percutaneous drainage in the treatment of Klebsiella pneumoniae lung abscess. Thorax 32:673–676.

105. Morin JE, Munro DD, MacLean LD (1972) Early thoracotomy for empyema. J Thorac Cardiovasc Surg 64:530–535.

106. Geha AS (1971) Pleural empyema. Changing etiologic, bacteriologic, and therapeutic aspects. J Thorac Cardiovasc Surg 61:626–635.

107. Mueller PR, Van Sonnenberg E (1990) Interventional radiology in the chest and abdomen. N Engl J Med 322:1364–1374.

108. Silverman SG, Mueller PR, Saini S, et al. (1988) Thoracic empyema: Management with image-guided catheter drainage. Radiology 169:5–9.

109. Westcott JL (1985) Percutaneous catheter drainage of pleural effusion and empyema. AJR 144:1189–1193.

110. O'Moore PV, Mueller PR, Simeone JF, et al. (1987) Sonographic guidance in diagnostic and therapeutic interventions in the pleural space. AJR 149:1–5.

111. Stavas J, Van Sonnenberg E, Casola G, et al. (1987) Percutaneous drainage of infected and non-infected thoracic fluid collections. J Thorac Imaging 2:80–87.

112. Brook I, Frazier FH (1993) Aerobic and anaerobic microbiology of empyema. Chest 103:1502–150.

113. Bartlett JC, Gorbach SL, Thadepalli HT, et al. (1974) Bacteriology of empyema. Lancet 1:338–340.

114. Van Sonnenberg E, Wittich GR, Goodacre W, et al. (1998) Percutaneous drainage of thoracic collections. J Thoracic Imaging 13:74–82.

115. Froelich JJ, Saar B, Hoppe M, et al. (1998) Real-time CT-fluoroscopy for guidance of percutaneous drainage procedures. J Vasc Inter J Radial 9:735–740.

116. Anzbock W, Mayrhofer R, Pichler L, et al. (1998) CT-fluoroscopy: Application and Advantages – first clinical experience. CIRSE '98 annual meeting and postgraduate course – Venice. Abstract book.

117. Hausheer FH, Yarbro JW (1985) Diagnosis and treatment of malignant pleural effusion. Semin Oncol 12:54–75.

118. Seaton KG, Patz EF, Goodman PC (1995) Palliative treatment of malignant pleural effusions: Value of small-bore catheter thoracostomy and doxycycline sclerotherapy. AJR 164:589–591.

119. Morrison MC, Mueller PR, Lee MJ, et al. (1992) Sclerotherapy of malignant pleural effusion through sonographically placed small-bore catheters AJR 158:41–43.

22 Pulmonary Atelectasis

J. Nishi, S. Tomiguchi and M. Takahashi

Introduction

Pulmonary atelectasis is one of the most commonly encountered abnormalities in chest radiology and remains a daily diagnostic challenge. At times atelectasis can be overlooked, particularly when pulmonary opacification is minimal or absent on radiographic films, and at other times it might be interpreted as being some other form of intrathoracic pathology.

In the current usage, atelectasis refers to acquired diminution in volume of part or all of a lung, with or without opacification of the affected portion of the lung (1–3). Acceptable synonyms for atelectasis are loss of volume and collapse; however, the term collapse is often reserved to denote total atelectasis of the affected part of the lung (3). Pulmonary atelectasis can be classified into six types: resorptive, passive, adhesive, cicatrization, compressive, and gravity-dependent (3). The purpose of this article is to review the pathogenesis of these types of atelectasis and to provide a broad overview of the radiographic signs and differential diagnoses.

Types of Atelectasis Based on Pathogenesis

Resorptive Atelectasis

Resorptive atelectasis is the most common (1). It stems from resorption of gas from the alveoli, which occurs when communication between alveoli and trachea is obstructed (1–3). For this reason, it is also referred to as obstructive atelectasis (2,4). Resorptive atelectasis can be divided into two groups cases are a group with a large-airway obstruction and cases with a small-airway obstruction.

When acute obstruction of a large airway occurs, resorption of air from the alveoli begins and results in progressive decrease in size of the alveoli (1). In the healthy lung, complete resorption of air will take place within 24 h after acute obstruction (2), since the diffusion rate for nitrogen is much slower than that of oxygen (1–2).

Radiographic appearances of the atelectatic lung are variable. The affected lobe usually loses volume and has increased density owing to resorption of air and retention of fluid (i.e., edema fluid from the capillary bed, some sequestration of blood in the lobe, secretions) distal to the obstruction. The amount of fluid present and the degree of collapse depends on the severity and duration of obstruction and on the presence or absence of collateral air drift (1–3).

The atelectatic lobe often appears very opaque on films even though its total volume is only slight (2). Two different pathophysiologic events, one acute and one chronic, are responsible for this increase in density (2). In the former, although the amount of trapped edema fluid and blood within the obstructed lung is often slight, the affected portion of the lung is filled predominantly with trapped edema fluid and blood rather than losing a significant amount of volume. This condition has been termed "drowned lung" (1–3). "Drowned lung" often remains a pathologic diagnosis. However, lobar enlargement distal to an obstructing lesion of the bronchus should be considered strong radiographic evidence of the diagnosis (3). The second and by far more common cause for the atelectatic lung to become opaque is the development within it of obstructive pneumonitis, which is often found distal to the obstructing lesion in the bronchus (3). It happens in many cases of bronchogenic carcinoma in which bronchial obstruction is of slow onset and atelectasis develops over a long period of time (1–3,5). In these cases the predominant pathologic features are those of a noninfectious process: bronchiectasis with distal mucoid impaction of the bronchi, alveolar volume loss, retention of edema fluid, and lymphocystic infiltration of the bronchial walls; polymorphonuclear leukocytes and parenchymal necrosis, features typical of acute bacterial pneumonia, are absent (3,5). This condition has been termed golden pneumonia, cholesterol pneumonia, or endogenous lipid pneumonia (2,5). If bacterial infection accompanies obstructive pneumonia, primarily it affects the airways and cannot be detected radiographically (5).

Resorptive atelectasis stemming from small-airway obstruction is a very common occurrence, developing as a result of obstruction of small bronchi and bronchioles in the face of inadequate collateral air draft (2). Impairment of mucociliary transport causes pooling of retained secretions in the smaller airways, with resultant bronchial and bronchiolar obstruction and distal resorptive atelectasis (6). In such conditions, the large airways are often patent and filled with air, resulting in the formation of air bronchograms within the atelectatic lung (1–2). However, rapid accumulation of secretions can cause filling of the bronchi all the way to the main bronchus, leading to complete disappearance of air bronchograms in the atelectatic lung (7). On plain films, air bronchograms are typically absent in the collapsed lung (1–2). Although the presence of air bronchograms within the atelectatic lung on plain films implies the absence of a central obstructing neoplasm ("patent or open bronchus sign") (Fig. 22.1) (8), this sign is not completely reliable (2), particularly on computed tomography (CT), where air bronchograms are not infrequently observed in atelectatic lung distal to a central obstructing neoplasm (3,9).

Passive Atelectasis

Passive atelectasis occurs when there is fault with pleural integrity, and lung collapse follows. The lungs have a natural tendency to collapse and do so when removed from the chest (1). Normally, the elastic recoil of the lung is opposed by the outward pull of the chest wall and downward pull of the diaphragm (1,10,11). These opposing forces make for negative intrapleural pressure. In the simple pneumothorax, intrapleural pressure becomes atmospheric, and intraalveloar pressure and intrapleural pressure are equalized. This situation allows the lung to

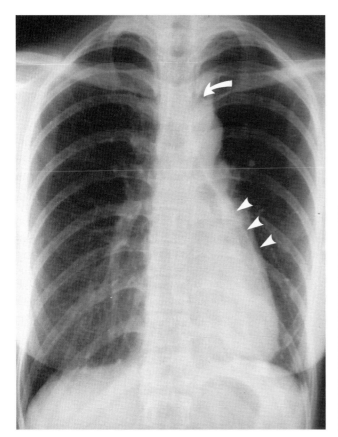

a

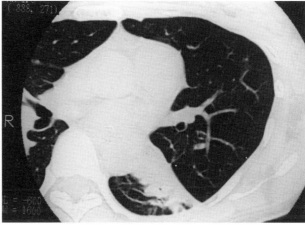

b

Figure 22.1. LLL atelectasis due to mucus plugging. On the posteroanterior view, the LLL is seen as an opacity behind the heart (a). The trachea shifts mildly to the left and the left hemidiaphragm elevates slightly. The descending aorta is also obscured. The shifted upper mediastinal soft tissues obscure the upper aspect of the aortic arch (top-of-knob sign) (*arrow*) and straightening of the left heart border is demonstrated (flat-waist sign) (*arrowheads*). Compensatory hyperexpansion of the LUL is clearly seen in the left lung. Some air bronchograms of the central bronchi are observed in the upper portion of the opacity. CT shows the anterior basal segment collapse (b). The shift of the major fissure and compensatory hyperexpansion are also demonstrated on CT. Furthermore, the air bronchograms are more clearly demonstrated on CT than on the posteroanterior view.

collapse and the thorax to spring out (10,11). Other causes of passive atelectasis are paralysis of the diaphragm, congenital eventration of the diaphragm and pulmonary hypoventilation (3).

Compressive Atelectasis

This term denotes pulmonary collapse in the presence of a space-occupying intrathoracic process such as pleural effusion, empyema, pleural tumors, large pulmonary masses, large emphysematous bullae, lobar emphysema or diaphragmatic hernias (3). In tension pneumothorax, positive intrapleural pressure forces all the air out of the alveoli, leaving the atelectatic lung completely airless (12). This finding is useful for distinguishing tension pneumothorax from a large simple pneumothorax, a condition in which the atelectatic lung remains partly aerated (12).

Adhesive Atelectasis

Adhesive atelectasis is the term used to describe a type of atelectasis, in which there is alveolar collapse in the presence of patient airways, stemming from surfactant deficiency (1,4,10). When there is a deficiency of surfactant, there is much greater tendency for the alveoli to collapse (1,4). Once collapsed, the alveolar walls tend to adhere, making reexpansion difficult (4). The diseases that have been shown to produce adhesive atelectasis are hyaline membrane disease, adult respiratory distress syndrome, smoke inhalation, uremia, pulmonary embolism, acute radiation pneumonitis, and pneumonia (3).

The opacity is characteristically homogeneous except for the air bronchogram that is almost always observed because the mechanism of adhesive atelectasis is surfactant deficit (13).

Cicatrization Atelectasis

The pathologic process in cicatrization atelectasis is localized or diffuse fibrosis, which produces the decrease in alveolar compliance (1,4,14). Diffuse pulmonary volume loss can be seen in a number of conditions that cause diffuse pulmonary fibrosis, including idiopathic pulmonary fibrosis, sarcoidosis, pneumoconiosis, asbestosis, and scleroderma and other collagen-vascular diseases (3). In these diseases, the increase in collagen leads to a decrease in air per unit lung volume as a result of both decreased lung compliance and increased tissue.

Localized cicatrization atelectasis can be seen in chronic bronchiectasis, chronic tuberculosis (Fig. 22.2), and fungal infections, and radiation fibrosis (3,15). Localized cicatrization atelectasis stemming from these diseases is also associated with demonstrable pleural thickening (4,14).

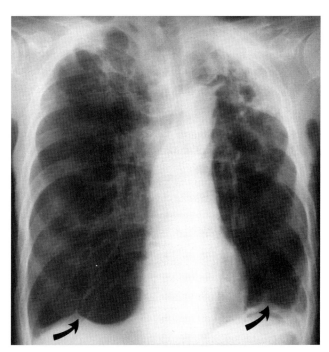

Figure 22.2. Bilateral upper lobe atelectasis due to tuberculosis. On the posteroanterior view, marked volume loss of bilateral upper lobes is shown. Elevation of the hilus and compensatory expansion is observed in bilateral lungs. The juxtaphrenic peak (*arrows*) is also demonstrated on the middle portion of the bilateral diaphragm.

Gravity-dependent Atelectasis

Gravity-dependent atelectasis is defined as atelectasis observed predominantly in the depending lung, and is often detected during anesthesia and the early postoperative period (16–20). CT demonstrates a gradient in attenuation between dependent and nondependent portions of the lungs, with gravity-dependent portions of the lung being of higher attenuation than nondependent areas (21). The increased attenuation in the dependent portions of the lungs reflects both greater perfusion and decrease alveolar expansion in the dependent areas and is greatest at low lung volume (21). Tomiyama et al. (22) reported that an inherent reduction in alveolar volume without small-airway collapse was the important causative factor for the development of gravity-dependent atelectasis. The reduction in alveolar volume is accentuated by disease processes that increase the lung weight, as in patients with pneumonia, increased blood volume, and pulmonary edema (3).

Radiographic Signs of Atelectasis

The radiographic signs of atelectasis may be both direct and indirect. Since we define atelectasis simply as loss of lung volume, a direct and highly dependable sign is displacement of the interlobar fissure (Fig. 22.1). This is considered further in relation to patterns of lobar and segmental collapse. Other direct signs of atelectasis are crowding together of the pulmonary vessels and crowded air bronchograms (3,23). If the collapsing portion of the lung still contains some air, crowding together of the pulmonary vessels is observed, and if the bronchi remain filled with air, crowded air bronchograms can be demonstrated on film (3,23). Crowding together of the pulmonary vessels is one of the earliest signs of atelectasis and is often appreciated when comparison is made with a normal baseline study (3). If the proximal bronchi are occluded or filled with secretions, air within the bronchi disappear. When this happens, displacement of the interlobar fissures could be the only direct sign of atelectasis (1–2).

Indirect signs of atelectasis include pulmonary opacification, elevation of the diaphragm, displacement of mediastinal structures, displacement of hilar structures, compensatory overinflation, and approximation of the ribs (1–2,8).

Pulmonary Opacification

Because of the large amount of air contained within the normal lung, when the lung loses volume, opacification of the collapsing lung may not be apparent until a considerable amount of volume loss has occurred (1,23). However, most cases do show a degree of local increase in density (1,23).

Elevation of the Diaphragm

Elevation of the diaphragm is an important indirect sign of atelectasis (1,3). However, not only is diaphragm elevation a common feature of many conditions unassociated with atelectasis, but it is also often encountered in the normal patient (8). This condition can be best appreciated when comparison is made with the normal baseline study (Fig. 22.3). Hemidiaphragmatic elevation is always a more prominent feature of lower than of upper lobe collapse (8).

In the diffuse atelectasis, elevation of the diaphragm is one of the earliest indications of volume loss in cases with diffuse surfactant deficiency, diffuse obstruction of the small airways and diffuse pulmonary fibrosis (1,3,6).

Displacement of Mediastinal Structures

The normal mediastinum is a mobile structure, and the degree of shift is usually greatest in the region of the major pulmonary collapse (1). Trachea and upper mediastinal displacement is a feature of upper lobe atelectasis, and inferior mediastinal shift is a feature of lower lobe atelectasis (1). For example, opacification ipsilateral is important where there is mediastinal displacement. When the mediastinum is displaced toward the lesion, the cause may be atelectasis. But if the displacement is contralateral to the normal lung the cause may be pleural effusion or massive mass in the hemithorax.

Displacement of Hilar Structures

The hilus is often displaced in the presence of atelectasis, and usually more markedly in the more chronic process (1). When atelectasis is bilateral, the trachea, heart, and mediastinum usually remain in the midline (1–3,23,24). Displacement of the hilus can be an important clue in diagnosing atelectasis (1–3,23,24).

It is important to assess the position of the air columns of the trachea and major bronchi in the lateral projection as an indication of collapse (25). On a well-aligned lateral view of the chest, the trachea, both main bronchi, and both upper lobe bronchi are in vertical alignment, and any alteration in this relationship should be considered abnormal (1).

Compensatory Hyperexpansion

Compensatory hyperexpansion or overinflation of the unilateral lung is sometimes a helpful indirect sign of atelectasis (8). As it occurs gradually, in the early stages of lobar collapse, it is less helpful than the other signs. In the period of collapse, however, hyperexpansion becomes more prominent and the other indirect signs regress (1). Radiographic evidence of hyperexpansion may be subtle. The reliable evidence of hyperexpansion is supplied by the alternation in vascular markings resulting from the increased lung volume; the vessels are more widely spaced and sparser than in the normal contralateral lung (1,8). The increase lung translucency might be difficult to appreciate on plain films but is usually easily seen on CT (1).

Approximation of the Ribs

Approximation of the ribs as a sign of the small size of a hemithorax occurs on the side of the collapsed lung and is a frequent indirect sign of atelectasis but it is difficult to evaluate unless present in considerable degree (8).

Role of Chest Radiograph and CT in the Diagnosis of Atelectasis

Although the cause of atelectasis may be apparent from the patient's medical history, clinical examination, and

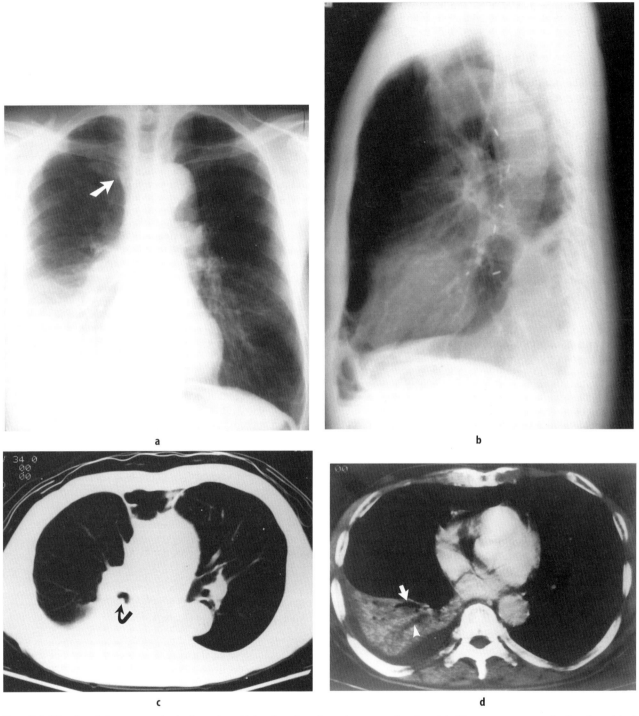

a

b

c

d

Figure 22.3. RLL atelectasis due to mucus plugging in a patient with bronchogenic carcinoma (squamous cell carcinoma). In this case, surgery was previously performed due to esophageal carcinoma. On the posteroanterior view, a homogeneous opacity with elevation of the right hemidiaphragm is shown. The upper triangular sign (*arrow*) is demonstrated in the right upper mediastinum and the right hilus shifts downward (**a**). There is no air bronchogram present in the atelectatic lung. On the lateral view, a typical triangular opacity lying in the posterior costophrenic angle is observed (**b**). CT shows the small intrabronchial tumor (*arrow*) in the right main bronchus (**c**). Postcontrast CT demonstrates an air bronchogram (*arrow*) and mucus bronchogram (*arrowhead*) (**d**).

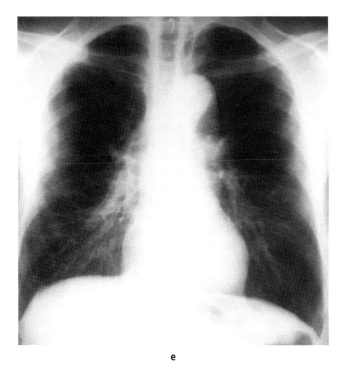

e

Figure 22.3. (*contd*) Some pleural effusion is also demonstrated. The elevation of the left hemidiaphragm and upper triangular sign on the posteroanterior view is more clearly recognized compared with the baseline study (**e**).

chest radiographic findings, further evaluation with CT is often useful. In CT, cross-sectional anatomic examination allows an unobscured view not only of the affected lobe and involved airways but also the mediastinum, hilus, pleura, and chest wall.

The findings of several radiographic investigations of atelectasis by chest radiograph and CT are described below.

Radiographic Forms of Atelectasis

Atelectasis can be divided into several types radiographically: segmental, lobar, or whole lung atelectasis; subsegmental atelectasis; plate-like atelectasis; round atelectasis; and generalized or diffuse atelectasis (1–3,10,23,26,27).

Lobar and Segmental Atelectasis

Lobar and segmental type atelectasis are concerned with obstructive atelectasis. Lobar atelectasis is common (3), and causes atelectasis are summarized in Table 22.1. Among inpatients, mucus plugging of the bronchus may necessitate bronchoscopic suctioning (7,23) and, in outpatients, an obstructing central bronchogenic carcinoma may be present (23).

Segmental atelectasis is invariably caused by airway obstruction, the resulting radiographic appearance being a combination of both loss of volume and obstructive pneumonitis. Radiographic signs of atelectasis of the

individual lobes, including segmental atelectasis, are described in the following sections and the main features are summarized in Table 22.2.

Right Upper Lobe Atelectasis

As the right upper lobe (RUL) loses volume, the minor fissure and the upper half of the major fissure approximate

Table 22.1. Causes of lobar atelectasis

Categories	Causes
Intrinsic mass	Primary neoplasm
	Metastatic neoplasm (renal cell breast carcinoma, melanoma)
	Lymphoma
	Adenoid cystic carcinoma
	Bronchial carcinoid
	Benign endobronchial tumors
	Eroding lymph nodes
Intrinsic stenosis	Inflammatory process (tuberculosis or fungal infection)
	Bronchial fracture
	Malpositioned endobronchial tubes
	Amyloidosis
	Tracheobronchopathia osteochondroplastica
Extrinsic pressure	Enlarged lymph nodes
	Mediastinal tumor
	Mediastinal fibrosis
	Aortic aneurysm
	Cardiac enlargement
Bronchial plugging	Foreign body
	Mucus accumulation

Table 22.2. Radiographic signs associated with lobar atelectasis

Location of atelectasis	Radiographic signs
Any lobe	Mediastinal wedge
	Golden's S sign
	Open bronchus sign
	Double lesion sign
Right upper lobe	*Luftsichel* sign
	Juxtaphrenic peak
Left upper lobe	*Luftsichel* sign
	Juxtaphrenic peak
	Tag on CT
Right lower lobe	Upper triangle sign
	Gatling gun sign
Left lower lobe	Top-of-the-knob sign
	Flat-waist sign
	Nordenström's sign

by shifting upward and forward, respectively (28). Both fissures become gently curved, as seen on the lateral view; the minor fissure assumes a concave configuration inferiorly, whereas the major fissure may be convex, concave, or flat (29). The minor fissure shows roughly the same curvature in the posteroanterior (PA) view. As the volume diminishes further, the visceral pleural surface sweeps upward over the apex of the hemithorax, so that the lobe comes to assume a flattened shape contiguous with the superior mediastinum (29).

As collapse causes the volume of the RUL to diminish, the right middle lobe (RML) and lower lobe (RLL) expand in compensation (8,23). Occasionally, the hyperexpanding superior segment of the RLL or the RML becomes insinuated between the mediastinum and the collapsing RUL (1–2,23,30), which has been referred to as the *Luftsichel* sign (30). On the PA view, the hyperexpanded lung forms a crescent-shaped lucency between the mediastinum and the opacity of the atelectatic RUL. The *Luftsichel* sign is more common in left upper lobe (LUL) than in RUL atelectasis (30). On the lateral view, the collapsed lobe may appear as an indistinctly defined triangular shadow with its apex at the hilus and its base contiguous with the parietal pleura. This triangular opacity on the lateral view has been called the "mediastinal wedge" (1–3,7–8,23).

When completely collapsed, its volume is so small that in the PA view its shadow creates no more than a slight widening of the superior mediastinum and can be mistaken for apical pleural thickening or a mediastinal mass (1–3,8,23). On the lateral view the mediastinal wedge becomes very small and inapparent (23). Extreme collapse may be very difficult to diagnose on only plain radiographs. Felson (8) has pointed out that the key radiographic findings of complete RUL collapse are hilar elevation, diminished right hilar size, and sparse pulmonary vessels in a hyperlucent right lung.

Mediastinal shift is usually less marked in upper lobe atelectasis than in lower lobe atelectasis (23). In RUL atelectasis there may be a detectable shift of the trachea to the right (8,23). In addition, there can be an elevation of the right hemidiaphragm (23), and, in some cases, also a peak-like shadow along the medial aspect of the hemidiaphragm (Fig. 22.2) (31). This sign, which was called "juxtaphrenic peak", is more common in LUL than in RUL atelectasis (31). Formation of the peak is considered to be related to traction on the basal pleura by the inferior pulmonary ligament, due to elevation of the right hilus (31). The appearance of the intercostal spaces in RUL atelectasis usually shows little or no change from normal (23).

In 1925, Golden (32) reported that tumor masses enveloped by RUL collapse could be detected by the convex bulge they produce against the adjacent aerated lung. This sign has come to be known as the "S line" of Golden or Golden's "S" sign because of the reversed S configuration of the minor fissure on the PA view (2,23) (Fig. 22.4). The concept of this sign can be applied to atelectasis of any lobe by noting a localized convex bulge of the displaced fissures near the hilus (2,23,33). The sign is highly suggestive of a bronchogenic carcinoma as the cause of atelectasis (33).

CT is more sensitive than plain films in distinguishing lobar atelectasis and detecting a centrally obstructing tumor as the cause of atelectasis (33–39). In the absence of a large central mass, the lateral margin of the atelectatic

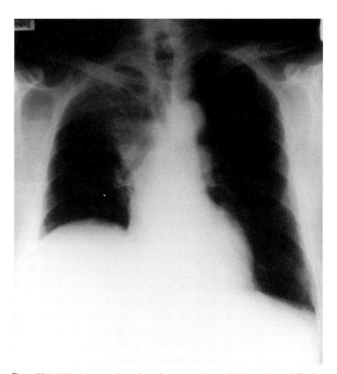

Figure 22.4. RUL atelectasis due to bronchogenic carcinoma (adenocarcinoma). On the posteroanterior view, the convex bulge and the reverse S configuration of the minor fissure is observed in the RUL field. The elevation of the right hemidiaphragm is also demonstrated.

RUL is usually smooth (34–36). In the presence of a large central mass, the lateral margin of the RUL broadens and has a pronounced lateral convexity (Golden's S sign) 34–36. Other signs of central tumor on CT are a luminal mass within the bronchus, narrowing or cutoff of the bronchial lumen, complete absence of air bronchograms, and mucinous bronchograms from mucoid impaction of the bronchi distal to the obstruction (33–39). Furthermore, CT may help to distinguish lobar atelectasis from pleural thickening, pleural effusion, or a mediastinal mass. In the differentiation between the central tumor and distal atelectatic lung, rapid-sequence CT with bolus injection of contrast medium has been recommended (40). With this technique, atelectatic lung is appreciably enhanced, but tumor enhancement is slow and minimal (40). This phenomenon may result from the difference in the amount of blood flow, which is more increased in the atelectatic lung than in the tumor due to crowding of relatively large pulmonary arteries within the atelectatic lung compared with tumor blood supply through small bronchial arteries (40).

In segmental RUL atelectasis, atelectasis of the apical segment stands out as an opacity against the mediastimun or thoracic apex (41). The minor fissure and right hilus are elevated on the PA view. The minor fissure usually remains visible as a thin white line outlined by the aerated anterior segment of the RUL above and the aerated RML below.

Atelectasis of the anterior segment produces an opacity that projects over the right hilus on PA view. This can be marginated inferiorly by the minor fissure, which may be mildly elevated (41). Hilar elevation is usually absent (41). On the lateral view, the opacity is often triangular in appearance. Because of its small size, the wedge-shaped opacity can be mistaken for an infarct or peripheral mass, but CT will provide the correct diagnosis (3). Atelectasis of the posterior segment resembles atelectasis of the anterior segment on the PA view (Fig. 22.5). However, it can be distinguished from atelectasis of the anterior segment on the lateral view. In atelectasis of the posterior segment the opacity is directed posteriorly (Fig. 22.5) (41), and in atelectasis of the anterior segment the opacity is directed anteriorly (41).

Left Upper Lobe Atelectasis

The principal difference between collapse of the LUL and that of the RUL is the absence of a minor fissure on the left; therefore, on the LUL atelectasis, all the lung tissue anterior to the major fissure is involved (1). When the LUL is collapsed, this fissure is displaced forward in a plane roughly parallel to the anterior chest wall on the lateral view (Fig. 22.6) (1,8). In cases with incomplete atelectasis,

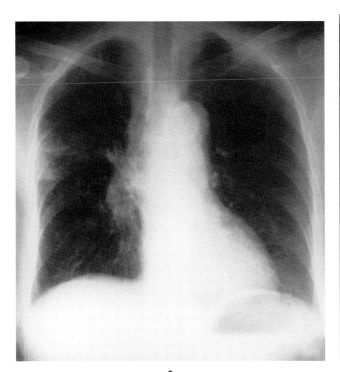
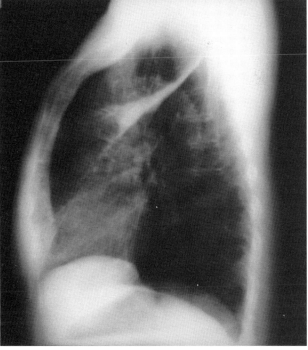

a   b

Figure 22.5. Atelectasis of the posterior segment of RUL due to bronchogenic carcinoma. On the posteroanterior view, an enlargement in the right hilus and a heterogeneous opacity in the lateral side of the right upper lung field upper are demonstrated (**a**). The mild elevation of the right hemidiaphragm is also shown. On the lateral view, a mediastinal wedge directed posteriorly, with the convex bulge in the hilar portion of the mediastinal wedge, is shown (**b**). The heterogeneous opacity observed on the posteroanterior view may represent the partial atelectasis of the anterior segment of RUL.

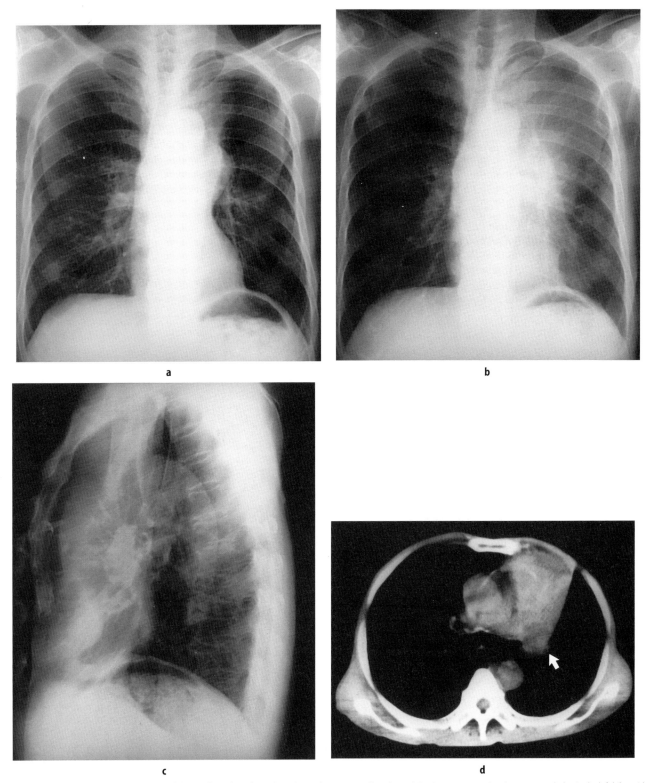

a

b

c

d

Figure 22.6. Atelectasis of the upper division of the LUL due to bronchogenic carcinoma (squamous cell carcinoma). On the posteroanterior view, a convex bulge in the left hilus with the reverse S configuration along the lateral margin of the atelectasis is demonstrated (Golden's S sign) (**a**). Crowded pulmonary vessels are shown in the mediastinal side of the left upper lung field. Compensatory hyperexpansion and mild elevation of the left hemidiaphragm are also observed. The left upper mediastinal border is obliterated by the atelectatic lung. However, the border of the aortic arch and the left cardiac border still remain. A few days later, atelectasis extends to the entire LLL in this case. On the PA view, a veil-like shadow of increased density is seen extending from the level of the clavicle downward. Atelectatic lung obliterates the left upper mediastinal border, aortic arch and the left cardiac border (**b**). On the lateral view, the left major fissure with an opacity is displaced forward in a plane roughly parallel to that of the anterior chest wall (**c**). CT shows a central mass (*arrow*) and a triangular density in the left mediastinal aspect (Golden's S sign) (**d**).

a veil-like shadow of increased density is seen extending from the level of the clavicle downward on the PA view (Fig. 22.6) (1,8). Unlike the RUL atelectasis, ordinarily the density diminishes toward the diaphragm, largely due to the fact that the thorax is bell shaped (1,8). Similarly the density of the partially collapsed LUL diminishes laterally (1,8,23). The contiguity of the collapsed lobe with the anterior mediastinum obliterates the left upper mediastinal border, aortic arch and the left cardiac border on the PA view; the positive of the silhouette sign (Fig. 22.6) (1-2,8,23,24). As collapse causes the volume of the LUL to diminish, the left lower lobe (LLL) expands upward behind the collapse, often to fill the apex of the chest. The vacancy of the apex is occupied by the hyperexpanding superior segment of the LLL; the apex thus contains aerated lung (Fig. 22.6) (1). Commonly, the LLL lies lateral to the collapse as well (1,8). Occasionally it will be found medial to the collapse because the hyperexpanding superior segment of the LLL becomes insinuated between the upper mediastinum and the upper portion of the opacity of the atelectasis: the *Luftsichel* sign (23,24,30). This results in the aortic arch being clearly discernible on the PA view (26). Complete collapse of the LUL is often more difficult to identify than is incomplete collapse of the LUL. Because of the relatively large volume of the LUL, compensatory hyperexpansion of the LLL is usually obvious (23,24,42). Diminutive parallel or divergent vessels coursing superiorly from the left hilus can be a clue to compensatory hyperexpansion of the LLL (24,42). In addition, elevation of the left hilus and left main bronchus can assist in the recognition of marked LUL atelectasis (1-2,8,23,24). Shift of the upper mediastinum and trachea to the left are usually apparent (24,41). The left hemidiaphragm is frequently elevated, and a juxtaphrenic peak is often seen (31). In addition to this peak on the left hemidiaphragm, the posterior aspect of collapsed LUL may show a prominent peak or "tag" (1). This feature is best seen on CT but can be evident as a vertical white line on the PA view. The cause of the tag is unknown. Close approximation of the ribs, although uncommon, can occur (43).

Golden's S sign may also be present when LUL collapse stems from a large hilar mass (Fig. 22.6) (2,23,24,32). The S sign is often best appreciated on the lateral view. CT is very useful for demonstrating Golden's S sign in LUL atelectasis (Fig. 22.6) (32).

Atelectasis of the entire LUL is more common than isolated atelectasis either of the lingula or of the upper division of LUL excluding the lingula (23,24). LUL atelectasis sparing the lingula results in a picture that closely resembles that of RUL atelectasis (23). In most respects atelectasis of the lingula resembles RML atelectasis (23,24). On the PA view, lingular atelectasis produces opacification of the lung below the left hilus, with obscuration of the left heart border (silhouette sign). On the lateral view, it produces a triangular opacity with its apex at the hilus and its base directed against the anterior chest wall (23,24). Atelectasis of the apicoposterior segment of the LUL produces a wedge-shaped opacity that is located against the upper left mediastinum and has its apex at the left hilus and its base against the lung apex on the PA view (Fig. 22.6) (41). On the lateral view the atelectatic apicoposterior segment produces a triangular opacity that is directed superiorly. There may be mild shift of the upper mediastinum to the left and superior displacement of the left hilus (41). Elevation of the left hemidiaphragm, which is typically absent in atelectasis of the apicoposterior segment, suggests that there is atelectasis of the entire upper division of the LUL (41). Atelectasis of the anterior segment of the LUL produces a round opacity on the PA view that is located against the upper left cardiac border and projects over the hilus (41). On the lateral view, this atelectasis produces a triangular opacity with its apex at the hilus and its base against the left anterior chest wall (41).

Right Middle Lobe Atelectasis

The RML can be thought of as a three-dimensional wedge, rather than a simple triangle (2,23,24). As collapse progresses, the minor fissure and the lower half of the major fissure approximate because the hyperexpanding RUL and RLL push the collapsed RML inferiorly, medially, and superiorly (1-2,8,23,24). This configuration is best demonstrated on the lateral view (1-2,8,23,24). RML atelectasis typically appears as a triangular opacity with its apex directed toward the hilus on the lateral view (1-2,8,23,24). This finding is very important (2). If a lateral radiograph shows RML collapse with the apex directed away from the hilus, a central mass lesion should be strongly suspected as a cause for the atelectatic process (Fig. 22.7) (2). On the PA view, there may be slight opacification of the lung below the right hilus and obscuration of a short portion of the right heart border (1-2,8,23,24). However, it is a common experience that when RML collapse is severe, but partly aerated, the PA radiographs will more likely be normal (23,24). The RLL expands forward to contact the right atrium by the progression of RML atelectasis, which therefore remains sharply outlined on the PA view. In addition, the RML usually is considerably smaller than the other lobes of the lungs. As a result, such indirect signs of collapse as hilar depression, diaphragmatic elevation, and mediastinul shift are infrequently present with RML atelectasis (2,8,23,24). When the diagnosis of RML atelectasis cannot be made with certainty from the standard PA and lateral views, an apical lordotic view can be diagnostic (24). The atelectatic RML will be seen on the apical lordotic view as a sharply defined triangle with its apex directed laterally and its base against the right heart border (2,8,23,24). In some cases, the RML will collapse in a "tipped up" configuration so that the collapsed lobe lies

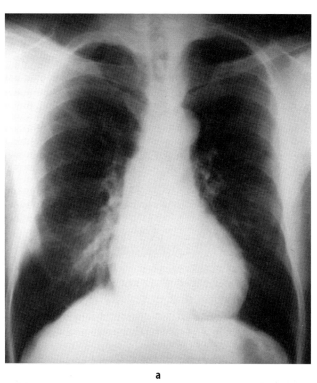

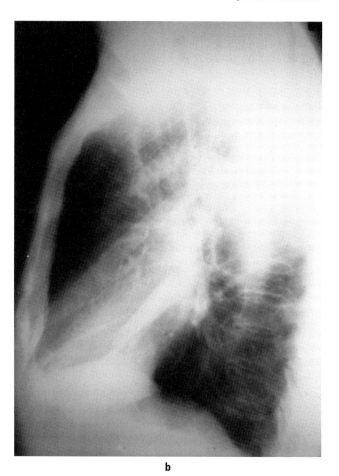

a

b

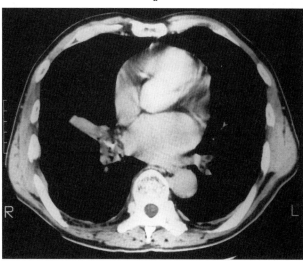

c

Figure 22.7. Atelectasis of the lateral segment of RML due to bronchogenic carcinoma. On the posteranterior view, an inhomogeneous opacity is observed below the right hilus. However, the right heart border is not obscured (**a**). On the lateral view, a triangular opacity with the apex directed away from hilus is demonstrated (**b**). CT shows the atelectasis of the lateral segment of RML with a convex bulge in its central side (**c**).

horizontally (8,24). Apical lordotic view also demonstrates the triangular opacity in this case (8,24).

At the end stage of RML atelectasis, the two fissures may be only a few millimeters apart, and the opacity produced by the atelectatic RML can be mistaken for pleural effusion or pleural thickening in the lower portion of the major fissure (23,24). An atelectatic RML usually abuts the anterior chest wall, whereas pleural effusion or pleural

thickening in the major fissure usually abuts the right hemidiaphragm (23,24). Loculated effusion in the major fissure may be distinguished from RML atelectasis by its typical biconvex shape (23).

CT visualizes more than the plain radiograph (24). The CT finding of the RML atelectasis is characteristic and consists of a broad triangular or trapezoidal opacity with the apex directed toward the hilum (34–36). Frequently

RML atelectasis is asymptomatic (2). The RML bronchus is the longest of the lobar bronchi from point of origin to bifurcation and at the same time has the smallest diameter of any of lobar bronchus (2). It is therefore less rigid than the other major bronchi (2). Atelectasis and segmental collapse of the RML is common on CT; so this is so-called middle lobe syndrome (2).

Segmental atelectasis of the RML is more common than atelectasis of the entire RML (44). Atelectasis of the medial segment is most common and closely resembles atelectasis of the entire lobe, except that the minor fissure remains visible as a thin line (23,44). True silhouetting of the right heart border should indicate medial segmental involvement; however, absolute distinction often requires CT examination (2). Atelectasis of the lateral segment has a characteristic appearance. The lateral segment is the only portion of the RML that lies posterior to the hilus (2,34, 44). Therefore, RML atelectasis that extends posterior to the right pulmonary artery on the lateral view must involve the lateral segment. On the PA view, the opacity from the atelectasis abuts the inferior aspect of the minor fissure; however, since the medial segment remains aerated, the right heart border is not obscured (23,44).

Lower Lobe Atelectasis

The left lower lobe is longer and more slender than the right (2). However, both lobes are similar in configuration (2). As the lower lobes lose volume, they swing posteriorly and medially like a door on a hinge (2). The hinge is the inferior pulmonary ligament (2). On the lateral view, with progressive loss of volume, the characteristic appearance of lower lobe atelectasis is that of a triangular shadow lying in the posterior costophrenic angle (Fig. 22.3) (2). When atelectasis is severe, the lobe becomes only a thin tongue of tissue lying in a paravertebral site (2). This wedge is not usually identified on the lateral view (2). On the PA view, the major fissure faces more and more laterally as collapse increases in degree, and so it may be visible (2). It is demonstrated as a vertical line on the PA view, which is called the vertical fissure line (2,45). When the atelectatic lobe is partially aerated, the displacement of the major fissure is an important diagnostic finding. Once opacification of the collapsing lower lobe appears, the atelectatic lower lobe has a convex superolateral margin that may extend laterally to the chest wall and lie in the lateral costophrenic angle (1-2,8,23,24). The entire length of the diaphragm and paraspinal interface are obscured (24). In LLL atelectasis, the descending aorta is also obscured (Fig. 22.1) (8,24). The heart border, however, remains visible, since it is outlined by the aerated RML or LUL. The opacity of the atelectasis begins to assume a characteristic triangular shape when a moderate amount of lower lobe volume loss has occurred (24). The

descending branch of the pulmonary artery becomes incorporated into the opacity of the atelectatic lower lobe and disappears, resulting in a small hilus (2,24). In cases of marked collapse, it is difficult to identify the atelectatic lobe even on the PA vew. In this case, the small hilus may be the most prominent clue to the diagnosis (2).

Owing to the large volume of the lower lobes, compensatory signs of lower lobe atelectasis are common (1-2,8,23,24). Compensatory hyperexpansion of the other lobes is usually obvious (1-2,8,23,24). Elevation of the hemidiaphragm is common, and there may be close approximation of the ribs (1-2,8,23,24). Shift of the heart and trachea to the affected side are also common (1-2,8,23,24).

Some radiographic signs are noticeable in lower lobe atelectasis. Kattan (46) has emphasized two additional signs of upper mediastinal shift seen in LLL atelectasis; "top-of-the-knob sign" and the "flat-waist sign". The top-of-the knob sign is demonstrated when the mediastinal soft tissues shift over upper aspect of the aortic arch and obscure its upper margin (Fig. 22.1). The flat-waist sign is the result of left lateral shift and posterior rotation of the heart into the left hemithorax (46). Initially this situation causes straightening of the left heart border, resulting in the flat-waist sign (Fig. 22.1). An additional diagnostic sign of LLL atelectasis is linear atelectasis in the lingula. Nordenström and Novek (49) noticed that linear atelectasis in the lingula often accompanies LLL atelectasis. This has been called "Nordenström's sign". They believed that the lingular – bronchial kinking, caused by the LUL hyperexpansion in response to LLL atelectasis, occluded the bronchial lumen and caused linear atelectasis in the lingula. Nordenstrm's sign is apparently not seen in RLL atelectasis.

In RLL atelectasis, shift of the upper anterior mediastinum to the right may occur, giving the upper right mediastinum a triangular appearance, continuous with the mediastinum and with its apex pointing toward the right hilus (Fig. 22.3). It may be mistaken for RUL atelectasis or an infiltrate by the unwary observer. Katten (48) refers to this as the "upper triangle sign" of RLL atelectasis.

A common variant in the appearance of RLL atelectasis is called as the "Gatling gun sign" (49). When there is marked elevation of the right hemidiaphragm, which is the primary response to volume loss of the RLL in some cases, the hilus is only mildly depressed in position, and the RLL is rotated posteriorly so that it comes to lie on the right hemidiaphragm in a horizontal plane. If air bronchograms are present in the atelectatic RLL, they will be demonstrated end-on as a cluster of round lucencies below the right hilus (49). This is an important sign, since the degree of RLL volume loss is often much more severe than might be implied by the small opacity that is visible (49).

Lower lobe atelectasis can be mistaken for pleural effusion, particularly when the lateral margin of the atelectasis forms a concave interface with the lower lobe in the lateral costophrenic angle on the PA view or when the anterior margin of the atelectasis forms a concave interface with the lower lobe in the posterior costophrenic angle on the lateral view (24). Lower lobe atelectasis can be distinguished from pleural effusion in several ways. In lower lobe atelectasis, the hilus is inferiorly displaced and a mediastinal wedge is often formed, whereas in the pleural effusion, the hilus is not displaced and there is no mediastinal wedge (24). Furthermore, the opacity of atelectasis expands higher medially near the hilus than it does laterally against the chest wall, whereas the opacity produced by pleural effusion typically extends higher laterally against the chest wall than it does medially near the hilus (24).

Segmental atelectasis of the LLL is common, with atelectasis of the basal segments seen more often than isolated atelectasis of the superior segment (2,23,24). Atelectasis of the basal segment resembles atelectasis of the entire LLL, except that the superolateral portion of the major fissure remains visible (2,23,24). Atelectasis of the superior segment of the LLL has a characteristic appearance (2,23,24). The superolateral portion of the major fissure moves medially and inferiorly, forming a wedge-shaped opacity on the PA view that projects over the hilus, with its apex at the hilus and its base directed inferiorly (2,23,24). On the lateral view, the atelectatic superior segment is typically seen as a broad band of opacity that extends posteriorly from the hilus to the posterior chest wall (2,23,24). Segmental atelectasis of the RLL is common and, in all respects, resembles segmental atelectasis of the LLL (2,23,24).

Multiple Lobar Atelectasis

Atelectasis of multiple lobes reflects the sum of the signs of collapse of the individual lobes (8), the most common being that of combined RLL and LLL atelectasis (24). When the bronchi of two collapsed lobes are in close anatomic proximity to each other, including a combination of RUL and RML or RML and RLL, it is easy to explain combined lobar collapse on the basis of a single bronchogenic carcinoma (8). If collapse of two or more pulmonary segments cannot be explained by a single bronchial lesion, one has reasonable assurance that a neoplasm is not present ("double lesion sign") (8). However, there are some exceptions, including the presence of multiple primary tumors, ie., atelectasis in one lobe stemming from a primary tumor and in another lobe from metastasis (3).

Whole Lung Atelectasis

Whole-lung atelectasis is not common; collapse of the left lung occurs more often than collapse of the right lung (23,24).

In whole-lung atelectasis, the affected hemithorax is opacified, the hemidiaphragm is elevated, the trachea, heart, and mediastisnum are displaced to the affected side, and there is often close approximation of the ribs (50). Compensatory hyperexpansion of the opposite lung is common (50). To make a correct diagnosis of whole-lung collapse, the differentiation of whole-lung atelectasis from massive unilateral pleural effusion and diffuse unilateral pneumonia is necessary. In diffuse unilateral pneumonia, the lung remains normal in size (50). As a result, elevation of the hemidiaphragm, shift of the heart and mediastinum, and close approximation of the ribs are absent. Massive unilateral pleural effusion is a space-occupying process characterized by enlargement of the involved hemithorax (50).

Subsegmental Atelectasis

Subsegmental atelectasis is a very common occurrence, developing as a result of obstruction of small bronchi or bronchioles in the face of inadequate collateral air drift (2,23). However, the radiographic identification of subsegmental atelectasis can be difficult (2). In such cases the volume loss can be very slight, and the radiograph may evidence only patchy opacities that resemble bronchopneumonia (2). Therefore, this type of atelectatic change cannot be distinguished radiographically from bronchopneumonia (2). Plate-like atelectasis and round atelectasis are also classified as other forms of subsegmental atelectasis (2).

Plate-Like Atelectasis

Plate-like atelectasis is one of the most common types of the segmental atelectasis, also referred to as linear or discoid atelectasis (2,10). The densities are also known as Fleischner's line (51). It can be limited to a bronchopulmonary segment or subsegment, or extend over a greater distance to involve a lobe, or even across fissures to affect several lobes; it always extends to the pleura (Fig. 22.8) (2). Plate-like atelectasis can be oriented in a horizontal, oblique, or vertical plane; it is usually oriented horizontally or slightly obliquely (2,10). The pathogenesis of the plate-like atelectasis is controversial. Westcott and Cole (10) found that bronchial and bronchiolar obstruction was not present in any cases of plate-like atelectasis. They stated that in a persistent low-volume state, plate-like atelectasis developed as the subpleura buckled and folded in along lines of acquired or preexisting pleural invagination (10). Gravity-dependent alterations in alveolar volume, coupled with surfactant deficiency and hypoventilation, appeared to be the main predisposing factors to the development of plate-like atelectasis.

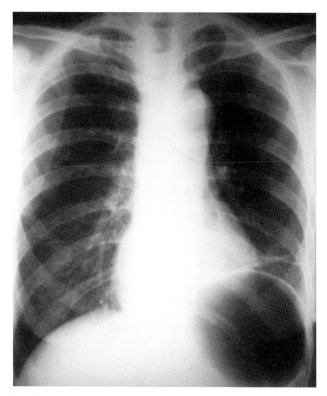

Figure 22.8. Plate-like atelectasis due to left abdominal distension. On the posterante-rior view, horizontal and oblique linear shadows are demonstrated, with elevation of the left hemidiaphragm in the left lower lung field.

Plate-like atelectasis can accompany a variety of thoracic and abdominal conditions, including pulmonary thromboembolism and infarction, pneumonia, pulmonary edema, prolonged shallow breathing, diaphragmatic dysfunction, thoracic or abdominal pain, trauma or surgery, general anesthesia, pregnancy, abdominal masses and distension, and morbid obesity (10). It should be clinically important that plate-like atelectasis frequently indicates more widespread peripheral atelectasis than is is radiologially apparent and can be associated with significant disturbances in ventilation and hypoxemia (10).

Round Atelectasis

Round or helical atelectasis is most commonly associated with exudative pleural disease, but any pleural inflammatory reaction can cause round atelectasis. Typically, round atelectasis is seen with benign pleural disease caused by exposure to asbestos. Many other causes have been noted, including tuberculosis, trauma, pulmonary infarction, cardiac failure, uremia, Dressler syndrome, aortocoronary bypass surgery, and therapeutic pneumothorax.

Round atelectasis is another form of subsegmental atelectasis associated with folding of the lung and an area of pleural invagination (1,26,27). Two theories about the

pathogenesis of round atelectasis have been proposed. The first theory involves resolution of a pleural effusion, with the atelectatic portion of lung failing to reexpand. The mass of round atelectasis is adjacent to a residual area of pleural thickening (52). The second theory, the "fibrosing theory," was proposed because free pleural effusion is seldom seen before round atelectasis has been demonstrated (53,54). This theory suggests that the area of pleuritis is the primary event, leading to pleural fibrosis (53,54). As the fibrous tissue matures, the lung becomes folded and collapsed in this area. However, the precise mechanism of formation of round atelectasis has not been completely clarified (55). In patients with asbestos exposure there is extensive pleural plaque formation and pleural calcification. Pleural effusion and pleural thickening may be important cofactors in the development of round atelectasis (55).

The radiographic appearance of round atelectasis is distinctive (55). The chest radiograph shows a rounded, oval, lobulated, or sometimes irregular peripheral mass, with curvilinear opacities extending from the hilus to the pleural mass (Fig. 22.9) (55). The size is usually 2.5–5 cm in greatest diameter (55). By far the most common site is along the posterior surface of the lower lobe (55). Occasionally it is located at the lung base directly on the diaphragm. The blood vessels and bronchi near the mass converge toward the base of the lung and then curve up to enter the mass along its anteroinferior margin ("comet tail sign" (56) or "vacuum cleaner effect" (57). CT permits confirmation of the diagnosis of round atelectasis made by conventional radiography. CT examination of this atelectasis demonstrates a characteristic curving ("comet tail sign") of bronchi and vessels entering a peripheral rounded or oval-shaped mass (Fig. 22.9) (58). The largest area of pleural thickening or fibrosis is usually adjacent to the lesion (58), but not always (59). O'Donovan et al. (60) reported that the presence of converging bronchovascular markings was the best discriminator on CT between round atelectasis and other lung masses, including neoplasms, pulmonary infarction, and pneumonia, but radiographic diagnosis was imperfect. The decision to forego biopsy necessitates close clinical follow-up to avert the possibility of misclassifying lung neoplasms as round atelectasis. Free pleural effusion is either minimal or nonexistent (55,58). Although round atelectasis is usually associated with benign pleural disease, an obvious pleural effusion associated with round atelectasis suggests a malignant process such as malignant mesothelioma (61).

Diffuse Atelectasis

Generalized or diffuse atelectasis is a term employed to describe widespread volume loss in the lungs without specific evidence of segmental or lobar atelectasis (24). In

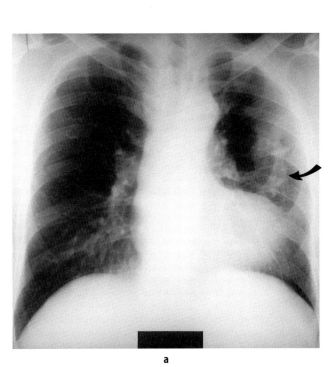

a

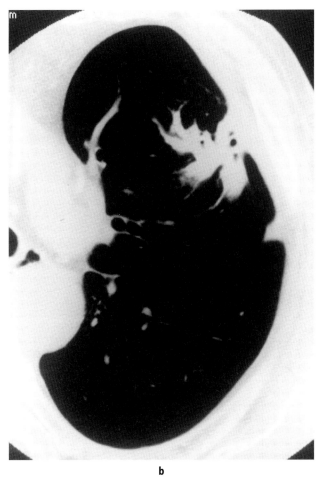

b

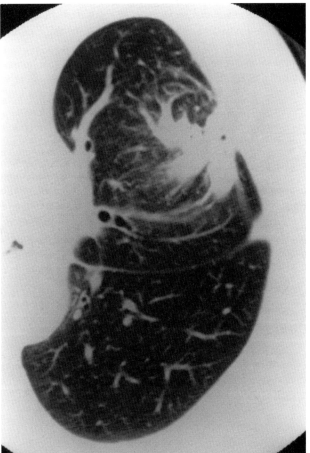

c

Figure 22.9. Round atelectasis due to previous pleuritis. On the posteranterior view, an irregular opacity is shown in the left middle lung field. A blood vessel in the LLL curves up (*arrow*) and enters the opacity along its lateroinferior margin (comet-tail sign) (**a**). Pleural thickening is demonstrated at the pleural side of the opacity on CT (**b**). CT also shows the comet-tail sign more clearly than does the posteranterior view (**c**).

diffuse atelectasis, there can be marked arteriovenous shunting; however, opacification of the lungs may be mild or inapparent, and elevation of the diaphragm may be the sole radiographic clue to the diagnosis of diffuse atelectasis (1). When pulmonary opacification is diffuse, most cases are probably interpreted as diffuse pneumonia or pulmonary edema. However, elevation of the diaphragm is still the clue to the correct diagnosis (24).

Role of MRI in the Diagnosis of Atelectasis

In comparison with CT, the role of magnetic resonance imaging (MRI) in patients with atelectasis is relatively limited, because CT is superior to MRI in its high spatial resolution. Although MRI may not be a good tool for precisely evaluating intrapulmonary and endobronchial lesions (62), it may be still provide information comparable to that given by CT regarding peribronchial tumor extension and associated mediastinal or pleural disease (63). MRI is useful in differentiating central obstructing tumor from peripheral collapsed lung, especially when intravenous contrast material cannot be administered on CT. Similar to CT, MRI appearances of obstructive atelectasis are largely dependent on underlying pathologic changes within the collapsed lung. In the atelectasis due to bronchogenic carcinoma, cholesterol pneumonitis and brochiectasis with mucus plugs are always hyperintense relative to tumor on heavily T_2-weighted images, and organizing pneumonitis and atelectasis are isointense and indistinguishable from tumor (64). Gadolinium-labeled diethylenetriaminepentaacetic acid (Gd-DTPA)-enhanced T_1-weighted images are superior to T-weighted images in separating tumor from collapsed lung (65,66). Kono et al. (67) reported that hilar tumors can be differentiated from obstructive pneumonitis or collapse in 85% of 27 cases on Gd-DTPA-enhanced T_2-weighted images. Signal intensity of the tumor was lower than the obstructed lung in 67% of cases and higher in 18% of cases. The optimal scan time for differentiation is 3–10 min after Gd-DTPA administration (66). When delineation of extrabronchial tumor extent is important, MRI can provide comparable and/or complementary information.

Yamaguchi et al. (67) reported that magnetic resonance imaging (MRI) was superior to CT in demonstrating several features of round atelectasis. First, the infolded visceral pleura was identified in more cases on MRI than on CT. Second, the presence of converging bronchovascular markings was sometimes better demonstrated by sagittal or oblique sagittal MRI than by CT. Third, round atelectasis and thickened visceral pleura were clearly separated on MRI. These findings may be helpful in the diagnosis of round atelectasis, distinguishing round atelectasis from bronchogenic carcinoma or other lung disease. MRI may be a useful complement to CT in the diagnosis of round

atelectasis. However, the role of MRI in the diagnosis of round atelectasis has not yet been well established.

Acknowledgment

We thank Masayuki Ando, Takeshi Yoshinaga and Hideaki Uozumi for their contributions to this article.

References

1. Fraser RG, Paré JAP (1988) Diagnosis of disease of the chest. WB Saunders Philadelphia.
2. Heitzman ER (1993) The lung: Radiologic pathologic correlations, 3rd edn. Mosby, St. Louis, MO.
3. Woodring JH, Reed JC (1996) Types and mechanisms of pulmonary atelectasis. J Thorac Imaging 11:92–108.
4. Reed JC (1991) Chest radiology: Plain film patterns and differential diagnosis, 3rd edn. Mosby, St. Louis, MO.
5. Burke M, Fraser R (1976) Obstructive pneumonitis: A pathologic and pathogenetic reappraisal. Radiology 166:699–704.
6. Gamsu G, Singer MM, Vincent HH, et al. (1976) Postoperative impairment of mucous transport in the lung. Am Rev Respir Dis 114:673–679.
7. Harris RS (1985) The importance of proximal and distal air bronchograms in the management of atelectasis. J Can Assoc Radiol 36:103–109.
8. Felson B (1978) Chest roentgenology. WB Saunders, Philadelphia.
9. Woodring JH (1988) Determing the cause of pulmonary atelectasis: A comparison of plain radiography and CT. AJR 150:757–763.
10. Westcott JL, Cole S (1985) Plate atelectasis. Radiology 155:1–9.
11. West JB (1979) Respiratory physiology: the essentials, 2nd edn. Williams and Wilkins, Baltimore, MD.
12. Milne ENC, Pistolesi M (1993) Reading the chest radiograph: A physiologic approach. Mosby, St. Louis, MO.
13. Stunick AI, Soloff LA (1964) Atelectasis with pneumonia. A pathophysiologic study. Ann Intern Med 60:39.
14. Naidich DP, MacCauley GL, Khouri NF, et al. (1983) Computed tomography of lobar collapse. Collapse in the absence of endobronchial obstruction. J Comput Assist Tomogr 7:758–767.
15. Westcott JI, Cole SR (1986) Traction bronchiectasis in end-stage pulmonary fibrosis. Radiology 161:665–669.
16. Strandberg A, Tokics L, Brismar B, et al. (1986) Atelectasis during anaesthesia and in the postoperative period. Acta Anaesthesiol Scand 30:154–158.
17. Morimoto S, Takeuchi N, Imanaka H, et al. (1989) Gravity-dependent atelectasis: Radiologic, physiologic and pathologic correlation in rabbits on high-frequency oscillation ventilation. Invest Radiol 24:522–530.
18. Tokics L, Strandberg A, Brismar B, et al. (1987) Computerized tomography of the chest and gas exchange measurements during ketamine anaesthesia. Acta Anaesthesiol Scand 31:684–692.
19. Strandberg A, Tokics L, Brismar B, et al. (1987) Constitutional factors promoting development of atelectasis during anaesthesia. Acta Anaesthesiol Scand 31:21–24.
20. Klingstedt C, Hedenstierna G, Lundquist H, et al. (1990) The influence of body position and differential ventilation on lung dimensions and atelectasis formation in anaesthetized man. Acta Anaesthesiol Scand 34:315–322.
21. Verschakelen JA, Van Fraeyenhoven L, Laureys G, et al. (1993) Differences in CT density between dependent and nondependent portions of the lung: Influence of lung volume. AJR 7:713–717.

22. Tomiyama N, Takeuchi N, Imanaka H, et al. (1993) Mechanism of gravity-dependent atelectasis: Analysis by nonradioactive xenon-enhanced dynamic computed tomography. Invest Radiol 28:633–638.

23. Proto AV, Tocino I (1980) Radiographic manifestations of lobar collapse. Semin Roentgenol 15:117–173.

24. Woodring JH, Reed JC (1996) Radiologic manifestations of lobar atelectasis. J Thorac Imaging 11:109–144.

25. Whalen JP, Lane EJ, Jr. (1969) Bronchial rearrangements in pulmonary collapse as seen on the lateral radiograph. Radiology 93:285.

26. Hanke R, Kretzschmar R (1980) Round atelectasis. Semin Roentgenol 15:174–182.

27. Woodring JH (1987) Round atelectasis. Australas Radiol 31:144–151.

28. Robbins LL, Hale CH (1945) The roentgen appearance of lobar and segmental collapse of the lung. II. The normal chest as it pertains to collapse. Radiology 44:543–547.

29. Khoury MB, Godwin JD, Halvorsen RA, et al. (1985) CT of obstructive lobar collapse. Invest Radiol 20:708.

30. Webber M, Davies P (1981) The Luftsichel: an old sign in upper lobe collapse. Clin Radiol 32:271–275.

31. Kattan KR, Eyler WR, Felson B (1980) The juxtaphrenic peak in upper lobe collapse. Semin Roentgenol 15:187–193.

32. Golden R (1925) The effect of bronchostenosis upon the roentgen ray shadows in carcinoma of the bronchus. AJR 13:21–30.

33. Reining JW, Ross P (1984) Computed tomography appearance of Golden's "S" sign. CT. J Comput Tomogr 8:219–223.

34. Raasch BN, Heitzman ER, Carsky EW, et al. (1984) A computed tomographic study of bronchopulmonary collapse. Radiographics 4:195–232.

35. Naidich DP, McCauley DI, Khouri NF, et al. (1983) Computed tomography of lobar collapse. I. Endobronchial obstruction. J Comput Assist Tomogr 7:745–757.

36. Naidich DP, Ettinger N, Leitman BS, et al. (1984) CT of lobar collapse. Semin Roentgenol 19:222–235.

37. Woodring JH (1988) Determining the cause of pulmonary atelectasis: A comparison of plain radiography and CT. AJR 150:757–763.

38. Woodring JH (1988) The computed tomography mucous bronchogram sign. J Comput Tomogr 12:165–168.

39. Glazer HS, Anderson DJ, Sagel SS (1989) Bronchial impaction in lobar collapse: CT demonstration and pathologic correlation. AJR 153:485–488.

40. Onitsuka H, Tsukuda M, Araki A, et al. (1991) Differentiation of central lung tumor from postobstructive lobar collapse by rapid sequence computed tomography. J Thorac Imaging 6:28–31.

41. Robbins LL, Hale CH (1945) The roentgen appearance of lobar and segmental collapse of the lung. VI. Collapse of the upper lobes. Radiology 45:347–355.

42. Proto AV, Moser ES, Jr. (1987) Upper lobe volume loss: Divergent and parallel patterns of vascular reorientation. Radiographics 7:875–887.

43. Mintzer RA, Sakowicz BA, Blonder JA (1988) Lobar collapse: Usual and unusual forms. Chest 94:615–620.

44. Robbins LL, Hale CH (1945) The roentgen appearance of lobar and segmental collapse of the lung. Collapse of the right middle lobes. Radiology 45:260–266.

45. Davis LA (1960) The vertical fissure line. AJR 84:451–453.

46. Kattan KR (1980) Upper mediastinal changes in lower lobe collapse. V. Semin Roentgenol 15:183–186.

47. Nordenstöm B, Novek J (1960) The atelectatic complex of the left lung. Acta Radiol 53:56–60.

48. Kattan KR, Felson B, Holder LE, et al. (1975) Superior mediastinal shift in right-lower-lobe collapse: the "upper triangle sign". Radiology 116:305–309.

49. Milne ENC (1986) A physiological approach to reading critical care unit films. J Thorac Imaging 1:60–90.

50. Robbins LL, Hale CH (1945) The roentgen appearance of lobar and segmental collapse of the lung. III. Collapse of an entire lung or the major part thereof. Radiology 45:23–26.

51. Fleischner FG, Hampton AO, Castleman B (1941) Linear shadow in the lung. AJR 46:610–618.

52. Hanke R, Kretzshmar R (1980) Round atelectasis. Semin Roentogenol 15:174–182.

53. Dernevik L, Gatzinski P, Hultman E, et al. (1982) Shrinking pleuritis with atelectasis. Thorax 37:252–258.

54. Menzies R, Fraser R (1987) Round atelectasis: Pathologic and pathogenetic features. Am J Surg Pathol 11:674–681.

55. Batra P, Brown K, Hayashi K, et al. (1996) Rounded atelectasis. J Thorac Imaging 11:187–197.

56. Schneider HJ, Felson B, Gonzalez LL (1980) Rounded atelectasis. AJR 134:225–232.

57. Sinner WN (1980) Pleuroma: A cancer mimicking atelectasis pseudotumor of the lung. Rofo Fatschr Get Rontyenstr Neurol Bildgeb Verfahr 133:578–585.

58. Doyle TC, Lawler GA (1984) CT features of rounded atelectasis. AJR 143:225–228.

59. McHugh K, Blaquire RM (1989) CT features of rounded atelectasis. AJR 153:257–260.

60. O'Donovan PB, Schenk M, Lim K, et al. (1997) Evaluation of the reliability of computed tomographic criteria used in the diagnosis of round atelectasis. J Thorac Imaging 12:54–58.

61. Munden RF, Libshitz HI (1998) Round atelectasis and mesothelioma. AJR 170:1519–1522.

62. Mayr B, Heywang SH, Ingrisch H, et al. (1987) Comparison of CT and MR imaging of endobronchial tumors. J Comput Assist Tomogr 11:43–48.

63. Webb WR, Gatsonis C, Zerhouni EA, et al. (1991) CT and MR imaging in staging non-small cell bronchogenic carcinoma. Report of the Radiologic Diagnostic Oncology Group. Radiology 178:705–713.

64. Bourgouin PM, MacLoud TC, Fitzgibbon JF, et al. (1991) Differentiation of bronchogenic carcinoma from postobstructive pneumonitis by magnetic resonance imaging: Histopathologic correlation. J Thorac Imaging Radiol 6:22–27.

65. Stiglbauer R, Schurawitzki H, Klepetko W, et al. (1991) Contrast-enhanced MRI for the staging of bronchogenic carcinoma: Comparison with CT and histopathologic staging: preliminary results. Clin Radiol 44:293–298.

66. Kono M, Adachi S, Kusumoto M, et al. (1993) Clinical utility of Gd-DTPA-enhanced magnetic resonance imaging in lung cancer. J Thorac Imaging 8:18–26.

67. Yamaguchi T, Hayashi K, Ashizawa K, et al. (1997) Magnetic resonance imaging of round atelectasis. J Thorac Imaging 12:188–194.

23 Pulmonary Thromboembolism

R. Sheehan and M. B. Rubens

Introduction

Pulmonary thromboembolism is a common cause of mortality in hospitalized patients. Accurate figures of incidence are difficult to obtain, primarily because clinical manifestations of the disease are extremely variable and depend on the size of the embolus and burden of clot. Small emboli are frequently subclinical, whereas large central emboli may result in sudden death.

Postmortem studies of hospitalized patients have shown pulmonary emboli in up to 64% (1). However, clinically diagnosed pulmonary thromboembolism is far less common, in the order of 1% or fewer in hospital patients. Conversely, pulmonary thromboembolism is the sole or major cause of death in approximately 10% of hospitalized patients (2). Approximately 30% of patients with pulmonary embolism will die if untreated, but the timely institution of anticoagulant therapy will reduce this number to 8% (3). On the other hand, anticoagulation therapy is not without risk, with an incidence of hemorrhage of 6.8% (4), although fatal hemorrhage is very uncommon.

No single test can be regarded as entirely satisfactory in the diagnosis of this important disease and there has been considerable debate and controversy in the literature regarding the development of a practical diagnostic algorithm. Laboratory tests, although widely used, suffer from low specificity in the diagnosis of acute pulmonary embolism, and heavy reliance has been placed on imaging techniques. This has traditionally involved ventilation-perfusion (*V/Q*) scanning and pulmonary angiography. In the wake of the Prospective Investigation of Pulmonary Embolism Diagnosis (PIOPED) study (5), which showed that in excess of 70% of *V/Q* scans are nondiagnostic for pulmonary embolism, there has been a search for a more specific and noninvasive method of diagnosing acute pulmonary embolism. This has conveniently coincided with the development of rapid helical computed tomography

(CT) scanners, which have revolutionized the diagnostic approach to pulmonary embolism.

Etiology

Over 90% of pulmonary emboli arise from thrombosis of the deep veins of the lower limbs. The remainder arise within pelvic, renal or hepatic veins, or within the right heart chambers. Unless related to indwelling cannulae, thromboemboli from upper limbs are too small to produce clinical symptoms. The predisposing factors for formation of thrombus within a vessel, known as Virchow's triad are:

1. Venous stasis.
2. Injury to the venous intima.
3. A change in the coagulability of blood.

Not all factors need to be present for thrombus to form and the presence of all three does not inevitably result in the development of thrombus. The exact pathogenesis of thrombus formation is incompletely understood but several risk factors are recognized as predisposing an individual to development of deep venous thrombosis (Table 23.1). Once a thrombus has formed within the venous system, there are three possible consequences. The thrombus may lyse, become organized into the vessel wall, or may embolize to the lungs. Not all venous thrombi of the lower limbs have the same potential for embolization. Thrombi within the deep veins of the calf are much less likely to result in pulmonary emboli than those which develop within or above the popliteal veins. This is probably a consequence of the larger size of more proximal veins.

The diagnosis and treatment of deep venous thrombosis is therefore the most important step in the prevention of pulmonary embolism. The clinical assessment of symptomatic deep vein thrombosis is inaccurate (6), and

Table 23.1. Risk factors for the development of venous thrombosis

1. Surgery. Particularly orthopedic and pelvic
2. Trauma. Particularly pelvic trauma and lower limb fractures
3. Prolonged immobilization. Paraplegic patients, lower limb fractures, long air flights
4. Obesity
5. Diabetes
6. Pregnancy 5.5 times increased risk
7. Oral contraceptives. Small increased risk with estrogen-containing pills
8. Smoking
9. Malignancy 2–3 times increased risk; more in pancreatic carcinoma
10. Heart disease. Particularly atrial fibrillation, myocardial infarction and heart failure
11. Previous history of DVT/PE, varicose veins
12. Coagulopathy
13. Age. Linear relationship with increasing age beyond age 40 years
14. Venous cannulation

DVT, deep vein thrombosis; PE, pulmonary embolism.

the diagnosis rests heavily on imaging. Contrast venography has traditionally been accepted as the gold standard for diagnosis but it does have several limitations including difficulties with venous access, incomplete filling of deep veins, discomfort to the patient, side-effects from the injection of contrast medium (including the development of deep vein thrombosis in up to 8% (7)), and interobserver variation in interpretation. These problems have led to the search for more acceptable, noninvasive diagnostic tools. Compression ultrasonography (± pulsed/color Doppler) has now become widely accepted as the investigation of choice for the detection of femoropopliteal deep vein thrombosis, with sensitivity and specificity rates as good as contrast venography. This high accuracy is, however, limited to femoropopliteal thrombus, and sensitivity and specificity figures drop for calf and pelvic vein thrombus, where the vessels are small and more difficult to visualize. The inability to accurately diagnose calf deep vein thrombus has not proved to be such a problem in clinical practice, since isolated calf thrombus rarely causes clinically significant pulmonary embolism (8). It has been shown venographically that 40% of calf clots remain isolated, 40% quickly lyse, and 20% extend upwards (9). It is this last 20% that have the potential to cause clinically significant pulmonary embolism. These can be easily identified by rescanning the leg over intervals of several days to detect the proximal extension of the clot.

Clinical Features

The clinical manifestations of pulmonary embolism are diverse and frequently nonspecific, ranging from no symptoms to sudden death. The classic presentation of chest pain, sudden dyspnea, hemoptysis, signs of a deep vein thrombus, and a normal or near normal chest radi-

ograph occur in the minority. The commonest symptom is acute dyspnea, with chest pain and hemoptysis occurring slightly less frequently. The majority of patients have an underlying disorder such as congestive heart failure, recent surgery, malignancy, or are immobilized. Because of the variable and nonspecific presentation, the diagnosis is easily overlooked and the first step in making the diagnosis is an awareness of the possibility of a pulmonary embolus in any susceptible patient who suddenly deteriorates.

Physiologic Consequences

The physiologic consequences of acute and complete occlusion of a pulmonary artery are both respiratory and hemodynamic. The respiratory consequence of pulmonary artery occlusion is the creation of alveolar dead space – that is, an area of ventilated lung that is not being perfused (10). In general, the diameter of the pulmonary artery lumen must be occluded by more than 80% to cause a reduction in distal blood flow. The affected lung parenchyma remains viable as a result of collateral blood supply through the bronchial circulation. In patients with impaired cardiovascular function, the bronchial circulation may be insufficient to maintain pulmonary parenchymal viability, resulting in infarction and ischemic necrosis of the lung parenchyma supplied by the occluded pulmonary artery. However, pulmonary infarction is uncommon and fewer than 15% of emboli cause true infarction (11). There is a slight reduction in the volume of the part of the lung affected by the pulmonary arterial occlusion. This loss of volume differs from the slightly delayed development of atelectasis of the affected lung, which usually occurs about 24 h after the embolic episode, and is thought to be due to depletion of alveolar surfactant. Pulmonary edema is a rare consequence of pulmonary embolism and usually occurs in patients with coexisting left ventricular dysfunction.

Arterial hypoxaemia is frequently observed in significant pulmonary embolism. Factors contributing to this hypoxemia include:

1. Shunting of blood from the part of lung obstructed by the embolus to the relatively overperfused remaining lung where ventilation is insufficient to fully oxygenate the perfusing blood.
2. Right to left intrapulmonary shunting.
3. Decreased cardiac output due to right ventricular decompensation. Hypoxemia is not invariable and is frequently transient, probably due to compensatory hyperventilation.

The hemodynamic consequence of pulmonary embolism is an acute reduction in the pulmonary vascular cross-sectional area resulting in an immediate increase in pulmonary vascular resistance. Due to the large reserve in normal patients, it is estimated that at least 50% of the pulmonary vasculature needs to be obstructed before there is an increase in pulmonary arterial pressure. Beyond this, right ventricular afterload rises significantly, ultimately resulting in right heart failure. Since the normal right ventricle cannot develop pressures greater than 45 mmHg, a mean pulmonary arterial pressure of greater than 50 mmHg indicates right ventricular hypertrophy due to a chronic process, either previous pulmonary emboli or other underlying cardiopulmonary disease. The severity of the hemodynamic consequences depend not only on the burden of clot load, but also on the presence of cardiopulmonary comorbidity, where even a moderate sized embolus can be fatal. Most emboli either lyse, fragment, or become organized and undergo recanalization (12). Uncommonly, repeated thromboembolic episodes may lead to chronic pulmonary arterial hypertension, a condition important to recognize as it may be treatable.

Laboratory Investigations

Laboratory tests are routinely performed in the evaluation of patients with suspected pulmonary embolism. Although none is able to make a definitive diagnosis of pulmonary embolism, they may provide useful, additional supportive evidence of the diagnosis.

The most interesting development in recent years has been the emerging role of the D-dimer test in the evaluation of this group of patients. D-dimer is a specific degradation product of cross-linked fibrin and is therefore elevated with intravascular thrombosis. However, the test is extremely nonspecific and many conditions including trauma, infection and inflammation will result in an elevated D-dimer level (13). The real value of the D-dimer test is in its high sensitivity. Several studies have shown the D-dimer test to have sensitivity and negative predictive values of, or close to, 100% (14–23). Therefore a normal D-dimer test is an extremely reliable way of excluding pulmonary embolism. Unfortunately, due to the low specificity of the test, and the frequent comorbidity in this group of patients, a positive result is all too common, and its extremely poor positive predictive value means a positive result is of no diagnostic value. Compounding this problem is the limited availability and time-consuming nature of the enzyme-linked immunosortent assay (ELISA), which was thought to be the only reliable way of performing the test. However, recent studies have demonstrated some of the more rapid quantitative methods to have an efficiency comparable to that of ELISA (15,23). Studies have also been performed to compare the performance of similar tests such as the fibrin monomer test

(20). The D-dimer test has therefore become a simple, noninvasive and cost-effective way of excluding the diagnosis of pulmonary embolism in patients with no comorbidity and a low clinical suspicion of the diagnosis (19).

The classic electrocardiogram (ECG) findings of tachycardia, right axis deviation, $S_1Q_3T_3$, pattern and ST changes are seen only in severe right ventricular overload and are therefore not present in the majority of patients with acute pulmonary embolism. Arterial blood gas analysis is similarly unreliable. However, although normal arterial blood gases do not exclude the diagnosis, the presence of a reduced arterial P_{O_2} and reduced P_{CO_2} (due to hyperventilation), provide additional supportive evidence of the diagnosis, increasing the overall level of clinical suspicion.

Imaging of Pulmonary Embolism

Chest Radiography

The imaging work-up of patients with suspected pulmonary embolus usually begins with a plain chest radiograph, despite its widely recognized limitations in the context of this disease. In the PIOPED study (5), the percentage of patients with an abnormal chest radiograph was not significantly different in the group with proven pulmonary embolism from the group who were subsequently proved not to have pulmonary embolism. Indeed, even in patients with life-threatening pulmonary embolism, the plain chest radiograph may appear completely normal. The major role of the chest radiograph is to exclude other diagnoses that can mimic the clinical picture of pulmonary embolism, such as pneumothorax, pneumonia, dissecting aortic aneurysm and rib fractures. The chest radiograph also provides a baseline, assisting in the interpretation of a subsequent V/Q scan.

Historically, many plain chest radiographic signs of pulmonary embolus have been described. These are best described by separating them into two groups: pulmonary embolism without infarction, and pulmonary embolism with infarction.

Pulmonary Embolism Without Infarction

As already discussed, even large central emboli may not result in any acute abnormality on the chest radiograph. The focal vasoconstriction of pulmonary vessels distal to an embolus, known as the Westermark sign, is often seen as an early plain radiographic finding, but is difficult to appreciate unless comparison can be made with previous radiographs. Dilatation of an individual left or right pulmonary artery, either by back pressure from a peripheral embolus or distension of the vessel by clot (Fleischner sign) with associated oligemia and transradiancy of the corresponding lung is rare. The plain radiograph findings of cardiomegaly and enlargement of the central pulmonary arteries with peripheral oligemia due to pulmonary arterial hypertension and cor pulmonale are rarely seen in acute pulmonary embolism. These findings are more typical of chronic thromboembolic disease where progressive occlusion of the pulmonary vasculature has resulted in symptomatic pulmonary arterial hypertension.

The commonest signs of volume loss are shift of the fissures, elevation of the hemidiaphragm and associated areas of linear atelectasis. Pleural effusions occur in approximately 50% of cases of pulmonary embolism. Those that occur in the absence of a radiographically demonstrable pulmonary infarction are typically small, unilateral and tend to reach a maximal size early in the course of the disease (24). Whether these small effusions are due to small infarcts that are not visible on the chest radiograph is uncertain.

Pulmonary embolism with infarction

Parenchymal consolidation is the radiographic feature that distinguishes pulmonary embolism with infarction from pulmonary embolism without infarction. This consolidation may be due to infarcted lung, pulmonary hemorrhage, or both. Consolidation most commonly occurs in the lower lobes, is frequently multifocal, and usually occurs 12–24 h after the embolic episode. The consolidation can assume a variety of shapes, depending on its location, the underlying architecture of the lung and the amount of surrounding hemorrhage. Infarcts are virtually never truly triangular or wedge shaped. Indeed, the classic appearance of a Hampton's hump (25) (Fig. 23.1) or truncated pyramid with its base applied to the pleural surface is unusual. Moreover, true lobar or segmental consolidation and air bronchograms as seen in infective consolidation are unusual. The subsequent behavior of this consolidation depends on whether or not true infarction is associated with the hemorrhage. In the absence of true infarction, radiographic clearing occurs fairly quickly, often within a few days, and is usually complete. A true infarct on the other hand, will take several months to resolve and frequently leaves a permanent linear scar. The only reliable way of distinguishing these two is by following them with serial radiographs. Pulmonary infarcts tend to resolve by "melting away" from the periphery toward the centre. This feature helps to distinguish it from a resolving pneumonia, which tends to clear in a patchy fashion resulting in an inhomogeneous opacity prior to complete resolution. At this late stage, however, the distinction is usually of academic interest only. Cavitation within an infarct is rare and when seen is

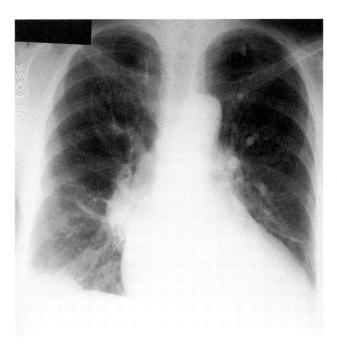

Figure 23.1. Plain film of pulmonary infarction in this patient with acute on chronic thromboembolic disease. There is bilateral lower lobe consolidation. That at the right base has the classic appearance of a Hampton's hump. The enlarged central pulmonary arteries reflect pulmonary arterial hypertension due to chronic thromboembolic disease.

usually the result of secondary infection or an infarct that has occurred as a consequence of a septic embolus. When aseptic cavitation occurs, the infarct is usually greater than 4 cm in diameter and the cavitation usually occurs within 2 weeks of the radiographic appearance of the infarct (26).

Pleural effusions are commonly associated with infarcts, occurring in approximately two thirds of patients (24) (Fig. 23.2). They may be bilateral, are more likely to be large and bloodstained, and are slow to resolve (24).

Radionuclide Imaging

Following chest radiography, a V/Q scan has traditionally been the next imaging investigation in the evaluation of patients with suspected pulmonary embolism. Perfusion scintigraphy is performed following intravenous injection of [99mTc]-labeled microspheres or macroaggregated albumin particles. These particles undergo microembolization, and become transiently lodged in the precapillary arterioles of the pulmonary vascular bed. Static images in anterior, posterior, right posterior oblique and left posterior oblique projections are obtained following injection. Concurrent ventilation images are obtained following the inhalation of a radioactive gas. The two most commonly used agents have traditionally been [81mKr] and [133Xe]. Due to the overwhelming superiority of [81mKr] in all respects other than

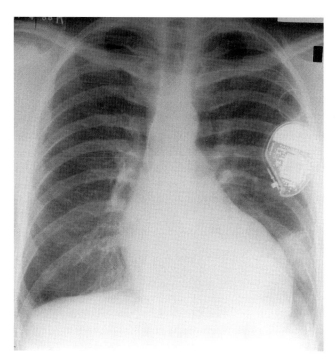

Figure 23.2. Plain film of pulmonary infarction. There is a peripheral wedge-shaped area of consolidation in the left lower zone and a right pleural effusion in this patient with an indwelling pacemaker.

cost, it has now largely replaced ^{133}Xe as the agent of choice. The more recent introduction of ^{99m}Tc-labeled aerosols such as carbon particles (Technegas) have met with some favor, although the slow biologic clearance requires some modification for the acquisition of the subsequent perfusion images.

The diagnostic feature of pulmonary embolism is a perfusion defect in a region of normally ventilated lung – the so-called mismatched perfusion defect (Fig. 23.3). A well-performed perfusion scan is extremely sensitive and is able to reliably detect small defects at a subsegmental level. However, even in the presence of a well-performed ventilation scan and a recent chest radiograph for comparison, the overall specificity of the test fails to match its sensitivity.

The generally accepted system of interpreting V/Q scans involves assigning a probability value to the scan. This system stratifies the probability into categories of normal, low, intermediate, and high probability of pulmonary embolism. While normal or high probability scans will reliably exclude or diagnose pulmonary embolism respectively, the majority of patients fall into the indeterminate (low or intermediate probability) probability group and will usually require further imaging.

In a patient with a high clinical suspicion of pulmonary embolism and no history of cardiopulmonary comorbidity, a positive perfusion scan showing multiple defects (particularly if they are segmental) with an accompanying normal ventilation scan and chest radiograph that reveals no abnormality, will be categorized as "high probability" for pulmonary embolism. Similarly, a completely normal perfusion scan is very specific, virtually excluding pulmonary embolism. Unfortunately, these situations occur in the minority of patients, and, depending on the prevalence of pulmonary embolism in the population studied (the pretest probability), more than 60% of patients will have an indeterminate scan (5), and up to 33% of these patients may have pulmonary embolism (27).

If the pulmonary embolus results in an area of pulmonary infarction, then the perfusion defect will be matched to a defect on the ventilation scan. The ventilation defect is usually smaller than the perfusion defect because the lung around the periphery of the defect continues to ventilate. Therefore the diagnosis of a pulmonary infarct relies on an incompletely matched perfusion defect and an appropriate radiographic abnormality. This requires high quality ventilation scanning in multiple projections, a requirement frequently not met, and pulmonary infarcts therefore often fall into the indeterminate group. There are several other causes of matched defects, including emphysema, fibrosing alveolitis, obstructive airways disease, and any pathologic process causing destruction of the lung parenchyma.

In many pulmonary conditions, the hypoxic vasoconstriction (which causes the matched perfusion defect) is incomplete, resulting in a reversed mismatched defect;

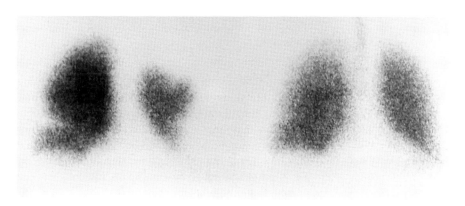

Figure 23.3. High probability radionuclide scan. There are multiple segmental and subsegmental defects on the perfusion scan on the left. These are not matched on the ventilation scan on the right, which is normal.

that is, there is relatively more perfusion than ventilation. Reversed mismatching is a characteristic feature of several chest diseases including pleural effusion, lobar pneumonia, collapsed and consolidated lung, bronchiectasis, gross cardiomegaly, and acute partial bronchial obstruction.

Various conditions other than acute pulmonary embolism can cause mismatched defects on *V/Q* scanning (see Table 23.2) and, although they may be apparent on a chest radiograph, their presence does not exclude the possibility of coexisting pulmonary embolism.

Radiolabeled Components of the Clotting System

It is possible to provide a positive image of thromboembolism by using radiolabeled components of the clotting system such as ^{111}In-labeled platelets and radiolabeled monoclonal antibodies to platelets, fibrin and other components of the clotting system. While in theory these agents offer attractive advantages over standard *V/Q* scanning, they have failed to achieve wide acceptance in clinical practice, due to their limited availability, short half-life, and expense.

Pulmonary Angiography

Although the last few years have seen major advances in the imaging evaluation of patients with acute pulmonary

Table 23.2. Causes of ventilation–perfusion mismatching

Pulmonary embolism
  Acute
  Chronic
External compression of pulmonary artery
  Carcinoma of bronchus
  Lymphoma
  Fibrosing mediastinitis
Primary pulmonary hypertension
Pulmonary venoocclusive disease
Vasculitis of medium-sized arteries
Focal obliteration of pulmonary capillaries
  Fibrosing alveolitis
  Emphysema
  Tuberculosis
  Irradiation
Congenital pulmonary arterial hypoplasia
Sequestered segment
Upper lobe blood diversion
Intraluminal obstruction
  Catheter
  Parasite
Pulmonary arteriovenous malformations

embolism, pulmonary angiography remains, for the time being, the recognized "gold standard" for diagnosis. Pulmonary angiography allows direct visualization of the pulmonary arterial tree and a well-performed study is highly accurate in the detection or exclusion of pulmonary embolism. Contrary to popular opinion, pulmonary angiography is a very safe procedure, with mortality rates of approximately 0.5% and major morbidity rates of about 1% (28). Even in patients with increased pulmonary arterial pressure (the subgroup said to be most at risk), there was no significant increase in mortality in the PIOPED study (28).

Indications

As the diagnostic gold standard, pulmonary angiography is logically indicated where clinical suspicion remains high and other less invasive tests have failed to make the diagnosis. The following situations have traditionally been used as specific indications.

1. An indeterminate *V/Q* scan.
2. Patients in whom anticoagulation therapy would carry a higher than normal risk (for example, gastrointestinal hemorrhage) and other tests are suggestive of pulmonary embolism.
3. When the *V/Q* scan result does not correlate with the degree of clinical suspicion.
4. Massive embolism where embolectomy, thrombolytic therapy, or vena cava filter insertion is being considered.

In reality, the majority of these situations are now dealt with by performing a CT pulmonary angiogram and the role of pulmonary angiography is limited to those cases requiring subsequent interventional procedures (situation 4 above), or where the CT is nondiagnostic and clinical suspicion remains high or the exclusion of small subsegmental emboli is clinically important.

Angiographic Signs of Pulmonary Embolism

There are two main angiographic signs and a number of minor signs.
  Major signs:

1. *Filling defect within the opacified arterial tree.* Filling defects are very variable in size, shape and number. Contrast flowing around the thrombus in incomplete occlusion may produce a faint ghost-like appearance when the vessel is seen side on (Fig. 23.4). The contrast may flow downstream beyond the thrombus to opacify the distal vascular bed depending on how much of the arterial lumen the thrombus occupies.

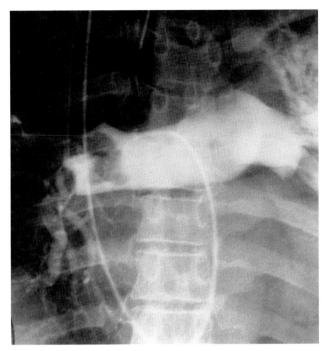

Figure 23.4. Pulmonary angiogram showing the two main signs of acute thromboembolism. There is a large filling defect within the right main pulmonary artery, extending as a tongue into the lower lobe artery and completely occluding the upper lobe artery.

2. *Occlusion of a pulmonary arterial branch.* Complete occlusion of an arterial branch (Fig. 23.4) is a less specific sign and may be seen in a variety of other conditions including congenital malformations, fibrosing mediastinitis, direct involvement by neoplasm and organized thrombus from previous embolism.

The *minor signs* include absent or reduced opacification of small arterial branches, which is analogous to the defect seen on perfusion scanning and therefore, in isolation, is no more specific than this. In patients with chronic thromboembolic disease, additional signs may be seen. These include webs, pouchings of partially occluded vessels, and in patients with chronic pulmonary arterial hypertension, abnormal tapering of vessels, tortuosity of remaining vessels and delayed filling and emptying of vessels.

Although pulmonary angiography is the recognized gold standard, it is not a foolproof method of detecting pulmonary embolism and false negatives can occur despite extensive intravascular thrombus (29). Because pulmonary angiography is the final arbiter, false positives are difficult to prove but likely to be rare. Nevertheless, several large studies have shown that life-threatening emboli are not missed by pulmonary angiography (5,30,31).

Perhaps the most important factor limiting the effectiveness of pulmonary angiography in the diagnostic algorithm is its limited availability. For example, pulmonary angiography is available in only one third of acute hospitals in the United Kingdom. This is further compounded by the fact that in order to maintain its lofty status as the

gold standard, a well-performed pulmonary angiogram requires a high degree of technical skill – a situation requiring a reasonable amount of practice in order to develop and maintain such abilities. These skills would appear to be becoming an ever-decreasing commodity.

Computed Tomography

The serendipitous detection of central pulmonary emboli on a contrast-enhanced CT scan was recognized as early as 1978 (32). However, it was not until the advent of rapid, continuous volume helical scanning that the pulmonary arteries could be reliably and consistently demonstrated with good contrast opacification. The first description of the continuous volume single breath-hold technique was in 1990 (33). CT pulmonary angiography as a technique capable of rivalling standard pulmonary angiography in the detection of proximal pulmonary embolism was first reported in the prospective study of Rémy-Jardin et al. in 1992 (34). Since that time, there has been considerable improvement in both technical factors and interpretative skills, and the technique is now considered as reliable as standard pulmonary angiography in the detection of pulmonary emboli at least to the segmental level. Furthermore, the reliability of standard pulmonary angiography beyond the segmental level is limited, with up to one third of cases being misdiagnosed (35).

An important advantage of CT over conventional pulmonary angiography is the ability to evaluate the lung parenchyma and pleural space. This allows the identification of secondary features supporting the diagnosis of pulmonary embolism, such as, peripheral wedge-shaped opacities, atelectasis, pleural effusions, and dilatation of central or segmental pulmonary arteries (CT correlate of the Fleischner sign on plain radiography) (36). However, these signs are supportive rather than diagnostic, and in a recent study, peripherally based wedge-shaped opacities were the only CT finding significantly associated with pulmonary embolism but were only present in 25% of cases (37). The real value of being able to image the lungs and pleura is the ability to provide an alternative diagnosis that may mimic the clinical picture of pulmonary embolism when there is no evidence of a pulmonary embolus on the CT (38,39).

Since the area of the thorax included in the contrast-enhanced scan is focused on the central pulmonary arteries, the entire thorax is not shown. It is therefore important to perform a precontrast scan of the entire thorax. In addition to the benefits already described, it provides a convenient method of accurately localizing the anatomic volume of interest to be scanned with contrast and may demonstrate areas of lymph node calcification that may be confusing on the contrast-enhanced scan. A widely interspaced thin section scan not only reduces radiation dose but the narrow collimation gives better details of subtle bronchial and parenchymal changes that may be missed on thick sections.

Before the imaging findings are described, several technical factors are worth considering.

Volume of Interest

CT pulmonary angiography can reliably demonstrate emboli within pulmonary arteries down to the segmental level. Therefore, the upper aspect of the aortic arch to the level of the inferior pulmonary veins (a z-axis distance of approximately 10–12 cm) is scanned, all pulmonary arteries large enough to allow a confident diagnosis will be included. Limiting the volume of the contrast-enhanced scan allows most scans to be performed during a single breath-hold, thereby minimizing misregistration artefacts, as well as minimizing radiation dose. Once the volume of interest has been chosen, two other factors have to be taken into consideration – the collimation and speed of table feed (pitch). These factors must be weighed against the patients' ability to hold their breath.

Collimation and Table Feed

The initial descriptions used 5 mm collimation with a 5 mm per second table feed at 1 second per revolution scan time (pitch of 1.0) (34,40). This technique was well tolerated by patients, with the area of interest able to be scanned in a single breath-hold by the majority of patients. However, the main disadvantage of this technique is the significant partial volume effects at the level of the smaller vessels, limiting the detection of segmental filling defects. By reducing the collimation to 3 mm and maintaining the same table feed (effectively increasing the pitch to 1.7) the same z-axis volume is covered in a single breath-hold but visualization of segmental arteries improves significantly (41). The introduction of subsecond scan times now enables an equivalent z-axis coverage with even thinner collimation. Using 2 mm collimation at a table speed of 4 mm per 0.75 sec revolution (pitch of 2.0) the evaluation of segmental and subsegmental arteries improves considerably (42). The recent introduction of multiring scanners that can scan multiple slices during a single subsecond revolution offers the potential for even more rapid data acquisition, which will be particularly beneficial for dyspneic patients with a limited breath-hold capacity.

Acquisition Protocols

In order to complete the above protocols in a single breath-hold, the patient must be capable of holding their breath for approximately 20 s. With hyperventilation prior to the start of the examination, most patients are able to hold their breath for the required duration of the scan – however dyspneic they appear. If the patient is incapable of a 20 s breath-hold, a shorter duration scan can be performed to cover the same z-axis by increasing collimation and pitch, but at the expense of spatial resolution. In the ventilated patient, ventilation can usually be suspended for the required duration of the scan without difficulty. Patients can be scanned during quiet respiration as a last resort, but diagnostic information is limited to the central pulmonary arteries. It is vital to the accurate interpretation of the scan that the technical factors involved in the acquisition of the images are known before the scan is interpreted.

Contrast Enhancement

The timing and delivery of intravenous contrast plays a vital role in determining the diagnostic quality of the scan. The aim is to establish excellent contrast opacification of the target vessels at the beginning of the scan and to maintain a consistent degree of contrast opacification throughout the scan duration. Several techniques have been studied in order to develop an ideal system of contrast administration. In general terms, there are two options: low concentration contrast material injected at a high flow rate, and high concentration at a low flow rate. The main problem with injecting high concentration contrast material (350–370 mg ml^{-1}) is streak artefacts at the level of the subclavian and brachiocephalic veins as well as the superior vena cava. This can cause severe degradation in image quality. The superior vena cava artefact, in particular, may hamper detection of intraluminal changes in the adjacent right pulmonary artery. In order to minimize these difficulties, the concentration of contrast material can be reduced and the flow rate increased. Various protocols have been evaluated by Rémy-Jardin et al. and their current recommendation is 120–140 ml of 150–240 mg iodine ml^{-1} concentration (24–30%) at a rate of 4–5 ml per sec (41).

Using a 20-gauge cannula in an antecubital fossa vein, a 10–20 s scan delay usually provides good opacification of the pulmonary arteries in most patients with normal right ventricular outflow (43). Patients with right-sided heart failure require a longer delay, but, perhaps surprisingly, pulmonary hypertension does not significantly alter the transit time of contrast through the lungs (44). Time density curves can be performed to determine the ideal timing for maximum contrast opacification (45). However, unless the patient's clinical condition suggests some alteration in pulmonary circulation time, the empiric determination of delay seems to work very well in the majority of patients. Nevertheless, it is not uncommon for a small part of the pulmonary arterial tree to be sub-optimally opacified on the first attempt, and a limited second scan targeted to this area, with an appropriate change in the timing of the contrast, will usually rectify this.

Image Reconstruction

The optimal scanning protocol involves a pitch of greater than 1.0 and therefore data should be reconstructed with a 180° linear interpolation algorithm (46). The reconstruction of overlapping sections is also recommended to improve longitudinal resolution and diminish partial volume effects (47). Vessels running obliquely through the plane of section may be poorly demonstrated. This is particularly problematic with the right middle lobe and lingular vessels. Reformatted images through the longitudinal axis of the vessel can overcome some of these interpretative problems (48). This is more of a problem with thicker sections, and when 2 mm collimation is used, multiplanar reformats are claimed to be almost completely unnecessary (43).

Images should not be reconstructed on a high spatial frequency algorithm as this can produce an artefactual high attenuation rim around vessels, mimicking a pulmonary embolus (49). Modification of window settings from standard mediastinal settings may be useful in the detection of pulmonary emboli (50).

Interpretation

CT Signs of Acute Pulmonary Embolism

The most reliable CT sign of acute pulmonary embolism is the demonstration of intravascular clots (34,41,51–53). A partial filling defect is seen as a central (floating freely within the vessel lumen) or marginal (attached to the wall of the vessel) area of low attenuation within the vessel lumen and surrounded by contrast (Fig. 23.5). If the artery lies parallel and within the plane of section, contrast can be seen surrounding a longitudinal area of central low attenuation giving the so-called "railway track sign". The same phenomenon in a vessel running perpendicular to the plane of section is seen as a central area of low attenuation surrounded circumferentially by high attenuation contrast. Mural thrombus is seen as peripheral areas of low attenuation. If thrombus completely occludes the vessel lumen, the vessel will be identified as a low attenuation vascular structure. This can usually be identified as thrombus rather than unopacified blood by examining the other vessels at that level to determine whether contrast opacification is optimal, and by tracing the vessel in question to determine the proximal extent of

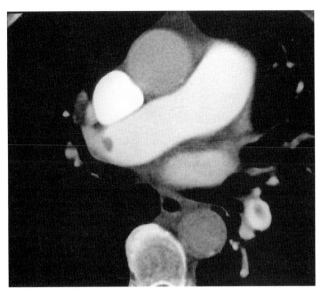

Figure 23.5. Acute pulmonary embolism on CT. There is a central filling defect surrounded by contrast in the left lower lobe artery. Central thrombus is also seen within the right main pulmonary artery.

thrombus. The vessel may be expanded by thrombus, which provides additional evidence in support of the diagnosis (Fig. 23.6). As described previously, ancillary signs of thromboembolic disease, such as a small pleural effusion or a pulmonary infarct may be seen (Fig. 23.7). There may be evidence of right heart strain, with an enlarged right ventricle and straightening or bowing of the interventricular septum (Fig. 23.8). Although these signs in

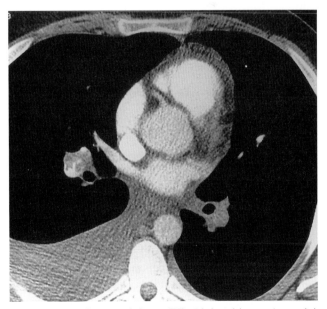

Figure 23.6. Acute pulmonary embolism on CT. The right lower lobe artery is expanded and partially occluded by thrombus. The left lower lobe artery is completely occluded and is also slightly expanded. Contrast within the pulmonary veins and the right ventricle indicate this is a thrombus rather than unopacified blood. Note also the right pleural effusion.

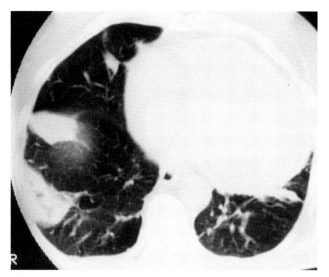

Figure 23.7. CT of pulmonary infarction. There are several pleurally based, wedge-shaped areas of consolidation. There are also small bilateral pleural effusions.

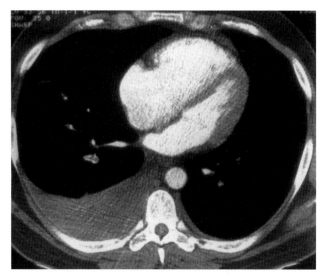

Figure 23.8. CT of acute pulmonary embolism. There are filling defects within the segmental arteries of both lower lobes. The right ventricle is enlarged and there is straightening of the interventricular septum, indicating right heart strain.

isolation are relatively nonspecific, in this context, they do provide important additional supportive evidence of pulmonary embolism.

CT Signs of Chronic Pulmonary Embolism

The distinction between acute and chronic pulmonary embolism on CT is not always possible. Dilatation of the proximal pulmonary arteries, narrowing of the peripheral pulmonary vessels and tortuosity of the segmental arteries are all signs of pulmonary arterial hypertension and suggest recurrent pulmonary embolism (54). However, the most specific vascular finding on CT is direct visualization of organized intravascular thrombus. This is

adherent to the vascular wall, irregularly marginated and may contain calcification. Without evidence of recanalization or calcification, complete vascular obstruction does not allow assessment of thrombus age (55). These vascular changes are frequently accompanied by attenuation changes in the lung parenchyma. Regional, sharply demarcated areas of high attenuation related to redistribution of bloodflow are often seen (54,56) (Fig. 23.9). Dilated bronchial arteries in areas of chronically reduced pulmonary arterial blood flow may also be seen (56).

Interpretative Pitfalls

Scans may be misinterpreted for a number of reasons, including technical factors such as motion artefact, slice thickness and poor contrast opacification, and anatomic factors such as lymphadenopathy and anatomic variants. These may result in false positive or false negative interpretation (as outlined in Table 23.3). False negatives are usually the result of technical factors, whereas false posi-

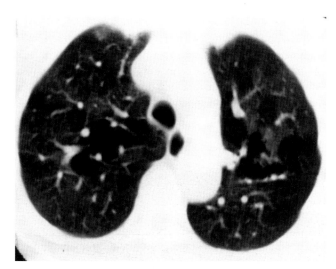

Figure 23.9. Patient with chronic thromboembolic disease. There is a mosaic perfusion pattern in this section through the upper lobes. The areas of decreased attenuation are not being perfused and are analogous to perfusion defects on a V/Q scan.

Table 23.3. Causes of false negative and false-positive diagnoses of pulmonary embolism on spiral CT

False negatives
Inadequate opacification of pulmonary arteries
Emboli confined to subsegmental pulmonary arteries
Unfavorable patient hemodynamics
Motion artefacts degrading image
Partial volume effect
Low signal-to-noise ratio
False positives
Hilar and bronchopulmonary lymph nodes
Partial opacification of pulmonary arteries or veins
Partial volume effect
Any cause of focal reduced pulmonary perfusion

tives are usually due to anatomic variants or other pathology.

Hilar lymph nodes lying immediately adjacent to central and segmental pulmonary arteries are a potent cause of misdiagnosis as they mimic pulmonary emboli. Therefore, a precise knowledge of the location of these nodes is important to avoid falling into this trap. The reader is referred to the excellent article by Rémy-Jardin et al. describing the location, appearance and incidence of these nodes (57). The most commonly identified and convincing mimic of an intravascular filling defect is the fibrofatty node lying on the superolateral aspect of the right main pulmonary artery, which occurs in up to 80% of patients. Incomplete opacification of pulmonary veins may mimic a pulmonary embolism but these can usually be identified as veins by analyzing contiguous sections on lung window settings.

Magnetic Resonance Imaging

In common with CT, magnetic resonance imaging (MRI) has the advantage of being able to directly and noninvasively image emboli within the lumen of pulmonary arteries (Fig. 23.10). In addition, MRI is capable of imaging vascular structures without the administration of iodinated contrast material and its associated hazards, and does not use ionizing radiation. There are several other theoretical advantages of MRI, such as: the ability to acquire multiplanar images – a particular

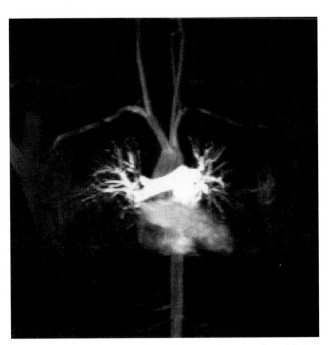

Figure 23.10. Gadolinium-enhanced MR pulmonary angiogram performed during a single breath-hold, showing acute thromboembolic disease. There is narrowing and attenuation of the right upper lobe vessels and complete occlusion of the right lower lobe artery.

problem with CT when vessels are orientated in the plane of section; the ability to image the pelvic and deep veins of the legs in a single examination (although CT protocols have been successfully developed to achieve this (58)); and the ability to estimate the hemodynamic effects of the embolus on the circulation. Despite these rather attractive advantages, MRI has, as yet, failed to rival CT in terms of diagnostic ability. Although this is partly due to the significant improvements in CT with the introduction of subsecond scanners, the main reason has been MRI's inability to overcome two problems: relatively poor spatial resolution, limiting the size of vessels that can be adequately visualized; and lengthy acquisition times resulting in artefacts from both breathing and cardiac motion (59).

Several techniques have been developed in an attempt to overcome these limitations. Ultrafast sequences such as inversion recovery turbo FLASH with ultrashort time-to-echo (TE) have been evaluated (60). ECG cardiac gating allows images to be obtained during a specific part of the cardiac cycle, usually diastole. A technique for respiratory gating allows the patient to breathe normally during image acquisition without causing breathing motion artefacts. This involves the patient breathing freely and a navigator echo pulse being applied for each cardiac cycle; data are accepted only if the diaphragm position falls within a narrow (3–7 mm) window around end expiration (61). Other techniques such as breath-hold three-dimensional contrast-enhanced MR angiography have been investigated and found to produce reliable images of the large to medium-sized pulmonary vessels (62). The use of gadolinium-based extracellular fluid contrast agents has been gaining increasing clinical application but the short intravascular half-life of the agents and the rapid redistribution into the extracellular space make them less suitable for imaging of the pulmonary vasculature, where the overall study time may be slow due to respiratory and cardiac gating, and where repeat acquisitions may be required if the initial images are nondiagnostic for technical reasons. The recent evaluation of ultrasmall superparamagnetic iron oxide particles (USPIO) as a blood pool agent have provided encouraging preliminary results on normal healthy subjects (63). The USPIO particles were originally developed as T_2 contrast agents for imaging of the reticuloendothelial system but have also been found to decrease T_1 and have been used for MR angiography (64,65). The major advantage of blood pool agents is the possibility of longer and repeated imaging (for up to several hours) because imaging is not restricted to the first pass. Longer imaging times are particularly valuable as they allow significant improvement in spatial resolution. In addition, the ability to investigate other vascular territories such as the inferior vena cava, pelvic and leg veins to search for the source of the pulmonary emboli is facilitated. The use of cardiac and respiratory gating helps to reduce motion artefacts. Whether these techniques evolve

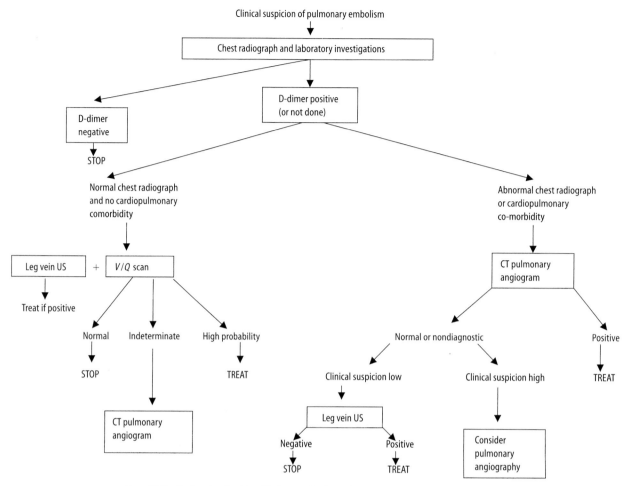

Figure 23.11. The imaging algorithm. *US*, ultrasound; *V/Q*, ventilation/perfusion; *CT*, computed tomography.

to challenge or replace CT or standard pulmonary angiography in clinical practice remains to be seen.

Conclusion

The diagnosis of pulmonary embolism remains one of the most controversial and hotly debated topics in the medical literature. An imaging algorithm is provided (Fig. 23.11) which is a reasonable reflection of the current state of the literature. You will note that MRI is not included in the algorithm. That is because its role as a clinically acceptable alternative to CT or angiography remains controversial and, as yet, unproven. There are as many different approaches to the problem of diagnosing pulmonary embolism as there are clinical manifestations of the disease. To a large extent, the diagnostic approach is a reflection of patient demographics (the pretest probability of pulmonary embolism), the availability of imaging modalities and the expertise of the radiologist, and the opinion and experience of the referring clinicians. Whether this complex topic is able to be simplified by the development of a single test which will provide the diagnosis in a reliable, noninvasive and cost-effective manner remains unclear.

References

1. Freiman DG, Suyemoto J, Wessler S (1965) Frequency of pulmonary thromboembolism in man. N Engl J Med 272:1278–1280.
2. Uhland H, Goldberg LM (1964) Pulmonary embolism: A commonly missed clinical entity. Dis Chest 45:533–536.
3. Dalen JE, Alpert JS (1975) Natural history of pulmonary embolism. Prog Cardiovasc Dis 17:257–270.
4. Coon WW, Willis PW (1974) Haemorrhagic complications of anticoagulant therapy. Arch Intern Med 133:386–392.

5. The PIOPED investigators (1990) Value of ventilation/perfusion scan in acute pulmonary embolism. Results of the prospective investigation of pulmonary embolism diagnosis. JAMA 263:2753–2759.

6. Sander A, Mitchell JR (1989) How do we know who has DVT? Postgrad Med J 65:16–19.

7. Bettmann MA, Robbins A, Braun SD, et al. (1987) Contrast venography of the leg: Diagnostic efficiency, tolerance and complication rates with ionic and non-ionic contrast media. Radiology 165:113–116.

8. Kakkar VV, Flanc C, Howe CT, et al. (1969) Natural history of postoperative deep-vein thrombosis. Lancet 2:230–232.

9. Cronan JJ (1993) Venous thromboembolic disease: The role of US. Radiology 186:619–630.

10. Burki NK (1986) The dead space to tidal volume ratio in the diagnosis of pulmonary embolism. Am Rev Resp Dis 133:679–685.

11. Moser KM (1977) Pulmonary embolism: State of the art. Am Rev Resp Dis 115:829–852.

12. Moser KM, Guisan M, Bartimmo EE, et al. (1973) In vivo and post mortem dissolution rates of pulmonary emboli and venous thrombi in the dog. Circulation 48:170–178.

13. Perrier A, Bounameaux H, Morabia A, et al. (1996) Diagnosis of pulmonary embolism by a decision analysis-based strategy including clinical probability, D-dimer levels and ultrasonography: a management study. Arch Intern Med 156:531–536.

14. de Moerloose P, Minazio P, Reber G, et al. (1994) D-dimer determination to exclude pulmonary embolism: A two step approach using latex assay as a screening tool. Thromb Haemost 72:89–91.

15. Freyburger G, Trillaud H, Labrouche S, et al. (1998) D-dimer strategy in thrombosis exclusion – a gold standard study in 100 patients suspected of deep vein thrombosis or pulmonary embolism: 8DD methods compared. Thromb Haemost 79:32–37.

16. Perrier A, Desmarais S, Goehring C, et al. (1997) D-dimer testing for suspected pulmonary embolism in outpatients. Am J Respir Crit Care Med 156:492–496.

17. Tardy B, Tardy-Poncet B, Viallon A, et al. (1998) Evaluation of D-dimer ELISA test in elderly patients with suspected pulmonary embolism. Thromb Haemost 79:38–41.

18. Turkstra F, van Beek EJ, Buller HR (1998) Observer and biological variation of the rapid whole blood D-dimer test. Thromb Haemost 79:91–93.

19. van Beek EJ, Schenk BE, Michel BC et al. (1996) The role of D-dimer concentration in the exclusion of pulmonary embolism. Br J Haematol 92:725–732.

20. Reber G, Bounameaux H, Perrier A, et al. (1999) Performance of fibrin monomer test for the exclusion of pulmonary embolism in symptomatic outpatients. Thromb Haemost 81:221–223.

21. Bournameaux H, Moerloose P, Perrier A, et al. (1994) Plasma measurement of D-dimer as a diagnostic aid in suspected venous thromboembolism: An overview. Thromb Haemost 72:488–490.

22. Michiels JJ (1998) Rational diagnosis of pulmonary embolism (RADIA PE) in symptomatic outpatients with suspected PE: An improved strategy to exclude or diagnose venous thromboembolism by the sequential use of a clinical model, rapid ELISA D-dimer test, perfusion lung scan, ultrasonography, spiral CT, and pulmonary angiography. Semin Thromb Haemost 24:413–418.

23. Egermayer P, Town GI, Turner JG, et al. (1998) Usefulness of D-dimer, blood gas, and respiratory rate measurements for excluding pulmonary embolism. Thorax 53:830–834.

24. Bynum LJ, Wilson JE (1978) Radiographic features of pleural effusions in pulmonary embolism. Am Rev Respir Dis 117:8229–834.

25. Hampton AO, Castleman B (1940) Correlations of post mortem chest teleroentgenograms with autopsy findings with special reference to pulmonary embolism and infarction. AJR 43:305–326.

26. Wilson AG, Joseph AE, Butland JRA (1986) The radiology of aseptic cavitation in pulmonary infarction. Clin Radiol 37:327–333.

27. Gottschalk A, Sostman HD, Coleman RE, et al. (1993) Ventilation perfusion scintigraphy in the PIOPED study. Part II. Evaluation of the scintigraphic criteria and interpretation. J Nucl Med 34:1119–1126.

28. Stein PD,. Athansoulis CA, Alavi A, et al. (1992) Complications and validity of pulmonary angiography in acute pulmonary embolism. Circulation 85:462–468.

29. Brown KT, Bach (1992) Paucity of angiographic findings despite extensive organised thrombus in chronic thromboembolic pumonary hypertension. J Vasc Intervent Radiol 3:395–399.

30. Novelline RA, Baltarowich OH, Athanasoulis CA, et al. (1978) The clinical course of patients with suspected pumonary embolism and a negative pulmonary angiogram. Radiology 126:561–567.

31. Cheely R, McCartney WH, Perry JR, et al. (1981) The role of non-invasive tests versus pulmonary angiographyint he diagnosis of pumonary embolism. Am J Med 70:17–22.

32. Sinner WN (1978) Computed tomorgraphic patterns of pulmonary thromboebolism and infarction. J Comput Assist Tomogr 2:395–399.

33. Kalender WA, Seissler W, Klotz E, et al. (1990) Spiral volumetric CT with single-breath-hold technique, continuous transport and continuous scanner rotation. Radiology 176:181–183.

34. Rémy-Jardin M, Rémy J, Wattinee L, et al. (1992) Central pulmonary thromboembolism: Dagnosis with spiral volumetric CT with the single-breath-hold technique – comparison with angiography. Radiology 185:381–387.

35. Diffin DC, Leyendeeker JR, Johnson SP, et al. (1998) Effect of anatomic distribution of pulmonary emboli on interobserver agreement in the interpretation of pumonary angiography. AJR 171:1085–1089.

36. Coche EE, Müller NL, Kim KI, et al. (1998) Acute pulmonary embolism: Ancillary findings at spiral CT. Radiology 207:753–758.

37. Shah AA, Davis SD, Gamsu G, et al. (1999) Parenchymal and pleural findings in patients with and patients without acute pulmonary embolism detected at spiral CT. Radiology 211:147–153.

38. Van Rossum AB, Treuniet FE, Kieft GJ, et al. (1996) Role of spiral volumetric computed-tomographic scanning in the assessment of patients with clinical suspicion of pulmonary embolism and an abnormal ventilation/perfusion lung scan. Thorax 51:23–28.

39. Kim KI, Müller NL, Mayo JR (1999) Clinically suspected pumonary embolism: Utility of spiral CT. Radiology 210:693–697.

40. Goodman LR, Curtin JJ, Mewissen MW, et al. (1995) Detection of pulmonary embolism in patients with unresolved clinical and scintigraphic diagnosis: Helical CT versus angiography. AJR 164:1369–1374.

41. Cauvain O, Rémy-Jardin M, Rémy J, et al. (!996) Diagnosis of acute pulmonary embolism with spiral CT: Comparison with pulmonary angiography and scintigraphy. Radiology 200:699–706.

42. Rémy-Jardin, Rémy J, Artaud D, et al (1997) Peripheral pumonary arteries: Optimisation of the sprial CT acquisition protocol. Radiology 304:157–163.

43. Remy-Jardin M, Remy J, Artaud D, et al. (1997) Spiral CT of pulmonary embolism: Technical consideration and interpretative pitfalls. J Thorac Imag 12:103–117.

44. Sostman HD, MacFall JR, Foo TK, et al. (1993) Pulmonary arteries and veins. In: Potechen EJ, Haacke EM, Siebert JE, Gottschalk A (Eds) Magnetic resonance angiography: concepts and applications. Mosby, St. Louis, MO, pp 546–572.

45. Kuzo RS, Goodman LR (1997) CT evaluation of pulmonary embolism: Technique and interpretation. AJR 169:959–965.

46. Polacin A, Kalender WA, Marchal G (1992) Evaluation of section sensitivity profiles and image noise in spiral CT. Radiology 185:29–35.

47. Kalender WA, Polacin A, Suss C (1994) A comparison of conventional and spiral CT: An experimental study on the detection of spherical lesions. J Comput Assist Tomogr 18:167–176.

48. Rémy-Jardin M, Rémy J, Cauvain O, et al. (1995) Diagnosis of central pulmonary embolism with helical CT: Role of two dimensional multiplanar reformations. AJR 5:1131–1138.

49. Swensen ST, Morin RL, Aughenbaugh GL, et al. (1995) CT reconstruction algorithm selection in the evaluation of solitary pulmonary nodules. J Comput Assist Tomogr 19:932–935.

50. Brink JA, Woodard PK, Horesh L, et al. (1997) Depiction of pulmonary emboli with spiral CT: Optimisation of display window settings in a porcine model. Radiology 204:703–708.

51. Mayo J, Rémy-Jardin M, Müller NL, et al. (1997) Pulmonary embolism: Prospective comparison of spiral CT and ventilation-perfusion scintigraphy. Radiology 205:447–452.

52. Goodman LR, Curtin JJ, Mewissen MW, et al. (1995) Detection of pulmonary embolism in patients with unresolving clinical and scintigraphic diagnosis: Helical CT versus angiography. AJR 205:447–452.

53. van Rossum AB, Pattynama PM, Ton ER, et al. (1996) Pulmonary embolism: Validation of spiral CT angiography in 149 patients. Radiology 201:467–470.

54. Tardivon AA, Musset D, Maitre S, et al. (1993) Role of CT in chronic pulmonary embolism: Comparison with pulmonary angiography. J Comput Assist Tomogr 17:345–351.

55. Roberts HC, Kauczor H, Schweden F, et al. (1997) Spiral CT of pulmonary hypertension and chronic thromboembolism. J Thorac Imag 12:118–127.

56. Rémy-Jardin M, Rémy J, Louvegny S, et al. (1997) Airway changes in chronic pulmonary embolism: CT findings in 33 patients. Radiology 203:355–360.

57. Rémy-Jardin M, Duyck P, Rémy J, et al. (1995) Hilar lymph nodes: Identification with spiral CT and histologic correlation. Radiology 196:387–394.

58. Loud PA, Grossman ZD, Klippenstein DL, et al. (1998) Combined CT venography and pulmonary angiography: A new diagnostic technique for suspected thromboembolic disease. AJR 170:951–954.

59. Woodard PK, Sostman DH, MacFall JR, et al. (1995) Detection of pulmonary embolism: Comparison of contrast enhanced CT and time-of-flight MR techniques. J Thorac Imag 10:59–72.

60. Hatabu H, Gaa J, Kim D, et al. (1996) Pulmonary perfusion: Qualitative assessment with dynamic contrast-enhanced MRI using ultra-short TE and inversion recovery turbo FLASH. Magn Reson Med 36:503–508.

61. Wang Y, Rossman P, Grimm R, et al. (1996) Navigator-echo-based real-time respiratory gating and triggering for reduction of respiratory effects on 3-dimensional coronary MR angiography. Radiology 198:55–60.

62. Leung DA, Debatin JF (1997) Three dimensional contrast enhanced magnetic resonance angiography of the thoracic vasculature. Eur Radiol 7:981–989.

63. Ahlström KH, Johansson LO, Rodenburg JB, et al. (1999) Pulmonary MR angiography with ultrasmall superparamagnetic iron oxide particles as a blood pool agent and a navigator echo for respiratory gating: Pilot study. Radiology 211:865–869.

64. Anzai Y, Prince MR, Chenevert TL, et al. (1997) MRI angiography with an ultrasmall superparamagnetic iron oxide blood pool agent. J Magn Reson Imaging 7:209–214.

65. Mayo-Smith WW, Saini S, Slater G, et al. (1996) MR contrast for vascular enhancement: Value of superparamagnetic iron oxide. AJR 166:73–77.

24 Pulmonary Edema

M. Pistolesi, F. Lavorini, G.A. Fontana, M. Mascalchi, and E.N.C. Milne

Pathophysiology of Pulmonary Edema

Liquid and Solute Exchange in the Normal Lung

Pulmonary edema, an increased amount of fluid and solute in the extravascular space of the lung, is to be considered as an extension of normal fluid dynamics rather than a condition of static pathology (1). Pulmonary edema results from an imbalance between physiologic mechanisms regulating filtration and removal rates of pulmonary fluid and protein.

In physiologic terms, as proposed by Starling in 1896 (2) and recently refined, expanded and mathematically quantified (3), the net filtration across any semipermeable barrier can be described by the product of the driving pressure and the conductance, or permeability, of the barrier. In normal conditions, the lung microvascular endothelial barrier is virtually impermeable to proteins and, for this reason, the effective driving pressure for liquid exchange is set by the balance between hydrostatic and oncotic pressures in the microcirculation and the surrounding interstitium. The hydrostatic gradient (i.e., the difference between microvascular and interstitial hydrostatic pressure) favors filtration toward the interstitium, whereas the oncotic gradient (i.e., the difference between the microvascular and interstitial oncotic pressures) acts to retain fluid in the microvessels. There is general agreement that the result of the interaction between hydrostatic and oncotic forces is a net filtration pressure from the microvessels to the interstitium (1,4,5–7). This physiologic imbalance does not result in pulmonary edema formation, since the lymphatic system of the lung is able to handle the small amount of liquid continuously filtered. It is important to recall that terminal lymphatic vessels are not distributed to the alveolar wall intersitium, but are confined to the loose connective tissue of the peribronchovascular sheaths, the interlobular septa and the pleura (1,4,5–7). Direct measurements of interstitial

hydrostatic pressure indicate the existence of a fluid pressure gradient between the septal space and that containing the lymphatics (8). As a consequence, the fluid that normally leaks out of the capillaries located in the alveolar walls moves through the septal interstitium toward the lymphatic endings. The very tight intercellular junctions of the normal alveolar epithelium prevent liquid filtered in the septal interstitium from flooding the airspaces. Fluid entering the peripheral lymphatics is drained, through funnel-shaped valves, toward the larger collecting lymphatic vessels of the hilar regions and, eventually, returned to the bloodstream. Lymph propulsion takes place both passively by respiratory motion and cardiovascular pulsation, and actively by intrinsic contraction of lymphatic walls (6,7).

1.2 Formation and Reabsorption of Pulmonary Edema

In most instances, pulmonary edema is the result of either an increase in the net driving pressure (increased hydrostatic pressure and/or a reduced oncotic pressure in the microcirculation) for fluid filtration across the microvessels or an increase in the permeability of the microvascular and/or the alveolar barrier. We will consider the two main forms of pulmonary edema separately here, even though it should be remembered that they are frequently combined. Indeed, increased hydrostatic pressure and increased permeability of the capillary/alveolar barrier coexist in the pathogenesis of many specific syndromes of pulmonary edema. A modern view of edema must recognize the natural barriers to the formation and spread of edema, the capillary endothelium and the alveolar epithelium (8). Varying degrees of damage to them can account for the varying radiographic and clinical manifestations of lung edema.

The commonest cause of an increase in transvascular driving pressure is a rise secondary to left heart dysfunction. The filtered fluid that cannot be cleared by lymphatics spreads along hydrostatic pressure gradients toward the connective tissue sheaths surrounding extraalveolar vessels and terminal airways, and progressively recruits the interstitial space around larger vessels and bronchi at the hilum of the lung. Therefore, the loose connective tissue spaces act as sumps, draining edema fluid in parallel with lymph vessels (5,7,9,10). It is accepted that these sumps can increase in volume by approximately 35% before fluid begins to flood the alveoli (7). The recruitment of the interstitial tissue space helps to remove fluid from the gas exchange portion of the lung and to preserve respiratory function, at least in the early phases of pulmonary edema accumulation. When the capacity of the loose interstitial space is exceeded, the alveolar wall interstitium begins to swell; eventually the alveolar barrier breaks down and the edema fluid collects in the airspaces.

In increased permeability (injury) pulmonary edema, elevated transvascular filtration of fluid and protein occurs as a consequence of microvascular endothelial loss of integrity. Hence, unlike hydrostatic pulmonary edema, in which the edema fluid has a low protein content, the extravasated fluid in this condition has a protein concentration close to that of plasma (7). Furthermore, morphometric studies in humans with injury lung edema demonstrate a concomitant disruption of the alveolar epithelium (11). The increased permeability of the alveolar barrier will thus favor a direct shift of fluid and protein from the interstitium to the airspaces, which represent a low resistance path for fluid accumulation (7). It has been demonstrated that, for comparable amounts of extravascular fluid, hydrostatic edema causes greater distension of the peribronchovascular space, whereas injury edema causes a greater degree of alveolar flooding (12). Alveolar filling with proteinaceous fluid is characteristic of the acute phase of injury edema, which correlates with the clinical finding that patients with injury edema have a greater and earlier impairment of respiratory function than patients with hydrostatic pulmonary edema.

The different extent, location (interstitial or alveolar), and protein composition of the extravascular fluid markedly influence even the recovery phase. The rate of reabsorption of interstitial pulmonary edema is quicker than that of alveolar edema; furthermore, in injury pulmonary edema, the high protein concentration in edema fluid and the presence of inflammatory elements and cellular debris further delay the process of resolution (13). Interstitial edema could simply resolve if the filtrate is returned to the pulmonary vascular space directly across the vascular wall or via the lymphatics to the systemic venous circulation. Although the lymph flow can increase dramatically in response to increased hydrostatic pressure experimentally, the extent to which lymphatic function increases in clinical forms of pulmonary edema is unknown. Furthermore, increases in lymph flow per se seem

to play little role in the clearance of either alveolar or interstitial edema (14). The paths by which alveolar edema is cleared are also not certain. Experimentally, with unchanged Starling forces, fluid instilled directly into the airspace is cleared predominantly into the pulmonary blood flow, with no increase in lymphatic function or changes in pulmonary blood flow (14). However, these observations are not necessarily relevant for clinical forms of pulmonary edema, especially when the development of pulmonary edema is the result of anatomic abnormalities in the alveolocapillary barrier. Pulmonary edema can also be cleared into the pleural space (15). The pathways by which fluid moves from the alveolar or interstitial spaces into the pleural space are unknown. However, it is conceivable that peripheral extension of interstitial edema could result in subpleural edema and eventually in pleural effusion (15). While the pathways for resolution are not well defined, it seems clear that the movement of edema out of the alveoli is an active, energy-requiring process, at least in lungs with an intact alveolar epithelium. Fluid is reabsorbed from the airspace at a faster rate than protein, leaving the protein concentration of the remaining alveolar fluid to rise progressively. As a result further clearance takes place against an increasing oncotic pressure gradient (14).

1.3 Clinical Forms of Pulmonary Edema

Elevation of the microvascular pressure in the microcirculation, reduction in oncotic pressure, and injury to the alveolocapillary barrier are the three commonest pathogenetic mechanisms causing clinical pulmonary edema. The commonest counterpart of the first mechanism (elevated hydrostatic pressure) is cardiogenic pulmonary edema. Fluid overload secondary to renal failure (16), and iatrogenic overhydration (17), are the counterparts of reduced plasma colloid oncotic pressure, which predisposes to pulmonary edema even if the microvascular pressure is only slightly elevated (18). Elevated left atrial pressure, secondary to either left ventricular failure or left heart valvular disease, is transmitted backward to the pulmonary veins and capillaries, resulting in an increased rate of fluid filtration in the lung.

The third mechanism, endothelial injury, is the common basis for all of the clinical disorders unified under the term adult respiratory distress syndrome (ARDS). ARDS can be defined as a sudden, progressive disorder characterized by pulmonary edema with normal pulmonary artery wedge pressure, severe dyspnea, hypoxemia refractory to supplemental oxygen, decreased lung compliance, and radiographic evidence of diffuse pulmonary infiltrates (19).

This clinical syndrome is associated with many predisposing factors, among which the most common are sepsis, pneumonia (viral or bacterial), trauma (long bone, thorax, head, surface burn), hypertransfusion, cardiopulmonary bypass, liquid inhalation (aspiration of gastric contents, drowning), toxic gas and fume inhalation, drug overdose, and disseminated intravascular coagulopathy (19–21). Various cellular (leukocytes and platelets) and humoral inflammatory mediators are thought to be involved in the development of the syndrome, but the exact mechanism leading to massive lung injury is still debated (22,23).

In the remainder of this chapter we focus on the two most common clinical categories of pulmonary edema, hydrostatic and injury. However, there are other forms of pulmonary edema that may be occasionally observed in clinical practice.

Pulmonary venoocclusive disease, either congenital or secondary to mediastinal disease, may lead to pulmonary edema of the hydrostatic type (24). The clinical, physiologic and radiographic manifestations of pulmonary edema are usually indistinguishable from those of pulmonary venous hypertension from cardiac causes, except that in most causes the heart is of normal size and, in cases in which only one or two veins are affected, the edema may be localized to a specific portion of the lungs (24).

Malignant infiltration of the lymphatics of the lung, lung transplantation, and obstructive lymphangitis in the course of silicosis may interfere with the efficiency of the lymphatic pump. The reduced removal of fluid and protein that are filtered across the microvascular bed may facilitate, in these conditions, pulmonary edema formation.

Rapid reexpansion of a pneumothorax or a pleural effusion may result in pulmonary edema, usually ipsilateral, whose pathogenetic mechanisms could be composite (25). Indeed, in this condition pulmonary edema seems to be secondary to both a rapid reduction of the interstitial hydrostatic pressure and an increased permeability of the alveolocapillary membrane (25).

Pulmonary edema after upper airways obstruction can occur sporadically and unexpectedly in circumstances characterized by temporary upper airway obstruction (near-hanging, epiglottitis, thyroid goitre, upper airways tumors, acromegaly, mediastinal tumors, foreign-body aspiration, or difficult insertion of an endotracheal or tracheotomy tube, among others) (26). The high transmural capillary pressure are generated by very negative intrapleural pressures that develop when vigorous breathing is attempted to overcome the airway obstruction. The negative pleural pressure, when transmitted to the interstitial space, increases the capillary transmural pressure. An increase in pulmonary vascular permeability is also implicated in the pathogenesis according to the relatively high protein concentration in the edema fluid (26).

Finally, high altitude and neurogenic pulmonary edema, although usually not classified with the groups of disorders collectively known as ARDS because of their peculiarities, share with these disorders the characteristic of an increased permeability of the alveolocapillary barrier. Indeed, in both conditions recovered pulmonary edema fluid has a high protein content (27–29). However, in high altitude edema, exaggerated regional pulmonary vasoconstriction secondary to hypoxia results in overperfusion and elevation of pressure in the nonconstricted segments of the lung, leading to high pressure edema in these areas. The concept that increased pulmonary vascular pressures are central to the pathogenesis of high altitude edema is also supported by remarkable and salutary responses to treatment based on reducing pulmonary pressure (27,28). In neurogenic pulmonary edema sympathetic discharge causes an increase, sometimes massive, in pulmonary microvascular pressure, causing a similar high pressure edema that may disrupt the endothelial cell junctions, giving a mixed picture of pressure and injury edema (29).

Assessment of Pulmonary Edema

Pulmonary edema is a very common event in critically ill patients. Clinical symptoms and signs are usually the hallmarks of far-advanced recruitment of the extravascular space of the lung. In consideration of the clinical relevance of pulmonary edema and of the relative insensitivity and inaccuracy of physical examination, it is not surprising that a large body of work has been addressed to the development of methods for the detection and measurement of lung edema (30). However, none of the methods based on either changes of the physical properties of the lung (transthoracic electrical impedance (31), microwave radiation (32), Compton-scatter densitometry (33) and transthoracic gamma-ray attenuation (34)), or equilibrium of tracers (inhalation of soluble inert gas (35), double indicator dilution (36), low molecular weight radio-aerosol clearance (37), protein external radioflux detection (38)) have been widely incorporated into clinical practice, mainly because of their complexity and poor reproducibility.

Any clinical method of assessing pulmonary edema must have two major goals: (a) to institute proper treatment, which is entirely different in hydrostatic versus injury edema; and (b) to follow objectively the effect of therapy and the evolution of the disease process. A National Institutes of Health Workshop (39) defined the "ideal" method for the clinical assessment of lung water as meeting the following criteria. It should be *sensitive* enough to detect small increases of extravascular lung water before clinical symptoms and signs become evident and, it should be *accurate* in measuring the actual amount of extravasated fluid. Since serial measurements are required, the method should be *reproducible, noninvasive,* and, if possible, *inexpensive*. Finally, the method should be *practical* enough to give readily available on-line data in an intensive care environment. According to the above workshop report (39), "the chest x-ray film remains the reference standard against which other lung water content methods are compared. Its advantages include moderate accuracy, fair sensitivity, good reproducibility, non-invasiveness, practicability, availability, portability, ease of use in the emergency care setting, and relatively low cost. It also provides excellent information about edema distribution" (39). All imaging techniques can provide information about the regional distribution of lung edema. Besides conventional chest radiography, other imaging techniques may be applied in the detection and measurement of pulmonary edema. Very low practicability and high cost are the major drawbacks limiting the clinical use of sophisticated techniques such as computed tomography (40–44), positron emission tomography (45–49), and magnetic resonance imaging (50–55). As a consequence, In the clinical assessment of lung edema, chest radiography is still the method of choice (6,39,56–66). In the following sections of this chapter we consider the main features of chest imaging techniques in patients with hydrostatic and injury lung edema.

Chest Radiography in Pulmonary Edema

Standardization of the Chest Radiographic Technique

The amount of information that can be extracted from a chest roentgenogram is dependent primarily on the film-reader's skill and knowledge of cardiopulmonary physiology, and secondarily on the quality of the roentgenogram, which in turn is largely dependent on the skill and specific training of the X-ray technician (much more than on the quality of the equipment). Two much has been said of the difficulties of taking intensive care unit (ICU) films. The condenser discharge units now commonly used permits reasonable high kilovoltages and currents to be used, with short exposure times. Most patients in an ICU are on mechanical ventilation and if the technician is trained to watch the ventilator dials and trigger the X-ray exposure at maximal inspiration, respiratory artefacts are rare and partially expiratory films not a problem.

A much more serious problem is that the film-reader often does not know the patient's exact position (i.e., erect, supine or partially erect), the anode-to-film distance, the exposure factors used on successive films, and, of major importance, whether the patient is on mechanical ventilation, and, if so, what the peak and positive end-expiratory pressure (PEEP) was at the time of the exposure. If the film-reader has not arranged to have this information supplied (e.g., in the form of a small label attached to the film (Fig. 24.1), it is almost impossible to extract valid hemodynamic information from the film or to make serial comparisons in the same patient (67,68).

Furthermore, many technical and environmental factors may interfere with the achievement of good-quality, reproducible roentgenograms in patients with pulmonary edema. Indeed, ICU chest films are usually taken at the bedside, with portable, low power, large focal spot X-ray machines on patients who may not be able to cooperate. Furthermore, radiographic signs of pulmonary edema can be simulated or obliterated to various degrees by circulatory or respiratory movements, if the exposure time is too

Mode of ventilation	Peak inflation pressure	Type of ventilation
❑ spontaneous	.... cmH₂O	❑ C-PAP .... cmH₂O
❑ assisted		❑ Bi-PAP .... cmH₂O
❑ controlled		❑ PEEP .... cmH₂O
Patient's position	**Tube to film distance**	**Technique**
❑ supine	.... cm	❑ mAs: ....
❑ semi-recumbent		❑ kV: ....
❑ sitting		
❑ upright		

Figure 24.1. Adhesive label that can be attached to each intensive care unit film. *C-PAP*, continuous positive airway pressure; *Bi-PAP*, bi-level positive airway pressure; *PEEP*, positive end-expiratory pressure; *mAs*, milli-ampere per second; kV, kilovolt.

long. The clinical usefulness of ICU chest radiography has been evaluated in a series of 200 consecutive portable chest roentgenograms (69). Only 6% of the films were of such poor quality as to be of no diagnostic utility. On the other hand, 43% of the radiographs showed "unexpected findings or findings on which changes in therapy were based" (69). In view of the wide utilization of the chest roentgenogram and its importance in assessing the clinical status of patients with pulmonary edema (39,70,71) it seems reasonable, instead of rejecting a priori the information that can be derived from bedside chest films, to set up simple arrangements that standardize the taking of the film and make it easier and more reliable to interpret (72).

The technologist performing the examination must be aware of the great importance of its contribution to the diagnosis and management of the critically ill patient. To avoid motion blurring, the radiographic technique should be directed toward the maximum tube output with the shortest exposure possible. The technical conditions should be kept constant when serial examinations are performed on the same patient. All of this information can be recorded on the X-ray film (Fig. 24.1), including the type of ventilation, and the peak and PEEP (72). With these data the film-reader can immediately increase the objectivity of the radiographic reading and can compare the patients' hemodynamics day by day and even hour by hour. It should be re-emphasized that standard training is not sufficient for interpreting ICU films, this necessitates a high level of physiologic knowledge (68,72).

Standardization of the Chest Radiographic Reading

The radiologic aspects of pulmonary edema have been extensively described (16,56,57,67,72–83), but the reading of the chest radiograph is still customarily based on a subjective judgment of the overall radiographic appearance. The lack of informed systematic analysis of all individual radiographic findings and of their characteristics and prevalence has generated the widespread erroneous belief that the chest X-ray interpretation in the ICU is too subjective to permit clinically accurate evaluation. There are many individual factors to be looked for, weighted and integrated in the detection, evaluation, and quantification of pulmonary edema and in the determination of its etiology (82). If these factors are not known to the film-reader, or are forgotten during the analysis, the interpretation may be quite incorrect. It is helpful when beginning to interpret ICU films to have a checklist (Table 24.1). The use of a checklist reduces both inter- and intraobserver variability.

Standardized and informed reading of the chest roentgenogram may permit the integration of various X-ray findings into specific patterns indicating the underlying cause of edema (30,57–59,71,72,82,84–86). Furthermore, it may enable the clinician to grade the severity of both hydrostatic and injury pulmonary edema by using numerical X-ray scoring techniques (30,57,58,71,72,82,84).

The radiographic features that we used initially to detect and quantify hydrostatic pulmonary edema included hilar abnormalities, septal lines, micronoduli, thickening of fissures, peribronchial and perivascular cuffings, blurring of vessel margins, subpleural effusions, and diffuse increase of density (Table 24.2) Our initial method of

Table 24.1. Format for the standardized reading of chest radiography in patients with pulmonary edema

Radiographic features
1. Heart size and hilar abnormalities
2. Size of the vascular pedicle and azygos vein
3. Size of the intrapulmonary vessels
4. Pleural effusion
5. Interstitial edema
   Blurring of intrapulmonary vessels
   Peribronchial cuffs
   Kerley's lines (A, B, C)
   Widening of fissures
   Increased lung density (hazy)
6. Alveolar edema
   Air bronchograms
   Increased lung density (patchy)
   Extensive white density

Table 24.2. Radiographic scoring list of pulmonary edema

Hydrostatic		Injury[b]	
X-ray finding	Score[a]	X-ray finding	Score[a]
Hilar vessels abnormalities		Right-sided cardiac enlargement with bulging of main pulmonary artery	2,4
Size	1,2,3		
Density	2,4,6		
Blurring	3,6,9		
Blurring of intrapulmonary vessels	4,8,12	Hilar vessel abnormalities (size and density)	1,2
Peribronchial cuffing	4,8,12	Air bronchogram	2,4
Kerley's lines		Increased lung density (hazy)	
A	4,8		
B	4,8	Central	1,2
C	4,8	Peripheral	2,4
		Central and peripheral	3,6
Widening of fissures	4,8	Increased lung density	
		Central	2,4
		Peripheral	5,10
		Central and peripheral	7,14
Increased lung density (hazy)	5,10,15	Extensive white density	20

[a] Each X-ray finding is scored when present, the higher the intensity of the X-ray finding, the higher the score attributed; [b] each lung is scored separately.

Table 24.3. Rapid quantification of hydrostatic pulmonary edema

1. Clarity of vessel margins
2. Peribronchial cuffing
3. Change in lung lucency
4. Visibility of subsegmental vessels

grading hydrostatic pulmonary edema utilized eight of these factors and attached a weighted "score" to each sign, the level of the score depending upon the observer's estimate of the severity of that sign (Table 24.2). The scores were added to give a total numerical index of the severity of the edema and the actual quantity of lung water present. This rigorous approach is of particular value in physiologic/radiologic correlation experiments (30,56–58, 87) but is time consuming. Consequently, we have developed a quicker approach (Table 24.3) for use in daily clinical practice, embodying only four factors and allowing us to grade hydrostatic pulmonary edema on the basis of their prominence (30,88,89). Comparison between the two film-reading methodologies demonstrates a significant correlation in quantifying pulmonary edema on 210 chest films obtained in cardiac patients (30). This finding confirmed that the simplified rapid assessment technique is quite accurate for clinical purposes.

The radiographic appearance of injury and hydrostatic edema differ in many respects (2,9,11,12,90), and the criteria for quantifying injury edema must therefore differ from those for hydrostatic edema. It is important to realize that the scores reported in the table cannot be directly related to absolute quantities of pulmonary edema because, first, no satisfactorily non-radiological method presently exists for the accurate in vivo quantification of injury edema that would calibrate with the radiographic estimate. Second, in ARDS the radiographic changes are caused not only by injury but also by areas of atelectasis, vascular occlusion, hemorrhage, hyaline membranes and fibrosis. Finally, in ARDS the increase in lung water does not develop gradually, as in hydrostatic edema, beginning with a clear interstitial phase and progressing in recognizable and quantifiable alveolar edema, but instead tends to appear quite abruptly. It is usually difficult to identify a separate interstitial phase but it appears from its onset to be a mixture of interstitial and alveolar edema and, usually, to assume its final degree of severity almost immediately. For these reasons any method, whether radiologic or not, aimed at assessing the quantity of pulmonary edema in ARDS is unlikely to be of much value in either the early detection or the later follow-up of the syndrome (30). In addition, in the early stage of lung injury, the turnover of fluid and solutes through the interstitial/lymphatic system may be increased substantially before any increase in extravascular lung water can be detected (30).

The radiographic score for injury edema (Table 24.2) is based on the presence, regional distribution, extent, and intensity of features including right-sided cardiac enlargement and bulging of the main pulmonary artery, changes in the size and density of the hila, the presence of air bronchograms, changes in lung density and the regional distribution of these density changes. Indeed, some of these features (i.e., right-sided cardiac enlargement, enlarged main pulmonary artery) may actually precede the onset of radiologically detectable edema (30). Each of the radiologic features in the Table 24.2 carries a set of weighting numbers, according to its severity, and the sum of all these numbers gives an index to the severity of the injury edema. The terms reported in the Table 24.2 to describe qualitatively the patterns of radiographic increase in lung density match with three degrees of lung involvement: (a) mixed interstitial and alveolar edema ("hazy", i.e., ill-defined, partially radioopaque densities that still allow the underlying vascular structures to be seen); (b) alveolar edema ("patchy", i.e., scattered radioopaque densities that completely obscure the underlying vascular structures locally); and (c) extensive lung consolidation ("extensive white density"). A peripheral distribution of increased lung density is given a higher score than central distribution because it represents a more severe degree of involvement of the gas exchange sites (30). It is important to point out that in the scoring procedure each lung must be considered separately, since lung injury edema is often asymmetric or even unilateral (30).

Heart and Hilar Vessel Abnormalities

The radiographic appearances of the heart and hilar vessels may constitute important clues for the understanding of cardiopulmonary pathophysiology in patients with cardiogenic edema or ARDS. Heart shape and size can be characterized in terms of right heart enlargement, left heart enlargement, and joint right and left heart enlargement. Hilar vessel abnormalities can be described radiographically by the size, density, and sharpness of the large vessels radiating from the lung hilum.

In patients with hydrostatic lung edema, the heart is usually enlarged and the hilar vessels are increased in size and density with loss of sharpness (blurring) of their borders (57,58) (Figs. 24.2, 24.3, 24.4). Whereas increased size and density of the hilar vessels may reflect, together with heart enlargement, the underlying central hemodynamic alteration, blurring of the hilar (and intrapulmonary) vessels can be considered a specific sign of interstitial pulmonary edema. For this reason, blurring of hilar vessels is assigned a higher numerical value in the hydrostatic edema scoring table (Table 24.2).

Normality in size and shape of the heart is widely reported in injury lung edema (19,30,67,81,82,86,91,92).

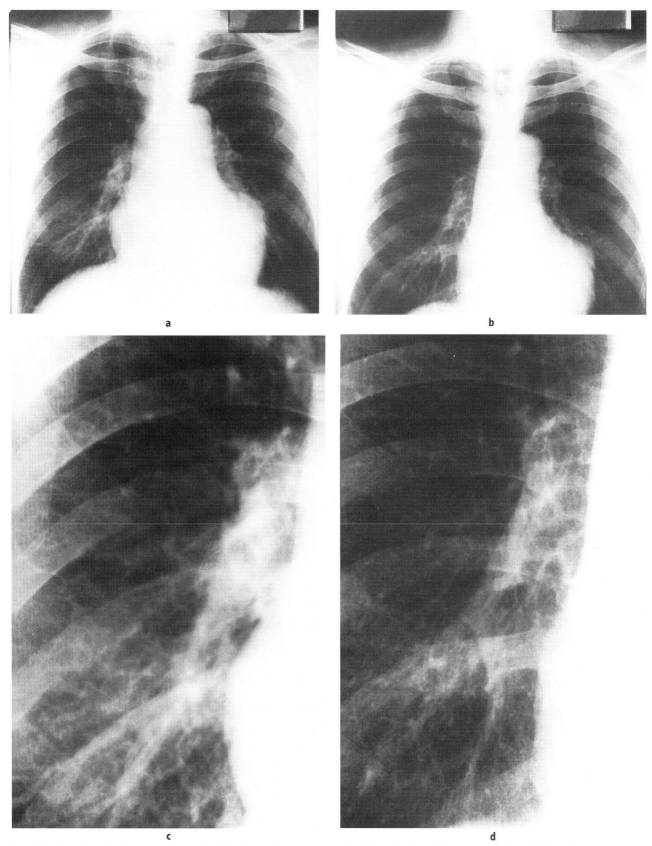

Figure 24.2. Chest radiographs of a 71 year old man affected by chronic ischemic cardiomiopathy. **a** Radiograph obtained during an episode of acute left heart decompensation shows enlargement of the right and left heart cavities. Bulging of the left ventricle is due to aneurysmatic dilatation. The main radiographic findings are: enlargement of the vascular pedicle and azygos vein; increased size, density, and blurring of the hilar vessels; peribronchial cuffings in both perihilar regions; blurring of the intrapulmonary vessels; Kerley's B lines at the right lung base; and increased lung density (hazy) in the mid–lower regions of the right lung. **b** Radiograph obtained 5 days later (with the same technical factors as **a**) showing striking reduction of all radiographic findings described in **a**. Particularly evident is the reduction in size of the heart, the vascular pedicle, and the azygos vein. **c** and **d** Close-up views of **a** and **b**, respectively, showing marked reduction of size, density and blurring of hilar vessels. A concomitant reduction of blurring of intrapulmonary vessels can be seen. The radiographic scoring of pulmonary edema (see Table 24.2, hydrostatic) in the original film was as follows: hilar vessels abnormalities: size 2, density 4, blurring 6; blurring of intrapulmonary vessels 4; peribronchial cuffs 4; Kerley's B lines 8; increased lung density (hazy) 5. Total score: 33.

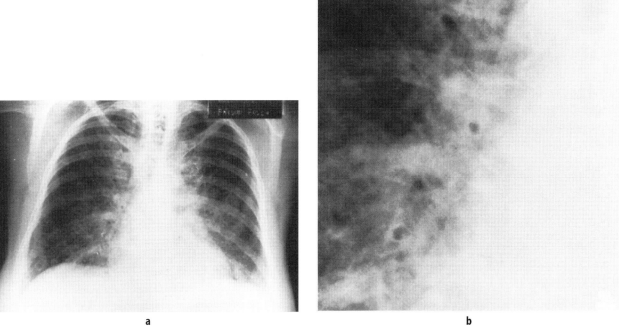

Figure 24.3. Chest radiographs of a 61 year old woman with angina pectoris. **a** The chest radiograph, obtained while the patient was experiencing chest pain and dyspnea, shows blurring of hilar vessels with widespread peribronchial cuffing (showed in detail in **b**), and Kerley B lines in the right lung.

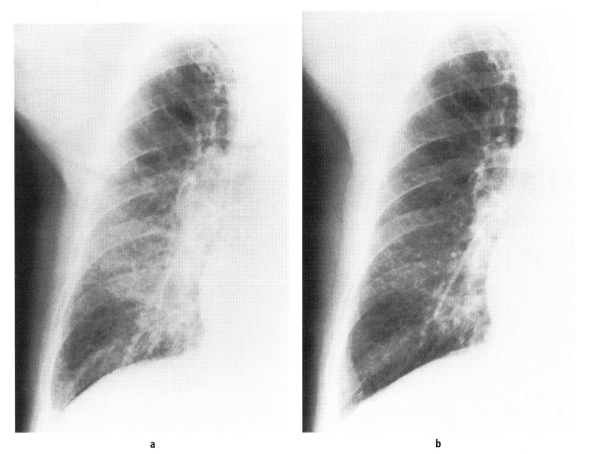

Figure 24.4. Right lung of a patient with chronic ischemic cardiomyopathy, radiographed during acute left heart decompensation (**a**), and 24 h later (**b**). The radiographs were obtained with the same technical factors. During decompensation (**a**) hilar vessels are increased in size and density and blurred. Upper lobe pulmonary vessels (arteries and veins) are increased in size. Lung density is increased. The pulmonary wedge pressure, obtained at the same time, was 31 mmHg. The day after (**b**), upper lobe vessels are still dilatated while the radiographic findings of pulmonary interstitital edema are markedly reduced and the wedge pressure had returned to within normal limits (8 mmHg).

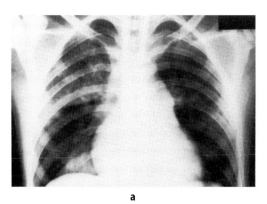 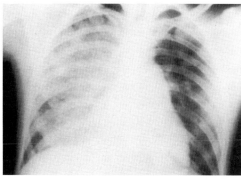

a   b

Figure 24.5. Chest radiographs of a 14 year old male with adult respiratory distress syndrome following head trauma and long bone fractures. **a** Main feature of the chest radiograph obtained 2 days after trauma is the right-sided cardiac enlargement with bulging of the main pulmonary artery. The radiographic scoring of pulmonary edema (see Table 24.2. injury) is as follows: right-sided cardiac enlargement with bulging of the main pulmonary artery 4. Right lung: hilar vessels abnormalities 2: air bronchogram 2: increased lung density (patchy) 7. Left lung: hilar vessels abnormalities 1: increased lung density (hazy) 2. Total score (right + left lung) 18. **b** In the chest radiograph obtained 2 days later the radiographic picture of adult respiratory distress syndrome is fully developed. Right-sided cardiac enlargement with bulging of the main pulmonary artery 4. Right lung: hilar vessels abnormalities 2: air bronchogram 4: extensive white density 20. Left lung: hilar vessels abnormalities 1: increased lung density (hazy) 6. Total score (right + left lung) 37.

However, in these patients we frequently observed a right-sided heart enlargement with bulging of the second arch on the left cardiac border (i.e., the main pulmonary artery) (30,58,82,85,86) (Fig. 24.5). Bulging of the main pulmonary artery is the most reliable sign of right-sided cardiac involvement, being less influenced by such factors as supine position, loss of lung volume, and increased circulating blood volume, than the right heart border (82). This radiographic finding, which generally occurs together with increased size and density of the hilar vessels, indicates elevated pulmonary artery pressure and vascular resistance, both frequently reported in patients with ARDS (93–98). The highest prevalence of right-sided cardiac enlargement was found in patients with ARDS after trauma and was sometimes observed before the development of radiographic changes in the lung fields (58,85,86). As a matter of fact, early pulmonary hemodynamic alterations may precede the increase of lung microvascular permeability in experimental and clinical ARDS (99–104), and this could be particularly relevant in patients with trauma, in whom massive sympathetic discharge (105–107) and bone marrow microemboli (108,109) could trigger an increase in pulmonary vascular resistance.

Right-sided cardiac enlargement and hilar vessels abnormalities (size and density) (Fig. 24.5) have been included in the injury edema radiographic score (Table 24.2) because of their value in the early detection of ARDS, but have been assigned a low numerical value, since they cannot be considered, per se, specific signs of the syndrome. Loss of definition of the hilar borders (blurring) and other radiographic signs of interstitial pulmonary edema are not considered in the injury scoring table because, as is discussed later, they are relatively seldom encountered in the chest roentgenograms of patients with ARDS.

Size of the Vascular Pedicle and Azygos Vein

In addition to the pulmonary vessels some of the largest systemic arteries and veins in the body can be seen on the chest radiograph. The right and left boundaries of the upper mediastinum on the frontal chest roentgenogram are formed, respectively, by the superior vena cava draining into the right atrium and the left subclavian artery arising from the aortic arch. The vena azygos can be seen, within the shadow of the superior vena cava, as an ovoid opacity lying just above the right main bronchus (Fig. 24.6).

The "vascular pedicle" of the heart is a term introduced to indicate the great vascular structures from which the heart is virtually suspended within the thorax (30,82, 110–112). It has been shown that changes in the width of the vascular pedicle correlate very closely with changes in systemic blood volume, while the width of the azygos vein can be used as a rough estimate of the right atrial pressure (30,82,112) (Fig. 24.2, 24.6). This information, which can be easily and accurately extracted from the chest radiograph, is of great assistance in evaluating fluid balance in ICU and renal patients (30,58,59,72,82).

The vascular pedicle and azygos vein are usually enlarged in overhydrated patients (113) or in the presence of renal failure with liquid and salt retention. Furthermore, an estimate of the amount as well as of the changes with time of the systemic blood volume may help in determining the correct therapeutic approach in cardiac patients, in whom a wide range of alterations in circulating blood volume, from reduced to highly increased, are known to occur (112–116). Vascular pedicle width can therefore be usefully integrated with other clinical and instrumental data to establish whether excess in body fluids is to be considered or excluded as a concomitant factor in pulmonary edema development.

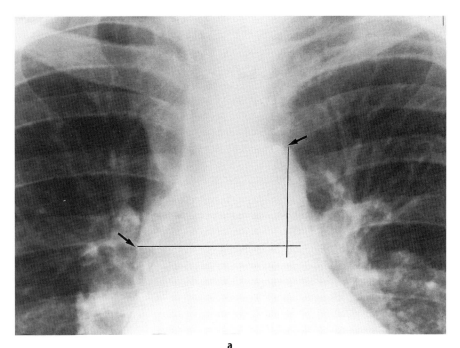

a

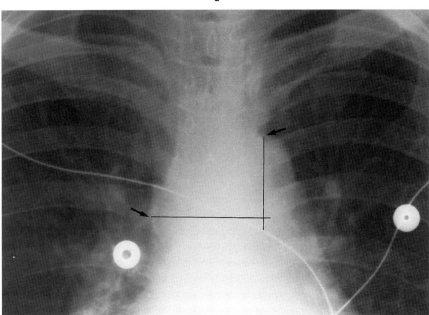

b

Figure 24.6. Close-up views of a chest radiograph of a 56 year old patient with renal failure. Vascular pedicle width and azygos vein size before (**a**) and after (**b**) dialysis. Measuring point for vascular pedicle width are: *1*, the point where the superior vena cava crosses the right main bronchus, and *2*, the take-off point of left subclavian artery from the aortic arch. Vascular pedicle width is measured from point *1* to a perpendicular dropped from point *2*. In the original radiographs, vascular pedicle width was 70 and 56 mm before and after dialysis, respectively. Azygos vein width was 12 and 5 mm, respectively.

Vascular pedicle and azygos vein dimensions, together with the size of intrapulmonary vessels, are not considered in the quantification tables. These findings are very important for evaluating the patient's hemodynamic status and in determining the cause of the patient's edema, but cannot be directly correlated with the severity of pulmonary edema.

Size of the Intrapulmonary Vessels

The radiographic pattern of the normal lung is formed almost entirely by arteries and veins. Although it is impos-

sible to quantify pulmonary blood flow in absolute terms from chest radiographs, the qualitative information that can be derived from general and regional variations in the calibre of pulmonary arteries and veins is of great value in detecting and specifying pathophysiologic alterations in the pulmonary circulation (83,117–119).

The relative size of upper and lower lobe vessels can be used as a qualitative index of pulmonary blood flow distribution, which can be classified as normal, balanced, or inverted (82,117–119). In order to perform a correct evaluation of the relative calibre of upper and lower lung vessels, it is of particular relevance to know the patient's exact position at the time the film was taken.

A visual estimate of pulmonary blood volume, both general and regional, from reduced (oligemic) to increased (hyperemic), can be given by looking at the size, density, and peripheral visibility of the vascular markings.

Chronic elevation of pulmonary venous pressure causes a reduction in flow through the bases of the lungs, with redistribution of flow to the upper lobes resulting in an inversion of the normal base to apex gravitational gradient (Fig. 24.4). It bas been suggested that redistribution of blood flow in left heart failure is due to compression or reduced traction of lower lung vessels by interstitial pulmonary edema (120). This is at variance with both experimental (121–123) and clinical (57,124–127) observations, showing that this pattern of flow inversion does not take place simply because of the presence of interstitial pulmonary edema (witness the absence of any flow inversion even with severe edema in renal failure or overhydration), but requires that there be elevation of left heart pressure and that this be longstanding. In patients with acute myocardial infarction, the distribution of pulmonary blood flow is usually normal or balanced, whereas, in left heart valvular disease and chronic ischemic heart failure, inversion of flow occurs almost invariably. Redistribution of blood flow as assessed by lung perfusion scan is closely correlated with pulmonary vascular resistance (126,127) and it is observed frequently in the absence of radiographic signs of interstitial pulmonary edema (57) (Fig. 24.4). Once organic changes of the pulmonary circulation, such as those often occurring at the lung bases in chronic obstructive lung disease, have been excluded, flow inversion can be used as a reliable sign of central hemodynamic dysfunction. The degree of redistribution can be correlated to the severity and duration of the hemodynamic alterations.

It is evident that the older theory that interstitial edema at the lung bases was the cause of flow inversion is incorrect. Flow inversion in chronic elevation of left heart pressure could reflect the well-documented organic changes in the basal lung microvasculature occurring with longstanding elevation of left heart pressure (128–131). A different mechanism for flow inversion has recently been postulated that appears to fit all of the clinical, temporal and radiologic findings (132). The theory proposed is that vasoconstriction of the lower lobe vessels occurs to prevent the increasing reflux of blood into the pulmonary veins, which would normally occur as left atrial outflow resistance is increased. This vasoconstriction, mediated by a reflex arc from the left atrium to the pulmonary vessels, increases the resistance to backflow and permits the left atrium to continue to pump an adequate amount of blood into the left ventricle. The theory fits well with the observation that inversion does not occur with acute left heart failure (where the left atrium is still strong and capable of overcoming the raised left ventricular end-diastolic pressure), and does not usually occur until the left atrium weakens and dilatates (well seen in mitral stenosis), and cannot otherwise maintain flow into the left ventricle. This theory fits also with the observation that flow inversion does not occur even with severe pulmonary edema in renal failure or overhydration, where there is no significant elevation in left heart pressure, and by the fact that flow inversion has never been reported to occur following cardiac transplantation (which severs all the nerve connections), no matter how severe or longstanding the failure (132).

Increased vascularity (size, density, and peripheral visibility of vessels) of the lung fields, without inversion of the normal gravitational pulmonary vascular pattern, can be often observed in patients with renal failure or overhydration (58,59). In these patients the radiographic findings of increased pulmonary blood volume indicating elevated circulating blood volume are usually associated with the enlargement of the vascular pedicle.

Assessment of pulmonary blood volume as well as distribution are affected by high inter-observer variability (59). The reader's training and expertise are of utmost importance in the evaluation of these findings.

Pleural Effusion

Pleural effusions are commonly seen in the chest roentgenograms of patients with both cardiac and overhydration pulmonary edema (Fig. 24.4), but are much rarer in injury edema (58,59,85,86).

There is clinical evidence that pleural fluid accumulation in patients with left heart failure is closely correlated with the elevation of left atrial pressure and with the quantity of pulmonary edema present (82,133,134). Increased pressure in the visceral subpleural capillaries, secondary to elevated pulmonary venous pressure, results in increased fluid filtration, particularly at the bases where the pulmonary venous pressure is highest. This edema will increase the subpleural interstitial pressure of the lung causing transudation of edema across the pleura into the pleural space. In contrast, in injury edema, due to damage of the alveolar epithelium, the extravasated liquid with a high protein content recruits the alveolar space rather than the pleura. As a consequence, pleural effusions are seldom encountered and, if present, they are of smaller size than those observed in hydrostatic edema (15).

Pleural effusion does not arise from an isolated increase in right heart pressure (133–135), unless the elevation in pressure is associated with low plasma protein oncotic pressure (136), or with ascites, which very frequently transgresses the right diaphragm to cause a right pleural effusion.

Contrary to the common belief that in left heart failure effusions are predominantly right sided, it has been observed that pleural liquid accumulation is usually bilateral and in some cases it may be more evident on the left hemithorax (72). The quantity of pleural effusion increases with the severity of the radiographic aspects of pulmonary edema (82,134). However, both formation and

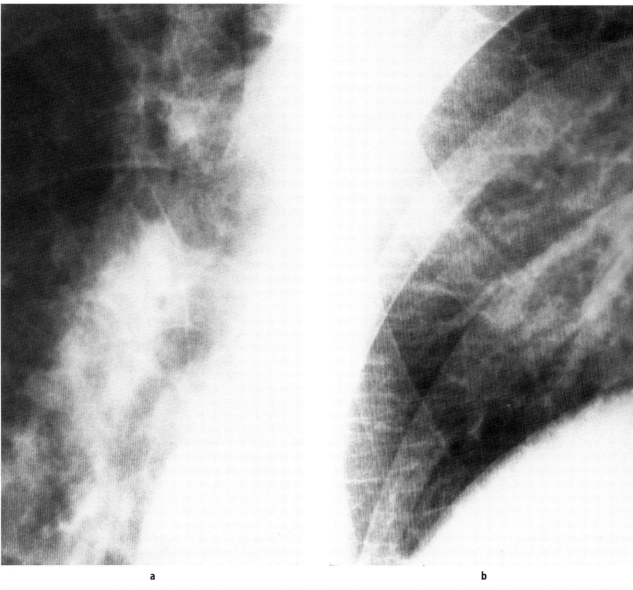

a   b

Figure 24.7. Close-up views of radiographs obtained in three patients with acute left heart decompensation showing Kerley's septal lines A in the right perihilar region (a), Kerley's septal lines B on the lower right costophrenic angle (b), (contd)

clearance of effusion "lag" behind the development and clearing of edema; therefore changes in size of the pleural effusion do not always temporally parallel changes in the quantity of pulmonary edema (137).

Interstitial Pulmonary Edema

As fluid begins to fill the loose connective tissue of the peribronchovascular sheaths, the vessels margins become progressively blurred and, where the peribronchial sheaths can be seen end-on (usually at the center of the lungs), the sheaths begin to increase in thickness, causing peribronchial cuffs to appear (Fig. 24.3). Excess fluid within interlobular and interlobar septa causes the formation of Kerley's lines (Fig. 24.7) and the widening of the fissures, respectively. Blurring of the intrapulmonary vessels is

often observed together with loss of definition of hilar borders (Fig. 24.2) (57). A micronodular pattern may be seen when cuffing of medium-sized vessels is seen end-on (57,75).

Peribronchial cuffs are one of the most frequent radiographic findings in patients with hydrostatic pulmonary edema (30,56–59,75,138). In addition to the cuffing seen around the larger bronchi, increasing density of the peribronchial connective tissues may make end-on smaller bronchi, which are not usually seen, stand out (Fig. 24.3).

Septal lines were first described by Kerley (73,139,140), who subdivided them into those more frequently seen radiating from the hila in the upper and midportion of the lungs (A lines), those usually seen at right angles to the pleural surface in the basal regions (B lines), and those, less frequently seen, forming a reticular pattern in the central and basal portions of the lungs (C lines)

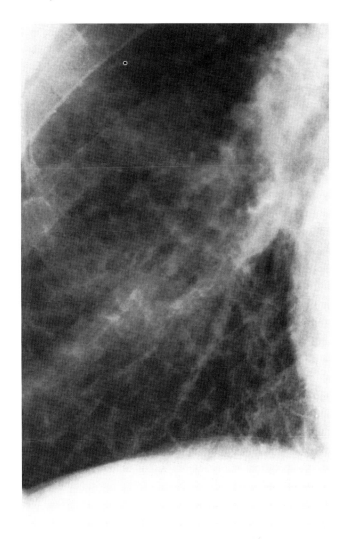

c

Figure 24.7. (*contd*) and Kerley's septal lines C on the right cardiophrenic angle (c).

(Figs. 24.2, 24.3, 24.7). The different radiographic appearance of the lines may be due to the different anatomic arrangement of the interlobular septa in different portions of the lung (141). Kerley's lines can disappear after improvement of left heart function. A and C lines are more commonly associated with acute or recent fluid collection, and B lines are seen in more chronic interstitial engorgement (57,76,142–145,82).

The horizontal fissure of the right lung is frequently denser and thicker during pulmonary edema than in normal conditions. Additionally, accessory fissures not usually seen may become widened and visible, in particular the right basal medial accessory fissure (57,146).

When water accumulates diffusely throughout the interstitial space of the lung, a hazy pattern of increased lung density can be observed (Figs. 24.2, 24.3, 24.4, 24.7) (56,57,75,147). Since there is still air in the alveoli, the lung vessels can still be seen, whereas with alveolar edema no air is present in the affected area of the lung and no lung structure (vessels) can be seen, i.e., the principal difference between interstitial and alveolar edema is that in the latter no lung structure can be seen. Haziness of lung fields may occur immediately prior to the development of alveolar edema (148) and sometimes it may be associated with scattered radiographic findings of airspace involvement (57). In hydrostatic lung edema the hazy texture of the lung fields is usually bilateral and gravitationally distributed to the basal regions (56–58,75,76,148– 151). Considering the horizontal axis of the lung, the increased lung density is evenly distributed from the periphery to the central regions in cardiac patients, whereas in overhydration or renal failure the central regions tend to be more involved and the periphery clearer (58,59,82).

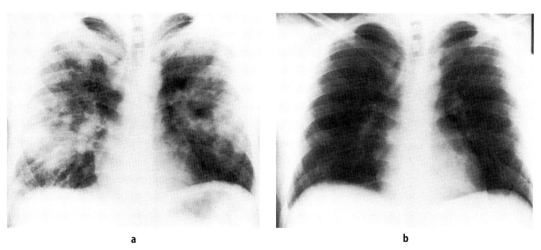

Figure 24.8. Chest radiographs of a 21 year old male who developed adult respiratory distress syndrome in the course of viral pneumonia. **a** The chest radiograph obtained in the acute phase shows right-sided cardiac enlargement (score 2), increased size and density of the hilar vessels (score 2 + 2), and patchy, bilateral, predominantly peripheral increase of lung density (score 10 + 10). Total score (right + left lung) 26. **b** One week later the chest radiograph (obtained with the same technical factors) demonstrates complete recovery. Of particular relevance is the striking decrease in size and density of the hilar vessels, as compared with the acute phase.

Radiographic findings of fluid accumulation in the interstitial space are invariably present in patients with hydrostatic lung edema and can be used for the early diagnosis of interstitial edema and for grading its severity (30,57,58,70,82). In patients with pulmonary edema secondary to injury to the alveolocapillary barrier, the chest radiographic pattern does not usually follow the characteristic sequence observed in hydrostatic edema (i.e., beginning as an interstitial process and later becoming alveolar); rather, alveolar space involvement develops abruptly, forming a patchy, randomly distributed pattern (with a tendency toward peripheral location), usually not associated with hilar blurring, peribronchovascular cuffs, and Kerley's lines (Figs. 24.5, 24.8, 24.9,) (57,58,70,85, 86,90).

For this reason the injury lung edema scoring list, with the exception of heart and hilar vessel abnormalities, is mostly made up of radiographic findings of alveolar edema and is of more value for the grading of lung involvement in the course of ARDS than for the early detection of the syndrome.

Alveolar Pulmonary Edema

Filling of airspaces by edema fluid causes the formation on the chest roentgenogram of patchy confluent areas of consolidation and air bronchograms (Figs. 24.5, 24.8, 24.9). A patchy increase of density can be defined as a shaped density obscuring the underlying lung structures. When consolidation entirely involves the lung fields it can be described as extensive white density (Fig. 24.9b). An air bronchogram can be defined as the cast of the intra-

parenchymal airways made visible by the increased density of the surrounding lung tissue (Fig. 24.9c) (152).

In the injury scoring table, patterns of increased lung density (hazy and patchy) are scored according to their regional distribution (Table 24.2). Peripheral distribution is given a higher score than central distribution, since it represents a more severe degree of involvement of the gas exchange sites (57–59). Extensive consolidation (white density) is assigned the highest score (Table 24. 2). Unlike in patients with hydrostatic pulmonary edema, lung involvement is often unilateral and asymmetric in patients with ARDS (58,85,86). For this reason, each lung has to be considered separately in the injury scoring system.

Radiographic Differentiation between Hydrostatic and Injury Lung Edema

From what has been discussed in the previous sections it appears that the different pathophysiologic mechanisms underlying hydrostatic and injury lung edema may explain the different radiographic patterns observed (58,59,72,82,85,86,90). The whole spectrum of pulmonary edema, with few exceptions of rare clinical occurrence, is included in three main categories: (a) left heart decompensation, (b) renal failure with fluid and salt retention or iatrogenic overhydration, and (c) injury to the alveolocapillary barrier. Although no single radiographic criterion allows an accurate differentiation among pulmonary edema etiologic categories, several findings can be combined in radiographic patterns which may be helpful in defining the predominant etiopathogenetic factor. The chest radiographic features encountered in the above described three categories of

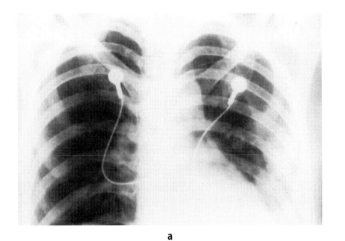
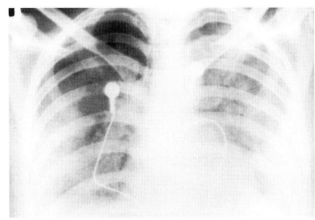

a

b

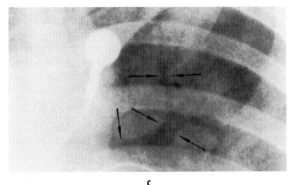

c

Figure 24.9. Chest radiographs of a 28 year old woman with adult respiratory distress syndrome after head trauma. **a** Chest radiograph showing patchy increase of density in the peripheral regions of the left lung. Total score 10. **b** One week later, the chest radiograph shows extensive white density in both lungs (score 20 + 20) and air bronchograms (score 4 + 4), especially in the upper regions of the left lung. Total score 48. **c.** Close-up view of the upper regions of the left lung showing air bronchogram (*arrows*). Note the difference between air bronchogram and peribronchial cuffing seen in Fig. 24.3.

patients with pulmonary edema may be summarized as follows. Patients with ARDS are characterized by a higher incidence of normal heart size, few hilar abnormalities, normal pulmonary blood flow distribution, absence of septal lines, rare occurrence of peribronchial cuffs and pleural effusions, and very frequent air bronchograms. Unlike cardiac or renal/overhydration patients, whose radiographs often feature a mild generalized haziness of the lung fields, increased lung density in patients with ARDS could have a nongravitational patchy appearance and a peripheral distribution. The peripheral distribution of pulmonary edema in ARDS has been sporadically reported (153–155) and has been confirmed by computed tomography in a canine model of ARDS (156). In cardiac patients, inversion of pulmonary blood flow and a trend toward an "even" (from the chest wall to the heart) distribution of edema occurs compared with renal/overhydration and injury patients. The distinctive features of renal/overhydration patients with pulmonary edema are an enlarged vascular pedicle, a balanced pulmonary blood flow distribution, increased pulmonary blood volume, and a central distribution of edema. This latter finding is in agreement with various reports in which the inner regions of the lungs were found to be affected to a greater extent than the outer regions (77–79,157).

The scoring lists of Table 24.2 reflect the different radiographic patterns of hydrostatic and injury lung edema. After the main cause of pulmonary edema has been identified by integrating standardized reading of the chest roentgenogram with history and other clinical and instrumental examinations, each roentgenogram should be scored according to the presence and the intensity of the various X-ray findings listed. The assignment of a number to the presence of each specific X-ray finding tends to make the scoring procedure relatively independent from the reader's subjectivity, since appreciating the presence or the absence of a sign is mostly a matter of training. On the other hand, the evaluation of the intensity of each sign renders the procedure more sensitive to the degree of edema, even if more dependent on the reader's interpretation (57,58). Variability about the mean value of the scores given by two independent observers has been found to be very low when the film-readers were trained to recognize the various radiographic findings (57–59). The total score of each roentgenogram is derived from the summation of the individual scores assigned to the presence and the intensity of each of the X-ray findings encountered and can be used to evaluate the severity of pulmonary edema and to correlate the chest radiographic appearance with other physiologic measurements (30,57,58,87).

Other Imaging Techniques

The chest radiography, if it is of adequate quality (taken by a technologist trained in ICU radiology, and interpreted by a film-reader trained in physiologic interpretation) remains the fundamental imaging procedure for the assessment of pulmonary edema. However, several more recently developed imaging modalities, such as computed tomography, positron emission tomography, and magnetic resonance imaging, can provide additional information in selected cases.

Computed Tomography

Computed tomography (CT) has the capacity to provide a quantitative estimate of the amount of pulmonary edema; because air has an attenuation of –1000 Hounsfield units, (HU) and water of 0 HU, CT densitometry and area measurements can be used to calculate the changes in lung water, lung weight, lung density, and distribution of pathology in both hydrostatic and injury edema (41–43, 158). By using CT, Slutski and co-workers (159) were able to demonstrate an excellent correlation between dependent lung density and left ventricular end-diastolic pressure in patients with cardiac failure. In one study performed in patients with ARDS, objective measurements of lung density were found to be highly correlated with parameters of severity of the syndrome, including the chest radiograph (87). CT scan can also be used to calculate the vertical gradient in lung inflation in patients who have ARDS (160). In general, the clinical use of both CT and high resolution CT in hydrostatic edema seems limited to only those patients in whom diagnosis is in question or in whom complications are suspected (41). Topographic information obtained by CT reveals that hydrostatic edema and renal pulmonary edema tends to be associated with a perihilar and gravitational distribution, whereas injury edema tends to be distributed in the peripheral portions of the lung (156,161). This information has led to a better understanding of the distinguishing characteristics of hydrostatic and injury pulmonary edema as visualized by conventional chest X-ray. As on conventional radiography, in hydrostatic pulmonary edema there is a disproportionate enlargement of nondependent arteries and veins, smooth thickening of the interlobular septa, subpleural connective tissue and peribronchial connective tissue (Fig. 24.10). Areas of ground-glass attenuation can result from interstitial or airspace edema, whereas consolidation reflects the presence of airspace edema and bronchial flooding (41,42,162) (Fig. 24.10). Pleural and pericardial effusions are more easily detected than on standard radiographs (Fig. 24.10) (43, 162). Recently, the sensitivity of high resolution CT in detecting heart failure

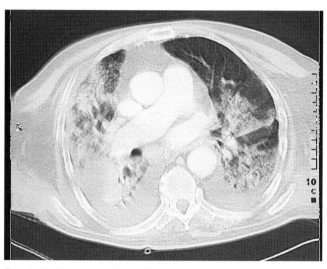

Figure 24.10. High resolution CT scan of the lung obtained in a 86 year old patient with chronic left heart failure during an acute episode of decompensation with massive pulmonary edema. Bilateral pleural effusion and right perihilar consolidation associated to gravitationally distributed ground-glass opacification are the more relevant findings. No air bronchogram is visible.

was tested by one group who performed scans at rest and after treadmill exercise in 10 normal subjects, in 10 patients who had mild heart failure (NYHA 1), and in 10 who had moderate failure (NYHA 2 and 3) (163). After exercise, they found that patients who had moderate heart failure developed signs of interstitial pulmonary edema, including the presence of a pulmonary artery-to-bronchial diameter ratio greater than 1 in the upper lobes, a peripheral increase in vascular markings, interlobular septal thickening, and peribronchial cuffing (163). In another study, pulmonary diffusion capacity and CT were performed in a group of elite athletes after a triathlon; the diffusion capacity decreased and the CT showed evidence of increased interstitial attenuation consistent with edema (164). Pulmonary interstitial edema has also been revealed in the chest radiograph of trained cyclists after prolonged high intensity exercise at altitude (165).

The CT scan, when combined with a measurement of lung gas volume, is very useful to assess lung weight in vivo in patients with severe ARDS (166) and may then be of value to grade the severity of ARDS.

In ARDS, CT findings are dependent on the stage at which the examination is performed. As a general rule, within the first few hours after injury, the CT scan often shows predominantly peripheral consolidation or mild ground-glass opacification (diffuse or patchy) and an exaggeration of the gravity-dependent lung density gradient (43,158) (Fig. 24.11). During the second and third day of the exudative phase, CT usually shows more uniform opacification and limited pleural effusions. Unlike severe left heart failure, there is usually no perihilar or basilar predominance. The heart and pulmonary

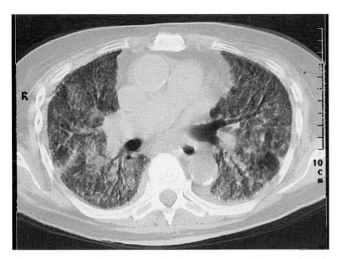

Figure 24.11. High resolution CT scan of the lung in an 84 year old patient who had suffered intracerebral hemorrhage 4 days earlier. Diffuse nongravitationally evenly distributed ground-glass opacification with evident air bronchograms are the more relevant findings. Subtle left pleural effusion is visible.

vessels are normal and there are frequent air bronchograms (Fig. 24.11). After several weeks CT evidence of fibrosis includes linear bands, distortion cysts, and traction bronchiectasis. During the fibrotic phase there is often a decrease in overall lung density and the appearance of interstitial reticulation (43).

As with conventional chest radiography, mechanical ventilation can markedly alter the CT features of ARDS (43,167). Because the involvement of the lung is often patchy, PEEP tends to inflate the uninvolved normally compliant regions but does not alter the volume of the densely consolidated regions. Less consolidated (ground-glass) or atelectatic areas of the lung may show an increase in aeration if the applied PEEP exceeds a critical opening pressure (167). This patchy inflation is the reason why application of high levels of PEEP and/or high tidal volumes frequently result in barotrauma in these patients (167).

Positron Emission Tomography

A number of investigative procedures, entailing the use of positron emission tomography (PET), have been described and validated for the study of the pathophysiology of pulmonary edema (45–49). By combining PET scanning of injected or inhaled positron-emitting isotopes with transmission scanning, it is possible to derive sensitive and accurate quantitative regional measurements of water, blood flow, hematocrit, extravascular density and vascular permeability of the lung (46–49, 168, 169). Compared with CT, which depicts the regional distribution of whole lung density and is unable to separate out the intra- and extravascular components, PET has the advantage of displaying intra- and extravascular lung density separately (45,170,171). Meyer and colleagues (172) described a technique for measuring the volume for extravascular lung water based on the constant infusion of radioactive water to label the water pool, and the subsequent inhalation of ^{11}C-labelled carbon monoxide to label the blood pool. A validation was made by comparing the regional extravascular water measurements with global lung water measurements by an indicator dilution technique as well as with global gravimetric measurements (172). Schuster and colleagues (161) described a technique for measuring the volume of extravascular lung water by injection of a bolus of radioactive water followed by equilibration of the tracer. They found a good correlation between gravimetric measurements and values for extravascular lung water calculated by PET (161). Noticeably, in this study and others (161,168–172), the tomographic technique tended to slightly underestimate the actual volume of extravascular lung water. Wollmer and associates (170) reported the use of PET to evaluate patients with acute cardiogenic pulmonary edema. In patients with radiologic evidence of interstitial pulmonary edema and moderately elevated pulmonary vascular pressure, extravascular lung density was uniformly increased throughout the lungs. In patients with radiographic evidence of alveolar edema and significantly elevated pulmonary vascular pressure, extravascular lung density was significantly increased in the dependent regions of the lungs (170). Although the introduction of PET has made it possible, non-invasively, to derive, information from humans, similar to that obtained with destructive methods in experimental animals, the technique is expensive and available in only a few selected clinical centers; its role, therefore, is still limited to investigative studies.

Magnetic Resonance Imaging

Studies based on various experimental animal models that take into account proton density, T_1 and T_2 relaxation times have indicated that magnetic resonance imaging (MRI) techniques can detect, quantify and, to some extent, characterize pulmonary edema (50–55,173–178). MRI techniques are particularly attractive because, unlike other methods for measuring lung water, they are not invasive. However, MRI techniques cannot discriminate between intravascular and extravascular lung water. In this respect, the use of sodium MRI, in combination with proton imaging and the administration of an intravascular paramagnetic agent, has been suggested as a possible means for assessing the distribution of lung water between the two compartments (179). In particular, in this technique, hydrostatic pulmonary edema tended to distribute homogeneously throughout the lung, while noncardiogenic pulmonary edema tended to occur predominantly in the peripheral portions of the lung (179). Recently, Caruthers and coworkers (54), in an animal model, developed a three-dimensional gradient-echo MRI technique to measure pulmonary edema and lung microvascular permeability and compared it with other conventional methods. The authors demonstrated that this method not only visualizes edema but also quantifies it and measures the time course of its development in vivo without using contrast agents or ionizing radiation (54).

At present, lack of mobility and the effects of the magnetic field on monitoring instruments and support equipment restrict the use of MRI in patients who are at high risk for pulmonary edema.

References

1. Staub NC (1974) Pulmonary edema. Physiol Rev 54 1:678–811.
2. Starling EH (1896) On the absorption of fluids from the connective tissue spaces. J Physiol (Lond) 19:312–326.
3. Renkin EM (1994) Cellular aspects of transvascular exchange: A 40-year perspective. Microcirculation 1:157–167.
4. Fishman AP (1972) Pulmonary edema. The water exchanging function of the lung. Circulation 46:390–408.
5. Staub NC (1980) The pathogenesis of pulmonary edema. Progr Cardiovasc Dis 23:53–80.
6. Murray JF (1985) The lungs and heart failure. Hosp Pract 4:55–68.
7. Taylor AE, Parker JC (1985) Pulmonary interstitial spaces and lymphatics. In Fishman AP, Fisher AB (eds) Handbook of physiology. The respiratory system I. American Physiological Society, Bethesda, MD, pp 167–230.
8. Ketai LH, Gowin JD (1998) A new view of pulmonary edema and acute respiratory distress syndrome. J Thorac Imaging 13:147–171.
9. Bhattacharya J, Gropper MA, Staub NC (1984) Interstitial fluid pressure gradient measured by micropuncture in excised dog lung. J Appl Physiol 56:271–277.
10. Gee MH, Spath JA, Jr (1980) The dynamics of the lung fluid filtration system in dogs with edema. Circ Res 46:796–801.
11. Bachofen M, Weibel ER (1982) Structural alterations of lung parenchyma in the adult respiratory distress syndrome. Clin Chest Med 3:35–36.
12. Montaner JSG, Tsang J, Evans KJ, et al. (1986) Alveolar epithelial damage. A critical difference between high pressure and oleic acid-induced low pressure pulmonary edema. J Clin Invest 77:1786–1796.
13. Matthay MA, Folkesson HG, Campagna A, et al. (1993) Alveolar epithelial barrier and acute lung injury. New Horizons 1:613–622.
14. Matthay MA (1985) Resolution of pulmonary edema. Mechanisms of liquid, protein and cellular clearance from the lung. Clin Chest Med 6:521–545.
15. Pistolesi M, Miniati M, Giuntini C (1989) Pleural liquid and solute exchange. Am Rev Respir Dis 140:825–847.
16. Alwall N, Lunderquist A, Olsson O (1953) Studies on electrolyte-fluid retention. I. Uremic lung-fluid lung? On pathogenesis and therapy. Acta Med Scand 146:157–163.
17. Stein L, Beraud JJ, Morissette M, et al. (1975) Pulmonary edema during volume infusion. Circulation 52:483–489.
18. Guyton AC, Lindsey AE (1959) Effect of elevated left atrial pressure and decreased plasma protein concentration on the development of pulmonary edema. Circ Res 7:649–657.
19. Iannuzzi M, Petty TL (1986) The diagnosis, pathogenesis, and treatment of adult respiratory distress syndrome. J Thorac Imaging 1:1–10.
20. Fowler AA, Hamman RF, Good JT, et al. (1983) Adult respiratory distress syndrome: Risk with common predisposition. Ann Intern Med 98:593–597.
21. Matthay MA (1985) Pathophysiology of pulmonary edema. Clin Chest Med 6:301–314.
22. Andreadis N, Petty TL (1985) Adult respiratory distress syndrome: Problems and progress. Am Rev Respir Dis 132:1344–1346.
23. Rinaldo JE, Rogers RM (1986) Adult respiratory distress syndrome. N Engl J Med 315:578–580.
24. Veeraraghavan S, Koss MN, Sharma OP (1999) Pulmonary veno-occlusive disease. Curr Opin Pulm Med 5:310–313.
25. Tarver RD, Broderick LS, Conces DJ Jr (1996) Reexpansion pulmonary edema. J Thorac Imaging 11:198–209.
26. Kollef MH, Pluss J (1991) Non-cardiogenic pulmonary edema following upper airway obstruction. Seven cases and a review of the literature. Medicine 70:91–98.
27. Schoene RB (1985) Pulmonary edema at high altitude. Review, pathophysiology, and update. Clin Chest Med 6:491–507.
28. Vock P, Fretz C, Franciolli M, et al. (1989) High-altitude pulmonary edema: Findings at high-altitude chest radiography and physical examination. Radiology 170:661–666.
29. Simon RP (1993) Neurogenic pulmonary edema. Neurol Clin 11:309–323.
30. Milne ENC, Pistolesi M (1993) Detection and quantification of pulmonary edema In Reading the chest radiograph. A physiologic approach, Mosby Year-Book Inc., St. Louis, MO, pp. 51–79.
31. Severinghaus JW, Catron C, Noble W (1972) A focus electrode bridge for unilateral lung resisantce. J Appl Physiol 32:526–530.
32. Iskander MF, Maini R, Durney CH, et al. (1986) A microwave method for measuring changes in lung water content: A numerical simulation. IEEE Trans Biomed Eng 28:797–804.
33. Webber LE, Coates G (1982) A clinical system for the in vivo measurement of lung density. Med Phys 9:473–477.
34. Simon DS, Murray JF, Staub NC (1979) Measurement of pulmonary edema in intact dogs by transthoracic gamma ray attenuation. J Appl Physiol 47:1228–1233.
35. Kallay MC, Hyde RW, Fahey PJ, et al. (1985) Effect of the re-breathing pattern on pulmonary tissue volume and capillary blood flow. J Appl Physiol 58:1881–1894.
36. Lewis FR, Elings VB, Hill SL, et al. (1982) The measurements of extravascular lung water by thermal-green dye indicator dilution. Ann NY Acad Sci 384:394–410.
37. Effros RM, Mason GR (1983) Measurements of pulmonary epithelial permeability in vivo. Am Rev Respir Dis 127(Suppl):56–59.
38. Mason GR, Effros RM, Uszler JM, et al. (1985) Small solute clearance from the lungs of patients with cardiogenic and noncardiogenic pulmonary edema. Chest 88:327–334.
39. Staub NC (1986) Clinical use of lung water measurements. Report of a workshop. Chest 90:588–594.
40. Gattinoni L, Pesenti A, Torresin A, et al. (1986) Adult respiratory distress syndrome profiles by computed tomography. J Thorac Imaging 1:25–30.
41. Forster BB, Müller NL, Mayo JR, et al. (1992) High-resolution computed tomography of experimental hydrostatic pulmonary edema. Chest 101:434–437.
42. Primack SL, Müller NL, Mayo JR, et al. (1994) Pulmonary parenchymal abnormalities of vascular origin: High-resolution CT findings. Radiographics 14:739–746.
43. Goodman LR (1996) Congestive heart failure and adult respiratory distress syndrome. New insights using computed tomography. Radiol Clin North Am 34:33–46.

44. Kato S, Nakamoto T, Iizuka M (1996) Early diagnosis and estimation of pulmonary congestion and edema in patients with left-sided heart diseases from histogram of pulmonary CT number. Chest 109:1439–1445.

45. Wollmer P, Rhodes CG (1988) Position emission tomography in pulmonary edema. J Thorac Imaging 3:44–50.

46. Velasquez M, Schuster P (1988) Effect of regional pulmonary blood flow on extravascular lung water measurements with PET. J Appl Physiol 65:1267–1273.

47. Schuster DP, Haller J (1990) Regional pulmonary blood flow during acute pulmonary edema: A PET study. J Appl Physiol 69:353–361.

48. Velazquez M, Haller J, Amundsen T, et al. (1991) Regional lung water measurements with PET: Accuracy, reproducibility, and linearity. Magn Biol Eng Comput 36:461–466.

49. Schuster DP (1998) The evaluation of lung function with PET. Seminar Nucl Med 28:341–351.

50. Hayes CE, Case TA, Ailion DC, et al. (1982) Lung water quantitation by nuclear magnetic resonance imaging. Science 18:1313–1315.

51. Cutillo AG, Morris AH, Ailon DC, et al. (1986) Determination of lung water content and distribution by nuclear magnetic resonance imaging. J Thorac Imaging 1:39–51.

52. Cutillo AG, Morris AH, Ailion DC, et al. (1988) Assessment of lung water distribution by nuclear magnetic resonance. A new method for quantifying and monitoring experimental lung injury. Am Rev Respir Dis 137:1371–1378.

53. Phillips DM, Allen PS, Man SFP (1989) Assessment of temporal changes in pulmonary edema with NMR imaging. J Appl Physiol 66:1197–1208.

54. Caruthers SD, Paschal CB, Pou NA, et al. (1997) Relative quantification of pulmonary edema with non-contrast-enhanced MRI. J Magn Reson Imaging 7:544–550.

55. Caruthers SD, Paschal CB, Pou NA, et al. (1998) Regional measurements of pulmonary edema by using magnetic resonance imaging. J Appl Physiol 84:2143–2153.

56. Milne ENC (1973) Correlation of physiologic findings with chest roentgenology. Radiol Clin North Am 11:17–47.

57. Pistolesi M, Giuntini C (1978) Assessment of extravascular lung water. Radiol Clin North Am 16:551–574.

58. Pistolesi M, Miniati M, Milne ENC, et al. (1985) The chest roentgenogram in pulmonary edema. Clin Chest Med 6:315–344.

59. Milne ENC, Pistolesi M, Miniati M, et al. (1985) The radiologic distinction of cardiogenic and noncardiogenic edema. AJR 144:879–894.

60. Casaburi R, Wasserman K, Effros RM (1978) Detection and measurement of pulmonary edema, In Staub NC (ed) Lung water and solute exchange. Marcel Dekker Inc., New York, pp 323–375.

61. Snashall PD, Hughes JMB (1981) Lung water balance. Rev Physiol Biochem Pharmacol 89:5–62.

62. Prichard JS (1982) Edema of the lung, Charles C Thomas, Springfield, IL, pp 227–252.

63. Staub NC (1983) The measurement of lung water content. J Microwave Power 18:259–263.

64. Hogg JC (1985) The assessment of pulmonary microvascular permeability and edema. In Said SI (ed) The Pulmonary Circulation and Acute Lung Injury, Futura Publishing Co, Mount Kisco, NY, pp 209–224.

65. Cutillo AG (1987) The clinical assessment of lung water. Chest 92:319–325.

66. Miniati M, Pistolesi M, Milne ENC, et al. (1987) Detection of lung edema. Crit Care Med 15:1146–1155.

67. Milne ENC (1980). Chest radiology in the surgical patient. Surg Clin North Am 60:1503–1518.

68. Milne ENC, Pistolesi M (1993) Intensive care unit radiology. In Reading the chest radiograph. A physiologic approach, Mosby-Year Book Inc., St. Louis, MO, pp 311–342.

69. Greenbaum DM, Marschall KE (1982) The value of routine daily chest x-rays in intubated patients in the medical intensive care units. Crit Care Med 10:29–30.

70. Pistolesi M, Milne ENC, Miniati M, et al. (1986) Detection and measurement of pulmonary edema: The chest radiographic approach. Intens Crit Care Dig 5:34–36.

71. Pistolesi M, Miniati M, Giuntini C (1988) A radiographic score for clinical use in the adult respiratory distress syndrome. Intens Crit Care Dig 7:2–4.

72. Milne ENC (1986) A physiological approach to reading critical care unit films. J Thorac Imaging 1:60–90.

73. Kerley P (1957) Lung changes in acquired heart disease. AJR 80:256–263.

74. Heitzman ER, Ziter FN (1966) Acute interstitial pulmonary edema. AJR 98:291–299.

75. Chait A (1972) Interstitial pulmonary edema. Circulation 45:1323–1330.

76. Meszaros WT (1973) Lung changes in left heart failure. Circulation 47:859–871.

77. Doniach I (1947) Uremic edema of the lung. AJR 58:620–628.

78. Bass HE, Singer E (1950) Pulmonary changes in uremia. JAMA 144:819–823.

79. Gibson DG (1966) Hemodynamic factors in the development of acute pulmonary edema in renal failure. Lancet 2:1217–1220.

80. Dick DR, Zylak CJ (1973) Acute respiratory distress in adults. Radiology 106:497–501.

81. Joffe N (1974) The adult respiratory distress syndrome. AJR 122:719–731.

82. Milne ENC, Pistolesi M (1993) Radiologic appearances of pulmonary edema. In Reading the chest radiograph. A Physiologic Approach, Mosby Year-Book Inc., St. Louis, MO, pp 9–51.

83. Fraser RS, Müller N, Colman N, et al. (1999) Pulmonary edema. In Diagnosis of diseases the chest, 4th edn. WB Saunders, Philadelphia, pp 1946–2018.

84. Halperin BD, Feeley TW, Mihm FO, et al. (1985) Evaluation of the portable chest roentgenogram for quantitating extravascular lung water in critically adults. Chest 88:649–652.

85. Pistolesi M, Miniati M, Ravelli V, et al. (1982) Injury versus hydrostatic lung edema: Detection by chest x-ray. Ann NY Acad Sci 384:364–380.

86. Miniati M, Pistolesi M, Paoletti P, et al. (1988) Objective radiographic criteria to differentiate cardiac, renal and injury lung edema. Invest Radiol 23:433–440.

87. Bombino M, Gattinoni L, Pesenti A, et al. (1991) The value of portable chest roentgenography in adult respiratory distress syndrome: Comparison with computed tomography. Chest 100:762–769.

88. Milne ENC, Pistolesi M (1990). Pulmonary edema – Cardiac and noncardiac. In Putman CE (ed) Diagnostic imaging of the lung. Marcel Dekker Inc., New York, pp 253–336.

89. Milne ENC, Pistolesi M (1993) Radiology of pulmonary edema. In Potchen EJ, Grainger RG, Greene R (eds) Pulmonary radiology, WB Saunders, Philadelphia, pp 113–124.

90. Milne ENC, Pistolesi M (1993) Differentiating increased pressure from injury pulmonary edema. In Reading the chest radiograph. A physiologic approach. Mosby Year-Book Inc., St. Louis, MO pp 242–267.

91. Johnson TH, Altman AR, McCaffree RD (1982) Radiological considerations in the adult respiratory distress syndrome treated with positive end expiratory pressure. Clin Chest Med 3:89–100.

92. Petty TL, Ashbaugh DG (1971) The adult respiratory distress syndrome. Chest 600:233–239.

93. Zapol WM, Snider MT (1977) Pulmonary hypertension in severe acute respiratory failure. N Engl J Med 296:476–480.

94. Czer LS, Appel P, Shoemaker WC (1980) Pathogenesis of respiratory failure (ARDS) after hemorrhage and trauma: II. Cardiorespiratory patterns after development of ARDS. Crit Care Med 8:513–518.

95. Zimmerman GA, Morris AH, Gengiz M (1982) Cardiovascular alterations in the adult respiratory syndrome. Am J Med 73:25–34.

96. Snow RL, Davies P, Pontoppidan H, et al. (1982) Pulmonary vascular remodelling in adult respiratory distress syndrome. Am Rev Respir Dis 126:887–892.

97. Tomashefski JF, Jr, Davies P, Boggis C, et al. (1983) The pulmonary vascular lesions of the adult respiratory distress syndrome. Am J Pathol 112:112–126.

98. Pistolesi M, Miniati M, Di Ricco G, et al. (1986) Perfusion lung imaging in the adult respiratory distress syndrome. J Thorac Imaging 1:11–24.

99. Brigham KL, Woolverton WC, Bland LH, et al. (1974) Increased sheep lung vascular permeability caused by pseudomonas bacteremia. J Clin Invest 54:702–804.

100. Porcelli R, Foster WM, Bergofsky ME, et al. (1974) Pulmonary circulatory changes in the pathogenesis of shock lung. Am J Med Sci 268:251–261.

101. Gee MH, Havill AM (1980) The relationship between perivascular cuff fluid and lung lymph in dogs with edema. Microvasc Res 115:209–216.

102. Shoemaker WC, Appel P, Czer LSC, et al. (1980) Pathogenesis of respiratory failure (ARDS) after haemorrhage and trauma: I. Cardiorespiratory patterns preceding the development of ARDS. Crit Care Med 8:504–512.

103. Greene R, Zapol WM, Snider MT, et al. (1981) Early bedside detection of vascular occlusion during acute respiratory failure. Am Rev Respir Dis 124:593–601.

104. Demling RM (1982) Role of prostaglandins in acute pulmonary microvascular injury. Ann NY Acad Sci 384:517–534.

105. Theodore J, Robin ED (1976) Speculations on neurogenic pulmonary edema. Am Rev Respir Dis 118:783–786.

106. Smith WS, Matthay MA (1997) Evidence for a hydrostatic mechanism in human neurogenic pulmonary edema Chest 111:1326.

107. Ingram RH, Szidon JP, Skalak R, et al. (1968) Effects of sympathetic nerve stimulation on the pulmonary arterial tree of the isolated lobe perfused in situ. Circ Res 22:801–815.

108. Jacob RR, McClain O (1979) The role of embolic fat in post-traumatic pulmonary insufficiency. Int Orthop 3:71–75.

109. Barie PS, Minnear FL, Malik AB (1981) Increased pulmonary vascular permeability after bone marrow embolization in sheep. Am Rev Respir Dis 123:648–653.

110. Milne ENC, Pistolesi M, Miniati M, et al. (1984) The vascular pedicle of the heart and the vena azigos. Part I: The normal subject. Radiology 152:1–8.

111. Pistolesi M, Milne ENC, Miniati M, et al. (1984) The vascular pedicle of the heart and the vena azygos. Part II: Acquired heart disease. Radiology 152:9–17.

112. Milne ENC, Imray TJ, Pistolesi M, et al. (1984) The vascular pedicle and the vena azygos: Part III: In trauma, the "vanishing" azygos. Radiology 153:25–31.

113. Haponik EF, Adelman M, Munster AM, et al. (1986) Increased vascular pedicle width preceding burn-related pulmonary edema. Chest 90:649–655.

114. Schreiber SS, Bauman A, Yalow RS, et al. (1954) Blood volume alterations in congestive heart failure. J Clin Invest 33:578–586.

115. Samet P, Fritts HW, Jr, Fishman AP, et al. (1958) The blood volume in heart disease. Medicine 36:211–235.

116. Figueras J, Weil MH (1978) Blood volume prior to and following treatment of acute cardiogenic pulmonary edema. Circulation 57:349–355.

117. Simon M (1963) The pulmonary vessels: Their hemodynamic evaluation using routine radiographs. Radiol Clin North Am 2:363–371.

118. Simon M (1968) The pulmonary vasculature in congenital heart disease. Radiol Clin North Am 6:303–317.

119. Milne ENC (1978) Some new concepts of pulmonary blood flow and volume. Radiol Clin North Am 16:515–536.

120. West JB, Dollery CT, Heard BE (1965) Increased pulmonary resistance in the dependent zone of the isolated lung caused by perivascular edema. Circ Res 17:191–206.

121. Ritchie BC, Schauberger G, Staub NC (1969) Inadequacy of the perivascular edema hypothesis to account for distribution of pulmonary blood flow in lung edema. Circ Res 24:807–814.

122. Naimark A, Kirk BW, Chernecki W (1971) Regional water volume, blood volume, and perfusion in the lung. In Giuntini C (ed) Central hemodynamics and gas exchange. Minerva Medica, Torino, pp 143–160.

123. Hogg JC (1978) Effect of pulmonary edema on distribution of blood flow in the lung. In Staub NC (ed) Lung water and solute exchange. Marcel Dekker Inc., New York, pp 167–182.

124. Kazemi H, Parson EF, Valencia LM, et al. (1970) Distribution of pulmonary blood flow after myocardial ischemia and infarction. Circulation 41:1025–1030.

125. Al Bazzaz FJ, Kazemi H (1972) Arterial hypoxemia and distribution of pulmonary perfusion after uncomplicated myocardial infarction. Am Rev Respir Dis 106:721–728.

126. Giuntini C, Mariani M, Barsotti A, et al. (1974) Factors affecting regional pulmonary blood flow in left heart valvular disease. Am J Med 57:421–436.

127. Pistolesi M, Miniati M, Bonsignore MR, et al. (1988) Factors affecting pulmonary blood flow in chronic ischemic heart disease. J Thorac Imaging 3:65–72.

128. Parker F, Weiss S (1936) The nature and significance of the structural changes in the lungs in mitral stenosis. Am J Pathol 12:573–598.

129. Smith RC, Burchell HB Edwards JE (1954) Pathology of the pulmonary vascular tree. IV. Structural changes in the pulmonary vessels in chronic left ventricular failure. Circulation 10:801–808.

130. Spencer H (1977) Pathology of the lung, 3rd edn. Pergamon Press, Oxford, pp 616–624.

131. Giuntini C, Pistolesi M, Miniati M (1989) Pulmonary venous hypertension – mechanisms and consequences. In Wagenvoort CA, Denolin H (eds) Pulmonary circulation. Advances and controversies. Elsevier, Amsterdam, pp 131–147.

132. Milne ENC, Pistolesi M (1993) Quantification of pulmonary blood volume, flow, and pressure. In Reading the chest radiograph. A physiologic approach, Mosby Year-Book Inc., St. Louis, MO, pp 164–202.

133. Wiener-Kronish JP, Berthiaume Y, Albertine KH (1985) Pleural effusions and pulmonary edema. Clin Chest Med 6:509–519.

134. Wiener-Kronish JP, Matthay MA, Callen PW, et al. (1985) Relationship of pleural effusions to pulmonary hemodynamics in patients with congestive heart failure. Am Rev Respir Dis 132:1253–1256.

135. Light RW (1983) Transudative pleural effusions. In Light RW (ed) Pleural diseases. Lea & Febringer, Philadelphia, pp 69–76.

136. Mellins RB, Levine DR, Fishman AP (1970) Effect of systemic and pulmonary venous hypertension on pleural and pericardial fluid accumulation. J Appl Physiol 29:564–569.

137. Milne ENC, Pistolesi M (1993) Pleural effusion. In Reading the chest radiograph. A physiologic approach. Mosby Year-Book Inc., St. Louis, MO, pp 120–163.

138. Gleason DC, Steiner RE (1966) The lateral roentgenogam in pulmonary edema. AJR 98:279–290.

139. Kerley P (1933) Radiology in heart disease. Br Med J 2:594–597.

140. Kerley P (1962) Cardiac failure. In Shanks SC, Kerley P (eds) A textbook of X-ray diagnosis. Lewis, London, pp 97–108.

141. Heitzman ER, Ziter FM, Markarian B, et al. (1967) Kerley's interlobular septal lines: Roentgen–pathologic correlation. AJR 100: 578–582.

142. Fleischner FG, Reiner L (1954) Linear x-ray shadows in acquired pulmonary hemosiderosis and congestion. N Engl J Med 250:900–905.

143. Grainger RG (1958) Interstitial pulmonary edema and its radiological diagnosis: A sign of pulmonary venous and capillary hypertension. Br J Radiol 31:201–217.

144. Jordan SC, Hicken P, Watson DA, et al. (1966) Pathology of the lungs in mitral stenosis in relation to respiratory function and pulmonary hemodynamics. Br Heart J 28:101–107.

145. Paré JAP, Fraser RG (1983) Synopsis of diseases of the chest. WB Saunders, Philadelphia, pp 206–208.

146. Trapnell DH (1973) The differential diagnosis of linear shadows in chest radiographs. Radiol Clin North Am 11:77–92.

147. Harley HRS (1966) The radiological changes in pulmonary venous hypertension, with special reference to the root shadows and lobular pattern. Br Heart J 23:75–87.

148. Harrison MO, Conte PJ, Heitzman ER (1971) Radiological detection of clinically occult cardiac failure following myocardial infarction. Br J Radiol 44:265–272.

149. Short DS (1956) Radiology of the lung in left heart failure. Br Heart J 18:233–240.

150. Logue RB, Rogers JV, Jr, Gay BB, Jr (1963) Subtle roentgenographic findings of left heart failure. Am Heart J 65:464–473.

151. Barden RP (1964) Pulmonary oedema: Correlation of roentgenologic appearance and abnormal physiology. AJR 92:495–500.

152. Felson B (1973) Chest roentgenology. WB Saunders, Philadelphia, pp 60–70.

153. Berrigan JJ, Carsky EW, Heitzman ER (1966) Fat embolism: Roentgenographic–pathologic correlation in three cases. AJR 96:967–971.

154. Kangarloo M, Beechley MC, Ghahremani GG (1977) The radiographic spectrum of pulmonary complications in burns victims. AJR 128:441–445.

155. Morrison VT, Wetherill S, Zyroff J (1970) The acute pulmonary edema of heroin intoxication. Radiology 97:347–351.

156. Hedlund LW, Effman EL, Bates W, et al. (1982) Pulmonary edema: A CT study of regional lung changes in lung density following oleic acid injury. J Comput Assist Tomogr 6:939–946.

157. Roubier C, Plauchu M (1934) Sur certain aspects radiographiques de l'oedeme pulmonaire chez le cardio-renaux azotemique. Arch Med Chir Appl Resp 9:189–200.

158. Gattinoni L, Bombino M, Pelosi A, et al. (1994) Lung structure and function in different stages of severe adult respiratory distress syndrome. JAMA 271:1772–1775.

159. Slutski RA, Peck WW, Higgins CB, et al. (1984) Pulmonary density distribution in experimental and clinical cardiogenic pulmonary edema evaluated by computed transmission tomography. Am Heart J 108:401–408.

160. Pelosi A, D'Andrea L, Vitale G, et al. (1994) Vertical gradient of regional lung inflation in adult respiratory distress syndrome Am J Respir Crit Care Med 149:8–13.

161. Schuster DP, Markin GF, Mintun MA, et al. (1986) PET measurement of regional lung density. J Comput Assist Tomogr 10:723–729.

162. Storto ML, Kee ST, Golden JA (1995) Hydrostatic pulmonary edema: High resolution CT findings. AJR 165:817–820.

163. Brasileiro FC, Vargas FS, Kavakama JI, et al. (1997) High-resolution CT scan in the evaluation of exercise-induced interstitial pulmonary edema. Chest 111:1577–1582.

164. Caillaud C, Serrecousine O, Anselme F, et al. (1995) Computerized tomography and pulmonary diffusion capacity in highly trained athletes after performing a triathlon. J Appl Physiol 79:1226–1232.

165. Anholm JD, Milne ENC, Stark P, et al. (1999) Radiographic evidence of interstitial pulmonary edema after exercise at altitude. J Appl Physiol 86:503–509.

166. Gattinoni L, Pesenti A, Baglioni G, et al. (1988). Inflammatory pulmonary edema and positive end-expiratory pressure: Correlations between imaging and physiological studies. J Thorac Imaging 313:59–64.

167. Gattinoni L, D'Andrea L, Pelosi A, et al. (1993) Regional effects and mechanism of positive end-expiratory pressure in early adult respiratory distress syndrome. JAMA 269:2122–2127.

168. Schuster DP, Mintun MA, Green MA, et al. (1985) Regional lung water and hematocrit determined by positron emission tomography. J Appl Physiol 59:860–868.

169. Calandrino FS, Anderson, DJ, Mintun MA, et al. (1988) Pulmonary vascular permeability during adult respiratory distress syndrome: A positron emission tomographic study. Am Rev Respir Dis 138:421–428.

170. Wollmer P, Rhodes CG, Deanfield J, et al. (1987) Regional extravascular lung density of the lung in patients with acute pulmonary edema J Appl Physiol 63:1890–1895.

171. Wollmer P, Rhodes CG, Allan RM, et al. (1983) Regional extravascular lung density and fractional blood volume in patients with chronic pulmonary venous hypertension. Clin Physiol 3:241–256.

172. Meyer GJ, Schober O, Bossaler C, et al. (1984) Quantification of regional extravascular lung water in dogs with positron emission tomography using constant infusion of ^{15}O-labeled water. Eur J Nucl Med 9:220–228.

173. Carrol FE, Jr., Loyd TE, Nolop KB, et al. (1985) NMR imaging parameter in the study of lung H_2O. Invest Radiol 20:381–387.

174. Wexler HR, Nicholson RL, Prato FS, et al. (1985) Quantitation of lung water by nuclear magnetic resonance: A preliminary study. Invest Radiol 20:583–590.

175. Podgoski GT, Carrol FE, Parker RE (1986) NMR evaluation of pulmonary interstitial and extravascular fluids. Invest Radiol 21:478–482.

176. Cutillo AG, Morris AH, Ailion DE, et al. (1988) Quantitative assessment of pulmonary edema by nuclear magnetic resonance. J Thorac Imaging 3:51–58.

177. Cutillo AG, Morris AH, Ganesan K, et al. (1989) regional effects of repetition time on MRI quantitation of water in normal and edematous lungs. Magn Reson Med 12:137–144.

178. Cutillo AG, Goodrich KC, Ganesan K, et al. (1995) Alveolar air/tissue interface and nuclear magnetic resonance behaviour of normal and edematous lungs. Am J Respir Crit Care Med 151:1018–1026.

179. Berthezene Y, Vexler V, Jerome H, et al. (1991) Differentiation of capillary leak and hydrostatic pulmonary edema with a macromolecular MR imaging contrast agent. Radiology 181:773–777

Drug-Induced Pulmonary Reactions

D.A. Lynch

Introduction

The diagnosis of drug-induced lung disease is difficult for the radiologist. Because we are usually not provided with the details of treatment, the diagnosis of drug toxicity does not come to mind as often as it should. Pulmonary drug toxicity occurs with a large number of drugs, making it difficult to remember which drug is associated with which pattern. Since the histologic features of drug-induced lung injury, like the imaging features, are usually nonspecific, a definitive diagnosis of drug toxicity can be made only by documenting resolution of the abnormality on withdrawal from the drug, with recurrence on rechallenge. Since rechallenge is rare, the diagnosis is usually made by excluding other causes of the abnormality. However, the entity of drug toxicity should always be considered in patients with unexplained parenchymal abnormalities.

The world wide web site www.pneumotox.com, developed by Dr. Pascal Foucher, Dr. Philippe Camus, and the Groupe d'Études de la Pathologie Pulmonaire Iatrogène, details the enormous variety of drugs that can cause pulmonary toxicity. This site, supported by thousands of references, identifies 11 separate clinical/imaging patterns of lung disease: interstitial lung disease, pulmonary edema, pulmonary hemorrhage, airways disease, pleural changes, vascular changes, mediastinal changes, major airways involvement, muscle and nerve abnormalities, constitutional/systemic symptoms and variegated effects. Interstitial lung disease is subdivided into 14 categories: acute hypersensitivity pneumonitis and respiratory failure, subacute cellular interstitial pneumonitis, pulmonary infiltrates and eosinophilia, organizing pneumonia ± bronchiolitis obliterans (BOOP), desquamative interstitial pneumonia (DIP), lymphocytic interstitial pneumonia (LIP), pulmonary fibrosis, subclinical cytologic changes in bronchoalveolar lavage (BAL) cell profile, diffuse pulmonary calcification, mineral oil pneumonia with basilar or more diffuse chronic lung changes, and lung nodules. The site is an invaluable resource for the radiologist or clinician seeking to define whether a specific pattern of lung disease has previously been described with a specific drug.

Although the topic of drug-induced lung disease almost defies attempts to superimpose a classification system, the radiologist can begin by considering the following:

The clinical context in which drugs were administered (cytotoxic drug, noncytotoxic drug, drug overdose, and illicit drug use)

The acuity of presentation (acute, subacute or chronic)

The presence of symptoms and signs of hypersensitivity reaction (e.g. fever, eosinophilia)

The imaging pattern

In most cases it is not possible for the radiologist to identify the offending drug, but, by integrating the radiologic pattern with the clinical situation, a relatively small list of suspects can often be identified.

Patterns of Lung Disease Associated with Drug Toxicity

The site www.pneumotox.com lists over 250 drugs that cause radiographically apparent disease in the lung, pleura, and mediastinum. Since a complete listing of drugs associated with pulmonary toxicity is well beyond the scope of this book, this chapter discusses only the commoner causes of each pattern likely to be encountered in clinical practice. For more detailed information, the reader is referred to the comprehensive website given above. Tables 25.1 and 25.2 list the common patterns of parenchymal abnormality related to cytotoxic and noncytotoxic drug treatment, with a highly selected list of potential causes. Several of the drugs listed cause more than one

Table 25.1. Radiologic patterns of lung toxicity in patients receiving cytotoxic drugs

Radiologic pattern	Drug
Noncardiac edema	Interleukin-2
	Mitomycin C
	BCNU
	Cytosine arabinoside
	Blood and blood products
Acute diffuse lung injury/ARDS	BCNU
	Retinoic acid
	Ara-C
	Bleomycin ± oxygen
	Mitomycin C
	Cyclophosphamide
Hypersensitivity	Methotrexate
	Procarbazine
Subacute alveolitis/lung fibrosis	Bleomycin
	Mitomycin C
	Cyclophosphamide
	Busulfan
	BCNU
	Methotrexate
Upper lobe lung fibrosis	BCNU
Pulmonary hypertension	Mitomycin C
Nodules	Bleomycin
Pulmonary hemorrhage	Autologous bone marrow transplantation
	Mitomycin C

BCNU, carmustine; ARDS, adult respiratory distress syndrome.

Table 25.2. Radiologic patterns of lung toxicity in patients receiving noncytotoxic drugs

Radiologic pattern	Common etiologic agents
Noncardiac edema	Tocolytic therapy (beta-agonists)
	Iodinated contrast
	OKT3
	Blood and blood products
	Methotrexate
	Aspirin (usually in overdose)
	Narcotic drugs (usually in overdose)
	Penicillin
	Sulfonamides
Acute hypersensitivity pneumonitis/ARDS	Gold
	Nitrofurantoin
	Carbemazepine
	Methotrexate
Subacute alveolitis/lung fibrosis	Gold
	Methotrexate
	Amiodarone
	Nitrofurantoin
Pulmonary infiltrates with eosinophilia	Amiodarone
	Nitrofurantoin
	L-tryptophan
	Sulfonamides
	Nonsteroidal antiinflammatory drugs
	Sulfasalazine
Bronchiolitis obliterans organizing pneumonia	Amiodarone
	Nitrofurantoin
	Minocycline
	Phenytoin
Lipoid pneumonia	Paraffin oil
	Nose drops
Obliterative bronchiolitis	Penicillamine
Vasculitis	L-tryptophan
	Zafirlukast (see text)
	Nitrofurantoin
Pulmonary hypertension	Fenfluramine/dexfenfluramine
Pulmonary thromboembolic disease	Oral contraceptives
	Estrogens
Nodules/conglomerate masses	Amiodarone
Pulmonary hemorrhage	Coumadin, thrombolytics
	Penicillamine

ARDS, adult respiratory distress syndrome.

type of pulmonary toxicity. Methotrexate is included in both tables, because it is commonly given in noncytotoxic doses to patients with autoimmune disease.

Drug toxicity can be classified clinically as acute, subacute, and chronic. The three acute patterns of pulmonary drug toxicity are noncardiac pulmonary edema, acute hypersensitivity pneumonitis and diffuse alveolar damage or adult respiratory distress syndrome (ARDS). These acute abnormalities must be distinguished from hydrostatic pulmonary edema due to fluid overload or heart failure, and from opportunistic infection. Noncardiac pulmonary edema is characterized radiologically by homogeneous, predominantly perihilar pulmonary opacity, often associated with peribronchial cuffing and septal lines (1–3) (Figs. 25.1, 25.2). It often resolves rapidly following withdrawal of the drug. It can usually be distinguished from cardiac edema by the absence of cardiomegaly.

The parenchymal opacity of drug-induced hypersensitivity pneumonitis is often patchy. It is important to note that drug-related hypersensitivity pneumonitis differs histologically and radiologically from hypersensitivity pneumonitis related to inhalation of organic antigens (extrinsic allergic alveolitis). Drug-related hypersensitivity is often associated with systemic symptoms such as fever. Its

occurrence is unrelated to the total dose of drug that has been ingested. Radiologically, drug hypersensitivity reactions may be associated with patchy, poorly defined consolidation (Fig. 25.3) (4), or may be associated with diffuse ground-glass attenuation (5,6). Hypersensitivity reactions generally have an excellent prognosis when the drug is withdrawn.

Diffuse alveolar damage differs from noncardiac edema in that it is usually associated with hypoxemic respiratory failure requiring mechanical ventilation. The radiographic

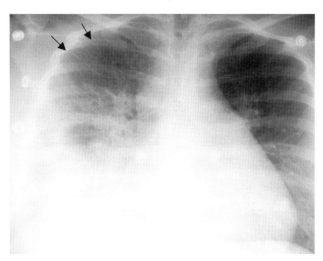

Figure 25.1. Twenty-two year old woman with premature labor who became short of breath while on tocolytic therapy with ritodrine. Anteroposterior portable chest radiograph shows extensive airspace opacity in the right lung, associated with Kerley A lines (*arrows*). The abnormality resolved within 24 h. The marked asymmetry of the edema may be related to the fact that the patient was lying on her right side.

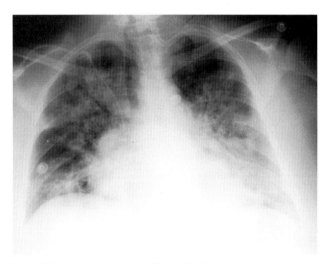

Figure 25.2. Forty year old woman with non-Hodgkin lymphoma, who developed bilateral lung edema 24 h after treatment with antithymocyte globulin. Chest radiograph shows bilateral, predominantly perihilar opacities. The opacities cleared within 24 h.

opacities of diffuse lung injury are usually more extensive than those of edema, and demonstrate rapid progression to alveolar consolidation on serial radiographs (Fig. 25.4).

Subacute or chronic drug injury is typically due to a direct toxic effect on lung cells, typified by the well-described entity of bleomycin toxicity. This type of toxicity is usually dose related, with a threshold dose below which injury is rare. The clinical presentation is usually insidious, and systemic symptoms are uncommon. Physiologic impairment is often significant.

Subacute patterns of drug toxicity include alveolitis, BOOP and pulmonary eosinophilia. In subacute drug toxic-

ity, ground-glass opacity usually indicates an alveolitis pattern (Fig 25.5). Patchy consolidation usually represents either a BOOP pattern (Fig. 25.6), or a pulmonary eosinophilic infiltrate (Fig. 25.7). The alveolitis pattern must be distinguished from extrinsic allergic alveolitis, from desquamative interstitial pneumonitis, and nonspecific interstitial pneumonitis. The patchy consolidation pattern should be distinguished from the many other causes of eosinophilic pneumonia and BOOP. Most, but not all, patients with eosinophilic pulmonary infiltrates have associated blood eosinophilia.

Chronic pulmonary drug toxicity is usually manifested on the chest radiograph and computed tomography (CT) as reticular abnormality, often relatively coarse and associated with ground-glass opacity and lung consolidation (6) (Fig. 25.8). The abnormality often predominates at the lung bases. Honeycombing is relatively uncommon. When the drug is stopped, the radiologic abnormality may remain stable, or may regress over 3–5 years (7). Corticosteroid treatment may speed resolution. This pattern must be distinguished from chronic extrinsic allergic alveolitis, nonspecific interstitial pneumonitis, idiopathic pulmonary fibrosis, and lung fibrosis due to collagen-vascular disease.

High resolution CT (HRCT) scanning may help in early detection of drug toxicity and in classification of the parenchymal abnormality. In a study by Padley et al. of 23 patients with drug toxicity (6), six patients had a normal chest radiograph, but HRCT scans were abnormal in all patients. The commonest abnormality was fibrosis with or without consolidation, found in 12 patients. The other patients had ground-glass attenuation, and widespread bilateral consolidation. Two patients with rheumatoid arthritis treated with penicillamine had a bronchiolitis obliterans pattern, which may have been due either to the penicillamine or, more likely, to the underlying rheumatoid arthritis. In general, the HRCT pattern reflected the underlying histology, but appearances were often nonspecific, apart from the hyperattenuating lesions of amiodarone, and three patients with peribronchovascular fibrosis and consolidation due to nitrofurantoin. However, CT can be useful in confirming the clinical suspicion of drug toxicity, particularly in patients with normal chest radiographs.

Uncommon forms of pulmonary drug toxicity include drug-induced lupus, alveolar hemorrhage, pulmonary hypertension related to appetite suppressants (fenfluramine) (Fig. 25.9), constrictive bronchiolitis related to penicillamine, and lipoid pneumonia (Fig. 25.10). Drug-induced lupus is usually milder than systemic lupus, and usually reverses when the drugs are withdrawn. The commonest agents to cause lupus are procainamide and hydrallazine. Isoniazid is a less common cause. Pleural effusions are the commonest manifestation of drug-induced lupus, but parenchymal abnormalities may be seen.

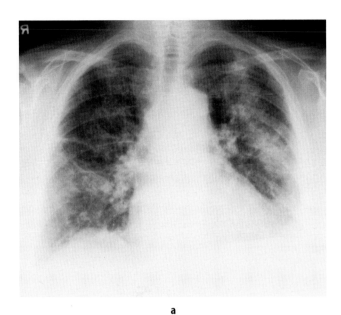

a

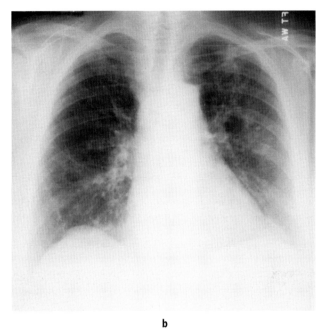

b

c

Figure 25.3. Sixty-seven year old woman who became short of breath while on treatment with a nonsteroidal anti-inflammatory drug (sulindac). **a** Chest radiograph shows bilateral airspace opacity. **b** The opacities cleared when she was admitted to hospital and the drug was stopped. **c** The opacities recurred when the drug was restarted. (From ref 36, with permission.)

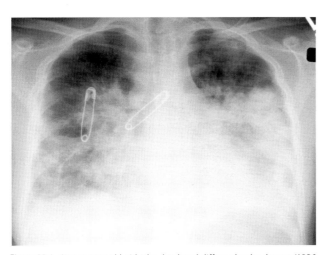

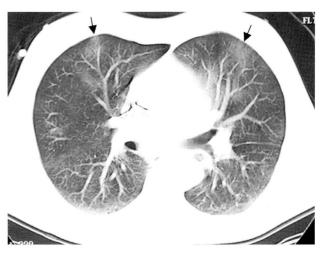

Figure 25.4. Sixteen year old girl who developed diffuse alveolar damage/ARDS 2 weeks after high dose chemotherapy with allogeneic bone marrow transplant for acute lymphatic leukemia. Chest radiograph shows extensive bilateral lung consolidation. The patient was intubated for hypoxemic respiratory failure shortly after this chest radiograph.

Figure 25.5. Delayed lung toxicity in 59 year old man who received high dose chemotherapy (including BCNU) with autologous bone marrow transplant for refractory non-Hodgkin lymphoma. Chest radiograph was normal. CT shows patchy areas of ground-glass attenuation (*arrows*). The patient responded well to corticosteroid treatment.

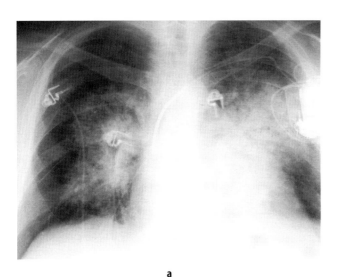

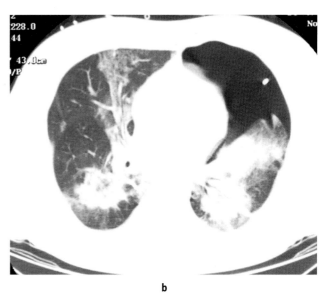

a   b

Figure 25.6. Fifty-four year old man who presented with shortness of breath 1 month after starting on amiodarone 400 mg daily for intractable ventricular tachycardia. **a** Chest radiograph shows automatic implantable cardiac defibrillator, and bilateral asymmetric lung consolidation. **b** Chest CT obtained after the patient had sustained a large left pneumothorax shows peribronchovascular consolidation and ground glass abnormality. The consolidation was of soft tissue attenuation. Histology showed bronchiolitis obliterans organizing pneumonia.

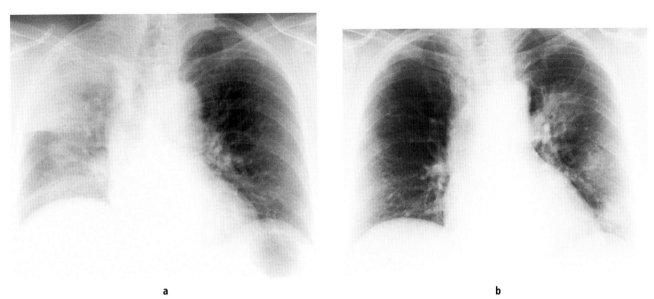

a   b

Figure 25.7. Fifty year old man with migratory eosinophilic pulmonary infiltrates thought to be due to acetaminophen. **a** Initial chest radiograph shows right upper lobe consolidation and more patchy right lower lung opacity. **b** Chest radiograph 3 months later shows resolution of the right upper lobe opacity, but new consolidation in the left lung.

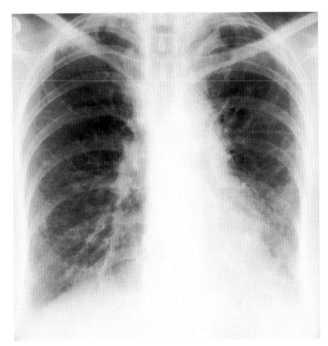

Figure 25.8. Sixty-one year old woman who developed lung fibrosis after 5 years of nitrofurantoin use. Chest radiograph shows basal predominant coarse reticular opacity.

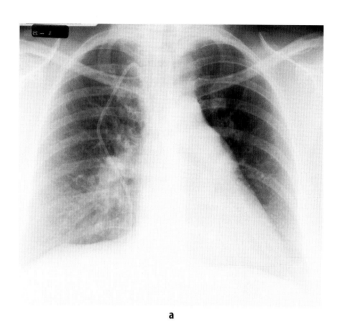 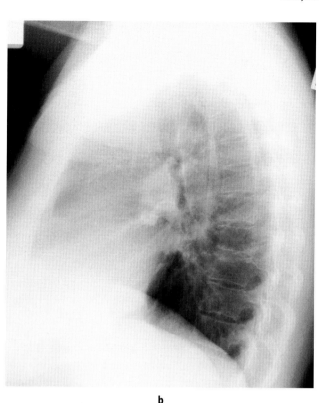

a

b

Figure 25.9. Fifty-one year old woman who developed severe pulmonary hypertension while being treated with the fenfluramine–phentermine combination for obesity. **a** and **b** Frontal and lateral chest radiographs show marked enlargement of the main, right and left pulmonary arteries.

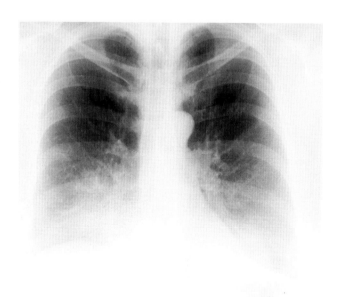 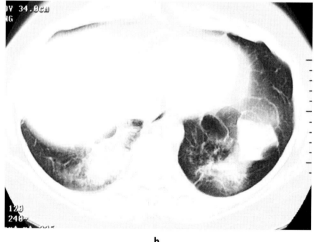

a

b

Figure 25.10. Fifty year old woman who developed lipoid pneumonia due to chronic ingestion of paraffin oil. **a** Chest radiograph shows bilateral lower lobe consolidation. **b** Chest CT (lung windows) shows the mass-like nature of the consolidation.

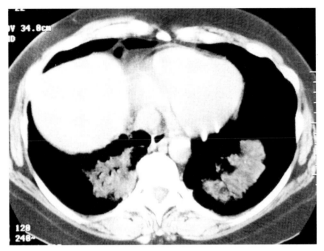

Figure 25.10c. Chest CT (mediastinal windows) shows that the consolidated areas contain a significant proportion of low attenuation material due to the combination of fat and soft tissue attenuation.

Table 25.3. Nonpulmonary manifestations of drug toxicity evident on the chest radiograph

Toxic manifestation	Drug
Heart failure	Daunorubicin
	Beta-blockers
	Calcium channel blockers
Pleural effusion	Amiodarone
	Interleukin 2
	Nitrofurantoin
Ovarian hyperstimulation syndrome	Genadotrophic hormones
Drug-induced lupus	Procainamide
	Hydrallazine
	Isoniazid
	Phenytoin
Tracheobronchial calcification	Warfarin
Extrapleural, and mediastinal fat deposition	Corticosteroids
Osteoporosis	Corticosteroids
Lymphadenopathy	Phenytoin

The radiologist can often identify nonpulmonary drug toxicity on the chest radiograph (Table 25.3). Patients treated with large doses of corticosteroids are frequently osteoporotic, and may have abundant mediastinal and extrapleural fat (Fig. 25.11). They may also show decreased lung volumes due to diaphragmatic muscle weakness caused by steroid myopathy. Patients treated with phenytoin may uncommonly develop hilar adenopathy, which may be due to benign reversible lymphoid hyperplasia, pseudolymphoma, or malignant lymphoma.

Pleural effusions may be due to a prominent feature in drug-induced lupus, or in reactions to nitrofurantoin, or to amiodarone. The ovarian hyperstimulation syndrome, a complication of ovulation induction with gonadotrophic

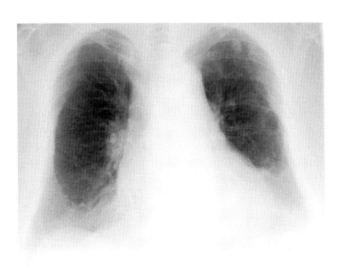

a

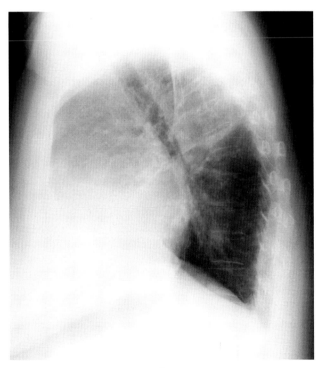

b

Figure 25.11. Seventy-three year old woman who had long-term treatment for asthma with high dose corticosteroids. **a** and **b** Frontal and lateral chest radiograph shows abundant deposition of fat in the mediastinum, paracardiac region, and extra pleural. There are multiple vertebral compression fractures due to osteopenia.

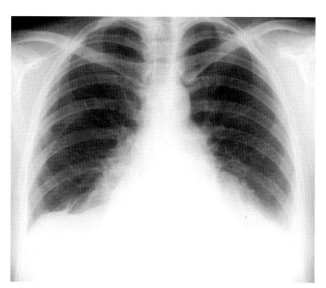

Figure 25.12. Thirty-four year old woman with infertility, treated with gonadotrophic hormones to induce ovulation. She developed respiratory distress. Chest radiograph shows bilateral pleural effusions and bilateral basal atelectasis.

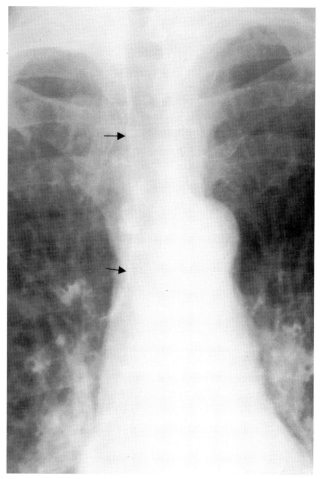

Figure 25.13. Seventy year old female with longstanding mitral valve disease, anti-coagulated because of a prosthetic valve. Detail of frontal chest radiograph shows marked tracheal calcification (*arrows*).

hormones used in fertility treatments, may present with ascites and bilateral effusions (Fig. 25.12), and may culminate in hypovolemic shock.

Progressive calcification of tracheobronchial cartilaginous rings is seen in patients undergoing prolonged anticoagulant treatment with warfarin sodium (coumadin) (8). This is seen most commonly in older female patients with prosthetic cardiac valves (Fig. 25.13), but may also be seen in children with prosthetic valves and in infants with warfarin embryopathy (9).

Drug Toxicity due to Chemotherapy

Many cytotoxic drugs have been implicated in the development of lung toxicity. In contrast to the noncytotoxic drugs, drug toxicity related to cytotoxic drugs is often mediated by a direct cytotoxic effect, and the risk of toxicity increases with increased cumulative dose. The cytotoxic effect is potentiated by other risk factors such as irradiation and oxygen administration.

Bleomycin is by far the best-studied cause of subacute and chronic lung toxicity. It is widely used in laboratory animals (often in combination with oxygen) to create a model of lung fibrosis (10). The incidence of lung toxicity in patients treated with bleomycin ranges from 2% to 40% (7). The incidence of toxicity increases dramatically after the patient has received a total cumulative dose of 450–500 units. Factors associated with increased risk of bleomycin toxicity include supplemental high dose oxygen administration, irradiation, renal failure and use of additional toxic chemotherapeutic agents. Patients who have been treated with bleomycin in the past may develop significant

lung disease if they subsequently receive radiotherapy or chemotherapy, or if they inhale increased concentrations of oxygen. Supplemental oxygen administration during anesthesia resulted in postoperative ARDS in five patients who had previously received bleomycin, in a series described by Goldiner et al. (11).

A study of CT scans in 100 patients receiving bleomycin for treatment of malignant testicular tumors showed that the lung parenchyma became abnormal in 38% (12). Minimal CT changes included basal linear and nodular opacities. Moderate changes of bleomycin injury were characterized by coarse reticular and nodular shadowing, while severe bleomycin-related lung damage was characterized by confluent irregular opacities extending through the lung, though the lung apices were relatively spared. Follow-up CT examinations showed that many or all of the pulmonary changes reversed over several months after withdrawal of therapy. However, those with severe lung damage tended to remain unchanged. Bleomycin may cause peripheral nodules that are difficult to distinguish from metastases (13).

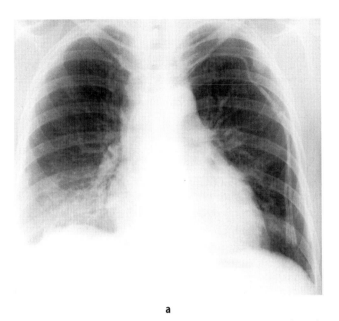
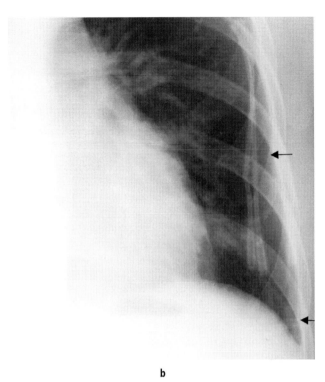

a   b

Figure 25.14. Thirty-six year old woman who developed pulmonary venoocclusive disease following high dose chemotherapy and bone marrow transplantation for breast cancer. Chest radiograph shows moderate cardiac enlargement. There is basal reticular abnormality with bilateral interlobular septal thickening (*arrows*).

Other important cytotoxic drugs that cause lung toxicity include mitomycin C, cyclophosphamide, methotrexate, and BCNU (carmustine). Cytosine arabinoside causes an acute, usually reversible toxicity due to noncardiac edema within 20 days after treatment (14). BCNU has been associated with a particularly insidious form of lung toxicity in which upper lobe fibrosis developed 13–17 years after treatment for brain tumors in children (15). The chest radiograph shows upper lobe volume loss with hilar elevation and pleural thickening. Pneumothorax may occur. On CT, the pattern of fibrosis is peripheral and linear, sometimes with subpleural cysts.

Lung toxicity is a particularly feared complication in patients receiving high dose chemotherapy associated with bone marrow transplantation or bone marrow salvage. Patients with solid malignancies (typically breast cancer) receive high dose chemotherapy with autologous bone marrow transplantation being used to regenerate the bone marrow after treatment. Patients with hematologic malignancy usually receive allogeneic bone marrow transplantation. Three distinct types of toxicity occur: acute alveolar hemorrhage, idiopathic pulmonary syndrome, and delayed pulmonary toxicity (16). Acute alveolar hemorrhage is the earliest complication, usually occurring within the first 2 weeks. It presents with a radiologic pattern of patchy airspace disease. Idiopathic pulmonary syndrome presents with a radiologic and clinical pattern of diffuse lung injury, usually occurring weeks to months after chemotherapy (Fig. 25.4). This syndrome is attributed mainly to BCNU, but other risk factors include graft versus host disease (in allogeneic transplants) and whole body irradiation. Its mortality is at least 50%. Pulmonary venoocclusive disease is a rare complication of high dose chemotherapy and bone marrow transplantation (Fig. 25.14).

Delayed lung toxicity has been described in patients receiving high dose cyclophosphamide, cisplatinum, and BCNU with an autologous bone marrow transplant. Delayed toxicity is typically maximal 15–18 weeks following bone marrow transplantation (Fig. 25.5). It may be treated with steroids, and its mortality is low. In a recent study, only 5 of 18 patients with delayed lung toxicity had marked changes on conventional CT at the time of diagnosis of toxicity, while two had minor changes, and two developed changes on follow-up scans. Ground-glass attenuation was the commonest type of abnormality seen. HRCT might have been more sensitive for early ground-glass attenuation, but was not used in this study. HRCT cannot usually distinguish changes of drug toxicity from changes due to opportunistic infection in immunocompromised patients. Usually, bronchoscopy with lavage and/or biopsy is required to exclude infection in patients in whom drug toxicity is considered.

In addition to the complications described above, allogeneic transplantation may be complicated by constrictive bronchiolitis. Constrictive bronchiolitis is characterized by bronchial dilatation and a mosaic pattern of lung attenuation, with air-trapping on expiratory scans (17).

Drug Toxicity due to Noncytotoxic Drugs

Acute noncardiac edema related to iodinated contrast administration is important for the radiologist. This complication appears to be relatively rare, but has been described with intravenous and intraarterial injection of most types of iodinated contrast medium, including nonionic contrast. It may be due to a direct toxic effect of the contrast material on the pulmonary basement membrane.

Amiodarone is one of the most effective drugs for suppression of ventricular arrhythmias. Its use is limited chiefly by the relatively high prevalence of pulmonary toxicity, occurring in 1–6% of patients (4). Toxicity is seen most commonly in patients treated with more than 400 mg daily, after 5–6 months of treatment, and appears uncommon in patients receiving lower doses. The radiologist should suspect amiodarone toxicity in patients with patchy lung consolidation, with or without effusions, particularly if the patient also has evidence of cardiac disease (Fig. 25.6). Pulmonary toxicity due to amiodarone is often associated with high attenuation parenchymal lesions on CT (18). This rather specific CT appearance, seen in 8 of 11 cases in one study, is thought to be due to the high concentration of iodine-containing amiodarone present in alveolar macrophages and type 2 pneumocytes in these lesions. The increased attenuation of the liver or spleen seen in these subjects is probably due to a similar mechanism. Associated pleural effusions are often increased in attenuation. Recognition of the high attenuation opacities may be helpful in distinguishing between amiodarone pulmonary toxicity and congestive heart failure (19). However, the absence of hyperintensity does not exclude amiodarone lung (Fig. 25.5). Gallium scans may show increased uptake in the lungs of patients with amiodarone toxicity (20).

Patients with chronic diseases such as rheumatoid arthritis are particularly prone to drug-induced complications. Many of the available treatments for rheumatoid arthritis, including gold, methotrexate and D-penicillamine have been implicated in the development of infiltrative lung disease. On the chest radiograph, gold-induced lung disease differs radiographically from rheumatoid lung because the infiltrates are most commonly diffuse, although about 30% of cases have basal predominance (21). On chest CT scans, gold-induced lung disease was characterized in 12 of 20 reported cases by alveolar opacities extending along bronchovascular bundles. This

CT finding, when present, is strongly suggestive of gold lung (21). Administration of low dose methotrexate may be associated with subacute hypersensitivity pneumonitis in about 5% of cases. Preexisting radiographic evidence of interstitial lung disease probably predisposes to the development of methotrexate pneumonitis in patients with rheumatoid arthritis (22). In a case of methotrexate pneumonitis, (5), HRCT showed widespread ground-glass attenuation and reticular abnormality. Treatment with D-penicillamine is associated with the development of constrictive bronchiolitis, and with pulmonary hemorrhage. In patients with constrictive bronchiolitis, the chest radiograph is commonly normal, but HRCT may show air-trapping and bronchial dilatation. Nonsteroidal anti-inflammatory drugs may be associated with hypersensitivity reactions (Fig. 25.3), while unintentional therapeutic overdoses of salicylate may result in pulmonary edema.

Nitrofurantoin causes a wide variety of pulmonary reactions. Acute nitrofurantoin toxicity, occurring within 1 month of start of treatment, accounts for 90% of reported cases of nitrofurantoin toxicity (4). Acute toxicity is associated with basal diffuse or patchy interstitial or airspace abnormalities. Unilateral pleural effusion is commonly present. Eosinophilia is present in most cases. In chronic nitrofurantoin lung, basal reticular abnormality is the commonest abnormality (Fig. 25.8), again often associated with pleural effusion.

Noncardiac edema develops in a significant number of women who are treated with beta adrenergic drugs (ritodrine or salbutamol) to inhibit preterm labor (Fig. 25.1). The mechanism is unclear, and may be related to the unique physiology of pregnancy.

Exogenous lipoid pneumonia occurs when lipid material is aspirated into the lungs. It occurs predominantly in children and in the elderly. Common etiologic agents include liquid paraffin or mineral oil (used to treat constipation) petroleum-based nasal drops, and, in Asian countries, shark oil. About 75% of patients who develop exogenous lipoid pneumonia have some underlying disorder predisposing them to aspirate (e.g., gastroesophageal reflux, chronic neurologic or psychiatric illness) (23). In industrial environments, chronic inhalation of cutting mist or oily vapor may also cause exogenous lipoid pneumonia.

Presentations of lipoid pneumonia include asymptomatic chest radiographic abnormalities, progressive dyspnea and cough, or a subacute development of cough, sputum, and fever. In the correct setting, macrophages laden with fat or lipid, found on sputum analysis or BAL support the diagnosis. Since recognition of lipid droplets may require special stains, the radiologist should prompt the clinician to consider this diagnosis when appropriate. The prognosis of lipoid pneumonia is good if the offending agent is identified and the exposure is stopped.

On the chest radiograph, lipoid pneumonia may present either with a focal area of consolidation (usually in a dependent region of lung), or with a mass (Fig. 25.10). Most (though not all) cases of lipoid pneumonia studied by CT have at least some areas in which the CT attenuation of the lung is less than that of water (24,25). This negative CT attenuation, which may be missed if the scans are photographed using lung window settings only, can be very useful in establishing a diagnosis. However, the absence of this sign does not exclude lipoid pneumonia. Because negative CT density can be simulated by partial volume averaging of the attenuations of aerated and consolidated lung within a region of interest, an area of homogeneously negative attenuation is necessary to be confident of the diagnosis. Magnetic resonance imaging (MRI) has no significant role in the diagnosis of lipoid pneumonia (26).

Patients treated with leukotriene antagonists such as zafirlukast, a new type of anti-inflammatory treatment for asthma, may develop a syndrome of vasculitis similar to Churg–Strauss syndrome (27–29). This syndrome is characterized by pulmonary infiltrates, cardiomegaly and eosinophilia, occurring within 4 months of starting treatment with the new drug and weaning from corticosteroids. It is characterized radiologically by patchy parenchymal airspace abnormality (Fig. 25.15). The relationship between this syndrome and the drug is controversial, with some authors suggesting that vasculitis might have been present prior to treatment, but unmasked by the decrease in steroid dose. Cardiac involvement may result in cardiomegaly.

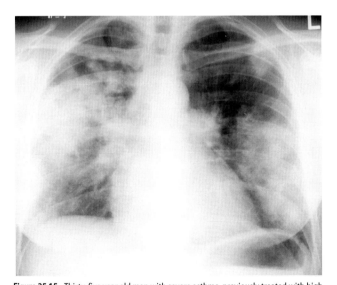

Figure 25.15. Thirty-five year old man with severe asthma, previously treated with high dose steroids, now on treatment with leukotriene antagonist. The patient had significant eosinophilia. Chest radiograph shows cardiomegaly and bilateral airspace opacities. Histology showed Churg–Strauss vasculitis. The cardiomegaly was due to a myocardial infarction caused by the vasculitis.

Some preparations of L-tryptophan (an over-the-counter nutritional supplement) were associated with an outbreak of an eosinophilic myalgia syndrome in 1536 patients in the USA between 1989 and 1990. Associated histologic features included pulmonary vasculitis and chronic interstitial pneumonitis. The radiologic manifestations included basal-predominant irregular linear opacities, with progression to confluent opacities in more severely affected cases (30). Chest radiographs were normal in about 50% of cases. This eosinophilic myalgia syndrome was attributed to chemical contamination of the batch of L-tryptophan. Although the offending preparations of L-tryptophan have now been withdrawn, similar syndromes may occur in the future in relation to other chemical compounds. A similar syndrome occurring in Spain in 1981 was attributed to toxic oil.

Drug Toxicity Associated with Drug Overdose

Noncardiac edema occurs with overdoses of a wide variety of drugs (Table 25.4). Lung edema due to salicylates and narcotic analgesics is due to increased capillary permeability, and usually has a good outcome. In the study (31), ARDS developed in 9% of 30 patients who had overdoses of tricyclic antidepressants, with typical appearances of diffuse parenchymal airspace opacity.

Paraquat is a widely used herbicide, sometimes employed for suicide attempts. Toxicity and death may occur even following accidental ingestion of small amounts of this substance. It is not available in the USA. It causes acute lung edema/ARDS, with subacute and chronic lung fibrosis in survivors. A series of 42 patients described by Im et al provided valuable information regarding the time course of the radiologic changes (32). In the first 7 days after paraquat ingestion, the chest radiograph commonly showed lung consolidation. Pneumomediastinum and pneumothorax were also commonly seen. Over the subsequent 1 or 2 weeks, the radiographic pattern evolved to cystic and tubular shadows. In the chronic phase of lung injury, the radiographs showed multifocal interstitial abnormality with honeycombing. On CT scanning in one patient, the distribution of abnormality was patchy, and tended to involve the central portions of the lung. The presence of pneumomediastinum

Table 25.4. Causes of noncardiac edema in drug overdoses

Narcotic drugs (heroin, morphine, etc.)
Aspirin and other salicylates
Phenothiazines
Tricyclic antidepressants
Paraquat

during the acute phase of injury was associated with 100% mortality: in some cases this may have been related to esophageal perforation.

Drug Reactions Associated with Illicit Drug Use

Illicit drug use is associated with a wide range of pulmonary complications, listed in Table 25.5. In a series of 97 cases (33), the commonest complications of illicit drug use were related to HIV infection. Noninfectious complications include noncardiac edema due to heroin overdose or cocaine use.

Inhalation of crack cocaine is associated with an extraordinary range of pulmonary and cardiac complications, ranging from thermal airway injury to diffuse lung edema and pulmonary hemorrhage to barotrauma (34). Chest pain in these patients may be due to bronchial irritation, myocardial ischemia, pneumothorax, or pneumomediastinum. Pulmonary hypertension may result from a direct vasoconstrictive effect on pulmonary vessels. The syndrome of crack lung may include any or all of the following features: pulmonary hemorrhage, chest pain, pulmonary edema, and interstitial lung abnormality. Other complications include pulmonary atelectasis, pulmonary eosinophilia and BOOP. Chest radiographs are therefore important in elucidating the cause of the patient's symptoms (35) (Fig. 25.16).

When intravenous drug abusers grind up, dissolve, and inject drugs in tablet form intended for oral use, the insoluble binding agents present in the tablets result in microscopic pulmonary emboli. This may cause significant pulmonary hypertension. If the binding agent is talc, a granulomatous inflammatory reaction to the talc may progress to pulmonary talcosis, with interstitial fibrosis, emphysema, and chronic respiratory failure.

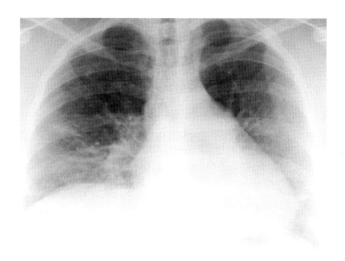

Figure 25.16. Thirty-five year old woman who developed shortness of breast and chest pain following inhalation of crack cocaine. Chest radiograph shows mild lung edema, with basal atelectasis. These abnormalities resolved overnight.

Pulmonary talcosis is radiologically similar to silicosis or sarcoidosis, being characterized by profuse fine nodules that coalesce to form perihilar mass-like opacities with marked anatomic distortion. The perihilar opacities usually contain areas of high attenuation (6). Progression of mass-like fibrosis may occur even when the patient has discontinued intravenous drug abuse. One case of talcosis described by Padley et al (6) showed diffuse ground-glass attenuation, thought to be due to microscopic talc granulomas. Talcosis may be associated with emphysema.

Intravenous injection of methylphenidate (Ritalin) may cause panlobular emphysema (36). This emphysema is thought to be due to microvascular occlusion.

Summary

The diagnosis of drug-induced lung disease can be reached only by careful consideration of the clinical and imaging features. The radiologist should consider this possibility in any patient with unexplained parenchymal abnormalities, particularly in illicit-drug users and in patients undergoing chemotherapeutic treatment for malignancy or other chronic diseases. Specific clinical contexts should suggest the possibility of drug-induced disease (e.g., premature labor should suggest ritodrine-induced lung edema, or rheumatoid arthritis should suggest lung disease due to aspirin, nonsteroidal anti-inflammatory drugs, gold, methotrexate or penicillamine). By integrating the imaging pattern with the clinical presentation, the radiologist may be able to suggest the possibility of drug-induced disease. Of all of the patterns of drug-induced disease, only lipoid pneumonia and amiodarone lung have imaging features that are sufficient to

Table 25.5. Radiologic patterns of lung injury in illicit drug use

Radiologic pattern	Drug
Noncardiac edema	Cocaine
Cardiac edema	Cocaine
Acute diffuse lung injury/ARDS	Crack cocaine
Hypersensitivity	Cocaine
Bronchiolitis	Cocaine
Vasculitis	Cocaine
Pulmonary hypertension	Chronic i.v. drug abuse/talcosis Crack cocaine
Nodules/conglomerate masses	Talcosis
Emphysema	Methylphenidate (Ritalin) abuse Talcosis
Pulmonary hemorrhage	Crack cocaine

ARDS, adult respiratory distress syndrome; i.v., intravenous.

allow a confident diagnosis. Access to a database such as the website www.pneumotox.com can help the radiologist and clinician to define the likelihood of drug-induced lung injury in an individual patient.

References

1. Saxon RR, Klein JS, Bar MH, et al. (1991) Pathogenesis of pulmonary edema during interleukin-2 therapy: Correlation of chest radiographic and clinical findings in 54 patients. AJR 156:281–285.

2. Mann H, Ward JH, Samlowski WE (1990) Vascular leak syndrome associated with interleukin-2: chest radiographic manifestations. Radiology 176:191–194.

3. Milos M, Aberle DR, Parkinson BT, et al. (1988) Maternal pulmonary edema complicating beta-adrenergic therapy of preterm labor. AJR 151:917–918.

4. Cooper JA, Jr, White DA, Matthay RA (1986) Drug-induced pulmonary disease. Part 2: Noncytotoxic drugs. Am Rev Respir Dis 133:488–505

5. Leduc D, De Vuyst P, Lheureux P, et al. (1993) Pneumonitis complicating low-dose methotrexate therapy for rheumatoid arthritis. Discrepancies between lung biopsy and bronchoalveolar lavage findings. Chest 104:1620–1623.

6. Padley SP, Adler B, Hansell DM, et al. (1992) High-resolution computed tomography of drug-induced lung disease. Clinical Radiology 46:232–236.

7. Cooper JA, Jr, White DA, Matthay RA (1986) Drug-induced pulmonary disease. Part 1: Cytotoxic drugs. Am Rev Respir Dis 133:321–340.

8. Moncada R, Venta L, Venta E (1992) Tracheal and bronchial cartilaginous rings: Warfarin sodium-induced calcification. Radiology 184:437–439.

9. Taybi H, Capitanio M (1990) Tracheobronchial calcification: An observation in three children after mitral valve replacement and warfarin sodium treatment. Radiology 176:728–730.

10. Hirose N, Lynch DA, Cherniack RM, et al. (1993) Correlation between high resolution computed tomography and tissue morphometry of the lung in bleomycin-induced pulmonary fibrosis in the rabbit. Am Rev Respir Dis 147:730–738.

11. Goldiner PL, Carlon GC, Cvitkovic E, et al. (1978) Factors influencing postoperative morbidity and mortality in patients treated with bleomycin. Br Med J 1:1664–1667.

12. Bellamy E, Nicholas D, Husband J (1987) Quantitative assessment of lung damage due to bleomycin using computed tomography. Br J Radiol 60:1205–1209.

13. Santrach PJ, Askin FB, Wells RJ, et al. (1989) Nodular form of bleomycin-related pulmonary injury in patients with osteogenic sarcoma. Cancer 64:806–811.

14. Tjon A, Tham R, Peters W, et al. (1987) Pulmonary complications of cytosine arabinoside therapy: Radiographic findings. AJR 149:23–27.

15. Taylor PM, O'Driscoll BR, Gattamaneni HR, et al. (1991) Chronic lung fibrosis following carmustine (BCNU) chemotherapy: Radiological features. Clin Radiol 44:299–301.

16. Wilczynski SW, Erasmus JJ, Petros WP, et al. (1998) Delayed pulmonary toxicity syndrome following high-dose chemotherapy and bone marrow transplantation for breast cancer. Am J Respir Crit Care Med 157:565–573.

17. Worthy SA, Flint JD, Müller NL (1997) Pulmonary complications after bone marrow transplantation: High-resolution CT and pathologic findings. Radiographics 17:1359–1371.

18. Kuhlman J, Teigen C, Ren H, et al. (1990) Amiodarone pulmonary toxicity: CT findings in symptomatic patients. Radiology 177: 121–125.

19. Nicholson A, Hayward C (1989) The value of computed tomography in the diagnosis of amiodarone-induced lung toxicity. Clin Rad 40:564–567.

20. Dake MD, Hattner R, Warnock ML, et al. (1985) Gallium-67 lung uptake associated with amiodarone pulmonary toxicity. Am Heart J 109:1114–1116.

21. Tomioka R, King TE, Jr (1997) Gold-induced pulmonary disease: Clinical features, outcome, and differentiation from rheumatoid lung disease. Am J Respir Crit Care Med 155:1011–1020.

22. Golden MR, Katz RS, Balk RA, et al. (1995) The relationship of pre-existing lung disease to the development of methotrexate pneumonitis in patients with rheumatoid arthritis. J Rheumatol 22:1043–1047.

23. Freidman DG, Engelberg H, Merritt WH (1940) Oil aspiration (lipoid) pneumonia in adults: a clinical pathological study of 47 cases. Arch Intern Med 66:11–38.

24. Gondouin A, Manzoni P, Ranfaing E, et al. (1996) Exogenous lipid pneumonia: A retrospective multicentre study of 44 cases in France. Eur Respir J 9:1463–9.

25. Lee K, Müller N, Hale V, et al. (1995) Lipoid pneumonia: CT findings. J Comput Assist Tomogr 19:48–51.

26. Brechot JM, Buy JN, Laaban JP, et al. (1991) Computed tomography and magnetic resonance findings in lipoid pneumonia. Thorax 46:738–739.

27. Holloway J, Ferriss J, Groff J, et al. (1998) Churg-Strauss syndrome associated with zafirlukast. J Am Osteopath Assoc 98:275–278.

28. Knoell DL, Lucas J, Allen JN (1998) Churg–Strauss syndrome associated with zafirlukast. Chest 114:332–334.

29. Wechsler ME, Garpestad E, Flier SR, et al. (1998) et al. (1998) Pulmonary infiltrates, eosinophilia, and cardiomyopathy following corticosteroid withdrawal in patients with asthma receiving zafirlukast. JAMA 279:455–457.

30. Williamson MR, Eidson M, Rosenberg RD, et al. (1991) Eosinophilia–myalgia syndrome: Findings on chest radiographs in 18 patients. Radiology 180:849–852.

31. Varnell R, Godwin J, Richardson M, et al. (1989) Adult respiratory distress syndrome from overdose of tricyclic antidepressants. Radiology 170:667–670.

32. Im JG, Lee KS, Haw MC, et al. (1991) Paraquat poisoning-Findings on chest radiography and CT in 44 patients. AJR 157:697–701.

33. O'Donnell A, Selig J, Aravamuthan M, et al. (1995) Pulmonary complications associated with illicit drug use: An update. Chest 108:460–463.

34. Haim DY, Lippmann ML, Goldberg SK, et al. (1995) The pulmonary complications of crack cocaine. A comprehensive review. Chest 107:233–240.

35. Eurman D, Potash H, Eyler W, et al. (1989) Chest pain and dyspnea related to "crack" cocaine smoking: Value of chest radiography. Radiology 172:459–462.

36. Stern EJ, Frank MS, Schmutz JF, et al. (1994) Panlobular pulmonary emphysema caused by i.v. injection of methylphenidate (Ritalin): Findings on chest radiographs and CT scans. AJR 162:555–560.

Environmental Lung Disorders: Mineral Pneumoconioses

M. Sperber and K. McConnochie

Introduction

The progress of humans has always been dependent on minerals, most of which must be extracted from the earth. Wherever this occurs, the work force is at risk of developing mineral pneumoconiosis. In the 16th century, two physicians, Agricola (1) and Paracelsus (2), working independently, recognized that fatal respiratory disease often occurred in miners. They were ahead of their time, for by the end of the 18th century very little more was known. The necessary diagnostic tools had not yet been developed. It was not until specialties such as pathology, radiology, pulmonary function, epidemiology, and statistics had come of age that our understanding of pneumoconioses improved, Today, we have a comprehensive range of resources that include computers, sophisticated lung imaging techniques, electron microscopy, and particulate mineralogic analysis.

Before considering the effect of individual minerals on the lung, some general points merit attention. Dust, regardless of its composition, can only damage the lung if it manages to evade or overwhelm the respiratory defense mechanisms. These have evolved to protect the lung against naturally occurring hazards, but they are equally effective when the invasion is occupational in origin. Large particles are deposited in the nose and the bronchi and removed by the mucociliary escalator. Some particles will be deposited in the alveoli, where they may be ingested by macrophages, and some particles will remain suspended in the airstream and will therefore be exhaled. It has been estimated that about 7% of all particles inhaled will enter the lung parenchyma (3). The behavior of particles in the lungs is related to their size, shape, surface characteristics, and density. This aerodynamic property is more important than apparent size, but, for general reference, the particles of most relevance in mineral pneumoconioses have a diameter between 0.5 and 10 μm (4).

The amount of respirable dust that reaches the lungs also depends on the quantity of airborne dust in the atmosphere. In many situations (e.g., the coal mining industry) it has been possible to construct a dose-response relationship where one can predict the amount of disease likely to be caused by exposure to a given amount of dust (5). This is achieved by combined use of epidemiology, radiology, and physiology. However, it is not always practical and possible to do the necessary studies, in which case estimates based on knowledge of particle behavior in the lung must be used and the effect on the work force carefully monitored.

Radiology plays a vital role not only in the recognition, investigation, and management of patients with mineral pneumoconioses but also as a epidemiologic tool.

The International Labour Organization (ILO) Classification of Radiographs of Pneumoconioses

The ILO classification (6) provides a means of turning the information on a chest X-ray into semiquantitative data. Radiographs read in this way are the cornerstone of epidemiologic studies of mineral pneumoconioses. In order to be successful, there must be careful attention to technical detail. Radiographs used should be of the highest quality. Each film should be read independently by two, preferably three, experienced readers (7) who need not necessarily be medically qualified so long as the films have been scrutinized by a clinician who will recognize treatable disease. Films should be read in random order and all identifying marks, except a code number, should be hidden. Other films, up to 2% of the total number to be read, whose readings have been agreed upon by readers beforehand, can be inserted into the series. Once read in the usual manner, their agreed reading is disclosed so that a reader may judge whether his or her performance is consistent. Equipment required for this exercise includes a set of ILO standard films and a copy of their *Guidelines*, a viewing box with capacity for a minimum of three or four films, reading sheets, and, if possible, an assistant to record the readings. In this way, it is possible to comfortably read up to 400 films in a day.

Small Opacities

Small opacities are graded for profusion, extent, size, and shape. The category of profusion is based on a comparative assessment between the film to be read and the standard films. The four major categories are 0, 1, 2, and 3, for which there are standard radiographs. However, the classification has been refined by allowing the reader to extend this to a 12-point scale. Thus the radiograph is classified in the usual way into one of the four major categories using the standard radiographs. If one of the major categories above or below is seriously considered then this is recorded. A reading of category 2/1 indicates that the major category is 2 but category 1 was seriously considered. If there was no doubt that the major category was 2, then the reading would be 2/2. Thus the complete 12-point scale becomes: 0/–, 0/0, 0/1, 1/0, 1/1, 1/2, 2/1, 2/2, 2/3, 3/2, 3/3, 3/+. 0/– is recorded if the absence of small opacities is particularly obvious (not frequently seen in urban dwellers), and 3/+ is recorded if there is markedly higher profusion than would be classified as 3/3.

There will be circumstances when small opacities are not equally distributed throughout all six lung zones. When this occurs, the category of profusion is determined from those zones that are affected, and any zone whose profusion differs by at least three minor categories is ignored.

The classification recognizes both round and irregular opacities but it is not possible in the convention to record these separately. Round opacities are denoted by the letters *p*, *q*, and *r*, irregular opacities by the letters *s*, *t*, and *u* (Table 26.1).

While the written definitions of these small opacities may be helpful, it is better to use the standard films for reference. Two letters are used for each reading, with the first letter indicating the predominant shape and size. As an example, *q*/*t* indicates that round shadows of size *q* are

Table 26.1. ILO classification of small opacities

p = diameter up to about 1.5 mm
q = diameter exceeding about 1.5 mm and up to about 3 mm
r = diameter exceeding about 3 mm and up to about 10 mm
s = width up to about 1.5 mm
t = width exceeding 1.5 mm and up to about 3 mm
u = width exceeding 3 mm and up to about 10 mm

Table 26.2. ILO classification of large opacities

Category A	An opacity having a greatest diameter exceeding about 10 mm and up to and including about 50 mm, or several opacities each greater than about 10 mm, the sum of whose greatest diameters does not exceed about 50 mm
Category B	One or more opacities larger or more numerous than those in category A whose combined area does not exceed the equivalent of the right upper zone
Category C	One or more opacities whose combined area exceeds the equivalent of the right upper zone

the main type of opacity present but there are significant numbers of irregular opacities as well. A reading of *q*/*q* would indicate that virtually all opacities seen were of one size and shape.

Large Opacities

Large opacities are defined in terms of their size (Table 26.2). Problems arise when it is considered that large opacities present are not due to pneumoconiosis. The *Guidelines* give clear instructions that if pneumoconiosis is a serious possibility then the opacity should be classified but a note should be made of alternative etiologies. However, if it is probable that the appearance is due to some other condition, then the opacity should not be classified, and use should be made of appropriate symbols (see later) and comments.

Pleural Abnormalities

Pleural thickening and pleural calcification are recorded separately. There are difficulties with this part of the classification that are discussed briefly in the *Guidelines*. The major problem is differentiating thickening of visceral and parietal pleura on the posteroanterior radiograph. This is not always possible but may be a desirable goal because evidence suggests that their etiology and natural history may be different. Pleural thickening on the chest wall is described as diffuse and/or circumscribed (plaque). Both of these may occur together and provide problems in interpretation for the novice. Circumscribed shadows are usually the result of parietal pleural thickening and they may go on to calcify. Both width and extent should be recorded (see Table 26.3), but it can readily be appreciated that both of these measurements are influenced by the actual position of the plaque on the chest wall. Diffuse shadows probably result from thickening of the visceral pleura. They are called "diffuse" because they generally are seen as an indistinct veiling of the lung

Table 26.3. ILO classification of pleural thickening and calcification

Pleural Thickening

Width: On the lateral chest wall, the measurement of the maximum width of the shadow is made from the inner line of the chest wall to the inner margin of the shadow seen most sharply at the parenchymal-pleural boundary.

a = maximum width up to about 5 mm
b = maximum width over about 5 mm and up to about 10 mm
c = maximum width over about 10 mm

If pleural thickening can be seen face on, this should be recorded, even if it can also be seen in profile. Pleural thickening that can only be seen face on generally has no measurable width.

Extent: This means maximum length, or sum of maximum lengths either in profile or face on.

1 = total length equivalent to up to one quarter of the projection of the lateral chest wall
2 = total length exceeding one quarter but not one half of the projection of the lateral chest wall
3 = total length exceeding one half of the projection of the lateral chest wall

Pleural Calcification

Site and extent are recorded for each lung separately.

1 = an area of calcified pleura with greatest diameter up to about 20 mm, or a number of such areas the sum of whose greatest diameters does not exceed about 20 mm.
2 = an area of calcified pleura with greatest diameter exceeding about 20 mm and up to about 100 mm, or a number of such areas the sum of whose greatest diameters exceeds about 20 mm but does not exceed about 100 mm.
3 = an area of calcified pleura with greatest diameter exceeding about 100 mm, or a number of such areas the sum of whose greatest diameters exceeds about 100 mm.

Table 26.4. Symbols for ILO classification comments

ax — coalescence of small opacities
bu — bulla(e)
ca — cancer of lung or pleura
cn — calcification in small opacities
co — abnormal cardiac size or shape
cp — cor pulmonale
cv — cavity
di — marked distortion of intrathoracic organs
ef — effusion
em — definite emphysema
es — egg-shell calcification of lymph nodes
fr — fractured rib(s)
hi — enlargement of hilar or other nodes
ho — honeycomb lung
id — ill-defined diaphragm
ih — ill-defined heart outline
kl — septal (Kerley) lines
od — other significant abnormality
pi — pleural thickening in the interlobular fissure or mediastinum
px — pneumothorax
rp — rheumatoid pneumoconiosis
tb — tuberculosis (not the calcified primary complex)

parenchyma. Sometimes, when this type of thickening is seen edge on, there will be a distinct line along the chest wall. When this occurs, width is recorded, along with extent (Table 26.3). Plaque on the diaphragmatic pleura is recorded separately, as is costophrenic angle obliteration. There is a standard radiograph (I/I *t/t*) that can be used to assess the lower limit for this obliteration.

Pleural calcification is recorded as present or absent on the chest wall, diaphragm, and "other" sites, which include the mediastinum and pericardium. The extent of this should also be measured (Table 26.3).

Comments

Other abnormalities seen in the chest radiograph are recorded using the symbols given in Table 26.4. While their use is obligatory, it is suggested in the *Guidelines* that each is assumed to be preceded by some such phrase as "changes are suggestive of . . ."

The ILO classification has proved itself to be a powerful tool in epidemiologic studies, but it must be used with care. Film quality can have a marked effect on the category attributed to the radiograph, emphasizing the need for technical excellence to obtain meaningful results. As with any form of radiology, there is no substitute for experience, so whenever possible each team of film-readers should include at least one person who is well versed in all the problems and pitfalls.

Silica

Background

Silicon is one of the most abundant elements in the earth's crust; therefore any operation that involves upheaval of this crust potentially can result in silicosis. Crushed siliceous rocks have a multitude of uses (8), which include cleaning and polishing, incorporation in ceramics, fillers in paper and plasters, and use as lubricants. This by no means exhaustive list shows the variety of manufacturing processes whose workers may be at risk of silicosis. The diagnosis can be missed easily if inquiry into the patient's exact occupation is not thorough. The risk of silicosis increases as the amount of respirable silica dust particles present in the atmosphere increases. People at greatest risk are those who work without adequate protection in confined spaces (e.g., tunnelers).

Crystalline silicone dioxide comes in many shapes and forms, such as granite, sandstone, flint, slate, and shale. It can also be found in lesser amounts in china and fire clays, feldspar, bentonite, and diatomite.

Pathology

In order to reach the alveolus, inhaled particles of silicon dioxide (quartz) are likely to have a diameter of less than

7 μm, usually between 1 and 5 μm. The majority of these particles will be engulfed by macrophages. This may kill the macrophages, which will then lyse; alternatively, if a sublethal dose is ingested, the macrophagelise may be stimulated to release a substance that activates fibroblasts (9). These activated fibroblasts produce hydroxyproline, which in turn leads to the formation of collagen. Reticulin fibers, which subsequently convert to collagen, are laid down in a concentric fashion to form the silicotic nodule. This may have a hyalinized or calcified center and the fibers at the outer edge may form a capsule (10–12). There is a clear relationship between the presence of silicotic nodules and round opacities on the chest radiograph (13,14).

Silicotic nodules can coalesce to form conglomerate lesions. While these may cavitate, they do not do so as readily as the lesions of progressive massive fibrosis found in coal workers. Fibrosis of the pleura certainly occurs and may extend into the mediastinum (15). Another major complication is tuberculosis that at one time was so prevalent that it obscured the true natural history of silicosis (16,17).

Clinical Features

There are no specific features in the clinical history or physical examination to indicate the diagnosis. Patients may complain of breathlessness, but unless their exposure has been particularly heavy, this may well be dismissed as part of the aging process, particularly if they are cigarette smokers. Chronic cough and phlegm are common but should nonetheless always alert the physician to the possibility of tuberculosis. Resistance to tuberculosis is low and radiologic evidence of disease is not always apparent, making it necessary to retain a high index of suspicion even when supporting evidence is scant.

The rate at which the disease progresses depends on the amount of dust originally inhaled. Those with high exposures are likely to have more rapid progression, which may continue after exposure has ceased (18). Coalescence of silicotic nodules may cause some areas of the lung to shrink and others to stretch. This is the best current explanation for the phenomenon of so-called compensatory emphysema that is seen so often both radiologically and pathologically, and the signs of which can be identified clinically. In extreme cases patients may complain of dysphagia, but this is rare.

In a typical case, there may be very few physical signs despite a grossly abnormal chest radiograph. However, extensive disease is likely to be associated with gradually progressive breathlessness, recurrent chest infections, and hypoxemia. Treatment is symptomatic but usually is sufficiently effective to allow the patient to die from some other cause, such as ischemic heart disease. There is no known connection between the inhalation of silica dust and lung cancer.

Lung Function

The changes in lung function in simple silicosis are so unobtrusive that they are generally only recognized in epidemiologic studies. When nodules conglomerate, it is more usual to find abnormalities, although these have no characteristic pattern. A recent study assessing the influence of silicosis on deteriorating lung function in gold miners in Canada employed underground for a mean period of 29 years has demonstrated that lung function deteriorated more rapidly in the men with silicosis and the deterioration increased in proportion to the degree of silicosis at the start of the study. Additionally, it has been found that the loss of lung function during the period of follow-up was directly in proportion with the nodule profusion on their initial chest radiographs (19).

A similar study checking the impairment of pulmonary function in 220. Chinese workers exposed to silica, has shown that radiographic hyperinflation was strongly associated with decreases in forced expiratory volume (FLV_1) and FEV_1/FVC (forced viral capcity). Comparison between workers with and without hyperinflation showed that the former had significantly lower pulmonary function values. The conclusion was that emphysema associated with silicosis is likely to be responsible for pulmonary obstruction and decreased diffusing capacity occurring in silica-exposed workers (20).

Radiology

The X-ray appearance of simple silicosis is that of diffuse, small, round opacities initially in the outer half of the upper zone of both lung fields (Fig. 26.1); as time progresses they may occupy all lung zones. At the start, opacities may be quite soft, but eventually they become more easily distinguished from background lung, particularly when they calcify (Fig. 26.2). As mentioned before, studies have demonstrated an exposure–response relationship between cumulative exposure to crytalline silica and radiographic opacities. In addition it has been shown that the relationship is substantially steeper among workers exposed at the highest average concentrations of crystalline silica (21).

Lung opacities in silicosis may coalesce. These lesions differ from the progressive massive fibrosis that occurs in coal workers' pneumoconiosis in that the coalescence often retains a nodular character. Cavitation may occur, but, when it does, it should immediately alert the physician to the possibility of tuberculosis. Pleural thickening in the apices and upper zones is common, particularly in association with conglomerate lesions. Compensatory emphysema may be obvious in the lower zones. Lymph node enlargement is often accompanied by egg-shell calcification (Fig. 26.3). This calcification is not pathognomonic of silicosis, as has been reported with tuberculosis, sarcoidosis, and histoplasmosis (22). Usually the natural history of the disease serves to distinguish these other etiologies, but diagnostic prob-

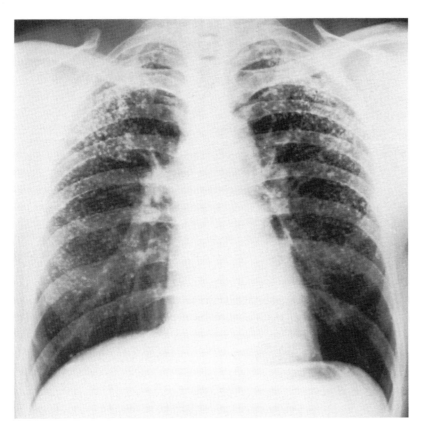

Figure 26.1. Silicosis in a metalliferous miner who worked underground for 22 years in a variety of jobs – a miner, a laborer, an ore sorter, and an axeman.

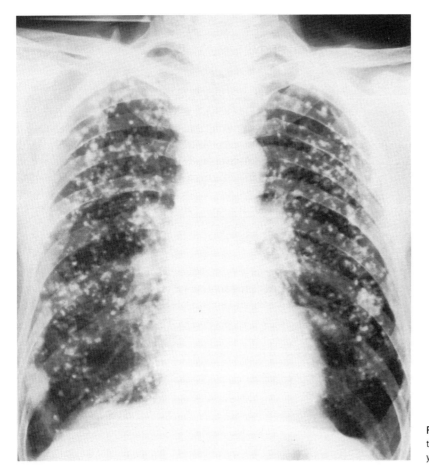

Figure 26.2. Silicosis in a stonemason showing calcified opacities. This film was taken just before he retired; he had spent 50 years in the same job.

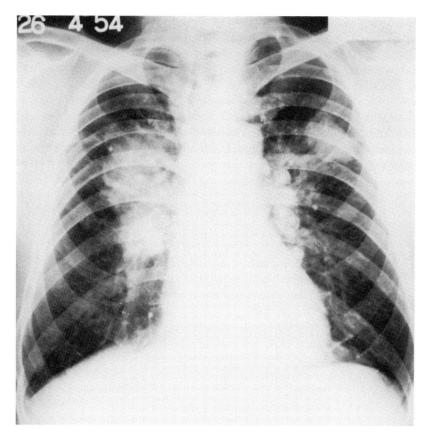

Figure 26.3. Silicosis in a gold miner. The conglomerate lesions are not typical of silicosis, which often has a more nodular appearance with definite areas of calcification within. There is, however, classical eggshell calcification of the hilar nodes. Note the paucity of background opacities.

lems can occur. For example, solitary massive lesions, known as silicomas, have been reported (23), although it would be wise to regard all solitary lesions as lung cancer until proved otherwise.

There may be radiologic changes associated with the development of tuberculosis, such as the rapid appearance of new infiltrates in the apices, unexpected progression, or cavitation of conglomerate lesions. However, if there is a background profusion of ILO category 2 or more, it may be impossible to identify new changes of tuberculosis and the diagnosis must rest on clinical suspicion supported by bacteriologic evidence.

The new radiologic techniques, computed tomography (CT) and high resolution CT (HRCT) have proven their benefit in the diagnosis of silicosis (14,24–26). Typical findings on high resolution scans in this disease will be that of tiny, short, branching opacities corresponding to irregular fibrosis around and along the respiratory bronchiole, as well as focal dust emphysema. A small, central fibrotic nodule can usually be identified, which makes the difference from true centrilobular emphysema. CT clearly identifies the rounded and diffuse lung opacities characteristic for silicosis as well as changes related to the confluent type. magnetic resonance imaging (MRI) has been used among other mentalities to identify signal characteristics of progressive massive fibrosis in patients with silicosis and silicotuberculosis and has shown that the most common MRI appearance of progressive massive fibrosis is isointensity on T_1-weighted images and hypointensity on T_2-weighted images

when compared with skeletal muscle, with internal high signal intensity areas on T_2-weighted images and either rim enhancement or no enhancement (27).

Diagnosis and Management

The diagnosis of silicosis is made by a combination of occupational history and radiology. There is no specific treatment, although various agents thought to modify fibrogenesis have had therapeutic trials, so far without success. The emphasis of management is therefore on maintaining adequate lung function by treating coexistent airway disease, on prompt therapy for chest infections, and, when necessary, on correction of hypoxia with supplemental oxygen. With this approach most patients do well, the only exceptions being those who have far-advanced conglomerate disease. Tuberculosis should be treated in a conventional manner with triple or, preferably, quadruple chemotherapy.

Prevention

As with all industrial hazards, a balance must be achieved between acceptable risk to workers and manageable working practice. As recent publications in this domain state, the morbidity and mortality due to pulmonary silicosis and other effects resulting from exposure to silica dust, such as nephrotoxicity, demonstrate that health effects of work exposure to silica are still marked (28,29). The potential of silica to cause serious disease means that all efforts must be made to keep the concentration of silica in the air below accepted threshold limit values. This can occur only if the risk is recognized and good occupational hygiene is undertaken. The work situation should be monitored by regular dust sampling, and, if dust is present, this surveillance should be supplemented by regular chest X-rays of the work force.

Coal

Background

In the 18th century, technical advances in engineering allowed deep coal mines to be exploited. This expansion in the industry led to coal becoming the most important source of energy for the first industrial revolution. In 1826 Laennec (30) described a specific condition in the lungs of coal miners that he called melanosis. Over the next hundred years there was much debate about the true nature of the condition, but it was not until 1937 that any real progress was made. At the request of the Medical Research Council (MRC), Hart and Aslett (31) reported on the health of coal workers in South Wales. In response to this report, the MRC Pneumoconiosis Research Unit was formed in South Wales to investigate problems encountered in the coal industry. Much of our present knowledge of this condition is a result of the work of this Unit.

Coal has an organic origin, being formed from compressed, decomposed trees and other vegetation. Its structure is dependent on local conditions at the time of formation. Thus it may occur in seams of varying thickness with layers of sandstone and shale, the whole lot being distorted by subsequent earth folds. The purest coal (anthracite) contains approximately 92–94% carbon; bituminous coal contains up to 92% carbon, but peat, the precursor of coal, contains only 54–75% carbon. Coal high in carbon is said to be of high rank. This kind of coal often produces more dust during extraction and therefore workers are more at risk of pneumoconiosis. The structure of coal seams often means that quartz-containing rock must be removed in order to gain access to the coal. Miners who work with rock as well as coal have the added risk of developing silicosis (32).

At the same time, epidemiological studies have shown that the prevalence of coal worker's pneumoconiosis (CWP) differs remarkably between different coal mine regions despite comparable exposure to respirable dust. In a study performed in the USA it has been found that CNP pneumoconiosi is more common among coal miners from Pennsylvania than in those from Utah., for example. One of the explanations offered is that the buffering capacity of coal is lower in Pennsylvania and its acid-soluble Fe^{2+} content higher than in Utah, possibly exercising a role in the development of the disease (33). In addition, a German study performed in vitro suggested that high concentrations of phenolic compounds can be extracted from coal mine dust generated by low rank coals. Adapted to physiologic conditions, leaching fluids showed that coal mine dust with varying content of different ranks can be seen as a parameter reinforcing its cytotoxic effect (34).

Pathology

As with quartz, coal particles that reach the alveolus are less than 7 μm. Here the similarity ends because coal does not have the same effect on macrophages. The primary lesion in CWP is the macule, which consists of dust, reticulin, macrophages, and fibroblasts (35). These macules tend to enlarge slowly in size and may eventually be associated with adjacent emphysema. Dust can also be found beneath both visceral and parietal pleura but does not cause pleural thickening. It can also be seen in lymph nodes at the hil and in the mediastinum. With increasing dust loads, progressive massive fibrosis (PMF) occurs. This is a confluent black lesion, often with a necrotic center and an irregular edge. These lesions have been shown to contain fibronectin rather than collagen (36). There may be associated endarteritis and thrombosis (37). When cavitation occurs, the patient expectorates black viscid material that has been inappropriately called melanoptysis. As in silicosis, compensatory emphysema may occur, and, indeed, emphysema may obscure the radiologic evidence of background simple pneumoconiosis. The association of the rheumatoid diathesis and discreet large nodular lesions in the chest radiographs of coal miners was first described by Caplan (38) in 1953.

Clinical Features

It is important to take an accurate occupational history even from those known to have worked underground all of their lives, because different jobs result in different exposure to dust. When simple pneumoconiosis consists only of coal macules it gives rise to very little, if any, respiratory impairment (39). In many instances, however, there will be accompanying emphysema, which results in progressive breathlessness (40). Complicated pneumoconiosis (PMF) is almost invariably associated with some degree of respiratory disability (41). Many miners complain of cough and sputum that may be attributed to cigarette smoking; however, there is evidence that heavy coal dust inhalation per se can cause chronic bronchitis (42).

PMF takes time to develop. When this radiologic appearance is seen for the first time, the differential diagnosis may include tuberculosis and lung cancer, particularly if the background lung opacities are not obvious. Whenever possible, old radiographs should be obtained for comparison. The expectoration of large quantities of inky black material signals cavitation of a PMF lesion. It is important to look for infection, especially tuberculosis (43), but this need not be present. Hemoptysis can occur but is usually self-limiting, and *Aspergillus* can invade residual cavities.

Lung Function

As with silicosis, the pattern of lung function abnormality cannot help to make the diagnosis of CWP. Of interest is the fact that p shadows are often associated with low gas transfer and with emphysema at postmortem (44). When comparing the respiratory impairment due to dust exposure in workers exposed to coal mine, silica, and coal mine dust, studies showed that all three groups of dust-exposed workers, even those without radiographic signs of pneumoconiosis, had decreased spirometric parameters and diffusing capacity in both smokers and nonsmokers. Pulmonary function was further decreased when pneu-

moconiosis was present in these groups. The major impairment pattern discovered was obstructive in exposure to coal mine dust, mixed in silica workers, and restrictive and mixed in asbestos workers, changes which have been demonstrated to precede the radiographic changes of pneumoconiosis (45).

Radiology

The first radiologic evidence of CWP is soft, discrete, round opacities that may be present in all lung zones. These round opacities may be predominantly classified as p, q (Fig. 26.4), or r shadows, but, equally, combinations of different round opacities and round and irregular opacities are frequently seen. The q shadow is probably most common. In some cases, the only opacities present are irregular in character. At present, there is speculation that these irregular opacities reflect either emphysema or interstitial fibrosis that may or may not be related to dust exposure (46). The opacities of CWP may look similar to opacities found in silicosis; however, they rarely become as dense and they are usually more evenly distributed throughout the lung. These often quoted generalizations can be useful in identifying the

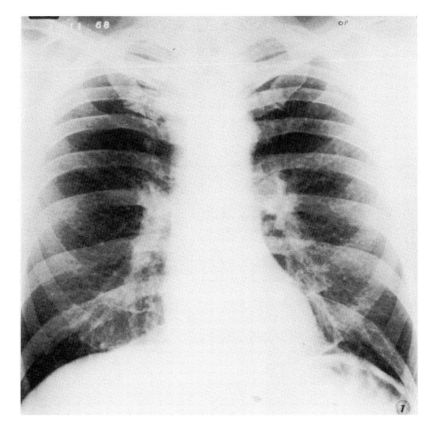

Figure 26.4. q Shadows in a coal worker with simple pneumoconiosis.

coal worker who has been exposed to a significant amount of stone dust.

As PMF develops, it usually slowly forms a sausage-shaped opacity or opacities (Fig. 26.5). These are found predominantly in the middle and upper zones. Compensatory emphysema may be well developed. Classically, PMF does not occur until there is at least a category 2 or more background, but this is not a rigid requirement. In most cases of category B or C PMF, it is difficult, sometimes impossible, to categorize the background shadows. An exception to this description is Caplan syndrome (47). Here the opacities tend to be smaller and peripheral, and tend to develop in a relatively short space of time (Fig. 26.6). However, this classical appearance can quickly progress to a picture that is difficult to differentiate from PMF or, in this instance, conglomerate silicosis. The lesions of PMF are more likely to cavitate than those of conglomerate silicosis. Cavitation is particularly common in Caplan syndrome (Fig. 26.7).

Recent studies comparing the findings on conventional radiography, CT, scintigraphy and pathologic samples concluded that irregular opacities usually identified on chest radiographs represent interstitial fibrotic changes associated with the accumulation of birefringent particles together with emphysematous changes, all confirmed on histologic studies (48–49). As the ILO classification of small and large opacities is the basis for the compensation of patients with pneumoconiosis, in order to validate radi-ologic findings the ILO classification was compared with the grading of pneumoconiosis on postmortem investigations. When the chosen threshold ILO value was 1/0 the sensitivity was 100% and the specificity 2%. With a value of 2/3, the sensitivity decreased to 60% and specificity increased to 74%. The grading of large opacities in the radiograph correlated well with the postmortem findings (50). The diagnosis of CWP has been continuously improved by the use of CT and especially of HRCT, which identifies typical pathologic changes earlier and with greater detail, including linear and reticular opacities or thickening of the interlobular septa and of the intralobular interstitium (51–53).

Diagnosis

CWP will develop only when a relatively large amount of coal dust has been retained in the lungs. Category 3 simple pneumoconiosis requires between 20 and 40 g of coal dust to accumulate despite efficient pulmonary defense mechanisms (54). How long this takes depends on the amount of atmospheric dust and the length of exposure. It seems likely that there is also individual variation, but this has a relatively minor role. The diagnosis therefore generally requires a history of coal dust exposure over many years. Exceptions may be coal workers exposed to large quantities of dust in mines where occu-

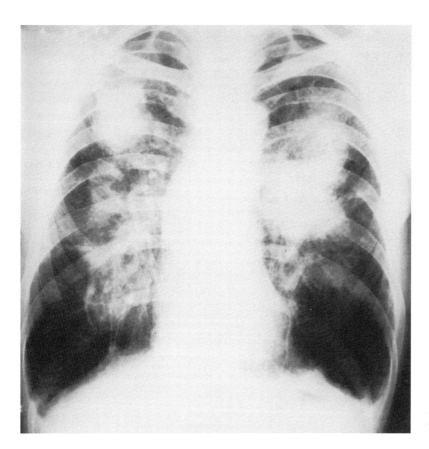

Figure 26.5. Category C PMF (progressive massive fibrosis) in a coal miner. Note the relative lack of background opacities and the compensatory emphysema.

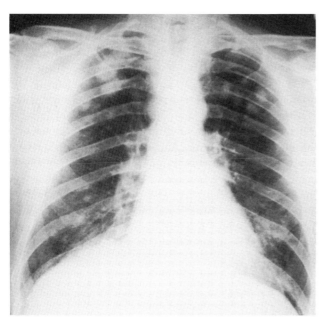

Figure 26.6. Caplan syndrome. The suggestion that this looks like the mark of white fingerprints is very apt.

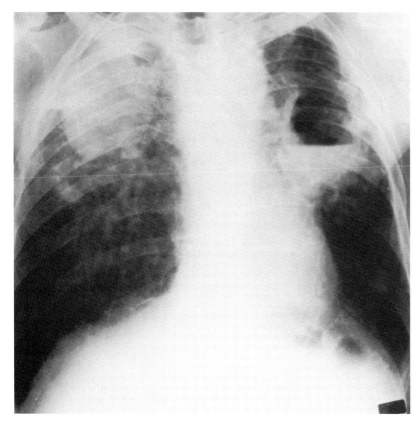

Figure 26.7. Cavitating PMF. This man first presented with breath-lessness when 27 years old. His radiograph then showed category A PMF. He had worked underground for 13 years on the coal face. This film was taken 32 years later.

pational hygiene is poor. In the United Kingdom, category 2, predominantly nodular opacities are usually present before compensation is awarded for occupational injury. Thus we tend to reserve the term "coal-worker's pneumo-coniosis" for these cases. Early studies had shown that progression rarely occurred without the degree of dust retention associated with category 2 pneumoconiosis (55). While this is true, improved conditions in the mines have meant that there are more cases with category one or less background opacities, some of whom undoubtedly progress to develop PMF (56). This is a growing area of research interest.

Management

There is no specific treatment. The principles employed in the management of silicosis apply equally to CWP. Cavitation of a PMF lesion can require symptomatic measures to help with difficult expectoration. Hemoptysis may occur but is usually self-limiting. A PMF cavity, as with any cavity, may be invaded by *Aspergillus*, and management is no different. Tuberculosis is not uncommon but there is no specific association except in those workers who have had significant exposure to rock dust. Men with this disease can have many years of active life and it is of paramount importance that they and their physicians maintain a positive approach.

Prevention

This depends mainly on dust suppression. Epidemiologic studies have made it possible to predict how many will develop disease given exposure to known dust levels over a presumed working life of 35 years (57). Adoption of work practices that keep dust levels below those estimated to produce no more than category one disease is the basis of prevention, but must be backed up by biologic monitoring of the work force.

Asbestos

Background

This rock, which can be woven into cloth, has been used since ancient times. In many instances it can be easily obtained without sophisticated mining techniques. It was produced on a small scale until the demands of the 20th century turned it into an almost indispensable mineral. Now, there are literally thousands of uses for asbestos and it is proving difficult in many cases to find adequate substitutes. Brake linings, lagging, cement products, floor tiles, building materials, and fire-resistant cloth all may contain asbestos, which means that, as with silica, workers in a wide range of industries may be at risk.

The word "asbestos" is used to describe a family of related minerals that share a similar fibrous form. Chrysotile, commonly called "white" asbestos, is a sheet silicate derived from serpentine rock. It occurs throughout the world, with the largest known deposits in Canada, the former USSR, and Southern Africa. The other types of asbestos are derived from amphibole rock. The best known is crocidolite or "blue asbestos," found in Southern

Africa and Western Australia. Amosite, or "brown asbestos," tremolite, actinolite, and anthophyllite are other forms of amphibole asbestos, of which only amosite is used commercially.

Asbestos exposure can cause pleural thickening and calcification, fibrosing pleurisy, pulmonary fibrosis, and malignant disease of the pleura, lung, and peritoneum (58–60). The cellular and molecular mechanisms of asbestos-induced fibrosis have been reviewed in a recent article (61). It seems that the pathogenesis in this disorder involves the participation of a number of cell types and is characterized by an early and persistent inflammatory response that involves the generation of oxidants, growth factors, chemokines and cytokines. These mediators may also contribute directly to cell injury, proliferation, and fibrogenesis.

Pathology

Pleural Thickening

Pleural plaques are areas of hyaline fibrous tissue that occur in up to 40% of people exposed to any form of asbestos (62). This exposure may be from an occupational or an environmental source, such as naturally occurring asbestos-contaminated soil. Plaques are found in the parietal pleura bilaterally and often symmetrically. The diaphragm is often affected. Plaque can also occur on the parietal pericardium. It takes about 20 years for sufficient calcium to accumulate to make plaque readily visible on the radiograph (63). Very occasionally plaque can envelop the lung.

Fibrosing Pleurisy

Fibrosing pleurisy can first manifest as a pleural effusion that resolves spontaneously. In its wake comes diffuse pleural thickening, which may involve the visceral surface. There may be associated plaque.

Pulmonary Fibrosis

Pulmonary fibrosis is the condition for which the term "asbestosis" is generally reserved. Inhaled asbestos fibers are trapped in alveoli that arise directly from the respiratory bronchioles. Those fibers that are coated are seen as asbestos bodies. Fibers longer than 10 μm are retained and may lie loose or may be engulfed by macrophages. When these macrophages lyse, they promote fibrosis, which is progressive. Initially only respiratory bronchioles are affected, but with time these discrete lesions become confluent and, eventually, fibrous tissue contracts, forming thick-walled cystic spaces. The distribution of this disease is initially subpleural, predominantly in the lung bases, but it spreads to affect virtually all areas of the lung (64).

Lung Cancer

Tumors are usually squamous in origin, but both oat cell tumors and adenocarcinomata can occur.

Pleural and Peritoneal Mesotheliomas

The relationship of asbestosis to the development of malignant mesothelioma is well established Although considered a rare neoplasm, a certain increase in its incidence has been noticed in recent years, not only as an occupational hazard of people involved directly in the production and industrial use of asbestos, but also in people living in the proximity of industrial plants, as well as in people in whom a history of exposure cannot be documented (65–68).

Pleural mesothelioma is far more common than peritoneal mesothelioma. Pleural mesothelioma appears to originate in the parietal pleura with nodules of tissue that exfoliate at an early stage. This leads to seeding of the pleural cavity. Nodules increase in size to involve both pleural surfaces. Mesothelial cells can differentiate into spindle-type sarcomatous cells or epithelial-like cells (64). As it progresses, tumor will invade the chest wall, the mediastinum, and the pericardium. Hematogenous spread occurs but is rare. Seeding of the opposite pleural surfaces also occurs. The origin of peritoneal mesothelioma is uncertain. Nodules occur along the serosal surface of the gut and the inferior surface of the diaphragm. Eventually the whole peritoneal cavity becomes full of tumor.

Clinical Features and Lung Function

Pleural Thickening

In most cases, pleural thickening is symptomless. Problems arise rarely when diffuse disease is associated with mild breathlessness, and then airflow restriction may be detectable on lung function tests.

Fibrosing Pleurisy

Asbestos pleurisy can present acutely with severe pain, fever, and leukocytosis. More often, it is symptomless or detected on a routine chest X-ray (70). Diffuse pleural fibrosis is more likely to be associated with breathlessness. Lung function may show airflow restriction with small lung volumes. Gas transfer may be slightly reduced. If it is significantly low, then associated disease of the lung parenchyma should be suspected.

Pulmonary Fibrosis

Pulmonary fibrosis occurs only in people who have had moderate or heavy exposure to asbestos and usually takes at least 10 years to develop (71). The major symptom is breathlessness, which progresses gradually but inexorably. Cough and sputum production may occur even in nonsmokers. Clubbing sometimes occurs but is not a helpful sign as it bears little relationship to the severity of disease. Late, crisp inspiratory crackles are usually audible at the lung bases but can be missed in the early stages. Lung function tests classically show airflow restriction with small lung volumes and low gas transfer. However, there may be evidence of airflow obstruction.

Lung Cancer

This presents in the same way as lung cancer from any other cause. The main features are pain, weight loss, and hemoptysis, but other less common manifestations, such as endocrine and metabolic disturbances, also occur. The prerequisites necessary for attributing lung carcinoma to asbestos, remain a controversial issue. A recent study (72) investigated 414 patients (353 men and 61 women) with lung cancer, recording the occupational history and the presence of pleural plaques and asbestos bodies. Depending on these criteria it has been found that in the male patients about 60% of the lung carcinomas could be plausibly attributable to asbestos.

Another study of 1376 Finnish patients with asbestosis and 4887 patients with benign asbestos-related pleural disease looked for the risk of cancer according to the histologic type of cancer, the time since diagnosis of asbestosis, the asbestos-associated risk for cancers other than lung cancer and mesothelioma, and the predictive value of asbestos-related abnormalities as regards the risk of cancer (73). Compared with the total incidence in Finland, men with asbestosis had a higher risk of lung cancer (standardized incidence ratio (SIR) 6.7), mesothelioma (SIR 32) and cancer of the larynx (SIR 4.2). The risk of lung cancer was similarly raised in all histologic types of lung cancer (the highest in insulators) and did not change markedly over time of notification or duration of follow-up. Men with benign pleural disease had a higher risk of mesothelioma (SIR 5.5), and a slightly elevated risk for lung cancer (SIR 1.3). Among women with asbestosis, a significant increase was found in the risk for lung cancer and mesothelioma.

Pleural and Peritoneal Mesotheliomas

The classical presentation of pleural mesotheliorna is dull chest or shoulder pain. There is often a pleural effusion with accompanying breathlessness. Hemoptysis is not a feature. Peritoneal mesotheliornas generally present late with ascites and cachexia.

Radiology

Pleural Thickening

Large calcified plaques are easily identified. Difficulties arise when plaques are small with little calcium. For this reason, the incidence of plaque noted at postmortem is far higher than the incidence seen in life on the chest X-ray. There are techniques that will help with visualization of plaque. The most useful are lateral (Fig. 26.8) and anterior oblique views. Plaque may only be visible on the diaphragm (a usual site) if an oblique film is taken. CT scanning is the most efficient way to visualize pleural thickening and plaque, much earlier than on conventional chest radiography (83,84,91). Nevertheless, CT evidence of pleural thickening does not necessarily indicate the presence of asbestosis (74,77).

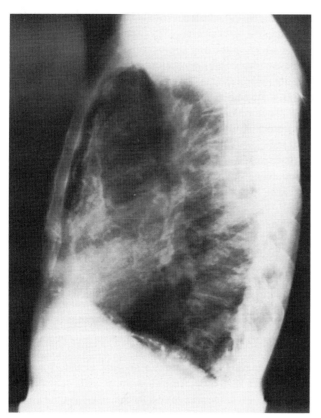

Figure 26.8. Lateral film showing both diaphragmatic and pleural plaque.

Fibrosing Pleurisy

The pleural effusion that often heralds the onset of diffuse pleural fibrosis may have no distinguishing features, but a careful search should always be made for any other radiologic evidence of asbestos exposure. As this effusion subsides it may leave a blunt costophrenic angle. Ultrasound examination is the best way to demonstrate that this residuum is solid and likely to be due to thickened pleura. Diffuse pleural fibrosis can occur in association with pulmonary fibrosis or extensive pleural plaque, or on its own.

Pulmonary Fibrosis

The radiologic hallmark of this condition is bilateral, irregular, initially basal shadows with associated evidence of pleural disease. If there is no pleural disease, the condition is indistinguishable from other forms of pulmonary fibrosis that have the same distribution. CT is very good at demonstrating underlying pulmonary disease when the parenchyma is veiled by pleural shadow. In general the findings range from early interstitial changes demonstrated by HRCT and late generalized changes, such as honeycombing and cystic abnormalities (74,75,78,79). The type of fibrotic changes described are usually centrilobular, peribronchiolar, which include irregular interfaces, pleural-based opacities, traction bronchiectasis, parenchymal bands, septal thickening and subpleural lines (80–82) (Fig. 26.9).

It has been checked whether the parenchymal abnormalities discovered by HRCT have a functional significance (83). A subjective semiquantitative scoring approach has been compared with a cumulation of the various high resolution features of asbestosis. Additionally, all patients had histologic confirmation of their disease and HRCT results were also compared with conventional chest radiographs. Both scoring modalities have been shown to give similar results in suggesting the presence of disease, with the observation that asbestosis can present with minimal histopathologic changes and a normal HRCT.

Pleural Mesothelioma

Due to the increased risk of developing mesothelioma, people known to have been exposed to asbestos should undergo routine radiographic examinations of the thorax, which may suggest the presence of a malignant lesion by demonstrating the presence of a unilateral pleural effusion or irregular pleural surfaces. Pleural mesothelioma often presents with a large pleural effusion. The nature of the underlying pleura may not be revealed until this effusion has been tapped. Even then it may be difficult to make a confident diagnosis. It is uncommon to find bilat-

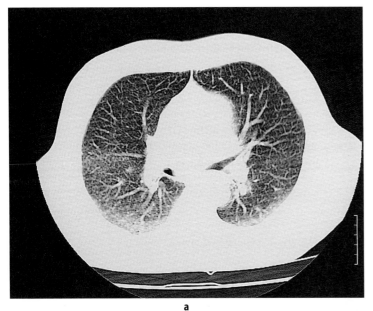

a

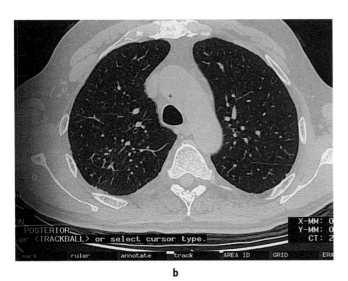

b

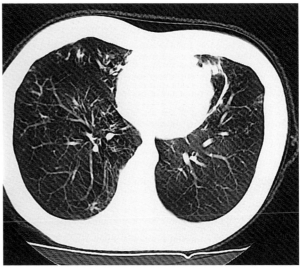

c

Figure 24.9. Chest radiographs of a 28 year old woman with adult respiratory distress syndrome after head trauma. **a** Chest radiograph showing patchy increase of density in the peripheral regions of the left lung. Total score 10. **b** One week later, the chest radiograph shows extensive white density in both lungs (score 20 + 20) and air bronchograms (score 4 + 4), especially in the upper regions of the left lung. Total score 48. **c** Close-up view of the upper regions of the left lung showing air bronchogram (*arrows*). Note the difference between air bronchogram and peribronchial cuffing seen in Fig. 24.3.

eral pleural plaque in this situation, but when present it clearly indicates previous exposure to asbestos.

The occurrence of massive lobular pleural thickening is suggestive, but not pathognomonic, of mesothelioma. Similar radiologic abnormalities can be found in metastatic processes or in extensive asbestos involvement. Careful differentiation should therefore be made by electron microscopy and histochemical studies.

When contralateral extension or involvement of adjacent organs occurs, they are better demonstrated by CT than by conventional radiography, as CT provides detailed information on the existence of nodular involvement of

the pleural fissures, parenchymal abnormalities, pericardial thickening, chest wall invasion, and lymph node involvement (84,85). MRI has added a new dimension to the diagnosis of this entity when tumoral masses are visualized as having a high signal intensity, and fibrotic changes can be seen as areas of low or intermediate signal intensity. There is also a capability of three-dimensional representation of the pathologic process, permitting an overall view and enhancing the diagnostic capabilities (86,87). In general for asbestos-related pleural lesions two types of magnetic resonance signal intensity patterns have been described: one which is low signal intensity on unenhanced and enhanced T_1-weighted and proton density and T_2-weighted images for benign plaques, and the other, a nonhomogeneous hyperintensity in T_2-weighted and enhanced T_1-weighted images for malignant mesothelioma (88).

When compared with CT, it appears that MRI is better at demonstrating spread of tumor into the interlobar fissures, tumor invasion of the diaphragm and through the diaphragm, and invasion of bony structures. While CT is more efficient in demonstrating inactive pleural calcifications, MRI is a sensitive modality for the visualization of the characteristic growth pattern and extension of this tumor, especially when one is attempting to assess resectability (89).

Diagnosis and Management

Pleural Thickening

Pleural thickening due to asbestos exposure occurs only when there has been inhalation of a moderate amount of fiber over a period of years. Plaque acts as a marker of exposure to asbestos and therefore may be associated with other asbestos-related diseases. In its own right pleural thickening seldom causes symptoms, although many patients require reassurance that it is not a premalignant condition.

Fibrosing Pleurisy

In its acute stages this may be impossible to differentiate from other causes of pleurisy. The diagnosis is often made in retrospect when evidence of diffuse pleural disease becomes more apparent. If asked, however, the patient should be able to give a good history of asbestos exposure. It is possible to surgically remove the thickened pleura but symptoms of breathlessness are only rarely sufficiently severe to warrant such a procedure.

Pulmonary Fibrosis

The diagnosis should be obvious from the occupational history and physical findings. Asbestosis does not occur unless there has been substantial exposure to asbestos fiber. If there is doubt, then examination of biopsy material for fibers using the electron microscope may be justified. Asbestos fibers can also be found in bronchoalveolar lavage fluid and in sputum but are more difficult to quantify. In most cases these investigations are not necessary. Treatment is supportive. Coexisting airflow obstruction may respond to conventional therapy. There is no evidence that corticosteroids are of any value. The most important task for the physician is to ensure that cigarette smoking is abandoned (see below). The disease normally progresses slowly over 20 years or so and thus has a better prognosis than cryptogenic fibrosing alveolitis (90).

Lung Cancer

Smoking increases the risk of lung cancer in asbestos-exposed subjects by approximately 50-fold when compared with nonsmoking, nonasbestos-exposed individuals (91). The diagnosis is made as for other forms of lung cancer, and management is similar.

Pleural Mesothelioma

Pleural mesothelioma usually occurs after exposure to amphibole fiber (92). The diagnosis can be made by identifying malignant mesothelial cells in pleural fluid. However, this requires considerable expertise so in practice the diagnosis is usually made from examination of solid tissue. One of the most efficient ways to achieve this is by biopsy at thoracoscopy. There has been reluctance in the past to perform this because of the risk of tumor tracking. It could be argued that the undoubtedly small chance of this occurring is far outweighed by the advantage of positive diagnosis. In particular, the risk of missing potentially treatable disease, such as tuberculous empyema, is avoided. Surgery and chemotherapy are offered in some centers but as yet there is no conclusive proof that either materially improve the very poor prognosis. Most patients die within 2 years of diagnosis.

Environmental Exposure

Most cases of asbestos-related disease occur in those who use the material in the course of their work. However, it is well known that the families of such workers can develop mesothelioma (93) and even pleural plaque from inhalation of fibers brought home on work clothes. Children who played on asbestos dumps are at risk of disease, as are people who lived in the vicinity of the mines before regulations on dust levels were enforced. Less well known is the fact that there is much naturally occurring asbestos throughout the world that can cause plaque and mesothelioma (94). Whether inhalation of this natural fiber increases lung cancer rates is the subject of much speculation and little fact.

Prevention

Asbestos is ubiquitous, making it virtually impossible to remove totally from our environment. Workers can be protected by employing strict occupational hygiene measures. Domestic exposure can be limited by ensuring that no free fiber gets into the atmosphere. On occasions this will be best achieved by total removal of fiber but the same effect can often be obtained by good fabric maintenance. Where possible, substitute materials should be used, although sometimes this is not practical for economic reasons. Chrysotile appears to be much less likely to cause disease than amphibole fiber and therefore should always be used in preference.

Artificial Mineral Fibers

One solution to the "asbestos problem" is to substitute materials that have similar capabilities but whose structure makes it unlikely that they will cause disease. Materials such as glass fiber, rock wool, and slag wool have a fibrous form, making them suitable substitutes for asbestos. In many cases these fibers are too large to penetrate far into the lung and this is corroborated by epidemiologic studies that, show no excess risk of mesothelioma (95) or pulmonary fibrosis. However, there does appear to be a slightly increased risk (1%) of lung cancer, which must be further evaluated (96).

Other Dusts

Metals

Aluminum

It is clear that aluminum fumes from welding may cause pulmonary granulomas and diffuse fibrosis (97), but previous reports that the metal powder caused pulmonary fibrosis are now thought to represent cases due to associated materials present during manufacturing processes.

Beryllium

Beryllium causes a granulomatous disease that is clinically, pathologically, and radiologically similar to sarcoidosis. It only affects a small percentage of those exposed. Beryllium can enter the body by inhalation or through cut skin to cause multisystem disease (98). The diagnosis is made from the occupational and clinical history, although care must be taken because slight exposure may have occurred some years before development of symptoms. Biopsies will show granulomas indistinguishable from those found in sarcoidosis, although it may be possible to identify beryllium within them. The lymphocyte transformation test (99), which identifies sensitivity to beryllium, should be positive and the Kveim test negative. Beryllium disease responds well to corticosteroid therapy.

Barium

Barium as barium sulfate (barytes) causes simple pneurnocomosis after prolonged inhalation (100). While this is easily seen radiologically (Fig. 26.10), it causes little limitation of pulmonary function.

Hard Metals

Hard metals (sintered metal carbides) are so called because of their extreme durability, which makes them

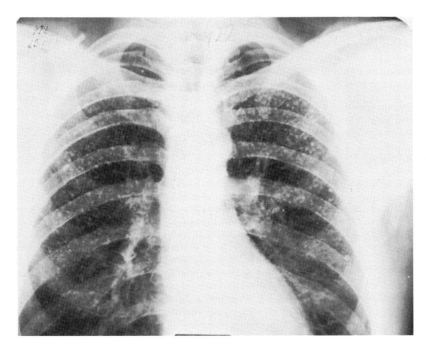

Figure 26.10. Barium pneumoconiosis. This man spent 6 years grinding and bagging barytes. When seen 5 years later, his X-ray was gradually clearing.

excellent cutting materials in, for example, drills. Tungsten carbide is the main constituent but titanium, vanadium, and tantalum are also used. Workers exposed to these dusts are at risk of developing interstitial fibrosis (101).

Iron

Iron is highly radiopaque, and thus easily seen on the radiograph. Fortunately it causes little reaction in the lung so that even if extensive siderosis (iron deposition) is present, the patient will usually be asymptomatic (102).

Tin

Tin is similar to iron in that it is highly radiopaque, but despite the dramatic X-ray appearance (Fig. 26.11) there will be no associated pulmonary symptoms (103). The condition is known as stannosis and is now rare. It should be distinguished from pneumoconiosis due to silica exposure found in some tin miners.

Other Substances

Kaolin

Kaolin can cause simple and, very rarely, complicated pneumoconiosis. There are no typical radiologic features (104).

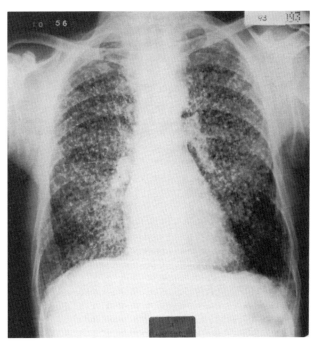

Figure 26.11. Stannosis in a man who spent 42 years working for a tin smelting firm.

Talc

Talc, when pure, may cause an innocuous simple pneumoconiosis, but it must be remembered that it can be contaminated with asbestos, in which case the range of asbestos-related diseases may be seen in those exposed (105).

Conclusion

In order to cause occupational lung disease a material must fulfill certain criteria. It must be present in the atmosphere in sufficient quantity, it must have respirable dimensions, and it must provoke some adverse response in the lung. To reduce risk, care should be taken to ensure that new materials are low in respirable particles and, if respirable particles are present, their level should be rigorously controlled using standards obtained from epidemiologic studies. Much information can be obtained from cell culture and from animal experimentation, but the final test of safety must always be the effect on a human population. New radiologic modalities such as CT and MRI have been proven to provide valuable information in the growing effort to diagnose and efficiently manage this group of important disorders.

References

1. Agricola G (1912) De re metallica, Hoover HC, Hoover LC 22 (trans). The Mining Magazine, London.
2. Paracelsus T (1567) Von der Bergsucht und anderen Bergkrankheiten. Dilinger, Frankfart.
3. Cotes JE, Steel J (1987) Work-related lung disorders. Blackwell Scientific Publications, Oxford, pp 61–77.
4. Hatch TF, Gross P (1964) Pulmonary deposition and retention of inhaled aerosols. Academic Press, Inc. New York.
5. Jacobsen M, Rae S, Walton WH, et al. (1971) The relation between pneumoconiosis and dust exposure in British coal mines. In Walton WH (ed) Inhaled particles III, Vol 11, Old Working, Surrey. pp 903–917.
6. International Labour Office (1980) Guidelines for the use of ILO International Classification of Radiographs of Pneumoconioses. Occupational Safety and Health Series No. 22. ILO Geneva.
7. Yerushalmy J (1955) Reliability of chest radiography in diagnosis of pulmonary lesions. Am J Surg 89:231–240.
8. Ziskind M, Jones RN, Weill H (1976) State of the art. Silicosis. Am Rev Respir Dis 113:643–665.
9. Heppleston AG, Styles JA (1967) Activity of a macrophage factor in collagen formation by silica. Nature 214:521–522.
10. Silicosis and Silicate Disease Committee (1988) Diseases associated with exposure to silica and nonfibrous silicate minerals. Arch Pathol Lab Med 112:673–720.
11. Heppleston AG (1982) Silicotic fibrogenesis: A concept of pulmonary fibrosis. Ann Occup Hyg 26:449–462.
12. Lowrie DB (1982) What goes wrong with the macrophage in silicosis? Eur J Resp Dis 63:180–182.

13. McConnochie K, Gibb A, Campbell MJ, et al. (1988) Pathology and radiology correlations in Welsh slate workers. Thorax 43:261P.

14. Bergin CJ, Müller NL, Vedal S, et al. (1986) CT in silicosis: Correlation with plain film and pulmonary function tests. AJR 14:477–483.

15. Hunter D (1975) The diseases of occupations. English Universities Press Ltd, London, p 926.

16. Royal Commission on Metalliferous Mines and Quarries (1914) Second report. Minutes of evidence. His Majesty's Stationery Office, London, vols II and Ill.

17. Chadgidakis CB (1963) Silicosis in South African white gold miners: A comparative study of the disease at its different stages. Med Proc 9:383.

18. Hughes JM, Jones RN, Gilson, JC, et al. (1982) Determinants of progression in sandblasters' silicosis. 26:701–712.

19. Cowie RL (1998) The influence of silicosis on deteriorating lung function in gold miners. Chest 113:340–343.

20. Wang X, Yano E (1999) Pulmonary dysfunction in silica-exposed workers: A relationship to radiographic signs of silicosis and emphysema. Am J Ind Med 36:299–306.

21. Hughes JM, Weill H, Checkoway H, et al. (1998) Radiographic evidence of silicosis risk in the diatomaceous earth industry. Am J Respir Crit Care Med 158:807–814.

22. Lillington GA (1987) A diagnostic approach to chest diseases. Williams & Wilkins, Baltimore MD, pp 283–284, 332–339.

23. Fiumicelli A, Fiumicefli C, Pagni M (1964) Contributo allo studio della silicosi massiva unilarale isolata. Medna Lav 5:516–530.

24. Akira M, Higashihara T, Yokoyama K, et al. (1989) Radiographic type P pneumoconiosis: High resolution CT. Radiology 171:117–123.

25. Raithel HJ, Valentin H (1983) Computed tomographic examination of patients with asbestosis and silicosis. Prac Clin Pneumol 37:1119–1129.

26. Begin R, Filion R, Ostigny G (1995) Emphysema in silica and asbestos exposed workers seeking compensation. A CT study. Chest 108:647–655.

27. Matsumoto S, Mori H, Miyake H, et al. (1998) MRI signal characteristics of progressive massive fibrosis in silicosis. Clin Radiol 53:510–514.

28. Merler E, Barchielli A, Sorso B, et al. (1998) The mortality due to pulmonary silicosis in the Tuscany region in the last decade demonstrates that the health effects of work exposure to silica are still marked. Epidemiol Prev 22:221–225.

29. Rapiti E, Sperati A, Miceli M, et al. (1999) End stage renal disease among ceramic workers exposed to silica. Occup Environ Med 56:559–561.

30. Laennec RTH (1819) Traité de l'auscultation médiate. Paris.

31. Hart PD'A, Aslett EA (1942) Chronic pulmonary disease in South Wales coalminers, Part 1, Section B, Medical Research Council Special Reports Series No 243. His Majesty's Stationery Office, London.

32. Banks DE, Wang ML, Lapp NL II (1998) Respiratory health effect of open cast coalmining: A cross-sectional study of current workers. Occup Environ Med 55:287–288.

33. Huang X, Fournier J, Koenig K, et al. (1998) Buffering capacity of coal and its acid-soluble Fe^{2+} content: Possible role in coal workersí pneumoconiosis. Chem Res Toxicol 11:722–729.

34. Schultz HM (1997) Coal mine workers pneumoconiosis (CWP): In vitro study of the release of organic compounds from coal mine dust in the presence of physiological fluids. Environ Res 74:74–83.

35. Heppeston AG (1947) Essential lesion of pneumoconiosis in Welsh coal workers. J Pathol Bacteriol 59:453–460.

36. Wagner JC, Burns J, Munday DE, et al. (1982) Presence of fibronectin in pneumoconiotic lesions. Thorax 37:54–56.

37. Wells AL (1954) Cor pulmonale in coal worker's pneumoconiosis. Br Heart J 16:74–78.

38. Caplan A (1953) Certain unusual radiological appearances in the chest of coal miners suffering rheumatoid arthritis. Thorax 8:29–37.

39. Cotes JE (1976) Serial data over 10–22 years for detailed lung function of working men. Scand J Respir Dis 57:764–768.

40. Cockcroft AE, Seal RME, Wagner JC, et al. (1982) Post-mortem study of emphysema in coal workers and non-coal workers. Lancet 2:600–603.

41. Gilson JC, Hugh Jones P (1965) Lung function in coalworkers pneumoconiosis. Medical Research Council, Special Reports Series No. 290. Her Majesty's Stationery Office. London.

42. Rae S, Walker DD, Attfield MD (1971) Chronic bronchitis and dust exposure in British coalminers. In Walton WH (ed) Inhaled particles III. vol II, Old Woking, Surrey, pp 883–896.

43. Marks J (1970) New mycobacteria. Health Trends 3:68–69.

44. Morgan WKC, Lapp NL (1976) Respiratory disease in coalminers. Am Rev Respir Dis 113:531–559.

45. Wang X, Yano E, Nonaka K, et al. (1997) Respiratory impairments due to dust exposure: A comparative study among workers exposed to silica, asbestos, and coalmine dust. Ann J Ind Med 31:495–502.

46. Cockcroft AE, Wagner JC, Seal RME, et al. (1982) Irregular opacities in coalworkers' pneumoconiosis – correlation with pulmonary function and pathology. Ann Occup Hyg 26:767–787.

47. Parkes WR (1982) Occupational lung disorders. Butterworths, London, pp 201–260.

48. Shida H, Chiotani K, Honma K, et al. (1996) Radiologic and pathologic characteristics of mixed dust pneumoconiosis. Radiographics 16:483–498.

49. Rukley VA, Fernie JM, Chapman JS, et al. (1984) Comparison of radiographic appearance with associated pathology and lung dust content in a group of coalworkers. Br J Ind Med 41:459–467.

50. Bauer TT, Merget R, Schmidt EW, et al. (1997) Correlation of radiologic and pathologic–anatomical findings in dust induced pneumoconiosis in former coal miners. Pneumologie 51:1093–1097.

51. Rémy-Jardin M, Degreef JM, Beuscart L, et al. (1990) Coalworkers' pneumoconiosis: CT assessment in exposed workers and correlation with radiographic findings. Radiology 177:363–371.

52. Webb WR, Stein MG, Finkbeiner WE, et al. (1988) Normal and diseased isolated lungs: High resolution CT. Radiology 166:81–87.

53. Meziane MA (1992) High-resolution computed tomography scanning in the assessment of interstitial lung disease. J Thorac Imaging 7:13–25.

54. Ruckley VA, Fernie JM, Chapman JS, et al. (1984) Comparison of radiographic appearances with associated pathology and lung dust content in a group of coalworkers. Br J Industr Med 41:459–467.

55. Cochrane AL (1962) The attack rate of progressive massive fibrosis. Br J Ind Med 19:52–64.

56. Shennan DH, Washington JS, Thomas DJ, et al. (1981) Factors predisposing to the development of progressive massive fibrosis in coalminers. Br J Ind Med 38:321–326.

57. Cotes JE, Steel J (1987) Work-related lung disorders. Blackwell Scientific Publications, Oxford, p 194.

58. Parkes WR (1973) Asbestos-related disorders. Br J Dis Chest 67:261.

59. Becklake MR (1976) Asbestos-related diseases of the lungs and other organs: Their epidemiology and implications for clinical practice. Am Rev Resp Dis 114:187–227.

60. Chung A, Warnock ML (1981) Asbestos and other ferruginous bodies: Their formation and clinical significance. J Pathol 102:447–456.

61. Robledo R, Mossman B (1999) Cellular and molecular mechanisms of asbestos-induced fibrosis. J Cell Physiol 180:158–166.

62. Jones JSP, Sheers G (1973) Pleural plaques. In Bogovski P, et al (eds) Biological effects of asbestos, vol. 8. International Agency for Research on Cancer, Lyons, pp 243–248.

63. Selikoff IJ (1965) The occurrence of pleural calcification among asbestos insulation workers. Ann NY Acad Sci 132:351–367.

64. Morgan A, Holmes A (1983) Distribution and characteristics of amphibole asbestos fibres measured with the light microscope in the left lung of an insulation worker. Br J Ind Med 40:45–50.

65. Strankinga WFM, Sperber M, Kaiser M, et al. (1987) Accuracy of diagnostic procedures in the initial evaluation and follow-up of mesothelioma patients. Respiration 51:179–187.

66. McCaughey WTE, Wade OL, Elmes PC (1962) Exposure to asbestos dust and diffuse pleural mesothelioma. Br Med J 2:1397.

67. Antman KH (1980) Current concepts: Malignant mesothelioma. N Engl J Med 303:200–202.

68. Lerner JJ, Schoenfeld DA, Martin A, et al. (1983) Malignant mesothelioma. The Eastern Cooperative Oncology Group (ECOG) experience. Cancer 52:1985–1995.

69. Davis JMG (1984) The pathology of asbestos-related disease. Thorax 39:801–808.

70. Robinson BWS, Musk AW (1981) Benign asbestos pleural effusion: Diagnosis and course. Thorax 36:896–900.

71. Allison AC (1974) Pathogenic effects of inhaled particles and antigens. Ann NY Acad Sci 221:299–308.

72. Bianchi C, Brollo A, Ramani L, et al. (1999) Asbestos exposure in lung carcinoma: A necropsy-based study of 414 cases. Am J Ind Med 36:360–364.

73. Karjalainen A, Pukkala E, Kauppinen T, et al. (1999) Incidence of cancer among Finnish patients with asbestos-related pulmonary or pleural fibrosis. Cancer Causes Control 10:51–57.

74. Bergin R, Ostigny G, Filion R, et al. (1993) Computed tomography in the early detection of asbestosis. Br J Ind Med 50:689–698.

75. Sperber M, Mohan K (1984) Computed tomography – a reliable diagnostic modality in pulmonary asbestosis. J Comput Assist Tomogr 8:125–132.

76. Staples CA (1992) Computed tomography in the evaluation of benign asbestos-related disorders. Radiol Clin North Am 30:1191–1207.

77. Ren H, Lee DR, Hruban RH, et al. (1991) Pleural plaques do not predict asbestosis: High resolution computed tomography and pathology study. Mod Pathol 4:201–209.

78. Akira M, Yokoyama K, Yamamoto S, et al. (1991) Early asbestosis – evaluation with high resolution CT. Radiology 178:409–416.

79. Aberle D, Gamsu G, Ray C, et al. (1988) Asbestos-related pleural and parenchymal fibrosis detection with high-resolution CT. Radiology 166:729–34.

80. Akira M, Yamamoto S, Yokoyama K, et al. (1990) Asbestosis – high resolution CT - pathologic correlation. Radiology 176:389–394.

81. Murray K, Gamsu G, Webb WR, et al. (1995) High resolution CT sampling for detection of asbestos-related lung disease. Acad Radiol 2:11–15.

82. Al-Jarad N, Strickland B, Oearson MC, et al. (1992) High resolution computed tomographic assessment of asbestosis and cryptogenic fibrosing alveolitis: A comparative study. Thorax 47:645–650.

83. Gamsu G, Salmon CJ, Warnock ML, et al. (1995) CT quantification of interstitial fibrosis in patients with asbestosis: A comparison of two methods. AJR 164:63–68.

84. Alexander E, Clark RA, Colley DP et al. (1981) CT of malignant pleural mesothelioma. Am J Roent Rad Ther Nucl Med 137:287–291.

85. Rabinowitz JC, Efremidis SC, Cohen B, et al. (1982) A comaparative study of mesothelioma and asbestosis using computed tomography and conventional chest radiography. Radiology 144:453–460.

86. Sperber M, Kaiser M (1987) Magnetic resonance imaging of the thorax. Warren Green Publishers, St Louis, MC.

87. O'Donovan PB, Ross JS, Sivak ED, et al. (1984) Magnetic resonance imaging of the thorax. The advantages of coronal and sagittal planes. AJR 143:183–188.

88. Knuuttila A, Halme M, Kivisaari L, et al. (1998) The clinical importance of magnetic resonance imaging versus computed tomography in malignant pleural mesothelioma. Lung Cancer 22:215–225.

89. Boraschi P, Neri S, Braccini G, et al. (1999) Magnetic resonance appearance of asbestos-related benign and malignant pleural diseases. Scan J Work Environ Health 25:18–23.

90. Turner-Warwick M, Barrows B, Johnson A (1980) Cryptogenic fibrosing alveolitis: Clinical features and their influence on survival. Thorax 35:171–180.

91. Saracci R (1977) Asbestos and lung cancer: An analysis of the epidemiological evidence on the asbestos-smoking interaction. Int J Cancer 20:323–331.

92. Wagner JC, Berry G, Pooley FD (1982) Mesotheliomas and asbestos type in asbestos textile workers: A study of lung contents. Br Med J 285:603–660.

93. Newhouse ML, Thompson H (1965) Mesothelioma of pleura and peritoneum following exposure to asbestos in the London area. Br J Ind Med 22:261–269.

94. McConnochie K, Simonato L, Mavrides P, et al. (1987) Mesothelioma in Cyprus. The role of tremolite. Thorax 42:342–47.

95. International Agency for Research on Cancer (1988) Man-made mineral fibers and radon, IARC monographs on the evaluation of carcinogenic risks to humans., No.43 IARC, Lyons.

96. Morgan RW, Bratsberg JA (1981) Mortality study of fibrous glass production workers. Arch Environ Health 36:179–183.

97. Parkes WR (1982) Occupational lung disorders. Butterworths, London, pp 454–457.

98. DeNardi JM, Van Ordstrand HS, Curtis GH, et al. (1953) Berylliosis. Summary and survey of all clinical types observed in a 12 year period. Arch Indust Hyg 8:1–24.

99. Jones Williams W, Williams WR (1983) Value of beryllium lymphocyte transformation tests in chronic beryllium disease and in potentially exposed workers. Thorax 38:41–44.

100. Doig AT (1976) Baritosis: A benign pneumoconiosis. Thorax 31:30–39.

101. Coates EO, Watson JHL (1971) Diffuse interstitial lung disease in tungsten carbide workers. Ann Intern Med 75:709–716.

102. Morgan WKC (1978) Magnetite pneumoconiosis. J Occup Med 20:762–763.

103. Robertson AJ, Rivers D, Nagelschmidt G, et al. (1961) Stannosis: Benign pneumoconiosis due to tin dioxide. Lancet 1:1089–1095.

104. Sheers G (1964) Prevalence of pneumoconiosis in Cornish kaolin workers. Br J Ind Med 21:218–225.

105. Gamble JF, Fellner V, Dimeo MJ (1979) An epidemiologic study of a group of talc workers. Am Rev Respir Dis 119:741–753.

27 Environmental Lung Disorders Induced by Organic (Nonmineral) Agents

M. Sperber

Introduction

A large variety of precipitating organic agents can be inhaled as fine particles or aerosols, including proteins of animal origin, pathogenic microorganisms, fungal spores, mineral oils, and several organic chemicals. Specific occupational disorders have been found to result from exposure to these offending substances. In addition to these exogenous antigens, endogenous antigens may be released from infectious agents invading the bronchopulmonary area, such as *Aspergillus fumigatus*.

Some pneumonic or granulomatous reactions can result from mineral or vegetable oil inhalation; however, in most cases the lung tissue reacts to inhaled organic material in the form of a hypersensitivity disorder recognized under the name of extrinsic allergic bronchioloalveolitis or hypersensitivity pneumonia.

The pathogenesis of extrinsic allergic "alveolitis" (because not only alveoli are involved, but also small airways, the term "bronchioloalveolitis" seems to be more appropriate) includes immunologic mechanisms induced by the contact of inhaled substances with the peribronchial lymphoid tissue and resulting in sensitization. Stimulation of mucosal lymphocytes induces the formation of immunoglobin (Ig) E or reaginic antibodies whose presence is typical for type I hypersensitivity reactions, such as extrinsic asthma or hay fever. Secretory immunoglobulins, or IgAs, are also formed by the sensitized submucosal lymphocytes. While IgA is binding the antigens to the mucosa surface, macrophages are ingesting the antigens, which initiates a process of T-cell and B-cell activation and antibody production. CD8 + lymphocytosis can usually be found in bronchoalveolar lavage (1,2).

An acute or subacute form of the disease can be recognized, when complement-fixing precipitating antibodies (IgA and IgM) are formed by plasma cells in the tissue or lymph nodes and can be identified. Also, in the same phase, accumulation of lymphocytes and other mono-nuclear cells takes place, resulting in a granulomatous reaction and the deposition of sarcoid-like granulomas in the walls of the alveoli and small airways. The chronic phase is characterized by the presence of disabling progressive diffuse interstitial fibrosis.

Pathology

Because reactions vary greatly in their acuteness and severity, pathologic changes are accordingly complex and varied. Initially, there is edema of the lungs, with thickening of the alveolar walls and lymphocytic and plasma cell infiltration. Accumulation of histiocytes, fibroblasts, and multinucleated giant cells results in the formation of numerous epitheloid granulomas, similar to those seen in other disorders, including sarcoidosis, tuberculosis and various fungal infections. It seems that, in contrast to sarcoidosis, inhalational hypersensitivity does not result in enlarged hilar glands (3,4), although hypertrophy of lymph nodes may be visualized radiologically.

Bronchiolitis with granulomatous infiltration of the small airways is a common finding. Vasculitis as a severe allergic reaction has not been reported. Bronchiolar plugging with mucus or inflammatory cells takes place in many kinds of inhalation reactions, because the granulomatous thickening of the interstitium can ultimately result in progressive interstitial fibrosis and honeycombing (5).

Clinical Features

Clinical manifestations may be mild or severe and are often difficult to differentiate from those of intercurrent bacterial or viral infections. They include fever, anorexia, nausea, and vomiting, together with persistent breathlessness. Repeated exposure may result in recurrent episodes of acute symptoms, and this can also serve as a diagnostic indicator for occupational hazard. If the exposure to the offending agent continues, dyspnea on effort, coughing, and mucus production become permanent, paralleling the widespread fibrotic changes occurring in the lung fields.

Radiologic Appearance

Radiologic findings in extrinsic allergic "alveolitis" vary with the degree of the disease and, often, the amount of radiographic changes correlate poorly with the severity of symptoms and the clinical picture. Earliest changes can range from fine basal opacities such as those in pigeon-breeder's disease, to more prominent, well-defined densities in the middle and lower zones of the lungs. Patchy airway infiltration can be quite extensive and pronounced, as in cases with allergic bronchopulmonary aspergillosis (Fig. 27.1).

Chronic inhalation of organic agents results in radiographic changes that are often indistinguishable from diffuse fibrotic end-stage pictures of various lung disorders. Computed tomography (CT), and especially high resolution CT (HRCT) are useful in demonstrating the ill-defined opacities, together with coarse interstitial thickening, which occupy mainly the upper and middle lung zones, enabling the differentiation of chronic from acute stages, during which the pulmonary abnormalities are located mainly at the lung bases (6) (Fig. 27.2). It can also help to visualize air-trapping, for which the best method is inspiratory and expiratory volumetric HRCT (7). Advanced disease is associated with loss of parenchymal volume, mediastinal deviation or distortion, and formation of parenchymal bullae and blebs.

Because the radiographic picture is not specific in either the acute or the chronic form, there is a need to distinguish extrinsic allergic "alveolitis" in the acute form from the variety of infectious respiratory disorders and that in the chronic form from widespread fibrosis, part of such conditions as fibrocavernous tuberculosis, chronic sarcoidosis, fungal disease in chronic stages, or asbestosis. In most cases diagnosis must therefore be based on detailed and careful occupational history and information on hobbies and the presence of house pets, as well as on the finding (in acute cases and some of the chronic cases) of specific precipitins and persistent radiographic abnormalities. Lung biopsy is rarely indicated, but may be needed in acute cases in which precipitins are not present, or in chronic cases in order to exclude other causes of diffuse interstitial pulmonary fibrosis (5,8–10).

Farmer's Lung

Extrinsic allergic "alveolitis" due to exposure to moldy hay and straw is known "farmer's lung" and is associated with inhalation of spores of thermophilic actinomycetes, a group of filamentous, Gram-positive bacteria. The disorder is common in farmers, poultry workers, and attendants of zoo and circus animals who handle moldy straw, hay, and grain (11,12). To be mentioned here is the fact that farmers are notoriously exposed to a variety of noxious organic or chemical substances, and this is one of the reasons why agriculture seems to be one of the occupations where prevalence of respiratory disorders is the highest. To allergic alveolitis, allergic asthma, silo filler's disease or pesticide-related lung pathology, some newly described entities have to be added, such as agricultural chronic bronchitis and organic dust toxic syndrome. Often the clinical presentation is a complex one in which there is a mixture of respiratory tract inflammation, bronchial hyperreactivity and chronic bronchial obstruction (13).

There are numerous descriptions of the disease in the literature, all underlying the importance of the presence of suitable conditions for the growth of fungi (hay type, water content, maximum temperature, etc.). Farmer's lung appears to be a disorder associated with cold and humid weather conditions, an increased percentage of water content in the hay, and a relative high temperature of the stored plant material (14,15). A study was performed in Ireland in order to investigate the epidemiology of the disease in the entire republic (population 3.5 million) and assess the relationship between the incidence of farmer's lung disease and the climatic conditions in South West Ireland. The study covered a period of 13 years, until 1996, and showed that during this period the incidence remained the same both on a national and on a regional basis. This constant level is highly suggestive of the fact that, much as elswhere in the world, farmers' working environments and farming practices need to be improved (16).

The long-term outcome of farmer's lung patients and matched control farmers has been evaluated by using HRCT. Aside from the latter, spirometry and pulmonary diffusing capacity were also performed. Emphysema was found significantly more often in patients with farmer's lung (23%) than in the control group (7%). Fibrotic changes were also discovered in farmer's lung patients (17%), as well as a miliary pattern (12%). Both emphysematous and fibrotic, but not miliary changes, correlated well with an impaired pulmonary function (17).

Because farmers can seldom change their profession, appropriate preventive measures must be instituted in order to avoid in such workers the development of respiratory disease caused by grain dust. They include good ventilation of storage areas and drying of stored hay or grain to prevent molding and reduce heating.

Bird Fancier's/Breeder's Disease

Bird raising is an occupation that is also often performed as a hobby, and the lung condition encountered

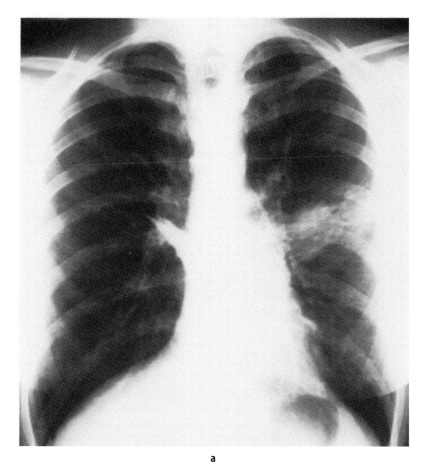

a

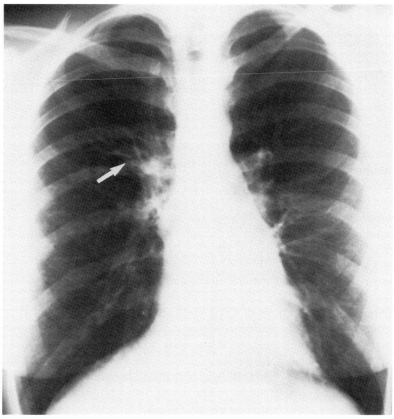

b

Figure 27.1. Allergic bronchopulmonary aspergillosis. **a** Posteroanterior radiograph showing right and left perihilar infiltrates. **b** Follow-up posteroanterior radiograph 3 weeks later demonstrates resorption of the perihilar infiltrates and strongly suggests the development of right suprahilar bronchiectasis (*arrow*). The proximity of the bronchiectasis to the hiluns and the labile character of the infiltrates are typical for bronchopulmonary aspergillosis. (Courtesy of Dr. J.P. Trigaux.)

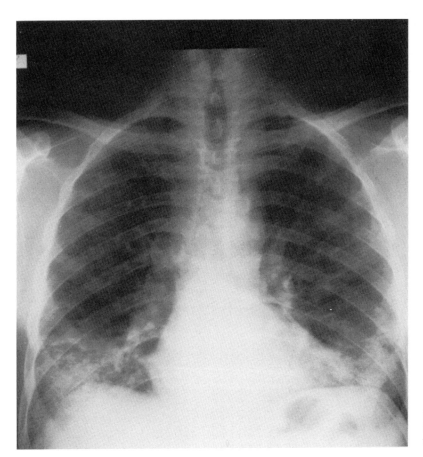

Figure 27.2. Acute farmer's lung. Diffuse shadowing at both lung bases in a farm worker complaining of morning respiratory troubles.

in people who are in contact with birds has been called "bird fancier's disease" or "bird breeder's disease" (18,19). The exposed population includes petshop workers, pigeon breeders, poultry farmers, and children or adults who are bird fanciers and keep only one or two pet birds.

Exposure to avian dust occurs while cleaning bird cages or hen houses. Also there is a possibility of continuous and chronic exposure to dropping dust. Studies have shown that the mucin antigen is present in pigeon droppings and pigeon bloom (20,21). The clinical presentation, therefore, can be either in the form of an acute respiratory illness or an insidious onset with progressively increasing dyspnea on effort. Patients usually recover rapidly when contact with the bird is interrupted, and their lung function returns to normal; however, irreversible chronic disease may develop if the contact with the allergen is maintained. Therefore, identification of the disorder is of major importance, especially in children, in whom permanent lung damage can occur unless all contact with birds is stopped (22,23).

An important difference to emphasize is that between the above condition and ornithosis (psittacosis), which is also encountered in people who are in contact with birds.

In the latter there is an acute pulmonary infection caused by an organism of the *Chlamydia* or Bedsoniae group. In this condition, aside from lung consolidation, lymphadenopathy, jaundice, and myocarditis have also been described (24).

Various Organic Pneumoconioses

Roentgenographic changes in organic pneumoconioses vary with the stage of the disease from total absence of abnormalities to the presence of fine, ill-defined densities predominantly in the middle and lower lung zones (Fig. 27.3). In other cases, a linear or diffuse reticulonodular pattern can be encountered radiating from both hili (Fig. 27.4). In the more advanced conditions, the formation of cysts and bullae can be identified, with loss of pulmonary volume (Fig. 27.5). Bagassosis, mushroom worker's lung, malt worker's lung, byssinosis, suberosis, water droplet antigen disease, furrier's lung, and cheese washer's hypersensitivity pneumonitis are additional examples of conditions that present the features of acute extrinsic allergic "alveolitis" in affected workers (25–32).

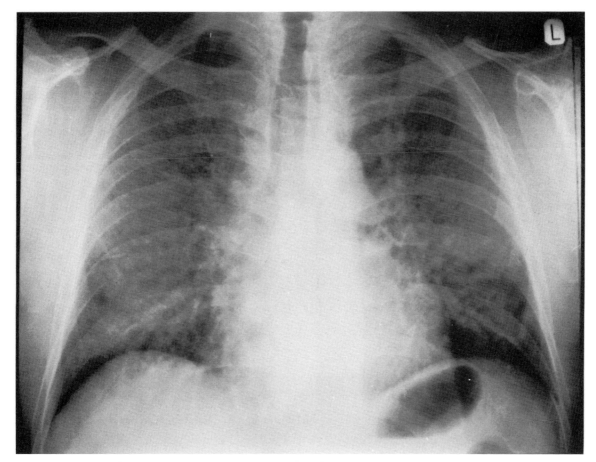

Figure 27.3. Diffuse increase in the pulmonary interstitial markings, mainly in the middle and lower lung zones, in a patient who raised pigeons for 5 years. Complete resolution of these changes occurred when the patient was removed from his environment.

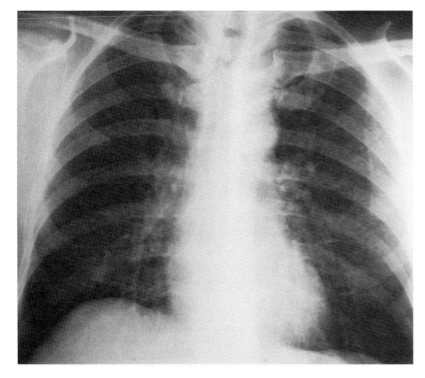

Figure 27.4. Chest radiograph of a young man training to work as a furrier and presenting with an influenza-like illness. A fine, diffuse pulmonary reticular pattern can be seen on the radiographic examination of this patient.

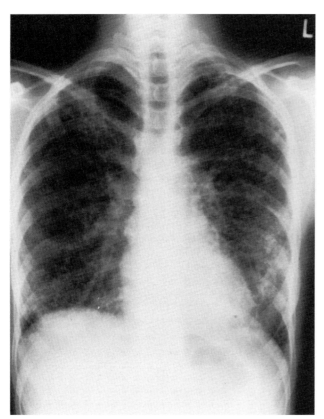

Figure 27.5. Permanent fibrotic changes demonstrated on the chest radiograph of a 46 year old man who worked on a farm for 14 years. The patient complained of cough, dyspnea on effort, and malaise.

Bagassosis

Bagassosis typically affects workers who handle bagasse, the fibrous cellulose residue of sugarcane stalk, after the juice has been extracted. Clinical presentations are similar to those of farmer's lung, with a greater incidence of an acute form that usually follows exposure to dry and moldy bagasse. Radiographically, ill-defined opacities can be identified, often in the midlung fields. The finding of a normal chest radiograph is not common (25,26).

Byssinosis

Byssinosis is a disease observed in workers exposed to cotton dust. Clinical characteristics of this disorder have been described, with the specific appearance of symptoms such as dyspnea on effort and cough after long periods of apparent good health (27,28). As in other disorders caused by exposure to organic antigenic materials, the best treatment involves first the control of the amount of the textile dust generated and the removal of the afflicted patient from the dusty atmosphere. Steroids administered during acute episodes have proven to dramatically improve the clinical conditions and reduce the duration of the pulmonary infiltrates.

"Humidifier Fever"

Respiratory symptoms consistent with extrinsic allergic "alveolitis" have been also reported in connection with air-conditioning systems contaminated with microorganisms. This condition, named "humidifier fever," was first described in the USA in 1970 (32), and repeatedly described afterward as an acute disorder consisting of fever, malaise, cough, and myalgia (33,34). These symptoms seem to be worst at the beginning of the working week ("Monday morning fever") and usually resolve in 24 h. Studies have suggested that an increased awarness has to exist concerning the possibility of patients presenting with hypersensitivity pneumonitis due to humidifier disease (35). In general, polluted indoor air has been associated with health problems that include sick building syndrome, multiple chemical sensitivity, and hypersensitivity pneumonitis, due to air-borne contaminants which include chemicals, vehicular exhaust, microbial microorganisms, fibrous glass particles, and dust. Clinical symptoms are often nonspecific and include headache, eye and throat irritation, coughing, chest tightness, shortness of breath and fatigue (36).

Food Production Alveolitis

Rare causes of extrinsic allergic alveolitis include "cheese washer's lung," in which respiratory symptoms develop in workers involved in washing molds off the surface of cheeses. Precipitins of IgE class against *Penicillium casei* have been found in the sera of these patients (30). In "malt worker's disease" there are clinical and radiologic signs of allergic alveolitis in involved workers due to inhalation of spore dust, especially *Actinomyces clavatus* (37), whereas exposure to thermophilic and thermotolerant actinomycetes causes, in workers involved in mushroom cultivation, symptoms such as persistent cough and heavy mucus production ("mushroom worker's disease"). In this condition, prominent radiographic changes can be found, including diffuse miliary opacities or, sometimes, ill-defined densities in the mid and lower lung areas (31).

Suberosis

Suberosis (29) is a condition with the same clinical and radiographic features as farmer's lung, occurring in cork workers and resulting from the inhalation of dust that contains the spores of numerous fungi, especially in damp warehouses. Rarely, exposure to sawdust may result in the development of a granulomatous alveolitis in affected patients (sequoiosis) (38).

Conclusion

In general, most of the antigens causing extrinsic allergic "alveolitis" consist of bacteria and protozoa growing on different substrates in the presence of heat and moisture (39,40). They often present an occupational hazard, and therefore various modalities of prevention have been proposed, including purification of contaminated areas and good ventilation of working places. These goals are quite difficult to achieve, since many industrial processes involve molding of various products, with consequent production of antigens and sensitization of exposed workers. Even more problematic seems to be the prevention of sensitization to animal residue in people involved in rearing of birds and animals (22,41,42).

Great progress is being made nowadays toward the understanding of the basic pathologic and physiologic changes occurring in lung disorders caused by organic agents (43,44). This knowledge, together with the prescription of effective preventive measures (personal protective clothing and masks, installation of good farming practices, etc.), is expected to significantly improve the management of the above disorders.

References

1. Delacourt C (1999) Extrinsic allergic alveolitis. Arch Pediatr 1:83S–86S.
2. Ando M, Suga M, Kohrogi H (1999) A new look at hypersemsitivity pneumonitis. Curr Opin Pulm Med 5:299–304.
3. Hapke EJ, Seal RMF, Thomas GO, et al. (1968) Farmer's lung: A clinical, radiographic, functional and serological correlation of acute and chronic stages. Thorax 23:451–468.
4. Kawanami O, Basset F, Barrios R, et al. (1983) Hypersensitivity pneumonitis in man. Light and electron microscopic studies of 18 lung biopsies. Am J Pathol 110:275–289.
5. Cotes JE, Steel J (1987) Work-related lung disorders. Blackwell Scientific Publications, Oxford, pp 320–345.
6. Webb WR, Müller NL, Naidich DP (1995) High-resolution CT of the lung. Lippincot-Raven, New York.
7. Honda O, Johkoh T, Ichikado K, et al. (1998) Vizualization of air-trapping area with expiratory CT in hypersensitivity pneumonitis. Radiat Med 16:293–295.
8. Burrell R, Rylander R (1981) A critical review of the role of precipitins in hypersensitivity pneumonitis. Eur J Respir Dis 62:332–343
9. Avila R (1983) Some aspects of occupational asthma. Clin Allergy 13:191–195.
10. Hensley GT, Gararicis JC, Cherayil GD (1969) Lung biopsies of pigeon breeders' disease. Arch Pathol 87:572–579.
11. Cross T, Maciver AM (1968) The thermophilic actinomycetes in mouldy hay. J Gen Microbiol 50:351–359.
12. Dickie HA, Rankin J (1958) Farmer's lung: An acute granulomatous interstitial pneumonitis occurring in agricultural workers. JAMA 167:1069.
13. Dalphin JC (1998) Respiratory pathology in the agricultural environment. Rev Prat 48:1313–1318.
14. Reyes CN, Wenzel FJ, Lawton BR, et al. (1982) The pulmonary pathology of farmers' lung disease. Chest 81:142–146.
15. Braun SR, do Pico GA, Tsiatis A, et al. (1979) Farmers' lung disease: Long-term clinical and physiologic outcome. Am Rev Respir Dis 119:185–191.
16. McGrath DS, Kiely J, Cryan B, et al. (1999) Farmer's lung in Ireland (1983–1996) remains at a constant level. Ir J Med Sci 168:21–24.
17. Erkinjuntti-Pekkanen R, Rytkonen H, Kokkarinen JI, et al. (1998) Long-term risk of emphysema in patients with farmer's lung and matched control farmer's. Am J Resp Crit Care Med. 158:662–665.
18. Christensen LT, Schmidt CD, Ribbins L (1975) Pigeon breeder's disease – a prevalence study and review. Clin Allergy 5:417–430.
19. British Thoracic Society (1984) A national survey of bird fancier's lung including its possible association with jejunal villous atrophy. Br J Chest 78:75–87.
20. Baldwin CI, Stevens B, Connors S, et al. (1998) Pigeon fancier's lung: The mucin antigen is present in pigeon droppings and pigeon bloom. Int Arch Allergy Immunol 117:187–193.
21. Calvert JE, Baldwin CI, Allen A, et al. (1999) Pigeon fancier's lung: a complex disease? Clin Exp Allergy 29:166–175.
22. Allen- DH, Williams GV, Woolcock AJ (1976) Bird breeder's hypersensitivity pneumonitis: Progress studies of the lung function after cessation of exposure to the provoking antigen. Am Rev Respir Dis 114:555–566.
23. Andersen P, Christensen KM, Jensen BE, et al. (1982) Antibodies to pigeon antigens in pigeon breeders. Eur J Respir Dis 63:113–121.
24. Schaffner W, Drutz DJ, Duncan GW, et al. (1967) The clinical spectrum of endemic psittacosis. Arch Intern Med 119:433.
25. Hearn CED (1968) Bagassosis. An epidemiological, environmental and clinical survey. Br J Ind Med 25:267–282.
26. Well H, Buechner HA, Gonzalez E, et al. (1966) Bagassosis: A study of pulmonary function.in 20 cases. Ann Intern Med 64:737–747.
27. Bouhuys A, Heaphy LJ, Jr, Schilling RSF, et al. (1967) Byssionosis in the United States. N Engl J Med 277:170.
28. Bouhuys A, Van de Woestijne KP (1970) Respiratory mechanics and dust exposure in byssinosis. J Clin Invest 49:106.
29. Pimentel JC, Avila R (1973) Respiratory disease in cork workers (suberosis). Thorax 28:409–423.
30. Campbell, JA, Kryda MJ, Treuhaft MW (1983) Cheese worker's hypersensitivity monitis. Am Rev Respir Dis 127:495–496.
31. Stewart CJ, Pickering CAC (1974) Mushroom worker's lung. Lancet 1:317.
32. Babaszak EF, Thiede WH, Fink JN (1970) Hypersensitivity pneumonitis due to contamination of an air conditioner. N Engl J Med 283:271–276.
33. Belin L (1980) Prevalence of symptoms and immunoresponse in relation to exposure to infected humidifiers. Eur J Respir Dis 61:155–162.
34. Fink JN, Banaszak EF, Baroriak JJ, et al. (1976) Interstitial lung disease due to contamination of forced air system. Ann Intern Med 84:406–413.
35. Patterson R, Mazur N, Roberts M, et al. (1998) Hypersensitivity pneumonitis due to humidifier disease: Seek and ye shall find. Chest 114:931–933.
36. Oliver LC, Shackleton BW (1998) The indoor air we breath. Public Health Rep 113:398–409.
37. Grant JWB, Blackadder ES, Greenberg M, et al. (1976) Extrinsic allergic alveolitis in Scottish maltworkers. Br Med J 1:490–493.
38. Cohen H1, Merigan TC, Kosek JC, et al. (1967) A granulomatous pneumonitis associated with red wood sawdust inhalation. Am J Med 43:785–794.

39. Coombs RRA, Gell PGH (1968) Classification of allergic reactions responsible for clinical hypersensitivity and disease. In Gell PGH, Coombs RRA (eds) Clinical aspects of immunology. Blackwell Scientific Publications, Oxford.

40. Parkes WR (1983) Occupational lung disorders, 2nd edn. Butterworth, London.

41. Wuthe H, Bergmann K, Vogel J (1981) Frequency of lung function disturbances and immunological status of industrial poultry farmers. Eur J Respir Dis 62:38–39.

42. Lee TH, Wraith GD, Bennett CO, et al. (1983) Budgerigar fancier's lung: The persistence of budgerigar precipitins and the recovery of lung function after cessation of avian exposure. Clin Allergy 13:197–202.

43. Scibner GH, Barboriak JJ, Fink JN (1980) Prevalence of precipitins in groups at risk of developing hypersensitivity pneumonitis. Clin Allergy 10:91–95.

44. Turton CWG, Firth G, Grundy E, et al. (1981) Raised enzyme markers of chronic inflammation in asymptomatic farmer's lung. Thorax 36:122–125.

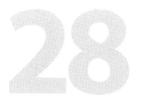

28 Environmental Lung Disorders Secondary to Inhalation of Toxic Gases, Fumes, and Aerosols

D. Novak

Inhalation lung injuries comprise fewer than 1% of total occupational injuries (1,2) and among chemically caused lung injuries they occupy only second place. Inhalation lung injuries are, however, of primary importance where morbidity, mortality, and cost of treatment are concerned (3).

There are several classifications of toxic gases, fumes, and aerosols (4–6). Noxious gases, vapors, and aerosols may be classified as simple asphyxiants, chemical asphyxiants, irritants, organometabolic gases, and vapors. A practical classification into lipid-soluble and water-soluble gases, vapors, and aerosols is summarized in the literature (3,4,7,8).

Intoxication with lipid-soluble gases is caused by interaction of two factors: (a) primary damage of the alveolar and capillary endothelium with consecutive increase of the capillary permeability and accumulation of exudate in the alveoli, and (b) blockade of enzymatic systems of the lung with secondary damage of the capillary endothelium and pathologically increased capillary permeability. The combination of these two pathologic processes leads to an increase in the lung water content, and to early radiographic signs of lung edema (5,7–9). Water-soluble gases, vapors, and aerosols, in contact with the moisturized mucosa of the respiratory tract, form acids and alkali compounds that produce erosions and ulcerations. There are also mixtures of different toxic gases, vapors, and aerosols (e.g., smoke) that produce damage to the upper airways, tracheobronchial tree, lung alveoli, and capillaries.

Mechanisms of Injury

Toxic gases, fumes, and aerosols cause injury through asphyxiation, systemic toxicity, immunologic mechanisms or direct mucosal and alveolar damage (4,6).

Asphyxiation is caused by displacement of oxygen by other inhaled gases (e.g., carbon monoxide or nitrogen dioxide). Tissue asphyxia results from altered oxygen-carrying capacity of blood (e.g., carboxyhemoglobinemia after carbon monoxide inhalation, methemoglobinemia after carbon monoxide inhalation, methemoglobinemia following oxides of nitrogen poisoning, and sulfhemoglobinemia due to hydrogen sulfide intoxication). Another cause of tissue asphyxia is the poisoning of cellular respiratory enzyme systems, for example after inhalation of phosgene or hydrogen sulfide.

Systemic toxicity results from the inhalation of minute particles of oxides of metals, particularly zinc, cadmium, and nickel.

Immunologic mechanisms are induced by a variety of inhaled gases and fumes, which act not only as respiratory irritants, but also as sensitizers.

Direct injury to the mucosa of the respiratory tract is the most common mode of injury in the survivors of acute inhalation poisoning. Pathologic changes may occur at all levels of the respiratory tract. The localization of toxic injury is determined primarily by (a) the physical and chemical properties of the inhaled gas, (b) the concentration of the agent, (c) the duration of exposure, and (d) the rate and pattern of breathing of the exposed person. The highly water-soluble agents (e.g., ammonia) tend to produce maximal injury in the upper airways. Less water-soluble gases (e.g., phosgene, oxides of nitrogen) cause injury to bronchioles and alveoli (4,5). Acute exposure to high concentration of almost any gas leads to severe injury at all levels of the respiratory tract (10–12).

Lipid-Soluble Inhalation Agents Causing Primary Damage to the Lung Parenchyma

Phosgene

Phosgene, or carbonyl chloride ($COCl_2$) is a colorless gas, 100 times more toxic than carbon monoxide and about

800 times more toxic than the equivalent amount of hydrochloric acid. Phosgene was commonly used in chemical warfare, and more than 80% of gas fatalities in the First World War were caused by phosgene. At the present time, phosgene is used in the chemical industry as an agent for direct chlorination. Cases of phosgene poisoning occur as a result of accidental leakage of containers, pipes, or valves.

Inhalation of phosgene in low concentrations causes only mild irritation of the upper respiratory tract, so that a dangerous amount may be inhaled before its presence is recognized. As phosgene reaches the lung parenchyma before it begins to act, workers proceed to work and inhale more of the noxious gas. Injuries caused by phosgene are significantly increased by physical exertion.

Phosgene inhalation is potentially lethal because of the resulting severe pulmonary edema with a decrease in the plasma volume and severe hypoxemia (13,14). There is a dose–effect relationship. Depending on the concentration of phosgene, alveolar edema may become histologically manifest only a few minutes following inhalation. Lymph drainage from the lung increases substantially (13,15). When a sufficiently large amount of fluid has collected in the lung, edema becomes apparent. At this stage, gas exchange becomes insufficient, with edema fluid gradually rising from the alveoli into the proximal segments of the respiratory tract (14).

At very high doses (e.g., 200 ppm) phosgene passes through the blood–air barrier, reaches the lung capillaries, and reacts with blood constituents, causing hemolysis that results in hematin formation in the pulmonary capillaries. Capillary circulation is stopped by obturation with erythrocyte fragments. Death occurs within a few minutes from acute cor pulmonale (14,16).

Radiologic Findings

The first radiologic signs in phosgene poisoning are recognized as a result of the increase of lung water by 30–80%. It is strongly recommended that a chest radiograph be made immediately on admission of the patient in order to provide a basis for subsequent comparison and early detection of initial signs of toxic edema (Fig. 28.1). The duration of the radiographic latent period is inversely proportional to the inhaled phosgen dose (4,7,8,17). If the suspected inhalation dose is low, a follow-up chest radiograph should be made about 8 h after inhalation. In cases with high or moderate inhalation doses, a follow-up radiograph should be made much earlier. A high kilovoltage technique does not seem to be suitable for the detection of minimal radiographic changes in these cases, and the recommended range for a chest radiograph is 50–80 kV (13,14).

Complications and Prognosis

Complications of phosgene poisoning are mostly bronchopneumonia and bronchiolitis obliterans. Rarely, mediastinal and subcutaneous emphysema as well as thromboembolic pneumonia are observed. There is a general consensus that the vast majority of phosgene poisoning cases have a good prognosis. Diller (18) demonstrated in a well-documented study that nearly all patients complain of exertional dyspnea and reduced physical fitness for several months to years after exposure to phosgene. Lung function parameters remain pathologic for several years. The impairment of pulmonary function appears to depend on preexisting chronic bronchitis and smoking habits. Also chronic inflammatory changes such as bronchiolitis, bronchiectasis, emphysema, and lung abscesses may be observed. Asthma bronchiale is a rare late complication (18).

Oxides of Nitrogen

Nitrogen dioxide is one of the best-studied noxious gases (19–21). It is a poorly water-soluble, reddish-brown gas with a pungent odor. Because of its low water solubility, nitrogen dioxide is more likely to penetrate to the distal airways and alveoli (22). The low water solubility also explains the time lag from the initial exposure to the onset of significant clinical and radiologic abnormalities (19,21,23).

Acute poisoning occurs accidentally during the manufacturing and use of nitric acid (22), in the manufacturing of dyes and lacquers (24), in agriculture as a result of exposure to fresh silage (silo filler's disease) (20,21), in fire fighters as a result of combustion of nitrogenous compounds (25), and even in astronauts (26).

Sudden death may occur after inhalation of high concentrations of NO_2 because of bronchiolar spasm, laryngospasm, reflex respiratory arrest, or simple asphyxiation (27). Nitrogen dioxide in contact with moist mucous membranes forms a mixture of nitric and nitrous acid, which are very irritating and corrosive to the epithelial layer of mucosal membranes. Nitric acid dissociates in the lungs into nitrates and nitrites, which react with hemoglobin, resulting in formation of methemoglobin. Methemoglobinemia was observed following exposure to high concentration of nitrogen dioxide (27).

Clinical Symptoms and Signs

The toxic disease that follows moderate to marked exposure to oxides of nitrogen is basically triphasic. The first phase is characterized by severe breathlessness with central cyanosis and sinus tachycardia. Death may occur in this phase

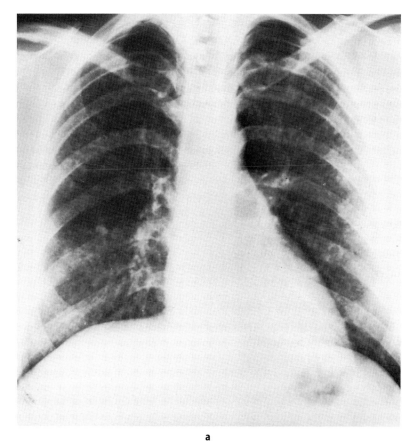

a

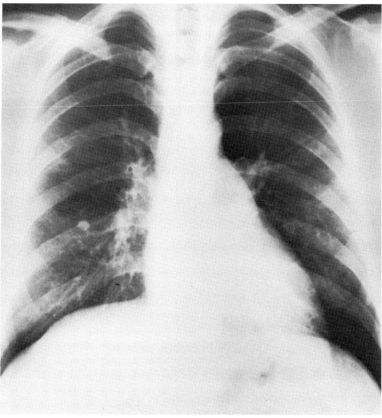

b

Figure 28.1. Phosgene low dose inhalation poisoning. **a** Following a latent phase of 48 h a chest radiograph reveals hazy perihilar shadows with patchy alveolar consolidations. **b** Toxic pulmonary changes resolved mainly in the peripheral regions in 72 h.

because of acute pulmonary edema. However, the onset of pulmonary edema may be delayed for up to 36 h from the time of exposure. During the second phase, lasting for 2–5 weeks, patients have minimal dyspnea or no symptoms. In the third phase, pyrexia, recurrence of cough, breathlessness, and cyanosis are observed. Reduced carbon monoxide transfer factor and hypocapnia are also found (19). Follow-up studies in patients developing lung edema demonstrated in all cases persistent pulmonary dysfunction (27).

Radiologic Findings

Following exposure to high concentrations of oxides of nitrogen, acute pulmonary edema may occur in a short period of time or up to 24 h later, with the typical radiographic signs of perihilar haziness in the early stages and diffuse alveolar shadowing in the more severe cases (7,8) (Fig. 28.2).

The radiologic lung findings following accidental poisoning in industrial settings do not differ from lung changes in silo filler's disease (20,21,23). If there is no secondary bacterial infection, acute pulmonary edema usually resolves within a few days to a week (7,8).

Dimethyl Sulfate

Dimethyl sulfate is an organic ester. It is used as a solvent and as a methylating agent in the chemical and pharma-

ceutic industries. Dimethyl sulfate is highly toxic as a liquid and as a vapor. In the presence of water or moisture, dimethyl sulfate hydrolyzes readily to sulfuric acid and methyl alcohol. The toxic effects of dimethyl sulfate are comparable to those of phosgene in causing severe damage to small airways and alveoli, resulting in pulmonary edema (1,3).

The radiographic picture is mainly that of pulmonary edema, similar to that caused by poisoning with phosgene or oxides of nitrogen. Initial roentgenologic signs are perihilar shadows and fine patchy consolidation of the lungs. Alveolar pulmonary edema follows. Roentgenologic diagnosis and differential diagnosis is identical to inhalation poisoning with phosgene or oxides of nitrogen (9,10).

Water-Soluble Inhalation Agents Causing Damage to the Upper Respiratory Tract and the Tracheobronchial Tree

Chlorine Gas

Chlorine is a highly toxic irritant gas. Its characteristic sharp odor can be detected in the air at 0.1 ppm. However, irritation of mucous membranes occurs only at 1.0 ppm. The potential risk for exposure to chlorine gas is widespread, since chlorine is used or generated during many industrial processes, which include the manufacture of plastics and the

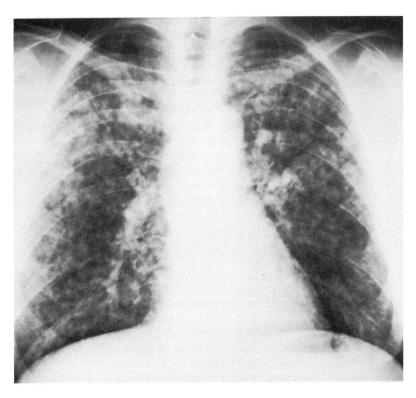

Figure 28.2. Acute pulmonary edema following inhalation of nitrogen dioxide in high concentration. Extensive involvement of both lungs by diffuse alveolar pulmonary edema 5 h after inhalation.

production of hydrochloric acid, alkali compounds, and bleaching powders. One of the major uses of chlorine has been in water purification (18,19). Exposure to chlorine gas may occur during the manufacturing process, from leakage of pipes or tanks, from accidental spillage during transportation, from mixing chlorine bleach with an acid cleaner, or as a swimming pool hazard (7,28–30).

Pathogenesis

The toxic action of chlorine gas on respiratory mucous membranes upon exposure is due to its potent oxidative properties, which lead to liberation of nascent oxygen, a protoplasmic poison, and formation of hydrochloric acid. The nascent oxygen as well as the hydrochloric acid possess severe toxic properties. Chlorine is nearly 20 times as toxic as hydrochloric acid (31).

Clinical Symptoms and Signs

Immediate symptoms of chlorine inhalation are a choking, suffocating sensation associated with acute anxiety. There is retrosternal burning pain, with burning of the nose and mouth and increased salivation.

Radiologic Findings

Radiologic findings in the initial stages of poisoning with chlorine resemble those found in "status asthmaticus": hyperinflation of the lung fields with lowered diaphragm. A preedema stage may follow when fine interstitial changes can be seen in the lung fields. Pulmonary edema usually resolves within a few days; however, severe chlorine gas poisoning with lung edema is often complicated by the development of bronchopneumonia, lung abscesses, and emphysema (32).

Chest radiology plays an important role not only in the early detection of the first signs of incipient lung edema caused by chlorine gas inhalation, but also in the demonstration of preexisting lung disease (e.g., emphysema and fibrosis), which determines the lung response to noxious gas, the duration of the toxic disease, and development of complications, as well as the prognosis (32,33).

Ammonia

Ammonia is a colorless, highly water-soluble, extremely irritant alkaline gas (34,35). Ammonia gas is widely used in the manufacturing of fertilizers, plastics, and synthetic fibers, in the production of nitric acid and explosives, in oil refining

processes, and in refrigeration plants. Exposure to ammonia gas is usually due to an industrial accident. In most cases, poisoning occurs as a result of rupture or leakage of containers, fractured pipes, or valve failures. The general public may also be affected by occasional accidents involving transportation of ammonia in containers (34,36).

Ammonia gas per se is not poisonous, but, because of its high solubility in water, the toxic action takes place in the moist mucous membranes of the airways (34). Ammonia as an alkaline compound produces liquefaction of the tissue with which it comes into contact. Tissue liquefaction allows deeper penetration of the toxic agent with increased damage. Therefore ammonia burns are very often severe and may be fatal (37).

Clinical Symptoms and Signs

Ammonia gas has an immediate irritating effect on the eyes, mouth, throat, and upper respiratory tract. This primary irritation usually prompts the exposed person to escape from the dangerous zone, avoiding inhalation of higher doses of noxious gas. Symptoms include acute pharyngitis and tracheitis, hoarseness, dysphagia, respiratory distress, cyanosis, pulmonary edema, and shock (35).

Radiographic Findings

The inhaled ammonia gas directly irritates and erodes bronchial mucosa almost at all levels. Thus the chest roentgenogram initially shows slightly enlarged pulmonary markings at the hila. Also, perihilar vascular and bronchial wall prominence is found. At this stage the main lung changes are therefore interstitial. In cases of severe poisoning, alveolar edema and segmental atelectasis can develop (38).

Sulfur Dioxide

Sulfur dioxide is an intense respiratory irritant and a commonly encountered toxic gas. It is used extensively in the chemical and paper industries and in bleaching, fumigation, and preserving. It has also been widely used in the liquefied state as a refrigerant. It occurs in combustion of sulfur and in burning of coal containing sulfur.

On contact with moist mucosal surfaces sulfur dioxide is hydrated and subsequently oxidized, forming sulfuric acid, which causes severe injuries to the tracheobronchial mucosa. Acute exposure to a high concentration of sulfur dioxide results in injuries of eyes, nasopharynx, and respiratory tract. Accidental exposure to high concentrations occurs in pulp and paper factories and in refrigeration plants.

Pulmonary changes documented on chest radiographs are similar to inhalation injuries caused by other irritant gases such as chlorine or ammonia. Follow-up examinations in patients who inhaled sulfur dioxide may show signs of extensive fibrotic bronchitis and generalized bronchiectasis (39).

Hydrogen Sulfide

Hydrogen sulfide (H_2S) is a colorless gas with a powerful odor of rotten eggs. It is somewhat heavier than air and it therefore tends to accumulate in tunnels, caissons, vats, and cellars. Hydrogen sulfide is an asphyxiant as well as an irritant. It is encountered in the production of many chemicals and dyes, in the tannery and rubber industries, in petroleum refining, in mines with sulfide ores, in sewers, and in the fishing and fish meal industries (28).

Accidental exposure to concentrations of hydrogen sulfide greater than about 700 ppm causes death from respiratory failure due to depression of medullary centers before the irritant effects in the lung have time to develop (28). More prolonged exposure to concentrations of 300–600 ppm results in irritation of the mucosa of the nose, throat, and chest with cough, headache, and dizziness. Pulmonary edema follows, while absorption of hydrogen sulfide in the lungs results in respiratory paralysis due to the blockade of intracellular cytochrome oxidases.

Radiographic Manifestations

Severe intoxication with hydrogen sulfide causes diffuse pulmonary edema. The most frequent complication is bronchopneumonia (7,8).

Metal Vapors and Aerosols

Nickel Carbonyl

Nickel carbonyl ($Ni(CO)_4$) is a heavy, colorless, unstable liquid that is vaporized at room temperature. The vapor is highly toxic. The toxicity of nickel carbonyl is at least five times as great as that of carbon monoxide. Accidental exposure to nickel carbonyl vapors can occur during the nickel refining process in nickel factories. Nickel carbonyl is used as a catalyst. Nickel is also used extensively in the production of nickel-based alloys in the manufacture of steel, glass, enamels, and ceramics (28).

Nickel carbonyl causes severe toxic damage to bronchial mucosa and alveoli. The lungs are the main target of the toxic action (28,40). In the respiratory tract, nickel carbonyl breaks down, depositing nickel as a slightly soluble compound in a very fine state of subdivision over the immense respiratory surface of the lungs. This causes irriation, congestion, and edema.

An acute disorder caused by inhalation of nickel carbonyl vapors has two phases. The immediate phase consists of dizziness, slight dyspnea, nausea, vomiting, and severe headache. These symptoms disappear quickly when the exposed person reaches open air. The delayed phase is characterized by paroxysmal coughing, breathlessness, chest tightness, substernal pain, and extreme weakness. The onset of this intoxication phase may vary from 10 to 36 h, or occasionally up to 8 days (41). In fatal cases, delirium develops with death on the 4th to 12th day. The cause of death is usually edema of the lungs (41,42).

Radiographic Findings

Early radiologic signs in nickel carbonyl poisoning are widening and blurring of hilar structures and perihilar hazy shadows. In about 60% of patients patchy bilateral consolidation due to a toxic pneumonitis develops (Fig. 28.3a). This usually is followed by extensive pulmonary edema. As a sequela of nickel carbonyl poisoning, lung fibrosis may also develop in some patients (Fig. 28.3b) (7).

Zinc Chloride

Zinc chloride is employed in oil refining, in the production of dry batteries, and in galvanizing iron. It is also used in smoke bombs. Exposure to zinc chloride smoke in confined spaces may be lethal.

Zinc chloride is extremely caustic to mucous membranes because of its hygroscopic and astringent nature, leading to protein denaturation. Inhalation of zinc chloride fumes causes severe acute tracheobronchitis and a rapidly developing diffuse interstitial fibrosis, resulting in lung induration (43,44).

Chest radiography demonstrates initially a diffuse reticulonodular pattern that changes to more patchy irregular consolidation as a result of a chemical pneumonitis. This is followed by bilateral diffuse consolidation due to toxic pulmonary edema. Acute lung edema and toxic pneumonia may progress within a few weeks to diffuse interstitial pulmonary fibrosis. Among the complications, subpleural emphysematous blebs are common in zinc chloride inhalation, and may result in a pneumothorax. Also, the development of lung abscesses and generalized lung fibrosis have been reported (7,43,44).

Cadmium

Cadmium oxide and chloride dusts are soluble in body fluids. Damage to the mucous membranes of the respiratory tract causes "chemical pneumonia" with edema.

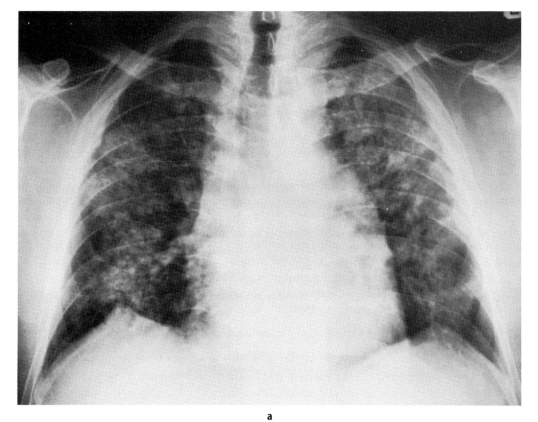

a

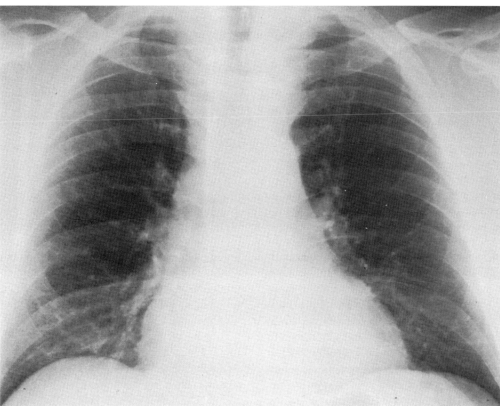

b

Figure 28.3. Nickel tetracarbonyl inhalation poisoning. **a** Thirteen days after inhalation, extensive patchy consolidations appear in both lung fields. **b** Signs of lung fibrosis are present 7 years after exposure.

Exposure to cadmium is especially dangerous, because concentrations of cadmium or fume dust sufficient to cause severe illness or death usually do not give rise to early warning symptoms (28,45,46).

The main radiographic feature in cadmium poisoning is pulmonary edema, which usually resolves in a week or two, but may not disappear completely for 2 or 3 months.

Cobalt

Cobalt is a silvery blue-white metal with magnetic properties. Cobalt is used for a variety of purposes in industry, medicine, and nuclear weapon production. Inhalation of particulate cobalt metal is strikingly toxic to the lungs. Poisoning results in hemorrhagic edema and obliterative bronchiolitis.

Acute pulmonary edema encountered in severe cases of cobalt inhalation shows the same typical radiographic pattern as described for toxic inhalations of other vapors. In the subacute type of poisoning, linear or ill-defined rounded opacities in the lung parenchyma with prominent hilar shadows develop within a year or less (28).

Organophosphates

Organophosphates are used as insecticides and have dozens of derivates. The most commonly used organophosphate compounds are parathion, malathion, and meoinphos. The most toxic organophosphate compounds have been stockpiled as "nerve gases" for possible use in chemical warfare and are available as powder, concentrate, and aerosol. Exposure to organophosphates is most common in agricultural workers during or shortly after spraying crops, and less common in industrial workers during manufacturing and transportation. Respiratory injuries are caused by (a) inhalation of organophosphate insecticides during spraying, (b) absorption through skin and mucous membranes, and (c) ingestion for suicide, homicide, or by mistake (acute poisoning in children).

The primary toxic effect of an organophosphate is the inhibition of the enzyme cholinesterase (47,48). As a result, a large amount of acetylcholine accumulates at nerve endings. The pulmonary edema observed in organophosphate poisoning has been attributed to the muscarinic effect of the organophosphates (48). Hypoxia may also play a role in the production of pulmonary edema by causing pulmonary capillary permeability (48).

Acute pulmonary edema induced by organophosphate poisoning can present either as diffuse pulmonary densities, basically of peripheral distribution with an enlarged cardiac shadow, or, a mixed pattern of alveolar and interstitial edema (Fig. 28.4). Pleural effusion can also be observed.

Smoke and Carbon Monoxide Inhalation

Smoke Inhalation Injury

Respiratory tract injury from smoke inhalation is one of the major causes of death in fire victims (49–52). There is a synergistic lethal relationship between body surface burns and the inhalation injury. The incidence of pulmonary complications in fire victims varies between 15% and 24%, with a mortality rate of 71–89%. The acute respiratory distress in burn patients is caused by smoke inhalation, carbon monoxide poisoning, and airway obstruction. To date, it is not possible to separate the respiratory effects of inhalation injury from the ventilatory effects of shock, massive fluid therapy, burn wound toxins, and sepsis (53).

The radiographic diagnosis of pulmonary edema in burn patients may be an early indicator of lung parenchymal injury and impending pulmonary insufficiency. Therefore the early diagnosis of pulmonary edema is crucial for the management of patients suffering from smoke inhalation (7). The initial radiologic findings appear in the first 24 h (54). Lung changes developing after 24 h are usually related to aspiration pneumonia, bacterial pneumonia, or a hemodynamic abnormality (55). The radiologic diagnosis of inhalation injury may be made at a time when results from other diagnostic tests are still equivocal or mildly abnormal, thus alerting the clinician to impending pulmonary failure. A single negative chest roentgenogram does not rule out respiratory tract damage. It is recommended therefore, to repeat chest examinations in patients with second- or third-degree flame burns of the face.

Early signs of alveolar and bronchial plugging and incipient alveolar edema are the appearance of patchy pulmonary densities. Atelectasis is suggested by the demonstration of linear densities, vascular crowding, elevation of the diaphragm, or displacement of a hilus. Atelectasis may shift from lobe to lobe or disappear according to the localized trapping of air caused by bronchial plugs. Widening of the vascular pedicle is a sign of increased circulating blood volume. Therefore the enlargement of the vascular pedicle is associated with early burn-related pulmonary edema and provides a useful radiographic predictor of this complication (56). Pulmonary edema may often be seen as a very faint haze or merely as lack of definition of the hilar and perihilar structures (54).

In general, chest radiologic findings in burn patients can be divided into three phases. In the acute intoxication phase during the first 24 h, patchy areas of chemical pneumonitis are often accompanied by diffuse pulmonary edema. In the subacute phase in the following 2–5 days, atelectasis, pulmonary microembolism, and adult respiratory distress syndrome (ARDS) develop. The relatively

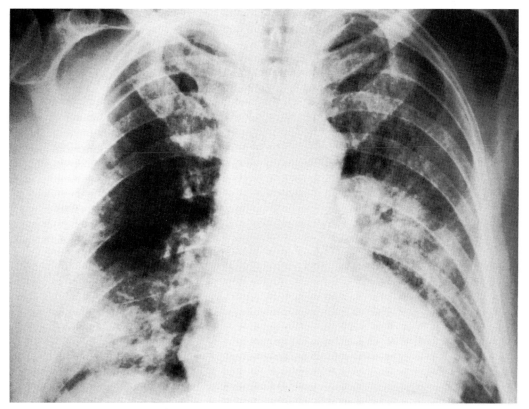

Figure 28.4. Lung changes following organophosphate poisoning with insecticide. A chest radiograph taken after hospital admission demonstrates a combination of alveolar and interstitial pulmonary edema. The heart shadow is markedly enlarged.

rapid change of size and location of pulmonary infiltrates strongly suggests the development of lung hemorrhage secondary to microembolism. In ARDS, moderate alveolar opacifications extending to the periphery of lungs without regard to lobar anatomic boundaries are demonstrated. This radiographic appearance of ARDS closely resembles diffuse pulmonary edema. However, it ordinarily does not spare the periphery of the lungs and is associated with volume loss leading to diminution of the vertical lung diameter. The third phase of radiologic findings is characterized by delayed complications such as pulmonary thromboembolism and pneumonia. Airborne pneumonia may also show alveolar densities that involve the basal areas of the lungs. Bronchiolitis obliterans, bronchostenosis, and bronchiectasis have been described as sequelae of smoke intoxication (57).

Carbon Monoxide Inhalation Injury

Smoke and carbon monoxide inhalation injuries are very often combined, but carbon monoxide intoxication has some specific characteristics. Carbon monoxide (CO) is a colorless, tasteless, and odorless gas with a specific gravity 0.97 times that of air. Carbon monoxide originates from the incomplete combustion of carbonaceous material (e.g., exhaust from automobiles, faulty heaters, mine explosives). Its toxic effects are caused by tissue hypoxia. The affinity of hemoglobin for carbon monoxide is 218 times greater than for oxygen. In addition, carbon monoxide may also have a direct toxic effect on the lung parenchyma when inhaled in high concentrations (58).

The most common finding on a chest radiograph of a patient with carbon monoxide inhalation is an increase in interstitial markings or a ground-glass appearance in both lung fields (Fig. 28.5). This pattern is attributed to interstitial edema, probably caused by a combination of tissue hypoxia and a direct toxic effect of carbon monoxide on the alveolocapillary membrane. Other findings include perihilar haze and perivascular and perihilar cuffing. Cardiac enlargement is usually encountered, suggesting myocardial damage secondary to carbon monoxide toxicity. Alveolar edema is another manifestation (58).

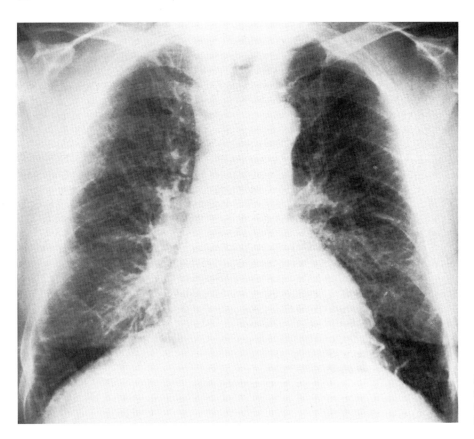

Figure 28.5. Combined inhalation intoxication with smoke, sulfur dioxide, and carbon monoxide. Bilateral increase in the interstitial markings is a sign of incipient pulmonary edema.

Lung Intoxication in Heavy Cigarettes Smokers ("Smoker's Lung")

Cigarette smoking is the most frequent source of indoor pollution affecting millions of people. Chest radiography remains an inexpensive method of evaluating pulmonary changes resulting from cigarette smoking (59–63). Computed tomography (CT), and especially HRCT (64–117), as well as CT with thin-slab maximum intensity projection (97) have increased the ability to identify specific abnormalities, especially in long-term, multiple packs day smokers. Most studies in these patients demonstrated proliferative lung changes, such as peribronchial thickening, interlobar thickening and ground-glass attenuation, as well as rarefication of lung vasculature and the presence of low attenuation areas (84,89,90,93,97–99,103,104) (Figs 28.6–28.9)

Conclusions

In general the radiologic input in the diagnosis and treatment of inhalation lung injuries can be summarized as follows:

1. Radiologic signs of pulmonary edema precede clinical manifestations for hours. The radiologic latent phase is inversely proportional to the dose and duration of exposure to a toxic gas. Recognition and exact interpretation of early radiographic signs of lung injury are vital in the timing of intensive care treatment.

2. Negative findings on the initial chest radiograph do not exclude respiratory injury. Repetition of chest examinations at short time intervals is therefore highly recommended. A chest radiograph should be performed also in asymptomatic patients. The lung response to an inhalation injury depends on preexisting lung disease. Complications and inhalation injury sequelae are also determined by the pulmonary status.

3. The most characteristic pattern of inhalation lung injury is pulmonary edema. Interstitial and alveolar edema, and very often a combination of both, are observed.

4. In the follow-up of patients with inhalation injuries of the lung, mostly chronic proliferative changes and lung fibrosis are observed. In such patients CT examination of the lung is the method of choice.

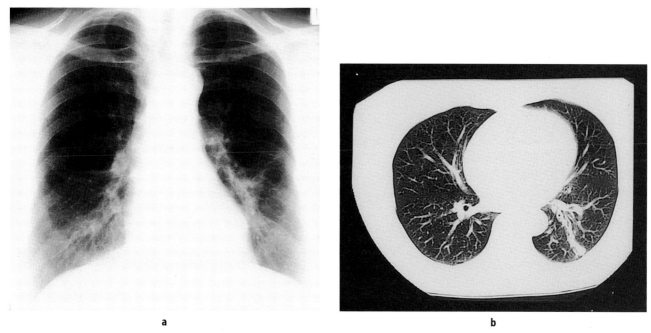

a   b

Figure 28.6. A 60 year old female smoking 20 cigarettes per day for 20 years. She became a nonsmoker for the 10 years prior to this radiograph. Chest radiograph (**a**) and CT (**b**) show heavy peribronchial and interlobar thickening.

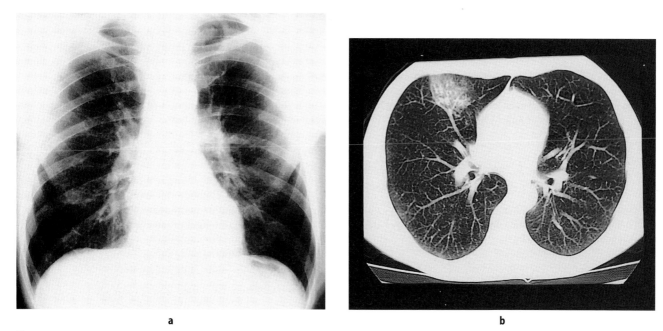

a   b

Figure 28.7. A 59 year old male patient smoking 20 cigarettes per day for 40 years. Radiograph (**a**), and CT (**b**), show the predominance of a triad of signs such as peribronchial thickening, interlobar thickening, and ground-glass attenuation.

References

1. Thiess AM (1969) Gewerbliche Vergiftunger mit Reizgazen. Arztl Prax 91:5074–5081.
2. Thiess AM (1974) Intoxikation in der werksärztlichen Praxis. Internist 15:424–431.
3. Thiess AM, Schmitz TH (1969) Gesundheitsschäden und Vergiftungen durch Einwirkung von Reizstoffen auf die oberen und mittleren Atemwege. Sich Arb 3:11–18.
4. Diller WF (1976) Radiologische Untersuchungen zur uerbesserten Frühdiagnose von Industriellen Inhalationsvergiftungen mit verzögertem wirkungseintritt. Verlag Dr. E. Fischer, Heidelberg.

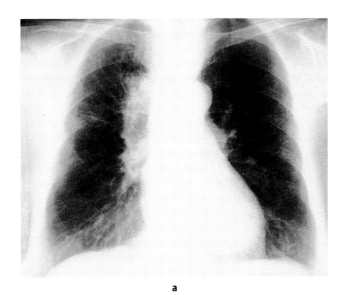
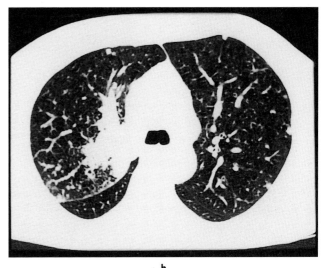

a   b

Figure 28.8. A 57 year old female smoking 15–20 cigarettes per day for 27 years. Radiograph (**a**), and CT (**b**), demonstrate the proliferative lung changes classified as a cluster of CT findings: peribronchial thickening, interlobular thickening, ground-glass attenuation, and bronchial carcinoma of the right lung.

5. Diller WF (1983) Inhalative Reizstoffvergiftungen. Arbeitsmedizin actuell, lieferung 13. Gustav Fischer Verlag, Stuttgart.
6. Ulmer WT. (1976) Inhalative Noxen. Internist 17:391–398.
7. Novak D, Rothenberger W (1979) Röntgenologische Lungenveränderungen, nach Inhalation von Reizgazen. Prakt Anästh 14:162–173.
8. Summer W, Haponik E (1981) Inhalation of irritant gases. Clin Chest Med 2:273–287.
9. Novak D (1988) Inhalationsschäden durch Gase. In Schinez H (ed): Radiologische Diagnostik, 7. Auflage, Band 1/2. Georg Thieme Verlag, Stuttgart.
10. Cordasco EM, Stone FD (1973) Pulmonary edema of environmental origin. Chest 64:182–185.
11. Cordasco EM, Demeter SR, Kester L, et al. (1980) Pulmonary edema of environmental origin – newer concepts. Angiology 37:440–447.
12. Evans MJ (1986) Oxidant gases. Environ Health Perspect 55:85–95
13. Diller WF (1984) Das toxische Lungenödem. Atemw Lungenkrankh 10:215–218.
14. Diller WF (1975) Radiologische Untersuchungen zur verbesserten Frühdiagnose von industriellen Inhalationsvergiftungen mit verzögertem Wirkungseitritt. Arbeitsschutz Arbeitsmed (Frankfurt) 8.
15. Diller WF (1985) Early diagnosis of phosgene overexposure. Toxicol Ind Health 1:73–80.
16. Seidelin R (1961) The inhalation of phosgene in a fire extinguisher accident. Thorax 16:91–93.
17. Diller WF (1974) Klinik und Pathologie der Phosgenvergiftung. Pneumonologie 150:139–148.
18. Diller WF (1985) Late sequelae after phosgene poisoning: A literature review. Toxicol Ind Health 1:129–136.
19. Horvath SM (1980) Nitrogen dioxide, pulmonary function, and respiratory disease. Bull NY Acad Med 56:835–846.
20. Ramirez RJ, Dowell AR (1971) Silo-filler's disease: Nitrogen dioxide-induced lung injury. Long-term follow-up and review of the literature. Ann Intern Med 74:569–576.
21. Morrissey WL, Gould JA, Carrington CB, et al. (1975) Silo-filler's disease. Respiration 32:81–92.
22. Fleming GM, Chester EH, Montenegro HD (1979) Dysfunction of small airways following pulmonary injury due to nitrogen dioxide. Chest 75:720–721.
23. Moskowitz RL, Lyons HA, Cottle HR (1964) Silo-filler's disease: Clinical, physiologic, and pathologic study of a patient. Am J Med 36:457–463.
24. Drake CS, Warrack AJN (1958) Bronchiolitis from nitrous fumes. Thorax 13:327–333.
25. Larcan A, Calamai H, Mentre B, et al. (1971) Pneumopathie par inhalation de vapeurs nitreuses (combustion de poupées de celluloide). Poumon 26:957–960.
26. Yockey CC, Edem BM, Byrd RB (1980) The McConnel missile accident. Clinical spectrum of nitrogen dioxide exposure. JAMA 244:1221–1223.
27. Norvath EP, doPico GA, Barbee RA (1978) Nitrogen dioxide-induced pulmonary disease: Five new cases and a review of the literature. J Occup Med 20:103–110.
28. Parkes WR (1983) Occupational lung disorders, 2nd edn. Butterworth, London.
29. Chester EH, Kaimal J, Payne CB, Jr et al. (1977) Pulmonary injury following exposure to chlorine gas. Possible beneficial effects of steroid treatment. Chest 72:247–250.
30. Decker WJ, Koch HF (1978) Chlorine poisoning at the swimming pool: an overheated hazard. Clin Toxicol 13:377–381.
31. Kaufman J, Burkons D (1971) Clinical, roentgenologic, and physiologic effects of acute chlorine exposure. Arch Environ Health 23:29–34.
32. Koenig H, Wolf HR (1975) Lungenbefunde nach akuter Chlorgasinhalation. Z Ärztl Fortbild 69:231–234.
33. Wheater RH (1974) Hazard of exposure to chlorine gas. JAMA 230:1064.
34. Walton M (1973) Industrial ammonia gasing. Br J Ind Med 30:78–86.
35. Montague TJ, Macneil AR (1980) Mass ammonia inhalation. Chest 77:496–498.
36. Percot C, Huriet C, Midon A, et al. (1972) L'intoxication aiguë professionelle par le gaz ammoniac. Á propos de quatre observations. Arch Mal Prof 33:5–12.

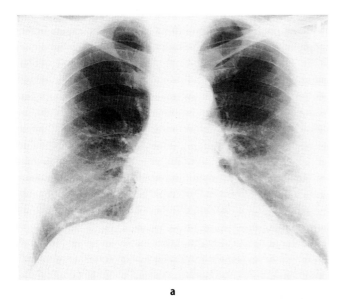

a

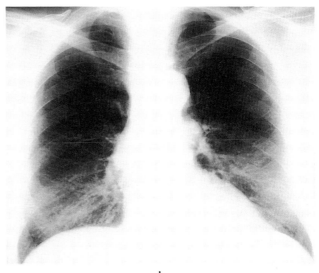

b

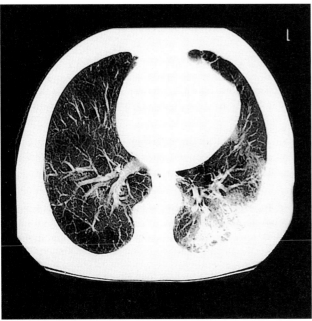

c

Figure 28.9. A 72 year old man smoking 20 cigarettes per day for 50 years. The radiograph (**a**) taken in 1988, and radiograph (**b**) taken 3 years later demonstrate the progression of proliferative lung changes. The CT (**c**) was performed 1998. It shows the further progression of proliferative lung changes as well as a bronchial carcinoma of the left lung.

37. Sobonya R (1977) Fatal anhydrous ammonia inhalation. Hum Pathol 8:293–299.
38. Kass J, Zamel N, Dobry CA, et al. (1972) Bronchiectasis following ammonia burns of the respiratory tract. A review of two cases. Chest 62:282–285.
39. Charan NB, Myers CG, Lakshminarayan S, et al. (1979) Pulmonary injuries associated with acute sulfur dioxide inhalation. Am Rev Resp Dis 119:555–560.
40. Hackett RL, Sunderman FW (1968) Pulmonary alveolar reaction to nickel carbonyl. Ultrastructural and histochemical studies. Arch Environ Health 16:349–362.
41. Viopala U, Huhti E, Takkunen J, et al. (1970) carbonyl poisoning. Ann Clin Res 2:214–222.
42. Jones CC (1973) Nickel carbonyl poisoning. Report of a fatal case. Arch Environ Health 26:245–248.
43. Mataresse SL, Matthews JI (1986) Zinc chloride (smoke bomb) inhalation lung injury. Chest 89:308–309.
44. Milliken JA, Waugh D, Kadish ME (1963) Acute interstitial pulmonary fibrosis caused by a smoke bomb. Can Med Assoc J 88:36–39.
45. Beton DC, Andrews GS, Davies HJ, et al. (1966) Acute cadmium fume poisoning. Br J Ind Med 23:292–301.
46. Townssend RH (1968) A case of acute cadmium pneumonitis: Lung function tests during a four-year follow-up. Br J Ind Med 25:68–71.
47. Namba T, Nolte CT, Jackrel J, et al. (1971) Poisoning due to organophosphate insecticides. Acute and chronic manifestations. Am J Med 50:475–492.
48. Bledsoe FH, Seymour EQ (1972) Acute pulmonary edema associated with parathion poisoning. Radiology 103:53–56.

49. Fein A, Leff A, Hopewell PC (1980) Pathophysiology and management of the complications resulting from fire and the inhaled products of combustion. Crit Care Med 8:94–98.

50. Achauer BM, Allyn PA, Furnas DW, et al. (1973) Pulmonary complications of burns: The major threat to the burn patient. Ann Surg 177:311–319.

51. Head JM (1980) Inhalation injury in burns. Am J Surg 139:508–513

52. Cathalane M, Demling RH (1986) Early respiratory abnormalities from smoke inhalation. JAMA 251:771–773.

53. Chu CS (1981) New concepts of pulmonary burn injury. J Trauma 21:958–962.

54. Teixidor HS, Rubin E, Novick GS, et al. (1983) Smoke inhalation: Radiologic manifestations. Radiology 149:383–387.

55. Traber DL, Schlag G, Redl H, et al. (1985) Pulmonary edema and compliance changes following smoke inhalation. J Burn Care Rehabil 6:490–494.

56. Haponik EF, Adelman M, Munster AM, et al. (1986) Increased vascular pedicle with preceding burn-related pulmonary edema. Chest 90:649–655.

57. McArdle CS: Finlay WEI (1975) Pulmonary complications following smoke inhalation. Br J Anaesth 47:618–623.

58. Kittredge RD (1971) Pulmonary edema in acute carbon monoxide poisoning. AJR 113:680–681.

59. Wittram C, Kenny JB (1994) The admission chest radiograph after acute inhalation injury and burns. Br J Radiol 67:751–754.

60. Wright JL (1993) Inhalation lung injuries causing bronchiolitis. Clin Chest Med 14:635–644.

61. Sperber M, Novak D (1998) Environmental lung disorders. Inhalation of In Sperber, M (ed) Diffuse lung disorders. Springer Verlag, London 1998 pp 158–184.

62. Navak D (1998) Inhalation of toxic gases and fumes In Sperber M (ed) Diffuse lung disorders. Springer Verlag, London, pp 000–000.

63. Terriff BA, Kwan SY, Chan-Yeung MM (1992) Fibrosing alveolitis: Chest radiography and CT predictors of clinical and functional impairment at follow-up in 26 patients. Radiology 184:445–449.

64. Rémy-Jardin M, Rémy J, Giraud F, et al. (1993) Computed tomography assessment of ground-glass opacity: Semiology and significance. J Thorac Imaging 8:249–264.

65. Bonelli FS, Hartman TE, Swensen SJ, et al. (1998) Accuracy of high-resolution CT in diagnosing lung diseases. AJR 170:1507–1512.

66. Katsuragawa S, Doi K, MacMahon H, et al. (1990) Quantitative computer-aided analysis of lung texture in chest radiographs. Radiographics 10:257–269.

67. Minnier-Cholley L, MacMahon H, Katsuragawa S, et al. (1995) Computerized analysis of interstitial infiltrates on chest radiographs: A new scheme based on geometric pattern features and Fourier analysis. Acad Radiol 2:455–462.

68. Morishita J, Doi K, Katsuragawa S, et al. (1995) Computer-aided diagnosis for interstitial infiltrates in chest radiographs: Optical-density dependence of texture measures. Med Phys 22:1515–1522.

69. Katsuragawa S, Doi K, MacMahon H, et al. (1996) Quantitative analysis of geometric-pattern features of interstitial infiltrates in digital chest radiographs. J Digital Imaging 9:137–144.

70. Kido S, Kuroda C, Tamura S (1998) Quantification of interstitial lung abnormalities with chest radiography: Comparison of radiographic index and fractal dimension. Acad Radiol 5:336.

71. Katsuragawa S, Doi K, MacMahon H, et al. (1997) Classification of normal and abnormal lungs with interstitial diseases by rule-based method and artificial neural networks. J Digital Imaging 10:108–114.

72. Ishida T, Katsuragawa S, Ashizawa K, et al. (1997) Artificial neural networks in chest radiographs: Detection and characterization of interstitial lung disease. Proc SPIE 3034:931–937.

73. Ishida T, Katsuragawa S, Kobayashi T, et al. (1997) Computerized analysis of interstitial disease in chest radiographs: Improvement of geometric-pattern feature analysis. Med Phys 24:915–924.

74. Rémy-Jardin M, Rémy J, Deffontaines C, et al. (1991) Assessment of diffuse infiltrative lung disease: Comparison of conventional CT and high-resolution CT. Radiology 181:157–162.

75. Leung AN, Miller RR, Müller NL (1993) Parenchymal opacification in chronic infiltrative lung diseases: CT–pathologic correlation. Radiology 188:209–214.

76. Müller NL, Miller RR (1995) Diseases of the bronchioles: CT and histopathologic findings. Radiology 196:3–12.

77. Leung AN, Staples CA, Müller NL (1991) Chronic diffuse infiltrative lung disease: Comparison of diagnostic accuracy of high-resolution CT and conventional CT. AJR 157:693–696.

78. Rémy-Jardin M, Giraud F, Rémy J, et al. (1993) Importance of ground glass attenuation in chronic diffuse infiltrative lung disease: Pathologic–CT correlation. Radiology 189:693–698.

79. Rémy-Jardin M, Rémy J, Artaud D, et al. (1996) Diffuse infiltrative lung disease: Clinical value of sliding-thin-slab maximum intensity projection CT scans in the detection of mild micronodular patterns. Radiology 200:333–339.

80. Adesina AM, Vallyathan V, McQuillen EN, et al. (1991) Bronchiolar inflammation and fibrosis associated with smoking: A morphological cross-sectional population analysis. Am Rev Respir Dis 143:144–149.

81. Meredith TJ, Vale JA, Proudfoot AT (1987) Poisoning by inhalation agents. In Weatherall DJ, Ledingham JGG, Warrel D (eds) Oxford textbook of medicine, 2nd edn. Oxford University Press, Oxford.

82. Murray VSG, Volans GN (1991) Management of injuries due to chemical weapons. Br Med J 302:129.

83. Gruden JF, Webb WR (1993) CT findings in a proved case of respiratory bronchiolitis. AJR 161:44–46.

84. Essadki O, Chartrand-Lefebvre C, Briere J, et al. (1998) Respiratory bronchiolitis: Radiographic and CT findings in proven case. Eur Radiol 8:1674–1676.

85. Hwang JH, Kim TS, Lee KS, et al. (1997) Bronchiolitis in adults: Pathology and imaging. J Comput Assist Tomogr 21:913–919.

86. Holt RM, Schmidt RA, Godwin JD, et al. (1993) High resolution CT in respiratory bronchiolitis-associated disease. J Comput Assist Tomogr 17:46–50.

87. Worthy SA, Müller NL (1998) Small airway diseases. Radiol Clin North Am 36:163–173.

88. Bankier AA, Fleischmann D, Mallek R, et al. (1996) Bronchial wall thickness: Appropriate window settings for thin section CT and radiologic–anatomic correlation. Radiology 199:831.

89. Garg K, Lynch DA, Newell JD, King TE, Jr (1994) Proliferative and constrictive bronchiolitis: Classification features. AJR 162:803–808

90. Bonelli FS, Hartman TE, Swensen SJ, et al. (1998) Accuracy of high-resolution CT in diagnosing lung diseases. AJR 170:1507.

91. Hartman TE, Tazelaar HD, Swensen SJ, et al. (1997) Cigarette smoking: CT and pathologic findings of associated pulmonary diseases. Radiographics 17:377–390.

92. Rémy-Jardin M, Rémy J, Boulenguez C, et al. (1993) Morphologic effects of cigarette smoking on airways and pulmonary parenchyma in healthy adult volunteers: CT evaluation and correlation with pulmonary function tests. Radiology 186:107–115.

93. Rémy-Jardin M, Rémy J, Gosselin B, et al. (1993) Lung parenchymal changes secondary to cigarette smoking: Pathologic CT correlations. Radiology 186:643–651.

94. Langford RM, Armstrong RF (1989) Algorithm for managing smoke inhalation. Br Med J 299:902.

95. Pelinkovic D, Lörcher U, Chow KU, et al. (1997) Spirometric gated quantitative computed tomography of the lung in healthy smokers and nonsmokers. Invest Radiol 32:335–343.

96. McAdams HP, Rosado de Christenson ML, Wehunt WD, et al. (1996) The alphabet soup revisited: The chronic interstitial pneumonias in the 1990s. Radiographics 16:1009–1033, discussion 1033–1034.

97. Worthy SA, Müller NL, Hartman TE, et al. (1997) Mosaic attenuation pattern on thin-section CT scans of the lung: Differentation among infiltrative lung, airway, and vascular disease as a cause. Radiology 205:465.

98. Brauner MW, Grenier P, Tijani K, et al. (1997) Pulmonary Langerhans' cell histocytosis: Evaluation of lesions on CT scans. Radiology 204:497.

99. Nakajima M, Manabe T, Niki Y, et al. (1998) Cigarette smoke-induced acute eosinophilic pneumonia. Radiology 207:829.

100. King MA, Pope-Harma AL, Allen JN, et al (1998) Cigarette smoke-induced acute eosinophilic pneumonia: Reply. Radiology 207:831.

101. Müller NL, Miller RR (1990) Computed tomography of chronic diffuse infiltrative lung disease. I. Am Rev Respir Dis 142: 1206–1215.

102. Müller NL, Miller RR (1990) Computed tomography of chronic diffuse infiltrative lung disease. II. Am Rev Respir Dis 142: 1440–1448.

103. Mathieson JR, Mayo JR, Staples CA, et al. (1989) Chronic diffuse infiltrative lung disease: Comparison of diagnostic accuracy of CT and chest radiography. Radiology 171:111–116.

104. Klein J, Gamsu G (1989) High resolution computed tomography of difuse lung disease. Invest Radiol 24:805–812.

105. Akira M (1995) Uncommon pneumoconioses: CT and pathologic findings. Radiology 197:403–409.

106. Giesen T, Zerlett G (1996) Berufskrankheiten und medizinischer Arbeitsschutz. Abschnitt C. Kohlhammer, Köln.

107. Bauer PC (1991) Obstruktive Atemwegserkrankungen durch allergisierende Stoffe. In Konietzko J, Dupuis (eds) Handbuch der Arbeitsmedizin, vol. IV, part 5 Loeblatl-Ausgabe.

108. Baur X (1995) Berufsbedingte bronchopulmonale Erkrankungen. In Fabel H (ed) Pneumologie. Urban und Schwarzenberg, Munich, pp ???.

109. Krieger HG, Woitowitz HJ (1990) Erkrankungen der Atemwege und Lungen durch chemische Substanzen. Medwelt 41:834–838.

110. Hering KG, Wiebe V (1990) Radiologische Diagnostik der Pneumokoniosen. Radiologe 30:574–580.

111. Hering KG (1992) Auswertung und Einordnung von CT-Befunden bei berufsbedingten Lungen und Pleuraveranderungen in Alehnung an die ILO-Staublungen-Klassifikation. Röntgenpraxis 45:304–308.

112. Hering KG, Tuergenthal S, Kraus TH, et al. (1994) CT Untersuchung und standardisierte Befundung bei berufsbedingten Lungen- und Pleuraveranderungen in Anlehnung an die ILO-Staublungen-Klassifikation. Röntgenpraxis 47:262–269.

113. Webb WR, Müller NL, Naidich DP (1993) Standardized terms for high-resolution computed tomography of the lung: A proposed glossary. J Thorac Imaging 8:167–175.

114. Krahe Th (1998) Bildgebende Diagnostik von Lunge und Pleura. Referenz-Reihe Radiologische Diagnostik. Thieme Verlag, Stuttgart.

115. Galanski M, Prokop M (eds) (1998) Ganzkörper-Computertomographie. Referenz-Reihe Radiologische Diagnostik. Thieme Verlag, Stuttgart.

116. Lörcher U, Schmidt H (1996) HR-CT der Lunge. Thieme Verlag, Stuttgart. Kullnig P (1990) High-resolution-CT bei interstitiellen Lungenerkrankungen. Rofo Furtschr Geb Rontgensh Neuen Bildbeg Verfahr 152:30–34.

117. Solomon A, Kreel L (eds.) (1989) Radiology of occupational chest disease. Springer, New York.

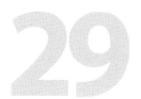

Carcinoma of the Lung

M.K. Wood and S.G. Spiro

Introduction

Lung cancer is the commonest cause of fatal malignancy worldwide, with over 900 000 deaths per year (1). The incidence is increasing in developing countries, where the rate was once relatively low. In eastern Asia and China, where the control of tobacco advertising and general public awareness is minimal, the mortality rates are higher than the world average. In developed countries the incidence among women has been rising steadily, matching the increased smoking habits of women since the 1950s (2,3). Smoking causes 85–90% of all lung cancers and it is only in countries with high profile anti-smoking lobbies where the incidence is decreasing. In America there has been a fall in the number of smokers, with a subsequent fall in the incidence of lung cancer in men every year for the last 5 years. The incidence among women, however, only began to plateau in the mid 1990s, which is a 10 year lag behind lung cancer rates in men and reflects smoking habits among American women (4).

Although smoking is by far the most important risk factor, there are other risk factors, which in combination with smoking produce an even higher risk. Asbestos exposure increases the chance of developing lung cancer by 50-fold compared with smoking alone.

Pathology

Lung cancers comprise four histological cell types, split into two groups for the purposes of treatment and prognosis. Small-cell lung cancer (SCLC) (20–30% of cases) metastasizes early and is usually disseminated at diagnosis. Thus treatment options are almost always nonsurgical. The other histologic groups are classified as non-small cell carcinoma (NSCLC) and consist of squamous cell carcinoma (30–40%), adenocarcinoma (30–40%) and large-cell

Table 29.1. Histological type associated with average doubling times[a] and incidence

Cancer cell type	Doubling time (days)	Incidence (%)
Adenocarcinoma	120–220	30–40
Squamous cell	90–115	30–40
Large cell	30–70	10–15
Small cell	30–85	20–30

[a] Data from ref. (5).

carcinoma (10–15%). Staging for possible resection is important, as these cell types tend to be slower growing and can be amenable to curative resection. Table 29.1 shows cell types with incidence and average doubling times.

Presentation

The growth rate of bronchial carcinoma is relatively slow. Doubling times can vary from between 1 and 18 months (6,7), which means tumors are present for several years before they become visible on a chest X-ray, usually at a size of about 1 cm. The tumor will have been growing for between 2.5 and 25 years (8), although may still not be diagnosed until even larger. Identification at 1 cm size is usually chance, for example via a preoperative chest X-ray or a general medical screen. Nevertheless most tumors present when larger, with either local or metastatic symptoms, or both. There have been several screening studies in high risk populations, using plain chest radiographs and both chest X-rays and CT scanning, with controversial outcomes due to overdiagnosis of innocent lesions (i.e., benign pulmonary nodules). However, some randomized clinical trials have found beneficial outcomes in terms of earlier stage at diagnosis, resectability and long-term survival using chest X-rays (9) and low dose CT scanning in high risk groups (10).

Table 29.2. Common symptoms and frequency at presentation

Symptom	Frequency (%)
Cough	55–65
Weight loss and/or anorexia	45–55
Chest pain	30–40
Dyspnea	30–40
Weakness	25–30
Hemoptysis	25–30
Pneumonia	10–15
Fever	5–10
Nausea and vomiting	5–10
Dizziness	1–5

Clinical presentation may be from direct involvement of intrathoracic structures, extrathoracic tumor spread, general tumor effects, or paraneoplastic symptoms. Eighty percent of primary lung cancers occur in the central airways. The most common presenting symptoms and their frequency are shown in Table 29.2.

Intrathoracic Symptoms and Signs

These are caused by the primary tumor and extrapulmonary invasion of other structures within the thoracic cavity:

Cough is common and may be caused by:

Narrowing of a major airway often with ulceration which can cause enough irritation to provoke cough before significantly impairing lung function.

Mediastinal involvement with recurrent laryngeal nerve paralysis causes a hoarse voice and can also cause coughing due to aspiration.

Collapse of the lung by tumor occluding an airway may also result in coughing.

A change in the nature of cough in a smoker with co-existent chronic bronchitis is a common complaint.

A chest infection or a pneumonia that is slow to resolve may indicate an underlying obstructing lesion, especially if the infection recurs.

Hemoptysis occurs when tumor erodes an airway. Hemoptysis in a smoker should be always treated with high suspicion, prompting further investigation.

Wheeze especially unilaterally can occur if tumor partially obstructs a large airway. Tumor in the trachea and proximal major bronchi causes *stridor*.

Mediastinal Invasion

The primary tumor or compression of structures by metastatic nodes can cause:

Superior vena caval obstruction (SVCO) by right paratracheal mediastinal lymph nodes, which presents with fullness within the face and head and progresses to distressing swelling of the face and upper limbs with non-pulsatile engorgement of the neck and superficial chest veins.

Involvement of the recurrent laryngeal nerve by metastatic invasion of the subaortic fossa – the commonest cause of unilateral vocal cord palsy producing *hoarseness* and a bovine cough.

Phrenic nerve palsy due to direct involvement of the primary tumor causing paralysis of the hemidiaphragm, which may cause breathlessness, or is only found on the chest X-ray.

Compression of the esophagus by direct invasion or by subcarinal nodes causing *dysphagia*.

A superior sulcus (Pancoast) tumor can juxtapose the sympathetic chain and erode into the brachial plexus. It lies posteriorly and close to the heads of the second to sixth ribs. It may present with Horner's syndrome, pain in the neck, shoulder, upper back or arm and wasting of the small muscles of the hand due to spinal region T1 involvement. There often is a history of shoulder or arm pain for many months before a chest X-ray is taken.

Other intrathoracic symptoms include:

chest pain caused by direct chest wall invasion

breathlessness, pleuritic pain and cough due to a *pleural effusion*, or rarely a *pneumothorax*

Extrathoracic Metastases

These can occur almost anywhere but the commonest sites include liver, adrenal glands, axial skeleton, skull and brain.

Liver metastases may cause jaundice if they obstruct the biliary drainage system but are usually asymptomatic at presentation and are thus screened for at diagnosis (see later), as are *adrenal metastases*, which do not cause symptoms unless they become very large. Unilateral adrenal adenomas are common and biopsy of an adrenal mass is recommended to exclude or confirm the malignancy if this is the only potential site of metastasis.

Bone metastases are lytic and cause pain or pathologic fractures, particularly of the long bones. Due to the high incidence of false positive bone scans, this investigation is recommended only in those presenting with symptoms suggestive of bony involvement, or in patients with non-specific malaise and greater than 5 kg weight loss. Bone pain in the thoracolumbar spine is associated with extension into the spinal canal causing compression and paraplegia. This can also occur due to interruption of the

Table 29.3. More common paraneoplastic syndromes, frequency and associated histologic cell type

Paraneoplastic syndrome	Incidence and predominant cell type
SIADH	10% of SCLC
Hypercalcemia	3% of all cases, mainly squamous
Cushing	1–2% of SCLC
Subacute peripheral neuropathy	Up to 5% of SCLC
LEMS	Up to 5% of SCLC
Encephalomyelitis	Less than 1% of SCLC
Clubbing	5–10% of NSCLC
HPOA	1–2% of squamous
Hematologic	20% with any type

SIADH, syndrome of inappropriate antidiuretic hormone, LEMS, Lambert–Eaton myasthenic syndrome; HPOA, hypertrophic pulmonary osteoarthropathy; SCLC, small-cell lung cancer; NSCLC, nonsmall-cell lung cancer.

anterior spinal artery. Symptoms due to compression are gradual whilst arterial invasion is usually more dramatic.

Brain metastases present as any space occupying lesion within the cerebrum, commonly causing headache, nausea and fits, with focal neurologic deficits or more subtle changes in mood or personality.

Paraneoplastic Syndromes

These may present earlier than symptoms directly due to tumor invasion but are in general a bad prognostic feature. They most commonly cause endocrine and neurologic disorders and can occur in up to 20% of lung cancer patients (11,12). They are summarized with frequency and associated cell type in Table 29.3 and include:

Endocrine, commonly:

Syndrome of inappropriate antidiuretic hormone (SIADH) production. This in general is limited to small-cell carcinoma. Fifty percent of patients with SCLC have increased levels of antidiuretic hormone but only 10% have symptoms directly attributed to the syndrome. The hyponatremia may cause confusion, seizures or a decreased level of consciousness. Treatment includes fluid restriction and cytotoxic chemotherapy. Refractory cases may respond to demeclocycline and occasionally lithium.

Hypercalcemia is most commonly associated with squamous cell carcinoma and is caused primarily by a parathyroid hormone-related peptide, including cases in which there are bone metastases. It occurs in approximately 3% of all lung cancers and may present with anorexia, nausea and vomiting, abdominal pain, lethargy, weakness, polyuria, polydipsia and confusion. Treatment is by rehydration and a forced saline diuresis with calciuric agents such as frusemide. The bisphosphonates, particu-

larly pamidronate are effective in reducing calcium levels. Reduction in calcium levels relieves symptoms but does not affect prognosis, which is usually very poor, with a median survival of approximately 1 month, as patients usually have advanced disease.

Excessive ACTH secretion occurs most commonly in small-cell lung cancer with an incidence of 1–2%. Increased corticotrophin levels are produced by enzymatic processing of ectopic adrenocorticotrophin hormone (ACTH) secretion, which can occur in up to 50% of patients with SCLC. Symptoms tend to be rapid in onset with weakness (specifically proximal myopathy), hyperglycemia, polyuria, and hypokalemic alkalosis. Diagnosis is with a 24 h urine collection and/or dexamethasone suppression testing showing a failure to suppress cortisol. Treatment is by direct treatment of the tumor by removal or chemotherapy. Adrenal inhibitors such as ketoconazole, aminoglutethimide, and metyrapone can give symptomatic relief.

Neurologic. These are most commonly associated with small-cell lung cancer. The primary lesion may not be detectable and symptoms are unrelated to tumor bulk. They are sometimes treated with plasmapheresis and immunosuppression using steroids and azathiaprine but responses are usually poor. They include:

Subacute peripheral neuropathies that are usually sensory and are associated with type 1 antineuronal nuclear antibody (ANNA-1) production, which is also known as "anti-Hu", a valuable serologic marker for the syndrome. ANNA-1 is not detected in normal persons, although it is rarely found in patients known to have SCLC without a neuropathy.

Lambert–Eaton myasthenic syndrome (LEMS) is characterized by proximal muscle weakness, which improves post-exertion. SCLC is the most commonly associated malignancy in patients with LEMS. On electromyography there is characteristic enhancement of a reduced amplitude muscle action potential 10–15 s after maximal voluntary contraction. Treatment, as with any paraneoplastic disorder, is of the primary tumor but specific treatments include anticholinesterases and 3,4-diaminopyridine, which enhances the release of acetylcholine from the nerve terminal.

Paraneoplastic encephalomyelitis is characterized by neuronal loss and perivascular lymphocytic infiltration of the cerebellum, brainstem, spinal cord, and dorsal root ganglia. This can present as cerebellar degeneration, limbic or brainstem encephalitis, myelopathy or sensory neuropathy (see above).

Other Common Paraneoplastic Syndromes

Musculoskeletal and cutaneous in the form of hypertrophic pulmonary osteoarthropathy (HPOA), polymyositis and myopathy, clubbing of the digits, which appears to share the same physiologic/pathologic process as HPOA, and dermatomyositis. There are numerous suggested mechanisms for HPOA and clubbing but the pathophysiology remains unknown. Clubbing most commonly involves the fingernails causing subungual thickening that is characteristic. HPOA is uncommon and usually presents with a symmetric arthropathy of the ankles, wrists and/or knees. There is proliferative periostitis, usually of the distal long bones with typical changes on plain films and on isotope bone scans (see later). Treatment of the bronchogenic carcinoma (usually non-small cell, predominantly squamous cell) may lead to a reversal of these changes. Other treatment includes nonsteroidal anti-inflammatory drugs, sometimes as a continuous infusion in severe cases.

Hematologic disorders includes anemia (20% of patients), venous thromboembolic disease, thrombophlebitis, eosinophilia, leukocytosis (in conjunction with leukemoid or leukoerythroblastic reaction) and thrombocytosis.

Clinical Investigations and Staging

In the majority of patients the initial history and examination will suggest inoperability – bone pains, neurologic symptoms, weight loss and malaise. Examination can reveal ill health, skin and lymph node metastases, a pleural effusion, hepatomegaly and bone tenderness. As many of these patients are elderly and also heavy smokers significant comorbidity (ischemic heart disease, chronic obstructive pulmonary disease, cerebral vascular disease, etc.) may prevent curative therapy.

Clinical Investigations

Blood Tests

These should include full blood count, urea and electrolytes, liver function tests and calcium.

Chest X-Ray

This is the most important investigation. Most tumors will lie at least in part in the lung on the chest X-ray. It can be very difficult to separate the anatomy and discriminate tumor from distal consolidation, and also from proximal mediastinal structures.

However, an intrapulmonary lesion will usually be identifiable. It may be the only abnormality and can be an asymptomatic finding representing a mass that may be

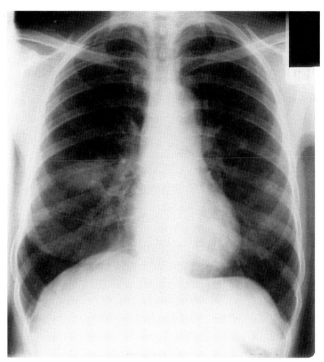

Figure 29.1. Chest X-ray showing an irregular-edged tumor mass in the right midzone.

benign or malignant. Most malignant tumors will be at least 1 cm in size, with irregular margins and spiculated edges (Fig 29.1). Most adenocarcinomas occur as peripheral masses, some squamous cell carcinomas do also and may cavitate (Fig. 29.2). Very few SCLC tumors appear as discrete masses – they are usually central in origin and radiologically form a homogeneous abnormal mass

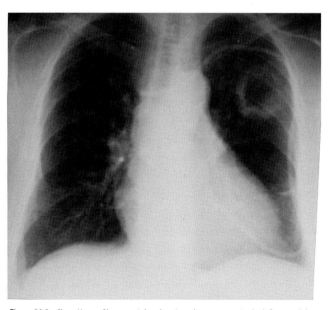

Figure 29.2. Chest X-ray of large peripheral cavitated tumor mass in the left upper lobe.

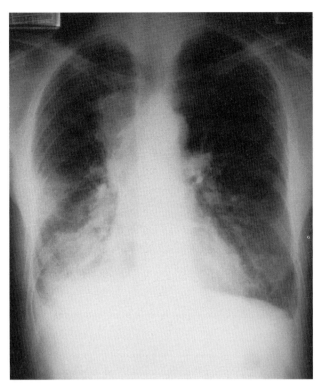

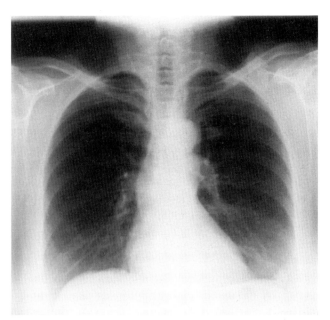

Figure 29.4. Chest X-ray of benign appearing small round lesion approximately 1.5 cm in diameter just to the left of the aortic knuckle.

Figure 29.3. Chest X-ray showing a huge mediastinal adenopathy on the right-hand side with abnormal tumor shadowing in the right lower zone.

contiguous from lung into the mediastinum (Fig. 29.3), often recognizable by the pattern of huge mediastinal adenopathy, often extending bilaterally.

Benign tumors tend to be small, smooth, round and may contain calcium (Fig. 29.4 and 29.5). The availability of previous chest x-rays is invaluable in attempting to decide whether a lesion is old and unchanged, or not

present 1–2 years previously – the latter making malignancy more probable.

As 70% of lung cancers occur centrally (at the carina or lobar bronchi), the primary tumor is often radiologically invisible, – but resultant pulmonary collapse or consolidation should arouse suspicion. Often careful examination of the mediastinum will reveal interruption of an air

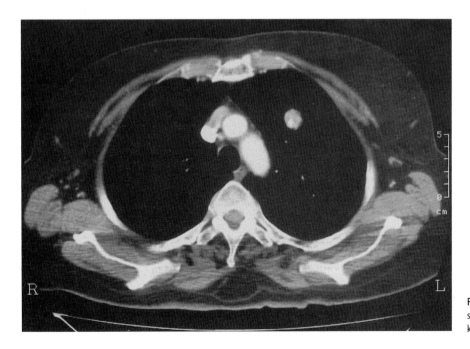

Figure 29.5. The lesion in Fig. 29.4 viewed with CT scanning demonstrating central calcification in keeping with, but not diagnostic of, a benign lesion.

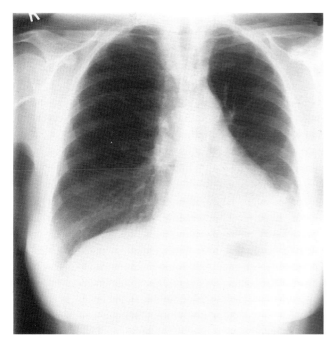

Figure 29.6. Chest X-ray of a collapse of the left lower lobe with loss of volume in the left lung field and increased density of shadowing behind the heart. There is an associated pleural effusion.

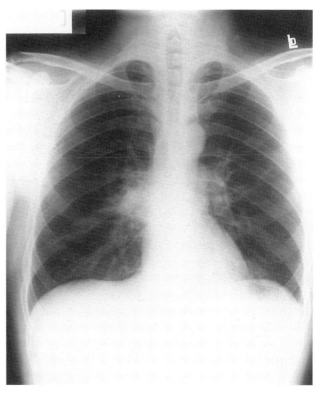

Figure 29.8. A chest X-ray showing an abnormally dense right hilum at which a tumor was detected on further investigation.

bronchogram by tumor, or mediastinal widening due to lymphadenopathy.

Sometimes the only abnormality is lobar collapse (Figs 29.6, 29.7); this can also occur in asthma, allergic bronchopulmonary aspergillosis, benign carcinoid tumors and with foreign bodies.

Examination of the chest X-ray should include careful scrutiny of "hidden areas". Tumors may not be easily visible in front or behind the dome of the diaphragm, hilar involvement may show only subtle increases in density,

and any difference in hilar shadowing should merit further imaging (Fig. 29.8). Often a lateral film will clearly demonstrate a mass near the diaphragm or within, or juxtaposed to, the hilus. Superior sulcus tumors can be missed until large and invading the upper ribs (Fig. 29.9).

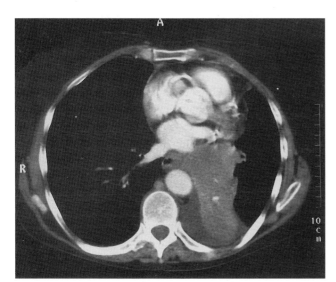

Figure 29.7. CT scan of the lower thorax in the patient seen in Fig. 29.6 showing the collapse of the lower lobe and the associated pleural effusion (darker area).

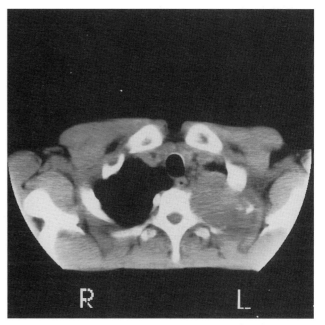

Figure 29.9. A CT scan showing a Pancoast tumor at the left apex with local bone and tissue invasion.

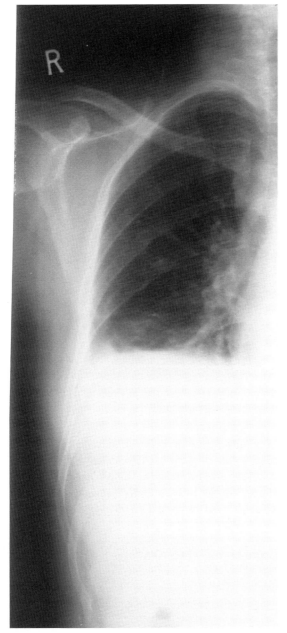

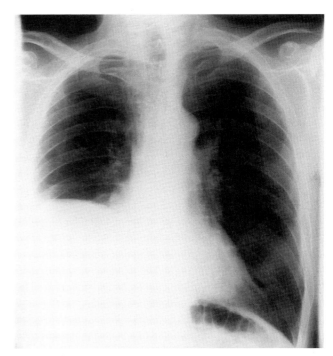

Figure 29.11. Chest X-ray of a large right pleural effusion.

Figure 29.10. Chest X-ray of a bone metastasis seen in the eighth rib posteriorly, just above the level of the effusion.

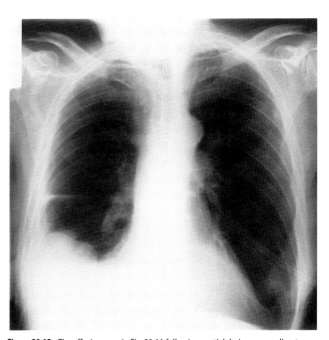

Figure 29.12. The effusion seen in Fig. 29.11 following partial drainage revealing tumor mass inferiorly (note the small iatrogenic pneumothorax).

The rib cage needs an organized search to identify a pathologic fracture, or early metastatic erosion (Fig. 29.10).

Pleural effusions in association with lung cancer are usually large and on aspiration bloody (Figs. 29.11, 29.12). However, small effusions need aspirated samples for cytologic evaluation – in general the detection of an effusion on a plain film on the side of the primary tumor indicates unresectability.

Lymphatic involvement by lung cancer is commonest in adenocarcinoma with peripheral lymph stasis lines, flaring perihilar shadowing, hilar adenopathy and often an effusion (Fig. 29.13).

Sputum Cytology

This has a sensitivity of 40–69% with an abnormal chest X-ray (13–15) and a better detection rate for squamous cell carcinoma than for other histologic cell types. It is an often-neglected test and may prevent a patient undergoing more invasive investigations, particularly in elderly patients and those whose fitness may make more invasive

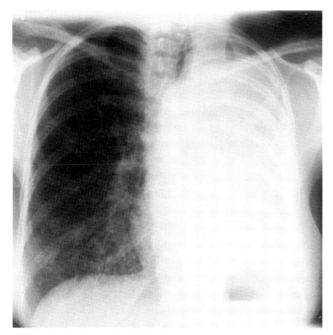

Figure 29.13. A previous pneumonectomy is seen on the left of the X-ray. There is now lymphangitis seen in the right lung field particularly in the mid and lower zones.

tests difficult. Induced sputum samples in elderly populations has shown sensitivity up to 84% (16). Specificity is high with virtually no false-positive results.

Fiber Optic Bronchoscopy (FOB)

This is the usual method of gaining histologic or cytologic diagnosis of lung cancer. It is a safe procedure used routinely as first-line investigation after, or instead of, sputum cytology if the chest X-ray is suspicious. Eighty percent of lung cancers arise in the central airways and therefore are visible. Provided that at least five biopsies are taken, the rate of successful diagnosis following bronchoscopy is 90–95%. The limitation of bronchoscopy is that it allows visualization only to the third subsegmental lobar division. Thus peripheral lesions are not seen and bronchoscopy is unlikely to yield positive histology. Washings and brushings taken from the segment involving the tumor may give positive cytology.

Bronchoscopy is also useful in assessing resectability of a tumor. Ideally the primary tumor should not involve the carina, – although minor involvement may be resectable. Most surgeons prefer at least 1 cm of normal main bronchus between the carina and the tumor to allow fashioning of a secure bronchial stump. Mediastinal lymphadenopathy can be recognized by splaying of the carina – particularly the main carina – by subcarinal nodal metastases, and also loss of its sharp edge. Stiffness of the trachea or main bronchi also suggests extrapulmonary nodal enlargement, and failure of the main airway wall to invaginate with coughing is a certain sign of invasion and unresectability. Vocal cord palsy should have been obvious before bronchoscopy, but, when seen, merely confirms advanced disease.

Percutaneous Transthoracic Lung Biopsy

There are an increasing number of imaging techniques and biopsy needles, allowing much more extensive and safe penetration into the chest and mediastinum. The most important decision is whether a percutaneous biopsy should be performed. There is no role for percutaneous lung biopsy in patients who are operable (17,18). In a fit patient with an abnormal chest X-ray containing a mass with a high suspicion of malignancy, a normal FOB and a CT scan showing no mediastinal abnormality (see later), provided the patient's pulmonary function tests are adequate, surgery is the next step. It is meddlesome to attempt a diagnosis that is extremely unlikely to change the treatment plan. The surgeon at operation is required to perform a frozen section of the mass to confirm cancer. In the small number of cases where the lesion is benign then only a limited resection will be required.

The majority of cases undergoing percutaneous transthoracic biopsy are those who have had a non-diagnostic FOB, and appear to have a tumor that is probably inoperable because of:

- more than one lesion
- pleural disease
- hilar or mediastinal adenopathy
- bone involvement
- liver involvement
- adrenal gland involvement. An adrenal mass or a possible liver metastasis should be the first choice biopsy site to make the diagnosis, or occasionally to exclude a metastasis, e.g., operable lung mass and enlarged adrenal gland. The biopsy may determine resectability.

Most percutaneous biopsies/fine needle aspirations (FNA) in the thorax are performed under ultrasound for pleural masses, or large intrapulmonary tumors (19), or by CT for small lesions, or central masses (Figs. 29.14, 29.15). There does not seem to be any advantage over sequential CT in using spiral scanning in performing percutaneous biopsies in terms of time taken, hit rate or complications, with sequential scanning involving less irradiation (20). The technique is safe, the main complication being pneumothorax. Normally these pneumothoraces are quick to resolve. Only in cases where the patient becomes breathless should an intercostal chest drain be inserted or simple aspiration performed. Rates of pneumothorax vary in different institutions usually depending on experience of the operator. For instance Cox et al. (21) showed pneumothorax to occur in 40.4% of cases with 17.4% requiring chest tube placement, which equated to 7% of all biopsies. Pneumothorax is more than three times less frequent if no aerated lung is traversed and more likely to occur in patients with emphysema or when the lesion is small. The sensitivity of percutaneous transthoracic needle aspiration biopsy is around 75%, with specificity approaching 100%.

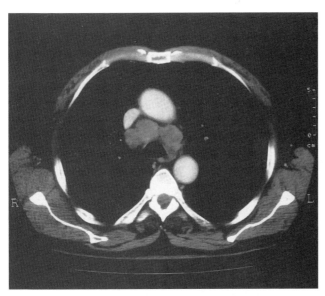

Figure 29.14. A CT scan showing subcarinal adenopathy of 2–2.5 cm diameter accessible for needle biopsy.

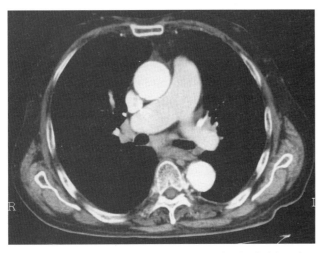

Figure 29.15. A CT scan showing right hilar and mediastinal nodes. The hilar node is accessible for needle biopsy.

Extrathoracic Biopsy Sites

These often yield cytologic diagnostic material – for instance metastatic supraclavicular lymph nodes. Bone metastases may be biopsied directly if palpable or under radiologic guidance with ultrasound or CT scanning for nonpalpable lesions such as rib metastases. Obtaining diagnostic material from these more superficial sites saves the patient more invasive tests. Most of these patients will not require a CT scan, as staging the disease with these distant metastases will not change the management.

Lung Function Tests

Such tests are performed in patients with potentially resectable tumors whose respiratory reserve or general fitness is in question. Patients with a forced expiratory volume in one second (FEV_1) of less than 40% predicted or less than 1200 ml are very high risk surgical candidates and not normally considered for resection. Patients with poor respiratory reserve and borderline spirometry are likely to require further assessment. The best method of predicting the postoperative lung function is with ventilation – perfusion scanning. Patients with marked respiratory limitations may still survive lobectomy as the resected lobe may have little or no respiratory function preoperatively due its tumor diseased state. Another method of predicting postoperative morbidity and mortality is with exercise testing (see below).

Exercise Testing and Ventilation/Perfusion Scanning

These have been shown to give good predictive measurements of postsurgical survival and complications in patients considered to be high risk (22). The use of lung scans allows a predicted postoperative FEV_1 to be estimated on the basis of the amount of lung expected to be resected. Anything less than 33% predicted normal contraindicates surgery as this predicts a high level of mortality and morbidity. Exercise testing gives the best prediction of postoperative morbidity and mortality. It can be performed on a treadmill or exercise cycle and allows the maximum oxygen consumption to be measured. If the maximum oxygen consumption is less than 15 ml kg/min^{-1} then a very high rate of postoperative mortality and morbidity can be expected.

Although exercise testing and ventilation–perfusion scans give valuable predictive information they are relatively infrequently used. This is particularly true of exercise testing, as the investigation is time-consuming and expensive.

Staging of Lung Cancer

If the patient appears fit for resection and the clinical evaluation of the patient, including chest X-ray and FOB suggest resection is possible by lobectomy or pneumonectomy then a CT scan of the thorax and upper abdomen should be performed. This is pointless if the X-ray clearly shows mediastinal lymphadenopathy, bone metastases or a significant pleural effusion. It is a vastly overused investigation and often only confirms what is already known, clogging the queue for scanning of more deserving cases.

CT scanning should be carried out for the following reasons:

To assess the mediastinum for direct invasion of the primary tumor or to identify enlarged mediastinal nodes. A lymph node of greater than 10 mm diameter is considered to be abnormal. The larger the lymph node the more likely it is to be involved by metastatic disease (Fig. 29.16). A node may still be smaller than 10 mm and yet have metastatic deposits within. These may be detected histo-

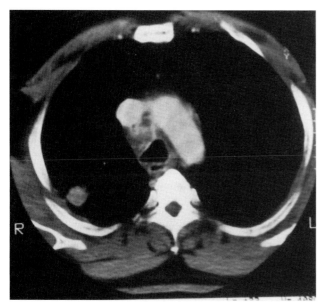

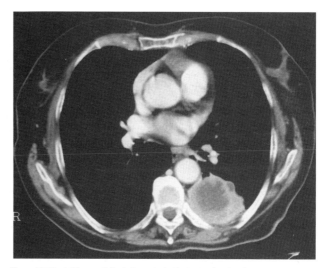

Figure 29.18. A CT scan of the lesion seen in Fig. 29.17 showing the posterior position and no direct invasion of the posterior chest wall.

Figure 29.16. A 1.5 cm tumor mass seen in the periphery of the right lung. The CT scan shows a 1.5–2 cm lymph node in the mediastinum.

logically only by node samples obtained at surgery or preoperatively by mediastinoscopy (see later). Intravenous contrast medium is used to help to differentiate between nodes and blood vessels.

To clarify the proximity of the tumor to the pleura and chest wall, as this information is unlikely to be gained from the chest X-ray when the tumor lies in close proximity to them. Involvement of these structures usually make the tumor inoperable (Figs. 29.17, 29.18)

To identify satellite lesions in the ipsi- or contralateral lung as the presence of an ipsilateral tumor may change a

potential lobectomy into a pneumonectomy. A contralateral nodule makes the tumor inoperable.

To attempt to discriminate the primary tumor from distal consolidation, again to allow correct staging of the tumor (see later) or to identify a tumor that cannot be discerned on the plain film when there is a suspicion of malignancy (Figs. 29.19, 29.20).

To examine the liver and adrenal glands for metastases (Fig. 29.21). Ultrasound examination is a useful adjunct to CT scanning, particularly if the liver lesion appears cystic in nature and may be benign.

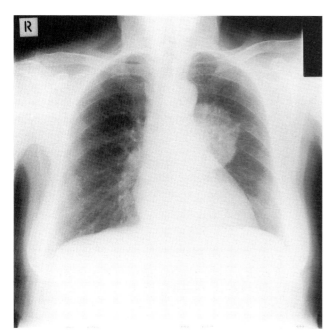

Figure 29.17. Chest X-ray of an obvious large tumor mass seen behind the left hilus.

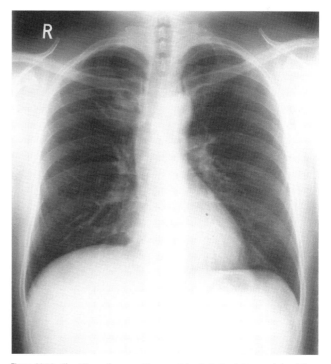

Figure 29.19. Chest X-ray of an area of increased density in the right upper lobe with an air bronchogram in keeping with consolidation.

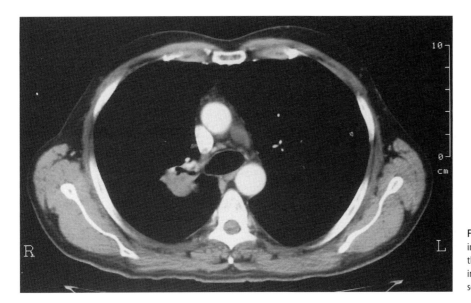

Figure 29.20. The same patient seen in Fig. 29.19 imaged with CT showing proximal tumor surrounding the right upper lobe bronchus. The consolidation is infection distal to this tumor mass (not seen on this section).

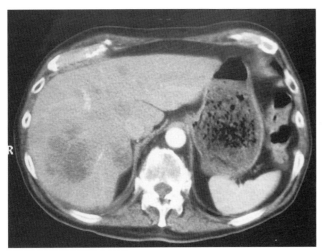

Figure 29.21. Multiple liver metastases seen on a staging CT scan.

CT Brain Scanning

CT brain scanning is performed when there is a suspicion of cerebral metastases, which are relatively common, particularly with small-cell carcinoma. Postmortem series have shown brain metastases in 25–40% of patients with lung cancer. It is found least frequently in squamous cell carcinoma. The detection rate for early cerebral metastases is relatively low with CT scanning and this is not performed as part of routine screening, unless there are suggestive symptoms. In patients with SCLC who survive longer than 2 years there is a 50% chance of developing central nervous system metastases and therefore some advocate prophylactic cranial irradiation at the end of initial radical treatment.

Isotope Bone Scanning

Bone scanning will identify areas likely to represent disease spread but false-positive scans can also occur due to other benign pathology including Paget's disease, and spontaneous and osteoporotic fractures. Because of a high false-negative rate bone scans are not performed as part of routine screening but only in patients with symptoms suggestive of bone metastases or those with malaise and weight loss of greater than 5 kg. Localizing bone metastases is important for therapeutic reasons as well as for staging as they respond well to palliative radiotherapy. It may be necessary to assess the bone scan in conjunction with other modalities to exclude false negatives (Figs. 29.22, 29.23). Bone scans may also be of use in assessing patients suspected of HPOA where there are characteristic changes within the distal long bones (Figs. 29.24, 29.25).

Magnetic Resonance Imaging

There is no overall advantage in staging the mediastinum using magnetic resonance imaging (MRI) instead of CT, as the overall accuracy is the same. CT scanning is more available and cheaper and so MRI is reserved only for cases where closer assessment of particular areas is thought necessary (see below). MRI can make a clear distinction between vessels and soft tissue, and is useful in patients with suspected vascular lesions. MRI is more accurate than CT in assessing nodal disease at the aorta-pulmonary window (23,24) and hilar regions (25,26).

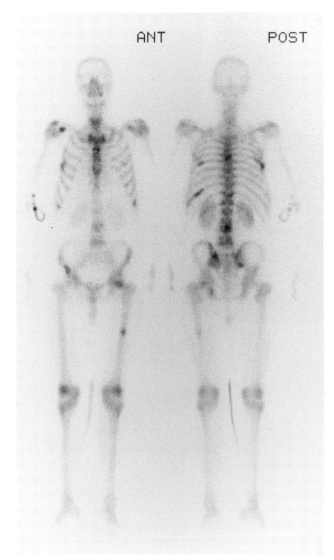

ANT   POST

Figure 29.22. An isotope bone scan showing multiple areas of increased isotope uptake consistent with metastases (left humerus, left sixth rib, right seventh and tenth ribs, the seventh thoracic and the third lumbar vertebrae).

However, there are disadvantages, including image degradation due to motion artefact from adjacent vessels and the fact that calcium deposition is not detected. Also the imaging of other mediastinal sites holds no improvement over CT.

MRI is the optimal modality for assessing invasion of soft tissues of the chest wall. This is due to its superior contrast resolution between muscle, fat and tumor, which is possible using T_1 and T_2 weighted sequences. The multiplanar imaging achievable with MRI, i.e., sagittal and coronal planes, allow better assessment of local invasion of the diaphragm, chest wall or neck (Figs. 29.26, 29.27). Superior sulcus tumors tend to be advanced at the time of diagnosis with bone destruction in approximately one third of cases (27). MRI has the advantage in assessing these tumors, as there is a lack of beam artefact from the shoulders, superior contrast between tissues as described

above and its multiplanar imaging capabilities allow more accurate assessments of local invasion (28–30) and can accurately assess tumor extent including three-dimensional reconstruction to improve surgical and radiation planning (31).

Positron Emission Tomography

The role of positron emission tomography (PET) in lung cancer is still emerging. Currently its main use has been in the assessment of solitary pulmonary nodules and in mediastinal staging using fluorodeoxyglucose positron emission tomography (FDG PET) (Fig. 29.28). The ability of FDG PET scanning to localize malignancy in tumors or nodes can guide further management when there is doubt about the presence of malignancy after conventional imaging has been performed. A malignant lesion usually becomes "hot" whereas a benign lesion remains "cold" (32). This modality is likely to become of increasing use as experience with PET scanning increases and availability of the technique becomes more widespread. Its use in identifying likely malignant tumors in the assessment of solitary lesions, identifying malignant nodal disease within the mediastinum, or identifying occult lesions in patients presenting with paraneoplastic syndromes is potentially important.

Recent studies have highlighted the ability of PET to identify malignant tissue in mediastinal lymph nodes of normal size. Compared with CT, which has a negative predictive value of 80% for mediastinal lymph node involvement, that of PET is as high as 97%. It probably will become a routine final investigation prior to surgery if a staging CT of the thorax and upper abdomen shows no signs of tumor dissemination. If the PET scan is equally reassuring then the patient could proceed to thoracotomy, but if a positive tissue signal is obtained then mediastinoscopy or appropriate biopsy would have to be done first.

Mediastinoscopy

Mediastinoscopy is used to sample mediastinal lymph nodes to stage bronchogenic carcinoma. CT scanning identifies potentially involved lymph nodes as being greater than 10 mm in transverse diameter, but only histologic information can confirm node involvement. Mediastinoscopy is indicated when CT scanning demonstrates ipsilateral mediastinal nodal enlargement as the only contraindication to resection. Its role in staging when the CT scan is negative is more controversial. In a comparison of mediastinal staging and CT staging using a 1 cm lymph node diameter as a cut-off for being positive in CT

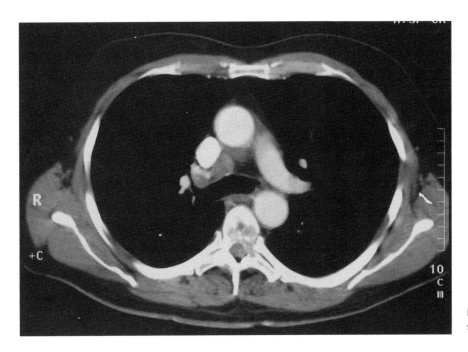

Figure 29.23. A CT scan showing a vertebral metastasis and mediastinal adenopathy.

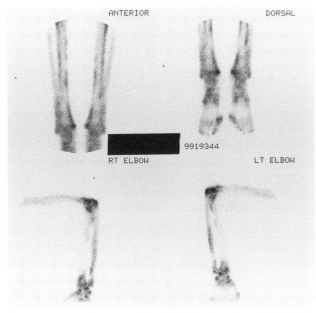

Figure 29.24. Increased isotope uptake in the distal long bones in a patient with HPOA. There is typical linear uptake along the medial tibial borders.

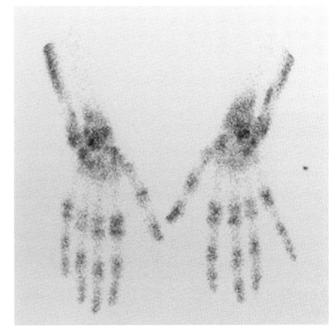

Figure 29.25. An isotope bone scan of the wrists and hands of the same patient seen in Fig. 29.24, showing increased uptake in the ulnar bones and wrists.

scanning, the sensitivity and specificity for CT were 63% and 57% and for mediastinoscopy 89% and 100% (33) i.e., relying on CT alone to stage ipsilateral mediastinal involvement will not give accurate staging of disease. It will understage in about 20% of patients with normal-size nodes. PET scanning as described above may help to resolve this issue. Correct pathologic disease staging with mediastinoscopy may offer the patient the best choice for

surgical treatment and a higher chance of cure. It should also prevent major surgery in those where it will not enhance their survival, and where node biopsy is positive.

The procedure is safe: the mediastinoscope is introduced 1 cm above the sternal notch and splits the strap muscles in the midline. It is advanced along the front of the trachea and a systematic search for lymph nodes and tumor tissue made at the different lymph node sites. Only

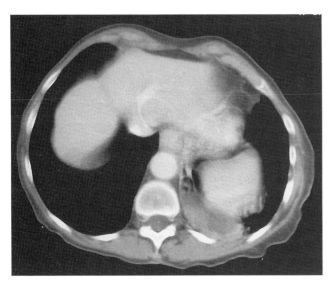

Figure 29.26. A CT scan of a large posterior tumor on the left with an area of possible chest wall invasion. The scan suggests that there is no invasion but is not conclusive.

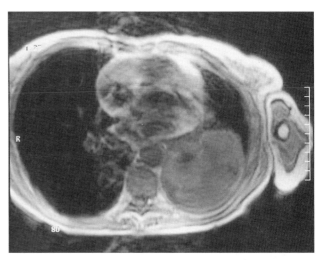

Figure 29.27. An MR scan of the same patient seen in Fig. 29.26 clearly showing the separation of tissue planes, indicating that there is no direct invasion of tumor.

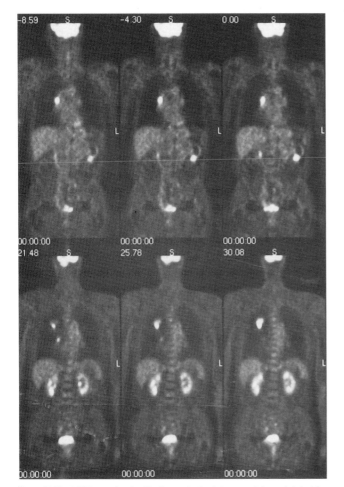

Figure 29.28. A PET scan showing "hot" areas in the right upper lobe and right hilus consistent with malignancy.

the right side is accessible to sampling – left-sided nodes in the subaortic fossa region can be approached via a separate incision in the second left anterior intercostal space, but should only be palpated; biopsy is hazardous due to the proximity of the major blood vessels.

Staging Classification

The International System for Staging Lung Cancer was most recently revised in 1997 and is described below. Staging is of the utmost importance in assessing a patient's suitability for surgical resection, but is also of importance in being universally standardized to allow comparison outcomes between different institutions and between different countries.

Staging is divided into an assessment of the primary tumor (T), regional lymph nodes (N) and distant metastasis (M) giving the TNM staging. This is summarized below (taken from ref. (34):

Primary tumor (T)

TX   Primary tumor cannot be assessed, or tumor proven, by the presence of malignant cells in sputum or bronchial washings but not visualized by imaging or bronchoscopy.

T0   No evidence of primary tumor.

T1   Tumor <3 cm in greatest dimension, surrounded by lung or visceral pleura, without bronchoscopic evidence of invasion more proximal than the lobar bronchus* (i.e. not in the main bronchus).

T2 Tumor with any of the following features of size or extent:

>3 cm in greatest dimension

Involves main bronchus, <2 cm distal to the carina

Invades the visceral pleura

Associated with atelectasis or obstructive pneumonitis that extends to the hilar region but does not involve the entire lung.

T3 Tumor of any size that directly invades any of the following: chest wall (including superior sulcus tumors), diaphragm, mediastinal pleura, parietal pericardium; or tumor in the main bronchus <2 cm distal to the carina, but without involvement of the carina; or associated atelectasis or pneumonitis of the entire lung.

T4 Tumor of any size that invades any of the following: mediastinum, heart, great vessels, trachea, esophagus, vertebral body, carina; or tumor with a malignant pleural or pericardial effusion[†], or with satellite tumor nodule(s) within the ipsilateral primary tumor lobe of the lung.

Regional lymph nodes (N)

NX Regional lymph nodes cannot be assessed

N0 No regional lymph node metastasis

N1 Metastasis to ipsilateral peribronchial and/or ipsilateral hilar lymph nodes, and intrapulmonary nodes involved by direct extension of the primary tumor

N2 Metastasis to ipsilateral mediastinal and/or subcarinal lymph node(s)

N3 Metastasis to contralateral mediastinal, contralateral hilar, ipsilateral or contralateral scalene, or supraclavar node(s)

Distant metastasis (M)

MX Presence of distant metastasis cannot be assessed

M0 No distant metastasis

M1 Distant metastasis present[‡]

Stage Grouping – TNM Subsets

Stage 0 (TisN0M0)

Stage IA (T1N0M0)

Stage IB (T2N0M0)

Stage IIA (T1N1M0)

Stage IIB (T2N1M0, T3N0M0)

Stage IIIA (T3N1M0), (T(1–3)N2M0)

Stage IIIB (T4, Any N, M0) (Any T, N3M0)

Stage IV (Any T, any N, M1)

Any stage from IA to IIIA may be considered for resection, although patients with stage IIIA disease are more carefully assessed and survival rates are worse with more advanced stages.

Treatment

Curative treatment is by surgical excision by lobectomy or pneumonectomy. As most lung cancers present at an advanced stage the number of potentially resectable cases is low – 15–25%. Surgery is accompanied by lymph node sampling from three or four draining lymph node sites, without which staging is incomplete.

Stage IA disease has a 5 year survival of 67%, whereas the 5 year survival for stage IIIA disease is approximately 25%. The 5 year cumulative survival for patients with stage IIIA, i.e., all patients at stage IIIA with or without surgery is approximately 10%. A summary of survival for the different stage groupings is in Fig. 29.29. Survival of patients with stage IIIB or stage IV disease is only 1–3% at 5 years.

SCLC can be staged using the TNM staging system but provides little prognostic information, and surgery is generally not possible due to the high incidence of metastatic disease. Surgical excision of SCLC occasionally happens if an isolated pulmonary nodule is excised and discovered to be a SCLC. The tumor is usually staged as "limited" or "extensive", with the limited stage being confined to one hemithorax and the ipsilateral supraclavicular lymph nodes. Approximately one third

---

[*] The uncommon superficial tumor of any size with its invasive component limited to the bronchial wall, which may extend proximal to the main bronchus, is also classified T1.

[†] Most pleural effusions associated with lung cancer are due to tumor. However, there are a few patients in whom multiple cytopathologic examination of the pleural fluid shows no tumor. In these cases, the fluid is nonbloody and is not an exudate. When these elements and clinical judgment dictate that the effusion is not related to the tumor, the effusion should be excluded as a staging element and the patient's disease should be staged T1, T2, or T3. Pericardial effusion is classified by the same rules.

[‡] Separate metastatic tumor nodule(s) in the ipsilateral nonprimary tumor lobe(s) of the lung also are classified M1.

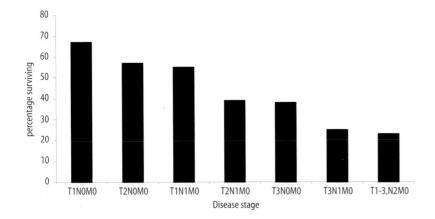

Figure 29.29. The 5 year survival of patients following surgery dependent upon surgical – pathologic stage (data taken from ref. (34)).

of patients will have limited stage disease at diagnosis. Treatment is with combination cytotoxic chemotherapy, as the tumor is highly responsive, with complete clinical remission obtained in 50% of limited disease and 25% of extensive disease. Unfortunately, relapse is common and further chemotherapy ineffective. The median survival is 15–18 months with 2 year survival rates of 20–30% for limited disease and 6–12 months median survival for extensive disease, with just 2% alive at 2 years.

Radiotherapy

Radiotherapy is used as both a palliative treatment and also potentially curative therapy. Patients with good performance status who have locoregionally advanced disease that is inoperable can be considered for radical radiotherapy. As conventional radiotherapy, it is given as 2 gray (Gy) per day for 30 days or if by continuous hyperfractionated accelerated radiotherapy (CHART), as 1.2 Gy 8 hourly over 12 continuous days. This latter protocol obtains better survival outcomes (35) particularly for squamous cell tumors compared with conventional radiotherapy. Also local control appears far better with CHART. Death is mostly due to distal metastases.

A recent meta-analysis of postoperative radiotherapy (PORT) showed no survival benefit for this modality. There appeared to be survival disadvantages for adjuvant radiotherapy in stage I and II disease, although the possible role of radiotherapy following resection of stage IIIA disease was less clear (36).

Palliative hypofractionated radiotherapy, for example one or two fractions given a week apart, is used for hemoptysis, bone pain, SVCO and cough with good relief.

In SCLC, radiotherapy to the primary site and mediastinum is recommended in those who respond very well to chemotherapy. It can also be given electively as prophylactic whole-brain irradiation to good responders at the end of chemotherapy to prevent brain relapse, although it has little effect on overall survival. Neurotoxicity can be a problem, with ataxia, poor concentration, memory problems, and occasional dementia.

Palliative Treatments

Good analgesia is an important part of palliation. Whilst radiotherapy and, to a lesser extent, chemotherapy can be very useful, opiates and nonsteroidal anti-inflammatory agents are an essential part of symptom control aiming to maintain quality of life. There is now a large range of fast and slower release morphine preparations that will control pain in almost every case. Attention to constipation, nausea and anorexia, all common side-effects of opiates is equally important. Corticosteroids (prednisolone 20 mg day^{-1} or dexamethasone 2–4 mg twice per day) are helpful and effective for 2–3 weeks, often in conjunction with radiotherapy. In patients with cerebral metastases the response to dexamethasone often predicts whether the patient is likely to respond to radiotherapy.

Endobronchial Treatments

These are used as palliation and can produce dramatic short-term improvements particularly in upper airway narrowing by tumor. The main indication is breathlessness due to a proximal obstructing lesion. It can also be used for hemoptysis and for local recurrence in a central airway, particularly when the patient has already received maximum doses of external beam radiotherapy. Approaches include laser treatment to tumors within an airway – particularly limited localized polypoid tumors, brachytherapy for extensive airway involvement or for hemoptysis, and stenting for external compression of central airways.

Treatment of lung cancer has become increasingly multidisciplinary and this includes the community nurses and doctors. Good communication between community and hospital staff is essential as most patients are dying of their disease and will wish to be cared for in or close to their home.

References

1. Pisani P, Parkin DM, Bray F, et al. (1999) Estimates of the worldwide mortality from 25 cancers in 1990. Int J Cancer 83:18–29.
2. Hill C (1998) Trends in tobacco smoking and consequences on health in France. Prev Med 27:514–519.
3. Devesa SS, Grauman DJ, Blot WJ, et al. (1999) Cancer surveillance series: Changing geographic patterns of lung cancer mortality in the United States, 1950 through 1994. J Natl Cancer Inst 91:1040–1050.
4. Garfinkel L, Mushinski M (1999) U.S. cancer incidence, mortality and survival: 1973–1996. Stat Bull Metrop Insur Co 80:23–32.
5. Arai T, Kuroishi T, Saito Y, et al. (1994) tumor doubling time and prognosis in lung cancer patients: Evaluation from chest films and clinical follow-up study. Japanese Lung Cancer Screening Research Group. Jpn J Clin Oncol 24:199–204.
6. Theros EG (1977) Caldwell Lecture: Varying manifestations of peripheral pulmonary neoplasms: A radiologic–pathologic correlative study. AJR 128:893–914.
7. Strauss MJ (1974) The growth characteristics of lung cancer and its application to treatment design. Semin Oncol 1:167–174.
8. Garland LH (1966) The rate of growth and natural duration of primary bronchial cancer. Am J Radiol 96:604–611.
9. Strauss GM, Dominioni L (1999) Lung cancer screening and the surgical oncologist: the controversy. Surg Oncol Clin North Am 8:372–387.
10. Henschke CI, McCauley DI, Yankelevitz DF, et al. (1999) Early Lung Cancer Action Project: Overall design and findings from baseline screening. Lancet 354:99–105.
11. Patel AM, Davila DG, Peters SG (1993) Paraneoplastic syndromes associated with lung cancer. Mayo Clin Proc 68:278–287.
12. Schiller JH, Jones JC (1993) Paraneoplastic syndromes associated with lung cancer. Curr Opin Oncol 5:335–342.
13. Kern WH (1988)The diagnostic accuracy of sputum and urine cytology. Acta Cytol 32:651–654.
14. MacDouggall B, Weinerman B (1992) The value of sputum cytology. J Gen Intern Med 7:11–13.
15. Sing A, Freudenberg N, Kortsik C, et al. (1997) Comparison of sensitivity of sputum and brush cytology in the diagnosis of lung carcinomas. Acta Cytol 41:399–408.
16. Khajotia RR, Mohn A, Pokieser L, et al. (1991) Induced sputum and cytological diagnosis of lung cancer. Lancet 338:976–977.
17. Larscheid RC, Thorpe PE, Scott WJ (1998) Percutaneous transthoracic needle aspiration biopsy: A comprehensive review of its current role in the diagnosis and treatment of lung tumors. Chest 114:704–709.
18. Odell MJ, Reid KR (1999) Does percutaneous fine-needle aspiration biopsy aid in the diagnosis and surgical management of lung masses? Can J Surg 42:297–301.
19. Sheth S, Hamper UM, Stanley DB, et al. (1999) US guidance for thoracic biopsy: A valuable alternative to CT. Radiology 210:721–726.
20. Ghaye B, Dondelinger RF, Dewe W (1999) Percutaneous CT-guided lung biopsy: Sequential versus spiral scanning. A randomized prospective study. Eur Radiol 9:1317–1320.
21. Cox JE, Chiles C, McManus CM, et al. (1999) Transthoracic needle aspiration biopsy: variables that affect risk of pneumothorax. Radiology 212:165–168.
22. Wyser C, Stulz P, Soler M, et al (1999) Prospective evaluation of an algorithm for the functional assessment of lung resection candidates. Am J Respir Crit Care Med 159:1450–1456.
23. Batra P, Brown K Steckel RJ, et al. (1988) MR imaging of the thorax: A comparison of axial, coronal and saggital imaging planes. J Comput Assist Tomogr 12:75–78.
24. Webb WR, Jensen BG, Gamsu G, et al. (1985) Sagittal MR imaging of the chest: Normal and abnormal. J Comput Assist Tomogr 9:471–479.
25. Webb WR, Gatsonis C, Zerhouni EA, et al. (1991) CT and MR imaging in staging non-small cell bronchogenic carcinoma: Report of the radiologic diagnostic oncology group. Radiology 178: 705–713.
26. Glazer GM, Gross BH, Aisen AM, et al. (1985) Imaging of the pulmonary hilum: A prospective comparative study in patients with lung cancer. Am J Radiol 145:245–248.
27. O'Connell RS, McLoud TC, Wilkin EW (1983) Superior sulcus tumor: Radiographic diagnosis and work up. Am J Radiol 140:25–30.
28. Castagno AA, Shuman WP (1987) MR imaging in clinically suspected brachial plexus tumor. Am J Radiol 149:1219–1222.
29. Salvatierra A, Baamonde C, Llamas JM, et al. (1990) Extrathoracic staging of bronchogenic carcinoma. Chest 97:1052–1058.
30. Heelan RT, Demas BE, Caravelli J, et al. (1989) Superior sulcus tumors. CT MR Imaging Radiol 170:637–641.
31. Bittner RC, Felix R (1998) Magnetic resonance (MR) imaging of the chest: State-of-the-art. Eur Respir J 11:1392–1404.
32. Sarinas PS, Chitkara RK, Buadu EO, et al. (1999) Usefulness of positron emission tomography imaging in the management of lung cancer. Curr Opin Pulm Med 5:201–207.
33. Gdeedo A, Van Schil P, Corthouts B, et al. (1997) Prospective evaluation of computed tomography and mediastinoscopy in mediastinal lymph node staging. Eur Respir J 10:1547–1551.
34. Mountain CF (1997) Revision in the International System for Staging Lung Cancer. Chest 111:1710–1717.
35. Saunders M, Dische S, Barrett A, et al. on behalf of the CHART steering committee (1997) Continuous hyperfractionated accelerated radiotherapy (CHART) versus conventional radiotherapy in non small cell lung cancer: A randomised multicentre trial. Lancet 350:161–165.
36. PORT Meta-analysis Trialists Group (1998) Postoperative radiotherapy on non-small cell lung cancer: Systematic review and meta-analysis of individual patient data from nine randomised controlled trials. Lancet 352:257–263.

30 Rare Tumors of the Lung

F. Laurent, V. Latrabe, and M. Montaudon

Introduction

Rare tumors of the lung encompass a large variety of benign and malignant lesions that can be understood as those that do not usually came under the heading bronchogenic carcinoma, i.e., small cell, large cell, squamous cell, and adenocarcinoma. Some of these conditions are very rare but other are simply uncommon. From a clinical and therapeutic point of view, we consider in this chapter the neoplastic conditions of the lung that are not usually described as nonsmall–cell or small-cell bronchogenic carcinomas. We use classification according to the type of cells from which they are derived So, neuroendocrine tumors, tumors of the tracheobronchial glands, epithelial tumors, lymphoproliferative disorders, mesenchymal neoplasms, tumors of uncertain histogenesis and lesions of uncertain neoplastic origin will be considered sequentially.

Whatever the histologic type the basis, the site of the lesion is for the clinical manifestations and the imaging features. Lesions may occur in the proximal bronchi or within the lung parenchyma. The latter are frequently asymptomatic and visible as "coin lesions" on imaging studies, whereas the former are often revealed by symptoms of bronchial obstruction and their appearances on imaging studies may be modified by the consequences of this obstruction.

Neuroendocrine Tumors: Bronchial Carcinoids

Several types of lung neoplasm show ultrastructural and immunohistochemical features similar to these of neuroendocrine cells. The tumors that can be included in this group are varied and their terminology is somewhat confusing. Most authors consider that are typical and atypical carcinoid types. But some also consider that small-cell carcinoma represents the most undifferentiated end of a spectrum of neuroendocrine tumors and should be included in that group, along with some large-cell carcinomas. In this chapter, we describe only bronchial carcinoids and pulmonary tumorlets.

Bronchial Carcinoids

The bronchi are the second most common location of carcinoids. The tumors show a spectrum of clinical behavior and microscopic appearance ranging from a slow-growing locally invasive tumor to a metastasizing tumor with a more or less fast growth rate. They are thought to derive from the neuroendocrine cells of the bronchial and bronchiolar epithelium. Neuroendocrine function has been demonstrated by means of ultrastructural studies and immunohistochemical markers. Bronchial carcinoids comprise 1–2% of all lung tumors and display a spectrum of clinical behavior and histologic differentiation in neuroendocrine tumors, ranging from the low grade typical carcinoids to the intermediate-grade atypical carcinoid (1–2).

Patients with bronchial carcinoid are younger and the population has a significantly lower male-to-female ratio than does the group with common primary pulmonary neoplasms. There is no documented association with cigarette smoking or exposure to other carcinogens. From 20% to 51% of patients are asymptomatic. Others present with recurrent pulmonary infection, cough, hemoptysis, wheezing, asthma of recent onset, chest pain or constitutional symptoms. Symptoms are related to the frequent central location of tumors. Two percent of patients present because of symptoms related to Cushing syndrome. In this case, the causative bronchial carcinoid is frequently occult on chest film or conventional computed tomography (CT) and may require repeated and advanced imaging for detection. The carcinoid syndrome is rarely seen in association with bronchial carcinoid, and is encountered only in patients metastatic to the liver (1–4).

Pathologically, a typical carcinoid is composed of uniform cells with an organoid growth pattern in a rich fibrovascular stroma. The cells are polygonal with an eosinophilic granular cytoplasm and round central nuclei. Necrosis is absent and mitoses fewer than two per 2 mm^2. They may show calcifications, ossification or amyloid deposition. Atypical carcinoid has the same morphologic features of typical carcinoid but displays increased mitotic activity (2–10 mitoses mm^{-2}) and areas of coagulative tumor necrosis (3). Ultrastructural analysis with electron microscopy demonstrates dense core granules. Immuno-histochemical markers such as chronogranin show diffuse staining, indicating their neuroendocrine nature. Typical and atypical carcinoids are indistinguishable on the basis of gross pathologic features. The majority of tumors are central and related to an airway, although 16–40% occur in the lung periphery. Macroscopically they are well-circum-scribed nodules or masses. Central lesions have a red-brown endoluminal polypoid component with a focal or broad attachment to the bronchial wall. The bronchial mucosa is often intact. Although some carcinoids grow exclusively within the bronchial lumen, invasion through the bronchial wall and its cartilaginous ring is the rule. Most of them exhibit a dumbbell shape and have extra-bronchial components of variable size. Some so-called "iceberg lesions" have a very small endoluminal compo-nent, which abuts the bronchial lumen whereas others completely occlude the bronchi. Carcinoids may also manifest as peripheral subpleural nodules without macro-scopic evidence of relationship with airways. They are well circumscribed but not encapsulated. Tumors rarely infiltrate into the adjacent parenchyma. Both typical and atypical carcinoids may metastasize to regional lymph nodes but atypical tumors do so more frequently. Metastases occur in 15% of bronchial carcinoids and affect the liver, bone, adrenal, and brain (5).

Typical and atypical carcinoid share similar radiologic features. The most frequent manifestation is a hilar or peripheral mass, which may represent an isolated finding or may be associated with distal parenchymal disease. The mass is characteristically well defined, rounded or ovoid, and typically ranges in size from 2 to 5 cm. Calcification may occur but the lesion never cavitates. The extraluminal components, the consequences of the bronchial obstruc-tion i.e., atelectasis, consolidation or mucoid impaction, are often the dominant or the sole feature. Tumors that are completely endobronchial may be visible within large central airways (5). Peripheral bronchial carcinoids lo-cated distal to the segmental bronchi, manifest as solitary sharply marginated nodules usually of less than 3 cm or masses surrounded by aerated lung parenchyma.

At CT, carcinoids are usually not distinguishable from carcinoma unless the lesion is demonstrably ossified. The incidence of calcification appears to be high, since about 30% of lesions exhibit punctuate or diffuse calcifications on CT (Fig. 30.1). Sometimes, it takes the recognizable form of ossification and occupies the whole of the tumor mass. Because they have a rich vascular stroma, carcinoids may demonstrate marked and homogeneous enhance-ment (Fig. 30.2). CT provides anatomic localization of both intraluminal and extraluminal components of the tumor in the major bronchi. Most bronchial carcinoid exhibit a small intraluminal component, with the bulk of the tumor extending into the adjacent lung parenchyma. Central lesions may partially or completely obstruct the bronchial lumen (Fig. 30.2). Contrast-enhanced CT allows visualization of the central enhancing carcinoid and allows differentiation from adjacent atelectatic or consoli-dated lung. CT may also reveal mucoid impactions (Fig. 30.3) or a distal pulmonary overinflation due to a ball-valve obstruction. Mucus-impacted bronchi are often of low attenuation, below 20 Housfield units (HU) (5–9). There is no difference between the appearance of typical and atypical carcinoids on imaging studies. Enlargement of hilar or mediastinal nodes may be related to hyperpla-sia resulting from associated recurrent or chronic distal infarction or to nodal metastases. Lymph nodes meta-stases are more frequently encountered in lesions with typical histologic characteristic (10).

A few carcinoids manifest as a focal masses or nodules located entirely within the lumen of bronchus. These patients are good candidates for conservative resection and CT allows visualization of these exclusively endo-bronchial lesions. Peripheral carcinoids manifest as well-defined, lobulated nodules or masses but a bronchial relationship may sometimes be demonstrated (11). In patients with Cushing syndrome, thin sections are useful for identifying these small lesions, which range in size from 0.4 to 2 cm. It has been recommended that negative cases undergo follow-up chest CT every 6 months to exclude an occult or recurrent carcinoid as the underlying cause (12,13).

Magnetic resonance imaging (MRI) of bronchial carci-noids has demonstrated lesions of high signal intensity on T$_2$-weighted images. Ultrafast contrast-enhanced studies have shown pronounced signal enhancement during the systemic phase of circulation (14). Nevertheless, no feature has been demonstrated to be specific for differentiating carcinoids from other lung tumors.

Octreotide scintigraphy has been used in the early and noninvasive recognition of carcinoids undetected with other imaging modalities. Lesions as small as 0.6 cm have been detected with somatostatin receptor scintigraphy Radionucleide imaging complements advanced cross-sectional imaging, allows identification of patients who may respond to octreotide therapy, and reveals previously unsuspected tumor sites or recurrent neoplasm (15).

Most bronchial carcinoids are central lesions within reach of bronchoscopy. They have a characteristic endo-scopic appearance as a smooth lobulated reddish endo-

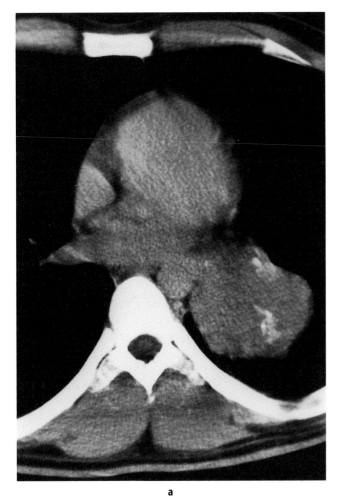

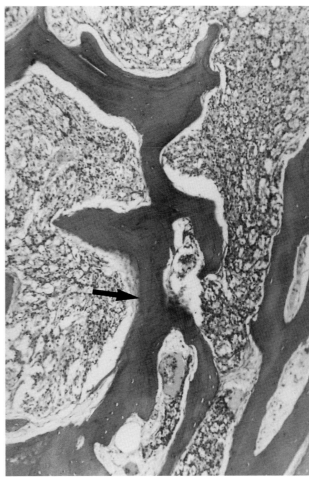

a   b

Figure 30.1. Typical carcinoid. **a** Unenhanced CT. Large hilar mas with calcifications. **b** Pathologic examination reveals osseous deposition (*arrow*) within the tumor.

bronchial lesion that may bleed at the time of visualization. Biopsies of these lesions are routinely performed but there are published reports of 25% of moderate-to-severe hemorrhage and a few emergent pulmonary resections.

Fine-needle aspiration is considered reliable in the diagnosis of typical carcinoid but there is a potential pitfall in the pathologic diagnosis between atypical carcinoid and carcinoma. The complete effective treatment for patients with bronchial carcinoid is complete surgical excision of the primary tumor mass. A few patients are candidates for conservative resection with bronchoplastic procedures. In the case of atypical carcinoid, an aggressive surgical approach is recommended. Patients with typical bronchial carcinoid have an excellent prognosis; those with atypical carcinoids have a less favorable one, with 5 and 10-year survivals of 69% and 24–52% respectively. Tumor size, histologic subtypes, nodal involvement at initial diagnosis are the factors that most influence recurrence and outcome (16,17).

Tumorlet

The term pulmonary tumorlet refers to a minute or nodular proliferation of neuroendocrine cells of the airways that extent beyond the epithelium into the adjacent wall or lung parenchyma. This condition has been observed in otherwise normal lung but most commonly in various conditions including bronchiectasies and carcinoid tumor itself. The fundamental nature of this neuroendocrine cell proliferation is controversial. It may represent an hyperplastic response to nonspecific airway injury. Because of their small size, tumorlets are usually not apparent on the radiograph or CT scan although some cases have been reported to be sufficiently large to be visible as minute nodules. The radiographic appearance depends on location, size and presence or absence of obstructive pneumonitis (18). On rare occasions, extensive disease may result in significant obliterative bronchiolitis (19).

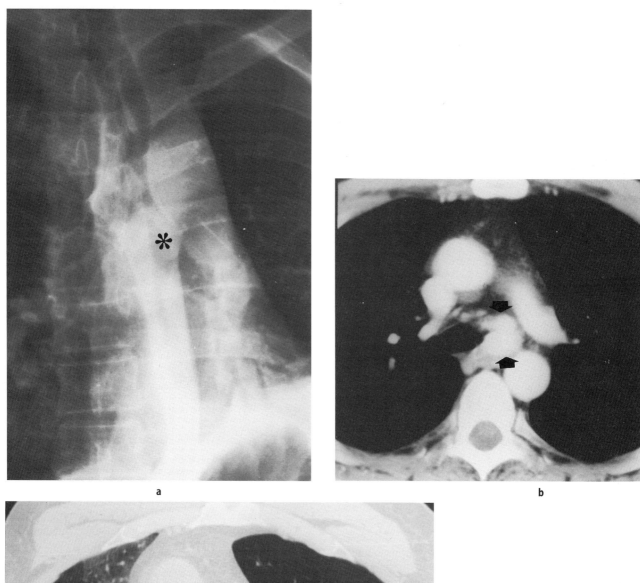

a

b

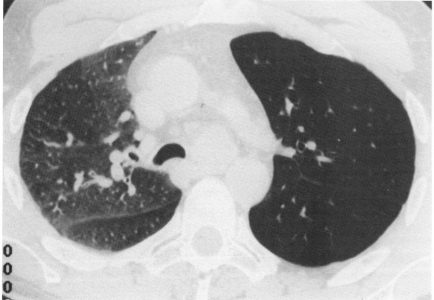

c

Figure 30.2. Typical carcinoid. **a** Chest X-ray: oval-shaped opacity projecting on the main left bronchus (*star*). **b** Enhanced CT: enhancing mass (*arrow*) obstructing the main left bronchus. **c** Expiratory CT showing air-trapping of the left lung.

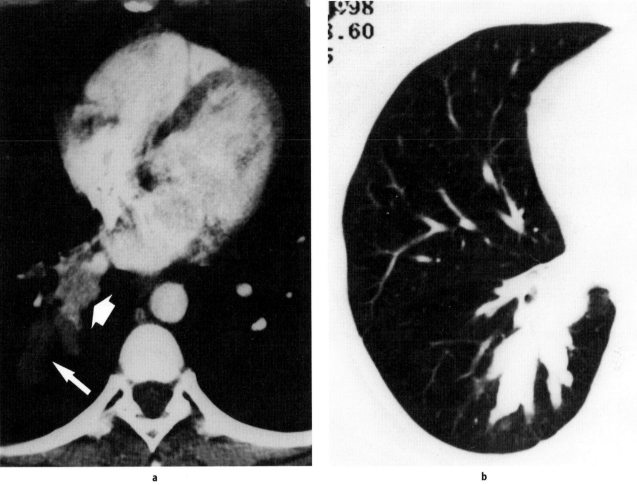

Figure 30.3. Typical carcinoid. **a** Enhanced CT showing 2 cm enhancing mass (*arrow*) developed in the posterobasal bronchus clearly separated from the dilatated mucus-filled bronchi (*long arrow*) seen well on lung window setting (**b**).

Neoplasms of the Tracheo Bronchial Glands

These neoplasms constitute a specific group characterized by their histologic pattern, their characteristic growth into the lumen of central airways, the lack of association with cigarette smoking, and their much better prognosis than that of neoplasms of surface airway epithelium. They can also be designated by the nonhistogenic term salivary-like tumor (20). These tumors are quite uncommon, accounting for no more than 0.1–0.2% of all tracheobronchial tumors, the majority being either adenoid cystic or mucoepidermoid carcinomas. The diagnosis should be considered in anyone with a polypoid intraluminal mass in the trachea or major bronchi. The symptoms are those of an airway obstruction, often simulating asthma when the lesion is situated in the thoracic portion of the trachea.

Conversely symptoms are inspiratory when it rises in the cervical portion of the trachea (21).

Pathologically, adenoid cystic carcinoma grows into the airway lumen, forming a polypoid tumor with submucosal extension, sometimes to a considerable distance from the main lesion. The histologic appearance is identical to that of salivary gland tumors (22–24). Mucoepidermoid carcinoma is the most common form after adenoid cystic carcinoma (25). Some forms have histologic similarities with adenosquamous carcinomas. Most are situated in the main bronchi but they may uncommonly involve the lung periphery or the trachea. Whatever the grade of the lesion, they are histologically composed of an association of mucus-secreting and epidermoid cells.

The lesions are often overlooked on chest radiograph. The radiographic features consist of an endotracheal or endobronchial lobulated mass that encroaches on the airway lumen to a variable degree. CT is superior to chest

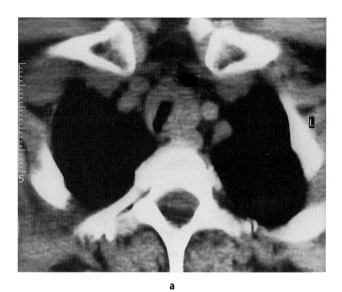

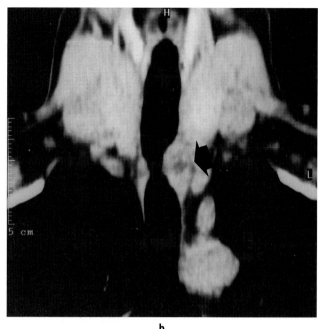

a

b

Figure 30.4. Adenoid cystic carcinoma. **a** Unenhanced CT: circumferential mass (*arrow*) of the thoracic trachea. **b** Oblique coronal reconstruction showing the craniocaudal extent (*arrow*) of the tumor.

radiograph in detecting the presence of the tumor and is particularly helpful in assessing the degree of extra-luminal and mediastinal invasion (Fig. 30.4) (21,26,27).

Epithelial Tumors

Papillomas

These tumors and are lobulated and composed of epithe-lium-lined fibrovascular papillae that arise from the epithelial surface. Solitary is less common than the multi-ple form. They are located in lobar or segmental bronchi, where they appear grossly as filiform or finely corrugated tumors 0.5–1.5 cm in diameter. Many are not detected on chest radiograph and are seen on CT as a polypoid mass in the airway. Multiple papillomas occur most commonly in the larynx of children of between 18 months and 3 years of age, but the disease may be present in adults. In the majority of patients, papillomas remain localized. Infrequently, they arise in the respiratory tract distal to the larynx. Tracheal and bronchial papillomas can be seen as small nodules projecting into the lumen of the airways. On CT, numerous papillomas may be seen as diffuse nodular thickening of the trachea. The papillomas may lead to bronchial obstruction resulting in atelectasis, obstructive pneumonitis, and bronchiectasis. The nodules may grow up to several centimeters in diameter, at which point they frequently cavitate (Fig. 30.5) (28).

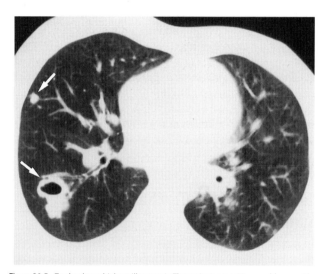

Figure 30.5. Tracheobronchial papillomatosis. The patient was a 25 year-old man with a longstanding papillomatosis. CT showing several nodules and cavities (*arrows*).

Pulmonary Adenomas

These tumors are believed to arise from tracheobronchial mucous glands and include mucinous cystic tumor, papil-lary adenoma, and alveolar adenoma. Radiological fea-tures are non-specific. Bronchioalveolar cell adenoma is considered to be a highly differentiated adenocarcinoma or a potentially malignant benign neoplasm. Lesions are often discovered incidentally at microscopic examination of surgically resected specimen but the CT findings have been recently described. They appear as small nodules with ground-glass attenuation (29).

Lymphoproliferative Disorders

Lymphoproliferative disorders constitute a large group of diseases, the prevalence of which is variable. In the chest, pulmonary manifestations of secondary non-Hodgkin's lymphoma and leukemia, mediastinal lymphomas, and Hodgkin disease are rather common and will be presented elsewhere in this volume as well as lymphoid interstitial pneumonia and follicular bronchiolitis that manifest as diffuse lung diseases. Some rare lymphoproliferative disorders manifest as focal diseases and can be grouped under this heading. They are focal lymphoid hyperplasia, primary pulmonary lymphomas and plasma cell neoplasms (30).

Focal Lymphoid Hyperplasia

This disorder is also called nodular lymphoid hyperplasia or pseudolymphoma. It is characterized by a localized polyclonal proliferation of mature mononuclear cells. The most common manifestation is a solitary nodule or a focal area of consolidation usually limited to one lobe. All lesions contain an air bronchogram. Less common manifestations include multiple nodules, sometimes cavitated, and infiltrates. As a rule, there is no associated adenopathy or pleural effusion. If present, this suggests the diagnosis of lymphoma. Patients are most of the time asymptomatic. The lesions are biopsied or resected and immunohistochemical and appropriate molecular analyses should exclude a low grade B-cell lymphoma. The prognosis of excised lesions is generally excellent but close follow-up is advisable (30).

Primary Pulmonary Lymphoma

This neoplasm represents only 3–4% of all extranodal lymphomas. The most widely accepted criteria for designating a lymphoma as primary is if it affects the lung and shows no evidence of extrathoracic dissemination for at least 3 months after the initial diagnosis. Most low grade B-cell lymphomas are derived from mucosa-associated lymphoid tissue (MALT). They appear pathologically as a single white or tan lesion that varies from a well-circumscribed nodule to a relatively ill-defined infiltrate in all or part of a lobe. Occasionally, they are multiple foci of disease (30–32). The most common radiographic manifestation consists of a solitary nodule or a poorly defined focal opacity (Fig. 30.6). Other patterns include a localized area of consolidation ranging from a segment to an entire

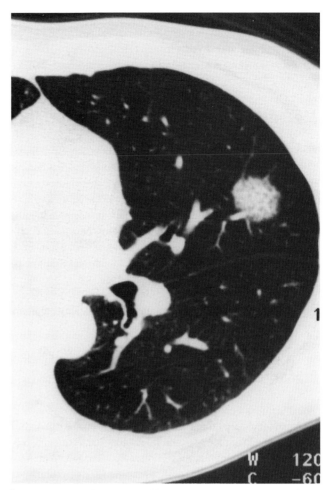

Figure 30.6. Primary low grade B-cell lymphoma. CT showing a 2 cm area of consolidation. The diagnosis was proven at percutaneous cutting needle biopsy and surgery.

lobe, and air bronchograms are visible in about 50% of cases. These abnormalities show an indolent course with slow growth over months or years (33–35). About 50% of patients are asymptomatic and others present with pulmonary or systemic symptoms. High grade primary pulmonary lymphomas are also of B-cell type. Some are derived from the low grade B-cell lymphomas and others occur in patients who have had organ transplantation. Pathologically, they tend to show a less prominent interstitial pattern and more frequent necrosis and vascular infiltration. Radiologic manifestations are nonspecific, including localized opacities, consolidation and diffuse reticulonodular pattern, which may progress to extensive consolidation with associated respiratory failure (32).

Multiple Myoloma and Plasmocytoma

Thoracic disease in multiple myeloma is common. Neoplastic infiltration of the skeleton is the most common by far. Pleural and pulmonary manifestations are less frequent, taking the form of one or multiple masses or an endobronchial or endotracheal tumor. Plasmocytoma, defined as a neoplastic proliferation of plasma cells in the absence of a generalized plasma cell disorder of the lung or major airways, is an exceedingly rare condition (36).

Mesenchymal Neoplasms

Neoplasms of the lung composed of mesenchymal tissue account for fewer than 1% of all lung tumors. They consist of various types of benign or malignant sarcomatous neoplasms arising from muscle, vascular, bone and cartilage, neural, adipose or fibrous tissues. When one is considering the diagnostis of sarcomas, it must be remembered that pulmonary carcinoma as well as some types of metastases such as renal cell and melanoma may have a sarcomatoid appearance. A definitive diagnosis of sarcoma on a bronchial biopsy or needle aspirate specimen should then be considered with caution. Most sarcomas of the lung, however, are metastases from extrathoracic primary tumors (37).

Primary Lung Sarcomas

These tumors occur once in every 500 cases of lung cancer and are usually fibrosarcomas and leiomyosarcomas (Fig. 30.7). Chondrosarcoma, fibroleiomyosarcoma, osteosarcoma, rhabdomyosarcoma, myxosarcoma, and neurofibrosarcoma synovial sarcomas may also arise primarily in the lung. Malignant fibrous histiocytoma is one of the most common soft tissue sarcomas in adults, usually occurring in the extremities, retroperitoneum and trunk. Metastasis to the lung is common. However, the primary lung localization is extremely rare. Endobronchial sarcomas generally exhibit a relatively benign behavior compared with tumors arising within the lung parenchyma, which showed great variability

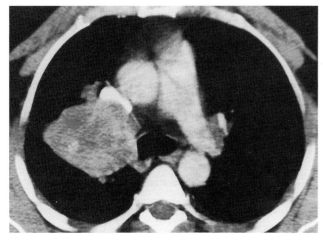

Figure 30.7. Primary leiomyosarcoma. Enhanced CT showing a large homogeneous right upper lobe mass with a slight compression of the superior vena cava.

in their degree of malignancy and a significance incidence of highly aggressive behavior (38).

In most cases, a solitary pulmonary mass or nodule is found on radiography. On CT, a soft-tissue density mass with or without central areas of lower attenuation is seen. CT is helpful in delineating involvement of the mediastinum, detecting subdiaphragmatic extension and identifying primary retroperitoneal tumor. Imaging features are indistinguishable from bronchial carcinomas, except that calcification is a feature of osteosarcoma and chondrosarcoma (39).

Mesenchymal tumors of vascular origin in the lung include epithelioid hemangioendothelioma, hemangiopericytoma, and the exceedingly rare angiosarcoma. Epithelioid hemangioendothelioma is best considered a low grade sarcoma. Radiographic manifestations simulate metastases or infarcts (40). Hemangiopericytoma is frequently asymptomatic, has the radiographic appearance of a solitary pulmonary nodule, and is often inhomogeneous at CT scan, with a central necrotic area and a peripheral enhancement (41).

Other Benign Mesenchymal Neoplasms

There include fibroma, chondroma, lipoma, hemangioma, neurofibroma and neurilemnoma, which may arise in the walls of the bronchi or in the lung parenchyma(42). Those located in the lung parenchyma are nonspecific solitary pulmonary nodules; those that arise in the larger bronchi are indistinguishable from the more common bronchial carcinoid, except that it may be possible to distinguish fat in a lipoma by CT. Pure chondroma is exceptional as compared with chondrohamartoma. It is an endobronchial tumor affecting the large bronchi of 1–2 cm diameter. It constitutes one the elements of Carney syndrome, together with gastric leiomyoma and extradural functional paraganglioma. This syndrome occurs most frequently in women and chondromas may be multiple (43).

Most lipomas arise extrapleurally from the chest wall, mediastinum or diaphragm. Other thoracic lesions are endobronchial. Bronchial lipoma originates in the bronchial wall in the submucosa and appears as a soft, deformable mass with a diameter 1–3 cm, sometimes pedunculated. The tumor is revealed by signs of bronchial obstruction or hemoptysis. CT makes possible presurgical diagnosis and highlights endoscopic excision, showing the endobronchial localization (Fig. 30.8) (44).

Leiomyoma of the lung may be a solitary lesion and is indistinguishable radiographically from the other benign connective tissue neoplasms. Multiple smooth muscle tumors in pulmonary parenchyma have been reported on rare occasions as benign metastasizing leiomyoma, multiple pulmonary fibroleiomyomatous hamartomas or pulmonary metastases from smooth muscle neoplasm.

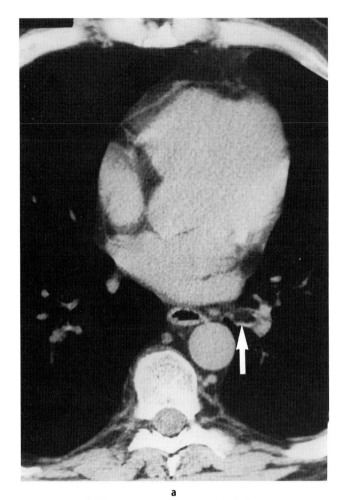

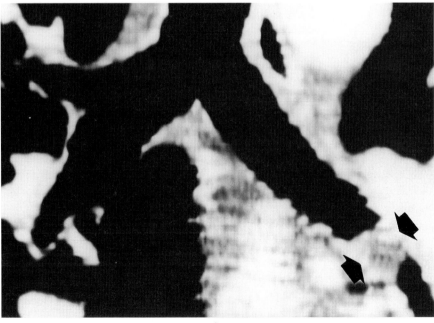

Figure 30.8. Endobronchial lipoma. **a** CT showing a small nodule of fatty attenuation (*arrow*) within the left inferior bronchus. **b** Oblique coronal reconstruction through the major airways tract delineates the lesion (*arrows*).

Benign metastasizing leiomyomas occur in women with known interine leiomyomas and have a long benign course. In men and children, the tumor has a quite different behavior. The growth pattern is much more invasive (45).

Hamartomas

A hamartoma is usually considered as a tumor-like malformation composed of tissues that are normally present in the organ in which the tumor occurs. The label hamartoma may be nosologically incorrect and these tumors may be more appropriately described by the term mesenchymoma. Hamartomas are uncommon tumors, representing about 5% of lung tumors. Endobronchial lesions are much less common than parenchymal lesions. The majority of them are solitary, usually peripheral in location and appear as well-circumscribed slightly lobulated tumors in a somewhat compressed surrounding lung. Most of them are less than 4 cm, composed of lobules containing a central area of well-developed cartilage, surrounded by a zone of loose fibroblastic tissue. Adipose tissue, smooth muscle, seromucinous tracheo bronchial glands, and mononuclear inflammatory cells may be present in variable proportions. Calcifications and ossification can be present. Entrapped epithelial cells are often seen at the periphery (46,47). Endobronchial hamartomas are fleshy polypoid tumors attached to the bronchial wall by a stalk (48).

Most hamartomas do not cause symptoms and, when they do, hemoptysis is the most common. The diagnosis can be done when typical imaging findings are present. Adequate surgical excision results in cure in the vast majority of patients (46,47).

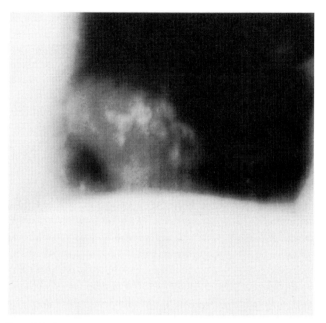

Figure 30.9. Hamartoma. Conventional tomography shows characteristic "popcorn" calcifications.

On chest radiograph, pulmonary hamartomas are well-defined smoothly marginated nodules without lobar predilection, usually smaller than 4 cm, calcified in about 10% of the cases. The radiographic pattern of calcification may resemble popcorn (Fig. 30.9), which is a very uncommon although virtually pathognomonic finding.

The thin-section CT findings that permit a diagnosis are a smoothly contoured nodule with a focal collection of fat (CT numbers between –40 and –100 HU) or fat alternating with areas of calcification (CT numbers >175 HU) (Fig. 30.10). CT was able to demonstrate this finding in

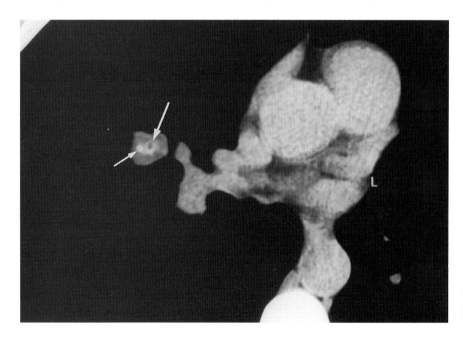

Figure 30.10. Hamartoma. Enhanced CT showing a 2 cm well-defined nodule with two small areas of calcium (*short arrow*) and fatty (*long arrow*) attenuation, respectively.

60% in a series of 47 hamartomas (49). Parenchymal hamartomas occasionally grow to a large size and slowly. They receive their blood supply from a systemic vessel and this explains the enhancement pattern that may occur.

Neoplasms of Uncertain Histogenesis

Clear Cell Tumors

These tumors are very rare pulmonary neoplasms occurring in adults. They are well-defined but nonencapsulated nodules measuring 1–3 cm in diameter. Microscopically, they are composed of sheets of polygonal cells with an abundant cytoplasm and a high glycogen content detectable on special stains. The lesion should be differentiated from the metastatic clear cell carcinoma of the kidney. Patients are asymptomatic and present with a radiologically nonspecific pulmonary nodule (50).

Sclerosing Hemangiomas

These tumors occur in patients in their 30s, 40s and 50s. They are well-defined round-to-oval, nonspecific nodules, from 1–4 cm, mostly in a subpleural location. Microscopically, they are composed of solid and papillary cellular areas, comprising round or oval cells with abundant eosinophilic cytoplasms admixed with inflammatory cells. Most behave in a benign fashion in asymptomatic patients. Radiologically, they present as homogeneous nodules or masses with a homogeneous enhancement at CT and rarely calcify (51).

Pulmonary Blastomas

Neoplasms of this type are malignant lesions of uncertain origin that recapitulate the developing lung in the fetal life. They appear at a somewhat younger age than carcinoma, with a small proportion found in children. They generally arise peripherally in the lung as a solitary well-defined mass or occasionally as multiple pulmonary masses. The 5-year survival has been reported to range between 15% and 50% (52,53).

Other Tumors

Tumors of uncertain origin have been reported to occur in the lung, including paragangliomas, germ cell tumors, thymomas, ependymomas, and meningiomas.

Lesions of Uncertain Tumoral Nature

Fibrous Histiocytoma

This is also called plasma cell granuloma, inflammatory pseudotumor or inflammatory myofibroblastic tumor. It is a group of lesions characterized by a mixture of fibroblasts, histiocytes, lymphocytes, and plasma cells. The variable proportion of cells constituting these lesions explains the variety of terms employed for designating this neoplasm. Radiologic manifestations consist of either a solitary pulmonary nodule or a focal area of consolidation that can mimic a primary or metastatic carcinoma. Long-term follow-up shows usually no change in size (54,55).

Hyalizing Granulomas

There are very rare lesions characterized by numerous regularly arranged lamellae of hyalinized collagen. Their pathogenesis is unclear. They manifest as several small well-defined nodules with a slow growth (56).

Thoracic Endometriosis

This is manifested clinically most often as pneumothorax but, on very rare occasions, has been reported as a pulmonary nodule (57).

References

1. Kramer R. Cited by Harpole DH, Jr, Feldman JM, Buchanan S, et al. (1992) Bronchial carcinoid tumors: A retrospective analysis of 126 patients. Ann Thorac Surg 54:50–55.
2. Warren WH, Faber LP, Gould VE (1989) Neuroendocrine neoplasms of the lung: A clinicopathologic update. J Thorac Cardiovasc Surg 98:321–332.
3. Travis WD, Rush W, Flieder DB, et al. (1998) Survival analysis of 200 pulmonary neuroendocrine tumors with clarification of criteria for atypical carcinoid and its separation from typical carcinoid. Am J Surg Pathol 22:934–944.
4. McCaughan BC, Martini N, Bains MS (1985) Bronchial carcinoids: Reviews of 124 cases. J Thorac Cardiovasc Surg 89:8–17.
5. Rosado de Christenson ML, Abbott GF, Kirejczyk WM (1999) Thoracic carcinoids: Radiologic–pathologic correlation. Radiographics 19:707–736.
6. Aronchick JM, Wexler JA, Christen B, et al. (1986) Computed tomography of bronchial carcinoid. J Comput Assist Tomogr 10:71–74.
7. Forster BB, Müller NL, Miller RR, et al. (1989) Neuroendocrine carcinomas of the lung: Clinical, radiologic and pathologic correlation. Radiology 170:441–445.
8. Zwiebel BR, Austin JH, Grimes MM (1991) Bronchial carcinoid tumors: Assessment with CT of location and intratumoral calcification in 31 patients. Radiology 179:483–486.

9. Magid D, Siegelman SS, Eggleton JC, et al. (1989) Pulmonary carcinoid tumors: CT assessment. J Comput Assist Tomogr 13:244–247.

10. Choplin RH, Kawamoto EH, Dyer RB, et al. (1986) Atypical carcinoid of the lung: Radiographic features. AJR 146:665–668.

11. David SD, Zirn JR, Govoni AF, et al. (1990) Peripheral carcinoid tumor of the lung: CT diagnosis. AJR 155:1185–1187.

12. Doppman JL, Nieman L, Miller DL, et al. (1989) Ectopic adrenocorticotropic hormone syndrome: Localization studies in 28 patients. Radiology 172:115–125.

13. Doppman JL, Pass HI, Nieman LK, et al. (1991) Detection of ACH-producing bronchial carcinoid tumors: MR imaging vs CT. AJR 156:39–43.

14. Douek PC, Simoni L, Revel D, et al. (1994) Diagnosis of bronchial carcinoid tumor by ultrafast contrast-enhanced MR imaging. AJR 163:563–564.

15. Christin-Maîre S, Chabbert-Buffet N, Mure A, et al. (1996) Use of somatostatin analog for localization and treatment of ACTH secreting bronchial carcinoid tumor. Chest 109:845–846.

16. Ducrocq X, Thomas P, Massard G, et al. (1998) Operative risk and prognostic factors of typical bronchial carcinoid tumors. Ann Thorac Surg 65:1410–1414.

17. Gould PM, Bonner JA, Sawyer TE, et al. (1998) Bronchial carcinoid tumors: Importance of prognostic factors that influence patterns of recurrence and overall survival. Radiology 208:181–185.

18. Benett GL, Chew FS (1994) Pulmonary carcinoid tumorlets. AJR 162:568.

19. Brown MJ, English J, Müller NL (1997) Bronchiolitis obliterans due to neuroendocrine hyperplasia: high-resolution CT-pathologic correlation. AJR 168:1561.

20. Moran CA (1995) Primary salivary gland-type tumors of the lung. Semin Diagn Pathol 12:106.

21. McCarthy MJ, Rosado de Christenson ML (1995) Tumors of the trachea. J Thorac Imaging 180:10.

22. Maziak DE, Todd TR, Keshavjee SH, et al. (1996) Adenoid cystic carcinoma of the airway: Thirty-two-year experience. J Thorac Cardiovasc Surg 112:1522.

23. Cleveland RH, Nice CM, Ziskind J (1997) Primary adenoid cystic carcinoma (cylindroma) of the trachea. Radiology 122:597.

24. Spizarny DL, Shepartd J-AO, McLoud TC et al. (1986) CT of adenoid cystic carcinoma of the trachea. AJR 146:1129.

25. Kim TS, Lee KS, Han J, et al. (1999) Mucoepidermoid carcinoma of the tracheobronchial tree: Radiographic and CT findings in 12 patients. Radiology 212:643–648.

26. Kwong JS, Adler BD, Padley SPG, et al. (1993) Diagnosis of diseases of the trachea and main bronchi: Chest radiography versus CT. AJR 161:519.

27. Newmark GM, Conces DJ, Jr., Kopecky KK (1994) Spiral CT evaluation of the trachea and bronchi. J Comput Assist Tomogr 18:552.

28. Kramer SS, Wehunt WD, Stocker JT, et al. (1985) Pulmonary manifestations of juvenile laryngotracheal papillomatosis. AJR 144:687.

29. Kushihashi T, Munechika H, Kyoushichi R et al. (1994) Bronchioalveolar adenoma of the lung: CT-pathologic correlation Radiology 193:789–793.

30. Bragg DG, Chor PJ, Murray KA, et al. (1994) Lymphoproliferative disorders of the lung: Histopathology, clinical manifestations and imaging features. AJR 163:273.

31. Lee KS, Kim Y, Primack SL (1997) Imaging of pulmonary lymphomas. AJR 168:339.

32. Cordier JF, Chailleux E, Lauque D, et al. (1993) Primary pulmonary lymphomas: A clinical study of 70 cases in nonimmunocompromised patients. Chest 103:201.

33. O'Donnel PG, Jackson SA, Tung KT, et al. (1998) Radiological appearances of lymphomas arising from mucosa-associated lymphoid tissue (MALT) in the lung. Clin Radiol 53:258.

34. Au V, Leung AN (1997) Radiologic manifestations of lymphoma in the thorax AJR 168:93.

35. Roggeri A, Agostini L, Vezzani G, et al. (1993) Primary malignant non-Hodgkin's lymphoma of the lung arising in mucosa-associated lymphoid tissue (MALT). Eur Respir J 6:138.

36. Logan PM, Miller RR, Müller NL (1995) Solitary tracheal plasmacytoma: Computed tomography and pathological findings. Can Assoc Radiol J 46:125.

37. Suster S (1995) Primary sarcomas of the lung. Semin Diagn Pathol 12:140.

38. Janssen JP, Mulder JJ, Wagenaar SS, et al. (1994) Primary sarcoma of the lung: A clinical study with long-term follow-up. Ann Thorac Surg 58:1151.

39. Stark P, Eber CD, Jacobson F (1994) Primary intrathoracic malignant mesenchymal tumors: Pictorial essay. Thorac Imaging 9:148–155.

40. Luburich P, Ayuso MC, Picado C, et al. (1994) CT of pulmonary epithelioid hemangioendothelioma. J Comput Assist Tomogr 18:562.

41. Yousem SA, Hochholzer L (1987) Primary pulmonary hemangiopericytoma. Cancer59:549.

42. Roviaro G, Montorsi M, Varoli F, et al. (1983) Primary pulmonary tumors of neurogenic origin. Thorax 38:942.

43. Schmutz GR, Fisch-Ponsot C, Sylvestre J (1994) Carney syndrome. Radiologic features. Can Assoc Radiol J 45:148.

44. Schraufnagel DE, Morin JE, Wang NS (1979) Endobronchial lipoma. Chest 75:97.

45. Martin E (1983) Leiomyomatous lung lesions: A proposed classification. AJR 141:269.

46. Hansen CP, Holtveg H, Francis D, et al. (1992) Pulmonary hamartoma. J Thorac Cardiovasc Surg 104:674.

47. Gjevre JA, Myers JL, Prakash UB (1996) Pulmonary hamartomas. Mayo Clin Proc 71:14.

48. Ahn JM, Im JG, Seo JW, et al. (1994) Endobronchial hamartoma: CT findings in three patients. AJR 163:49.

49. Siegelman SS, Khouri NF, Scott WW, et al. (1986) Pulmonary hamartoma: CT findings. Radiology 160:313.

50. Kung M, Landa JP, Lubin J (1984) Benign clear cell tumor ("sugar tumor") of the trachea. Cancer 54:517.

51. Im JG, Kim WH, Han MC, et al. (1994) Sclerosing hemangiomas of the lung and interlobar fissures: CT findings. J Comput Assist Tomogr 18:34.

52. Senac MO, Wood BP, Isaacs H, et al. (1991) Pulmonary blastoma: A rare childhood malignancy. Radiology 179:743

53. Majid OA, Rajendran U, Baker LT. (1998) Pulmonary blastoma. Ann Thorac Cardiovasc Surg 4:47.

54. Schwartz EE, Katz SM, Mandell GA (1980) Postinflammatory pseudotumors of the lung: Fibrous histiocytoma and related lesions. Radiology 136:609.

55. Agrons GA, Rosado-de-Christenson ML, Kirejczyk WM, et al. (1998) Pulmonary inflammatory pseudotumor: Radiologic features. Radiology 206:511.

56. Eschelman DJ, Blickman JG, Lazar HL, et al. (1991) Pulmonary hyalinizing granuloma: A rare cause of a solitary pulmonary nodule. J Thorac Imaging 6:54.

57. Hertzanu Y, Heimer D, Hirsch M (1987) Computed tomography of pulmonary endometriosis. Comput Radiol 11:81.

31 Congenital Malformations of the Lung

J.M. Mata, J. Cáceres, and J.R. Manzano

Introduction

A review of the published literature gives the impression that congenital pulmonary malformations are infrequent. We usually think of them as occurring only during childhood. However, the lack of symptoms in the majority of congenital pulmonary malformations makes them go undetected until adult age. It is not rare to discover abnormalities due to congenital malformations in chest radiographs of adults. If we ignore this possibility, important errors in diagnosis and management are bound to occur.

In the recent past, congenital lung malformations were diagnosed by invasive techniques, such as bronchography and/or angiography. New imaging techniques – computed tomography (CT), spiral CT, and magnetic resonance imaging (MRI) – allow us to easily detect and characterize such malformations, thus avoiding invasive techniques that are potentially harmful for the patient. CT and spiral CT provide the most extensive information for diagnosis. MRI should be used only in selected cases and the information is less complete than that given by CT.

Classification

The accurate classification of congenital malformations is not an easy task (1–4), considering that the underlying embryogenesis is not well defined in the majority of cases. We have chosen a radiologic classification based on the chest radiograph findings. From a radiologic point of view, we divide the malformations into two groups: *dysmorphic lung*, when an entire hemithorax is affected and *focal pulmonary malformations* when only part of one lung is affected.

Dysmorphic lung includes developmental anomalies of the entire lung and its blood drainage, divided into two categories: lung agenesis–hypoplasia complex, and lobar agenesis–aplasia complex. Focal pulmonary malformations include congenital bronchial atresia, bronchogenic cyst, adenomatoid malformation, pulmonary sequestration, and isolated systemic supply to normal lung.

Dysmorphic Lung

Dysmorphic lung (DL) is characterized by arrested development of either a whole lung or a lobe. Absence of a lobe may be associated with other abnormalities, some of them common and others highly unusual. DL can be recognized on chest radiographs when we are aware of its existence and it is sometimes possible to reach a diagnosis based solely on plain film evidence. In doubtful cases it is advisable to use CT (5,6) or, occasionally, MRI (7, 8) to confirm the diagnosis without resorting to more expensive and potentially dangerous invasive procedures such as angiography or bronchography. Spiral CT allows biplane and three-dimensional reconstructions of this anomaly, making invasive techniques unnecessary.

The term dysmorphic lung was first used by Partridge in 1988 (9). According to the appearance in the chest radiograph, we classify the dysmorphic lung into two groups. The first group encompasses agenesis, aplasia and hypoplasia of the entire lung (lung agenesis–hypoplasia complex). The second group encompasses agenesis or aplasia of one or two lobes (lobar agenesis–aplasia complex). This second group has several levels of complexity. Lobar agenesis–aplasia is a constant feature. According to whether or not there are associated anomalous veins, we distinguish the following four variants:

1. Lobar agenesis–aplasia and no anomalous veins present (*hypogenetic lung syndrome*)
2. Lobar agenesis–aplasia and single pulmonary vein (*anomalous unilateral single pulmonary vein*)
3. Lobar agenesis–aplasia and levo atriocardinal vein (*levo atriocardinal vein*)

4. Lobar agenesis–aplasia and partial venous drainage to systemic veins (*venolobar syndrome*)

Accessory diaphragm and/or *horseshoe* lung may be associated with any of these variants.

Lung Agenesis–Hypoplasia Complex

Arrested development of an entire lung (lung agenesis–hypoplasia complex) is uncommon and occurs equally often in either hemithorax. This anomaly was first described by De Pozzi in 1673 (10). Various theories have been postulated to explain lung agenesis-hypoplasia, but the exact reason for the stunted growth of one of the shoots arising from the primitive intestine and the causative mechanisms are unknown.

Although the terms agenesis (absence of bronchus and lung), aplasia (absence of lung with bronchus present) and hypoplasia (bronchus and rudimentary lung present) describe different anomalies (11), we group all three under the term agenesis–hypoplasia complex because they all have a similar radiologic appearance on the chest radiograph. These entities tend to be clinically asymptomatic and they are usually discovered accidentally on plain film studies carried out for unrelated reasons.

The characteristic appearance of lung agenesis–hypoplasia complex on the posteroanterior view is a diffuse opacity of one hemithorax with marked mediastinal shift, reminiscent of the appearance of whole-lung atelectasis (12,13).

Occasionally, lung agenesis–hypoplasia complex presents an atypical appearance, with a small hemithorax, aerated lung and apparent pleural thickening that simulates chronic pleural disease and is more difficult to recognize on plain film (14,15). This appearance results from the marked herniation of the contralateral lung. Typical and atypical cases show the same radiologic appearance on the lateral chest view: retrosternal hyperclarity with the heart and great mediastinal vessels displaced backward (5).

CT shows the reasons for the two distinct radiologic presentations. Pulmonary herniation takes place behind the sternum in both groups and accounts for the retrosternal hyperclarity. Mediastinal rotation explains the posterior displacement of the heart and mediastinum. If the herniation of the contralateral lung is not severe, plain film shows the typical appearance of a small opaque hemithorax. In atypical cases, the extensive herniation of the contralateral lung crosses the midline to penetrate deep into the malformed hemithorax, giving the appearance of aerated lung on plain film. The pseudo thickening of the pleura is produced by accumulation of fatty tissue in the subpleural space, where the herniation of the contralateral lung or the mediastinal shift has been unable to fill the space left by the absent or underdeveloped lung (5).

CT is able to differentiate among lung agenesis, aplasia, and hypoplasia, although this distinction has little clinical significance. CT reveals the presence or absence of bronchus or pulmonary tissue, and allows measurement of the homolateral pulmonary artery (16). Although lung agenesis–hypoplasia complex is said to go together with a small or absent homolateral pulmonary artery (17), a normal-sized pulmonary artery with substantial blood flow can be detected with CT and MRI in the majority of patients.

In some patients with lung agenesis, the new sectional techniques also reveal a small pleural space, which usually contains a small quantity of fluid. The presence of the pleural space is accounted for by the different embryologic origins of the lung and pleura.

Lung agenesis–hypoplasia complex is associated with malformations in other systems, including the skeletal, digestive, cardiac and urinary systems, and even in the other lung (5). The association of lung agenesis–hypoplasia with malformations in the skeleton or other organs is very high in some series (18). A common origin as an insult to the neural crest in the embryo has been postulated to explain these phenomena, giving rise to the VACTERL syndrome of anomalies (19).

Lobar Agenesis-Aplasia Complex

The term lobar agenesis–aplasia complex groups pulmonary malformations affecting, almost exclusively, the right hemithorax. All of these malformations present pulmonary anomalies in the form of one or more absent or underdeveloped pulmonary lobe.

Depending upon the associated venous malformation, we can look at this group as a continuum. At one extreme, the pulmonary malformation is isolated and the veins are normal (hypogenetic lung syndrome). The second step of the continuum includes the anomalous unilateral single pulmonary vein, which drains all the lung parenchyma into the left atrium (20). Next in line is the levo atrio-cardinal vein; in this malformation there is an anomalous vein that drains the entire lung and connects the left atrium with a systemic vein (21). Last in the continuum is an anomalous vein draining into the systemic venous system (venolobar syndrome).

Accessory diaphragm (part of the right lung trapped by a membranomuscular duplication of the diaphragm) (22) and horseshoe lung (tissue from the malformed lung crossing the mediastinum to meet or fuse with the left lower lobe) (23) can accompany any of these malformations.

Systemic supply from the thoracic aorta is almost always present, although it is hardly ever seen on plain film or CT scans. Sometimes the systemic artery can be thick, mimicking a scimitar vein (9).

Hypogenetic Lung Syndrome

In hypogenetic lung syndrome there is agenesis or aplasia of one or two pulmonary lobes together with anomalies in the blood supply to the lung. Patients are usually asymptomatic. This entity almost always occurs in the right hemithorax, and its appearance in the left hemithorax is exceptional (24).

The chest radiograph shows a small right hemithorax with mediastinal shift to the right and haziness of the right cardiac border. In some cases, the right hilus is hidden by the mediastinal rotation and cannot be seen, and in others the shape of the hilus is reminiscent of the left hilus. In most cases, lateral chest films show a retrosternal band. In the past, this band was interpreted as an accessory diaphragm or as fatty areolar tissue filling the empty space left by the underdeveloped lung (25,26). In 1984, Ang and Proto (27) demonstrated with CT that the dense retrosternal band is due to the decrease in the anteroposterior diameter of the underdeveloped lung, which also accounts for the haziness of the right heart border on the posteroanterior view.

CT provides a wealth of information (5,16,28) by demonstrating the size of the pulmonary artery, the branching of the bronchi, anomalous fissures and accompanying anomalies of the diaphragm (diaphragmatic hernias). If underdevelopment is very pronounced, one can observe extrapleural fat deposits along the thoracic wall, simulating pleural thickening; these are similar to, though not as striking as, those seen in lung agenesis–hypoplasia complex (5). The right upper lobe is most often affected. This gives a bronchial distribution of the right lung similar to that observed in the left lung in normal conditions (hypoarterial bronchus) (4). CT demonstrates the pulmonary veins draining into their normal location, ruling out venous anomalies.

Lobar Agenesis–Aplasia with Anomalous Unilateral Single Pulmonary Vein

The second step of the continuum is a symptom-free malformation that was first described by Benfield in 1971 (29). In the past it received different names: pulmonary varix, meandering right pulmonary vein, or scimitar sign with normal pulmonary venous drainage. It consists of a hypogenetic lung with a single anomalous vein draining all the lung parenchyma into the left atrium. The vein

follows an unusual pathway before it meets the left atrium (30,31).

In the chest radiograph anomalous unilateral single pulmonary vein has the same appearance as hypogenetic lung syndrome plus a tubular and serpiginous shadow due to the anomalous vein. In rare cases, the anomalous vein may mimic a scimitar vein (9,32–34). CT provides the right diagnosis, showing a serpiginous shadow running through the lung and ending in the left atrium (16). In all cases of anomalous unilateral single pulmonary vein, the vein goes to an extracardiac chamber located behind the left atrium (cor triatriatum).

Exceptionally, we can see atypical cases with an anomalous single pulmonary vein affecting both lungs. This entity has been described as idiopathic prominence of the pulmonary veins (35). The veins of both lungs follow an unusual pathway and drain into the extracardiac chamber.

Lobar Agenesis–Aplasia with Levo Atriocardinal Vein

The levo atriocardinal vein is defined as an anomalous vein that connects the left atrium and one vein of the systemic venous system. It was first described by Edwards and DuShane in 1950 (21). The systemic venous system derives from the embryologic system called cardinal veins. This malformation consists of a hypogenetic lung with the anomalous vein connecting a cor triatriatum and one of the main systemic veins. The levo atriocardinal vein would be the midpoint in the continuum between the anomalous unilateral single pulmonary vein and the venolobar syndrome. It is a very uncommon malformation with few descriptions in the literature, found mainly in angiographic journals. This may explain why many radiologists are unaware of this anomaly.

On chest radiograph the levo atriocardinal vein looks very similar to the anomalous unilateral single pulmonary vein. CT demonstrates the usual findings of hypogenetic lung syndrome and the vein joining the cor triatriatum and a systemic vein. The anomalous vein drains all the pulmonary veins, and MRI shows the pathway of the vein as well as the points where it meets with the systemic vein and the left atrium. By MRI we can demonstrate that there is no gradient between the left atrium and the systemic vein.

Congenital Venolobar Syndrome

In congenital venolobar syndrome (CVS), also known as scimitar syndrome, partial anomalous venous return (PAVR) is associated with the hypogenetic lung syndrome.

This malformation is one of the extremes of the dysmorphic lung continuum. This anomaly was first described by Chassinat (36) and Cooper (37) in 1836. Most patients are asymptomatic. The left–right shunt produced by the anomalous drainage is usually small with no clinical repercussions, though, on rare occasions, it can lead to pulmonary hypertension (38). Associated cardiac malformations may cause symptoms in pediatric patients (39). For all practical purposes, CVS occurs exclusively in the right hemithorax, with only one case reported in the left (40).

Plain film findings are similar to those of hypogenetic lung. The differential finding is the anomalous vein (41). The vessel is seen as a widening tubular shadow that extends toward the base of the lung, thus originating the term scimitar syndrome. The anomalous vein usually drains into the inferior vena cava or the right atrium. The fact there may be more than one vein or that a single vein may be hidden behind the displaced heart, is the reason why PAVR is not seen on plain film in half of the cases (Fig. 31.1).

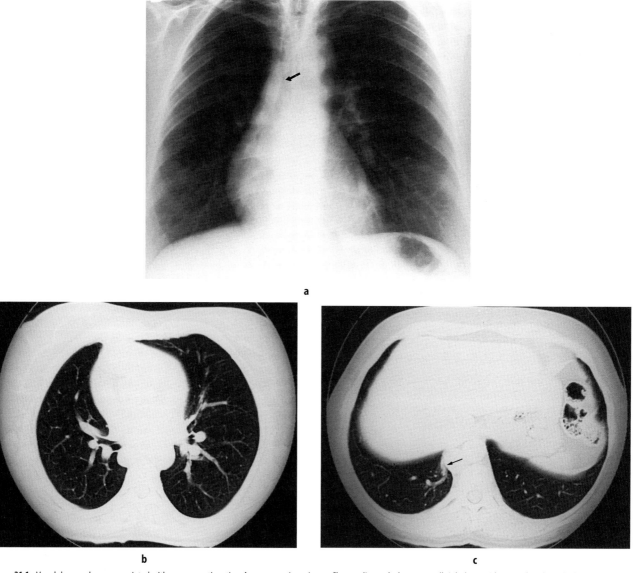

Figure 31.1. Venolobar syndrome, associated with azygos continuation. Asymptomatic patient. **a** Chest radiograph shows a small right lung with anomalous bronchial branching. The azygos vein (*arrow*) is increased in size. **b** CT shows that the right main bronchus bifurcates into two branches, one for the middle lobe and the other for the lower lobe. A large azygos vein is seen. **c** Caudal slice shows anomalous venous return (*arrow*) draining to the azygos vein. Abdominal CT (not shown) demonstrated absence of the intrahepatic segment of the inferior vena cava, with azygos continuation.

CT allows visualization of the anomalous vein and where it drains (5,6, 27,28). As a corollary, it also reveals the absence of the inferior pulmonary vein. In the majority of patients, PAVR is associated with an accessory pulmonary fissure that is visible on CT study (28).

The anomalous vein can be seen with MRI (8), and in some cases the entire course of the vessel can be followed in a single plane. MRI is less useful than CT in this malformation, as it cannot characterize the bronchial anomaly.

Horseshoe Lung

This uncommon malformation was first described by Spencer in 1962 (42). The horseshoe lung is associated with hypogenetic lung syndrome, and occurs when a small quantity of right pulmonary tissue arising from the lower lobe crosses the midline and joins the left lower lung. The right and left lower lobes may fuse, or be separated by a fissure. This isthmus of pulmonary tissue crosses the mediastinum behind the pericardium, in front of the aorta and the esophagus, and it is supplied by the right lower lobe vessels and bronchus (42, 43).

Chest radiograph shows hypogenetic lung syndrome or congenital venolobar syndrome together with an anomalous fissure in the base of the left lung. This finding suggests the correct diagnosis on the posteroanterior chest film (42). Sometimes the anomalous fissure can be seen as a thick opacity due to internal fat. CT shows typical findings of hypogenetic lung, with or without abnormal veins, plus two additional findings: mediastinal discontinuity behind the heart, with crossing of the midline by the vessels of the right lower lobe and, when present, an anomalous fissure located at the base of the left lung (44).

Accessory Diaphragm

Accessory diaphragm, also known as diaphragmatic duplication, is a rare congenital anomaly associated with the lobar agenesis–aplasia complex. It does not occur as an isolated malformation. It was first described by Drake et al. in 1950 (45). These authors postulated that the anomaly is produced in the initial stages of embryonic development when the septum transversum, which gives rise to the diaphragm, is in a very high position. If, for some reason, the descent of the septum transversum is arrested, part of the primitive lung could be trapped by it. The septum transversum would then remain anchored to the posterior wall, creating an additional diaphragmatic leaf (45).

Accessory diaphragm is a thin fibromuscular membrane fused anteriorly with the diaphragm and coursing posterosuperiorly to join the posterior chest wall. It produces two compartments in the right hemithorax, trapping part of the lung parenchyma (46,47). The vessels and bronchi that supply the trapped lung pass through a central hole in the accessory diaphragm.

The accessory diaphragm can have two different appearances in the chest radiograph. When the central hiatus is very narrow, the trapped lung is not aerated and it appears as a mass. When the trapped lung is aerated, the accessory diaphragm is visualized as a thin oblique line in the posteroanterior or the lateral chest view (48). In some patients there is a haziness where the duplicated diaphragm joins the normal one.

In CT scans, when the lung is aerated, the accessory diaphragm is seen as a fissure-like line with a hole in the center (6). Depending upon the size of the central hole, the CT appearance varies. When the hole is large, it may be difficult to identify the accessory diaphragm. When the hole is small, the trapped lung may be opaque or hyperlucent, due to air-trapping. Vessels and bronchi are crowded together when they go through the central hiatus.

Focal Malformations

Focal congenital malformations are a heterogeneous group whose boundaries are not well defined and whose radiologic and pathologic manifestations may vary and be difficult to classify, particularly when there is infection. They may cause symptoms in early life or be discovered incidentally. These malformations can be separated into different groups with the understanding that significant overlapping may occur.

Bronchial Atresia

Congenital bronchial atresia is an anomaly characterized by obliteration of the proximal lumen of a segmental bronchus, with preservation of the distal structures. Its pathogenesis is unknown. Air enters the affected segment via collateral channels, producing overinflation. The mucous secretions generated in the bronchi accumulate at the point of obstruction. The majority the patients are asymptomatic.

The radiographic findings mirror the pathologic changes: the affected area is hyperlucent, and, on radiographs obtained at expiration, obstructive emphysema is obvious. The accumulated secretions appeared as areas of mucus impaction with the typical branching pattern. The findings on CT scans are the same as those observed on chest radiographs, namely segmental overinflation and

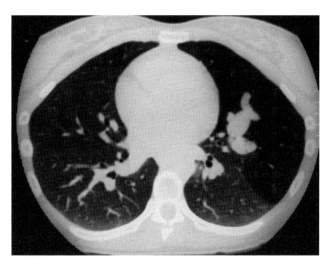

Figure 31.2. CT scan of congenital bronchial atresia. Hyperclarity of the lingula with a tubular branching image, representing mucus impaction.

Bronchogenic Cyst

Bronchogenic cyst is a congenital cystic anomaly containing mucus or clear fluid. It is commonly located in the mediastinum, but can occasionally occur in the lung (51,52). The patients are usually asymptomatic.

Radiographically, a bronchogenic cyst appears as a round mass that may have an air–fluid level. There are no specific features to differentiate it from other cystic lesions.

Adenomatoid Cystic Malformation

Congenital cystic adenomatoid malformation is characterized by anomalous fetal development of terminal respiratory structures, resulting in an adenomatoid proliferation of bronchiolar elements and cyst formation. The condition is classified into three types: type 1, the most common, is characterized by one or more cysts, some of which are over 2 cm in diameter; in type 2, the cysts are multiple and smaller than 2 cm, and type 3 consists of solid adenomatoid tissue (53).

The patients usually have symptoms, and in 90%, the condition is discovered in the first year of life. The typical radiographic finding is a multicystic opacity with entrapped air. Less often, the fluid-filled cysts may appear solid, but their true nature is discovered when the contents of the cysts are emptied (54,55). The lesion can be bilateral. Rare cases with systemic artery supply have been found.

By means of CT we can observe three basic patterns: a large solitary cyst (either air filled or fluid filled), multiple cysts (Fig. 31.3), and focal emphysematous changes

mucus impaction (Fig. 31.2) (49,50). When the apicoposterior segment of the left upper lobe is affected, the features are fairly typical on both radiographs and CT scans. CT demonstrates more clearly the extent of the emphysematous area and mucus impaction. When the bronchial atresia does not affect the left upper lobe, the plain radiographs show only nonspecific areas of focal emphysema, and CT is of great value, demonstrating the combination of emphysema and bronchial impaction that is the hallmark of this malformation.

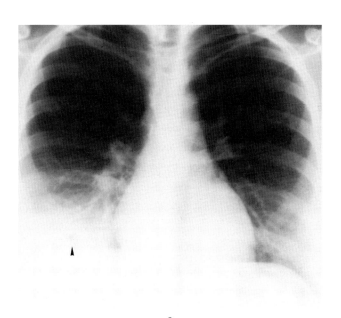

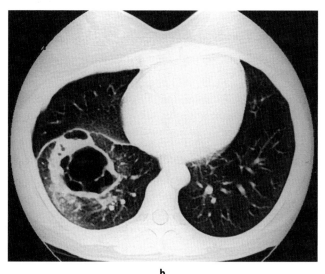

a   b

Figure 31.3. Cystic adenomatoid malformation. Twenty two year old patient with fever. **a** Chest radiograph shows an opacity in right lower lobe, with a small air fluid level (*arrowhead*). **b** CT after treatment shows a mass with multiple cysts up to 2 cm in size. Some of them have air–fluid levels. Surgery confirmed a type I adenomatoid malformation.

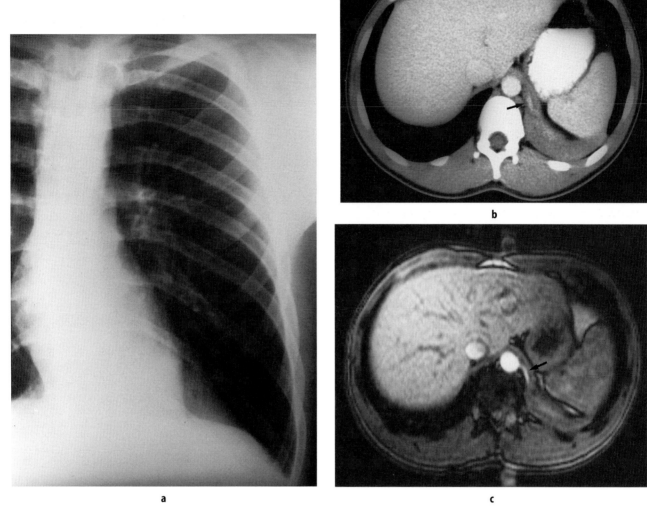

Figure 31.4. Intralobar sequestration. Sixteen year old with fever. **a** Chest radiograph shows a homogeneous opacity in the left lower life. **b** CT after treatment shows a mass with heterogeneous contrast enhancement and a systemic artery arising from the descending aorta (*arrow*). **c** Enhanced MRI confirms the origin of the anomalous artery (*arrow*).

(without mucous impaction) (5). CT can also identify rare cases of multifocal involvement, which is basic for a correct surgical approach to avoid recurrences.

Pulmonary Sequestration

Pulmonary sequestration is a congenital malformation in which a lung segment fails to communicate with the normal bronchial tree and remains isolated. The majority of cases are intralobar, and only a few are extralobar, i.e., surrounded by pleura with no contact with the adjacent lung. Characteristically, the sequestered lung is supplied by a systemic artery. Anatomically, the great majority of sequestrations are located in the basal segments of the

lower lobes and only rarely affect the middle or upper lobes (56).

The radiologic appearance of pulmonary sequestration is well known: recurrent pulmonary consolidation in a lower lobe that never clears completely. The diagnosis is confirmed by means of helical CT or MRI (57), which show the systemic arterial supply. Systemic arterial supply is an essential feature of pulmonary sequestration and differentiates it from other focal lesions with similar CT characteristics.

Intralobar sequestration is the most common form of pulmonary sequestration. On CT examination, it may appear as a homogeneous mass (Fig. 31.4) that shows internal cystic areas after contrast enhancement. It may also present as a nonhomogeneous mass with air–fluid levels, simulating an adenomatoid malformation. Rarely, it

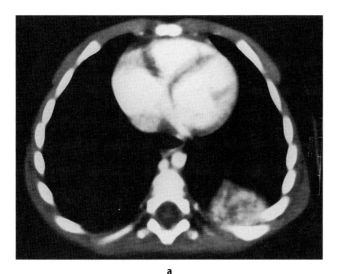

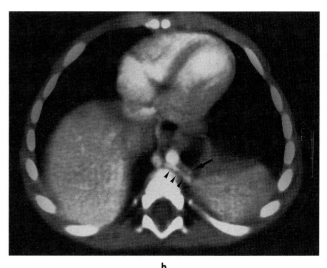

a   b

Figure 31.5. Extralobar sequestration. **a** CT shows a mass in the base of the left lung, which enhances heterogeneously. **b** Caudal slice identifies the systemic artery (*arrow*) and the draining vein (*arrowheads*), which crosses behind the aorta to end in the azygos vein.

may appear as an area of focal emphysema. Very infrequently, it may have calcification.

Extralobar sequestration usually appears in the paravertebral region at the thoracoabdominal inlet (56). In rare cases, it may be located in the retroperitoneum. On CT study it appears as a homogeneous mass that may be less dense than the surrounding soft tissues. With intravenous contrast it may enhance uniformly or in the periphery. In same cases, CT identifies not only the systemic artery, but the draining vein which, in extralobar sequestration, ends in a systemic vein (Fig. 31.5).

Isolated Systemic Supply to Normal Lung

Isolated systemic supply to normal lung is a rare congenital anomaly, first described by Huber in 1777 (58). In this malformation, aberrant systemic arterial supply to a lobe of the lung occurs as an isolated finding. The anomalous arteries perfuse normal pulmonary tissue. Chest radiography shows increased density in the affected lung and sometimes well-defined tubular or rounded images produced by the anomalous vessels can be recognized. The pulmonary parenchyma does not present any other changes. CT should be the initial method of study when isolated systemic supply to normal lung is suspected. CT provides rapid, noninvasive identification of the systemic vascularization and demonstrates the absence of pulmonary involvement, both characteristic signs of this entity (59).

References

1. Landing BH, Dixon LG (1979) Congenital malformations and genetic disorders of the respiratory tract. Am Rev Respir Dis 120:151
2. Reid L (1977) The lung: Its growth and remodeling in health and isease. AJR 129:777.
3. Panicek DM, Heitzman ER, Randall PA (1987) The continuum of pulmonary developmental anomalies. Radiographics 7:747.
4. Heitzman ER (1984) The lung: Radiologic–pathologic correlations. Mosby, St. Louis, MO.
5. Mata JM, C#aaceres J, Lucaya J, et al. (1990) CT of congenital malformations of the lung. Radiographics 10:651.
6. Woodring JH, Howard TA, Kanga JF (1994) Congenital pulmonary venolobar syndrome revisited. Radiographics 14:349.
7. Naidisch DP, Rumanik, Ettenger NA, et al. (1988) Congenital anomalies of the lung in adults: MR diagnosis. AJR 151:13.
8. Baxter R, McFadden PM, Gradman M, et al. (1990) Scimitar syndrome: Cine magnetic resonance imaging demonstration of anomalous pulmonary venous drainage. Ann Thorac Surg 50:121.
9. Partridge JB, Osborne JM, Slaughter RE (1988) Scimitar etcetera: The dysmorphic lung. Clin Radiol 39:11.
10. Rosenberg DML (1962) Pulmonary agenesis. Dis Chest 42:68.
11. Boyden EA (1955) Developmental anomalies of the lung. Am J Surg 89: 79.
12. Brünner S, Nissen E (1963) Agenesis of the lung. Am Rev Respir Dis 78: 103.
13. Yaghmai I (1970) Agenesis of the lung. AJR 108:564.
14. Nesbit WM, Paul LW, Middleton WS (1947) Congenital aplasia of the lung. Radiology 57:446.
15. Calenoff L, Friederici HH (1964) Unilateral pulmonary hypoplasia in an adult. AJR 91:265.
16. Mata JM, Cáceres J (1996) The dysmorphic lung: Imaging findings. Eur Radiol 6:403.
17. Valle AR (1955) Agenesis of the lung. Am J Surg 89:90.

18. Osborne J, Masel J, McCredie J (1989) A spectrum of skeletal anomalies associated with pulmonary agenesis: Possible neural crest injuries. Pediatr Radiol 19:425.

19. Knowles S, Thomas RM, Lindenbaum RH, et al. (1988) Pulmonary agenesis as part of the VACTERL sequence. Arch Dis Child 63:723.

20. Hasuo K, Numaguchi Y, Kishikawa T, et al. (1981) Anomalous unilateral single pulmonary vein mimicking pulmonary varices. Chest 79: 602.

21. Edwards JE, DuShane JW (1950) Thoracic venous anomalies. Arch Pathol 49: 517.

22. Nazarian M, Currarino G, Webb WR, et al. (1971) Accessory diaphragm: Report of a case with complete physiological evaluation and surgical correction. J Thorac Cardiovasc Surg 61:293.

23. Dische MR, Teixeira ML, Winchester PA, et al. (1974) Horseshoe lung associated with a variant of the "scimitar" syndrome. Br Heart J 36:617.

24. Remy J, Marache P, Duplouy E, et al. (1976) Agenesies, aplasies et hypoplasies lobaires. J Radiol Electrol 57:197.

25. Cremin BSJ, Bass EM (1975) Retrosternal density: A sign of pulmonary hypoplasia. Pediatr Radiol 3:145.

26. Davis WS, Allen AP (1968) Accessory diaphragm. Radiol Clin North Am 6: 253.

27. Ang JGP, Proto A (1984) CT demonstration of congenital pulmonary venolobar syndrome. J Comput Assist Tomogr 8:753.

28. Godwin JD, Tarver RD (1986) Scimitar syndrome: Four new cases examined with CT. Radiology 159:15.

29. Benfield JR, Gots RE, Mills D (1971) Anomalous single left pulmonary vein mimicking a parenchymal nodule. Chest 59:101.

30. Moro C, Marín E, Sánchez A, et al. (1978) Pulmonary varix: Report of a case with additional anomalies of the vascular pulmonary tree. Am Heart J 95:243.

31. Chilton SJ, Canpbell JB (1978) Pulmonary varix in early infancy: Case report with 8-year follow-up. Radiology 129:400.

32. Goodman LR, Jamshidi A, Hipona FA (1971) Meandering right pulmonary vein simulating the scimitar syndrome. Chest 62:510.

33. Morgan JR, Focker AD (1971) Syndrome of hypoplasia of the right lung and dextroposition of the heart: "Scimitar sign" with normal pulmonary venous drainage. Circulation 43:27.

34. Herer B, Jaubert F, Delaisements C, et al (1988) Scimitar sign with normal pulmonary venous drainage and anomalous inferior vena cava. Thorax 43:651.

35. Collins DR, Shea PM, Vieweg WVR (1982) Idiopathic prominence of pulmonary veins on chest x-ray. Angiology 33:613.

36. Chassinat R (1836) Observations d'anomalies anatomiques remarquables de l'appareil circulatoire avec hépatocèle, n'ayant donné lieu pendant la vie à aucun symptôme particulier. Arch Gen Med (Paris) 11:80.

37. Folger GM (1976) The scimitar syndrome. Angiology 27:373.

38. Haworth SG, Sauer U, Bühlmeyer K (1983) Pulmonary hypertension in scimitar syndrome in infancy. Br Heart J 50:182.

39. Carter CE, Martin TC, Spray TL, et al. (1986) Scimitar syndrome in childhood. Am J Cardiol 58:652.

40. D'Cruz IA, Arcilla RA (1964) Anomalous venous drainage of the left lung into the inferior vena cava. Am Heart J 67:539.

41. Roehm JOF, Jue KL, Amplantz K (1966) Radiographic feature of the scimitar syndrome. Radiology 86:856.

42. Frank JL, Poole CA, Rosas G (1986) Horseshoe lung: Clinical, pathologic, and radiologic features and a new plain film finding. AJR 146:217.

43. Freedom RM, Burrows PE, Moes CAF (1986) "Horseshoe" lung: Report of five new cases. AJR 146:211.

44. Beitzke VA, Gypser G, Sager WD (1982) Scimitarsyndrom mit Hufeisenlunge. Rofo Fortschr Get Rontganstr Neurn Bildget 136:265.

45. Drake EH, Portland ME, Lynch JP (1950) Bronchiectasis associated with anomaly of the right pulmonary vein and right diaphragm. J Thorac Surg 19: 433.

46. Wille L, Holthusem W, Willich E (1975) Accessory diaphragm: Report of 6 cases and a review of the literature. Pediatr Radiol 4:14.

47. Ikeda T, Ishihara T, Yoshimatsu H, et al. (1972) Accessory diaphragm associated with congenital posterolateral diaphragmatic hernia, aberrant systemic artery to the right lower lobe, and anomalous pulmonary vein. J Thorac Cardiovasc Surg 64:18.

48. Nigogosyan G, Ozarda A (1961) Accessory diaphragm. AJR 85:309

49. Putgatch RD, Gale ME (1983) Obscure pulmonary masses: Bronchial impaction revealed by CT. AJR 141:909.

50. Cohen AM, Salomon EH, Alfidi RJ (1980) Computed tomography in bronchial atresia. AJR 135:1097.

51. Rogers LE, Osmer JC (1964) Bonchogenic cyst. A review of 46 cases. AJR 91:273.

52. Baker EM (1989) Intrathoracic duplication cyst: a review of 17 patients. J Med Imaging 3:127.

53. Stocker JT, Madewell JE, Drake RM (1977) Congenital cystic adenomatoid malformation of the lung. Hum Pathol 8:155.

54. Blane CE, Donn SM, Mori KW (1981) Congenital cystic adenomatoid malformation of the lung. J Comput Assist Tomogr 5:418.

55. Hulnick DH, Naidich DP, McCauley DI, et al. (1984) Late presentation of congenital cystic malformation of the lung. Radiology 151:569.

56. Savic B, Birtel FJ, Tholen W, et al. (1979) Lung sequestration: Report of seven cases and review of 540 published cases. Thorax 34:96.

57. Pessar ML, Soulen RL, Kan JS, et al. (1988) MRI demonstration of pulmonary sequestration. Pediatr Radiol 20:4.

58. Pryce DM, Holmes Sellors T, Blair LG (1947) Intralobar sequestration of lung associated with an abnormal artery. Br J Surg 35:18.

59. Mata JM, Cáceres J, Lucaya X (1991) CT diagnosis of isolated systemic supply to the lung: A congenital broncho-pulmonary vascular malformation. Eur J Radio 13:138.

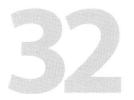

32 The Solitary Pulmonary Nodule: Radiologic Assessment

J.E. Takasugi and J.D. Godwin

Introduction

A solitary pulmonary nodule (SPN) is a discrete, rounded opacity without associated obstructive atelectasis, hilar or mediastinal lymphadenopathy or other significant lung abnormality (1,2). The accepted size limit of an SPN varies up to 6 cm (3), but most masses of this size are malignant and the discussion of whether or not to remove such a mass is inconsequential. Greater importance lies in the consideration of whether a smaller nodule represents a benign lesion that does not require surgical intervention versus an early malignancy that is potentially curable by local resection. We regard a nodule with a diameter less than 3 cm as an SPN; this size limit includes the majority of benign processes and also the lung cancers that are most likely to be curable.

Of all nodules detected by chest radiography, the majority are benign (4–6) (Table 32.1). Features useful in the discrimination of benign from malignant nodules fall into two categories: first, risk factors related to patient charac-

Table 32.1. Common causes of a solitary pulmonary nodule (SPN)

Benign
Granuloma (from tuberculosis, histoplasmosis, coccidiodomycosis)
Hamartoma, fibroma, lipoma
Infections (bacterial pneumonia, *Pneumocystis carinii* pneumonia, atypical mycobacterial infection)
Sarcoidosis, Wegeners' granulomatosis
Rheumatoid nodule
Arteriovenous malformation
Pulmonary infarction
Bronchogenic cyst
Bronchiolitis obliterans organizing pneumonia (BOOP)
Intrapulmonary lymph node

Malignant
Primary lung cancer (adenocarcinoma, bronchioloalveolar carcinoma, squamous cell, small cell, carcinoid tumor)
Metastasis (from primary site in head and neck, breast, colon, kidney, also from melanoma or sarcoma)

Table 32.2. Likelihood of malignancy patient factors

Patient factor	Greater likelihood of malignant diagnosis
Age	
<35 years	No
>50 years	Yes
Tobacco use	Yes
Known extrathoracic malignancy	Yes
Occupational exposure to carcinogens	Yes
Exposure to tuberculosis/fungi	No

teristics and habits (Table 32.2) and, second, imaging characteristics of the nodule. Compared to four decades ago, the percentage of resected nodules that are malignant has increased from about 15% (7) to over 50% (8,9), reflecting both improvements in preoperative distinction of benign from malignant nodules and the increasing incidence of lung cancer. Unfortunately, there is no single clinical or radiologic feature or group of features that will distinguish a benign nodule from a malignant nodule with 100% accuracy. In this chapter we review the radiologic studies commonly used in the evaluation of the SPN.

The Chest Radiograph

Technique

Currently, most chest radiographs are obtained using high energy photons (110–150 kilovolts kVp)), a wide-latitude film, and rare-earth phosphor screen. This technique provides excellent visualization of lung detail and penetration of mediastinal structures. A grid or air-gap is used to reduce scatter. A drawback of high kilovoltage is a reduction in the sensitivity to calcification within the nodule. This problem may be solved by using fluoroscopy at a lower kilovoltage or by using computed tomography (CT).

Nodule Detection

Chest radiography is the mainstay for detection of asymptomatic SPNs, but it has limitations. Nodules must be at least 9 mm in diameter before they are reliably detected on chest radiographs (10). Error rates in the identification of nodules are high, as many as 14% false-negative and 20% false-positive calls (11). On posteroanterior chest radiographs, up to 40% of the lung volume may be obscured by the heart, mediastinum, or diaphragm (12), limiting detection of nodules in these areas. Five percent to 10% of nodules may be visible only on the lateral view (1). It is possible that new techniques may aid in detection of nodules: digital radiolography helps to assure high quality of images, and scanning equalization radiolography (12) and computer processing of images (13) have promise.

Once a suspected nodule has been detected, a true nodule must be distinguished from a spurious one caused by extra-pulmonary structures. Up to 20% (14,15) of questioned lung nodules are produced by artefacts, skin nodules, or pleural or rib abnormalities (Figs 32.1, 32.2, 32.3). The cause of the spurious nodule can be determined through examination of the skin and external chest wall, or through fluoroscopy, rib films or, when necessary, by CT.

Nodule Characteristics

Two plain film criteria are helpful in distinguishing a benign from a malignant SPN. The first is calcification in one of a few specific patterns, and the second is the lack of growth over a long enough period of time. Other characteristics of the nodule – its margins and its size – will be considered, but they are not very helpful.

Calcification

Four patterns of calcification are associated with benign nodules (1,14,16) and essentially exclude malignancy if the nodule is single and well-defined and its margins are smooth or only slightly lobulated. Infectious granulomas

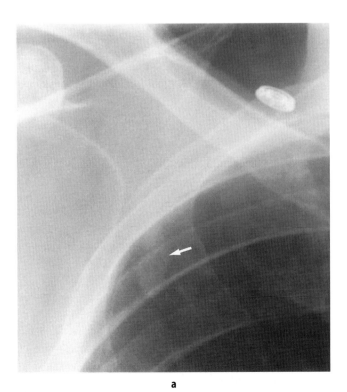

a

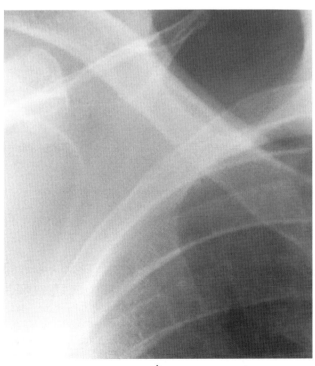

b

Figure 32.1. Radiograph of right upper lung (**a**) shows a button (*arrow*), mimicking a pulmonary nodule. With the button removed (**b**) it is obvious that the lung itself is clear. Notice small holes in button in (**a**).

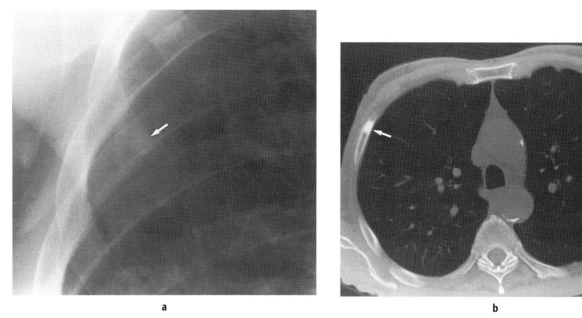

Figure 32.2. Radiograph (**a**) and axial CT scan using bone windows (**b**) show a sclerotic rib lesion – a bone island – (*arrows*) – mimicking a right upper lobe nodule.

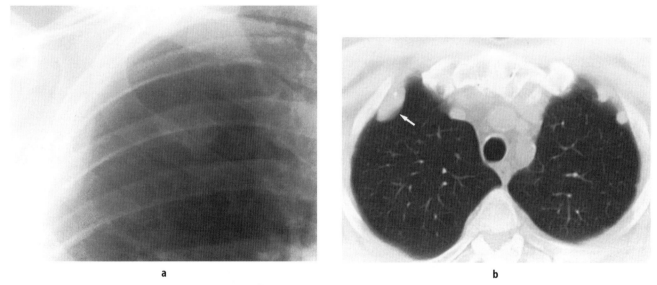

Figure 32.3. Radiograph (**a**) and CT scan (**b**) show an asbestos-related plaque (*arrow*) mimicking a right upper lobe nodule.

are the most common nodules with *diffuse* calcification (Fig. 32.4). Granulomas produced by histoplasmosis may also show *concentric or laminated* calcification (Fig. 32.5). The other two types of benign calcification are *dense, central* calcification and *popcorn* calcification (Fig. 32.6), both typically occurring in hamartomas.

Bronchogenic carcinomas and carcinoid tumors may also calcify, but the calcification is stippled or eccentric and the nodule often has irregular, lobulated, or spiculated margins. Typically, calcification in a lung cancer is not visible on plain radiographs, but only on CT.

Growth

In the 1960s and 1970s, the concept of doubling time, i.e., the time required for a nodule to double its volume (which requires an increase in diameter by a factor of only 1.26),

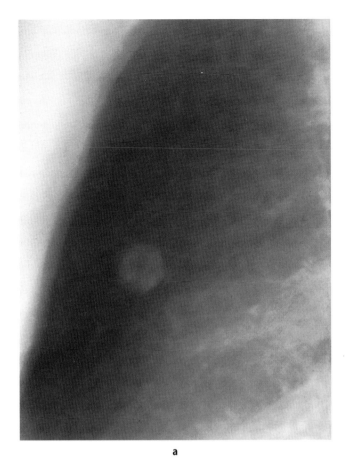

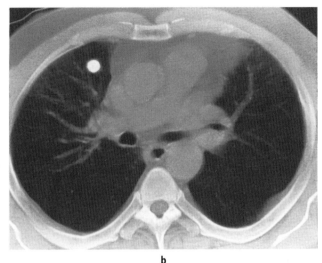

a

b

Figure 32.4. Lateral radiograph (**a**) and CT scan (bone window) (**b**) show a well-defined, smoothly marginated, diffusely calcified SPN, a granuloma caused by remote tuberculosis.

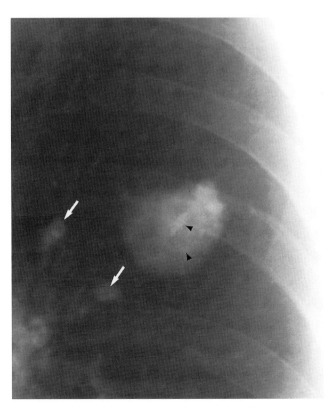

Figure 32.5. Radiograph shows concentric calcification (*arrowheads*) in a well-defined, fairly smooth, dominant nodule caused by histoplasmosis. Note two calcified, satellite nodules (*arrows*).

was proposed as a means to decide whether a nodule was benign or malignant (17). A nodule that doubles its volume in less than 1 month or longer than 18 months is usually benign. Exceptions occur on both ends of the time scale: lung cancers may double in less than 1 month and some nodules that remain unchanged for longer than 18 months may turn out to be cancers.

These days, doubling time is not used, but establishing stability by comparing current and old radiographs (preferably 2 or more years old) is used widely in predicting benignity. A recent analysis (18) examined the data behind the concept that 2 years of stability implies benignity. The predictive value was only 65%. Despite this low predictive value, the criterion of 2 years of stability continues to be considered useful.

If serial observation is to be used in managing an SPN, it is important that accurate measurements can be obtained and compared on follow-up examinations. When an SPN is small (less than 1.5 cm) or the margins are not clearly visible, serial chest radiography may not be accurate enough to detect the growth of an early malignancy and CT should be used instead to establish baseline dimensions and for follow-up.

Serial observation is particularly appropriate if the risk of cancer is low. A low risk might reflect patient factors, such as age less than 35 years in a nonsmoker who has no known extrathoracic malignancy, or it might reflect radio-

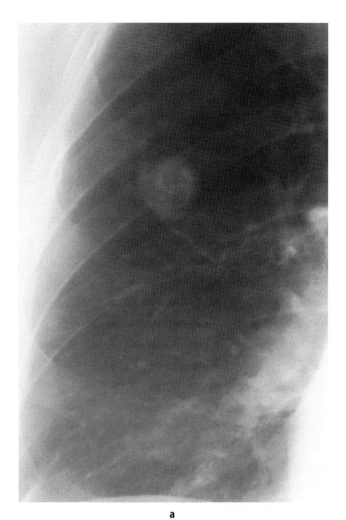

a

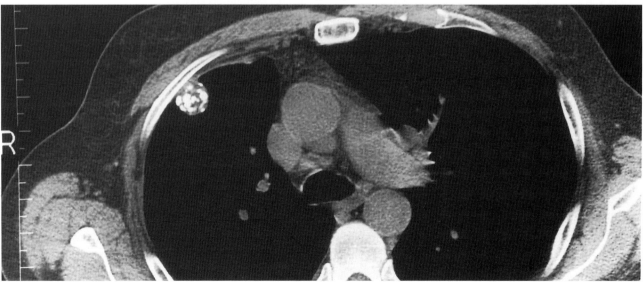

b

Figure 32.6. Radiograph (**a**) and CT scan (soft tissue window) (**b**) show a well-defined, smoothly marginated nodule with popcorn calcification typical of hamartoma.

logic factors, such as smooth margins of the nodule with a benign pattern of calcification or stability in size for 2 years.

The appropriate time interval between serial radiographs also varies depending on clinical setting. In a patient who presents with an acute process and some risk factors for malignancy, a nodular opacity on chest radiographs may be observed by serial films every 2 weeks for a total of 4 weeks (16). Inflammatory and infectious processes may shrink or completely resolve during this period, obviating further investigation. Waiting longer than four weeks in the hope that a nodule will decrease in size is inadvisable. In a young, asymptomatic patient with a low risk of cancer and a smoothly marginated, clearly visible and easily measurable, noncalcified nodule, serial

chest radiographs might be obtained at 3 month intervals for the first year and 6 month intervals for the second year (1). Once two years of stability have been established, longer observation is advocated by a number of authors (16,18–20), although a specified time interval has not yet been suggested. We propose that additional films be obtained every 2 years for a total of 5 years.

Margins

The characteristics of the margins of the nodule are not specific for malignancy or benignity, although a spiculated margin is worrisome. A spiculated margin is characteristic of bronchogenic carcinoma (Fig. 32.7); however, a benign

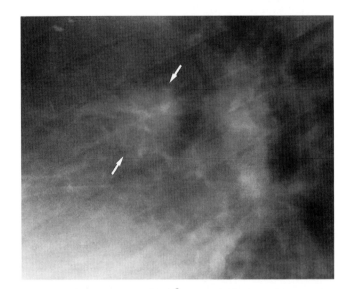

a

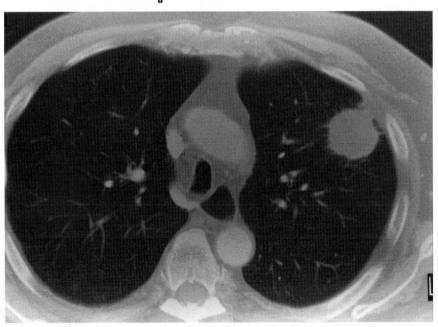

b

Figure 32.7. Lateral radiograph (**a**) and CT scan (**b**) show a 3 cm, spiculated, left upper lobe nodule (*arrows*) caused by non small-cell lung cancer.

lesion, such as a focal pneumonia, a septic or bland pulmonary embolus, or a lung abscess, may also have a spiculated margin. A smooth margin is typical for a benign lesion, such as a granuloma. However, it can occur with some lung cancers (Fig. 32.8) and it occurs with most metastases (Fig. 32.9). In one study (21) of 91 nodules with spiculated margins, 80 (88%) were malignant. In the same study, 78 of 128 (44%) nodules with smooth margins were also malignant.

Computed Tomography

CT has had a major impact on the evaluation of the SPN, not only in characterization of the nodule itself, but also in detection of additional nodules, staging of a nodule thought to be malignant, and in follow-up of an indeterminate nodule in selected patients. An indeterminate SPN is a noncalcified, smooth or minimally lobulated nodule less than 3 cm in diameter.

Nodule Characteristics

Specific patterns of calcification, the presence of fat, and lack of growth are reliable CT signs of benignity. CT, particularly high resolution CT (HRCT), is much more sensitive than radiography in the detection of both calcification and fat because of its greater contrast resolution. In order to avoid edge enhancement artefacts and achieve accurate densitometry, it is advisable to use a smooth or standard

Size

As we have already defined an SPN as being under 3 cm, the absolute size under this 3 cm limit does not have any further predictive value in determining whether the nodule is benign or malignant. Masses larger than 3 cm are often malignant (1), but smaller nodules can be benign or malignant. In a study of 177 lung cancers, 42% of the cancers were smaller than 2 cm (21).

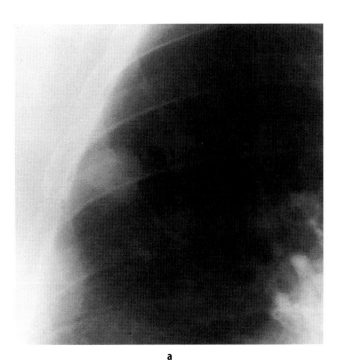

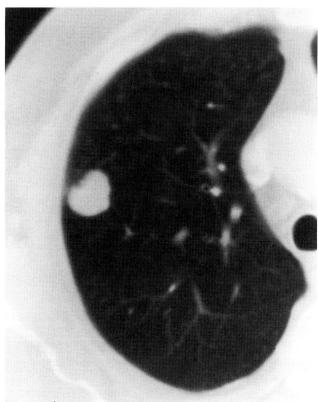

a   b

Figure 32.8. Radiograph (**a**) and CT scan (**b**) show a 2 cm, well-defined, smoothly marginated, right upper lobe nodule caused by a primary squamous carcinoma.

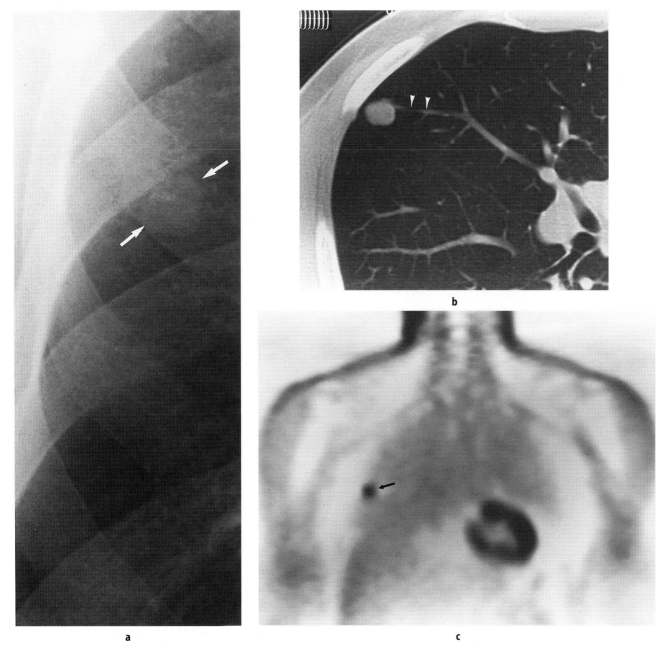

Figure 32.9. Radiograph **a**, and CT scan **b** and ^{18}F-FDG-PET scan (**c**), showing a 1.5 cm, well-defined, smoothly marginated, right middle lobe nodule (*arrows*) caused by metastatic melanoma. Note feeding vessel (*arrowheads*) on CT.

reconstruction algorithm instead of a sharp algorithm. CT is also more precise in the determination of nodule size than is plain radiography and this makes CT more reliable for determining growth or stability of the nodule.

Calcification

Benign patterns of calcification can be visualized in nodules on CT images just as on chest films

(Figs. 32.4,32.6). However, thin-section CT is more sensitive in the detection of calcification than is radiography or conventional tomography. Low grade diffuse (uniform) calcification may be detectable only by CT. In an early study by Siegelman et al. (6), 634 nodules, all thought to be noncalcified and thus indeterminate by conventional tomography, underwent CT densitometry. Ninety benign nodules (14%) were distinguishable by means of high attenuation values, thought to represent diffuse calcification. From this study, it initially

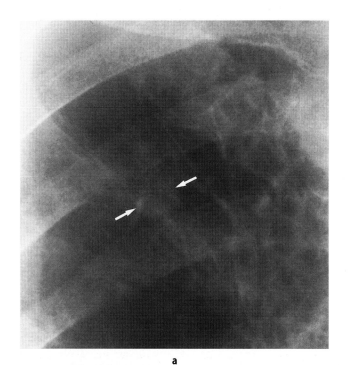

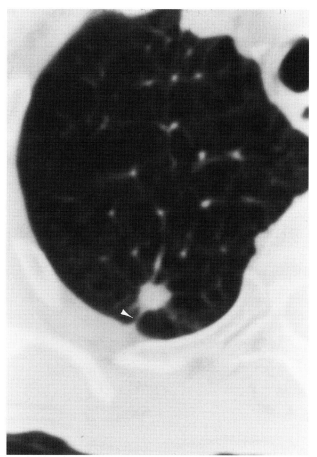

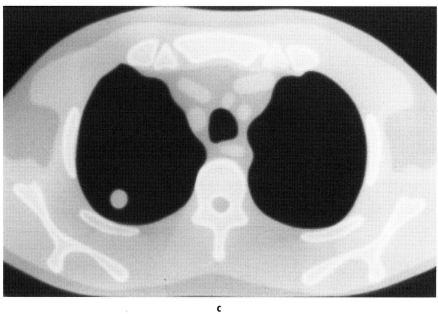

Figure 32.10. Radiograph (**a**) and CT scan (**b**) show a 1 cm, spiculated, right upper lobe nodule (*arrows*) caused by a primary adenocarcinoma. Note pleural tail on CT image (*arrowhead*). CT scan through the reference phantom (**c**) shows the selected "nodule" of similar size and location as the patient's nodule.

appeared that a numerical criterion based on attenuation values could objectively distinguish many benign nodules on the basis of their density. However, attempts to reproduce these results using this numerical criterion for calcification failed because of the variability of attenuation values among different scanners and even in the same scanner over time. For this reason a reference phantom (22) was created as a mean of standardization. The phantom could be adjusted to simulate the size of the patient, the size and location of the nodule and the presence of mediastinal structures on the CT slice of interest. A pulmonary nodule that showed greater attenuation than the reference nodule was considered to be calcified (Fig. 32.10).

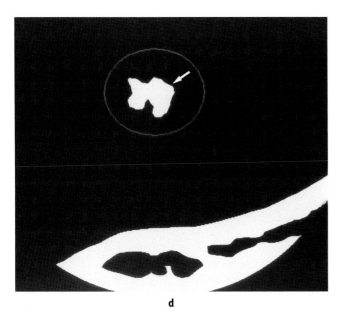

Figure 32.10. CT scan (**d**) through the patient's nodule shows the window and level settings at which the reference nodule disappears. All areas of the patient's nodule that remain visible at these settings (*arrow*) are more dense than the reference nodule and are thus considered to be calcified. The white ring indicates the margin of the nodule on standard lung windows. Although more than 10% of the patient's nodule is calcified and the calcification is central in location, the nodule was not smoothly marginated and therefore did not satisfy all the requirements for a benign nodule.

Although the phantom succeeded in removing some variability in CT densitometry, problems remained, including basic biology. One problem is that not all calcified nodules are benign. Up to 14% (23) of malignant nodules showed at least some calcification. Again, the patterns of malignant calcification, fine, speckled, or eccentric, are different from the patterns of benign calcification. The criteria for benignity used with the phantom include: nodule size less than 3 cm, relatively smooth margins, and attenuation values higher than those of the reference phantom; in addition, at least 10% of the nodule should be calcified, with a central, diffuse, laminated, or popcorn pattern. Even under these circumstances the nodule should be followed to demonstrate lack of growth for at least 2 years (14). Thus CT densitometry, even with the reference phantom, still requires careful consideration and follow-up. There is no simple numeric criterion that can replace judgment.

Fat

A pulmonary hamartoma is a benign tumor arising from the fibrous connective tissue within bronchial walls. Fat is visible histologically in 50% of hamartomas (14,24) and has been demonstrated by CT in 28 of 47 small hamartomas (24). Criteria for the CT diagnosis of hamartoma include a smooth margin with diameter of 2.5 cm or less, and the presence of fat, with or without calcification (24) (Fig. 32.11). Attenuation values between −40 and

−120 Hounsfield units (HU) are considered to reflect fat, whereas values greater than −10 HU might reflect central necrosis, and values less than −200 HU might reflect cavitation. The CT features of hamartoma were never found in lung cancers or metastases ($n = 133$) of the same size and margination. Nodules fulfilling the CT criteria for hamartomas should be observed and not resected unless they exceed 2.5 cm diameter, become symptomatic, or begin to grow rapidly (24).

Growth

In order to accurately determine growth, nodule dimensions must be measured and compared over time. The nodules most difficult to measure accurately are small (less than 1 cm in diameter), indistinct in margination, or obscured by the diaphragm, hilus, mediastinum, or bones. Chest radiography may be satisfactory in comparing sizes over time in larger nodules. However, in smaller nodules, changes in diameter of 1 or 2 mm may be significant, and these small changes are more easily appreciated on CT scans. With thin sections (1–3 mm collimation depending on the diameter of the nodule), accurate measurements can be obtained on all but the smallest nodules. A baseline CT is recommended for any small nodule that will be observed over time (18). A nodule should be measured on lung windows rather than mediastinal (soft tissue) windows (25).

Size

As with chest radiography, size (within the 3 cm limit used to define an SPN) is not an accurate means of distinguishing benign from malignant nodules by CT.

Margins

The margins of an SPN are better characterized by CT, particularly HRCT, than by conventional chest radiographs. Well-defined and ill-defined interfaces between the nodule and the adjacent lung (as distinct from smooth, lobulated or irregular margins) can occur with either benign or malignant nodules and are not discriminative (Figs. 32.7, 32.8, 32.9). Spiculated and lobulated margins are particularly suggestive of malignancy (16), but can be found with infectious and inflammatory diseases, such as tuberculosis, inflammatory pseudotumors, and postinflammatory scars. Smooth margins suggest benignity, but may occasionally occur in primary lung cancers and occur commonly in hematogenous metastases. The "CT halo sign," a border of ground-glass opacity

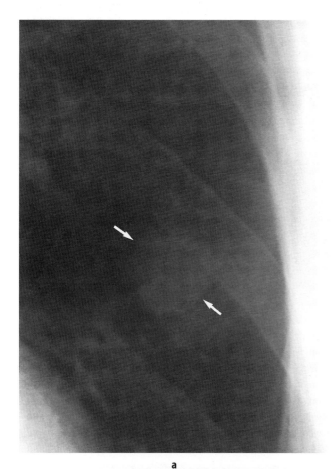

a

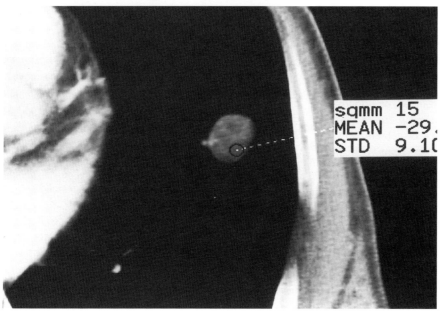

b

Figure 32.11. Radiograph (**a**) and contrast-enhanced, CT scan (**b**) show a 2 cm, smoothly marginated, left lower lobe nodule (*arrows*) in a patient with known colon carcinoma. The CT scan demonstrates inhomogeneous attenuation, with some areas near fat density (−29 HU), suggesting hamartoma, as was confirmed by percutaneous biopsy.

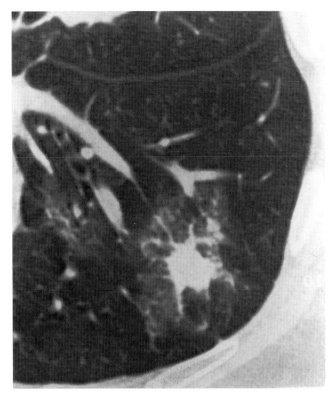

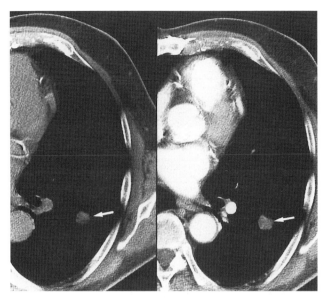

Figure 32.13. CT scan before (**a**) and after (**b**) the administration of intravenous contrast material in a male smoker shows a left lower lobe nodule (*arrows*). Nodule attenuation increased from –5 HU on precontrast scans to 28 HU on postcontrast scans. A 1.5 cm primary adenocarcinoma was found at thoracotomy.

Figure 32.12. CT scan shows an irregularly marginated, 1 cm, left lower lobe nodule with a halo of ground-glass opacity (CT halo) caused by invasive aspergillosis in a bone marrow transplant patient.

surrounding a denser central nodule (Fig. 32.12), is found in a number of benign lesions (26) such as invasive aspergillosis, cytomegalovirus infection, herpes simplex pneumonia, coccidioidomycosis, infarct, Wegener granulomatosis, *Pneumocystis carinii* pneumonia (27), and also in some cases of bronchioloalveolar cell carcinoma and metastases from vascular primary tumors, such as angiosarcoma or Kaposi sarcoma.

Contrast Enhancement

In 1992 Swensen et al. (28) reported preliminary results on the use of contrast enhancement as a means of distinguishing benign from malignant SPNs. Nonionic contrast given at a rate of 2 mls^{-1} for 50 s was preceded and followed by thin section scans through the nodule every minute for 5 mins. The degree of contrast enhancement, calculated as the mean postcontrast attenuation values minus the mean precontrast attenuation values, was greater than 20 HU during the first 2 min of scanning in all 23 of the malignant but only one of the seven benign nodules. Since then, a number of reports (29–34) have documented that malignant nodules enhance to a greater

degree than most benign nodules (Fig. 32.13). The sensitivity of this finding for diagnosis of malignancy ranges from 93% to 100% and the specificity from 73% to 85% (29,32). Granulomas and hamartomas show contrast enhancement greater than 20 HU only rarely (28,29,33). However, acute or subacute inflammatory lesions often show contrast enhancement (31). The pattern of nodule enhancement – whether complete, peripheral, or capsular – may prove useful in further discrimination of benign from malignant enhancing SPNs (33), but additional investigation is still needed.

Pleural Tail Sign

A pleural tail, i.e., a linear extension from the surface of a pulmonary nodule to the adjacent visceral pleural surface (Fig. 32.10b), is not useful in distinguishing a benign from a malignant SPN. A pleural tail represents a thickened, fibrotic connective tissue septum that may retract the visceral pleura inward. A pleural tail can be associated with a scar, a scar carcinoma, or a tuberculoma (35,36).

Air Bronchogram Sign

Air bronchograms may occur within an SPN caused by lung cancer, particularly by bronchioloalveolar cell carci-

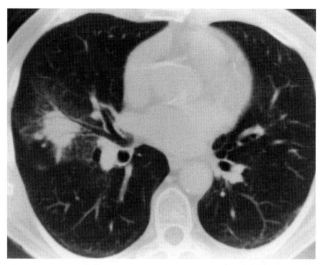

Figure 32.14. CT scan in a cigarette smoker shows a nonresolving, ill-defined, 3 cm, right middle lobe nodule caused by bronchioloalveolar carcinoma. Note airbronchograms.

noma (Fig. 32.14), or by lymphoma. Benign nodules, such as focal pneumonitis, radiation fibrosis, or nodular sarcoidosis (37), less commonly contain air bronchograms. In a retrospective review of 132 patients with SPNs (38), only one of 17 benign lesions had air bronchograms, whereas 33 of 115 lung cancers did.

Pseudocavitation

Small collections of air producing bubble-like lucencies or pseudocavitation (Fig. 32.15) may occur in a spiculated SPN. In the absence of clinical signs of infection, their presence suggests the diagnosis of bronchioloalveolar carcinoma or adenocarcinoma (39,40,41). The small gas collections may represent air within ectatic bronchioles or, in the setting of bronchioloalveolar carcinoma, air within cystic spaces in papillary regions of the tumor (39). The pseudocavitation in bronchioloalveolar carcinomas must be distinguished from the air trapped within a mycetoma (Fig. 32.16). Usually, the outer margins of the cavity containing the mycetoma is smoother than the spiculated margins of a bronchioloalveolar carcinoma, and there is often, although not always, a sliver of air separating the mycetoma from the cavity wall.

Feeding Vessel

Identification of a vessel leading to the medial margin of an SPN on HRCT images may be useful in distinguishing nonhematogenous from hematogenous dissemination and thus a primary lung tumor from a blood-borne metastasis (Fig. 32.9b). The presence of a feeding vessel is not specific

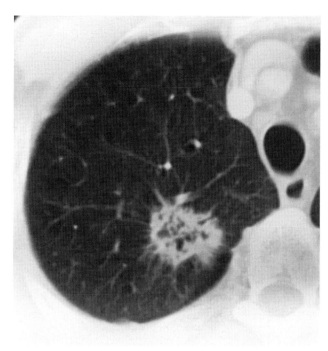

Figure 32.15. CT scan shows a spiculated, 2.5 cm bronchioloalveolar carcinoma with pseudocavitation and ectatic bronchioles.

for metastasis; it may also occur with a pulmonary infarct or septic embolus (42–44).

Other Lesions with Distinctive CT Characteristics

There are a few other nodules that have almost pathognomic appearances on CT scans. An arteriovenous malformation is a serpiginous lesion with a feeding artery and draining vein and maximum enhancement during the pulmonary arterial phase of scanning (Fig. 32.17). A mycetoma is a mobile, air-containing fungal nodule that arises in a preexisting cavity (Fig. 32.16). Round atelectasis is a homogeneously enhancing, subpleural mass of contracted lung with vessels or airways curving into it and with overlying pleural thickening (Fig. 32.18).

Helical CT

Helical or spiral CT makes it possible to scan through the entire lung more quickly and with fewer registration artefacts than with conventional (incremental) CT scanning. One problem with helical CT scanning in the evaluation of the small SPN (less than 10 mm) is that calcification is not as accurately depicted as with conventional CT unless narrow collimation is used. Further, edge-enhancing

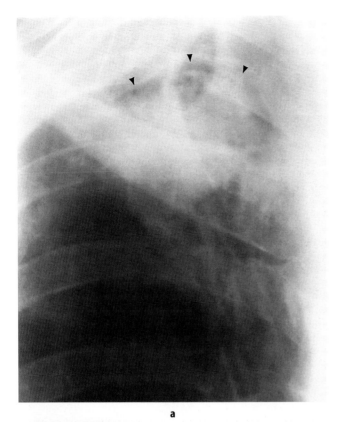

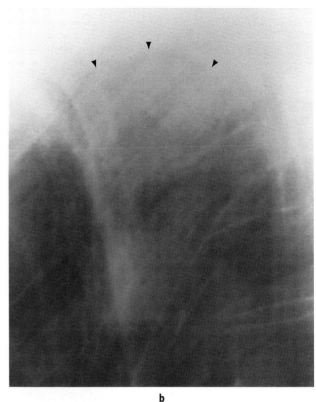

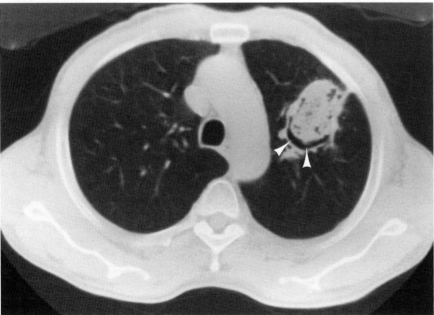

Figure 32.16. Frontal (**a**) and lateral (**b**) radiographs shows a 3 cm, right upper lobe mycetoma caused by Aspergillus, and a prone CT scan (**c**) shows a left upper lobe mycetoma in a different patient. Air trapped within the mycetoma may be mistaken for the pseudocavitation seen in bronchioloalveolar carcinoma. However, the outer margin of the mycetoma-containing cavity is smoother than the spiculated margin of a carcinoma; the mycetoma is often mobile; and non-dependent air (*arrowheads*) is usually present in the cavity containing the mycetoma.

reconstruction algorithms used in spiral CT do not render accurate CT numbers. Therefore, any evaluation of possible calcification within a nodule will require rescanning with narrow collimation and standard or smooth reconstruction algorithm.

Solitary versus Multiple Nodules

Whether a nodule is truly solitary or whether multiple nodules are actually present is important in the subsequent evaluation of the patient with an apparently solitary nodule

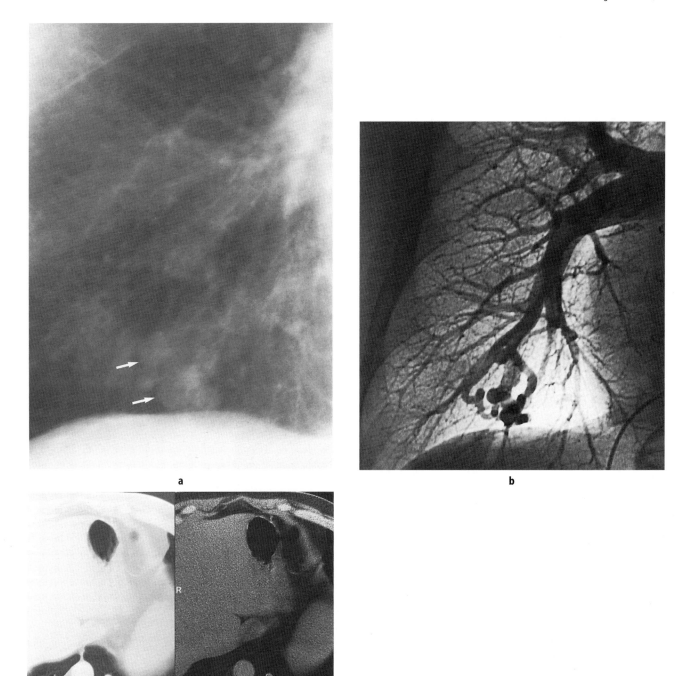

Figure 32.17. Radiograph (**a**) and pulmonary arteriogram (**b**) show a lobulated, 2 cm, right lower lobe nodule caused by an arteriovenous fistula (*arrows*). Contrast-enhanced CT scan (**c**) in a different patient with arteriovenous fistula shows serpiginous, enhancing blood vessels. Enlarged feeding artery and draining vein were visible on other images.

detected on chest radiographs. Multiple primary lung cancers are rare, occurring in only 1–3% of cases (16,45), although a recent article suggests they may be more common (46). A solitary lung cancer may coexist with multiple granulomata (Fig. 32.19) or the patient may not have

lung cancer at all, but rather multiple metastases from an extrathoracic source. Helical CT scanning with a single breath-hold detects a greater number of nodules than conventional CT (47,48) and is the preferred method for screening the lungs of a patient with an apparently solitary nodule.

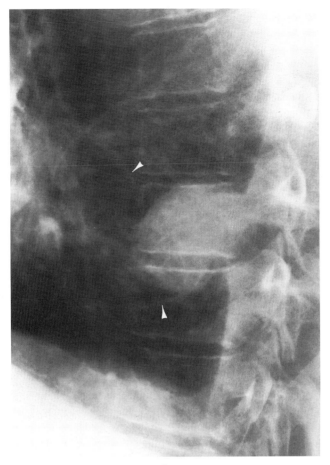

a

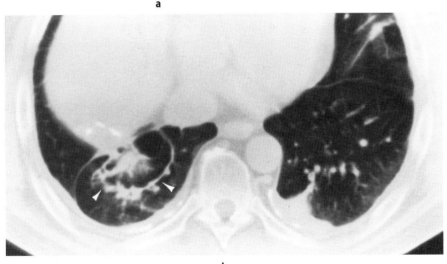

b

Figure 32.18. Lateral radiograph (a) shows a 3 cm, right lower lobe nodule caused by round atelectasis. Note associated pleural thickening and lung structures (*arrowheads*) curving toward the nodule. CT scan (b) in a different patient with right lower lobe round atelectasis shows asbestos pleural plaques, right lower lobe volume loss with displacement of fissures, and lung vessels curving toward the nodule (*arrowheads*).

Accuracy of CT in Detection of Lung Nodules

Until recently, CT has not been used to screen the lungs of patients at risk for primary lung cancer and therefore the accuracy of CT in lung cancer detection has not yet been evaluated. However, the accuracy of CT in the detection of multiple lung nodules has been assessed, using surgical findings as the standard. The sensitivity of conventional CT for the detection of lung metastases is between 51% and 73% (44). Nodules were missed because of motion artefacts (respiratory and cardiac), misregistration of CT slices between breath-holds, obscuration by other opacities in the lungs, misinterpretation of the nodule as a vessel, and small diameter of the nodule (less than 3 mm).

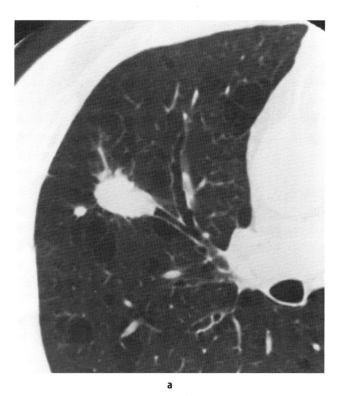
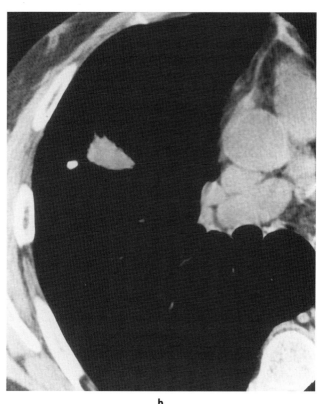

a   b

Figure 32.19. CT scans using lung (**a**) and mediastinal (soft tissue) (**b**) windows show a 2 cm, spiculated, nonsmall-cell carcinoma occluding the lateral segmental bronchus of the right middle lobe (CT bronchus sign). Note small calcified granuloma posterolateral to the dominant nodule.

With helical scanning, CT has improved even further in the detection of lung nodules (47,48). Nodules of 2–3 mm are frequently detected (49) and image degradation by respiratory or cardiac motion is less frequent. Radiologists have learned how to disregard partial-volume artefacts and may scroll through images on monitors in order to help to distinguish nodules from vessels.

Unfortunately, many of the additional nodules detected by current scanners will be false positives that may require some other test in order to exclude malignancy (44). The specificity of CT for the detection of malignancy will decline as CT is put into use for screening patients at risk for primary lung cancer. The decision of whether to observe or biopsy or remove one of these nodules will depend on the presence or absence or risk factors for malignancy, the results of physiologic tests (such as positron emission tomography (PET)), the expected operative morbidity and mortality, and the patient's own treatment preferences.

Positron Emission Tomography Using ^{18}F-FDG

Technique

The high metabolic rate of malignant tumors can be used to distinguish them from benign nodules. PET scanning uses 2-(fluorine-18) fluoro-2-deoxy-D-glucose (FDG), a positron-emitting glucose analog, to detect tumors with rapid glucose turnover (50). ^{18}F-FDG is transported across cell membranes by glucose transport receptors and phosphorylated to ^{18}F-FDG 6-phosphatase, in which form it accumulates within cells. Positrons emitted by ^{18}F are annihilated with the release of 511 keV photons, which are detected by coincidence and mapped by the scanner.

Images may be displayed in axial, coronal (Fig. 32.9c) or sagittal projections, and total body images may be generated for the purpose of cancer staging. Quantitative analysis of the SPN is based on calculation of the standard uptake value (SUV). The SUV is the mean activity of the region of interest divided by the injected dose over body weight.

Accuracy

An SUV over 2.5 is highly suggestive of malignancy with sensitivity ranging from 82% to 100% and specificity from 70% to 89% (51–59). False-positive scans can be caused by inflammatory nodules, as occur in tuberculosis (51,58,59), histoplasmosis (58), cryptococcosis (59), anthrasilicosis (51), and rheumatoid lung disease (50). False-negative scans may occur with bronchioloalveolar carcinoma (59,60), lung carcinoid (61), a tumor that is too small to be resolved (6–10 mm diameter on current scanners) (52,55,57), and in the presence of hyperglycemia, since FDG competes with glucose for entry into cells (58). A negative FDG-PET scan is associated with a 4.7% chance of malignancy (54).

Biopsy

Fiberoptic Bronchoscopy and Transbronchial Biopsy (TBB)

In a patient with evidence of central airway involvement by an SPN, TBB can provide tissue diagnosis. The CT-bronchus sign (i.e., an airway leading directly to the SPN) (Fig. 32.19) predicts successful diagnosis (90%) by TBB when the bronchus is a first subsegmental branch or larger (61). If the CT-bronchus sign involves a smaller bronchus, successful biopsy is less likely.

In a patient with a peripheral SPN, the likelihood of accurate diagnosis by TBB is lower (28–73%) (62–64) than by transthoracic biopsy (TTB), which is over 90% accurate (61,65–67), and the yield of TBB decreases with decreasing size of the nodule. Transbronchial biopsy of a peripheral SPN is performed under fluoroscopic guidance and pneumothorax is less common than with transthoracic biopsy.

Fluoroscopically Guided Transthoracic Biopsy (TTB)

Technique

For an SPN that is visible on both posteroanterior and lateral chest radiographs, fluoroscopically guided TTB is an excellent method to obtain tissue. The needle is aligned with the nodule in the frontal plane and advanced into the nodule under fluoroscopic observation in the lateral pro-

jection. Specimens may be obtained with a fine needle (20–22 gauge) to aspirate material for cytology and bacteriologic studies or with a cutting or a spring-loaded needle to obtain a core of tissue (18–22 gauge) for cytologic, bacteriologic or histologic assessment. Fluoroscopically guided needle biopsy is usually quicker than CT-guided biopsy and can sometimes be performed on a patient who is too large for the CT scanner (68).

Accuracy

In the hands of an experienced radiologist, the sensitivity of transthoracic needle aspiration in the diagnosis of malignancy is 70–96.5% (69–74). In the absence of a specific benign diagnosis, such as harmartoma or granuloma, a negative aspirate does not exclude malignancy, and further evaluation with a second aspirate, surgical resection, or close follow-up is indicated depending on the level of suspicion of malignancy (70).

Complications

Complications from this procedure are usually minor, consisting of minor hemoptysis (8%) and pneumothorax (5–27%); tube thoracostomy is required in 0–15% of cases of pneumothorax (68,70–74).

CT-Guided Transthoracic Biopsy

Currently CT is the most common method for guiding biopsy of the lung. CT can be used: (a) to biopsy nodules that are visible on only one view of orthogonal chest radiographs; (b) to avoid penetration of vessel, other vital structure, or a bulla; (c) to document that the tissue sampled is from the lesion and not from adjacent lung; (d) to obtain tissue from the margin of a necrotic or cavitary nodule; and (e) to guide a complex or angled approach to the lesion.

CT-guided biopsy usually takes longer than fluoroscopically guided biopsy, often requiring 45–90 mins.

Technique

The patient is positioned for access to the SPN via the shortest and straightest course that avoids bones, vital structures, vessels, and bullae. Multiple specimens may be obtained using a single lung puncture if a coaxial needle system is used. The outer needle of the coaxial system is planted in the tissue of the chest wall and angled appropriately at the nodule using CT guidance. When the patient has exhaled, the needle is advanced to the edge of the nodule and its position is documented by CT. A higher-gauge inner needle is passed into the nodule and tissue is obtained as the patient holds his or her breath at end-expiration.

Complications

Pneumothorax occurs at a slightly higher rate (0–60%) than with fluoroscopically guided biopsy (68) and requires treatment, usually only with a small-bore tube, in 0–15%. The risk of pneumothorax is independent of size of the biopsy needle (18–22 gauge) (75–77), but is related to the number of pleural punctures. Hemorrhage into the lung around the needle tract may be visible on postbiopsy images, but most patients who have this finding do not experience hemoptysis. Significant bleeding occurs in less than 5% (68). Cases of air embolism caused by TTB are rare, but they can lead to death, stroke, or myocardial infarction. Air is thought to be introduced through the inadvertent creation of a bronchovenous or alveolovenous fistula by the biopsy needle (68), sometimes during the deep inspiration preceding a cough. If air embolism is recognized early, the patient should be placed in the left lateral decubitus position to prevent air from exiting the left atrium and entering the systemic circulation. Transthoracic biopsies should not be performed in patients with intractable cough, those who cannot maintain the necessary position for at least 30 mins, or those who cannot control their respiratory rate and depth. Malignant seeding of the needle-tract is extremely rare (68).

Accuracy

For the diagnosis of malignancy, CT-guided TTB has a sensitivity between 70% and 100% and a false-positive rate of less than 1% (68). For the diagnosis of a benign condition that obviates further diagnostic evaluation for malignancy, TTB has a yield of 16–68% (65,70,78). Some suggestions to improve the yield of a specific diagnosis by TTB include having the expert cytopathologist immediately available to determine the adequacy of the tissue sample before the patient is released from the CT suite (79,80), obtaining the full complement of special stains and cultures of aspirated material, repeated sampling of various portions of the lung lesion, and using core specimens when aspirates are insufficient (68,75,77). When neither a malignant nor a specific benign diagnosis has been achieved by TTB, a significant number of SPNs (18–69%) have subsequently turned out to be malignant (11,66,71,81). As with fine-needle aspiration biopsy, a non-

specific diagnosis must be followed by additional biopsy, PET scanning, surgical resection, or close observation.

A minor difficulty is the subclassification of lung cancers based on TTB. Identification of the specific histologic type is only about 80% accurate on cytologic specimens, whereas it is much higher on resected or postmortem specimens (68). The greatest difficulty is in distinguishing the subtypes of nonsmall-cell cancer. Currently, treatment protocols distinguish only between small-cell and nonsmall-cell carcinomas. Should different kinds of non-small cell carcinomas eventually require different treatments, then biopsy and cytologic techniques will need to advance.

Video-Assisted Thoracoscopic Wedge-Resection

Video-assisted thoracoscopic surgery (VATS) and, in particular, video-assisted thoracoscopic wedge-resection (VATWR) have had an impact on the evaluation of the SPN (82–85).

Technique

In this procedure (82), three 1–2 cm incisions are made in intercostal spaces near the SPN. The scope and attached video camera are introduced through one incision and surgical instruments through the other two. The procedure is performed under general anesthesia, with unilateral ventilation of the opposite lung. When the lung containing the SPN collapses, the SPN may cause a visible or palpable abnormality of the visceral pleura. In the absence of either of these features, the SPN may be difficult to find, and the surgeon may rely on estimates of its position from the preoperative CT scan or on preoperative, CT-guided needle localization or methylene blue injection (86–88). A wedge of lung containing the SPN is isolated by an endoscopic stapling tool or by laser, placed in a bag, and removed through one of the incisions. If the nodule is malignant on frozen-section, an open thoracotomy may be performed for lobectomy and node sampling. If the nodule is benign, the patient is spared thoracotomy.

Complications

Prolonged air leak occurs in 5–10% and significant bleeding in 1.6% (89,90). Conversion from VATS to standard thoracotomy may be necessitated by difficulty in locating the nodule, which occurs in up to 14.4% of cases (82,84,91), or by technical problems with instrumentation, which occur in up to 6% (93). Compared with limited thoracotomy and wedge-resection, VATWR causes less pain and permits earlier discharge (85). Mortality is less than 1% in most series (84,91–93).

Accuracy and Limitations

VATWR is the most accurate means of diagnosing an SPN short of thoracotomy. A specific benign or malignant diagnosis is made in 97–100% of patients (66,82,85,94). There are some SPNs that are not amenable to VATWR, such as lesions that are too deep in the parenchyma or too near the hilum (82). For a deep nodule, biopsy or PET scanning assumes a more important role, since VATWR is not an

option. Extensive pleural adhesion precludes the use of the VATS in some patients.

Conclusion and Recommendations

Significant advances have been made in the evaluation of the SPN. In the last decade, helical CT, PET scanning, and VATS have emerged. Any current strategy for evaluation of the SPN must incorporate these new techniques and integrate them appropriately and flexibly in different clinical settings. We summarize our current approach in Tables 32.3A and 32.3B.

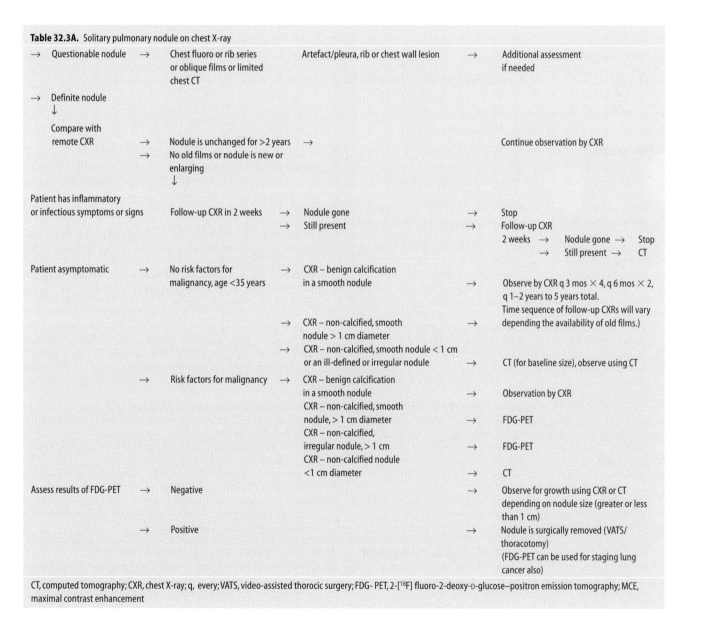

Table 32.3A. Solitary pulmonary nodule on chest X-ray

→ Questionable nodule	→	Chest fluoro or rib series or oblique films or limited chest CT	Artefact/pleura, rib or chest wall lesion	→	Additional assessment if needed
→ Definite nodule ↓					
Compare with remote CXR	→ →	Nodule is unchanged for >2 years No old films or nodule is new or enlarging ↓	→		Continue observation by CXR
Patient has inflammatory or infectious symptoms or signs		Follow-up CXR in 2 weeks	→ Nodule gone → Still present	→ →	Stop Follow-up CXR 2 weeks → Nodule gone → Stop → Still present → CT
Patient asymptomatic	→	No risk factors for malignancy, age <35 years	→ CXR – benign calcification in a smooth nodule	→	Observe by CXR q 3 mos × 4, q 6 mos × 2, q 1–2 years to 5 years total. Time sequence of follow-up CXRs will vary depending the availability of old films.)
			→ CXR – non-calcified, smooth nodule > 1 cm diameter	→	
			→ CXR – non-calcified, smooth nodule < 1 cm or an ill-defined or irregular nodule	→	CT (for baseline size), observe using CT
	→	Risk factors for malignancy	→ CXR – benign calcification in a smooth nodule	→	Observation by CXR
			CXR – non-calcified, smooth nodule, > 1 cm diameter	→	FDG-PET
			CXR – non-calcified, irregular nodule, > 1 cm	→	FDG-PET
			CXR – non-calcified nodule <1 cm diameter	→	CT
Assess results of FDG-PET	→	Negative		→	Observe for growth using CXR or CT depending on nodule size (greater or less than 1 cm)
	→	Positive		→	Nodule is surgically removed (VATS/thoracotomy) (FDG-PET can be used for staging lung cancer also)

CT, computed tomography; CXR, chest X-ray; q, every; VATS, video-assisted thoracic surgery; FDG- PET, 2-[18F] fluoro-2-deoxy-D-glucose–positron emission tomography; MCE, maximal contrast enhancement

Table 32.3B. Results of CT (CT used in place of FDG-PET if FDG-PET not locally available)

Nodule margins:	→ Smooth →	Nodule attenuation (use reference phantom if available) →		
			>10% of nodule calcified, benign type calcifications with or without fat →	Observe for growth by CXR or limited CT scans depending on nodule size
		→	< 10% of nodule calcified →	MCE determination
		→	Psammomatous or speckled calcification →	Surgical removal (VATS/thoracotomy)
	→ Noncalcified, fat present		→	Observe for growth by CXR or limited CT scans depending on nodule size
	→ Noncalcified, no fat		→	MCE determination
	Irregular, spiculated, lobulated		→	VATS resection if accessible

Results of MCE calculation

MCE <20 H.U.	→	Observe or VATS resection
MCE >20 H.U.	→	VATS resection if accessible

VATS resection not possible and tissue diagnosis is necessary

Nodule location/size →	Central/large →	Transbronchial biopsy	Specific benign diagnosis →	Stop
→	Central/small →	Transthoracic biopsy →	malignant diagnosis →	Treatment
→	Peripheral →	Transthoracic biopsy	nondiagnostic →	Repeat biopsies
			→	Close observation

For abbreviations, see Table 32.3A.

CT refers to visual inspection of finely collimated scans through the nodule, CT densitometry, CT performed with and without intravenous contrast material to help characterize the SPN (MCE determination) or full chest CT performed to document the presence of a single or multiple pulmonary nodule(s), or to help stage a suspected lung cancer.

References

1. Midthun DE, Swensen SJ, Jett JR (1993) Approach to the solitary pulmonary nodule. Mayo Clin Proc 68:378–85.
2. Swensen SJ, Jett JR, Viggiano RW, et al. (1990) An integrated approach to evaluation of the solitary pulmonary nodule. Mayo Clin Proc 65:173–86.
3. Higginson JF, Hinshaw DB (1955) Pulmonary coin lesions. JAMA 157:1607–1609.
4. Swensen SJ, Silverstein MD, Ilstrup DM, et al. (1997) The probability of malignancy in solitary pulmonary nodules. Application to small radiologically indeterminate nodules. Arch Intern Med 157:849–855.
5. Mori K, Ohta S, Yokoyama K, et al. (1995) Clinical evaluation of the small solitary pulmonary nodule. Nihon Kyobu Shikkan Gakkai Zasshi 33:695–699.
6. Siegelman SS, Zerhouni EA, Leo FP, et al. (1980) CT of the solitary pulmonary nodule. AJR 135:1–13.
7. Edwards WM, Cox RS Jr, Garland LH (1962) The solitary nodule (coin lesion) of the lung. AJR 8:1020–1041.
8. Lovich SF, Ostrow LB, Samples TL, (1990) The solitary pulmonary nodule: A recent military experience. Mil Med 155:266–268.
9. Turpin S, Marques H, Costa P, (1998) The solitary pulmonary nodule. A retrospective study of 119 cases. Acta Med Port 11:533–538.
10. Kundell HL (1981) Predictive values and threshold detectability of lung tumors. Radiology 139:25–29.
11. Kundel HL, Nodine CF, Carmody D (1978) Visual scanning pattern recognition and decision-making in pulmonary nodule detection. Invest Radiol 13:175–181.
12. Wandtke JC, Plewes DB, McFaul JA (1988) Improved pulmonary nodule detection with scanning equalization radiography. Radiology 169:23–27.
13. Giger M, MacMahon H (1996) Image processing and computer-aided diagnosis. Radiol Clin North Am 34:565–596.
14. Caskey CI, Templeton PA, Zerhouni EA (1990) Current evaluation of the solitary pulmonary nodule. Radiol Clin North Am 28:511–520.
15. Jain P, Kathwalla SA, Arroliga AC (1998) Managing solitary pulmonary nodules. Cleveland Clin J Med 65:315–326.
16. Webb WR (1990) Radiologic evaluation of the solitary pulmonary nodule. AJR 154:701–708.
17. Nathan MH (1974) Management of solitary pulmonary nodules: an organized approach based on growth rate and statistics. JAMA 277:1141–1144.
18. Yankeleitz DF, Henschke CI (1997) Does 2-year stability imply that pulmonary nodules are benign? AJR 168:325–328.
19. Midthun DE, Swensen SJ, Jett JR (1992) Clinical strategies for solitary pulmonary nodule. Ann Rev Med 43:195–208.
20. Viggian RW, Swenson SJ, Rosenow EC (1992) Evaluation and management of solitary and multiple pulmonary nodules. Clin Chest Med 13:83–95.
21. Zerhouni EA, Stitik FP, Siegelman SS, et al. (1986) CT of the pulmonary nodule: A national cooperative study. Radiology 160:319–327.
22. Zerhouni EA, Boukadoum M, Siddiky MA, et al. (1983) A standard phantom for quantitative CT analysis of pulmonary nodules. Radiology 149:767–773.
23. O'Keefe ME Jr, Good CA, McDonald JR (1957) Calcification in solitary nodules of the lung. AJR 77:1023–1033.
24. Siegelman SS, Khouri NF, Scott WW Jr, et al. (1986) Pulmonary hamartoma: CT findings. Radiology 160:313–317.
25. Harris KM, Adams H, Lloyd DCF, et al. (1993) The effect on apparent size of simulated pulmonary nodules using three standard CT window settings. Clin Radiol 47:241–244.
26. Primack SL, Hartman TE, Lee KS, et al. (1994) Pulmonary nodules and the CT halo sign. Radiology 190:513–515.
27. Kim Y, Lee KS, Jung KJ, et al. (1999) Halo sign on high resolution CT: findings in spectrum of pulmonary diseases with pathologic correlation. J Comput Assist Tomogr 23:622–626.

28. Swensen SJ, Morin RL, Schueler BA, et al. (1992) Solitary pulmonary nodule: CT evaluation of enhancement with iodinated contrast material – a preliminary report. Radiology 182:343–347.
29. Swensen SJ, Brown LR, Colby TV, et al. (1996) Lung nodule enhancement at CT: Prospective findings. Radiology 201:447–455.
30. Gaeta M, Volta S, Bartiromo G, et al. (1997) Contrast-enhanced study of solitary pulmonary nodules with thin-section computed tomography. Radiol Med Torino 94:189–192.
31. Matsuo H, Murata K, Takahashi M, et al. (1998) Benign pulmonary nodule: Morphological features and contrast enhancement evaluated with contiguous thin-section CT. Nippon Igaku Hoshasen Gakkai Zasshi 58:685–691.
32. Potente G, Guerrisi R, Iacari V, et al. (1997) The solitary pulmonary nodule: The preliminary results in differential diagnosis by high-resolution computed tomography with a contrast medium. Radiol Med Torino 94:182–188.
33. Yamashita K, Matsunobe S, Tsuda T, et al. (1995) Solitary pulmonary nodule: Preliminary study of evaluation with incremental dynamic CT. Radiology 194:399–405.
34. Zhang M, Kono M (1997) Solitary pulmonary nodules: evaluation of blood flow patterns with dynamic CT. Radiology 205:471–478.
35. Webb WR (1978) The pleural tail sign. Radiology 127:309–313.
36. Hill CA (1982) "Tail" signs associated with pulmonary lesions: Critical reappraisal. AJR 139:311–316.
37. Grenier P, Valyre D, Cluzel P, et al. (1991) Chronic diffuse interstitial lung disease: Diagnostic value of chest radiography and high-resolution CT. Radiology 179:123–132.
38. Kui M, Templeton PA, White CS, et al. (1996) Evaluation of the air bronchogram sign on CT in solitary pulmonary lesions. J Comput Assist Tomogr 20:983–986.
39. Zwirewich CV, Vedal S, Miller RR, et al. (1991) Solitary pulmonary nodule: High-resolution CT and radiologic–pathologic correlation. Radiology 179:469–476.
40. Kuhlman JE, Fishman EK, Kuhajda FP, et al. Solitary bronchiolo-alveolar carcinoma: CT criteria. Radiology 167:379–382.
41. Adler B, Padley S, Miller RR, et al. (1992) High-resolution CT of bronchioloalveolar carcinoma. AJR 159:275–277.
42. Milne EN, Zerhouni EA (1987) Blood supply of pulmonary metastases. J Thorac Imaging 2:15–23.
43. Webb WR, Müller NL, Naidich DP (1996) Diseases characterized primarily by nodular or reticulonodular opacities. In High-resolution CT of the lung. Lippincott-Raven, New York, pp 154–155.
44. Davis SD (1991) CT evaluation for pulmonary metastases in patients with extrathoracic malignancy. Radiology 180:1–12.
45. Stark P (1982) Multiple independent bronchogenic carcinomas. Radiology 145:599–601.
46. Zwirewich CV, Miller RR, Müller NL (1990) Multicentric adenocarcinoma of the lung: CT–pathologic correlation. Radiology 176:185–190.
47. Costello P, Ander W, Blume D (1991) Pulmonary nodule: evaluation with spiral volumetric CT. Radiology 179:875–876.
48. Rémy-Jardin M, Rémy J, Giraud F, (1993) Pulmonary nodules: Detection with thick-section spiral CT versus conventional CT. Radiology 187:513–520.
49. Diederich S, Lentschig MG, Winter F, et al. (1999) Detection of pulmonary nodules with overlapping vs non-overlapping image reconstruction at spiral CT. Eur Radiol 9:281–286.
50. Erasmus JJ, McAdams HP, Patz EF Jr, et al. (1998) Thoracic FDG PET: State of the art. Radiographics 18:5–20.
51. Bury T, Dowlati A, Paulus P, et al. (1996) Evaluation of the solitary pulmonary nodule by positron emission tomography imaging. Eur Respir J 9:410–414.
52. Dewan NA, Gupta NC, Redepenning LS, et al. (1993) Diagnostic efficacy of PET FDG imaging in solitary pulmonary nodules. Potential role in evaluation and management. Chest 104:997–1002.
53. Duhaylongsod FG, Lowe VJ, Patz EF Jr, et al. (1995) Detection of primary and recurrent lung cancer by means of F-18 fluorodeoxyglucose positron emission tomography (FDG PET). J Thorac Cardiovasc Surg 110:130–139.
54. Gupta NC, Maloof J, Gunel E (1996) Probability of malignancy in solitary pulmonary nodules using fluorine-18-FDG and PET. J Nucl Med 37:943–948.
55. Lowe VJ, Fletcher JW, Gobar L, et al. (1998) Prospective investigation of positron emission tomography in lung nodules. J Clin Oncol 16:1075–1084.
56. Prauer HW, Weber WA, Romer W, et al. (1998) Controlled prospective study of positron emission tomography using the glucose analogue [18F]fluorodeoxyglucose in the evaluation of pulmonary nodules. Br J Surg 85:1506–1511.
57. Worsley DF, Celler A, Adam MJ, et al. (1997) Pulmonary nodules: differential diagnosis using 18F-fluorodeoxyglucose single-photon emission computed tomography. AJR 168:771–774.
58. Hagberg RC, Segall GM, Stark P, et al. (1997) Characterization of pulmonary nodules and mediastinal staging of bronchogenic carcinoma with F-18 fluorodeoxyglucose positron emission tomography. Eur J Cardiothorac Surg 12:92–97.
59. Graeber GM, Gupta NC, Murray GF (1999) Positron emission tomographic imaging with fluorodeoxyglucose is efficacious in evaluating malignant pulmonary disease. J Thorac Cardiovasc Surg 117: 719–727.
60. Lee KS, Kim Y, Han J, et al. (1997) Bronchioloalveolar carcinoma: Clinical, histopathologic, and radiologic findings. Radiographics 17:1345–1357.
61. Gaeta M, Pandolfo I, Volta S, et al. Bronchus sign on CT in peripheral carcinoma of the lung: Value in predicting results of transbronchial biopsy. AJR 157:1181–1185.
62. Radke JR, Conway WA, Eyler WR, et al. (1979) Diagnostic accuracy in peripheral lung lesions: Factors predicting success with flexible fiberoptic bronchoscopy. Chest 76:176–179.
63. Chechani V (1996) Bronchoscopic diagnosis of solitary pulmonary nodules and lung masses in the absence of endobronchial abnormality. Chest 109:620–625.
64. Chin T, Yano T, Akusawa K, et al. (1996) Clinical evaluation of fiberoptic bronchoscopy for the diagnosis of solitary pulmonary nodules 2 cm or less in diameter of chest roentgenogram. Nihon Kyobu Shikkan Gakkai Zasshi 34:266–269.
65. Khouri NF, Stitik FP, Erozan YS, et al. (1985) Transthoracic needle aspiration biopsy of benign and malignant lung lesions. AJR 144:281–288.
66. Mitruka S, Landreneau RJ, Mack MJ, et al. (1995) Diagnosing the indeterminate pulmonary nodule: percutaneous biopsy versus thoracoscopy. Surgery 118:676–684.
67. Golfieri R, Sbrozzi F, de-Santis F, et al. (1998) Clinical role of CT-guided transthoracic needle biopsy in the diagnosis of solitary pulmonary nodules. Radiol Med Torino 95:329–337.
68. Klein JS, Zarka MA (1997) Transthoracic needle biopsy: An overview. J Thorac Imaging 12:232–249.
69. Westcott JL (1980) Direct percutaneous needle aspiration of localized pulmonary lesions: Results in 422 patients. Radiology 137:31–35.
70. Winning AJ, McIvor J, Seed WA, et al. (1986) Interpretation of negative results in fine needle aspiration of discrete pulmonary lesions. Thorax 41:875–879.
71. Penketh AR, Robinson AA, Barker V, et al. (1987) Use of percutaneous needle biopsy in the investigation of solitary pulmonary nodules. Thorax 42:967–971.
72. de Gregorio Ariza MA, Alfonso Aguiran ER, Vilavieja Atance JL, et al. (1991) Transthoracic aspiration biopsy of pulmonary and mediastinal lesions. Eur J Radiol 12:98–103.
73. Taber RE, Lupovitch A, Kantzler PJ (1986) Fine-needle aspiration biopsy of lung tumors. Ann Thorac Surg 42(Suppl. 6):S44–S47.

74. Poe RH, Tobin RE (1980) Sensitivity and specificity of needle biopsy in lung malignancy. Am Rev Respir Dis 122:725–729.

75. Rotte KH (1995) CT-assisted needle biopsy in pulmonary and mediastinal space-occupying lesions. The effect of spiral CT and various biopsy needles on results. Aktuelle Radiol 5:136–139.

76. Core F, Virapongse C, Saterfiel J (1989) Low-risk large-needle biopsy of chest lesions. Chest 96:538–541.

77. Arakawa H, Nakajima Y, Kurihara Y, et al. (1989) CT-guided transthoracic needle biopsy: A comparison between automated biopsy gun and fine needle aspiration. Clin Radiol 51:503–506.

78. Gardner D, van Sonnenberg E, D'Agostino HB, et al. (1991) CT-guided transthoracic needle biopsy. Cardiovasc Intervent Radiol 14:17–23.

79. Santambrogio L, Nosotti M, Bellaviti N, et al. (1997) CT-guided fine-needle aspiration cytology of solitary pulmonary nodules: A prospective, randomized study of immediate cytologic evaluation. Chest 112:423–425.

80. Austin JH, Cohen MB (1993) Value of having a cytopathologist present during percutaneous fine-needle aspiration biopsy of lung: Report of 55 cancer patients and metaanalysis of the literature. AJR 160:175–177.

81. Calhoun P, Feldman PS, Armstrong P, et al. (1986) The clinical outcome of needle aspirations of the lung when cancer is not diagnosed. Ann Thorac Surg 41:592–596.

82. Kaiser LR, Shrager JB (1995) Video-assisted thoracic surgery: The current state of the art. AJR 165:1111–1117.

83. Hazelrigg SR, Magee MJ, Cetindag IB (1998) Video-assisted thoracic surgery for diagnosis of the solitary lung nodule. Chest Surg Clin North Am 8:763–774.

84. Mack MJ, Hazelrigg SR, Landreneau RJ, et al. (1993) Thoracoscopy for the diagnosis of the indeterminate solitary pulmonary nodule. Ann Thorac Surg 56:825–830.

85. Santambrogio L, Nosotti M, Bellaviti N, et al. (1995) Video-thoracoscopy versus thoracotomy for the diagnosis of the indeterminate solitary pulmonary nodule. Ann Thorac Surg 59:868–870.

86. Schwarz RE, Posner MC, Plunkett MB, et al. (1994) Needle localization thoracoscopic resection (NLTR) of indeterminate pulmonary nodules: impact on management of patients with malignant disease. Ann Surg Oncol 2:49–55.

87. Shah RM, Spirn PW, Salazar AM, et al. (1993) Localization of peripheral pulmonary nodules for thoracoscopic excision: value of CT-guided wire placement. AJR 161:279–283.

88. Lenglinger FX, Schwarz CD, Artmann W (1994) Localization of pulmonary nodules before thoracoscopic surgery: value of percutaneous staining with methylene blue. AJR 163:297–300.

89. Lee JM, Lee YC, Huang CJ, et al. (1996) The role of video-assisted thoracoscopic surgery in the diagnosis and treatment of the indeterminate pulmonary lesion. Int Surg 81:327–329.

90. Landreneau RJ, Hazelrigg SR, Ferson PF, et al. (1992) Thoracoscopic resection of 85 pulmonary lesions. Ann Thorac Surg 54415–54419.

91. Allen MS, Deschamps C, Lee RE, et al. (1993) Video-assisted thoracoscopic stapled wedge excision for indeterminate pulmonary nodules. J Thorac Cardiovasc Surg 106:1048–1052.

92. DeCamp MM, Jr, Jaklitsch MT, Mentzer SJ, et al. (1995) The safety and versatility of video-thoracoscopy: A prospective analysis of 895 consecutive cases. J Am Coll Surg 181:113–120.

93. Gossot D, de Kerviler E, Paladines G, et al. (1997) Thoracoscopic approach in pulmonary nodules: A prospective evaluation of a series of 120 patients. Rev Mal Respir 14:287–293.

94. Celik M, Halezeroglu S, Senol C, et al. (1998) Video-assisted thoracoscopic surgery: Experience with 341 cases. Eur J Cardiothorac Surg 14:113–116.

33 Malignant Pulmonary Disorders other than Bronchogenic Carcinoma

T. Pirronti, R. Manfredi, and P. Marano

Introduction

Besides bronchogenic carcinoma, which represents the majority of primary pulmonary neoplasms, a great variety of tumors originate in the lung, benign and malignant, of very different histogenesis, but sharing anatomic site of origin. They account for 3–5% of all resected lung tumors and, with the exception of metastases, lymphomas, carcinoid tumors, and bronchoalveolar cell carcinoma, fewer than 100 cases of these unusual neoplasms have been reported in literature. Due to their disparate histogenesis and rarity, it is difficult to categorize them and with the introduction of electron microscopy and immunohistology the classifications have undergone continuous changes.

It is best to discuss them according to the cell of origin, as follows (1):

Tumors of APUD cells

Bronchial carcinoid tumor

Tumors derived from alveolar epithelium or bronchial mucous glands

Bronchoalveolar cell carcinoma
Adenoid cystic carcinoma of the bronchus
Bronchial mucoepidermoid carcinoma
Acinic cell tumors (Fechners' tumors)

Tumors of pulmonary connective tissue origin

Chondrosarcoma
Osteosarcoma
Soft tissue sarcomas of the lung

  Leiomyosarcoma
  Spindle cell sarcoma
  Rhabdomyosarcoma
  Angiosarcoma
  Malignant hemangiopericytoma

Fibrosarcoma
Neurogenic sarcoma
Synovial sarcoma
Kaposi sarcoma
Liposarcoma

Malignant lymphoreticular disorders of the lung

Hodgkin disease
Non-Hodgkin lymphoma
Plasmacytoma

Malignant germ cell tumors

Malignant teratoma
Choriocarcinoma

Miscellaneous

Carcinosarcoma
Epithelioid hemangioendothelioma (intravascular and sclerosing bronchoalveolar tumor)
Blastoma (embrioma)
Malignant melanoma of the bronchus
Malignant ependymoma
Ewing sarcoma
Lymphoepithelioma
Pseudomesotheliomatous carcinoma

Metastases

Bronchial Carcinoid Tumor

This tumor originates from APUD common precursor uptake and elecarboxylation) cells of the tracheobronchial walls. It represents approximately 2% of primary lung tumors and usually occurs in the fifth decade of life. At bronchoscopy it appears as a reddish polypoid mass, occurring in the main or lobar or segmental bronchi;

peripheral tumors occur in 20% of cases (2,3). Carcinoid tumors may be divided into two categories: typical, and atypical with more malignant histologic and clinical features. Half of the patients are asymptomatic at presentation (4). Hemoptysis, wheezing, postobstructive pneumonitis and dyspnea are the most common clinical manifestations. Rarely, atypical carcinoid may present with metastatic disease. Paraneoplastic syndromes occurs as: carcinoid syndrome, Cushing syndrome and acromegaly; occasionally they occur in multiple endocrine neoplasm (MEN) type I syndrome.

At chest X-ray, carcinoid tumors appear as central or peripheral solitary nodules; regional lymph node metastases are almost never present in typical carcinoids. Typical tumors occur as well defined round or slightly lobulated lesions. Often they produce intermittent lobar or segmental atelectasis and postobstructive pneumonitis. Diffuse or punctate eccentric calcifications in the lesion, especially in central tumors, are identified in 30% of computed tomography (CT) studies (Fig 33.1). These lesions are extremely vascular and show marked and homogeneous contrast enhancement following administration of intravenous contrast medium (5).

Cytologic examination of sputum is not productive, but microbiopsy using forceps through a fiberoptic bronchoscope has useful a diagnostic sensitivity of 60–80%. Conservative resection is indicated for peripheral small lesions, instead of central or atypical tumors that should be treated by lobectomy or pneumonectomy in the same way as one would treat a bronchogenic carcinoma.

Bronchoalveolar Cell Carcinoma

Bronchoalveolar cell carcinoma (BAC) is also called alveolar cell carcinoma, bronchiolar cell carcinoma, and pulmonary adenomatosis because of a controversy concerning the cell of origin. The production of mucus suggested bronchiolar cell origin, but recently it has been demonstrated that alveolar cells also can differentiate into cells capable of mucus secretion. The tumor arises from type II alveolar pneumocytes and Clara cells; however, the denomination remains because of growth modalities within alveoli and terminal bronchioles. The etiology is unknown, but histologically the BAC likened to an infectious disease of animals (primarily sheep) in South Africa, presumably viral, called "jaagsiekte". Histologically it is composed of flat or columnar malignant cells along alveolar and bronchiolar walls, with frequent intraalveolar projections, but preservation of the interstitial framework (6,7). Approximately 40% of patients present with advanced disease (III and IV TNM stages). Cough, copious watery sputum, dyspnea and general symptoms are the typical manifestations at diagnosis (8). The sputum cytology and more often bronchoscopic biopsy and fine needle alveolar biopsy can be diagnostic. Clinically and radiologically two entities have been described: focal and diffuse form, (9). Focal BAC presents as solitary peripheral nodule with slow growth and infrequent regional lymph node metastases; diffuse form is less common but more aggressive and characterized by multiple nodules or consolidation (Fig. 33.2). High

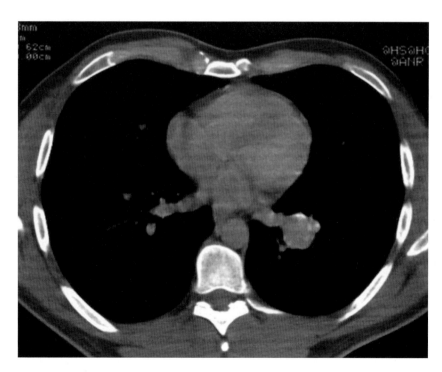

Figure 33.1. CT scan: round mass with sharp margins and internal, eccentric calcifications in the left hilus.

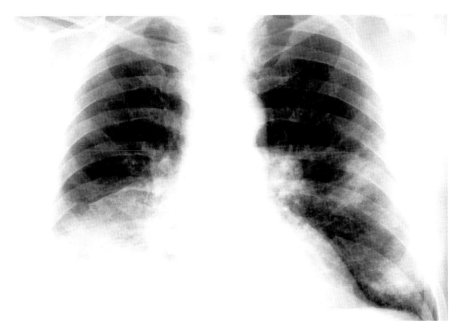

Figure 33.2. Chest radiograph shows parenchymal consolidation of the right lower lobe and fissure displacement due to associated atelectasis. We can also see parenchymal consolidations in the left lower lobe and bilateral hilar enlargement.

resolution computed tomography (HRCT) confirms a wide range of radiologic manifestations and shows numerous air bronchograms, pseudocavitation (10,11), focal ill-defined areas of ground-glass attenuation (12,13), halo sign (11). Defined as small oval areas of lucency in or around pulmonary masses, the pseudocavitation was interpreted as consistent with residual dilatated bronchioles and expanded airspaces, the result of preservation of pulmonary architecture. Pseudocavitations are more commonly in BAC (50%) than in acinar adenocarcinomas (31%) or other lung tumors (11%), making this sign highly suggestive of BAC (14).

HRCT studies also show a propensity toward subpleural localization in association with pleural retraction (a so-called pleural tag).

The tumor is not particularly responsive to chemotherapy or radiation therapy and, although it has slow growth, untreated lesions proceed to pulmonary insufficiency and death. The treatment is surgical and lobectomy is the procedure of choice.

Tumors Arising from Bronchial Mucous Glands

These tumors originate from mucous glands throughout the body, especially in salivary glands. *Adenoid cystic carcinoma* of the tracheobronchial tree occurs in the trachea or in mainstem bronchus as sessile obstructing lesions causing atelectasis or postobstructive pneumonias (15). Histologically the cells form duct-like tubules, cysts that contain mucin and glands (16). These tumors are low grade adenocarcinomas that metastasize to regional nodes through tracheobronchial walls. Perineural invasion is a hallmark. The diagnosis is established with a bronchoscopic biopsy. The treatment is surgical but radiotherapy is utilized for inoperable patients and incomplete resections.

Mucoepidermoid carcinomas are the malignant and highly lethal variety of a wide range of mucoepidermoid tumors. This tumor presents as pedunculated polypoid lesion arising from excretory duct cells of tracheobronchial mucous glands, usually in mainstem or lobar bronchi but can arise peripherally (17); this is coated with mucus, occasionally producing large and obstructing mucoceles. Characteristic symptoms are cough, wheezing, hemoptysis and recurrent pneumonias. In general these are benign in children, whereas in adults many of these are found to be highly malignant with a tendency to early metastases. At chest X-ray these lesions present as lobar or segmental consolidation or atelectasis. Bronchoscopic biopsy usually is diagnostic. Radiation therapy and chemotherapy are not effective. Conservative lung resection for low grade tumors has been suggested; high grade are typically unresectable.

Histologic diagnosis of *acinic cell tumors* suggest a search for an extrathoracic primary tumor (especially in the salivary glands) (18). Primary or secondary pulmonary tumors are endobronchial or peripheral. The microscopic pattern resembles that of a neuroendocrine tumor and it is necessary to differentiate it from the more common carcinoid tumor. The growth is slow and recurrence or metastases after surgery have not been reported.

Carcinosarcoma

This unusual pulmonary tumor account for 0.3% (19) and is composed of carcinomatous and sarcomatous elements. It is usually found in older men. At radiographs it occurs as central or peripheral nodule, especially in the upper lobes. Slow growth is characteristic (20) but metastases to the regional nodes and distant organs are not rare. The patients usually are symptomatic at diagnosis: chest pain, cough and hemoptysis. Surgery is the treatment of choice but the prognosis is poor.

Tumors of Pulmonary Connective Tissue Origin Sarcomas

Primary pulmonary sarcomas originate from the mesenchymal cells of pulmonary interstices and bronchial or vascular walls. The primary sarcomas are more rare than secondary, and are usually large (3 cm), solitary and asymptomatic. The most common types are malignant fibrous histiocytoma, fibrosarcoma, and leiomyosarcoma. As a result of the spread of acquired immune deficiency syndrome (AIDS), the incidence of Kaposi sarcoma is increasing (Fig. 33.3). The other types are most rare (21).

Malignant fibrous histiocytoma (MFH) occurs more frequently in patients who have undergone radiotherapy protocols, and approximately 50% have metastases at diagnosis. At radiography it presents as a central or peripheral nodule, often large, with frequent nodal involvment.

Fibrosarcoma and leiomyosarcoma are clinically and radiologically similar to MFH. Central occurrences have a much better prognosis because they become symptamatic earlier. In contrast, peripheral types are found only when they are large and metastatic (22,23).

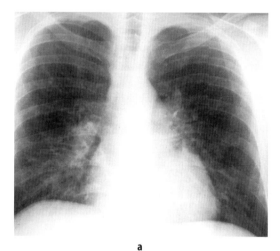

a

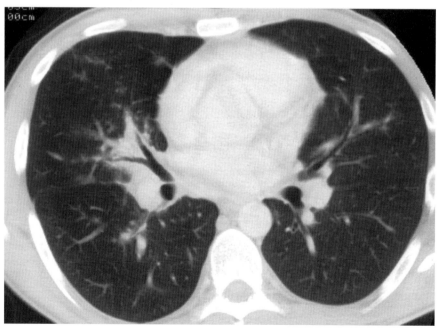

b

Figure 33.3. a and **b** Peribronchovascular thickening in Kaposi sarcoma.

Pulmonary chondrosarcomas are rarer and, despite radiographic calcifications, they are malignant, especially the peripheral types.

Pulmonary hemangiopericytoma is very rare, has no characteristic signs at radiograph, but occurs in older men, in the left lower lobe and has sharp contours, probably owing to a fibrous capsule (24) (Fig. 33.4). It arises from pericytes within the basement membranes of capillaries and is usually less than 5 cm. Necrosis or vascular, bronchial or pleural involvement are predictive of a poor prognosis. The differential diagnosis should include pulmonary fibromas, metastatic sarcomas and bronchial carcinoids. The other types do not have different clinico-radiologic features and for diagnosis it is always necessary to do a bronchoscopic biopsy for central lesions or percutaneous CT-guided biopsy for peripheral types.

Malignant Melanoma of the Bronchus

Many theories have been proposed to explain pulmonary melanomas including melanocytic metaplasia of bronchial epithelial cells, fetal migration of benign melanocytes to the bronchus, and neuroendocrine origin (25). It is necessary to exclude all other possible primary sites, especially cutaneous and ocular melanomas to make a diagnosis. At chest X-ray they generally present as solitary lung lesions centered on a bronchus and rarely in the trachea. Histologically the so called "junctional or lentiginous change" (in situ melanocytic change of bronchial mucosa adjacent to the lesion) is characteristic. Metastases are the most common cause of death.

Pulmonary Blastoma (*Embrioma*)

These tumors are very rare and originate from both malignant mesenchymal and epithelial cells that resemble the pseudoglandular stage of fetal lung. Koss et al. (26) suggested two categories based on histologic features: well-differentiated fetal adenocarcinoma (without a malignant stroma) and biphasic blastoma (without malignant epithelium). Central and peripheral asymptomatic lesions have characteristic features at routine chest radiographs. Usually they occur as sharply circumscribed lesions with sometimes extensive necrosis. Nodal metastases and the size of the lesion (< 5 cm) make, the prognosis worse. Most patients die of extrathoracic

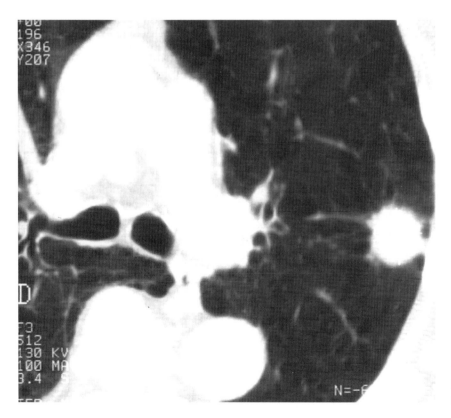

Figure 33.4. Small subpleural nodule representing primary malignant hemangiopericytoma.

metastases. All patients should undergo of surgical resection, and combination chemotherapy may be useful in children.

Epithelioid Hemangioendothelioma

Also named intravascular bronchioloalveolar tumor, this tumor has been demonstrated to be of endothelial origin (reactivity for factor VIII-related antigen) and is categorized as a low grade sarcoma. Usually multifocal, it occurs in young asymptomatic (<40) women. At radiograph it presents as small bilateral nodules (27,19). Intrapleural hemorrhage is rare but characteristic (28,29). Therapy is nonspecific: chemotherapy, hormonotherapy and radiotherapy are ineffective. Excision of the rare solitary tumor is recommended.

Malignant Germ Cell Tumors

Teratomas originate from remnants of all three germ cell layers. Primary intrapulmonary teratomas are very rare and it is necessary exclude all other primary locations (especially the testes) (30). Generally symptoms are aspecific (cough, chest pain, and hemoptysis). The most specific symptom, trychoptysis, is rare. Radiologically they may occur with calcifications and peripheral radiolucency, especially in the left upper lobe. They contain hair, sebum, pancreatic and other tissues. Growth is slow and only 30–40% of these tumors are malignant.

Choriocarcinomas, extraordinarily rare, are composed of syncytiotrophoblasts and cytotrophoblasts; they produce chorionic gonadotrophin (CG) and must be differentiated from a nonsmall-cell lung carcinoma that can also produce CG. These are frequently necrotic and hemorrhagic. Resection is recommended.

Malignant Pulmonary Lymphomas

They represent less than 1% of all primary lung cancers (31). The International Lymphomas Study Group has proposed a new classification of lymphoid disorders that recognizes different clinico-pathologic entities based on multiparametric studies including immunophenotyping and molecular genetics (32). Most primary pulmonary lymphomas are included within these categories:

A. Non-Hodgkin lymphomas of the lung

   1. Low grade, small B-cell
   2. High grade, large B-cell
   3. Angiocentric lymphoma (lymphomatoid granulomatosis)

B. Large B-cell lymphoma (not otherwise specified)
C. Primary pulmonary Hodgkin disease
D. Pulmonary plasmacytoma

Non Hodgkin Lymphomas of the Lung

Primary pulmonary lymphomas are those in which the lung is the major site of disease at the diagnosis. Non-Hodgkin lymphomas represent fewer than 10% of all extranodal lymphomas and are more common than primary Hodgkin disease of the lung. In most studies, primary pulmonary lymphomas have been confined to the lung radiographically; however, several studies have demonstrated hilar and mediastinal node involvement at microscopy in up to 20% of these cases (33).

The majority (75–90%) of primary pulmonary non-Hodgkin lymphomas are *low grade, small B-cell* and most of them originate from the bronchial mucosa-associated lymphoid tissue (BALT). Both sexes are equally affected with a peak incidence in the sixth decade of life. Half the patients are asymptomatic at diagnosis on routine chest radiograph. Local symptoms are aspecific and the presence of constitutional symptoms suggests extrathoracic involvement. On the basis of apparently benign clinicopathologic features they were originally designated as "pseudolymphomas" (34); today immunophenotyping and molecular biological studies have demonstrated a monoclonal origin, which is supported by long-term follow-up that documents progression to overt lymphoma. Typically they present as a solitary well-delineated mass but sometimes as multiple unilateral or bilateral nodules, less frequently as diffuse interstitial infiltrates. Radiographic features are variable: single or multiple lesions, located centrally or peripherally, with homogeneous and sometimes quite large densities (differentiation from lung carcinoma is often not possible!). Alternatively there is a reticulonodular infiltrate simulating lymphangitic spread of metastatic carcinoma or pneumonic consolidation. The air bronchogram is present but cavitation, atelectasis and hilar adenopathy are usually absent (35). The treatment for many of these lesions is surgical, but it is very important to do a clinicoradiologic follow-up because some of these cases can transform to high grade lymphoma.

Some of the *high grade lymphomas* develop from low grade BALT lymphomas, suggesting BALT origin. However, for most of these lesions specific markers are not available. They are solitary masses larger than 3 cm but sometimes occur as diffuse infiltrates or multiple nodules in the lymphatics (Fig. 33.5). In contrast to the low grade lymphoma, patients with high grade lymphomas are usually symptomatic. Chest radiographs and CT scans reveal nodular masses or diffuse pneumonic infiltrates with an air bronchogram. The nodules may cavitate secondary to necrosis (36). Rapid evolution suggests an infec-

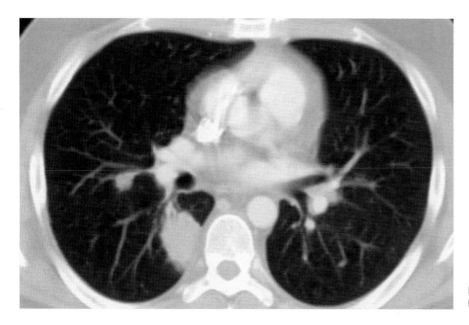

Figure 33.5. Homogeneous mass in the right lower lobe, adjacent to the vertebral body.

tious process or vasculitis. Pleural effusions are not rare, in contrast to nodal enlargement.

Angiocentric lymphoma was originally named lymphomatoid granulomatosis because it is similar to Wegner granulomatosis but with a propensity to progress to malignant lymphoma (37). It is characterized by polymorphic typical lymphoid infiltrates with vascular invasion, which can obliterate the lumen and result in ischemic necrosis. Most of these lesions have a preeminent monoclonal population of large atypical Epstein–Barr virus-positive B-cells with a high content of reactive T-cells. However, some lesions appear to be T-cell lymphomas, and Epstein–Barr virus negative (38). There is a considerable overlap in the clinical presentation with other forms of pulmonary lymphomas. The patients are asymptomatic at diagnosis. Extrathoracic manifestations are due to involvement of the central nervous system, kidneys, skin, and peripheral nerves. At radiography, depending on the stage of disease, there are bilateral nodules that may contain cavities with thick walls (36). The nodules may rapidly increase or decrease in size. Alternatively there are nonspecific reticulonodular infiltrates. Hilar nodes involvement is rare. More than half of patients have pleural effusion. The prognosis is related to the extrathoracic involvement and to the histologic grade (percentage of large atypical lymphocytes).

Pulmonary Hodgkin Disease

Over 50% of patients with Hodgkin disease have pulmonary involvement at autopsy. However, primary pulmonary Hodgkin disease is rare. Regardless of its origin, primary or secondary, these lymphomas occur as nodular infiltrates along the lymphatics (bronchovascular bundles, interlobular septa and visceral pleura), and may form masses (also with cavities) compressing adjacent airspaces. Infiltration of bronchial mucosa presents as diffuse thickening or endobronchial masses. Occasionally there is a miliary pattern due to numerous small nodules along the lymphatic Stemberg – Reed cells are diagnostic elements at microscopy in a reactive background of small a lymphocytes, scattered plasma cells, and eosinophils. Sometimes the nodular lesions are necrotic. Nonnecrotizing giant-cell granulomas may also be present but present an aspecific reaction to noninfectious antigenic stimuli. The majority of patients are symptomatic at diagnosis: fever, pruritus, weight loss, night sweat, and fatigue. Enlarged nodes are frequent (35). Pulmonary involvement causes cough and dyspnea. The radiographic apparence is a coarse reticulonodular or linear pattern (lymphatic routes involvement) often with pleural effusion. Confluent nodules form large opacities that may present with central cavitation (necrosis) (Fig. 33.6). Frequently regional nodes are enlarged. Extrinsic or endobronchial obstruction result in atelectasis. The most important prognostic factor is the stage, which is also important for therapy. Primary pulmonary Hodgkin disease is stage in the E (extranodal) in the second Ann Arbor classification. An "E" designation is also given to secondary pulmonary involvement from mediastinal or hilar nodal Hodgkin disease to distinguish it from pulmonary involvement secondary to disseminated stage IV. Thus contiguous lung involvement from regional nodes is designated stage I or II "E" rather than stage IV.

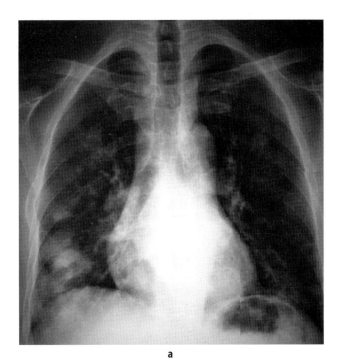

a

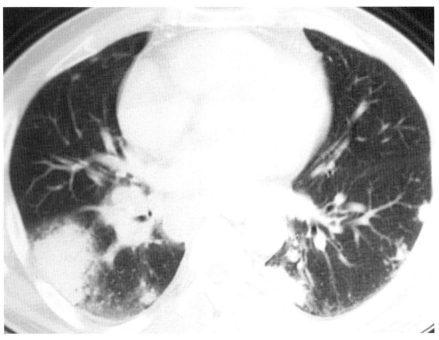

b

Figure 33.6. PA chest radiograph shows: multiple nodules without cavitation, predominantly in the right lower lobe (**a**); multiple subpleural nodules with irregular margins (**b**).

Plasmacytoma

It may present as a parenchymal or an endobronchial lesion. It is necessary to exclude any other primary sites of origin. Patients require careful monitoring because they may develop multiple melanoma. Surgery is the treatment of choice but they need radiotherapy if the tumor is identified prior to surgery by bronchoscopic biopsy.

Pulmonary Metastases

The lung is a common site of metastases. Approximately 30% of neoplastic patients develop pulmonary metastases. In tumors such as renal cell carcinoma, Wilm tumor, choriocarcinoma and osteosarcoma there is a high incidence of synchronous pulmonary metastases (60%) in choriocarinoma). The percentage is greater than 75% at autopsy in melanoma, choriocarcinoma, renal cell carci-

Table 33.1. Radiographic features of pulmonary metastases

Radiograph feature	Neoplasm
Multiple nodules	
Calcified	Osteogenic sarcoma, chondrosarcoma, thyroid, ovarian, breast
Military	Thyroid, melanoma, renal cell, ovarian
Cannon-ball	Sarcoma, colorectal, renal cell, ovarian
Slow growing	Adenoid cystic (salivary glands), thyroid
Cavitary	Squamous cell, melanoma, sarcoma, germ cell, transitional cell (bladder)
Poorly defined	Choriocarcinoma, liposarcoma, laryngeal, pancreatic
Solitary nodules	Nonspecific
Lymphangitic features	Adenocarcinoma of breast, lung, prostate, stomach, pancreas
Hilar or mediastinal adenopathy	Genito urinary, head and neck, melanoma, seminoma, renal cell
Endobronchial disease	Breast, colorectal, pancreas, renal cell
From ref. 44.	

noma, Ewing sarcoma, osteosarcoma, and germ cell carcinoma of the testes (39). Parenchymal metastases are asymptomatic in the absence of bronchial or pleural involvement, except for rapidly growing tumors such as choriocarcinoma in women or germ cell carcinoma of the testes in men. Most cases are discovered on routine chest radiograph either as synchronous or as metachronous lesions. Hemoptysis or fever are occasionally present at diagnosis. At radiography pulmonary metastases have variable features: solitary or multiple nodules, lymphangitic features, hilar or mediastinal adenopathy, and endobronchial disease (Table 33.1) (40) (Figs. 33.7, 33.8, 33.9, 33.10).

Several studies have demonstrated the same percentage of involvement of upper and lower lobes, which in greater than that of the middle lobe (41). Whereas bronchogenic carcinoma displays specific malignant signs at radiography (spiculated and irregular lesions), metastases often are aspecific and knowledge of the neoplastic state is very important.

Calcified nodules often indicate that a lesion may be benign (granuloma or hamartoma), but it is different in cancer patients (Fig. 33.11).

Cavitation of subpleural nodules may lead to pneumothorax.

Lymphangitic features result both from hematogenous spread (with extension from the capillaries to lymphatic vessels) and from retrograde lymphatic spread from mediastinal or hilar nodes into the lung.

Endobronchial metastases cause dyspnea and hemoptysis.

Pleural effusion is due to pleural involvement, especially with breast carcinoma, and occasionally to impaired lymphatic drainage and thus maybe cytologically negative.

There are no diagnostic problems in cancer patients with multiple pulmonary nodules, but the probability that a solitary nodule in these patients is a metastasis depends on the histology and site of the primary tumor; melanoma and sarcoma may present as solitary pulmonary metastases more after than other tumors (42,43).

Several methods are available for detecting metastases. Conventional chest radiograph is less sensitive, with a limiting resolution of 9 mm (however, it is the most specific: 90 of these nodules were determined to be true metastases after resection.

CT is accepted as the best imaging modality both in preintervention assessment and in evaluation of response to chemotherapy. HRCT scans detect nodules of 2–3 mm with 60–90% specificity. If there is a doubt concerning the nature of a nodule in a noncameras patient fine-needle biopsy CT-guided can be utilized for peripheral lesions, whereas flexible fiberoptic bronchoscopy has been successful in central ones.

Magnetic resonance imaging (MRI) spatial resolution (MRI) inferior to that of CT; however, it is superior in evaluating peripheral masses and vascular invasion.

The minimum criteria for resection of metastatic disease are the following (44):

- The primary tumor has been controlled.
- There are no extrathoracic metastases.
- Pulmonary metastases are deemed completely resectable.
- There is adequate pulmonary reserve.
- The patient's general medical condition permits the planned operation.
- Effective systemic therapy is not available.

The resection, if possible may significantly improve the prognosis.

References

1. Spencer H (1983) Pathology of the lung. Pergamon Press, Oxford.
2. Chapleau D, Page A, Verdant A, et al. (1991) Bronchial carcinoids: Longterm prognostic factors. Can J Surg 34:111.
3. Stamatis G, Freitag L, Greschuchna D (1990) Limited and radical resection for tracheal and bronchopulmonary carcinoid tumors. Report on 227 cases. Eur J Cardiothorac Surg 4:527.
4. Forster BB, Müller NL, Miller RR, et al. (1989) Neuroendocrine carcinomas of the lung: Clinical, radiological and pathologic correlation. Radiology 170:44.
5. Magid D, Siegelman SS, Eggleston JC (1989) Pulmonar carcinoid tumors: CT assessment. J Comput Assist Tomogr 13:244.
6. Greco RJ, Stemer RM, Gldman S et al. (1986) Bronchoalveolar cell carcinoma of the lung. Ann Thorac Surg 41:652.

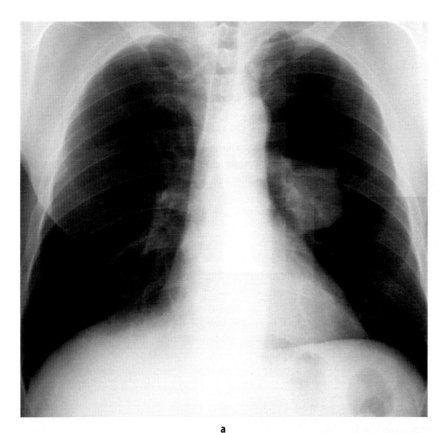

a

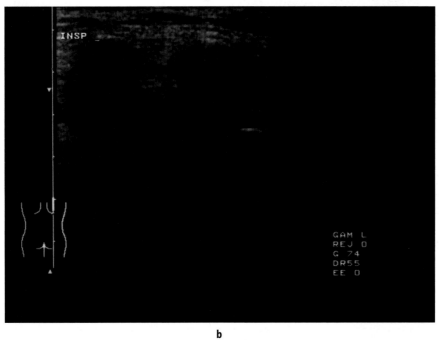

b

Figure 33.7. Round mass with sharp margins in the superior segment of the lower lobe (**a**). During inspiration and expiration the mass does not move at sonography: this sign is indicative of parietal pleural infiltration.

7. Schraufnagel D, Pelozuin A, Paré JA, et al. (1982) Differentiating bronchioloalveolar carcinoma from adenocarcinoma. Am Rev Resp Dis 125:74.

8. Harpole DH, Bigelow C, Young, WR Jr. et al. (1988) Alveolar cell carcinoma of the lung: A retrospective analysis of 205 patients. Ann Thorac Surg 46:502.

9. Epstein DM (1990) Bronchioloalveolar carcinoma. Semin Roentgenol 25:105.

10. Kuhlman JE, Fishman EK, Kuhajda FP (1988) Solitary bronchoalveolar carcinoma: CT criteria. Radiology 167:379.

11. Gaeta M, Barone M, Caruso R et al. (1994) CT pathologic correlation in nodular bronchoalveolar carcinoma. J Comp Assist Tomogr 18:229.

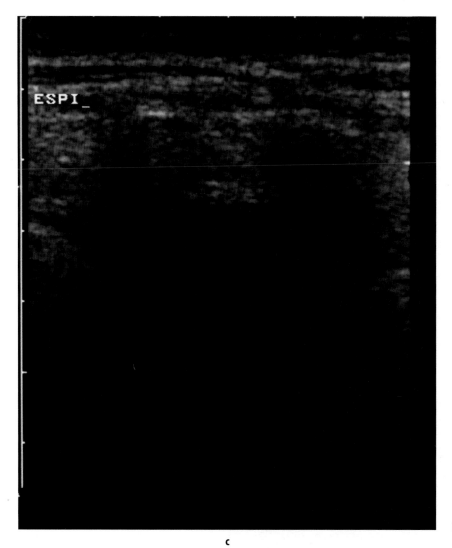

Figure 33.7c.

c

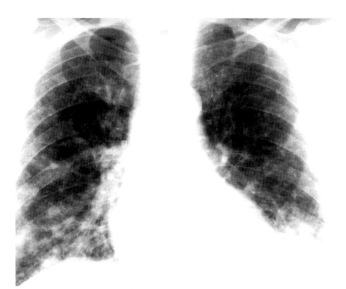

Figure 33.8. Hematogenous diffusion of metastases. Chest radiograph shows multiple nodular opacities in both lungs.

12. Kushihashi T, Munechika H, Ri K (1994) Bronchoalveolaer adenoma of the lung: CT–pathologic correlation. Radiology 193:789.
13. Jang HJ, Lee KS, Kwon OJ (1996) Bronchioloalveolar carcinoma: Focal area of ground glass attenuation at thin section CT as an early sign. Radiology 199:485.
14. Zwirewich CV, Vedal S, Miller RR, et al. (1991) Solitary pulmonary nodule: High resolution CT and radiologic–pathologic correlation. Radiology 179:469.
15. Felson B (1983) Neoplasms of the trachea and main stem bronchi. Semin Roentgenol 18:23.
16. Lozowski MS, Mishriki Y, Solitare GB (1983) Cytopathologic features of adenoid cystic carcinoma: Case report and literature review. Acta Cytol 27:317.
17. Yousem SA, Hochholzer I (1987) Mucoepidermoid tumors of the lung. Cancer 60:1346.
18. Moran CA (1995) Primary salivary gland type tumors of the lung. Semin Diag Pathol 12:106.
19. Dail DH, Hammar SP (1988) Pulmonary pathology. Springer Verlag, New York.
20. Cabarcos A, Gomez DM, Lobo BJ (1985) Pulmonary carcinosarcoma: A case study and review of the literature. Br J Dis Chest 79:83.
21. Fishman NH, Merrick SH (1994) Tumors of the lung other than bronchogenic carcinoma. In Baum GL, Wolinsky E (ed.) Textbook of

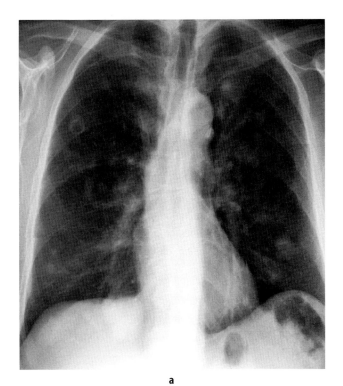

a

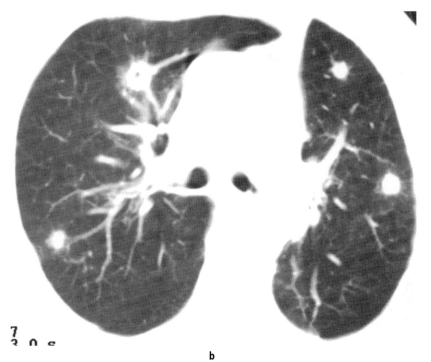

b

Figure 33.9. a–b Multiple nodules. Cavitations may be seen in some of them (**a**). Multiple parenchymal metastases are in connection with pulmonary vessels because of hematogenous spread.

pulmonary diseases, vol. II. Little, Brown and Co. New York Chapter 54, p. 1393.

22. Guccion JG, Rosen SH (1982) Bronchopulmonary leiomyosarcoma and fibrosarcoma. Cancer 30:836.

23. Pedersen VM (1984) Primary pulmonary leiomyosarcoma: Review of the literature and report of a case. Scand J Thorac Cardiovasc Surg 18:251.

24. Yousem SA, Hochholzer L (1987) Primary pulmonary hemangiopericytoma. Cancer 59:549.

25. Jennings TA, Axiotis CA, Kress Y, et al. (1990) Primary malignant melanoma of the lower respiratory tract. Report report of a case and literature review. Am J Clin Pathol 94:649.

26. Koss M, Hochholzer L, O'Leary T (1991) Pulmonary blastomas. Cancer 67:2368.

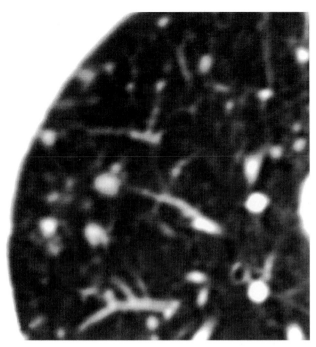

Figure 33.10. CT scan: the relationship between the vessels and the metastases is depicted.

27. Mackay B, Lukeman JM, Ordonez NG (1991) Tumors of the lung. Saunders, Philadelphia.
28. Carter EJ (1990) Alveolar hemorrhage with epithelioid hemangioendothelioma. A previously unreported manifestation of a rare tumor. Am Rev Resp Dis 142:700.
29. Struhar D (1992) Alveolar hemorrhage with pleural effusion as a manifestation of epithelioid hemangioendothelioma. Eur Respir J 5:592.
30. Morgan DE, Sanders C, McElvein RB (1992) Intrapulmonary teratoma: A case report and review of the literature. J Thorac Imaging 7:70.
31. Miller DL, Allen MS (1993) Rare pulmonary neoplasms. Mayo Clin Proc 68:492.
32. Harris NL, Jaffe ES, Stein H (1994) A revised European–American classification of lymphoid neoplasms: A proposal from the International Lymphoma Study Group. Blood 84:1361.
33. Yousem SA, Colby TV (1992) Pulmonary lymphomas and lymphoid hyperplasias In: Knowle DM (ed) Neoplastic hematopathology. Williams & Wilkins, Baltimore, MD, pp 170–77.
34. Saltzzstein SL (1963) Pulmonary malignant lymphomas and pseudolymphomas: Classification, therapy and prognosis. Cancer 16:928.
35. Pietra GG, Salhany KE (1998) Lymphoproliferative and hematologic diseases involving the lung. In Fishman's Pulmonary diseases and disorders. McGraw-Hill, New York, pp 123–28.
36. Jackson SA, Tung KT, Mead GM (1996) Multiple cavitating pulmonary lesions in non-Hodgkin's lymphomas. Clin Radiol 49:883.
37. Liebow AA, Carrington CB, Friedman PJ (1972) Lymphomatoid granulomatosis. Hum Pathol 3:457.
38. Myers JL, Kurtin PJ, Katzenstein ALA (1995) Lymphomatoid granulomatosis: Evidence of immunophenotypic diversity and relationship to Epstein–Barr virus infection. Am J Surg Pathol 19:1300.
39. Gilbert HA, Hagan AR (1976) Metastases: Incidence, detection, and evaluation without histologic confirmation. In Weiss L (ed) Fundamental aspects of metastases. Amsterdam, pp 84–96.
40. Whitesell P, Peters S (1993) Pulmonary manifestations of extrathoracic malignant lesions. Mayo Clin Proc 68:483.
41. Muller K, Respondek M (1990) Pulmonary metastases: Pathologic anatomy. Lung 168:1137.
42. Cahan W, Shah J, Castro E (1978) Benign solitary lesions in patient with cancer. Ann Surg 187:241.
43. Toomes H, Deephendahl A, Manke H, et al. (1983) The coin lesions of the lung. Cancer 51:534.
44. Burt M (1998) Pulmonary metastases. In Fishman's Pulmonary diseases and disorders, McGraw-Hill, New York, pp 238–49.

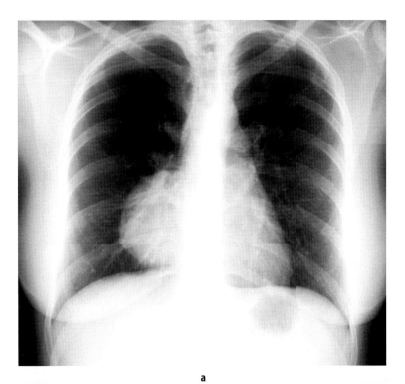

a

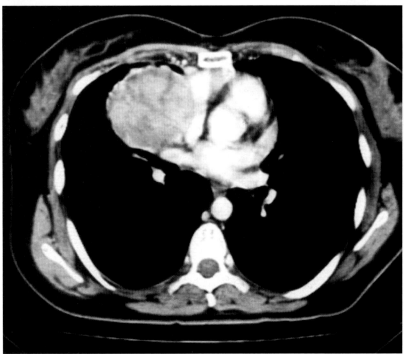

b

Figure 33.11. **a** and **b** Large pericardial metastasis with eccentric calcifications infiltrating the right atrium, due to malignant hemangiopericytoma.

34 Benign and Malignant Mediastinal Lesions

A.R. Wright

General Considerations

The mediastinum is that part of the thorax lying between the pleural cavities, and bounded superiorly and inferiorly by the thoracic inlet and diaphragm, and posteriorly and anteriorly by the thoracic spine and sternum. Conventionally, the mediastinum is divided into four compartments superior, anterior, middle, and posterior. The superior compartment is the portion lying above a plane between the manubrium and the lower border of spinal region T4. The lower mediastinum is divided into an anterior compartment, in front of the heart and pericardium, a middle compartment containing the heart, pericardium and hili, and a posterior compartment between the heart and pericardium and the thoracic spine. As the mediastinum contains so many different structures, it is home to a wide variety of lesions.

Division of the mediastinum in this way is of some value in that most mediastinal masses have a predilection for certain compartments (Table 34.1). Knowing the anatomic position of a lesion may therefore limit the differential diagnosis. However, this is less helpful with large masses that may occupy more than one compartment. The arbitrary division of the mediastinum is becoming less important now that evaluation of lesions with cross-sectional imaging is more common. Precise information about the location, size, shape, density (Computed Tomography, CT) and signal characteristics (Magnetic resonance imaging, MRI) of a mass is now available from imaging. Virtually all mediastinal masses are amenable to percutaneous image-guided biopsy. Complete assessment of a lesion is now possible in the radiology department before definitive treatment.

Table 34.2 shows the prevalence of different types of mediastinal mass in a recent surgical series of 230 patients

Table 34.2. Prevalence of different mediastinal masses in a recent surgical series of 230 patients

Mass	Prevalence (%)
Thymic tumors/cysts	24.3
Benign cysts (foregut cysts)	19.6
Neurogenic tumors	16.9
Lymphoma	15.7
Germ cell tumor	10.0
Thyroid/parathyroid masses	2.2
Vascular tumor/malformation	1.7
Miscellaneous	9.6
Data from ref. (1).	

Table 34.1. Common mediastinal masses by compartment

Superior	Anterior	Middle	Posterior
Thymic tumor	Thymic tumor	Lymphoma	Neurogenic tumors
Thymic cyst	Thymic cyst	Bronchogenic cyst	Esophageal mass
Lymphoma	Lymphoma	Pericardial cyst	Esophageal duplication cyst
Thyroid mass	Germ cell tumor		Neurenteric cyst
Parathyroid adenoma	Thyroid mass		Lateral thoracic meningocele
Lymphangioma	Parathyroid adenoma		
	Nerve sheath tumor		
	Lymphangioma		
	Hemangioma		
	Liposarcoma		
	Lipoma		

(1). The prevalence of specific types of mass differs between adult and pediatric populations. The neurogenic tumors are much more common in children, whereas lymphoma occurs more frequently in adults (2). Since around half of all mediastinal masses are asymptomatic (3), it is not uncommon for lesions to be picked up as an incidental finding on a chest radiograph or CT scan being performed for some other reason. Symptomatic masses are more likely to be malignant than benign (3).

High kilovoltage (kVp) chest radiographs (in the region of 140 kVp) are optimal for demonstrating mediastinal structures and lines (4). Special filters can be used to improve X-ray penetration of the mediastinum, without overexposing the lungs (5).

The majority of masses discovered on plain radiographs will nowadays be referred for CT evaluation. The examination should cover the whole chest, and can easily be extended to include the upper abdomen, if clinically appropriate. Intravenous contrast medium is helpful to define optimally the anatomic relations of any lesion, and to study patterns of enhancement. A precontrast scan will demonstrate any foci of calcification. A slice width of 5–10 mm is suitable for most mediastinal applications with spiral CT scanners.

CT can define most masses well, but usually histologic confirmation of disease will be required. Possible exceptions to this include mature teratoma, and other fatty masses such as mediastinal lipomatosis, fat herniation, liposarcoma, and lipoma, where the CT appearances are highly specific.

MRI is generally used as a problem-solving modality in the mediastinum. It shows the vascular relations of a mass well without the need for intravenous contrast medium, e.g., when contrast agents are contraindicated. The ability to image in any plane can help in assessment of lesions in the aortopulmonary window and subcarinal area. In a few cases MRI can give specific information that can narrow the differential diagnosis. It is particularly useful for confirming hemorrhage or the cystic nature of a mass, as well as chest wall invasion. It is also the modality of choice for neurogenic tumors because it can show the intraspinal component of the tumor better than CT scan (6).

Thymus

The Normal Thymus

The thymus is a lobulated, encapsulated organ with cortical and medullary portions, consisting mainly of epithelial cells and lymphocytes. The thymus is relatively large in infancy and childhood and undergoes fatty involution after puberty, but never disappears completely. Small islands of thymic tissue are consistently found at histology in the mediastinal fat in adults (7).

Differentiation of the large, normal thymus in the young from a thymic tumor may be difficult. A normal

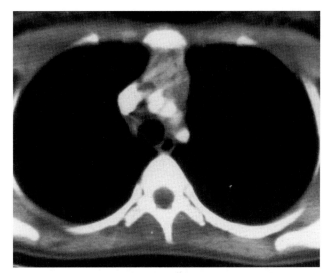

Figure 34.1. Normal appearance of the thymus in a 13 year old female.

thymus generally does not displace, encase or distort the great vessels, and is symmetric (Fig. 34.1). The epicentre of any mass is usually to one side of the midline. Invasive masses will show changes in the adjacent mediastinal fat on CT. The signal characteristics on MRI may be helpful: thymic masses tend to have heterogeneous signal on MRI, whereas the T_1 and T_2 signal of normal thymus is homogeneous (8). Small tumors may be extremely difficult to detect if they do not deform the contour of the thymus. Moreover, an angular contour to the thymus may be normal in those under 20 years of age (8,9). Fortunately, thymic tumors in the young are fairly rare.

Thymoma

The term thymoma should be reserved for thymic epithelial neoplasms, as distinct from other tumor types (seminoma, carcinoid tumor, Hodgkin and non-Hodgkin lymphoma) that can involve the thymus, but are not types of thymoma. Historically, there have been many attempted histologic classifications of thymoma, indicating the difficult and controversial nature of this undertaking. A new classification of thymic epithelial tumors into five categories has recently been proposed by Müller-Hermelink and coworkers, as follows: (a) medullary thymoma; (b) mixed thymoma; (c) predominantly cortical (organoid) thymoma; (d) cortical thymoma; and (e) well-differentiated thymic carcinoma (10). An advantage of this system is that it allows a good prediction of tumor behavior and prognosis and, broadly speaking, correlates well with the surgical staging system of Masaoka et al. (11). The medullary and mixed thymomas correlate with stage I (fully encapsulated) and Stage II (microscopic or limited macroscopic invasion) lesions; the cortical thymomas with stage II and stage III (macroscopic invasion into neighboring organs) lesions; and the carcinomas with

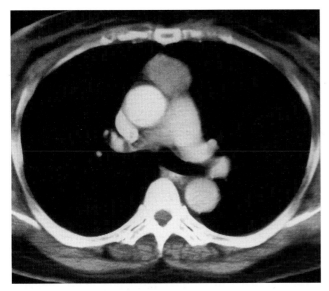

Figure 34.2. Thymoma. Small, well-defined anterior mediastinal mass discovered incidentally on CT scan. At surgery, fully encapsulated thymoma.

stage III and stage IV (pleuropericardial or distant dissemination) lesions (12,13).

Thymomas generally arise in the anterior mediastinum, but are occasionally seen in the neck or extending in to the middle and posterior mediastinum. They are unusual in the young, and tend to occur at an average age of 50–60 years, with equal sex predominance. They are asymptomatic and present as an incidental finding in 25% of cases (14). A small, encapsulated thymoma rarely produces symptoms directly, and is not commonly seen on the chest radiograph (Fig. 34.2). However, it may present indirectly, since thymoma is associated with a variety of autoimmune disorders, of which the most important is myasthenia gravis. Myasthenia is the commonest mode of presentation of thymoma, with symptoms from tumor compression next in frequency (14).

The relationship of thymic disease to myasthenia gravis is complex. In patients with myasthenia, around 10% will have a thymoma, 65% will have follicular hyperplasia of the gland, and 25% will have a normal thymus. Conversely, in a series of 283 patients with thymoma, 46% had myasthenia gravis (15,16). In patients who have not responded well to medical therapy, total thymectomy will improve symptoms of myasthenia irrespective of whether a thymoma is present. In general, patients with a thymoma should have surgery to prevent the complications of invasive thymoma (17). It is therefore important to seek a thymoma in patients with myasthenia gravis, even if they are responding well to medical therapy and would not otherwise be candidates for thymectomy on clinical grounds.

Invasive thymoma shows tumor growth through the thymic capsule into mediastinal fat or into neighboring organs or structures. More advanced lesions can affect the pleural space, either as pleural seeding, or as a more generalized pleural thickening that may resemble mesothe-

lioma. Direct transdiaphragmatic spread can occur, but true metastatic spread is rare (14,16).

CT is effective for detection and assessment of extent of thymoma. In the adult, thymoma appears as a smooth or lobulated soft tissue density mass, which may have low attenuation regions representing cyst formation or hemorrhage. Calcification may be present. These features are relatively nonspecific, and can be seen in other thymic masses. A smooth border and preserved fat plane around a thymoma indicates that it is encapsulated, although microscopic invasion will not be detected on CT. Conversely, stranding into the mediastinal fat around the tumor may be caused by associated inflammatory or fibrotic changes, leading to a false-positive diagnosis of invasion. Frank tumor invasion of adjacent structures and pleural deposits are easily detected with CT (18,19).

With MRI, thymoma has a higher intensity than muscle on T_1-weighted images, and increased signal intensity on T_2-weighted images. In malignant thymomas, heterogeneity of T_2 signal may be seen, and 50% show a distinctly lobulated architecture with prominent fibrous septa. There may also be areas of very high T_2 signal intensity due to the presence of areas of cystic degeneration and hemorrhage. In benign thymoma, there is only mild inhomogeneity of signal on T_2-weighted images, with absence of lobulated architecture (20).

Thymic carcinoma cannot readily be distinguished from other forms of invasive thymoma on imaging grounds. There are usually signs of locally aggressive behavior, and calcification and heterogeneity of the lesion are more prominent features (21). In a series comparing invasive thymoma and thymic carcinoma, mediastinal lymph node enlargement and distant metastases were a feature of carcinoma (22).

Thymic Carcinoid Tumor

Thymic carcinoid is a malignant tumor of neuroendocrine origin, which is pathologically distinct from thymoma. It may be associated with carcinoid tumors at other more typical sites such as bronchus or ileum, and may be part of multiple endocrine neoplasia syndromes, types I and IIa. Ectopic adrenocorticotrophic hormone (ACTH) production can occur in up to one third of cases, resulting in Cushing syndrome. In these patients, the tumor may have a more aggressive course. Generally, thymic carcinoid often invades locally and tends to metastasize (23,24). The CT imaging features are essentially those of thymoma.

Thymolipoma

Thymolipoma is a rare, benign thymic lesion consisting of mature adipose tissue with islands of normal thymus. Sex incidence is approximately equal, and the lesion affects children and adults. It may grow to a large size, and is invariably situated in the anterior mediastinum, in contact with thymus. On plain radiographs the lesion may resemble cardiomegaly. Appearances on CT and MRI are those of a predominantly fatty tumor with soft tissue strands representing the areas of normal thymus (25).

Thymic Follicular Hyperplasia and Rebound Hyperplasia

Thymic follicular hyperplasia is a histologic term referring to the presence of lymphoid follicles within the thymus. The gland may be normal in size, shape or weight in the presence of thymic hyperplasia. As previously stated, this condition is present in 65% of patients with myasthenia gravis (17), and is also seen in a variety of other autoimmune conditions, including thyrotoxicosis. Addison disease and systemic lupus erythematosus. Thymic hyperplasia may appear normal on CT and MRI, or the gland may show diffuse enlargement with density and signal characteristics of a normal gland (26).

The thymus may undergo rapid involution as a result of steroid therapy, Cushing syndrome, chemotherapy and other stresses. Following removal of the stressful stimulus, the thymus usually grows back to its normal size. In rebound thymic hyperplasia, the growing gland exceeds its original size by 50% of its previous volume (27). Histologically, overgrowth of normal thymus elements in normal proportions is seen, in contrast to follicular hyperplasia. In the study of Choyke et al. (27), this phenomenon was seen in 25% of the children and young adults studied, between 3 and 8 months following cessation of chemotherapy. Eventually the thymus returns to its normal size.

In patients being treated for malignancy that may involve or recur in the thymus, rebound hyperplasia after cessation of chemotherapy may suggest tumor recurrence. Where patients satisfy the criteria for rebound hyperplasia on imaging, it is reasonable to adopt a conservative approach and observe with CT or MRI to ensure that the thymus is returning to normal size.

Thymic Cysts

Thymic cysts may be developmental in origin, and in this case are usually unilocular, asymptomatic and occur most frequently in the young. They are thought to originate in remnants of the third branchial pouch, and present as a cystic lesion in the neck more often than a mediastinal cyst.

Other thymic cysts are multilocular in nature, and this is thought to represent an acquired process of a reactive nature as it is invariably accompanied by evidence of inflammation and fibrosis (28). Multilocular cystic changes in the thymus may be idiopathic, or may be associated with specific infections such as HIV in children (29). More importantly it can be seen in association with malignancy in the thymus, usually nodular sclerosing Hodgkin disease or seminoma, although thymoma and large-cell lymphoma are associated with lesser frequency.

Other cystic change in the thymus can result from cystic degeneration in tumors, and from cystic lymphangioma of the thymus (30a). Appearances on plain films and CT or MRI are similar to cysts elsewhere. MRI is useful for detecting hemorrhage within the cyst, which is seen as an area of high signal intensity on both T_1- and T_2-weighted images.

Lymphoma

Malignant lymphoma of the mediastinum may occur as a primary mediastinal disease, or it may be part of a widespread, disseminated process. The three main categories of lymphoma affecting the mediastinum are Hodgkin disease (usually of nodular sclerosing type), lymphoblastic lymphoma and large-cell lymphoma. All of these have a strong predilection for the thymus, and thus present primarily as anterior or superior mediastinal masses. Lymph node involvement may occur in addition to thymic infiltration, or as an isolated finding.

Mediastinal lymphoma tends to affect young adults, and is commoner in females. It may present incidentally on a chest radiograph, or may cause symptoms of chest pain, cough, dyspnea or superior vena cava (SVC) obstruction if sufficiently large. Systemic symptoms can occur in disseminated disease.

CT is used to stage disease extent prior to treatment, and to monitor treatment, and shows soft tissue density enlargement of the thymus and/or mediastinal lymph nodes groups. Cystic change may be present, particularly in Hodgkin disease. Calcification is unusual at presentation, but occurs quite commonly after treatment. In aggressive tumors, involvement of the pericardium, pleura, lung, or chest wall may be visible, as well as SVC obstruction (Fig. 34.3).

A common problem in the management of lymphoma is the residual anterior mediastinal mass after treatment. MRI may be helpful in determining whether such masses contain active tumor tissue or are merely fibrotic. The T_2 signal intensity is raised in tumor and low in mature fibrosis. There can be overlap in these appearances in the first 3–6 months after completion of treatment due to active fibrosis with cellular fibroblastic activity. MRI has a predictive value of approximately 75% and appears superior to erythrocyte sedimentation rate (ESR) and gallium scanning for this purpose (30b–d).

Germ Cell Tumors of the Mediastinum

Germ cell tumors (GCT) comprise approximately 20% of all mediastinal masses. They probably arise from extragonadal primitive germ cell rests within or closely related to the thymus, although they are histologically quite distinct from thymoma (31–33). The discovery of a mediasti-

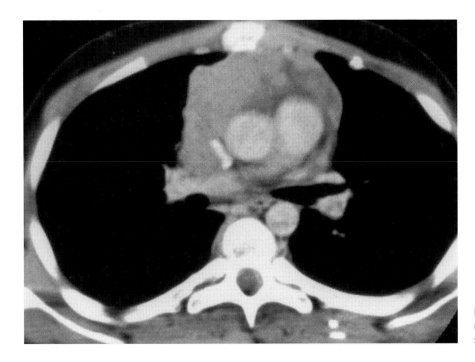

Figure 34.3. Lymphoma. Large, lobulated anterior mediastinal mass, causing marked compression of superior vena cava.

nal GCT should prompt investigation of testis or ovary as a possible primary site, although this is rare in the absence of retroperitoneal involvement (32,34).

Benign (mature cystic teratoma) and malignant (seminoma and nonseminoma) forms occur. The malignant tumors have a strong predilection for the male sex.

Mature Cystic Teratoma

This benign lesion accounts for the majority of mediastinal GCT, and occurs with approximately equal frequency in both sexes. Mature teratoma is often clinically silent,

and may be diagnosed incidentally. It can grow to a very large size, when symptoms occur due to compression of adjacent structures, sepsis or rupture into the pleural space or bronchial tree. In the latter case, the patient may cough up sebaceous material and hair. Histologically, the lesion is usually cystic and multilocular, and contains multiple elements including skin, sebaceous glands and hair follicles, fat (35), and foci of calcification or ossification (35).

Plain films show a well-defined anterior mediastinal mass with calcification and areas of soft tissue and fat density (Fig. 34.4). The CT features include the following: the wall is well defined and may contain calcification,

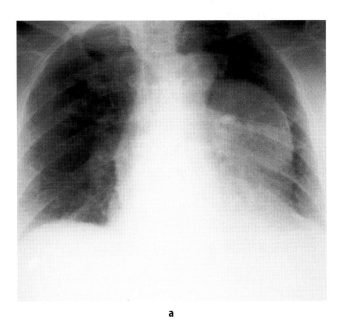

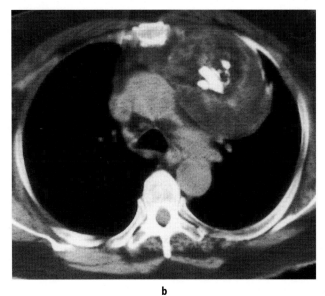

a   b

Figure 34.4. **a** Plain radiograph showing large anterior mediastinal mass. Faint rim and central calcification. **b** CT scan showing well-encapsulated mass containing fat and soft tissue density, with central calcification. Appearances are very specific for mature teratoma.

water or soft tissue attenuation is seen in the cystic regions; areas of fat attenuation are common, with occasional fat–fluid levels, and foci of calcification may be present within the mass (36,37). The presence of fat, soft tissue and calcification within a benign-looking lesion is highly specific for this diagnosis (Fig. 34.4).

Malignant Germ Cell Tumors

These are classified into seminoma, and nonseminomatous forms (teratocarcinoma, embryonal carcinoma, yolk sac tumor, choriocarcinoma and mixed GCT). Malignant GCT is predominantly a disease of young male adults and, unlike, benign cystic teratoma, most patients (about 70%) have symptoms at presentation (35,38). These include dyspnea, cough, chest pain and SVC obstruction, which occurs in 10% (38). However, up to 30% of patients may be asymptomatic, the mass being discovered as an incidental finding following chest radiography or CT (35,38). Most nonseminomatous GCT (and a few seminomas) cause high blood levels of tumor markers such as human chorionic gonadotrophin (HCG) and alpha-fetoprotein (AFP). These are helpful for diagnosis and follow-up, if present (35).

The plain film, CT and MRI features of malignant GCT are relatively nonspecific and are similar to those of other malignant tumors of the anterior mediastinum. Plain films show a lobular mass, in which fat density or calcification is absent. CT features are those of an asymmetric, lobulated or irregular soft tissue mass, with little enhancement, which may show areas of necrosis of hemorrhage. Capsular enhancement is occasionally seen, but calcification is rare. The lesion may show locally invasive behavior, with loss of fat planes and involvement of adjacent structures. Metastatic spread to lung and bone, and pleuropericardial effusions may be seen (Fig. 34.5) (39,40).

After treatment, a residual mass may be present which may be soft tissue density or cystic. This may represent fibrosis or residual benign mature teratoma. Cystic masses, despite being benign, may grow in size following successful therapy (41). It is impossible on imaging criteria to be certain whether lesions of this type are benign or malignant, and the tumor marker levels may be helpful in patients who are marker-positive.

Thyroid and Parathyroid Masses

Eighty percent of mediastinal thyroid masses are sited anterior to the trachea, the remainder lying between the trachea and esophagus. They are mostly due to nodular hyperplasia (multinodular goitre). Thyroid adenoma is less common and carcinoma occurs in 16% (42). On plain radiographs, the goitre is seen as a smooth, well-defined soft tissue mass causing displacement and possibly narrowing of the trachea. The direction of tracheal displacement will depend on the site of the goitre. Narrowing and displacement are easily assessed on thoracic inlet views or CT. In severe cases, cough, dyspnea or stridor may be present. The rationale for surgery is to relieve compressive symptoms on the trrachea and occasionally the great veins, and because of the possibility of occult carcinoma (42).

Calcification is common, particularly in benign disease where it is often of a focal, nodular pattern.

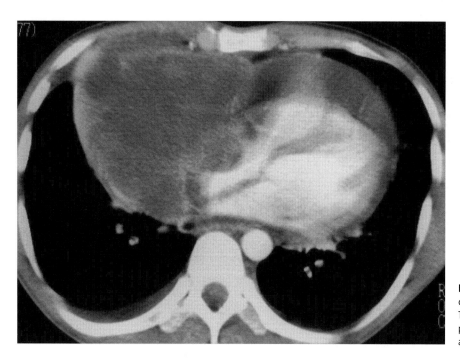

Figure 34.5. CT scan showing large mass with some capsular enhancement and extensive central necrosis. There is invasion of the pericardium and heart with pericardial effusion. Chest wall invasion is also seen anteriorly. Malignant germ cell tumor.

Calcification is also seen in thyroid malignancy (43). On CT, the normal thyroid is high attenuation due to its iodine content, and shows prolonged, intense enhancement with intravenous contrast medium (44–46). After enhancement, the multinodular gland appears heterogeneous with areas of low attenuation representing poorly enhancing nodules or cysts. The mediastinal component is usually connected to the thyroid in the neck, although true ectopic thyroid masses do rarely occur (45,46). Radioisotope imaging with ^{123}I or ^{131}I can be useful for confirming the thyroid nature of a mediastinal mass if there is sufficient functioning thyroid tissue in the lesion to take up the tracer. However, the CT appearances are usually sufficiently specific.

Overall, about 20% of parathyroid adenomas occur in the mediastinum, the majority in the anterior compartment, with about 10% in the superior mediastinum. They are more common in previously operated patients, and those with multiple endocrine neoplasia syndromes, types I and IIa (47,48). In patients with uncomplicated hyperparathyroidism, preoperative imaging is controversial as an experienced surgeon has a 95–98% chance of locating the abnormal parathyroid glands during surgical exploration (49,50). When an ectopic gland is suspected, imaging with either MRI or ^{99m}Tc-sestamibi radioisotope scanning is indicated, since prior localization facilitates surgery in these cases. Both imaging techniques are effective for orthotopic and ectopic mediastinal adenomas (51,52): On MRI, parathyroid adenomas show intermediate signal on T_1-weighted images, and high signal on T_2-weighted images and short-tau inversion recovery (STIR) sequences (Fig. 34.6). Typical sensitivities for adenoma detection with MRI are 64–88%, with specificities 88–95% (51,53).

Mesenchymal Tumors

A large number of mediastinal mesenchymal tumors have been described. They arise from adipose tissue, blood vessels, lymphatics, connective tissue and muscle, and are quite rare.

Fatty Tumors

Liposarcoma, although rare, is one of the commoner malignant mesenchymal neoplasms. In the mediastinum, the average age at presentation is 45 years, and the tumor may be large when diagnosed. Symptoms due to tumor compression occur in 63%. Like liposarcomas elsewhere in the body, it has a heterogeneous appearance on CT, with variable degrees of fat density interspersed with soft tissue elements. It may vary from a relatively benign, encapsulated tumor to an aggressive infiltrating lesion (54,55). Lipoblastoma is a benign neoplasm of infants and children that which may arise primarily in the mediastinum. It shows a variable amount of fat density, and may appear similar to liposarcoma (56). Angiolipoma, another benign tumor that can appear identical to liposarcoma, has been reported as arising in the mediastinum (57). Lipoma occurs rarely in the mediastinum, and on CT has the appearance of lipoma elsewhere in the body, namely well-circumscribed fat density with few, if any, soft tissue strands or septa.

The above fatty mesenchymal tumors may be confused with other fat-containing masses in the mediastinum. Mature teratoma should be easy to differentiate due to its well-defined wall, possibility of fat–fluid levels and

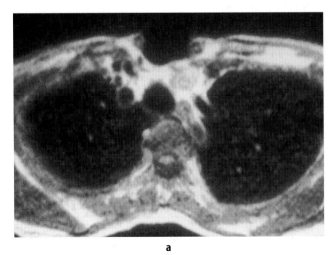

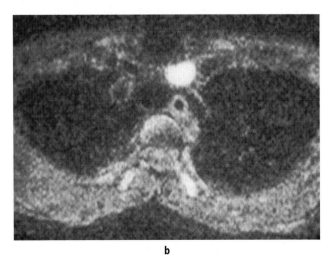

| a | b |

Figure 34.6. T_1-weighted (**a**) and STIR sequence (**b**) MRI scan in a patient with hypercalcemia. The left-sided superior mediastinal parathyroid adenoma shows high signal on the STIR image. (From ref. (51), with permission.)

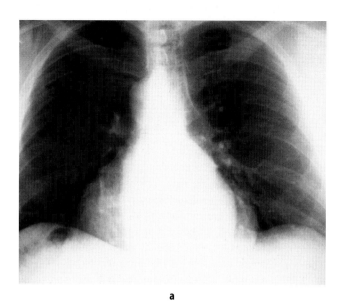

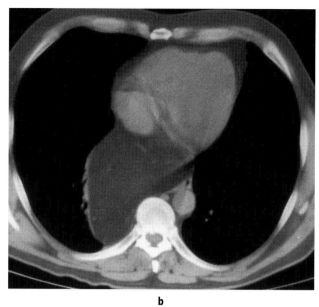

a

b

Figure 34.7. **a** Chest radiograph shows posterior mediastinal mass, probably of fat density. **b** CT scan confirms huge herniation of intraabdominal fat through esophageal hiatus.

calcification either within the mass or the wall. Thymolipoma, on the other hand, may be indistinguishable from liposarcoma on morphologic grounds. Thymolipoma favors an anterior mediastinal position, whereas liposarcoma tends to occur posteriorly. Mediastinal lipomatosis is a diffuse, benign infiltration of the mediastinum with histologically normal fat, usually seen in obese patients, or those taking steroids or with Cushing syndrome (58,59). The diagnosis is easily made from CT. Herniations of intraabdominal fat can occur into the mediastinum through the foramina of Morgagni or Bochdalek, acquired diaphragmatic defects or the esophageal hiatus (Fig. 34.7). Connection of these fatty masses with the intraabdominal fat is usually obvious on CT.

Vascular Tumors

Hemangiomas of the mediastinum occur in the anterior or (less commonly) the posterior mediastinum. In adults they are usually of the cavernous variety. In a recent series of 14 cases, the CT appearances were as follows: well-circumscribed mass, heterogeneous appearance on plain scan (60%), punctate calcifications or phleboliths (55%), heterogeneous, mainly central contrast enhancement (60).

Lymphangioma (cystic hygroma) is a cystic congenital malformation of the lymphatic system, generally presenting in infancy. It usually originates in the neck, but may extend into the superior mediastinum, or be wholly within

the mediastinum. Where present, symptoms are usually due to compression of adjacent structures. CT shows a water-density mass in the appropriate location, which may contain septa (61). If large, the lesion usually envelopes adjacent structures, but may compress or even invade locally in rare cases (62).

Neurogenic Tumors

Two main categories of mediastinal neurogenic tumor can be considered: the peripheral nerve sheath tumors (neurofibroma, Schwannoma and malignant peripheral nerve sheath tumor); and the tumors of the sympathetic nervous system (ganglioneuroma, neuroblastoma and ganglioneuroblastoma). They comprise the largest group of posterior mediastinal neoplasms, although they do occur rarely in other compartments, e.g., arising from the vagus or phrenic nerve (63). Neuroblastoma and ganglioneuroblastoma are childhood tumors, while the peripheral nerve sheath tumors are rare in patients under 20 years of age.

Tumors of Peripheral Nerves

These tumors are all more common in patients with neurofibromatosis. Usually asymptomatic when benign, they are often discovered incidentally on chest radiographs. The majority of intrathoracic nerve sheath tumors arise from intercostal nerves and form a usually well-rounded mass that may straddle an intervertebral foramen (dumb-bell tumor), or which may displace and thin adjacent ribs. Peripheral nerve tumors rarely calcify. Malignant change occurs most commonly in patients with neurofibromatosis (64).

A specific appearance has been reported at MRI in a proportion of neurofibromas (65,66). This consists of a target pattern, with an area of relatively high T_1 signal centrally in the lesion, and high T_2 signal in the periphery of the mass. With intravenous contrast medium, the central portion enhances. This pattern is thought to represent myxoid degeneration surrounding a central nidus of solid tumor tissue. Schwannomas may show a mildly inhomogeneous pattern due to areas of cystic degeneration (65).

Tumors of Sympathetic Nerves

Neuroblastomas are usually highly malignant, and ganglioblastomas of intermediate malignancy. Ganglioneuromas are benign and occur in an older age group than do the other sympathetic nerve lesions. The malignant tumors more commonly arise in the adrenal, where they are less well differentiated, and have a poorer prognosis. A mediastinal tumor may therefore represent either a primary manifestation or a secondary deposit. The benign lesions are said to have an elongated tapering shape rather than rounded. Calcification occurs frequently, approximately 10% overall on plain radiographic criteria (67), but in 25% on CT (68). In neuroblastoma, calcification is generally amorphous and fine in appearance, with fewer tumors showing punctate or rim clacification (68). However, the presence of calcification is not a reliable way of differentiating benign from malignant tumors. As with peripheral nerve tumors, bone changes are common, and bone destruction is a reliable sign of malignancy (Fig. 34.8). On CT, lesions may show areas of low density representing cystic degeneration and necrosis, as well as lipid deposition. Neurogenic tumors generally show intense enhancement with intravenous contrast media. MRI is superior to CT when there is involvement of the spinal canal (6).

Mediastinal Cysts

Table 34.3 shows the different types of cystic lesion that arise in the mediastinum. The majority of these are developmental in origin. The foregut cysts (bronchogenic, esophageal duplication, and neurenteric cysts) share certain histologic characteristics that may make it difficult to distinguish them in some situations.

Table 34.3. Cystic lesions of the mediastinum

Bronchogenic cyst
Esophageal duplication cyst
Neurenteric cyst
Pericardial cyst
Thymic cyst
Lateral thoracic meningocele
Thoracic duct cyst
Mediastinal pancreatic pseudocyst

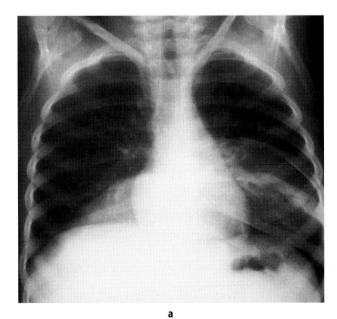
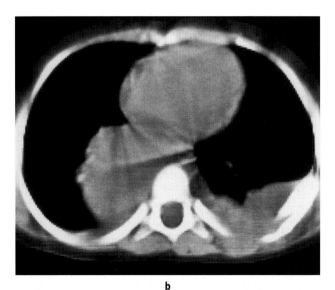

a   b

Figure 34.8. a Chest radiograph in a child with right-sided posterior mediastinal mass, with further left-sided component showing rib displacement and destruction. **b** CT scan shows minimal calcification in the mass and confirms left rib and chest wall involvement. Neuroblastoma.

Mediastinal cysts are frequently asymptomatic, and an incidental finding on imaging performed for another purpose. As with cysts elsewhere in the body, the essential imaging features are smooth outline, imperceptible or thin wall, low density and lack of contrast enhancement.

Bronchogenic Cysts

Formed from a developmental outpouching of the foregut, bronchogenic cysts are most frequently found in the right paratracheal region or near the carina. They can also occur at other mediastinal or intrapulmonary locations (69,70). The cyst wall is lined with ciliated columnar epithelium, and may contain cartilage, smooth muscle, bronchial glands and nerve trunks. Cysts are usually unilocular and spherical with a thin wall, and contain clear or gelatinous fluid.

A bronchogenic cyst is best evaluated with CT, where it appears as a well-defined, rounded mass in the appropriate position with an imperceptible wall. As with all cysts, there should be absence of enhancement following administration of intravenous contrast medium. The cyst should be of homogeneous density, although the Hounsfield value of bronchogenic cysts may vary from water density to as high as 120 HU due to protein hemorrhage or mucus within the cyst (Fig. 34.9). (71). This may make it difficult to differentiate the cyst from a solid lesion. In these cases, the signal characteristics of the cyst on MRI may be helpful. The T_1 signal intensity may be relatively high in cysts containing protein, blood or mucus, and layering of contents may be visible. The T_2-weighted images should show a very high signal (72,73).

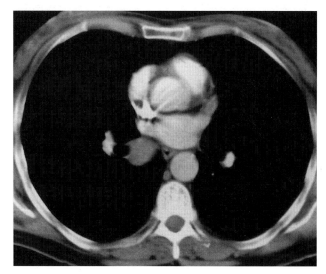

Figure 34.9. Well-defined soft tissue density lesion inferomedial to bronchus intermedius. Bronchogenic cyst.

Esophageal Duplication Cysts

Esophageal duplication cysts have a developmental origin similar to that of bronchogenic cysts, occur in similar sites in the mediastinum, and may even be difficult to distinguish histologically. Often clinically silent, they may present with dysphagia, pain or compressive symptoms. Barium swallow shows the typical appearances of a submucosal or extrinsic lesion with no irregularity of the mucosal surface. The CT features are of a smooth spherical or tubular structure, of water or soft tissue density, in close proximity to the esophagus.

Neurenteric Cysts

Neurenteric cysts are rare. They have a complex embryologic origin due to the close proximity of the notochord and the embryonic foregut. Imaging studies demonstrate a posterior mediastinal cyst often associated with an anomaly of the adjacent vertebrae, such as butterfly vertebra or hemivertebra (74).

Pericardial Cysts

Pericardial cysts are caused by failure of fusion of one of the multiple lacunae that form the pericardium in embryologic life. They are generally unilocular and contain clear fluid, unless infected or hemorrhagic. The cardiophrenic angles are the usual site, particularly the right. About one third of pericardial cysts are situated higher in the mediastinum (75).

Pericardial cysts are usually asymptomatic, but in 30% of patients can cause dyspnea or chest pain when large (75). They are often an incidental finding on the chest radiography where they typically appear as a well-defined soft tissue density lesion in one of the cardiophrenic angles. On CT, they are of water density, rounded or ovoid in shape, do not enhance and very rarely calcify (Fig. 34.10). Occasionally the density of the cyst may be in the soft tissue range (76). MRI shows the typical features of a benign cystic lesion.

Other Mediastinal Cystic Lesions

Lateral thoracic meningocele is an outpouching of the meninges through an intervertebral foramen. It is commonly associated with neurofibromatosis type I, and there may be local costovertebral abnormalities. The CT appearances are those of a posterior mediastinal mass of cerebrospinal fluid density density, which communicates

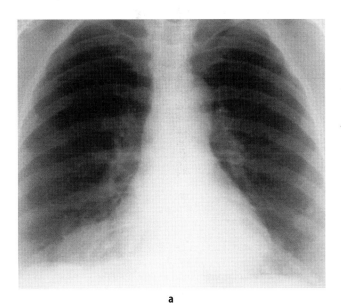

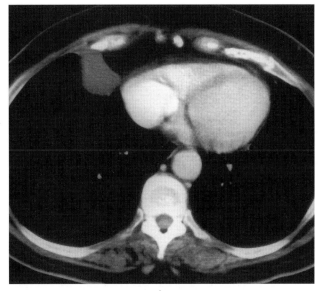

a

b

Figure 34.10. a Well-defined, soft tissue density mass in right cardiophrenic angle, consistent with pericardial cyst. **b** CT scan confirms water-density pericardial cyst in typical position.

with the spinal theca. This latter feature may be easier to appreciate on MRI (77).

Thoracic duct cysts are extremely rare, and are found in the posterior mediastinum where they have the imaging features of a chylous cyst. Diagnosis can be made by lymphangiography or needle aspiration of the cyst (78).

In cases of mediastinal pancreatic pseudocyst, there is usually associated abdominal symptomatology, as well as imaging signs of pancreatic inflammation in continuity with the mediastinal lesion (79).

References

1. Cohen AJ, Thompson L, Edwards FH, et al. (1991) Primary cysts and tumours of the mediastinum. Ann Thorac Surg 51:378–386.
2. Azarow KS, Pearl RH, Zurcher R, et al. (1993) Primary mediastinal masses. A comparison of adult and pediatric populations. J Thorac Cardiovasc Surg 106:67–72.
3. Benjamin SP, McCormack LJ, Effler DB, et al. (1972) Primary tumours of the mediastinum. Chest 62:297–303.
4. Revesz G, Shea FJ, Kundel HL (1982) The effects of kilovoltage on diagnostic accuracy in chest radiography. Radiology 142:615–618.
5. Wieder S, Adams PL (1981) Improved routine chest radiography with a trough filter. AJR 137:695–698.
6. Webb WR, Sostman HD (1992) MR imaging of thoracic disease: Clinical uses. Radiology 182:621–630.
7. Moore AV, Korobkin M, Olanow W, et al. (1983) Age-related changes in the thymus gland: CT-pathologic correlation. AJR 141:241–246.
8. Bothroyd AE, Hall-Craggs MA, Dicks-Mireaux C, et al. (1992) The magnetic resonance appearances of the normal thymus in children. Clin Radiol 45:378–381.
9. Heiberg E, Wolverson MK, Sundaram M, et al. (1982) Normal thymus: CT characteristics in subjects under age 20. AJR 138:491–494.
10. Müller-Hermelink HK, Marx A, Kirchner T (1994) Advances in the diagnosis and classification of thymic epithelial tumours. In Anthony PP, MacSween RNM (eds) Recent advances in histopathology, vol 16. Churchill Livingstone, London, pp 49–72.
11. Masaoka A, Monden Y, Nakahara K, et al. (1981) Follow-up study of thymomas with special reference to their clinical stages. Cancer 48:2485–2492.
12. Kuo TT, Lo SK (1993) Thymoma: A study of the pathologic classification of 71 cases with evaluation of the Müller-Hermelink system. Hum Pathol 24:766–771.
13. Quintanilla-Martinez L, Wilkins EW, Ferry JA, et al. (1993) Thymoma: Morphologic subclassification correlates with invasiveness and immunohistologic features in a study of 122 cases. Hum Pathol 24:958–969.
14. Le Golvan DP, Abell MR (1977) Thymomas. Cancer 39:2142–2157.
15. Wilkins EW, Edmunds LH, Castleman B (1966) Cases of thymoma at the Massachusetts General Hospital. J Thorac Cardiovasc Surg 52:322–330.
16. Lewis JE, Wick MR, Scheithauer BW, et al. (1987) Thymoma. A clinicopathologic review. Cancer 60:2727–2743.
17. Drachman DB (1994) Myasthenia gravis. N Engl J Med 330:1797–1810.
18. RL Baron, Lee JK, Sagel SS, et al. (1982) Computed tomography of the abnormal thymus. Radiology 142:127–134.
19. Rosado-de-Christenson ML, Galobardes J, Moran CA (1992) Thymoma: Radiologic–pathologic correlation. Radiographics 12:151–168.
20. Sakai F, Sone S, Kiyono K et al. (1992) MR imaging of thymoma: Radiologic–pathologic correlation. AJR 158:751–756.
21. Lee JD, Choe KO, Kim SJ, et al. (1991) CT findings in primary thymic carcinoma. J Comput Assist Tomogr 15:429–433.
22. Do YS, Im JG, Lee BH, et al. (1995) CT findings in malignant tumour of thymic epithelium. J Comput Assist Tomogr 19:192–197.
23. Wick MR, Rosai J (1991) Neuroendocrine neoplasms of the mediastinum. Semin Diagn Pathol 8:35–51.
24. Wang DY, Chang DB, Kuo SH, et al. (1994) Carcinoid tumours of the thymus. Thorax 49:357–360.

25. Rosado-de-Christenson ML, Pugatch RD, Moran CA, et al. (1994) Thymolipoma Analysis of 27 cases. Radiology 193:121–126.

26. Batra P, Herrmann C, Mulder D (1987) Mediastinal imaging in myasthenia gravis: Correlation of chest radiography, CT, MR and surgical findings. AJR 148:515–519.

27. Choyke PL, Zeman RK, Gootenberg JE, et al. (1987) Thymic atrophy and regrowth in response to chemotherapy: CT evaluation. AJR 149:269–272.

28. Suster S, Rosai J (1991) Multilocular thymic cyst: an acquired reactive process. Study of 18 cases. Am J Surg Pathol 15:388–398.

29. Mishalani SH, Lones MA, Said JW (1995) Multilocular thymic cyst. A novel thymic lesion associated with human immunodeficiency virus infection. Arch Pathol Lab Med 119:467–470.

30a. Dyer NH (1967) Cystic thymomas and thymic cysts. A review. Thorax 22:408–421.

30b. Webb WR (1989) MR imaging of treated residual Hodgkin disease. *Radiology* 170:315–316.

30c. Hill M, Cunningham D, MacVicar D et al. (1993) Role of magnetic resonance imaging in predicting relapse in residual masses after treatment of lymphoma. *J Clin Oncol* 11:2273–2278.

30d. Rahmouni A, Tempany C, Jones R, Mann R, Yang A, Zerhouni E (1993) Lymphoma: monitoring tumor size and signal intensity with MR imaging. *Radiology* 188:445–451.

31. Levine GD (1973) Primary thymic seminoma – a neoplasm ultrastructurally similar to testicular seminoma and distinct from epithelial thymoma. Cancer 31:729–741.

32. Cox JD (1975) Primary malignant germ cell tumors of the mediastinum. A study of 24 cases. Cancer 36:1162–1168.

33. Chaganti RSK, Rodriguez E, Mathew S (1994) Origin of adult male mediastinal germ cell tumours. Lancet 343:1130–1132.

34. Oberman HA, Libcke JH (1964) Malignant germinal neoplasms of the mediastinum. Cancer 17:498–507.

35. Nichols RD (1991) Mediastinal germ cell tumors: Clinical features and biologic correlates. Chest 99:472–479.

36. Brown LR, Muhm JR, Aughenbaugh GL, et al. (1987) Computed tomography of benign mature teratomas of the mediastinum. J Thorac Imaging 2:66–71.

37. Fulcher AS, Proto AV, Jolles H (1990) Cystic teratoma of the mediastinum: Demonstration of fat/fluid level. AJR 154:259–260.

38. Polansky SM, Barwick KW, Ravin CE (1979) Primary mediastinal seminoma. AJR 132:17–21.

39. Levitt RG, Husband JE, Glazer HS (1984) CT of primary germ-cell tumors of the mediastinum. AJR 142:73–78.

40. Lee KS, Im JG, Han CH, et al. (1989) Malignant primary germ cell tumors of the mediastinum: CT features. AJR 153:947–951.

41. Panicek DM, Toner GC, Heelan RT, et al. (1990) Nonseminomatous germ cell tumours: Enlarging masses despite chemotherapy. Radiology 175:499–502.

42. Wick MR, Allo MD, Thompson NW (1983) Rationale for the operative management of substernal goitres. Surgery 94:969–977.

43. Komolafe F (1981) Radiological patterns and significance of thyroid calcification. Clin Radiol 32:571–575.

44. Iida Y, Konishi J, Harioka T, et al. (1983) Thyroid CT number and its relationship to iodine concentration. Radiology 147:793–795.

45. Bashist B, Ellis K, Gold RP (1983) Computed tomography of intrathoracic goitres. AJR 140:455–460.

46. Glazer GM, Axel L, Moss AA (1982) CT diagnosis of medistinal thyroid. AJR 138:495–498.

47. Beazley RM, Costa J, Ketcham AS (1975) Reoperative parathyroid surgery. Am J Surg 130:427–429.

48. Edis AJ, Sheedy PF, Beahrs OH, et al. (1978) Results of reoperation for hyperparathyroidism, with evaluation of preoperative localisation studies. Surgery 84:384–393.

49. Satava RM, Beahrs OH, Scholz DA (1975) Success rate of cervical exploration for hyperparathyroidism. Arch Surg 110:625–628.

50. Thompson NW, Eckhauser FE, Harness JK (1982) The anatomy of primary hyperparathyroidism. Surgery 92:814–882.

51. Wright AR, Goddard PR, Nicholson S, et al. (1992) Fat-suppression magnetic resonance imaging in the preoperative localisation of parathyroid adenomas. Clin Radiol 46:324–328.

52. Nguyen BD (1999) Parathyroid imaging with Tc-99m sestamibi planar and SPECT scintigraphy. Radiographics 19:601–614.

53. Kang YS, Rosen K, Clark OH, et al. (1993) Localization of abnormal parathyroid glands of the mediastinum with MR imaging. Radiology 189:137–141.

54. Schweitzer DL, Aguam AS (1977) Primary liposarcoma of the mediastinum. Report of a case and review of the literature. J Thorac Cardiovasc Surg 74:83–97.

55. Standerfer RJ, Armistead SH, Paneth M (1981) Liposarcoma of the mediastinum: Report of two cases and review of the literature. Thorax 36:693–694.

56. Dudgeon DL, Haller JA (1984) Pediatric lipoblastomatosis. Two unusual cases. Surgery 95:371–373.

57. Kline ME, Patel BU, Agosti SJ (1990) Noninfiltrating angiolipoma of the mediastinum. Radiology 175:737–738.

58. Homer MJ, Wechsler RJ, Carter BL (1978) Mediastinal lipomatosis. CT confirmation of a normal variant. Radiology 128:657–666.

59. Teates CD (1970) Steroid-induced mediastinal lipomatosis. Radiology 96:501–502.

60. McAdams HP, Rosado-de-Christenson ML, Moran CA (1994) Mediastinal hemangioma: Radiographic and CT features in 14 patients. Radiology 193:399–402.

61. Pilla TJ, Wolverson MK, Sundaram M, et al. (1982) CT evaluation of cystic lymphangiomas of the mediastinum. Radiology 144:841–842.

62. Scalzetti EM, Heitzman ER, Groskin SA et al. (1991) Developmental lymphatic disorders of the thorax. Radiographics 11:1069–1085.

63. Dabir RR, Piccione W, Kittle CF (1990) Intrathoracic tumours of the vagus nerve. Am Thorac Surg 50:494–497.

64. Reed JC, Hallet KK, Feigin DS (1978) Neural tumours of the thorax: Subject review from the AFIP. Radiology 126:9–17.

65. Sakai F, Sone S, Kiyono K (1992) Intrathoracic neurogenic tumours: MR – pathologic correlation. AJR 159:279–283.

66. Suh JS, Abenoza P, Galloway HR, et al. (1992) Peripheral (extracranial) nerve tumours: Correlation of MR imaging and histologic findings. Radiology 183:341–346.

67. Eklof O, Gooding CA (1967) Intrathoracic neuroblastoma. AJR 100:202–207.

68. Armstrong EA, Harwood-Nash DC, Ritz CR, et al. (1982) CT of neuroblastomas and ganglioneuromas in children. AJR 139:571–576.

69. St-Georges R, Deslauriers J, Duranceau A, et al. (1991) Clinical spectrum of bronchogenic cysts of the mediastinum and lung in the adult. Ann Thorac Surg 52:6–13.

70. Wick MR (1990) Mediastinal cysts and intrathoracic thyroid tumors. Semin Diagn Pathol 7:285–294.

71. Mendelson DS, Rose JS, Efremedis SC, et al. (1983) Bronchogenic cysts with high CT numbers. AJR 140:463–465.

72. Nakata H, Egashira K, Watanabe H, et al. (1993) MRI of bronchogenic cysts. J Comput Assist Tomogr 17:267–270.

73. Lyon RD, McAdams HP (1993) Mediastinal bronchogenic cyst: Demonstration of a fluid–fluid level at MR imaging. Radiology 186:427–428.

74. Wilson ES (1969) Neurenteric cyst of the mediastinum. AJR 107:641–646.

75. Feigin DS, Fenoglio JJ, McAllister HA, et al. (1977) Pericardial cysts: A radiologic–pathologic correlation and review. Radiology 125:15–20.

76. Brunner DR, Whitley NO (1984) A pericardial cyst with high CT numbers. AJR 142:279–280.

77. Nakasu Y, Minouchi K, Hatsuda N, et al. (1991) Thoracic meningocele in neurofibromatosis: CT and MR findings. J Comput Assist Tomogr 15:1062–1064.

78. Morettin LB, Allen TE (1986) Thoracic duct cyst: diagnosis with needle aspiration Radiology 161:437–438.

79. Owens GR, Arger PH, Mulhern CB, et al. (1980) CT evaluation of mediastinal pseudocyst. J Comput Assist Tomogr 4:256–259.

35 Chest Trauma

K. Malagari and Ch. Roussos

Introduction

Chest trauma, as indicated by World Health Organization reports, is responsible for one fourth of trauma deaths and contributes in about the same percentage to a lethal outcome. Motor vehicle accidents represent the majority of causes and most commonly involve young people.

Accumulated knowledge and expertise from a variety of casualties from civilian and military trauma centers over the years have led to the emergence of *trauma medicine* as a new discipline on the medical field, one, that requires immediate and multidisciplinary involvement of several clinical specialties and radiologists for decision-making during primary survey, rescuscitation and stabilization, secondary survey, and definitive care.

In this chapter, imaging manifestations of chest trauma to different thoracic sites are discussed separately, focusing on initial and secondary imaging surveys, with all advocated imaging modalities.

Trauma to the Lung Parenchyma and Tracheobronchial Tree

Lung Parenchyma

Trauma to the lung parenchyma occurs in 17–70% (1,2) of blunt chest trauma, and results from direct high energy impacts through the chest wall (2) or sudden deceleration that causes shearing stresses, spallation, and explosion (3,4).

Initial injury may be followed by the development of a variety of superimposed conditions, such as posttraumatic atelectasis, aspiration, hydrostatic pulmonary edema, and alveolocapillary injury leading to adult respiratory distress syndrome (ARDS), and differential diagnosis is necessary.

Lung Contusion

It is the most common lung injury identified, accounting for 30–75% of severe blunt chest trauma (5). Depending on the extent of concurrent intrathoracic or extrathoracic injuries lung contusion may be associated with a mortality rate of 14–40% (6).

Lung contusion connotes a parenchymal injury resulting in hemorrhage and interstitial edema that gradually leads to alveolar collapse and lung consolidation. Increased permeability of the alveolar capillary membrane allows extravasation that continues for several hours after the impact. Edema accumulates and becomes detectable 1–2 h after injury and reaches a maximum after 24 h (2,7).

Radiologically, lung contusion presents as homogeneous or patchy airspace opacities (with or without an air bronchogram) that are present on admission Chest X-ray (CXR) or within 6 h from the accident and fully developed within 24 h (Fig. 35.1). It may coexist with other lung injuries such as laceration. As expected from the causal mechanism it has no lobar or segmental distribution. The absence of an air bronchogram is common and is associated with the presence of blood or secretions within the

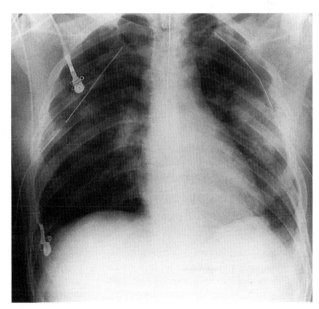

Figure 35.1. Bilateral contusions, appearing as airspace opacities of nonsegmental distribution. Rib fractures coexist on the left.

airways. CXRs almost always understimate the extent of injury (8).

Computed tomography (CT) demonstrates contusion at earlier phases than CXR. (9,10) and estimates the total volume of injured lung, which predicts the need for ventilatory support (11). In addition, the peripheral and geographic distribution adjacent to chest wall solid structures that reflects the sites of energy transfer is better shown on CT (Fig. 35.2). Furthermore, Wagner et al. correlated CT distribution and injury mechanism, identifying four distinct types of lesion (12). Sparing of subpleural parenchyma has been observed in children and has been proposed as a differential diagnostic sign from superimposed processes (13).

Despite the fact that there is no consistent relationship between the clinical and radiologic severity of chest wall injury and the extent of parenchymal trauma, it seems that lung contusion related to rib fractures and flail chest tends to be more localized, whereas, in the absence of identifiable chest wall injury, lung contusion is more diffuse. Bony thoracic cage trauma may be absent, especially in children, due to the elasticity of their chest walls.

Evolution, Imaging Follow-up and Differential Diagnosis

Time intervals of development and clearing are important for differential diagnosis. Aspiration is uncommonly seen before 6 h from the injury, whereas infection or fat embolism does not develop earlier than 24–48 h. Because opacification from edema resolves rapidly, initial clearing of contusion begins radiographically 48–72 h after the injury (14).

In any case, uncomplicated contusion clears radiologically within 4–7 days after injury (2) whereas the hemorrhagic component may take more than 10 days to clear (5). Presumed contusions that fail to resolve within this timeframe should be considered to be possible infection, atelectasis, aspiration, ARDS, lung lacerations, or preexisting lesions (15,16).

Pulmonary Laceration

Laceration consists of a traumatic disruption of lung tissue that forms a posttraumatic lung space. As shown by Santos and Moolten (17,18) the initially linear shape of the tear is not detectable radiologically until it converts to ovoid due to the elastic recoil of the lung. Penetrating wounds cause longitudinal hematomas that may not resolve for months (Fig. 35.3).

In most cases this traumatic space fills with blood (hematoma) or remains filled with air (pneumatocele, posttraumatic cyst – pseudocyst) (19–22). In the latter case, under high pressure mechanical ventilation, these may rapidly enlarge and cause pneumothorax via bronchopleural tears.

Roentenologically, on CXR, lacerations appear as ill-defined opacities or ovoid lucent lesions with or without an air – fluid level, depending on whether they contain blood or air or both. In the initial phase, CXR findings are covered by the almost-always surrounding contusion and are only detected when the latter starts to resolve .

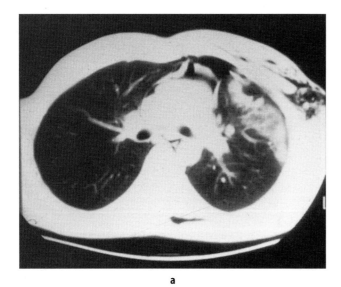

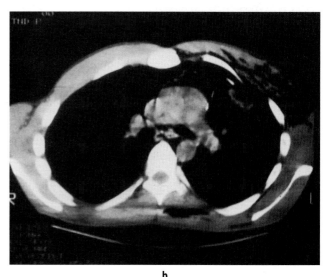

a   **b**

Figure 35.2. a and **b** CT appearances of lung contusion: peripheral nonsegmental distribution. Pneumothorax, pneumomediastinum and extensive subcutaneous emphysema coexist.

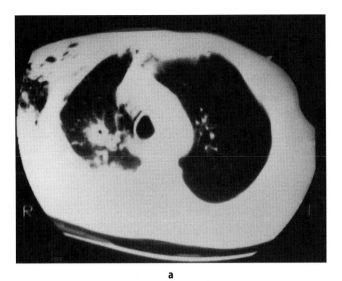
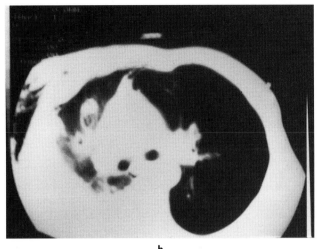

a   b

Figure 35.3. a and **b** Longitudinal laceration of the right lung from penetrating injury. Hemothorax and extraparenchymal air collections are also seen.

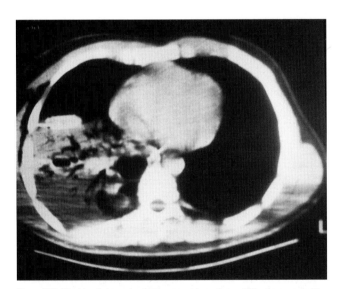

Figure 35.4. Ovoid radiolucencies that represent lacerations within airspace opacities (contusion) are revealed by CT in this patient.

CT is more sensitive at detecting pulmonary lacerations (12); they present as ovoid radiolucencies with a thin 2–3 mm pseudomembrane, surrounded by ill-defined areas of contusion (Fig. 35.4). Fresh intracavitary blood may be seen as on air–fluid level, while organized thrombus may present with a crescent sign (23).

Evolution, Imaging Follow-up and Differential Diagnosis

Lacerations resolve spontaneously (24–26) slowly over 3–5 weeks and may leave a residual nodule (hematoma)

for months (should clear within 6 weeks) (Fig. 35.5) (14). As mentioned above, due to positive pressures exerted on the cystic walls, lacerations in patients receiving mechanical ventilation persist for longer periods (27).

Complications of lacerations are not common, but should be recognized radiologically, since they may require surgical intervention. Infected lacerations are usually resistant to conservative treatment; bronchopleural fistulae with persistent air leak to the pleural space may not improve with chest tube placement. Compression of the adjacent lung impairing lung function may also be observed in large pneumatoceles. Bronchopleural fistulae that result from pneumatoceles may resolve spontaneously over a 2–3 month period after mechanical ventilation is discontinued.

Differential diagnosis in the trauma clinical setting includes pneumonia, abscess, localized pneumothorax (in pneumatoceles) or underlying tumor in cases of organized hematomas that remain unresolved after recovery.

Lung Torsion

Direct compression on the upper or lower hemithorax may result in lung torsion, i.e., rotation through 180° around the hilus. Children are more vulnerable because of the elasticity and compressibility of the thoracic cage.

Roentgenologically the diagnosis may be suggested by the inverted pulmonary vascular markings but this is not commonly achieved because vascular impairment of the affected lung rapidly causes exudation of hemorrhagic edema and the lung becomes radiopaque (14).

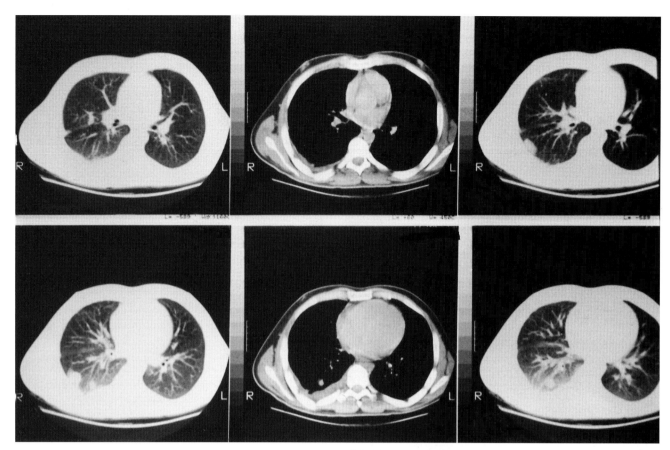

Figure 35.5. Residual hematomas presenting as small nodules are seen 4 weeks after chest trauma that had caused multiple right lower lobe lacerations.

Atelectasis

Unless the presence of pneumomediastinum suggests a fractured bronchus, atelectasis in the trauma setting is the result of bronchial obstruction (aspirated foreign body, mucus plugging).

Tracheobronchial Tree

Tracheobronchial Injury

Tracheobronchial rupture is a rare injury occurring in 1–5% of blunt trauma, severe enough to cause fractures to the first three ribs (28–31). Involvement of the bronchi is more common than that of the tracheal and represents 80% of all tracheobronchial injuries (29,30). Bronchial fractures occur 1–2 cm from the carina , the right bronchus being affected more frequently than the left.

Roentgenologically the most common CXR findings are pneumomediastinum combined with pneumothorax and associated with a variable extent of cutaneous thoracocervical emphysema. The presence of large persistent pneumothorax and pneumomediastinum unrelieved by chest tube drainage or large mediastinal emphysema in a patient not receiving mechanical ventilation are signs highly suggestive of tracheobronchial injuries with complete disruption. If the fracture is incomplete and the peribronchial connective tissue prevents air leakage, CXR may be false negative initially and demonstrate findings only later when atelectasis due to bronchial kinking develops (32). Non-rotated fractured bronchi do not cause ischemia of the lung peripherally, since the adjacent vascular bundle is not damaged (14).

CT demonstrates similar signs (pneumomediastinum, pneumothorax, and cutaneous emphysema) at earlier stages than CXR, but findings are not specific. After initial evaluation with CXR and CT, bronchoscopy and esophagoscopy are necessary to establish the diagnosis and make decisions concerning treatment (32,33).

Ectopic Locations of Air in the Chest

Pneumothorax

Pneumothorax is the commonest sequela of chest injury, reported in 40% of patients, with increasing iatrogenic incidence in the trauma setting after cardiovascular line placements and positive pressure ventilatory support (34).

Prompt diagnosis is vital, especially in those with decreased cardiopulmonary reserves and those under mechanical ventilation.

Roentgenologically, as intrapleural air collection has a gravity-dependent distribution, in the absence of pleural departmentalization, radiographic diagnosis is straightforward in the erect CXR views, with visualization of the thin visceral pleural line in the apices and absence of lung markings beyond it. As pneumothorax increases, the lucency extends laterally and is easier to recognize.

As stressed by Fraser et al. (35), the visceral pleura, in the absence of coexisting pleural fluid, should be visualized as a thin line and not as a stripe, since the degree of passive atelectasis of the subpleural lung is not enough to produce a radiographically increased opacity in the nondiseased parenchyma. Pitfalls therefore in misinterpeting skin folds, bandages, chest wall subcutaneous emphysema and chest tubes as pneumothorax can be avoided. Moreover, in some cases these stripes can be followed extrathoracically to some extent, being easier to distinguish from pneumothorax.

Atypical distributions of pneumothorax. Besides pleural adhesions, nongravity-dependent pneumothorax (subpulmonary, within the pulmonary ligament, paramediastinal) may be related to the presence of atelectasis, variations in the anatomy of the pulmonary ligament and large quantities of air.

In the supine patient, distribution of air is different as air extends to the nondependent pleural spaces, anteromedially and subpulmonically. In a thorough study, Tocino et al. identified the most frequent sites of air collection in the supine and semirecumbent patient (36): the *anterior costophrenic sulcus*, extenting from the 7th costal cartilage to the 11th rib in the midaxillary line, is the most common site, followed by *the anterior* and *paramediastinal sulcuses* (37). Therefore, CXR signs of pneumothorax in the supine view include (Fig. 35.6):

1. *Hyperlucency of the lower hemithorax and hemidiaphragm* (air collection in anterior costophrenic sulcus).
2. *Low position/flattening of the hemidiaphragm* (air in the anterior costophrenic sulcus).
3. The *"double diaphragm sign,"* visualized as an interface outlining the dome and anterior insertion of the affected hemidiaphragm (air in the anterior costophrenic sulcus.
4. The *"deep sulcus sign"* (air in the anterior costophrenic sulcus and laterally).
5. *Sharp outline and enhancement of the negative Mach band of the cardiac boarder* (air anteromedially),
6. The *"apical pericardial fat tag sign"* (air anteromedially outlining pericardial fat).

Tension pneumothorax is a medical emergency and is visualized as a contralateral mediastinal shift, flattening or

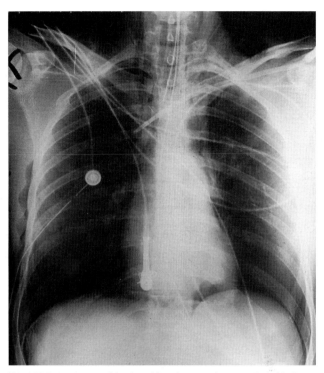

Figure 35.6. Supine view of the chest: bilateral pneumothorax is indicated by hyperlucency of lower hemithorax and hemidiaphragms, and deep costophrenic sulcuses. The thin pleural line of pneumothorax is seen only on the left. Subpulmonary distribution of pneumothorax and signs of pneumomediastinum with linear radiolucencies and continuous diaphragm may also be noted.

inversion of the hemidiaphragm and intercostal space widening. However, a moderate mediastinal shift occurs in most pneumothoraces with complete lung collapse and should not be mistaken for tension pneumothorax (35).

Erect CXRs are very accurate for pneumothorax detection and good-quality supine views are sensitive enough to detect most pneumothoraces requiring thoracostomy. Supine views though, even under ideal laboratory conditions (38), have a sensitivity of only 37% in the detection of moderate pneumothorax followed by erect (59%) and lateral decubitus (88%). Portable computed radiography has had slightly better results (39). In 30–50% of trauma patients pneumothoraces initially missed clinically and on admission CXR are first detected on CT of the chest or the abdomen.

CT is very sensitive, detecting even a few milliliters of air; CT depiction may suggest early prophylactic chest tube placement in patients that subsequently undergo surgery or mechanical ventilation, since one third of them will develop tension pneumothorax if untreated (40–41). CT may also assist in revealing malpositioned chest tubes, and residual pneumothorax.

Localized pneumothorax of paramediastinal distribution or pneumothorax within the pulmonary ligament can be easily distinguished from pneumomediastinum and pneumatoceles.

Even if no chest CT is performed, including the anterior costophrenic sulcus in the abdomen, CT protocols for trauma often reveal occult pneumothoraces (40–41). However, emergency management they be questioned in those cases, since they do not seem necessarily to progress, and enlarge regardless of the need for positive pressure ventilation (42).

Pneumomediastinum

Most commonly pneumomediastinum is the result of ruptured alveoli and subsequent passage of air into the interstitium along the bronchovascular bundle to the hilus and mediastinum. This interstitial dissection due to sudden chest compression and reexpansion has been described as the Macklin effect (43,44). Alveolar rupture may be the result of blunt or penetrating trauma, or a sequela of interstitial emphysema from barotrauma. Air in the mediastinum can also originate from (a) perforation or rupture of the mediastinal airways or esophagus, (b) the deep fascial planes of the neck in cases of upper airway injury, (c) the retroperitoneal soft tissues (in perforated duodenun, colon), and (d) rarely through diaphragmatic fissures from the peritoneal cavity (in pneumoperitoneum). The process can also occur in the reverse way.

Presistent severe pneumomediastinum, unrelieved by tube thoracostomy is an indication of thracheobronchial or, more rarely, esophageal rupture. The initially resulting interstitial emphysema and subsequent course of air along the peribronchovascular interstitium has recently been demonstrated by CT (45,46).

From the mediastinal connective tissue, air can extend peripherally and cause pneumothorax, which is often a concurrent finding, but the reverse does not happen (47).

The most common radiographic sign of pneumomediastinum is the presence of *linear radiolucencies* within it, often extending into the neck (Fig. 35.6). They are easily depicted in frontal views. Longitudinal radiolucencies may also be seen to extend inferiorly, parallel to the heart border, or outline the margins of the aortic knob, the descending aorta, and the extrapericardial parts of the pulmonary artery (left pulmonary artery and less often along part of the right peripheral to the truncus anterior branch) (Fig. 35.7). These linear lucencies are produced as air lifts the mediastinal pleura off the heart and the other mediastinal structures. Outlined by air, epicardial and pericardial fat tags (Fig. 35.8) can be observed as "irregular" cardiac borders (48).

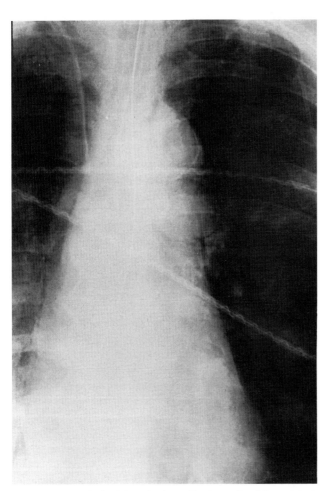

Figure 35.7. Longitudinal radiolucencies that outline the margins of the aortic knob and extrapericardial parts of the pulmonary artery indicate the development of pneumomediastinum in this patient.

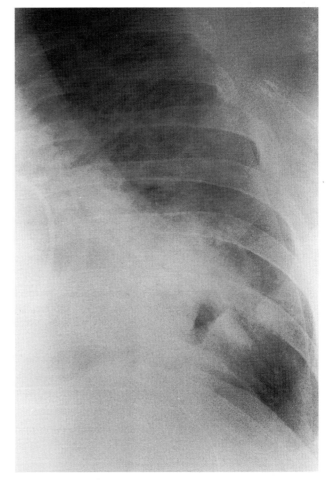

Figure 35.8. Epicardial fat tags presenting as gross irregularity of the left-hand border indicate the presence of pneumomediastinum. A pleural line is seen laterally (pneumothorax).

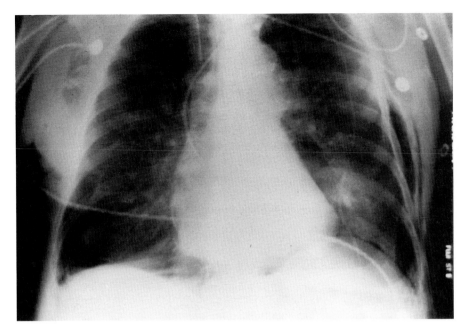

Figure 35.9. Clear visualization of the central portion of the diaphragm as air lifts the pericardium off the diaphragm; this is called the "continuous diaphram sign", and is diagnostic of pneumomediastinum.

Air interposed between the heart and the diaphragm allows visualization of the central portion of the diaphragm that is normally obscured by the heart. This has been described by Levin (49) as "the continuous diaphragm sign" (Fig. 35.6, 35.9). The concurrent visualization of paraspinal and extrapleural supradiaphragmatic air (Fig. 35.10), described as "V sign", is another finding of pneumomediastinum (50). However, the latter is difficult to distinguish from subpulmonary pneumothorax, or paramediastinal pneumatoceles in CXRs. Air in the perithymic fascia in children produces the "spinnaker sail sign" (51).

CT is very sensitive in the detection of pneumomediastinum (Fig. 35.11); it has the above-described distribution and can easily be distinguished from paramediastinal air collections.

Pneumopericardium

Pneumopericardium is almost always associated with direct trauma, especially if it is the only extrapulmonary air site, although reports exist that describe different mechanisms (52). In contrast to pneumomedinastinum, it never results from interstitial emphysema in adults (43, 47).

The mechanism that allows air to enter into the pericardium in mechanical ventilation-related barotrauma is tracking of air along the adventitia of the pulmonary veins. In this case, however, pneumomediastinum and pneumothorax always coexist.

In CXR, pneumopericardium is seen as a radiolucency outlining the serous pericardium that characteristically is

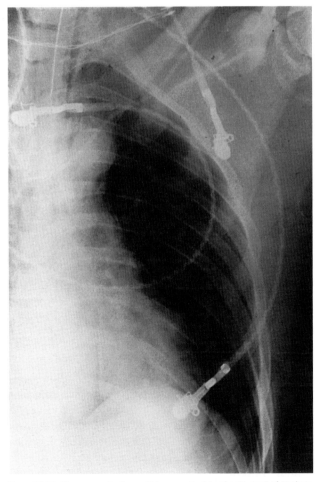

Figure 35.10. Pneumomediastinum. It is recognized by the "V sign" of Naclerio: paraspinal and extrapleural subdiaphragmatic air (not changing location with patient position).

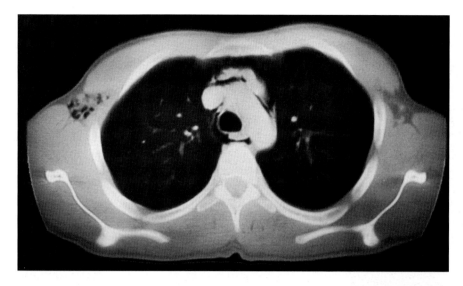

Figure 35.11. Pneumomediastinum: curvilinear radiolucencies outlining mediastinal structures.

dome-shaped upwards, and outlines the left ventricle laterally. Pneumopericardium is only an indicator of a pericardial tear and is usually benign. Tension pneumopericardium is extremely rare and small cardiac silhouette has been described in CXR (53).

Pleural Fluid Collections in Trauma

Hemothorax

Hemothorax of various quantities is present in as many as 50% of major trauma patients (54). A large hemothorax is usually the result of bleeding from intercostal or internal mammary arteries often associated with an extrapleural hematoma distinguished only on CT. Bleeding from lung parenchyma is of low pressure and therefore is almost always self-limiting (55), Large, gradually increasing hemothorax should raise suspicion of major vessel or cardiac injury. Coagulation of extravasated blood in the pleural space is rapid and loculation tends to occur early in hemothorax.

In the erect or semi-erect views, obliteration of the costophrenic sulcus and diaphragmatic contour, whether or not associated with a homogeneous opacity at the lower hemithorax, are standard findings (Fig. 35.12). However, differentiation from associated lung injuries or posttraumatic sequelae is frequently not possible in portable radiographs and the need for intervention cannot be predicted based on CXR findings only (56).

CT provides information regarding distribution, compartmentalization, and quantity that influence decision-making. The presence of clots (high attenuation values) is often detected on CT. Follow-up CXR and CT studies may be necessary to monitor posttraumatic residual hemothorax but thoracoscopic evacuation may be necessary to avoid fibrothorax (56).

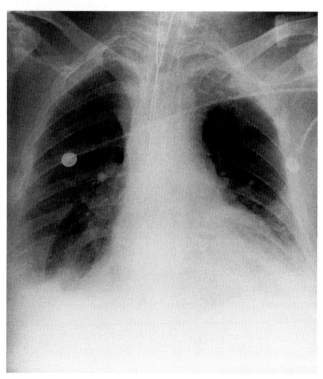

Figure 35.12. Homogeneous opacities at the dependent portions of both hemithoraces not obliterating lung markings indicate the presence of pleural effusions bilaterally. Obliteration of costophrenic sulcuses may also be noted, as well as extension of fluid within the fissures on the right.

Empyema – Infection

Undrained hemothoraces, occluded chest tubes, unexpanded lung and pneumonias are predisposing factors (57).

CT accuracy is 72% for empyema and 95% for lung abscess (57,58). The split pleura sign, lung compression, thin smooth enhancing walls and lenticular shape (Fig. 35.13) are signs recognized on CT (58,59).

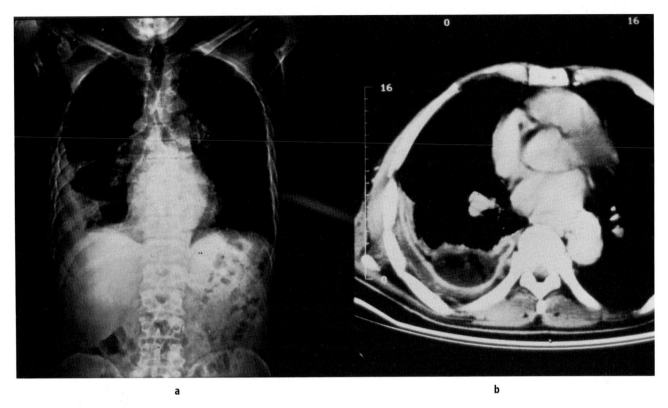

Figure 35.13. **a** and **b** Lenticular-shaped pleural fluid collection: enhancing pleura indicates empyema.

Esophageal Disruption

It is usually the result of penetrating injury, although it has been described also in major blunt trauma. Iatrogenic causes have also to be considered in the trauma setting.

CXR demonstrates signs of pneumomediastinum and/or left-sided pleural effusion but it is not diagnostic. Leakage of oral contrast medium into the mediastinum or pleural space may be detected on CT (60).

Aortic Trauma

Acute thoracic aortic injury accounts for 63% of deaths due to chest trauma (60) and 20% of high speed deceleration accidents (60–62).

The physical history of this injury can be seen from older data showing that, of the individuals sustaining aortic injury, 80–90% die at the scene – most of them from rupture of the ascending aorta (63). Of the remaining, if

undetected and untreated, 30% die within 6 h, 40–60% within the first day and 95% within 4 months (61–64). More recent data indicate that currently up to 50% of aortic injury cases may reach the hospital alive (65). Prompt treatment and surgery increases survival rates to 80% (66).

Sites and Types of Injury Related to Imaging

The rapid deceleration and shearing forces exerted on the aorta have their maximal impact at sites located near fixed portions of the vessel (64). In patients that survive to reach hospital these are the aortic isthmus (80–90%), the ascending aorta (5–9%), and diaphragmatic aorta (1–3%) (62,67). Multiple sites are involved in 6–20%, and concurrent brachiocephalic injuries are observed in 4–10% (68–71).

Impact forces cause injuries that vary in severity and extent from a subintimal/intramural hematoma due to ruptured vasa vasorum to lacerations/tears that extend from the intimal to deeper layers of the aorta. If the disruption extends to the adventitia, complete transmural transection occurs. Postmortem and surgical data indicate that the initial intimal tear is almost always circumferential, of small length (a few millimeters) and posteriorly located. The adventitia remains intact in about 60% of cases (72,73).

Imaging modalities demonstrate the aortic wall injury itself and the resulting pseudoaneurysm (direct signs), as well as indirect signs of aortic injury, the most significant of them being mediastinal hematoma.

Radiographic Findings

Because direct signs of aortic injury such as intimal or mural abnormalities cannot be seen, mediastinal hematoma is the most significant radiographic abnormality to look for on admission CXR during the initial patient survey. In addition, chronic pseudoaneurysms may also be detected on CXR (an incidental finding in missed cases).

Mediastinal hematoma even in confirmed aortic injury is rarely the result of aortic extravasation, but it indicates that impact forces, strong enough to cause vascular damage have been applied to the mediastinum.

CXR findings suggestive of mediastinal hematoma include (Fig. 35.14):

1. *Contour abnormalities:* irregular contour of the aortic knob and superior mediastinum (sensitivity 53–100%; specificity 21–42%); obscuration of the aortopulmonary window (sensitivity 40–100%; specificity 56–83%).

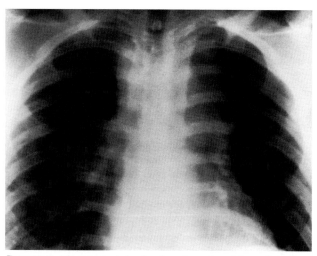

Figure 35.14. CXR anteroposterior view: irregular contour of the aortic knob and superior mediastinum, obscuration of the aortopulmonary window and widening of the mediastinum indicate the presence of mediastinal hematoma in this patient. Thickening of the left paraspinal stripe is also observed.

2. *Widening of the mediastinum* (> 8 cm) at the level of the origin of the left, subclavian artery (sensitivity 53–100%; specificity 1–60%).

3. *Deviation of mediastinal structures:* seen as actual shift of the trachea to the right, or outlined by the deviation of the endotracheal tube or nasogastric tube to the right of the T3 through T4 spinous process (sensitivity 12–100%; specificity 80–95%); depression of the left mainstem bronchus more than 40° below the horizontal plane (sensitivity 3–80%; specificity 80–100%).

4. *Thickening of the left paraspinal stripe* (sensitivity 12–83%; specificity 89–97%) (74–78).

Contour abnormalities have the higher positive predictive value, while widening of the superior mediastinum at the level of the origin of the left, subclavian artery, although present in more than 90% of cases of aortic injury, has a specificity as low as 10% (77–79).

Other CXR signs of aortic or mediastinal vessel injury include an apical cap, left hemothorax and a thick paratracheal stripe but have very low positive predictive value alone. Although a few reports to the contrary exist (80), isolated fractures of the first ribs and sternum may be associated with aortic trauma but alone they are not an indication for aortography (81,82).

Good-quality CXRs are a prerequisite for the evaluation of aortic or mediastinal vessel injury; although erect views are preferred, good-quality supine views (end-inspiratory, nonrotated, well-centered) may demonstrate signs of mediastinal hematoma with a positive predictive value reaching 96% (83). However, portable CXRs are very inaccurate in the depiction of mediastinal hematoma.

CXR as a Screening Method for Aortic Injury

In the past, the chest radiograph has been the main initial screening technique to select patients for further evaluation. When used in combination with other elements comprising the so-called "aortic triage" (clinical signs and high risk mechanism of injury) it has a sensitivity reaching 92.7% (73,74,78,79).

The importance of CXR lies on its negative predictive value that reaches 98% (74,78,83), provided that it is of good quality. In the multiple trauma patient, however, poor-quality films are quite often obtained and CT evaluation that will also detect other organ injuries is necessary.

The specificity of CXR for aortic injury is very low, ranging from 10–50% (73,75,84–86); false positives include true mediastinal hematomas but of venous or small-vessel origin or due to nontraumatic causes of mediastinal widening (lipomatosis, projection and positioning factors) (85).

In cases of strong clinical suspicion, and/or questionable or positive CXRs, further evaluation for aortic injury is required: traditionally the next step was angiography, now widely replaced for the stable patients, by CT.

CT Evaluation

CT studies demonstrate both direct as well as indirect signs of aortic injury: (a) intimal flap/aortic laceration; (b) mediastinal hematoma; (c) posttraumatic pseudo-aneurysm; (d) or pseudocoarctation; and (e) aortic wall changes, intramural hematoma (87–89).

1. Intimal flap/aortic laceration abnormalities. They are direct, virtually pathognomonic signs of aortic injury and are recognized in contrast-enhanced studies as a lucent line within the aortic lumen that represents an intimal flap or as peripheral irregular filling defects (confined aortic injury). They are seen in 3–17%, the higher rates being with contrast-enhanced spiral CT, even in the absence of mediastinal hematoma (90–92). CT aortography can demonstrate aortic lacerations more than 15 mm in length (88,93).

2. Mediastinal hematoma is an indirect sign of aortic injury, easily detected on CT even in noncontrast-enhanced studies (Fig. 35.15). It is seen as an obliteration of the normal mediastinal contours and replacement of the fat planes with the accumulation of increased density hematoma (90,91). Although aortic injury without mediastinal hematoma was thought to be rare (86–89), with the advent of contrast-enhanced spiral CT it is clear that intimal laceration may exist and be successfully demonstrated even without mediastinal hematoma in nearly 5–10% of cases. If conventional CT is used, it may be the only CT finding of aortic injury. Periaortic distribution is highly suggestive of aortic laceration (Fig. 35.15), while small hematomas of posterior location may be due to spinal trauma. Anterior distribution may be related to sternal, venous or internal mammary vessel trauma. Hemopericardium is another indication of aortic injury.

3. Posttraumatic pseudoaneurysm is a direct sign, most commonly located at the ligamentum arteriosum. Chronic forms can also be recognized by CT (only 2% of case, survive long enough to develop a chronic pseudoaneurysm) (85).

4. Pseudocoarctation. It is seen as an abrupt tapering of the diameter of the descending aorta distal to the injury site and is an indirect sign of posttraumatic pseudoaneurysm.

5. Aortic wall changes , intramural hematoma. Mural changes are a direct signs of aortic injury (87,88,90). Signs of intramural hematoma include:

    1. Aortic wall "thickening". Useful tips to distinguish it from atherosclerotic changes that are also seen as

wall thickening are the facts that the latter are rather diffuse (longitudinally and circumferentially), invariably irregular, and are rarely seen in the ascending aorta. Intramural hematoma is better evaluated with magnetic resonance imaging (MRI).

    2. Increased attenuation within the aortic wall is another sign of mural hematoma sometimes seen on unenhanced CT scans. Uncomplicated intra-mural hematoma (hematoma or noncommunicating dissection) is not a surgical emergency but should be carefully looked for, since it is of high risk for complications especially if located at the ascending aorta.

CT for Screening Aortic Injury: Diagnostic Accuracy

Overall, contrast-enhanced spiral CT has a 100% sensitivity, 82% specificity and 47% positive predictive value provided only that examinations are of good or acceptable quality. Contrast-enhanced spiral CT can virtually exclude aortic injury with a negative predictive value of 100%, while it nearly halves unnecessary aortographies (94,95).

Direct CT signs of aortic injury that can consistently be demonstrated in well-performed studies (intimal flap, mural changes, pseudoaneurysm) have 90% sensitivity and 99% specificity (90–92,94–96). As for mediastinal hematoma, CT has a sensitivity of 100% but a specificity for aortic injury not exceeding 87% and a positive predictive value of approximately 21% because it is often due to small vessel trauma (79,87,89,93,97).

CT Pitfalls

Ductus diverticulae and ectatic origins of brachiocephalic vessels are the most important and difficult to diagnose causes of false-positive studies. Transesophageal echocardiography may successfully complement CT in these cases to avoid aortography (that anyway has similar diagnostic problems in these cases). Visualization of vessel walls from prominent periaortic right bronchial and mediastinal vessels in contact with the aorta (left superior intercostal vein, brachiocephalic vein) and prominent atheromas may be mistaken for intimal flaps (101). Volume averaging of the pulmonary artery of thymus, paramediastinal hemothorax and lung contusion may also be erroneously taken for mediastinal hemorrhage (97–99).

Good-quality studies are required (99,100); however, poor-quality studies are quite often obtained especially in the multiple trauma patient. Suboptimal studies (motion,

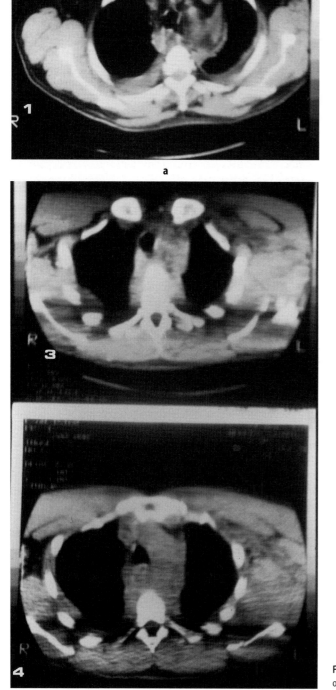

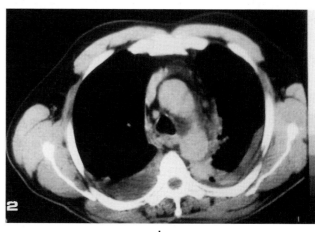

a

b

c and d

Figure 35.15. CT. **a–b** Mediastinal hematoma of periaortic distribution is an indirect sign of aortic injury, most probably at the isthmus. Bilateral hemothorax is also present.

beam-hardening artefacts) limit the diagnostic value of the study.

CT examination protocols should be tailored to demonstrate apart from mediastinal hematoma the luminal and vessel wall abnormalities described above

(99,101). Fast scanning is preferred; for spiral CT, image reconstruction every 2.5–3.5 mm with a 50% overlap (extending 2 cm above the aortic arch to the carina) and every 5–7 mm for the rest of the chest is required (5–7 mm collimation, pitch of 1:1–1,7). Contrast injection rates of 1.5–2 ml/sec with a 20–30 s scan delay are necessary (99,101,102).

Aortography

Aortography demonstrates direct signs of injury. Angiographic findings of aortic injury include (a) intimal irregularities, (b) pseudoaneurysm, (c) mural irregularities, and (d) free extravasation.

1. *Intimal irregularities.* These are shown as peripheral filling defects or linear intraluminal lucencies.
2. *Pseudoaneurysm.* It is seen as a local buldge of the aortic contour and represents a contained rupture (diverticular or fusiform). It may be confined to one side of the aortic wall or may be circumferential; pseudoaneurysms vary considerably in shape from small, multilobular, flask-shaped, or mushroom shaped to large and bulbous. The pseudocoarctation (decreased calibre of the descending aorta distal to the pseudoaneurysm) is another sign of the same condition (103).
3. *Mural irregularities,* These may be quite subtle and may represent intramural hematoma. They may be mistaken for intimal flap but in either case they indicate aortic injury.
4. *Free extravasation.* This is rarely seen in clinical practice, since it is rapidly lethal.

Angiography has so far been the gold standard imaging modality for aortic injury. A small mediastinal hematoma in the absence of direct CT signs of aortic injury is not an indication for aortography, unless hematoma is large or of periaortic distribution (104–106). It is also indicated in equivocal or questionable CT findings (differential diagnosis of pseudoaneurysm from ductus diverticulum) and in the presence of overt intimal changes and when the origins of brachiocephalic vessels are involved. Angiography provides surgical guidance with respect to the surgical approach, type of repair (location extent of injury) and promotes for a fast procedure (prolonged clamping has been associated with postoperative paraplegia) (60).

Angiography Diagnostic Accuracy

Although false-negative aortography has been reported, the sensitivity of the method reaches virtually 100%, and the specificity is approximately 98% (90,104,107,108).

Good technique is essential with imaging in at least two planes (preferably left aorta and right aorta at a rate of 35–40 ml s⁻¹). Pigtail catheters and J-tipped guidewires are used and carefully advanced under fluoroscopy through the femoral approach, unless a difference in pulses between the upper and lower limbs is present (brachial

approach preferred). The slightest resistance in advancing them should alert for aortic injury .

Angiographic Pitfalls

A ductus diverticulum, an aortic spindle (congenital narrowing of the aorta at the ligamentum arteriosum with distal dilatation), enlarged infundibulae of brachial-intercostal trunk (right third intercostal artery) or the brachiocephalic branches may look like pseudoaneurysms or pseudocoarctation. More uncommon sources of error include the diverticulum of Kommerell and other variations of the origins of the brachiocephalic vessels (105,109). Atherosclerotic plaques and, rarely, penetrating atherosclerotic aortic ulcers have been mistaken for pseudoaneurysms.

Intravascular ultrasound (IVUS) may be used during aortography in those cases and demonstrate directly intimal flaps and aortic wall hematoma.

Transesophageal Echocardiography

Transesophageal echocardiography (TEE) is highly sensitive for the stable patient with 88–100% and 75–91% sensitivity and specificity rates, respectively. The positive predictive value of the examination is approximately 98% (110–112). Suggestive findings include: (a) increased distance of the probe from the aortic wall, (b) double contour of aortic wall, (c) increased echogeneity between aortic wall and visceral pleura, (d) intimal flap, (e) intraluminal echogenic strips, and (f) aortic wall hematoma. TEE is of vital importance in CT findings that raise the question of differentiation of ductus diverticulum from aortic injury. However, it has the disadvantage of operator dependency and does not visualize the entire circumference of the aorta in 30–60% of cases (113). In addition, other sites besides the isthmus are not adequately seen (103–114) and brachiocephalic vessels are not demonstrated. Moreover, its use is further restricted by the fact that it is contraindicated in patients with unstable cervical spine injuries, severe maxillofacial fractures or esophageal disease.

MRI Evaluation

MRI is limited to the detection of aortic injury in the acute setting and at present it is only confined to, and suitable for, stable, alert and cooperative patients that have no other serious injuries that will anyway require CT. Diagnostic accuracy is very high and indicated if delayed surgery is done (115). It has also been used in delayed cases, i.e. patients suspected of having an old post

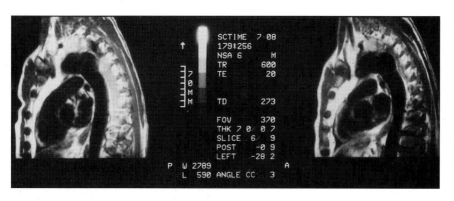

Figure 35.16. MRI, T_1-weighted image, sagittal plane. Posttraumatic pseudoaneurysm is demonstrated at the isthmus in a patient who sustained chest injury in the past.

(initially missed from traumatic injury) traumatic pseudoaneurysm (116) (Fig. 35.16).

MRI also contributes to the recognition of intramural hematoma, a traumatic noncommunicating aortic dissection that potentially may lead to communicating dissection and/or aneurysmal dilatation. Intramural hematoma may be missed in angiography. It is recognized by TEE as long as its location does not fall in the blind spots of the technique.

In intramural hematoma, MRI demonstrates well the smooth and crescent-shaped thickening of the aortic wall both longitudinally and circumferentially on sagittal and axial planes and identifies its nature. Pulse sequences that differentiate slow laminar flow or slow flow in a communicating dissection such as dynamic phase contrast or dynamic MRI tissue tagging should be used (117,118).

Although the MR signal of hematoma has been better studied in the central nervous system environment, the chronicity of the hematoma may also be suggested by MRI. Increased intramural signal at T_1- and T_2-weighted images indicates early subacute hematoma, while in chronic phases the signal at T_1 weighted images is low to intermediate and at T_2-weighted sequences is variable or very low (115) .

Imaging Algorithm

If CXRs are of good quality and without abnormalities, no further studies are required during the primary survey (119). If the CXR is positive or technically unacceptable, after hemodynamic stabilization, contrast-enhanced spiral CT is required (120). If CT is negative and of good quality no arteriography is done. In equivocal cases TEE or aortography with or without IVUS is necessary (121). Gavant's studies showed that direct signs of aortic injury have 90% sensitivity and 99% specificity (90,121,123). Surgeons however, are still reluctant to operate solely on the basis of CT findings and insist on angiographic confirmation (122,123). False-positive rates of CT (average of

different techniques) range from 0% to 39% and false negatives do not exceed 0.7% (123).

Chest Wall Trauma

Bony Cage

Although isolated fractures of the bony cage are seldom of major clinical significance; they serve as an index of the mechanical forces applied during the impact and should be carefully looked for, a an indication of further treatment planning. Bony fractures are often missed or underestimated in the acute phase, since no special projections can be obtained. In addition, the presence of immobilizing devices, especially in the neck and shoulder girdle, compromise the images, and CT is often necessary. The special projections required for orthopedic reduction are beyond the scope of this chapter and are not discussed.

Fractures of the Ribs

Fractures of the ribs are of little significance per se, but potential intrathoracic complications justify radiologic investigation.
Of the particular importance are:

Lower rib fractures may be associated with splenic, liver and renal injuries.

Fractures of the first three ribs may be associated with pleura, lung and mediastinal trauma especially if combined with sternoclavicular dislocation. At the level of the thoracic outlet they may cause damage to the brachial plexus and adjacent blood vessels in 3–15% of patients (124,125). Signs of extrapleural hematoma, brachial plexus neuropathy, and mediastinal hematoma or upper limb ischemia should prompt for emergency angiography but, on there own, rib fractures need no further investigation (126). Fractures of the upper ribs may are associated with

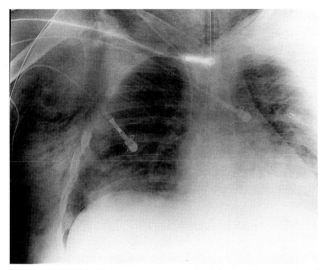

Figure 35.17. Multiple rib fractures are seen on the right. Resulting alteration of respiratory mechanics may add to impairment of lung function caused by the concurrent right lung contusion and pneumothorax.

tracheobronchial tree injuries; of all tracheobronchial ruptures, 91% are associated with fractures of the first three ribs (30,31).

Double or multiple rib fractures (Fig. 35.17) may affect wall instability and impair respiratory mechansins and drainage of secretions. Flail chest is a serious trauma entity and may have a 20% mortality rate.

Extrapleural hematomas, visualized as convex soft tissue bulges toward the lung, are most often related to rib fractures. Apical extrapleural hematomas that grow in size indicate active bleeding and require angiographic evaluation, especially if of apical location.

Roentgenologically, CXR has been found to detect only 18% of all fractures found at postmortem (34). Despite this low detection rate significant rib fractures are seldom missed. CT reveals lung mediastinum and pleural injuries related to them.

Fractures of the Sternum

Sternal fractures indicate severe impact and are associated with a 25–45% mortality rate due to associated aortic, cardiac, bronchial and head injuries that should be looked for in imaging studies (28,55,127).

Roentgenologically, sternal fractures are usually missed on frontal CXRs and revealed by CT.

In *CT* they are easily recognized unless horizontally oriented and parallel to the axial slice plain. Horizontally oriented sternal fractures may be overlooked in the absence of dislocation and reformatted images may be necessary. Retrosternal hematoma is an indirect sign of sternal fracture and if seen on the axial slices it may lead to fracture recognition. The visualization of a normal fat

plane between the hematoma and the aorta suggests that it is not due to aortic injury (97).

Fracture of the Clavicle and Sternoclavicular Dislocations

Fractures of the clavicle are easily detected and evaluated on CXR. Anterior dislocation of the clavicle is more common and of small clinical significance. Posterior dislocation, though, is more likily due to compression injury of the trachea, esophagus, supraaortic vessels and nerves (128). These latter injuries are more commonly seen in young adults and may lead to epiphyseal avulsions. CT better demonstrates dislocation and minimizes reduction injuries. Although the presence of gas in the sternoclavicular joints in young trauma patients was suspected to represent an index of significant extraction forces and hence significant mediastinal injury, a recent study did not confirm it (129).

Shoulder Girdle

Fractures and Dislocations of the Scapula

Roentgenologically they are often missed on CXRs and may be associated with significant blood loss. Lateral displacement of the scapula is recognized on frontal CXRs and concomitant fractures of the shoulder girdle are also observed. The ratio of the distance between the midline and the medial surfaces of the scapula should fall within the range of 1.07 ± 0.04 and certainly not exceed 1.4 (130).

CT reveals fractures missed on CXR and demonstrates extension of fractures into the shoulder joint.

Scapulothoracic dissociation is an important injury associated with sternoclavicular separation, distracted clavicular fracture and acromioclavicular joint separation. Injuries of upper arm vessels and nerve are very common and arteriography is indicated to evaluate subclavian and axillary vessel integrity. In the absence of upper arm ischemia the injury may be overlooked in multitrauma patients in the acute phase. MRI is indicated for the evaluation of nerve trauma and may demonstrate nerve avulsion, atrophy or pseudomeningoceles. Post traumatic meningoceles are easily detected on T_2-weighted images but can also be evaluated with contrast myelography.

Shoulder

Roentgenologically, shoulder dislocations can be recognized at plain CXR but usually localized views and projections are needed. *CT* is also helpful in questionable cases.

MRI is not used in the acute trauma setting but is reserved for later stages in the evaluation of soft tissue, muscular, tendon and joint capsule injuries (131).

Thoracic Spine Trauma

Thoracic spine injuries account for 25–30% of all spine fractures and they have a high prevalence of neurologic deficits reaching 62% (132).

The majority of thoracic spine injuries occur at the so-called functional thoracolumbar junction (T9–T11) (133). Five percent to 20% of spinal trauma is multiple (134) and nearly 5% of patients have injuries at multiple non-contigous levels (135). Hence, the detection of one spinal injury makes evaluation of the entire spine necessary.

Thoracic spine injuries often go undetected on CXRs and require frontal and lateral views collimated to the thoracic spine (Fig. 35.18). These views if possible to obtain demonstrate most (70–90%) spine fractures (136), and enable better targeting of CT. CXRs may suggest a diagnosis if there are bilateral paraspinal hematomas causing local bulging of the paraspinal lines. Thoracic spine trauma is an absolute indication for CT which is the imaging modality of choice for diagnosis and evaluation.

Burst fractures are easily recognized on CT; they are unstable injuries and may be associated with neurologic defici (137–139).

CXR may show decrease in the height of the vertebral body. Increased interpedicular distance indicates coexisting involvement of the posterior column that renders the fracture highly unstable. Interpedicular distance (horizontally and vertically) of contiguous vertebral bodies should not vary by more than 2.0 mm.

Chance fractures are stable injuries (unstable only in flexion), lap-belt-type injuries. They are horizontal fractures of the posterior elements extenting into the posterior aspect of the vertebral body.

Plain films, in the lateral view, show increased distance between contiguous spinous processes and increased height of the posterior vertebral body. The distance between spinous processes should not vary by more than 2.0 mm between adjacent levels. CT without reconstructions will not show these fractures well.

Fractures/dislocations (Figs 35.18, 35.19) are unstable injuries and are often associated (75%) (138) with neurologic deficit.

Anterior wedge compression fractures are easily detected on CT and are stable injuries, unless they are multiple or there is more than 50% compression deformity and disc space narrowing.

Early detection and evaluation of stability of the injury before removing initially placed stabilizing devices is pertinent to avoid or minimize trauma to the spinal cord and nerves (10% of patients develop neurologic deficit after admission) (132).

MRI assists in the evaluation of intervertebral discs and ligaments and demonstrates spinal cord, nerve and thecal post traumatic changes and their complications (spinal cord hematomas, syringes, meningoceles) (Fig. 35.18c). MRI is particularly helpful in evaluating patients with the SCIWORA syndrome (spinal cord injury without radiographic abnormality). Posttraumatic sequelae such as cord edema, hematoma or transection may be revealed in these cases (140,141).

Posttraumatic Lung Hernia

Protrusion of a portion of lung through a chest wall tear is uncommon. It can occur practically anywhere but the most vulnerable site is the parasternal region just medial to the costochondral junction (126). Unless imaged tangentially it is usually missed on CXR but easily detected on CT. Images obtained during the Valsalva maneuver may clarify obscure cases (142).

Diaphragmatic Trauma

From patients undergoing celiotomy for severe abdominal trauma, diaphragmatic tears are observed in 3–5% of blunt and 10–20% of penetrating injuries (143–145). Diaphragmatic trauma (DT) is often associated with other serious intrathoracic (45%) and abdominal (59–82%) injuries (145–147).

Diagnosis may be missed or delayed in 7–66% of admission, because of the presence of concurrent injuries and the absence of pathognomonic imaging findings (145,148,149) or first recognized only at celiotomy performed for accompanying injuries in 42% (149).

Although by itself not a life-threatening condition, the importance of early diagnosis is appreciated by the fact that diaphragmatic injury causes ventilatory impairement (tidal volume decreased 25–50%) and the high risk of strangulation of the herniated hollow abdominal viscera (150); 90% of strangulated diaphragmatic hernias are of traumatic origin (32) and associated with a high mortality (151). Visceral herniation is favored by transdiaphragmatic gradient and occurs in 90–95% (23).

Roentgenologically, CXR is the initial imaging modality for the evaluation of diaphragmatic integrity (Fig. 35.20): the diagnostic finding is the visualization of intrathoracic hollow viscera with or without a focal constriction ("collar sign") through the tear. Marked elevation of a hemidiaphragm, obliteration or distortion of its contour, with or without contralateral mediastinal shift and pleural effusions are findings suggestive but not specific for DT, present in 18–50% of the patients (152,153). Gastro-

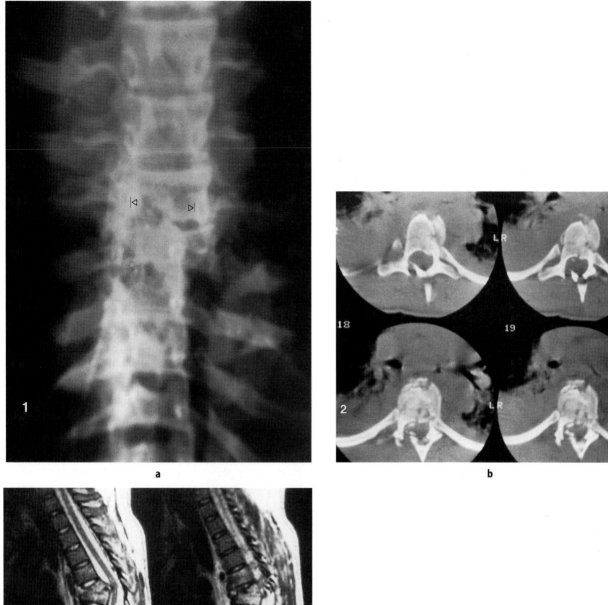

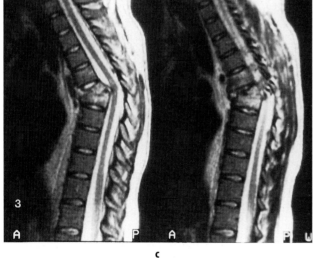

Figure 35.18. Fracture/dislocation: **a** AP collimated spot view: fractures of T6/T7 vertebrae with T6/T7 lateral dislocation. Note increased interpedicular distance at T7 (*arrows*). **b** CT: comminuted, burst fractures of T6/T7 with bone fragments into the spinal canal. Note the large paravertebral hematoma and bilateral pleural effusions. **c** MRI: kyphotic deformity at the fracture/dislocation level. There is no evidence of cord transection, although there are signs of cord trauma.

intestinal contrast studies demonstrate the herniated viscus (Fig. 35.21).

Unexplained persistence of an elevated diaphragmatic position is a subtle finding and should raise suspicions of DT after the acute trauma phase. In patients on ventilatory support, positive pressures may delay herniation and

detection of the diaphragmatic tear (154) and repeat studies are necessary (CXR, CT) to check on diaphragmatic integrity (155).

Radiographic demonstration of DT in the acute phase is impaired by concurrent findings from lung and pleural injuries. Collective reviews and clinical studies report that

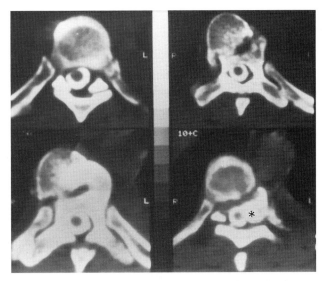

Figure 35.19. Fracture dislocation at T9–T10 level. CT myelography: spinal cord appears of normal caliber but there is a large pseudomeningocele on the left (*asterisk*) indicating root avulsion.

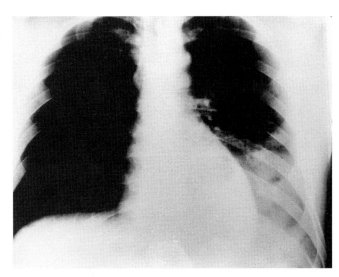

Figure 35.20. Posteroanterior view of the chest: obliteration of the contour of the left hemidiaphragm along with an elevated position that persists after the acute phase of the injury in this patient is highly suggestive of diaphragmatic trauma. The small lucency seen in the center raises suspicions of visceral herniation.

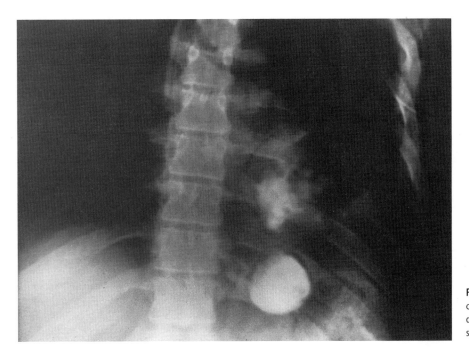

Figure 35.21. Herniation of the stomach with focal constriction through the diaphragmatic defect is demonstrated in this upper gastrointestinal barium study.

CXR diagnostic value ranges from 25% to 56% (143,144, 145) and diagnosis can be reached in only 46–49% (152,156).

False-negative CXRs range from 20% to 50%, the higher rates being observed in penetrating injuries (147). Moreover, phrenic nerve palsy, acute gastric distension and eventration may mimic or masque DT.

The radiologic detectability rate of blunt injury to the left hemidiaphragm is 75% far exceeding that of the right; however, surgical and postmortem data indicate that the frequency of injury is equal on both sides (143,157,158) or at least quite high on the right as well (12–52%) (157–159). Penetrating DT can occur anywhere (126).

CT signs of DT include localized defects of the diaphragmatic contour and intrathoracic herniation of abdominal organs (Fig. 35.22). Although detection rates of diaphragmatic discontinuity as high as 82% have been reported (160), mean CT sensitivity is below 70% (153).

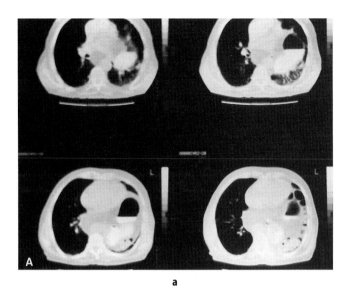
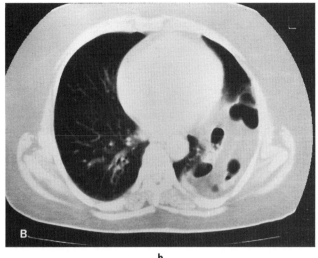

a   b

Figure 35.22. Diaphragmatic trauma: herniation of the stomach (**a**), left colic flecture (**a** and **b**) and abdominal fat are demonstrated in CT scans in these two cases.

Adjacent organ pathology, low contrast of diaphragm to adjacent parenchymal organs and in-plane artefacts are the main causes of the low detection rates (97).

Volumetric data acquisition of helical CT reduce motion artefacts and allow more accurate reconstructed images that may be necessary in subtle cases; because the medial and posterolateral portions of the left hemidiaphragm are more frequently torn (143,161) (at the junction of the tendinous portion and the posterior leave), sagittal reconstructions are necessary. Tears through the central tendon are shown better at coronal reconstructions (162).

MRI should be considered in stable patients with findings suggestive of DT. Small localized tears, particularly at the diaphragmatic dome, that are in question or missed on CT, can be seen to advantage. T_1-weighted images with sequence parameters that do not reduce the high signal from fat (to increase the contrast with the low signal of the diaphragm) are preferred. The pseudodiaphragm artefact from a chemical shift in the gradient echo sequences should not be confused with diphragmatic injury (163).

Ultrasound may occasionally demonstrate diaphragmatic injury as a localized defect or discontinuity. Adjacent organ pathology, however, often obscurates the diaphragmatic defect.

Accuracy of Imaging Modalities

Overall, presurgical imaging diagnosis in blunt DT does not exceed 75%, while DT from penetrating injuries is usually revealed at surgical exploration. Shortcomings of single imaging can be overcome by combining different imaging modalities. Radionuclide peritoneography, liver radionuclide scanning, thoracoscopy and laparoscopy are additional examinations used for occult injuries among patients without other indications for celiotomy.

References

1. Cohen MC (1997) Pulmonary contusion: Review of the clinical entity. J Trauma 42:973–979.
2. Greene R (1987) Lung alterations in thoracic trauma. J Thorac Imaging 2:1–11.
3. Schardin H (1950) The physical principles of the effects of a detonation. In Scheeley WF, (ed) German aviation medicine, World War II, vol 2, Government Printing Office, Washington DC.
4. Gerblich AA, Kleineman J (1977) Blunt chest trauma and the lung [editorial]. Am Rev Respir Dis 115:369–370.
5. Allen GS, Coates NE (1996) Pulmonary contusion: A collective review. Am Surg 62:895–900.
6. Kirsch MM, Sloan HH (1977) Blunt chest trauma. Little Brown, Boston, MA.
7. Fluton RL, Peter ET (1970) The progressive nature of pulmonary contusion. Surgery 67:499–502.
8. Blair E, Topuzlu C, Davis JH (1971) Delayed or missed diagnosis in blunt chest trauma. J Trauma 11:129–145.
9. Tocino I, Miller MH (1987) Computed tomography in blunt chest trauma. J Thorac Imaging 2:45–59.
10. Toombs BD, Sandler CM, Lester RG (1981) Computed tomography of chest trauma. Radiology 140:736–738.
11. Wagner RB, Jamieson PM (1989) Pulmonary contusion: Evaluation and classification by computed tomography. Surg Clin N Am 69:211–24.
12. Wagner RB, Crawford WO, Schimpf PP (1988) Classification of parenchymal injuries of the lung. Radiology 167:77–82.
13. Donnelly LF, Klosterman LA (1997) Subpleural sparing: A CT finding of lung contusion in children. Radiology 204:385–387.

14. Fraser RS, Pare JA, Fraser RG, et al. (1994) Synopsis of diseases of the chest (2nd edn); WB Saunders, Philadelhia.

15. Crawford W (1973) Pulmonary injury in thoracic and nonthoracic trauma. Radiol Clin North Am 11:527–541.

16. Mirvis SE, Rodriguez A, Whitley NO, et al. (1985) CT evaluation of thoracic infections after major trauma. Am J Roentgenol 144:1183–1187.

17. Santos GH, Mahendra T (1979) Traumatic pulmonary pseudocysts. Ann Thorac Surg 27:359–362.

18. Moolten SE (1935) Mechanical production of cavities in isolated lungs. Arch Pathol 19:825–832.

19. Hankins J, Attar S, Turney S, et al. (1973) Differential diagnosis of pulmonary parenchymal changes in thoracic trauma. Am Surg 39:309–318.

20. Parsai D, Nussle D, Cuendet A (1974) Presentation of two cases of pulmonary hematoma in child after closed chest trauma and review of literature. Ann Radiol 17:831–836.

21. Specht DE (1966) Pulmonary hematoma. Am J Dis Child 111:559–563.

22. Williams JR, Stembridge VA (1964) Pulmonary contusion secondary to non-penetrating chest trauma. AJR 91:284–290.

23. Mirvis SE, Templeton Ph (1992) Imaging in acute thoracic trauma. Semin Roentenol XXVII(3) 27:184–210.

24. Shirakusa T, Araki Y, Isutsui M, et al. (1987) Traumatic lung pseudocyst. Thorax 42:516–519.

25. Sivit CJ, Taylor GA, Eichelberger MR (1989) Chest injury in children with blunt abdominal trauma: Evaluation with CT. Radiology 171:815–818.

26. Ulstad DR, Bjelland JC, Quan SF (1990) Bilateral paramediastinal post-traumatic lung cysts. Chest 97:242–244.

27. Kato R, Hoirinouchi H, Maennaka Y (1989) Traumatic pulmonary pseudocyst. J Thorac Cardiovasc Surg 97:309–312.

28. Pratt LW, Guitee LA, Smith RJ, et al. (1984) Blunt chest trauma with trachobronchial rupture. Ann Otol Rhinol Laryngol 93:357–363.

29. Unger JM, Schuchmann G, Grossman JE, et al. (1989) Tears of the trachea and main bronchi caused by blunt trauma. Radiologic findings. AJR 158:1175–1180.

30. Burke JF (1962) Early diagnosis of traumatic rupture of the bronchus JAMA 181:682–688.

31. Woodring JF Woodring JH, Fried AM, et al. (1982) Fractures of the first and second ribs: Precictive value for arterial and bronchial injury. AJR 138:211–217.

32. Wiot JF (1975) The radiologic manifestations of blunt chest trauma JAMA 231:500–502.

33. Hager J, Gunkel AR, Riccabona U (1999) Isolated longitudinal rupture of the posterior tracheal wall following blunt neck trauma. Eur J Pediatr Surg 9(2):104–108.

34. Dougall AM, Paul ME, Finley RJ, et al. (1977) Chest trauma: Current morbidity and mortality. J Trauma 17:547–553.

35. Fraser RG, Paré JAP, Paré PD, et al. (1988) Diagnosis of diseases of the chest. WB Saunders, Philadelphia.

36. Tocino IM (1985) Pneumothorax in the supine patient. Radiographic anatomy. Radiographics 5:557–586.

37. Tocino I, Miller MH, Fairfax WR (1985) Distribution of pneumoththorax in supine and semirecumbent critically ill adult. AJR 144:901–905.

38. Carr JJ, Reed JC, Choplin RH, et al. (1992) Plain and computed radiography for detecting experimentally induced pneumothorax in cadavers: Implications for detection in Patients, Radiology 183:193–199.

39. Fajardo LL, Hillman BJ, Pond GD, et al. (1989) Detection of pneumothorax: Comparison of digital and conventional chest imaging. AJR 152:475–480.

40. Mirvis SE, Rodriguez A (1992) Diagnostic imaging of thoracic trauma. In Mirvis SE, Young JWR (eds) Imaging in trauma and critical care. William & Wilkins, Baltimore, MD, pp 93–144.

41. Wall SD, Federle MP, Jeffrey RB, et al. (1983) CT diagnosis of unsuspected pneumothorax after blunt intimal trauma. AJR 141:919–921.

42. Brasel K, Stafford RE, Weigelt JA, et al. (1999) Treatment of pneumothoraces from blunt trauma J Trauma, 46(6):987–991.

43. Marchaud P (1951) The anatomy and applied anatomy of the mediastinal fascia. Thorax 6:359–368.

44. Macklin CC (1939) Transport of air along seaths of pulmonic blood vessels from alveoli to mediastinum: Clinical implications. Arch Int Med 64:913–926.

45. Wintermark M et al. (1999) Blunt traumatic pneumomediastinum: Using CT to reveal the Macklin effect. AJR 172:129–130.

46. Kemper AC, Steinberg KP, Stern EJ (1999) Pulmonary interstitial Emphysema: CT Findings. AJR 172:1642.

47. Heitzman ER (1977) The mediastinum: radiologic–pathologic correlations with anatomy and pathology (2nd edn.) Springer Verlag, Berlin.

48. Lane EJ, Carsky E (1968) Epicardial fat: Lateral plain film diagnosis in normals and pericardial effusion. Radiology 91:1–5.

49. Levin B (1973) The continuous diaphragm sign – a newly recognized sign of pneumomediastinum. Clin Radiol 24:337–338.

50. Naclerio EA (1957) The "V" sign in the diagnosis of spontaneous rupture of the esophagus (an early clue). Am J Surg 93:291.

51. Swischuk L (1976) Two lesser known but useful signs of neonatal pneumothorax. Radiology 127:623–627.

52. Westaby S (1977) Pneumopericardium and tension pneumopericardium after closed chest injury. Thorax 32:91–97.

53. Mirvis SE, Indeck M, Schorr RM, et al. (1986) Posttraumatic tension pneumopericardium: The "small heart" sign. Radiology 158:663–669.

54. Stark P (1993) Pleura, In Stark P (ed) (1993) Radiology of Thoracic Trauma. Andover Medical Publishers, Boston, MA, pp 54–72.

55. Rutherford RB, Cambell DN (1985) Thoracic injuries in Zuidema GD, Rutherford RB, Ballinger WF (eds). The management of trauma, WB Saunders, Philadelphia.

56. Velmajos GD, Demetriades D, Chan L et al. (1999) Predicting the need for thoracoscopic evacuation of residual traumatic hemothorax. Chest radiography is insufficient J Trauma 46(1):65–70.

57. Vilealba M, Lucas CE, Ledgerwood AAM, et al. (1979) The etiology of post-traumatic empyema and the role of decortication. J Trauma 19:414–421.

58. Stark DD, Federle MP, Goodman PC, et al. (1983) Differentiating lung abscess and emphysema. Radiography and computed tomography. AJR 141:163–167.

59. Chan O, Hiorns M (1996) Chest trauma. Eur J Radiol 23:23–34.

60. Fabian TC, Richardson JD, Croce MA, et al. (1997) Prospective study of blunt aortic injury: Multicenter trial of the American Association for the Surgery of Trauma. J Trauma 42:374–380.

61. Kodali S, Jamieson WR, Leia SM, et al. (1991) Traumatic rupture of the thoracic aorta: A 20-year review – 1969–1989. Circulation 84(pt 2):140–146.

62. Sutorius DJ, Schreiber JT, Helmsworth JA (1973) Traumatic disruption of the thoracic aorta. J Trauma 13:583–590.

63. Bennett DE, Cherry JK (1967) The natural history of traumatic aneurysms of the aorta. Surgery 61:516–523.

64. Parmley LF, Mattingly TW, Manion WC, et al. (1958) Non-penetrating injury of the aorta. Circulation 17:1086–1101.

65. Townsend RN, Coletta JJ, Diamond DL (1990) Traumatic rupture of the aorta: Critical decision for trauma patients J Trauma 30:1169–1174.

66. Kieney YR, Champentier A (1991) Traumatic lesions of the thoracic aorta: A report of 73 cases. J Cardiovasc Surg 32:613–615.

67. Greendyke PM (1966) Traumatic rupture of the aorta. JAMA 195:119–122.

68. Feczko JD, Lynch L, Pless JE, et al. (1992) An autopsy case review of 142 nonpenetrating (blunt) injuries of the aorta. J Trauma 33:846–849.

69. Cimochowski GE, Barcia PJ, DeMeester TR, et al. (1973) Multiple transections of the thoracic aorta secondary to blunt trauma. Ann Thorac Surg 15:536–540.

70. Jennettoni MD, McCurry KR, Rodriguez JL, et al. (1994) Stimultaneous traumatic ascending and descending thoracic aortic rupture. Ann Thorac Surg 57:481–484.

71. Turney SZ (1992) Blunt trauma of the thoracic aorta and its branches. Semin Thorac Cardiovasc Surg 4:209–216.

72. Kirsh MM, Behrendt DM, Orringer MB, et al. (1976) The treatment of acute traumatic rupture of the aorta: A 10-year experience. Ann Surg 184:308–316.

73. Ayella RJ, Hankins JR, Turney Sz, et al. (1977) Ruptured thoracic aorta due to blunt trauma. J Trauma 17:199–205.

74. Woodring JH, Loh FK, Kryscio RJ (1984) Mediastinal hemorrhage: An evaluation of radiographic manifestations. Radiology 151:15–21.

75. Mirvis SE, Bidwell JK, Buddemeyer EU, et al. (1987) Value of chest radiography in excluding traumatic aortic rupture. Radiology 163:487–493.

76. Richardson JD, Wilson ME, Miller FB (1990) The widened mediastinum: Diagnostic and therapeutic priorities. Ann Surg 211:731–736.

77. Seltzer SE, O'Orsi C, Kirshner R, et al. (1981) Traumatic aortic rupture: Plain radiographic findings. AJR 137:1011–1014.

78. Sefczek DM, Sefczek RJ, Deeb ZI (1983) Radiographic signs of acute traumatic rupture of the thoracic aorta. AJR 141:1259–1262.

79. Woodring JH (1990) The normal mediastinum in blunt traumatic rupture of the thoracic aorta and brachiocephalic arteries. J Emerg Med 8:467–476.

80. Hsu YP, Chen RJ, Bullard MJ, et al. (1998) Traumatic thoracic aortic injury caused by sharp edge of left fractured rib on body position. A case report. Chang Keng I Hsueh Tsa Chih 21(3):343–346.

81. Albers JE, Rath RK, Glaser RS, et al. (1982) Severity of intrathoracic injuries associated with first rib fractures. Ann Thorac Surg 33:614–618.

82. Kirshner R, Seltzer S, D'Orsi C, et al. (1983) Upper rib fractures and mediastinal widening: Indications for aortography. Ann Thorac Surg 35:450–454.

83. Patel NH, Stephens KE, Jr, Mirvis SE, et al. (1998) Imaging of acute thoracic aortic injury due to blunt trauma: A Review. Radiology 209:335–348.

84. Mirvis SE, Shanmuganathan K, Miller BH, et al. (1996) Traumatic aortic injury: Diagnosis with contrast-enhanced thoracic TC–five year experience at a major trauma center. Radiology 200:413–422.

85. Kram HB, Appel PL, Wohlmuth DA, et al. (1989) Diagnosis of traumatic thoracic aortic rupture: A 10-year retrospective analysis. Ann Thorac Surg 47:282–286.

86. Marnocha KE, Maglinte DD, Woods J, et al. (1984) Mediastinal width/chest-width ratio in blunt chest trauma: A reappraisal. AJR 142:275–277.

87. Miller FB, Richardson JD, Thomas HA, et al. (1989) Role of CT in diagnosis of major arterial injury after blunt thoracic trauma. Surgery 106:596–602.

88. Gavant ML, Menke PG, Fabian T, et al. (1995) Blunt traumatic aortic rupture: Detection with helical CT of the chest. Radiology 197:125–133.

89. Brooks AP, Olson LK, Shackford SR (1989) Computed tomography in the diagnosis of traumatic rupture of the thoracic aorta. Clin Radiol 40:133–138.

90. Gavant ML, Flick P, Menke P, et al. (1996) CT aortography of thoracic aortic rupture. AJR 166:955–961.

91. Tomiak MM, Rosenblum JE, Messersmith RN, et al. (1993) Use of CT for diagnosis of traumatic rupture of the thoracic aorta. Ann Vasc Surg 7:130–139.

92. Wilson D, Voystock JF, Sariego J, et al. (1994) Role of computed tomography scan in evaluating the widened mediastinum. Am Surg 60:421–423.

93. Svenson LG, Labit SB, Eisenhauer AC, et al. (1999) Intimal tear without hematoma: An important variant of aortic dissection that can elude current imaging techniques. Circulation 99:1331–1336.

94. Kuhlman JE, Pozniak MA, Colins J, et al. (1998) Radiographic and CT findings of blunt chest trauma: Aortic injuries and looking beyond them. Radiographics 18:1085–1106.

95. Harris JHJ, Horowitz DR, Zelitt DL (1995) Unenhanced dynamic mediastinal computed tomography in the selection of patients requiring thoracic aortography for the detection of acute traumatic aortic injury. Emerg Radiol 2:67–76.

96. Ledbetter S, Stock JL, Kaufman JA (1999) Helical CT in the evaluation of emergent thoracic aortic syndromes. Traumatic aortic rupture, aortic aneurysm, aortic dissection, intramural hematoma, and penetrating atherosclerotic ulcer. Radiol Clin North Am 37:575–590.

97. Van Hise ML, Primack SL, Israel RS, et al. (1998) CT in blunt chest trauma: Indications and limitations. Radiographics 18:1071–1084.

98. Haesemeyer SW, Gavant ML (1999) Imaging of acute traumatic aortic tear in patients with an abberant right subclavian artery. AJR 172:117–120.

99. White CS, Mirvis SC (1995) Pictorial review: Imaging of traumatic aortic injury. Clin Radiol 50:281–287.

100. Raptopoulos V (1994) Chest CT for aortic injury: Maybe not for everyone. AJR 162:1053–1055.

101. Richardson P, Mirvis SE, Scorpio R, et al. (1991) Value of CT in determining the need for angiography when findings of mediastinal hemorrhage on chest radiographs are equivocal. AJR 156:273–279.

102. Tello R, Munden RF, Hooton S, et al. (1998) Value of spiral CT in hemodynamically stable patients following blunt chest trauma. Comput Med Imaging Graphics 22:447–452.

103. Fisher RG, Sanchez-Torres M, Thomas JW, et al. (1997) Subtle or atypical injuries of the thoracic aorta and brachiocephalic vessels in blunt thoracic trauma. Radiographics 17:835–849.

104. Gundry SR, Williams S, Burney RE, et al. (1982) Indications for aortography in blunt thoracic trauma: A reassessment. J Trauma 22:664–671.

105. Ahrar K, Smith DC, Bansal RC, et al. (1997) Angiography in blunt thoracic aortic injury. Trauma: Injury Infect Crit Care 42:665–669.

106. Stark P (1984) Traumatic rupture of the thoracic aorta: A review. Crit Rev Diagn Imaging 21:229–255.

107. Pozzato C, Fedriga E, Donateli F, et al. (1991) Acute posttraumatic rupture of the thoracic aorta: The role of angiography in a 7-year review. Cardiovasc Intervent Radiol 14:338–341.

108. Sturm JT, Hankins DG, Young G (1990) Thoracic aortography following blunt chest trauma. Am J Emerg Med 8:92–96.

109. Fisher RG, Sanhez-Torres M, Whigham CJ, et al. (1997) "Lumps" and "Bumps" that mimic acute aortic and brachiocephalic vessel injury. Radiographics 17:825–834.

110. Kearney PA, Smith DW, Johnson SB, et al. (1993) Use of transesophageal echocardiography in the evaluation of traumatic aortic injury. J Trauma 34:696–701.

111. Smith MD, Cassidy JM, Souther S, et al. (1995) Transesophageal echocardiography in the diagnosis of traumatic rupture of the aorta. N Engl J Med 332:356–362.

112. Treasure T (1997) Imaging the thoracic aorta in the injured patient. Heart 78:207–208.

113. Vignon P, Rambaud G, François B, et al. (1998) Transesophageal echocardiography for diagnosis of traumatic injuries to the major intrathoracic vessels in 150 patients. The effect of the learning curve. Ann Fr Anesth Reanim 17:1206–1216.

114. Goarin JP, Caloire P, Jacquens Y, et al. (1997) Use of transesophageal echocardiography for diagnosis of traumatic aortic injury. Chest 112:71–80.

115. Murray JC, Manisali M, Flam SD, et al. (1997) Intramural hematoma of the thoracic aorta: MR imaging findings and prognostic implications. Radiology 204:349–355.

116. Pattori R, Celletti F, Beertaccini P, et al. (1996) Delayed surgery of traumatic aortic rupture: Role of magnetic resonance imaging. Circulation 94:2865–2870.

117. Hughes JP, Ruttley MST, Musumeci F (1994) Case report: Traumatic aortic rupture: Demonstration by magnetic resonance imaging. Br J Radiol 67:1264–1267.

118. Bluemke DA (1997) Definitive diagnosis of intramural hematoma of the thoracic aorta with MR imaging. Radiology 204:319–321.

119. Banning AP, Pillai R (1997) Non-penetrating cardiac and aortic trauma. Heart 78:226–229.

120. Shackford SR (1995) The evolution of modem trauma care. Surg Clin North Am 75:147–153.

121. Greenberg MD, Rosen CL (1999) Evaluation of the patient with blunt chest trauma: An evidence-based approach. Emerg Med Clin North Am 17:41–62.

122. Trerotola SO (1995) Can helical CT replace aortography in thoracic trauma [editorial]? Radiology 197:13–15.

123. Gavant ML (1999) Helical CT grading of traumatic aortic injuries. Impact on clinical guidelines for medical and surgical management. Radiol Clin North Am 37:553–574.

124. Shannmuganathan K, Mirvis SE (1999) Imaging diagnosis of nonaortic thoracic injury. Radiol Clin North Am 37:533–552.

125. Deluca SA, Rhea JT, O'Malley TO (1982) Radiographic evaluation of rib fractures AJR 138:91–92.

126. Malagari K, Fraser RG (1995) Imaging of the chest wall and diaphragm. In (Ch. Roussos ed.) M. Roussos, C. (ed) The thorax, part C. Marcel Dekker, New York, pp. 1763–1837.

127. Benmenachem Y (1988) Avulsion of the innominate artery associated with fracture of the sternum. AJR 150:621–622.

128. Dec PM (1992) The radiology of chest trauma. Radiol Clin North Am 30:291–306.

129. Patten RM, Dobbins J, Gunberg SR (1999) Gas in the sternoclavicular joints of patients with blunt chest trauma: Significance and frequency of CT findings. AJR 172:1633–1635.

130. Klebel JM, Jardon OM, Huurman WW (1986) Scapulothoracic dislocation: A case report. Clin Orthop 209:210–214.

131. Tsai DW, Swiontkowski MF, Kottra CL (1996) A case of sternoclavicular dislocation with scapulothoracic dissociation. AJR 167:332.

132. Pal J, Mulder D, Brown R, et al. (1988) Assessing multiple trauma: Is the cervical spine enough? Trauma 28:1282–1284.

133. Meyer P (1989) Surgery of spine trauma. Churchill Livingstone, New York.

134. White A, Paujabi M (1978) Clinical biomechanics of the spine. Lippincott, Philadelphia.

135. Calenof L, Chesare JW, Rogers LF, et al. (1978) Multiple level spinal injuries: Importance of early detection AJR 130:655–699.

136. Murphey M, Batmitzky S, Bramble J (1989) Diagnostic imaging of spinal trauma. Radiol Clin North Am 27:855–872.

137. Kaye JJ, Nance PE (1990) Thoracic and lumbar spine trauma Radiol Clin North Am 28:361–377.

138. Denis F (1983) The three column spine and its significance in the classification of acute thoracolumbar spine injuries Spine 8:817–831.

139. McAfee PC, Yuan HA, Lasda NA (1982) The unstable burst fracture. Spine 7:365–373.

140. Pang D, Pollack I (1989) Spinal cord injury without radiographic abnormality in children: The SCIWORA syndrome. J Trauma 29:654–664.

141. Groskin SA (1992) Selected topics in chest trauma. Radiology 183:605–617.

142. Bhalla M, Leitman BS, Forcade C, et al. (1990) Lung hernia: Radiographic features AJR 154:51–55.

143. Root HD (1991) Injuries to the diaphragm. In Moore EE, Mattox KL, Feliciano DV (eds) Trauma, 2nd edn., Conn Appleton and Lange, Norwalk, CT, pp 427–439.

144. Shapiro MJ, Heiberg E, Durham RM, et al. (1996) The unreliability of CT scans and initial chest radiographs in evaluating blunt trauma induced diaphragmatic rupture. Clin Radiol 51:27–30.

145. Kearney PA, Rouhaba SW, Burney RE (1989) Blunt rupture of the diaphragm: Mechanism, diagnosis and treatment. Ann Emerg Med 18:1326–1330.

146. Morgan AS, Flancbaum L, Espositio T, et al. (1986) Blunt injury to the diaphragm: An analysis of 44 patients. J Trauma 26:565–568.

147. Wienecek RG, Wilson RF, Steiger Z (1986) Acute injuries of the diaphragms: An analysis of 165 cases. J Thorac Cardiovasc Surg 92:989–993.

148. Aoki AA, Mock CN, Talner LB (1998) Traumatic rupture of the right hemidiaphragm in an automobile accident victim. AJR 171:386.

149. Guth AA, Pachter HL, Kim U (1995) Pitfalls in the diagnosis of blunt diaphragmatic injury. Am J Surg 170:5–9.

150. Lucido JL, Wall CA (1963) Rupture of the diaphragm due to blunt trauma. Arch Surg 86:989–994.

151. Gourin A, Garzon AA (1974) Diagnostic problems in traumatic diaphragmatic hernia. J Trauma 14:20–31.

152. Gelman R, Mirvis SE, Gens D (1990) Diaphragmatic rupture due to blunt trauma: Sensitivity of plain chest radiographs. AJR 156:51–57.

153. Murray, JA, Demetriades D, Cornwell E III, et al. (1997) Penetrating Left thoracoabdominal trauma: The incidence and clinical presentation of diaphragm injuries. J Trauma: Injury, Infect Crit Care 43:624–626.

154. Rodriguez-Morales G, Rodriguez A, Shatney CH (1986) Acute rupture of the diaphragm in blunt trauma: Analysis of 60 patients. J Trauma 26:438–444.

155. Tarver RD, Godwin JD, Putman CE (1984) The diaphragm. Radiol Clin North Am 22:615–631.

156. Holm A, Bessy PQ, Aldrette JS (1988) Diaphragmatic rupture due to blunt trauma: Morbidity and mortality in 42 cases. South Am Journ 81:956–999.

157. Estera AS, Landay MJ, McClelland RN (1985) Blunt traumatic rupture of the right hemidiaphragm: Experience in 12 patients. Ann Thorac Surg 39:525–530.

158. Flancbaum L, Morgan AS, Esposito T, et al. (1985) Non left-sided diaphragmatic rupture due to blunt trauma. Surg Gynecol Obstet 161:266–270.

159. Boulanger BR, Milzman DP, Rosati C, et al. (1993) A comparison of right and left blunt traumatic diaphragmatic rupture. J Trauma 35:255–260.

160. Worthy SA, Kang EY, Hartman TE, et al. (1995) Diaphragmatic rupture CT findings in 11 patients. Radiology 194:885–888.

161. Shah R, Sabanathan S, Meams AJ, et al. (1995) Traumatic rupture of diaphragm. Ann Thorac Surg 60:1444–1449.

162. Murray JG, Caioli E, Gruden JF, et al. (1996) Acute rupture of the diaphragm due to blunt trauma: Diagnostic sensitivity and specificity of CT. AJR 166:1035–1039.

163. Shanmuganathan K, Mirvis SE, White CS, et al. (1996) MR imaging evaluation of hemidiaphragms in acute blunt trauma: Experience with 16 patients. AJR 167:397–402.

36 The Diaphragm

R.D. Tarver and D.J. Conces Jr.

Introduction

The diaphragm has two important functions: it provides most of the work of inspiration and it divides the thoracic and the abdominal cavities. Understanding these two functions of the diaphragm allows for a complete understanding of the normal and abnormal processes that involve the diaphragm and the spaces it divides. Most diaphragmatic abnormalities are asymptomatic and are usually detected on a chest radiograph obtained for other reasons. Various pathologic conditions may present as alterations in diaphragmatic shape, position, or movement. However, the radiographic abnormalities identified on the chest radiograph are often nonspecific and the chest radiograph only serves as a starting point for further evaluations. Diaphragmatic disorders are evaluated with fluoroscopy, ultrasound, computed tomography (CT), magnetic resonance imaging (MRI), and nuclear medicine scintigraphy.

In this chapter the anatomy, physiology, and pathophysiology of the diaphragm are discussed. A thorough discussion of the peridiaphragmatic regions are also included (1).

Anatomy and Physiology

The diaphragm is a dome-shaped, thin, musculotendinous structure that separates the thoracic and abdominal cavities (Fig. 36.1). The peripheral portion is composed of

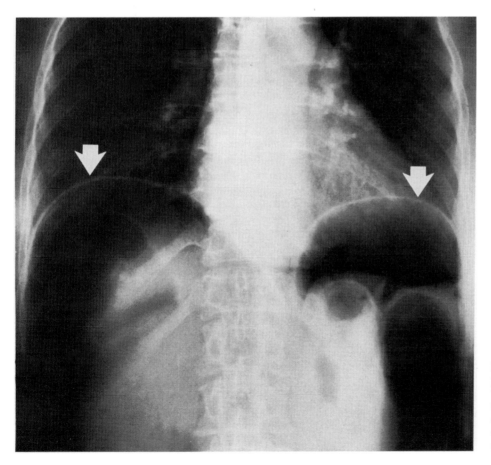

Figure 36.1. An upright radiograph in a patient with a large pneumoperitoneum. This is one of the ways that the diaphragm itself (*arrows*) can be visualized radiographically. Because it lies adjacent to the liver, which is of similar radiographic density it is usually not visualized.

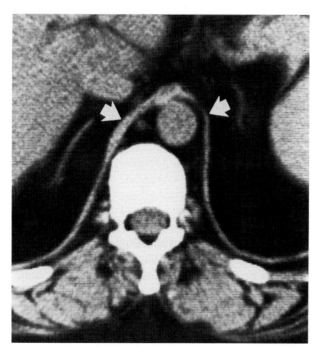

Figure 36.2. A CT scan showing the aorta passing through the aortic hiatus at the level of T12. The crura are the thin soft tissue density structures identified by the *arrows*.

three groups of muscular fibers on each side: the sternal portion, arising from the back of the xiphoid process; the costal portion, arising from the lower six ribs and their costal cartilages; and the lumbar portion, arising from the medial and lateral arcuate ligaments and the lumbar vertebral bodies. The portions arising from the vertebral bodies are the crura, which blend with the anterior longitudinal ligament of the spine. The central tendon is a thin aponeurosis at the convergence point of the muscular portions (2).

The diaphragm has three major openings: the aortic, the esophageal, and the vena caval. The aortic aperture, located behind the left median arcuate ligament at the level of T12, is the largest and lowest opening. It transmits the aorta, thoracic duct, lymphatic vessels, and the azygos and hemiazygos veins (Fig. 36.2). The esophageal aperture, lying at the level of T10, is formed by the splitting if the medial fibers of the right crus. It transmits the esophagus, the anterior and posterior vagal nerves, esophageal branches of the left gastric artery and vein, and some lymphatics. The vena caval opening is the highest opening, lying at the level of T8 or T9 at the junction of the right hemidiaphragm and the central tendon (3).

The motor nerve supply of the diaphragm is the phrenic nerve, which arises from C4 nerve roots, with lesser and variable contributions from the C3 and C5 roots. Sensory fibers are supplied by the phrenic nerve and the lower six intercostal nerves (2).

Blood vessels supplying the diaphragm ramify over its superior and inferior surfaces. The pericardiophrenic and musculophrenic branches of the internal thoracic artery and the superior phrenic branches of the thoracic aorta supply the superior surface. Veins draining the superior surface are the pericardiophrenic (draining into the internal thoracic or brachiocephalic vein), musculophrenic (draining into the internal thoracic vein), and small posterior branches (draining into the azygos and hemiazygos veins). The inferior surface is supplied by inferior phrenic branches from the abdominal aorta and drained by the inferior vena cava and the left suprarenal vein. Lymphatics of the superior surface drain into the anterior, middle, and posterior phrenic nodes. The inferior surface drains through the diaphragm into the superior system and also along the inferior phrenic veins into the lumbar lymphatic chains (4).

Understanding diaphragmatic embryology helps to explain both the physiology and congenital abnormalities of the diaphragm. Formation of the diaphragm occurs from the sixth to tenth fetal weeks. The first and most important component of the diaphragm is the septum transversum, a mesodermal plate that incompletely separates the thoracic and abdominal cavities. The persistent communications between the abdominal and thoracic cavities are the pericardioperitoneal canals. They close progressively as the pleuroperitoneal membranes grow anteromedially and eventually fuse to the esophageal mesentery and the septum transversum. As the pleural cavity enlarges, an additional rim of tissue is laid down peripheral to the pericardioperitoneal membranes by inward migration of myoblasts from the body wall, ultimately forming the muscular portion of the diaphragm. In the fourth intrauterine week, the septum transversum lies at the level of cervical somites and derives its nerve supply from C3, C4 and C5. By the sixth intrauterine week, the diaphragm is at the thoracic level, and the muscular ingrowth is accompanied by sensory branches from intercostal nerves (5–7).

In summary, the diaphragm is composed of four structures: (a) the central tendon, formed from the septum transversum; (b) the pleuroperitoneal membranes, constituting a small portion of the adult diaphragm; (c) the dorsal esophageal mesentery, from which the crura develop; and (d) the body wall component, forming the muscular portion.

The diaphragm is the vital pump for the respiratory system, just as the heart is for the circulatory system. Inspiration is an active process resulting from an increase in thoracic volume. At quiet inspiration, the diaphragm provides 75% of the increased volume (8). When larger intrathoracic volumes are needed, the accessory muscles – scalene, sternocleidomastoid, and external oblique muscles – provide progressively more help with inspiration. The expiratory muscles – internal intercostal muscles and muscles of the anterior abdominal wall – are used only for forced expiration. Normal diaphragmatic contraction in the upright position causes an outward expansion of the lower ribs and an increase in abdominal pressure, pushing the abdominal wall outward. In the supine position, most of the inspiratory motion is manifested by outward abdominal motion with very little chest wall motion.

Physiologically, the diaphragm acts as if composed of two muscles, the costal portion and the crural portion. The costal portion, attached to the lower ribs, both lifts these ribs and displaces the abdominal viscera outward. The crural portion, not attached to the ribs, only displaces the abdominal contents downward and outward (9,10).

Normal Radiographic Appearance

On the posteroanterior radiograph, the superior surface of the diaphragm forms a domed interface with aerated lung. The interface is lost where the heart obscures the medial third of the left hemidiaphragm, and the inferior surface is similarly obscured by the soft tissues of the abdomen. The lateral costophrenic angles are formed where the diaphragm meets the lateral chest wall. In deep inspiration, the right dome is located between the fifth and sixth ribs anteriorly and the tenth rib posteriorly. The left dome is one half interspace (1–3 cm) lower than the right dome in 90% of patients but can be even with the right or slightly higher in normal persons. The left hemidiaphragm is probably lower because the heart depresses it (11). In children, young adults, obese patients, or supine patients the diaphragm is higher. In asthenic patients, patients with emphysema, and some young men who take an exceptionally deep breaths, it may lie as low as the tenth posterior rib. A scalloped contour of the diaphragm is not uncommon, is usually seen on the right, and is of no clinical significance (12–17).

On the lateral radiograph, the top of the dome is anterior to the midaxillary line. The diaphragm intercepts the anterior chest wall at the level of the sixth rib or sixth interspace and the posterior chest wall at the level of the twelfth rib. The two hemidiaphragms are usually separable on the lateral view because they lie at slightly different levels. The entire right hemidiaphragm is usually visible, whereas the anterior portion of the left hemidiaphragm is obscured by the heart and mediastinal fat. The left hemidiaphragm may also be identified by underlying gas in the stomach or splenic flexure of the colon (15,16).

On fluoroscopy, the diaphragm moves down with inspiration and up with expiration, with an average excursion of 3.5 cm for the left hemidiaphragm and 3.2 cm for the right hemidiaphragm. Seventy-five percent of patients have 3–6 cm of excursion, 2% have greater than 6 cm, and 23% have less than 3 cm. The excursion of the left hemidiaphragm is not only slightly greater but slightly more rapid. Minimal asynchronous or paradoxic inspiratory motion is common (13–16, 18,19).

Fluoroscopy should be performed with the patient upright, and all respiratory motion must be voluntary, not assisted by a ventilator. Having the patient practice the maneuvers and commands before fluoroscopy helps to ensure a successful examination. First both hemidiaphragms are observed in the frontal projection during slow, deep inspiration and expiration. If no abnormalities are detected, more forceful respirations should be observed. During the respiratory cycle, the mediastinum should be observed for a shift in position: in young patients, the mediastinum typically shifts away from the paralyzed side during inspiration. In older patients the shift of the mediastinum is not as great because of its relatively fixed position in the thorax. Peripheral and central portions of the hemidiaphragm should be observed separately because some disorders involve one portion and not the other. Second, an oblique or lateral position is used to observe both hemidiaphragms simultaneously. If it is not clear which is the left hemidiaphragm when the patient is in the lateral position a small amount of effervescent drink or tablets can be given to distend the stomach. A sniff test-forceful, quick inspiration through the nose – is the best test for eliciting paradoxic hemidiaphragmatic motion.

Observing the diaphragms with the patient in the supine position can also elicit differences in the strength of the two hemidiaphragms. In the supine position the full weight of the abdominal contents rests against the hemidiaphragms. Any differences in the strengths of the two hemidiaphragms will be accentuated when they are loaded with the additional weight of the abdominal contents in the supine position. In the upright position, in which most fluoroscopy is done, gravity acts to unload the weight of the abdominal contents from the diaphragm. The supine position can be used to accentuate the differences in the strengths of the two diaphragms much like the sniff test does.

The diaphragm also can be imaged using ultrasonography. On ultrasound, the diaphragm has the echogenicity of skeletal muscle. The diaphragm can be differentiated from the liver, which has a similar echogenicity because the acoustic impedances are different. The diaphragm can also be differentiated from the subpleural fat and the intercostal muscles. Ultrasound can also be utilized to check diaphragmatic movement if fluoroscopy is not readily available (20).

On CT scans, the diaphragm is visible as a circular or oval soft tissue density with fat below and aerated lung above. The diaphragm has intermediate attenuation like skeletal muscle. The diaphragm is not visible where it is tangent to the scan plane or where there is no fat separating it from soft tissue structures such as the liver, spleen, stomach, or colon. The domes of the diaphragm and the peridiaphragmatic structures are well depicted using spiral CT and multiplanar reformations (21–24).

On MRI scans the diaphragm appears similar to is configuration on CT if the cuts are axial; however, the unique ability of MRI to visualize the body in all planes allows for coronal and sagittal depiction of the diaphragm. The main problem in visualizing the diaphragm and the peridiaphragmatic structures is the motion of the diaphragm during the scan times. Respiratory gating programs eliminate many of the problems associated with imaging the moving diaphragm. Newer techniques allow for imaging the motion of the diaphragm. The muscular diaphragm has signal intensity similar to that of skeletal muscle, liver, and spleen on all pulse sequences and is well depicted where it is separated from these structures by high signal intensity abdominal or mediastinal fat (25,26).

Diaphragmatic Disorders

Bochdalek Hernia

Bochdalek hernia is a congenital posterolateral defect occurring in 1 in 2200 live births (27). It results from failure of the pleuroperitoneal membrane to fuse with the other existing portions of the diaphragm prior to the intestines returning to the abdomen (6,28). Visceral herniation usually involves the stomach, spleen, colon, or small bowel. Over 80% of the hernias are left sided because the right pleuroperitoneal canal closes before the left at the time when the gut is returning to the abdominal cavity from the yolk sac. Fifteen percent are right sided and 5% are bilateral (28). A small defect may contain only retroperitoneal fat whereas larger defects may contain stomach, intestine, spleen, or kidney on the left and liver on the right. In fewer than 10% of cases a hernia sac is present (3–29,30).

In 1901, Aue performed the first successful repair of a congenital diaphragmatic hernia in a 9 year old boy who had presented with empyema. In 1902, Broman postulated that a defect in the embryogenesis of the diaphragm led to herniation of the bowel into the chest. Although Bonet first described the anatomy of the lesion in 1679, the failure of the primitive posterolateral portions of the diaphragm to fuse would become known as the Bochdalek hernia, after Vincent Bochdalek (28).

Bochdalek hernia can result in hypoplasia of the lungs. Hypoplasia is more severe in the ipsilateral lung but also affects the contralateral lung because of mediastinal shift. When herniation occurs early in fetal development, lung hypoplasia is more severe. Both the number of bronchial generations and the number of alveoli are reduced, and the pulmonary vasculature is often hypoplastic.

Bochdalek hernia is a common cause of respiratory distress in the newborn, usually presenting within 24 h of birth with severe respiratory distress, acidosis, absent left-sided breath sounds, scaphoid abdomen, and, rarely, bowel sounds in the left chest. Today the diagnosis is frequently made on prenatal sonography. The ultrasound diagnosis can be made as early as 15 weeks of gestation. Sonography is approximately 90% accurate in making the diagnosis prenatally. Serial radiographs initially show an opaque hemithorax with later aeration of the intrathoracic bowel loops as the infant swallows air (31). Barium studies usually are not needed to identify the bowel in the thorax. The differential diagnosis includes staphylococcal pneumonia and congenital adenomatoid malformation of the lung. In newborn infants, the mortality rate is 50%, even with surgical correction, with most patients dying of respiratory insufficiency caused by the lack of mature lung tissue and the high pulmonary vascular resistance (32,33). However, Bochdalek hernia presenting after 24 h of age usually causes only mild distress, and the mortality rate is only 5% with surgical correction. Children studied years after diaphragmatic repair may show emphysematous lung changes (34).

A newborn with a major congenital anomaly has a much higher incidence of associated malformations. Babies with congenital diaphragmatic hernias have 28% associated defects. The incidence of major anomalies, excluding pulmonary hypoplasia and intestinal malrotation ranges from 40% to 57%. Associated congenital defects include, central nervous system abnormalities, patent ductus arteriosus, ventriculo-septal defect, vascular rings, coarctations, and trisomies 13 and 18. Postmartem examinations on stillbirths with congenital diaphragmatic hernias reveal that 95% have associated defects (28,35).

Bochdalek hernia detected in an adult is usually seen on a chest radiograph as a variable-sized soft tissue mass bulging upward through the posterior aspect of the hemidiaphragm (Fig. 36.3). Barium studies identify any bowel within the hernia, and CT shows any herniated retroperitoneal fat and sometimes the diaphragmatic defect itself (36). Recent reviews of CT scans show that asymptomatic, small Bochdalek hernias are present in 6% of otherwise normal patients (37). The increasing incidence with age, emphysema, and obesity suggests that the vast majority of the adult abnormalities may be acquired defects rather than true Bochdalek hernias (25).

Morgagni Hernia

Morgagni hernia is caused by failure of fusion between the fibrotendinous elements of the sternal and costal parts of the diaphragm. Herniation occurs through the foramen of Morgagni, which normally contains fat, the superior epigastric arteries, and some lymphatic vessels. The hernia is surrounded by a sac of pleura and peritoneum. It usually contains omentum and transverse colon, but stomach, small bowel, and portions of the liver can also herniate.

Morgagni hernia typically presents in adults, often associated with obesity, trauma, or other causes of

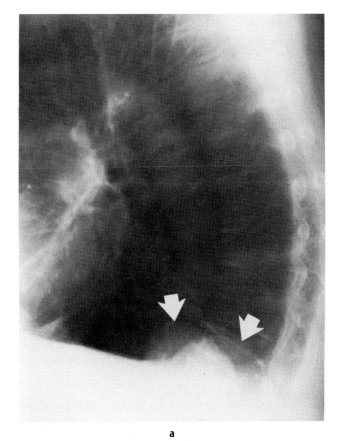

a

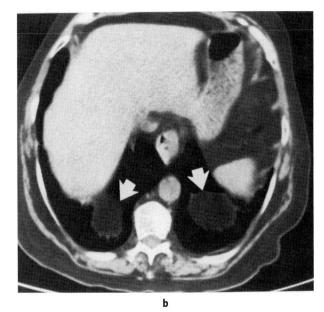

b

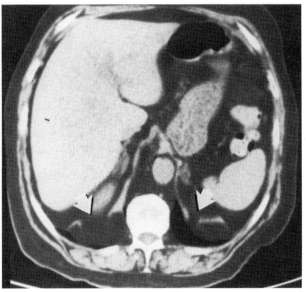

c

Figure 36.3. Bilateral Bochdalek hernias in an adult. **a** Lateral chest radiograph showing two semicircular masses in the posterior costophrenic sulcus (*arrows*). **b** CT scan showing the top of the two masses that were visible on the lateral chest radiograph (*arrows*). **c** CT scan lower in the thorax showing bilateral diaphragmatic defects (Bochdalek hernias) that allow the retroperitoneal fat to herniate into the chest (*arrows*).

increased intraabdominal pressure (Fig. 36.4). It is most often right sided, since the heart and pericardium cover left-sided defects (38). Although these hernia usually contain only omentum, a few will have a portion of colon to protrude. Incarceration or strangulation rarely occur in foramen of Morgagni hernia (39). Rarely, bilateral defects or total absence of the sternal portions of the diaphragm occurs (40). Either condition tends to

present early in childhood with large anterior defects that usually contain liver.

Radiographs typically show a right anterior costophrenic mass that can usually be distinguished from pericardial cyst, eventration, or tumor by barium examination. Occasionally, visible bowel gas is present. Hepatic scintigraphy, CT, or ultrasonography can identify herniated liver (41,42).

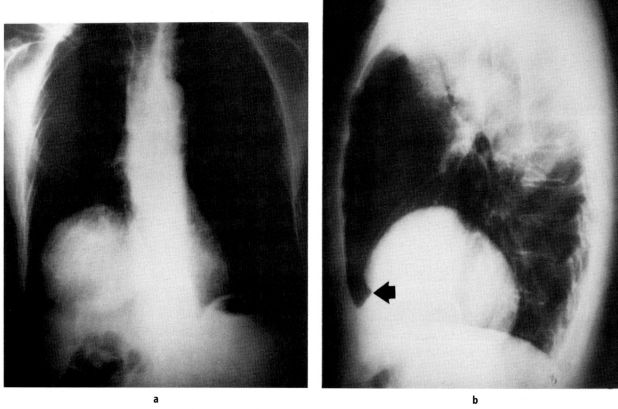

a

b

Figure 36.4. a Chest radiograph showing a large right Morgagni hernia in an adult. **b** Lateral radiograph showing the Morgagni hernia with the "mushroom-type" appearance where the liver is constricted by the rent in the hemidiaphragm (*arrow*).

Peritoneopericardial Diaphragmatic Hernia

Peritoneopericardial diaphragmatic hernias are rare and are congenital or traumatic in origin. The congenital ones present in infancy and probably occur as a result of the failure of the septum transversum to completely close the communication between the pericardium and the peritoneal cavity. The infant may present at birth with choking or later with cyanosis, dyspnea, regurgitation, and poor weight gain. Liver or bowel may herniate into the pericardium. Surgical correction is curative once the condition is diagnosed. Traumatic peritoneopericardial diaphragmatic hernias occur when the portion of the diaphragm adjacent to the pericardium is lacerated during blunt or penetrating trauma. They may present acutely or some time after the injury. Symptoms may be cardiovascular, gastrointestinal or pulmonary in nature. They include dyspnea, congestive heart failure, tamponade, tachyarrhythmias, intestinal obstruction and intestinal pain. CT, plain films and barium studies are often needed to make the diagnosis. Once the diag-

nosis is made the treatment is surgical correction (43,44).

Hiatal Hernia

Congenital hiatal hernia presents in childhood with symptoms of reflux: vomiting, failure to thrive, respiratory difficulty, and anemia (3). The diagnosis can be confirmed by an esophagram. The etiology is probably a weakness of the right crural musculature that allows the hiatus to widen. Rarely, a congenitally short esophagus is the cause.

Most often, hiatal hernia presents in adulthood and causes symptoms of reflux or no symptoms at all. It is the result of acquired widening of the esophageal hiatus and laxity of the phrenoesophageal ligament by increased intraabdominal pressure, such as occurs with obesity. The sliding variety of hernia is much more common that the paraesophageal type. Occasionally, the hernia is large and can cause incarceration or volvulus of the stomach (45). On radiographs, a hiatal hernia causes a retrocardiac soft

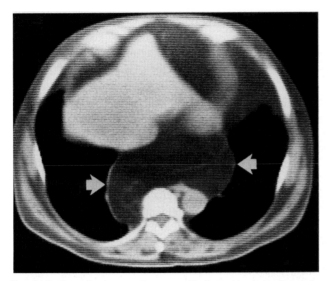

Figure 36.5. CT scan showing a massive amount of fat (*arrows*) herniating through the esophageal hiatus.

tissue mass, without or without an air – fluid level. A barium study clearly demonstrates the size and contents of the hernia and any complications such as reflux esophagitis or volvulus. Hiatal hernia is also visible on CT scans (Fig. 36.5).

Chilaiditi Syndrome

Chilaiditi's syndrome is the interposition of the right colon between the diaphragm and the liver (46). The diaphragm is normal in this disorder but the radiographic findings involve the diaphragm. The diaphragm is seen, outlined above by air in the right lower lobe of the lung and below by air in the right colon. Occasionally the right hemidiaphragm may appear slightly elevated in this disorder but at fluoroscopy there is normal motion and excursion. Chilaiditi syndrome is probably a normal variant, seen in approximately 0.1–0.2% of normal patients. However, some reports have linked the syndrome to as many as 8% of mentally deficient patients with abdominal pain.

Eventration

Congenital eventration is uncommon. It is caused by inadequate migration of myoblasts into the diaphragm, resulting in incomplete muscularization of the pericardioperitoneal membrane (3,47–49). The deficiency may be partial or complete; in either case, the peripheral portion of the diaphragm retains normal musculature. Lesions are most often unilateral. The pericardioperitoneal membrane is intact, but where muscularization has failed, the

diaphragm is abnormally thin and subject to stretching and upward displacement by the rapidly growing liver and viscera (7). Histologically, the thinned portion consists primarily of fibrous tissue, with little or no skeletal muscle (49). The increased incidence of eventration with age suggests that there is an acquired component in the development of an eventration (50).

Eventration presenting in childhood is most likely to be on the right side, but, in adults, it is most likely to be on the left side. Partial eventration is usually right sided, has no sex predilection, and almost always contains liver. Complete eventration is usually left sided and usually occurs in males. The most common eventration is partial, right sided, and anteromedial, and it affects both sexes equally (47,49).

A large eventration is more likely to cause symptoms than a small one. Symptoms result from respiratory insufficiency and are more common in children, probably because the mobility of the mediastinum in children prevents the unaffected, contralateral hemidiaphragm from functioning efficiently. Adults with eventration develop symptoms only if other thoracopulmonary disease has decreased their respiratory reserve. Only symptomatic eventrations that are unresponsive to medical therapy require plication (51).

On radiographs, an eventration causes a smooth elevation of the hemidiaphragm or a focal, broad-based, mass-like elevation. On fluoroscopy, there is little or no downward motion with inspiration. Initially, a small amount of apparently paradoxic motion may occur until the slack is taken out by the intact peripheral musculature (51). Ultrasonography can often identify the intact, but thin, diaphragm, thereby distinguishing eventration from hernia. It can also identify the contents of the eventration. Hepatic scintigraphy can also be used to identify the liver under the elevated hemidiaphragm.

Trauma

Traumatic Rupture

Traumatic rupture of the diaphragm from blunt trauma is due to a sudden, explosive increase in the pleuroperitoneal pressure gradient. Diaphragmatic rupture is recognized in 0.5–0.6% of blunt trauma survivors (50). The usual cause is a fall or automobile accident, but occasionally, the traumatic event is too minor to be recalled by the patient (52,53). In postmartem series of fatal injuries, the incidence of diaphragmatic rupture is 5%, with right- and left-sided rupture being equally common (54). However, in patients who survive to be evaluated for their injuries, the proportion of left-sided rupture is greater than 90%, either because the liver protects the right hemidiaphragm or because the left hemidiaphragm is inherently weaker

(3,55,56). In more recent reports the ratio of left-sided to right-sided ruptures has decreased, and the incidence of right-sided ruptures is now generally reported at between 20% and 30% (57,58). Rupture usually involves the posterior central portion of the hemidiaphragm and extends medially, but avulsions of the peripheral diaphragm from the chest wall also occur (31,59). The stomach is the organ most likely to herniate, but sometimes, colon, omentum, small bowel, spleen, liver, or gallbladder enters the thorax (60). A hernia resulting from blunt trauma is usually larger than that from penetrating trauma, and associated injuries are usually more severe (60). The concomitant severe injuries and the rarity of acute visceral herniation obscure the signs and symptoms of rupture and may delay its diagnosis. Only about one third of ruptures are diagnosed promptly, and the rest have delayed presentation. Rarely interruption of the diaphragm where it is attached to the pericardium results in a peritoneopericardial diaphragmatic hernia (43). Stomach, colon, jejunum, or liver may be found within the pericardium after this type of hernia occurs. Acute presentation and delayed presentation are discussed separately.

Acute Presentation

Symptoms of acute rupture are nonspecific – dyspnea, shoulder pain, and cyanosis (61). Chest radiographs currently are the most valuable simple test, but can be diagnostic or suggestive in only 28–70% of cases (62). Radiographic findings are also nonspecific – an opacity in the lower thorax could represent atelectasis, hemathorax, or lung contusion (56). The diagnosis of acute rupture is suggested by an unusual air – fluid level in the lower thorax, an abnormal diaphragmatic contour, a contralateral mediastinal shift greater than expected for the amount of basal opacity (71), or a higher than suspected position of the stomach as indicated by the course of the nasogastric tube (Fig. 36.6) (59,63). The radiologist should maintain a high level of suspicion of the possibility of rupture so that confirmatory studies with barium, water-soluble contrast material, fluoroscopy, ultrasonography, CT, or scintigraphy can be performed promptly (56,64,65).

Diaphragmatic tears can be seen on CT and several signs are indicative of traumatic disruption. Abrupt discontinuity of the diaphragm may be visible, with or

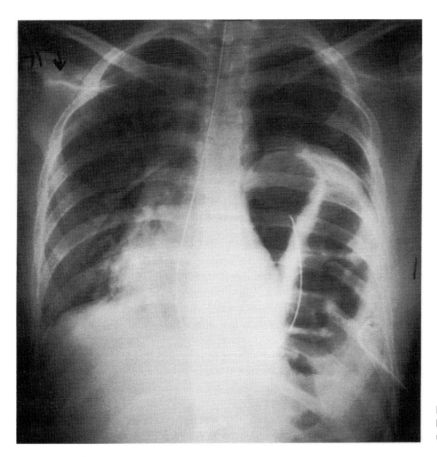

Figure 36.6. Portable chest radiograph showing an acute left hemidiaphragmatic rupture. The nasogastric tube takes the unusual but diagnostic turn upward.

without visceral herniation. Inability to identify the diaphragm in an expected location, the "absent diaphragm sign", may be noted. Identification of abdominal structures external to the diaphragm is a sign of intrathoracic herniation. Occasionally a focal constriction of the viscera at the site of herniation, the "collar or hourglass sign", can be seen. Spiral CT with reformation of the images in coronal and sagittal planes can be helpful in identifying a traumatic hernia. The sensitivity and specificity of CT in the diagnosis of acute rupture of the diaphragm are 61% and 87%, respectively. MRI can be helpful as well for the same reasons (24,50,62,66–70).

Delayed Presentation

Although late presentation of intrathoracic visceral herniation secondary to blunt trauma is a rare occurrence, it was one of the first types of diaphragmatic hernias to be reported. In 1541, Sennertus first described the delayed presentation of herniated viscus through an injured diaphragm. Similarly, Ambroise Paré in 1597 reported the case of a young artillery captain who died secondary to a gangrenous colon that had herniated through a bullet hole in the left diaphragm 8 months prior to the patient's death (39).

Although most diaphragmatic disruptions are recognized at the time of initial hospitalization, a small minority go undiagnosed, despite exploratory laparotomy (39). A diaphragmatic rupture may be asymptomatic or mildly symptomatic for years, causing only vague abdominal distress, chest or shoulder pain, or recurrent pneumonia. However, rupture does not heal spontaneously, and the constant transdiaphragmatic pressure gradient acts to force abdominal viscera into the chest, enlarging the defect (71). Serial radiographs may show a growing diaphragmatic mass that can be confused with eventration, large hiatal hernia, diaphragmatic or pleural tumor, lung abscess, or cyst. Eventually, most patients (85% by 3 years) develop symptoms of obstruction because of incarceration, which can progress to strangulation and necrosis (3). Mortality rates as high as 30% occur with strangulation, despite prompt surgical intervention.

Penetrating Trauma

Penetrating tear of the diaphragm is more common than blunt injury (54,72). Usually, the diaphragmatic defect is discovered incidentally during exploratory surgery for a knife or gunshot wound (73). Gunshot injuries affect both sides equally, but knife wounds predominate on the left because most assailants are right handed. Occult penetrating injury to the diaphragm may initially be asympto-

matic because of its small size but may present later as abdominal viscera eventually herniate through the defect. A stab wound is the most common cause of delayed traumatic hernia, and the risk of strangulation is high because the defect is small (60). Chest radiographs and clinical examination at the time of initial injury are often nonspecific, and only a high index of suspicion will lead to prompt surgical correction (72).

Tumors

Diaphragmatic tumors are rare. Benign tumors are more common than malignant tumors of the diaphragm (3,74–76). Of primary malignant tumors most are sarcomas of fibrous or muscular origin. Patients develop epigastric or pleuritic chest pain, and radiographs typically show a large mass. Of benign tumors, lipomas are most common. Lipomas are often asymptomatic and discovered only at autopsy or as a small diaphragmatic irregularity on radiographs (50).

Cysts of the diaphragm are congenital or acquired. Congenital ones include teratoid cysts, mesothelium-lined cysts, and cysts resembling bronchogenic cysts or sequestrations. Acquired cysts include simple cysts, fibrous-lined cysts, and cysts developing from degenerating traumatic hematomas.

CT is the most helpful radiographic technique for evaluating diaphragmatic masses. In cases of lipoma or cyst, CT attenuation values may provide a specific diagnosis. The CT distinction of a diaphragmatic discontinuity can be identified at the site of fat herniation.

Metastasis to the diaphragm is not uncommon; most cases represent direct spread from adjacent tumors of the lung, stomach, kidney, adrenal gland, colon, or retroperitoneum. Rarely, hematogenous metastasis occurs, but usually not until the primary tumor is widely disseminated. Lymphoma can also involve the diaphragm.

Other Abnormalities

Accessory Hemidiaphragm

Accessory hemidiaphragm is a rare congenital anomaly (12,77). Fewer than 30 have been reported in the world's literature. The abnormal diaphragm consists of a fibromuscular membrane that separates a portion of the lung from the rest of the parenchyma. It is predominately a right-sided anomaly that originates anteriorly from the regular diaphragm and extends posteriorly to insert on the posterolateral fifth to seventh ribs. Most patients have disordered ventilation to the portion of the lung distal to the abnormal diaphragm, which may result in respiratory distress or repeated infections. Radiographically the hemithorax affected by the accessory hemidiaphragm is smaller and often the incorrect diagnosis of right middle and upper lobe atelectasis is made. On the frontal views the mediastinal border is indistinct and on the lateral view there is an anterior dense opacity behind and paralleling the sternum that represents the mediastinal fat between the chest wall and the small lung.

Diaphragmatic Agenesis

Diaphragmatic agenesis is a particularly severe form of congenital diaphragmatic hernia. True agenesis or aplasia of the diaphragm is thought to result from failure of development of three of the four diaphragmatic anlagen (pleuroperitoneal membrane, septum transversum, and dorsal esophageal mesentery). Although a distinction from a large posteriolateral hernia has not always been made in the literature, true diaphragmatic agenesis results in the presence of a thin rim of muscular tissue anteriorly derived from the remaining anlage – body wall musculature. Agenesis or aplasia has been reported to be responsible for anywhere from 1% to 30% of all cases of diaphragmatic hernia. These cases appear to be autosomal recessive and have a poor prognosis (78).

Paralysis, Weakness and Fatigue

Paralysis

Paralysis of the diaphragm has many causes (79,80). In the newborn, it can be caused by birth trauma and can be difficult to distinguish from congenital eventration. Both conditions are usually unilateral. Concomitant Erb's palsy or a fractured clavicle helps to make the diagnosis of phrenic nerve injury rather than eventration (81). In an infant, causes of paralysis are viral infection, pulmonary or pleural infection, and surgical injury to the phrenic nerve during repair of tracheoesophageal fistula or congenital heart disease (81,82).

In the newborn period and in the first years of life, diaphragmatic paralysis is poorly tolerated for several reasons. First, the infant depends on the diaphragm because the accessory muscles of inspiration are weak. Second, the mobile mediastinum of the child interferes with the action of the functioning contralateral hemidiaphragm (48,83,84). Thus diaphragmatic paralysis may require prolonged ventilatory support or, alternatively, diaphragmatic plication.

In older patients, the causes of paralysis are infectious, iatrogenic, or malignant. Transient left phrenic nerve paralysis is commonly caused by cardioplegia during heart surgery. Older children and adults tolerate unilateral paralysis of the diaphragm and are often asymptomatic because of the relative fixity of the mediastinum and the strength of accessory muscles (48). Even with total paralysis of one hemidiaphragm, only a 20% loss of ipsilateral lung ventilation and perfusion occurs (83). Therefore surgical plication is rarely needed.

In unilateral paralysis, a paralyzed hemidiaphragm paradoxically moves upward on inspiration and downward on expiration. It moves passively following the changing intrapleural and intraabdominal pressure. In bilateral paralysis, both hemidiaphragms move upward with inspiration. A paralyzed hemidiaphragm may show a slight downward motion with slow deep inspiration from passive stretching as the rib cage expands. The sniff test is needed to confirm that poor diaphragmatic motion is due to paralysis and not weakness. As the patient forcefully inhales through the nose with the mouth closed there is a quick descent of both hemidiaphragms. Paradoxical upward motion of an entire hemidiaphragm of greater than 2 cm is consistent with paralysis of the hemidiaphragm (50).

Neurogenic Weakness

Weakness of the diaphragm can result from a neurologic lesion at any level from the motor cortex to the neuromuscular end-plate (85). A lesion of the motor cortex or descending pyramidal pathways affects voluntary control of respiration. A lesion in the medullary reticular formation affects involuntary control, and a high cord lesion disrupts both. A midcervical lesion destroys the phrenic nerve neurons, and ventilation must be maintained by accessory muscles. A lower cervical or upper thoracic lesion affects the inspiratory intercostal muscles. One rare central abnormality of ventilation is Ondine's curse, a defect in involuntary regulation of ventilation that leads to hypoventilation (86). The clinical syndrome consists of episodic apnea that occurs when the patient is asleep. While the patient is awake, there is sufficient sensory stimulation to maintain respiratory drive. The condition is presumably caused by injury to the medullary chemoreceptors with decreased CO_2 sensitivity and consequent CO_2 retention; with voluntary hyperventilation, the arterial CO_2 levels return to normal. Pulmonary arterial hypertension ultimately develops. Diaphragmatic pacing has helped in some patients (Fig. 36.7).

Peripheral neurologic abnormalities include poliomyelitis, amyotrophic lateral sclerosis, Guillain Barré neuropathy, and myasthenia gravis. Myopathies (e.g. polymyositis, acid maltase deficiency, thyrotoxicosis, hyperthyroidism, systemic lupus erythematosus (87), and alcoholism) can all cause similar clinical findings (85).

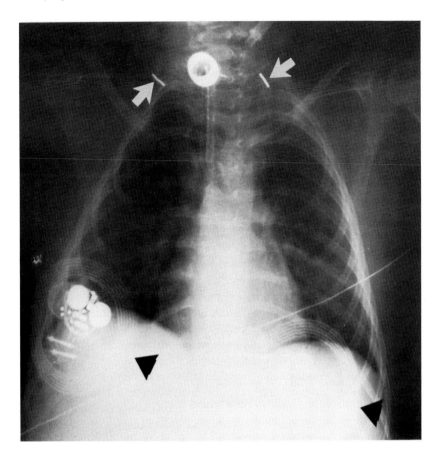

Figure 36.7. Chest radiograph of a child with bilateral diaphragmatic paralysis due to cervical spinal cord disease. The patient has bilateral phrenic nerve pacemakers. The subcutaneous radiofrequency pickups are over the lower chest (*arrowheads*). The electrical stimulus is carried by the wires to the electrodes (*arrows*) implanted in the neck.

Fatigue

Diaphragmatic fatigue is the inability to maintain the work required for adequate ventilation (9). Fatigue is now recognized as an important component of ventilatory limitation, contributing to hypercapnic respiratory failure in a variety of conditions (88). Respiratory fatigue should be considered by the radiologist in the differential diagnosis of diaphragmatic paralysis and weakness.

Fatigue occurs when the energy demand of the respiratory muscle exceeds the energy supply (9). The energy supply is decreased by reduced substrate delivery (low cardiac output, hypoxemia, anemia, or malnutrition). Demand is increased by increased respiratory work, decreased strength, or decreased efficiency. Respiratory work increases with airway obstruction (asthma, chronic bronchitis, emphysema), decreased lung compliance (lung fibrosis, pulmonary edema), inefficient respiratory pattern (rapid, shallow breathing), and hyperinflation (88,89). Hyperinflation increases the work of respiration by shortening the diaphragmatic muscle fibers and decreasing their maximal strength. Causes of decreased strength are neuromuscular disease, prematurity, and prolonged ventilatory assistance. Inefficient muscle action results from

airway obstruction. Often, there are many interrelated causes for respiratory fatigue in the same patient.

Untreated respiratory fatigue can progress to respiratory failure (88). Initially, respiratory rate is increased and breathing is shallow. Next, discoordinated respiratory motions occur, including both abdominal paradox and respiratory alternans (90). In abdominal paradox, diaphragmatic contraction is weak or absent, and the negative pleural pressure generated by the accessory muscles and transmitted to the abdomen causes an inward motion of the abdominal wall rather than the usual outward motion. In respiratory alternans, the normal motion of the diaphragm alternates after a few breaths, with motion generated only by the accessory muscles and manifested by inspiratory motion of the rib cage (9). Ultimately, respiratory rate and ventilation decline as respiratory failure ensues (90).

Treatment of fatigue requires ventilatory assistance, which rests the inspiratory muscles, and aminophylline administration, which increases diaphragmatic contractility (91). Inspiratory muscle endurance training can also help over the long term.

The radiologic evaluation of respiratory fatigue and diaphragmatic weakness or paralysis requires clinical information, adequate chest radiographs, and fluoroscopy. The finding of unilateral paralysis or weakness on chest radiographs is an elevated hemidiaphragm. Bilateral paralysis, weakness, or respiratory fatigue all cause low lung volumes on radiographs and are indistinguishable from each other.

Fluoroscopy can often distinguish between diaphragmatic paralysis, weakness, and fatigue. Unilateral paralysis results in a lack of motion on slow inspiration and paradoxic motion of the elevated hemidiaphragm on rapid inspiration or sniffing. Unilateral weakness can be missed on slow inspiration but becomes obvious on rapid, deep inspiration, because the weak hemidiaphragm lags behind the normal one. Unilateral weakness occasionally causes paradoxic motion on rapid, deep inspiration, or sniffing, just as unilateral paralysis does, but can be distinguished by the persistence of some delayed orthograde motion during less rapid inspiration. Bilateral weakness has the same radiographic and fluoroscopic findings as respiratory fatigue and bilateral paralysis. In all three conditions, there is often marked thoracic motion from the action of the accessory inspiratory muscles, but there is little diaphragmatic motion. In fatigue, fluoroscopy may show abdominal paradox or respiratory alternans, or no diaphragmatic motion at all.

Other Disorders of Diaphragmatic Motion

Hiccups

Hiccups are uncoordinated diaphragmatic and intercostal contractions which can occur at the rate of 6–100 times per minute (12,79,92). They are often unilateral and may last for prolonged times, up to 60 days. Fluoroscopy shows that all or portions of one or both hemidiaphragms may be involved. The etiologies of hiccups are varied and include psychogenic and organic causes. Organic etiologies include central nervous system (stroke, tumors, skull fractures, neurosyphilis, anesthesia, and encephalitis), the neck (tumors and aneurysm), the thorax (aneurysms, tumors, myocardial infarction, pericarditis, pneumonia, lung abscess and diaphragmatic hernia), and the abdomen (aneurysm, tumors, gall bladder diseases, pancreatitis, abscess, ulcer and gastritis). Herpes zoster has also been reported to cause hiccups. Uremia is a common predisposition for the occurrence of hiccups.

Flutter

Diaphragmatic flutter is due to rapid irregular contractions of the diaphragm occurring at a rate from 35 to 480 per minute, with an average of 150 (12,79,92). The first case to be

reported was that of Leeuwenhoek in 1723, who complained to his physician of epigastric pulsations. He determined that it was not cardiac palpations as his pulse was slow and regular and therefore he attributed the palpations to his diaphragm. These patient often complain of palpations or an abnormal feeling over their upper abdomen or lower chest. Fluoroscopically they can involve one or both hemidiaphragms. The rapid fluttering is superimposed upon the normal diaphragmatic motion. The etiology usually remains unknown but a search for any area of irritation of the diaphragms or phrenic nerve should be carried out.

The Peridiaphragmatic Regions

CT is the best radiographic technique for evaluating the retrocrural region (93). The normal retrocrural structures include fat, the azygos and hemiazygos veins, the aorta, nerves, lymph nodes, air, and the cisterna chyli and the thoracic duct (2,94). The right crus has a large lateral component and a small medial component, both of which originate from the anterior aspect of the first three lumbar vertebrae. The smaller left crus arises from the first two lumbar vertebrae. The medial tendinous margins of the crura meet in the midline to form an arch anterior to the aorta, called the median arcuate ligament (95). The proximal abdominal aorta is crossed anteriorly by the left crus and fibers of the medial right crus (96,97). The crura are usually thin, but nodularity is normal and should not be mistaken for lymphadenopathy (Fig. 36.8). The usual abnormality in the retrocrural region is adenopathy from metastatic cancer or from lymphoma. CT is thus essential in staging malignancies that could potentially extend into this space from the thorax or the abdomen.

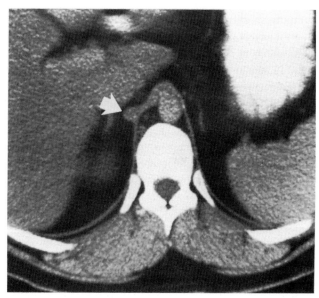

Figure 36.8. CT scan showing a normal amount of nodularity to the right crus (*arrow*). This should not be confused with adenopathy.

Lymph nodes anterior to the central diaphragm drain the diaphragm, adjacent liver, and anterior mediastinum. These prepericardial and cardiophrenic angle lymph nodes are located anterior to the diaphragm, posterior to the xiphoid and adjacent costal margins in the cardiophrenic angles. Normally up to two, less than 5 mm, nodes can be seen on CT. Anterior sternal attachments can simulate adenopathy in this region (50).

Peridiaphragmatic fluid collections or abscesses are common clinical problems. The diagnosis, treatment, and complications depend on accurate radiographic location of the collection above or below the diaphragm.

Chest films, including decubitus views, demonstrate the amount and mobility of any pleural fluid. A pleural empyema with abscess formation may contain visible air bubbles, as may a subdiaphragmatic abscess. Sometimes, a sympathetic pleural effusion on chest radiographs is a sign of a subdiaphragmatic abscesses.

Peridiaphragmatic fluid collections can often be identified as pleural, peritoneal, or retroperitoneal by their appearance on CT (98–102). Fluid within the rounded contour of the diaphragm is subphrenic or intraabdominal, whereas fluid outside the contour is pleural or thoracic. At the level of the crura, retroperitoneal and peritoneal fluid lies anterolateral to the crura (Fig. 36.9) and pleural fluid lies posteromedial to them. The interface with the liver (or spleen) is sharp for fluid in the abdomen, but hazy for fluid in the thorax (103). The displaced crus sign is another indication that the fluid is pleural rather than peritoneal (104). It is the lateral displacement of the posteromedial portion of the diaphragm by fluid above (Fig. 36.10).

Ultrasonography also helps in determining the location of peridiaphragmatic fluid collections. The right side is evaluated utilizing the liver as a window. The left side is harder to evaluate because of bowel gas, but a portion of the peridiaphragmatic region can be imaged through the spleen. Ultrasonography often images the diaphragm itself, which clearly helps to locate the fluid collections. Only direct coronal CT scanning or peritoneography (with gas or iodinated contrast medium) provides comparable visualization of the diaphragm. MRI may prove helpful in imaging peridiaphragmatic fluid collections.

Gallium or labeled-leukocyte scans are often utilized in the evaluation of infected peridiaphragmatic fluid collections. In the past, a nuclear liver–lung scan was commonly used to detect any fluid separating the lung from the liver. However, it has been largely supplanted by CT and ultrasonography.

Conclusion

Radiologic evaluation of the diaphragm is important in many clinical situations, but visualization of the diaphragm is difficult because of its thinness, its domed contour, and its contiguity with abdominal soft tissues. Each clinical situation involving the diaphragm presents its own imaging difficulties, and each radiographic technique has advantages and disadvantages. No one modality is best for all situations. Often, several imaging methods must be used to resolve the clinical question.

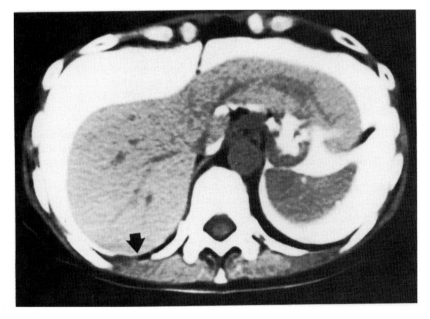

Figure 36.9. CT scan of a patient with intraperitoneal contrast which demonstrates that the bare area of the liver is on the upper posterior portion of the liver (*arrow*) and not over the apex of the liver. This is often a useful area to examine when trying to decide whether fluid is intraperitoneal or in the pleural space. Fluid posterior to the bare area is usually in the pleural space.

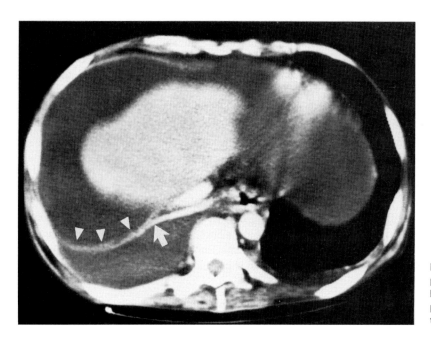

Figure 36.10. CT scan demonstrating the "displaced crus sign" of pleural fluid. Here the right crus is displaced away from the spine by pleural fluid (*arrow*). In addition to the pleural fluid this patient has ascites, allowing for the unique chance to visualize the hemidiaphragm itself (*arrowheads*).

The particular difficulties in diaphragmatic imaging are (a) distinguishing eventration from paralysis or hernia, (b) distinguishing lipoma from herniated omental fat, and (c) distinguishing unilateral paralysis from weakness and bilateral paralysis from respiratory fatigue. By selecting and applying appropriate radiographic techniques, the radiologist serves an essential role in assessing the disorders of the diaphragm.

References

1. Tarver RD, Godwin JD, Putman CE (1984) The diaphragm. Radiol Clin North Am 22:615–631.
2. Williams PL, Warwick R (eds) (1980) Gray's anatomy, 36th edn. Philadelphia WB Saunders, pp 547–551.
3. Pomerantz M (1983) The diaphragm. In Sabiston DC, Jr, Spencer FC (eds) Gibbon's surgery of the chest, 4th edn. Philadelphia WB Saunders, pp 833–838.
4. Woodburn RT (1983) Essentials of human anatomy. New York, Oxford University Press, pp 449–452.
5. Langman J (1981) Medical embryology 4th edn. Williams & Wilkins, Baltimore, MD, pp 282–317.
6. Pansky B (1982) Review of medical embryology. Macmillan, New York, pp 110–125.
7. Snell RS (1983) Clinical embryology for medical students, 3rd edn. Little, Brown, Boston, MA, pp 177–196.
8. Ganong WF (1977) Review of medical physiology, 8th edn. Lange Medical Publications, Los Altos, CA, pp 483–493.
9. Roussos C, Macklem PT (1982) The respiratory muscles. N Engl J Med 307:786–797.
10. Troyer AD, Sampson M, Sigrist S, et al. (1981) The diaphragm: Two muscles. Science 213:237–238.
11. Reddy V, Sharma S, Cobanoglu A (1994) What dictates the position of the diaphragm – the heart or the liver? J Thorac Cardiovasc Surg 108:687–691.
12. Dietrich P, Alsofrom G (1986) The Diaphragm. In Taveras JM, Ferrucci JT (eds) Radiology, Vol. 1, Lippincott, Philadelphia, Chapter 83.
13. Felson B (1973) Chest roentgenology. WB Saunders, Philadelphia, pp 421–435.
14. Fraser RG, Pare, JAP (eds) (1977) Diagnosis of diseases of the chest, 2nd edn. Philadelphia, WB Saunders, pp 156–159, 207–208.
15. Paul LW, Juhl JH (1972) The essentials of Roentgen interpretation, 3rd edn. Harper and Row, New York, pp 768–769, 963–970.
16. Sutton D (1975) A textbook of radiology Churchill Livingstone, New York, pp 295–303.
17. Wynn-Williams N (1954) Hemidiaphragmatic paralysis and paresis of unknown aetiology without any marked rise in level. Thorax 9:299–303.
18. Alexander C (1966) Diaphragm movements and the diagnosis of diaphragmatic paralysis. Clin Radiol 17:79–83.
19. Simon G, Bonnell J, Kazantzis G, et al. (1969) Some radiological observations on the range of movement of the diaphragm. Clin Radiol 20:231–233.
20. Gottesman E, McCool FD (1997) Ultrasound evaluation of the paralyzed diaphragm. Am J Respir Crit Care Med 155:1570–1574.
21. Gale ME (1986) Anterior diaphragm: Variations in the CT appearance Radiology 161:635–639.
22. Kleinman PK, Raptopoulos V (1985) The anterior diaphragmatic attachments: Anatomic and radiologic study with clinical correlates. Radiology 155:289–293.
23. Brink JA, Heiken JP, Semenkovich J, et al. (1994) Sagel, SS Abnormalities of the diaphragm and adjacent structures: Findings on multiplanar spiral CT scans. AJR 163:307–310.
24. Killeen KL, Mirvis SE, Shanmuganathan K (1999) Helical CT of diaphragmatic rupture caused by blunt trauma. AJR 173: 1611–1616.

25. Gierada DS, Curtin J, Erickson SJ, et al. (1995) Goodman LR Diaphragmatic motion: fast-gradient-recalled echo MR imaging in healthy subjects. Radiology 194:879–884.

26. Taylor AM, Jhooti P, Keegan J, et al. (1999) Pennell DJ. Magnetic resonance navigatorecho diaphragm monitoring in patients with suspected diaphragm paralysis. J Magn Reson Imaging 9:69–74.

27. Naeye RL, Shochat SJ, Whitman V, et al. (1976) Unsuspected pulmonary abnormalities associated with diaphragmatic hernia. Pediatrics 58:902–906.

28. Weinstein S, Stolar CJH (1993) Congenital diaphragmatic hernia and extracorporeal membrane oxygenation. Pediatric Clin North Am 40:1315–1333.

29. Thibeault DW, Sigalet DL (1998) Congenital diaphragmatic hernia from the womb to childhood. Curr Prob Pediatr 28:3–25.

30. Donnelly LF, Sakurai M, Klosterman LA, et al. (1999) Correlation between findings on chest radiography and survival in neonates with congenital diaphragmatic hernia. AJR 173:1589–1593.

31. Sabiston DC, Jr (ed) (1977) Davis-Christopher textbook of surgery, 11th edn. WB Saunders Philadelphia, pp 404–405, 1362–1365, 2071–2072.

32. Levin DL (1978) Morphologic analysis of the pulmonary vascular bed in congenital left sided diaphragmatic hernia. J Pediatr 92:805–809.

33. Nair UR, Entress A, Walker D (1983) Management of neonatal posterolateral diaphragmatic hernia. Thorax 38:254–257.

34. Omojola MF, Reilly BJ, Mancer K (1981) Emphysema associated with pulmonary hypoplasia in congenital diaphragmatic hernia. AJR 136:1007–1009.

35. Grmolijez PF, Lewis JE (1976) Congenital diaphragmatic hernia: Bochdalek type. Am J Surg 132:744–746.

36. DeMartini WJ, House AJS (1980) Partial Bochdalek's herniation Chest 77:702–704.

37. Gale ME (1985) Bochdalek hernia: Prevalence and CT characteristics. Radiology 156:449–452.

38. Baran EM, Houston HE, Lynn HB, et al. (1976) Foramen of Morgagni hernias in children. Surgery 62:1076–1081.

39. Naunheim KS (1998) Adult presentation of unusual diaphragmatic hernias. Chest Surg Clin North Am 8:359–369.

40. Robinson AE, Gooneratne NS, Blackburn WR, et al. (1960) Bilateral anteromedial defect of the diaphragm in children. AJR 135: 301–306.

41. Soucek DC (1975) Foramen of Morgagni hernia diagnosed by liver scan. J Nucl Med 16:261–263.

42. Merten DF, Bowie JD, Kirks DR, et al. (1982) Anteromedial diaphragmatic defects in infancy: Current approaches to diagnostic imaging. Radiology 142:361–365.

43. Adamthwaite DN, Snyders DC, Mirwis J (1983) Traumatic pericardiophrenic hernia: A report of 3 cases. Br J Surg 70:117–119.

44. Einzig S, Munson DP, Singh S (1981) Intrapericardial herniation of the liver: Uncommon cause of massive pericardial effusion in neonates. AJR 137:1075–1077.

45. Pearson FG, Cooper JD, Ilves R, et al. (1983) Massive hiatal hernia with incarceration: A report of 53 cases. Ann Thorac Surg 35:45–51.

46. Melester T, Burt ME (1985) Chilaiditi's syndrome. JAMA 254:944–945.

47. Hesselink JR, Chung KJ, Peters ME, et al. (1978) Congenital partial eventration of the left diaphragm. AJR 131:417–419.

48. Ravitch MD, Welch KJ, Benson CD, et al. (eds.) (1979) Pediatric surgery, 3rd edn. Year Book Medical Publishers, Inc., Chicago, pp 432–445.

49. Wayne ER, Campbell JB, Burrington JD, et al. (1974) Eventration of the diaphragm. J Pediatr Surg 9:643–651.

50. Gierada DS, Slone RM, Fleishman MJ (1998) Imaging evaluation of the diaphragm. Chest Surg Clin North Am 8:237–280.

51. Symbas PN, Hatcher CR, Waldo W (1977) Diaphragmatic eventration in infancy and childhood. Ann Thorac Surg 24:113–119.

52. Ball T, McCrory R, Smith JO, Clements JL, Jr (1982) Traumatic diaphragmatic hernia: Errors in diagnosis. AJR 138:633–637.

53. Bekassy SM, Dave KS, Wooler GH, et al. (1973) "Spontaneous" and traumatic rupture of the diaphragm. Ann Surg 177:320–324.

54. Estrera AS, Platt MR, Mills LT (1979) Traumatic injuries of the diaphragm. Chest 75:306–313.

55. Hegarty MM, Bryer JV, Angorn IB, et al. (1978) Delayed presentation of traumatic diaphragmatic hernia. Ann Surg 188:229–233.

56. Heiberg E, Wolverson MK, Hurd RN, et al. (1980) CT recognition of traumatic rupture of the diaphragm. AJR 135:369–372.

57. Reber PU, Schmied B, Seiler CA, et al. (1998) Buchler MW Missed diaphragmatic injuries and their long-term sequelae. J Trauma Injury Infect Clin Care 44:183–188.

58. Mansour KA (1997) Trauma to the diaphragm. Chest Surgery Clin North Am 7:373–383.

59. Symbas PN (1975) Blunt traumatic rupture of the diaphragm. Ann Thorac Surg 26:193–194.

60. Payne JH, Yellin AE (1982) Traumatic diaphragmatic hernia. Arch Surg 117:18–24.

61. Wise L, Connors J, Hwang YH, et al. (1973) Traumatic injuries to the diaphragm. J Trauma 13:946–950.

62. Athanassiadi K, Kalavrouziotis G, Athanassiou M, et al. (1999) Skrekas G, Poultsidi A Blunt diaphragmatic rupture. Eur J Cardiothorac Surg 15:469–474.

63. Perlman SJ, Rogers LF, Mintzer RA, et al. (1984) Abnormal course of nasogastric tube in traumatic rupture of left hemidiaphragm. AJR, 142:85–86.

64. Ammann AM, Brewer WH, Maull KI, et al. (1983) Traumatic rupture of the diaphragm: Real time sonographic diagnosis. AJR 140:915–916.

65. Kim EE, McConnell BJ, McConnell RW, et al. (1983) Radionuclide diagnosis of diaphragmatic rupture with hepatic herniation. Surgery 94:36–40.

66. Kulhman JE, Pozniak MA, Collins J, et al. (1998) Radiographic and CT findings of blunt chest trauma: Aortic injuries and looking beyond them. Radiographics 18:1085–1106.

67. Worthy SA, Kang EY, Hartman TE, et al. (1995) Diaphragmatic rupture: CT findings in 11 patients. Radiology 194:885–888.

68. Shanmuganathan K, Mirvis SE, White CS, et al. (1996) MR imaging evaluation of hemidiaphragms in acute blunt trauma: Experience with 16 patients AJR 167:397–402.

69. Shanmuganathan K, Mirvis SE (1999) Imaging diagnosis of nonaortic thoracic injury. Radiol Clin North Am 37:533–551.

70. Murray JG, Caoili E, Gruden JF, et al. (1996) Acute rupture of the diaphragm due to blunt trauma: Diagnostic sensitivity and specificity of CT. AJR 166:1035–1039.

71. Gourin A, Garzow AA (1974) Diagnostic problems in traumatic diaphragmatic hernia. J Trauma 14:20–31.

72. Aronoff RJ, Reynolds J, Thal ER (1982) Evaluation of diaphragmatic injuries. Am J Surg 144:671–675.

73. Fallazedeh H, Mays ET (1975) Disruption of the diaphragm by blunt trauma. Am Surg 41:337–341.

74. Anderson LS, Forrest JV (1973) Tumors of the diaphragm. AJR 119:259–265.

75. Olafsson G, Rausing A, Holen O (1971) Primary tumors of the diaphragm. Chest 59:568–570.

76. Weksler B, Ginsberg RJ (1998) Tumors of the diaphragm. Chest Surg Clin North Am 8:441–447.

77. Wille L, Holthusen W, Willich E (1975) Accessory diaphragm: Report of 6 cases and a review of the literature. Pediatr Radiol 4:14–20.

78. Gibbs DL, Rice HE, Farrell JA, et al. (1997) Familial diaphragmatic agenesis: An autosomal recessive syndrome with a poor prognosis. J Pediatr Surg 32:366–368.

79. Derenne JPH, Macklem PT, Roussos CH (1978) The respiratory muscles: Mechanics, control, and pathophysiology. Am Rev Resp Dis 118:581–601.

80. Riley EA (1961) Idiopathic diaphragmatic paralysis: A report of eight cases. Am J Med 32:416.

81. Mickell JJ, Oh KS, Siewers RD, et al. (1978) Clinical implications of postoperative unilateral phrenic nerve paralysis. J Thorac Cardiovasc Surg 76:297–304.

82. Otherson HB, Lorenzo RL (1977) Diaphragmatic paralysis and eventration: Newer approaches to diagnosis and operative correction. J Pediatr Surg 12:309–315.

83. Merav AD, Attai LA, Condit DD (1983) Successful repair of a transected phrenic nerve with restoration of diaphragmatic function. Chest 84:642–644.

84. Commare MC, Krustjens SP, Barois A (1994) Diaphragmatic paralysis in children: A review of 11 cases. Pediatr Pulmonol 18:187–193.

85. Rochester DF, Arora NS (1983) Respiratory muscle failure. Med Clin North Am 76:573–597.

86. Mellins RB, Balfour HH, Gerard MD, et al. (1970) Failure of autonomic control of ventilation (Ondine's curse). Medicine 149:487–504.

87. Martens J, Demedts M, Vanmeenen MT, et al. (1983) Respiratory muscle dysfunction in systemic lupus erythematosus. Chest 84:170–173.

88. Macklem PT (1980) Respiratory muscles: The vital pump. Chest, 78:753–758.

89. Roussos C, Grassino A, Macklem PT (1980) Inspiratory muscle fatigue and acute respiratory failure. Can Med Assoc J 122:1375–1377.

90. Cohen CA, Zagelbaum G, Gross D, et al. (1982) Clinical manifestations of inspiratory muscle fatigue. Am J Med 73:308–316.

91. Belman MJ, Speck GC (1982) The ventilatory muscles. Chest 82:761–766.

92. Rigatto M, DeMedeiros NP (1985) Diaphragmatic flutter: Report of a case and review of literature. Am J Med 132:103–109.

93. Shin MS, Berland LL (1985) Computed tomography of retrocrural spaces: Normal, anatomic variants, and pathologic conditions. AJR 145:81–86.

94. Silverman PM, Godwin JD, Korobkin M (1982) Computed tomographic detection of retrocrural air. AJR 138:825–827.

95. Brengle M, Cohen MD, Katz B (1996) Normal appearance and size of the diaphragmatic crura in children: A CT evaluation. Pediatr Radiol 26:811–814.

96. Callen PW, Filly RA, Korobkin M (1978) Computed tomographic evaluation of the diaphragmatic crura. Radiology 126:413–416.

97. Naidich DP, Megibow AJ, Ross CR, et al. (1983) Computed tomography of the diaphragm: Normal anatomy and variants. J Comput Assist Tomogr 7:633–640.

98. Alexander ES, Proto AV, Clark RA (1983) CT differentation of subphrenic abscess and pleural effusion. AJR 140:47–51.

99. Federle MP, Mark AS, Guillaumin ES (1986) CT of subpulmonic pleural effusions and atelectasis: Criteria for differentiation from subphrenic fluid AJR 146:685–689.

100. Halvorsen RA, Fedyshin PJ, Korobkin M, et al. (1986) CT differentiation of pleural effusion from ascites: An evaluation of four signs using blinded analysis of 52 cases. Invest Radiol 21:391–395.

101. Naidich DP, Megibow AJ, Hilton S, et al. (1983) Computed tomography of the diaphragm: Peridiaphragmatic fluid localization. J Comput Assist Tomogr 7:641–649.

102. Silverman PM, Baker ME, Mahony BS (1985) Atelectasis and subpulmonic fluid: A CT pitfall in distinguishing pleural from peritoneal fluid J Comput Assist Tomogr 9:763–766.

103. Teplick JG, Teplick SK, Goodman L, et al. (1982) The interface sign: A computed tomographic sign for distinguishing pleural and intra-abdominal fluid. Radiology 144:359–362.

104. Dwyer A (1978) The displaced crus: A sign for distinguishing between pleural fluid and ascites on computed tomography. J Comput Assist Tomogr 2:598–599.

37 Benign and Malignant Lesions of the Pleura and the Chest Wall

P. Vock

Extrapulmonary diseases of the chest consist of a wide spectrum of entities and may exist alone or accompany pulmonary and mediastinal lesions. This present chapter discusses specific abnormalities of the pleura and the chest wall, with special attention to the most reliable imaging techniques in this area.

For a long time, conventional radiography played a prominent and often the only role in imaging benign and malignant lesions of the pleura and the chest wall. In recent years, more sophisticated modalities, such as computed tomography (CT) and magnetic resonance imaging (MRI) but also ultrasound (US) and nuclear medicine (both bone scintigraphy and positron emission tomography) have become more important in the detection and evaluation of this group of pathologies. CT, due to the general introduction of volumetric (spiral/helical) data acquisition with thinner collimation, provides excellent images of the pleura and the bony chest wall and a much improved resolution in the longitudinal axis. MRI, with its excellent soft tissue contrast has overcome most problems due to motion artefacts, its major previous limitation in the chest, and often adds significant information about the chest wall.

The Pleura

The radiologic work-up of pleural disease usually starts with a pair of erect posteroanterior and lateral chest radiographs at maximum inspiration. Depending on the clinical problem, additional investigations may be added; ultrasound has mostly replaced the lateral decubitus view to demonstrate minimal amounts of pleural fluid, and it is clearly superior in offering additional information on loculated fluid collections as well as solid lesions (1,2). Therefore the supine radiograph or fluoroscopy have become less important in demonstrating the behavior of any particular certain lesion with a change in position. For a more accurate survey, CT and MRI are increasingly used,

with the ability both to differentiate between fluid, solid, and vascular lesions and to demonstrate extrapleural infiltration in the case of infection or malignancy (3–10). Of special interest is the capability of MRI to characterize pleural effusion by identifying components, for example in case of hemothorax (11).

The diagnostic approach to pleural disease reasonably differentiates three physical categories depending on the pathologic substrate of gas (pneumothorax), fluid (effusion), or solid tissue, respectively. Of course, one has to be aware of an overlap in several clinical situations, such as trauma with combined pneumothorax and effusion, or infection/neoplasm with a combination of effusion and solid tissue.

Pneumothorax

Air may enter the pleural cavity through the chest wall, the mediastinum, the diaphragm, or most often from the lung itself. Causes of pneumothorax include rupture of a subpleural bulla (typically in a young man), rupture of the esophagus, penetrating or blunt thoracic trauma, sequelae of diagnostic or therapeutic procedures, mechanical ventilation, airflow obstruction in chronic asthma, diffuse pulmonary disorders (e.g., Langerhan cell histiocytosis or cystic fibrosis), and occasionally pulmonary infection, neoplasms, or endometriosis (12).

Pneumothorax is detected on radiographs as a separation of the visceral pleural line from the parietal line adjacent to the chest wall by a transradiant zone without lung markings (13,14). Since the volume of pneumothorax increases relative to the lung volume, an expiration view was earlier thought to be superior to inspiration; recent work, however, has not been able to prove this superiority, and inspiration seems to be preferable due to the improved information about the lung (15,16). On a supine radiograph, air is less easily detected and must be carefully searched for above a depressed diaphragm and at the mediastinal border (13,14). Small amounts of air may be detected on a lateral decubitus or a supine cross-table lateral projection. CT is much more sensitive in detecting minimal amounts of pleural air (17), and high-resolution CT (HRCT) may establish the etiology of spontaneous pneumothorax and the location of the pulmonary air leak. Occasionally, even using this modality the differentiation between pneumothorax and pulmonary blebs and bullae may be difficult.

While pneumothorax may be accompanied by some degree of pleural effusion (seropneumothorax), tension is the major severe complication. In this situation, a valve mechanism prevents air from leaving the pleural space during expiration and causes pleural pressure to increase, with compromised systemic venous return and serious hemodynamic consequences. The presence of a tension pneumothorax is suggested by radiographic signs that include an upper concavity of the depressed diaphragm and a mediastinal shift to the contralateral side (18,19)

(Fig. 37.1). Tension pneumothorax requires immediate drainage.

Rapid reexpansion of the collapsed lung under drainage may be followed by the development of pulmonary edema. Delayed reexpansion and persistance of pneumothorax likewise may be due to the presence of adhesions, a broad communication between the pleura and peripheral pulmonary airspaces, or a preexisting pulmonary abnormality resulting in a bronchopleural fistula.

Pleural Effusion

According to the hydrostatic pressure levels in the pulmonary and the systemic circulation, pleural fluid is normally produced by the parietal pleura and measures less than 5 ml. Any additional fluid collection is called effusion. By composition, four major types of pleural effusion are distinguished:

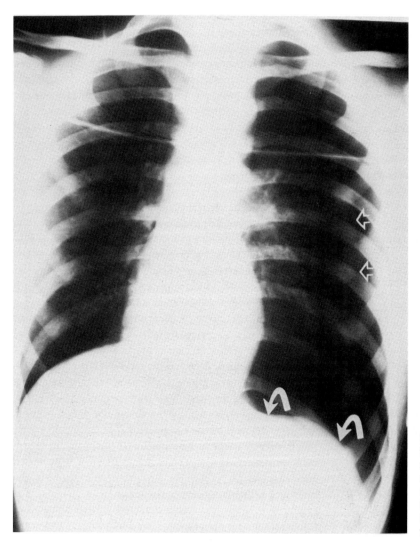

Figure 37.1. Tension pneumothorax. After several unsuccessful trials for left subclavian vein puncture, this young male developed respiratory problems. In the supine position, the presence of tension pneumothorax is strongly suggested by the diaphragmatic depression caused by subpulmonic air (*curved arrows*) and by the marked contralateral shift of the mediastinum. There is air between the visceral pleura (*open arrows*) and the lateral chest wall as well.

Transudates have a low protein content (of less than 20 g/l⁻¹) and are due to either elevated hydrostatic or lowered oncotic pressure. They are mostly seen in association with cardiac or renal failure, constrictive pericarditis, superior vena cava obstruction, or hypoproteinemia (e.g., liver cirrhosis); in other words, the normal pleura itself is involved secondarily by disease in this type of effusion.

Exudates have a high protein content (of more than 20 g l⁻¹) and usually result from direct involvement of the pleura by disease, such as empyema (Fig. 37.2), tuberculosis, and other inflammatory disorders (e.g., pancreatitis), or neoplasms.

Bloody pleural effusion is called hemothorax and is caused by trauma, surgery, anticoagulation, rupture of aortic aneurysms, thromboembolism, or neoplasms.

Chylothorax, i.e., chylous pleural effusion, has the lowest prevalence among all types of effusion. It may be encountered after thoracic trauma, surgery, in infections, neoplasms (e.g., lymphoma or bronchogenic carcinoma),

or lymphatic pathology (lymphangiomyomatosis). High thoracic obstruction or lesions of the thoracic duct tend to produce left-sided chylothorax; low obstruction usually results in right-sided chylothorax.

Since free pleural effusion distributes mainly according to hydrostatic pressure and surface tension, in the erect position it will prefer the subpulmonary diaphragmatic compartment and/or the posterior and lateral costophrenic angles of the pleural cavity before involving the costal compartment and the interlobar fissures (20).

Radiography, usually the first diagnostic tool, will often detect, but is unable to differentiate, the different types of pleural effusion, even under the best imaging conditions. Up to 250 ml may remain subpulmonary and undetected on the posteroanterior radiograph; a "pseudoelevated hemidiaphragm" with an unusually lateral "dome," or a separation of the gastric gas bubble and the apparent left hemidiaphragm are important signs in this situation (21,22). Larger quantities of fluid will cause a homogeneous shadow in the costophrenic angles that has more or less

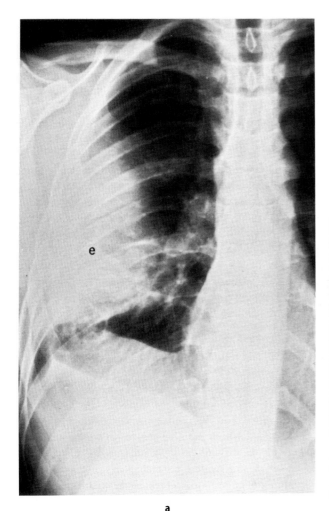

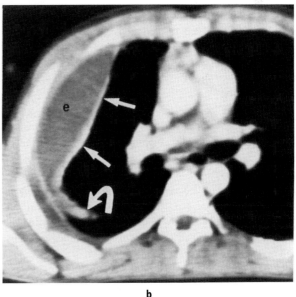

a   b

Figure 37.2. Pleural empyema. Radiographically (**a**), empyema presents as a loculated effusion (*e*) that may extend into the fissures (**b**, *curved arrow*), as better demonstrated by CT. The inflamed pleura around the hypodense collection enhances after intravenous contrast injection (*arrows*).

sharp, concave medial borders toward the lung. Recognition of pleural effusion is even more difficult on supine radiographs (23). For this reason, ultrasound is more and more used in the detection of small amounts of effusion (1,2); its superiority to the lateral decubitus radiograph with horizontal beam is based on the ease of performance and the independence of loculation and motility.

The larger the effusion, the more the pleural cavity is filled up from dependent to nondependent areas, and the more easily the corresponding opacification is detected by radiography. The increasing fluid volume first compresses the lung, then lowers the diaphragm, and finally shifts the mediastinum to the contralateral side (21,24). In contrast to pulmonary airspace disease, pleural pathology does not produce the air bronchogram sign, unless there is complete parenchymal collapse due to compression by the fluid.

Free mobility of pleural effusion is limited by the pulmonary ligament and mainly by preexisting pleural adhesions. Its distribution may therefore be atypical and pose diagnostic problems. Loculated pleural effusion, seen frequently in hemothorax and exudates, can be discovered along the chest wall and in an interlobar or retrocardiac position and may be difficult to differentiate from solid pleural lesions by conventional radiography. In acute heart failure, an interlobar localization of pleural effusion can sometimes cause the so-called phantom tumor, which according to the position of the fissure will appear biconvex on the lateral projection. Under medical treatment it will disappear more slowly than pulmonary transudation and it may recur.

Pleural empyema (Fig. 37.2) mostly appears as a loculated effusion (3,4). Enhancement of thickened adjacent pleural layers, as visualized by CT and MRI, is an important imaging sign that suggests superinfection. In contrast to a lung abscess, pleural empyema is of lentiform rather than rounded shape, with a different length of the frequent gas – fluid levels on different projections; it compresses and displaces adjacent lung parenchyma and has a thinner, more regular wall than an abscess.

CT and MRI reliably differentiate liquid from solid pleural pathology and quantify effusion; however, determination of the composition of a pleural effusion still remains a major challenge. CT, in spite of its theoretical ability to quantify protein concentration by densitometry, has failed to do so in vivo, mainly because of motion artefacts (7). MRI is able to identify hemothorax, but still faces problems related to the analysis of the protein content in vivo (8,11). Therefore, currently, in most cases one still has to aspirate pleural effusion in order to determine its content (5), and diagnostic puncture may easily be combined with image-guided drainage. When US is not successful, CT and occasionally MRI may be very helpful in guiding the aspiration needle into loculated or very small amounts of fluid and provide a nonsurgical means of treatment (1,25–27).

Benign Solid Pleural Pathology

In the subacute phase pleural effusion is organized and will often be replaced by shrinking solid tissue. Lack of fluid detected with imaging methods does not exclude the presence of active pleural disease, for instance chronic infection. Pleural thickening is very common and mostly a sequela of previous pleural disease. It includes a spectrum that goes from discrete costophrenic or cardiophrenic adhesions to severe fibrothorax, a thick, often widespread scar formation that may contain calcification and mechanically impair ventilation. Detection of pleural thickening generally poses no problem; however, flat, regular pleural adhesions and scars with concave borders must be differentiated both from active disease and from asbestos-induced pleural plaques.

Pleural plaques are the most frequent radiographic finding of asbestos exposure, and may therefore indicate persons at risk to develop more serious asbestos-induced changes (Fig. 37.3) (28). Pleural plaques are usually bilateral and mainly located in the parietal diaphragmatic and posterolateral pleura. They often calcify, and early calcifications are easily discovered by CT, which may help also in differentiating plaques from ordinary pleural thickening (3,20). Rounded atelactasis, due to invagination of the visceral pleura and concomitant curled retraction of the contiguous lung, is also a sequela of asbestos exposure (29).

Characterized by a lobulated soft tissue mass and periodic hemothorax and/or pneumothorax, pleural endometriosis is a complication of diaphragmatic defects (30). Benign pleural neoplasms are rare lesions. Pleural and subpleural lipoma has a lower density than soft tissue and partly adapts to the shape of the pleural surface. Mostly parietal, it has a smooth, regular convex contour (31). Its density on CT scans and its signal intensity on MR images are identical to subcutaneous fat and provide the diagnosis. Benign localized mesothelioma or fibroma (32,33), usually of visceral pleural origin, tends to produce a nodular, sometimes pedunculated mass lesion whose position changes with respiration. Hypertrophic osteoarthropathy may accompany this condition.

Malignant Pleural Disease

Malignant pleural disease, listed by increasing prevalence, includes primary malignant mesothelioma, direct tumor infiltration from neighboring structures, and pleural metastases, which may be present at the same time and therefore be difficult to separate. In spite of its increasing frequency during the past 20 years, malignant pleural mesothelioma remains a rare entity with poor prognosis (3,9,29,34,35). The tumor invades the whole pleural cavity, including interlobar and mediastinal portions; early on, it infiltrates the lung, chest wall, diaphragm, and medi-

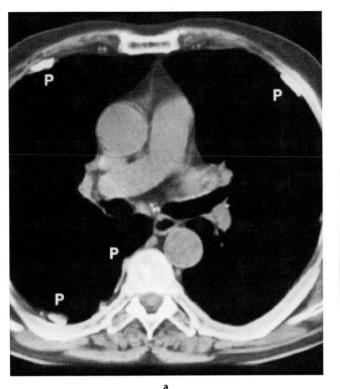

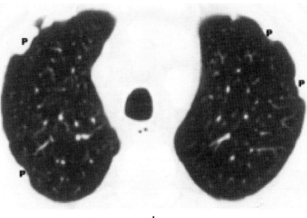

a   b

Figure 37.3. Pleural plaques due to asbestos exposure. **a** CT scan at the level of the hila: note partial calcification of the multifocal pleural areas of thickening, representing plaques (*P*). **b** The pulmonary window, at a slightly higher level, demonstrates the typical flat indentation of peripheral lung parenchyma by plaques (*P*).

astinum; and often further disseminates to involve other mesothelial cavities, such as the contralateral pleura, the peritoneum, and the pericardium (Fig. 37.4). Similar to the wide histologic variation, the radiographic presentation of malignant mesothelioma may be dominated by relapsing effusion, irregular nodular pleural masses, or diffuse pleural thickening that is often combined with a reduced volume of the hemithorax. Attempts to differentiate malignant from benign pleural disease have been made using sonography (36), CT (37), and MRI (38). Extrapleural infiltration, unless gross and obvious, can hardly be determined by radiography. While ultrasound is excellent in showing local mass lesions and, during respiration, the fixation of an infiltrating tumor to the chest wall, CT and MRI give a better overall estimation of tumor extent (34); MRI, due to its flexible scanning planes and the contrast between fat-saturated normal tissue and contrast-enhanced tumor, usually offers the best clinical staging of malignant mesothelioma (Fig. 37.4b), and it has mostly been superior to CT in recent publications for estimating invasion of the chest wall, the thoracic inlet, and the diaphragm.

The pleura is often involved with *malignancies of the neighboring structures*, above all the lung, but also the breast, thymus, and peritoneal cavity. While local infiltration of the pleura and even the chest wall by lung cancer (T3 category) (39) no longer excludes curative surgery, the presence of malignant pleural effusion (T4 category)

(36,38) usually indicates the need for palliative treatment. The nonspecificity of pleural effusion and local pleural thickening for malignant involvement reduces the staging accuracy of imaging modalities, despite their usefulness in planning the surgical approach. In breast cancer, unless clearly iatrogenic, any homolateral pleural thickening or effusion suggests malignant involvement. Malignant thymoma deserves to be mentioned because of its high propensity for pleural dissemination. The combination of uni- or bilateral convex solid pleural mass lesions and an anterior mediastinal mass may indicate the thymic origin radiographically. Peritoneal carcinomatosis, whether due to ovarian cancer, carcinoma of the colon, or cancer at another site, tends to propagate by diaphragmatic lymphatics to the superior diaphragmatic lymph nodes (40), causing lymphatic obstruction and, as a result, malignant pleural effusion.

Pleural metastases from other primary tumors and malignant lymphoma are common; they are discovered by pleural effusion and/or solid pleural mass lesions and need bioptic verification.

The Chest Wall

Conventional chest radiography is a prerequisite for any further evaluation of chest wall disorders. Some skeletal

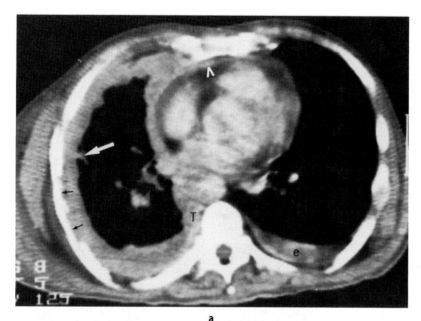

a

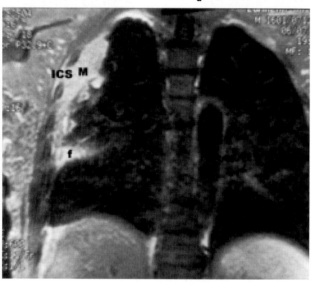

b

Figure 37.4. Malignant mesothelioma. **a** CT section showing a right-sided pleural soft tissue mass (*T*) involving the mediastinum and the interlobar surface (*white arrow*). Malignancy is suggested by osseous infiltration (*short black arrows*) and by pericardial thickening (*white arrowhead*). Contralateral dissemination, as suggested by pleural effusion (*e*), arises mainly from posterior mediastinal propagation. **b** In another patient, coronal gadolinium-enhanced MRI demonstrates infiltration of mesothelioma (*M*) through the intercostal space (*ICS*) into the chest wall. There is interlobar fissure involvement as well (*f*).

lesions, such as displaced rib fractures, are easily discovered on radiographs or on oblique rib views. Other pathologic changes, such as localized bone destruction, will be better demonstrated with low kilovoltage projections or CT. Skeletal infections and neoplasms mostly require the performance of isotope studies and the use of modern investigative techniques, such as ultrasound, CT, and MRI. Bone scintigraphy, a sensitive detector of increased bone metabolism, easily evaluates the activity and distribution of osseous lesions. When there is no acoustic barrier between the skin and the lesion, ultrasound represents an inexpensive and often satisfactory approach to a circumscribed area, offering, for instance, important details on shoulder anatomy, especially the rotator cuff, on fluid col-

lections and even the respiratory mobility between the parietal and the visceral pleura, thus ruling out chest wall involvement in case of intrathoracic infections or neoplasms (41). The need to control a larger field of view will call for the use of the other two techniques, CT and MRI, which permit superior visualization of the various anatomic structures and pathologic changes. Technical refinements, such as motion suppression, scanning during apnea and the use of surface coils, together with a superior soft tissue contrast, enable MRI to compete with and often to excel CT in this area. However, CT still offers better bony structural details and a rapid simultaneous evaluation of all compartments of the chest (42), a significant advantage in emergency situations.

Thoracic Inlet, Shoulder Girdle, and Axilla

The most superior portion of the chest wall includes the musculoskeletal connection between the body trunk and the superior extremity (the clavicles, scapulae, scapulo-humeral joints with their muscles and tendons, and loose tissue in between them) and the vertebral column, sternum, and rib cage. In fact, the thoracic inlet is a transitional zone from the mediastinum to the neck and the axillae, rather than a real anatomic area (43). Its narrow space forces any space-occupying lesion to threaten the crossing important functional connections, such as arteries, veins, nerves, the trachea, and the esophagus (Fig. 37.5) (44). More laterally, the brachial plexus and the subclavian vessels run to the axillae, which contain important groups of lymph nodes. Congenital anomalies include isolated rib modeling variations and cervical ribs, which may cause thoracic outlet syndrome (43,44), and also defective or absent clavicles as part of generalized syndromes, such a cleidocranial dysostosis.

During birth or later in life, trauma may cause bony fractures or dislocations, endangering the nearby vessels and nerves. Radiographic soft tissue signs of thoracic injury, such as the apical cap, are often nonspecific. The performance of US, CT, or MR scanning may be necessary to detect hematomas and to visualize lacerated vessels or nerves.

Degenerative disease is another cause of thoracic outlet syndrome, in which conventional, CT or MR angiographic studies may need to be performed to show vascular impingement (44). Ectatic vessels can cause pulsating pseudotumors of the thoracic inlet (43), and vascular obstruction may result in the formation of collaterals. In chronic painful syndromes of the shoulder, soft tissue calcifications are detected on plain radiographs, while high resolution ultrasound noninvasively demonstrates the rotator cuff and is likely to overtake some of the indications for arthrography in the study of the joint capsule (41,45). CT arthrography for chondral structures and, increasingly, MRI are used in the study of the humeroscapular joint.

Infectious osteomyelitis or arthritis may involve any of the joints. Sternoclavicular arthritis must be differentiated from sternocostoclavicular hyperostosis, a rare condition of unknown origin that features a more generalized inflammation (Fig. 37.6).

Benign neoplasms of the thoracic inlet include diffuse or nodular goiters, which are evaluated by ultrasound or isotope scanning and, when they extend into the thorax, by CT or MRI (43). Less frequently, neurogenic tumors can be found, mostly associated with neurofibromatosis; also, parathyroid adenomas, tracheal papillomas, and, in children, cervicothoracic lymphangiohemangiomas (46) are seen. Aside from lipomas, benign tumors of the shoulder girdle include osteochondromas (47), mesenchymomas, and aneurysmal bone cysts (46,48).

Primary malignant lesions are much less common in the upper thorax than secondary tumors. Thyroid, esophageal, and tracheal carcinoma may arise within the thoracic inlet. More laterally, soft tissue sarcomas and bone tumors of the clavicle and the scapula are found, in particular Ewing sarcoma, multiple myeloma, osteosarcoma, chondrosarcoma, fibrosarcoma, malignant fibrous histiocytoma, and malignant lymphoma (46–50).

Hematogenous metastases spread mainly to the red marrow of the clavicle and the scapula. Malignant lymphadenopathy of the thoracic inlet, the supraclavicular, or axillary station is due mainly to malignant lymphoma (49–51), metastatic breast (52) or lung cancer, but may also be caused by infradiaphragmatic primaries with lymphatic drainage to the thoracic duct (e.g., testicular or ovarian tumors), by primaries in the upper extremity or the head and neck area. Pancoast syndrome includes a superior sulcus tumor with the involvement of the sympathetic trunk (Horner syndrome), the subclavian vessels, and the brachial plexus (ulnar pain, waisting of small hand muscles). CT and MRI are diagnostic modalities for the demonstration of the typical pathologic changes related to this condition, with clear advantages for MRI thanks to the excellent demonstration of the brachial plexus in the sagittal and coronal planes (44,53).

The Sternum and its Neighborhood

While the anterior and posterior contours of the sternum are well displayed on lateral chest radiographs, the lateral contours and the sternocostal articulations are hard to identify on posteroanterior or oblique chest radiographs and may require the use of CT (54). Among sternal deformities, *funnel chest* (pectus excavatum), either alone or in combination with cardiac or musculoskeletal anomalies, is the most common. In this condition, the xiphoid process with the lower part of the anterior chest wall is depressed toward the spinal column. This compresses the heart and rotates it to the left; it may simulate cardiomegaly or right middle lobe disease. Rarely, functional disturbances may occur and be associated with chronic bronchitis and bronchiectasis. *Pigeon chest* (chicken chest, pectus carinatum), a *midline foramen* (55), or a *bifid sternum* with partial or complete lack of fusion are more rare sternal anomalies.

Unilateral painful enlargement of one or more costosternal cartilaginous junctions, mostly of the second to fourth ribs, is called Tietze syndrome. It may include redness and swelling of the area and be confused with other, more serious causes of chest pain. Conventional radiography and eventually CT may be needed in order to exclude other pathologic changes; they may occasionally demonstrate an enlargement of the costal bridge.

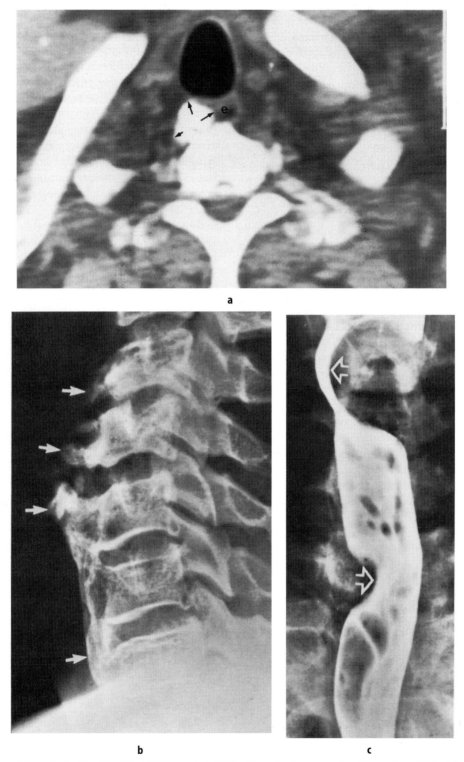

Figure 37.5. Esophageal pseudotumor due to diffuse idiopathic skeletal hyperostosis (DISH). **a** CT scan showing compression of the esophagus (*e*) due to hyperostosis near the thoracic inlet (*small arrows*). **b** Lateral radiograph showing cervical hyperostosis (*arrows*). **c** Compression and lateral displacement of the esophagus by hyperostotic cervical vertebrae (*arrows*).

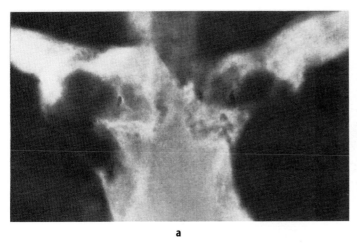
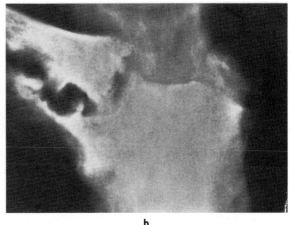

a

b

Figure 37.6. Sternocostoclavicular hyperostosis versus osteomyelitis. **a** Sternocostoclavicular hyperostosis is often bilateral and typically involves both the sternoclavicular joint and the anterior ends of the uppermost ribs, causing intensive sclerosis, enlargement, and destruction. **b** Sternoclavicular osteomyelitis, whether rheumatoid or infectious, is unilaterally limited to these two bones and centered around the joint. Destruction and sclerosis are seen as well.

Traumatic changes at the level of the costal cartilages do not necessarily give radiographic signs; even sternal fractures are difficult to image with conventional radiography. At the level of tenderness, a lateral projection will usually discover a retro- and presternal hematoma in these cases and, less consistently, a thin fracture line. A bony fragment may rarely injure the pericardium and even cause cardiac tamponade.

Because of a better patency rate when compared with venous bypasses, internal mammary arteries are routinely employed for coronary bypass surgery. Postoperative retro- and parasternal hematomas occur, but fortunately are seldom of sufficient hemodynamic importance to require reintervention.

Inflammatory pathology of the sternum and the parasternal area includes manubriosternal rheumatoid arthritis, osteomyelitis, and mainly postoperative infections of the bone and parasternal soft tissues after sternotomy. Heroin addicts are at high risk for developing septic arthritis of the sternochondral and sternoclavicular joints. Fluid collections and the extent of soft tissue and bony lesions are best demonstrated by MRI or CT, and direct connections of chronic fistulae by contrast injection into the sinus under fluoroscopic control.

Aside from chondroma, *neoplasms* of the sternum and sternocostal junctions are mostly malignant (47,48,56). Large lobulated masses with bone destruction and scattered calcifications are typical for chondrosarcoma. Exact location and extension are preoperatively evaluated with CT and MRI in the above and other malignant lesions, such as lymphoma, multiple myeloma, and bony metastases. Radiation-induced neoplasms (e.g., fibrosarcoma) may be detected many years after radiotherapy for Hodgkin disease (56). Extraosseous neoplasms arise from the skin, subcutaneous, and parasternal soft tissues.

Parasternally, the most important finding to discover is *internal mammary adenopathy*, as seen in malignant lymphoma (49–51) and in metastases of breast cancer (57). Three to five of these lymph nodes are located bilaterally within 3 cm of the sternal edge, mainly in the first three intercostal spaces. They drain the lymph from the medial quadrants and central portion of the breast and from the superior diaphragmatic lymph nodes. Enlargement due to malignant involvement pushes the adjacent anterior parietal pleura posteriorly, causing a convex bulge toward the lung on the lateral chest radiograph.

The Lateral Chest Wall

The breast *gland* is the single most important organ in the anterolateral part of the chest wall that is supported by bony ribs and is not in contact with the vertebral column. In both sexes, physiologically asymmetric breast and nipple shadows may give rise to diagnostic pitfalls, as do supernumerary breast glands and nipples or the congenital absence of the pectoralis major muscle. In general, mammography and ultrasonography complement the clinical examination and are increasingly important screening methods for breast diseases, especially cancer (58). Other imaging modalities, such as CT and MRI (57), have shown their value mainly in the assessment of extramammary extent of the disease (Fig. 37.7) and of multifocal malignancy.

The wide spectrum of isolated or combined *rib abnormalities* comprises hypoplastic, splayed, bifid, and fused variants. In cases of asymmetry, nomenclature is simplified by the constant landmark of the second rib inserting into the sternomanubrial junction. Bone marrow disorders (e.g., thalassemia) and primary skeletal

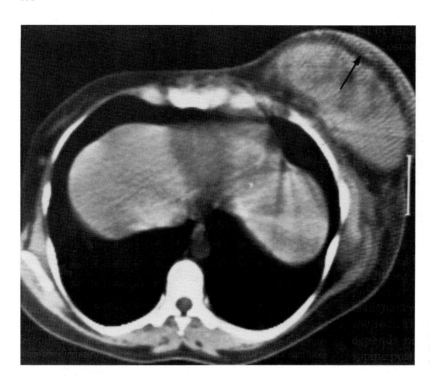

Figure 37.7. Non-Hodgkin lymphoma of the breast gland. CT scan demonstrating a voluminous mass of the left breast gland with skin (*arrow*) and subcutaneous infiltration in a 35 year old woman.

disorders (e.g., achondroplasia or osteogenesis imperfecta) diffusely distort both the shape and the structure of ribs. Inferior *rib notching* may be arterial in cases of aortic obstruction, subclavian artery obstruction, or pulmonary oligemia; venous in cases of chronic superior vena cava obstruction; arteriovenous in pulmonary and chest wall malformations; or neural in neurofibromatosis. Superior marginal rib defects are less common and have a different spectrum of mostly acquired etiologies.

Trauma to the chest wall is often combined with deeper, more serious lesions of the pleura, lungs, and mediastinum. Chest wall emphysema is easily detected by the typical configuration of air collections paralleling muscle fibers and surpassing the outer borders of the bony rib cage on chest radiographs.

Rib fractures are detected on conventional chest radiographs by systematically searching for tiny angulations, cortical discontinuities, or displacement. Fractures of the first two ribs are uncommon and prove a severe trauma with elevated risk of intrathoracic damage. Serial fractures, especially when double, may result in a "flail chest," with chest wall instability, paradoxical movement, and respiratory failure. Aside from trauma, osteomalacia, osteoporosis, cough, alcohol abuse, and multicentric neoplasms (e.g., metastases or multiple myeloma) are specific causes of multiple widespread rib fractures.

Iatrogenic changes include postoperative rib defects and regeneration, osteonecrosis, and multiple pseudarthrosis after chest wall irradiation for breast cancer. Unilateral radical mastectomy is detected by a unilateral trans-

lucency of the pulmonary field and a medially rising straight anterior axillary fold. Reductive or reconstructive surgery and breast implants are sometimes responsible for diagnostic problems that can be solved by an adequate patient history.

Infections of the chest wall are either local, originating in skin lesions and wounds, rarely hematogenous, or propagated from the pleura (59), as typically seen with pleuropulmonary actinomycosis (60,61). Fluid collections can be aspirated and drained using ultrasound or CT. MRI is indicated for planning surgery in complex multicompartmental infections.

Primary chest wall tumors, beside those arising from the breast gland, include benign lesions, such as transmural lipoma (31), desmoid tumor, hemangioma or neurofibroma, and malignant ones, such as lipo- and fibrosarcoma (46,48,62). When growing externally, they are surrounded by air and well demarcated, or have one sharp edge and one that fades off. When growing internally, they indent the pleura, causing the typical local bulge of extrapulmonary disease. Hematogenic metastases, scar implantation, or infiltration from the neighboring structures in case of lung cancer, malignant mesothelioma (34,35,37), and lymphoma (49–51) are responsible for *secondary chest wall tumors*.

Enchondroma and osteochondroma (47) along the chostochondral junctions and, more posteriorly, fibrous dysplasia, eosinophilic granuloma, and aneurysmatic bone cyst form the group of benign rib tumors. Their malignant counterparts, chondrosarcoma, lymphoma, osteosarcoma,

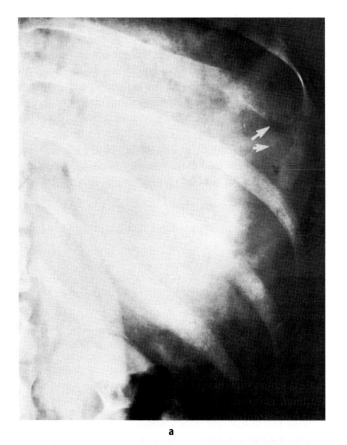

a

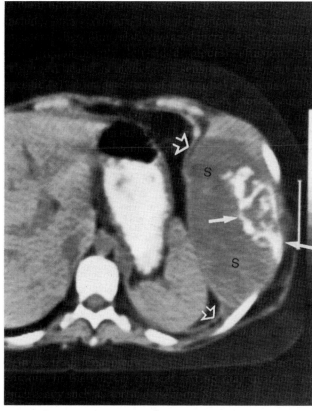

b

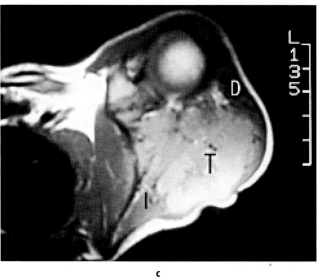

c

Figure 37.8. Ewing sarcoma of the chest wall. **a** Destruction of the left eighth rib and tiny matrix calcifications (*arrows*), detected on plain radiograph. **b** CT scan reveals a huge soft tissue tumor (*S*), located in the chest wall and displacing the diaphragm (*open arrows*) medially. Extensive intratumoral calcifications (*white arrows*). **c** In another patient, a girl of 9 years of age studied by MRI, Ewing sarcoma of the left scapula not only destroys cortical bone but also infiltrates into adjacent soft tissue (*T*), mainly the infraspinatus muscle (*I*), displacing the deltoid muscle (*D*).

and round cell tumors (Fig. 37.8), are seen less frequently than metastases and multiple myeloma (46,48,62). MRI is going to replace CT as the diagnostic modality of choice for the above lesions (Fig. 37.8b), facilitating the recognition of the primary mass and also of associated bone marrow infiltration. In cases in which tumoral presence is not signalled by rib destruction or intercostal penetration, diagnosis may still remain difficult (39,63).

The Spine and the Paraspinal Chest Wall

Kyphoscoliosis with *vertebral defects*, such as hemivertebrae, is the most common congenital anomaly of this area. As in acquired paralytic or idiopathic forms, severe congenital kyphoscoliosis may cause pulmonary arterial hypertension. Spinal dysraphism and diastematomyelia are other abnormalities of the spine.

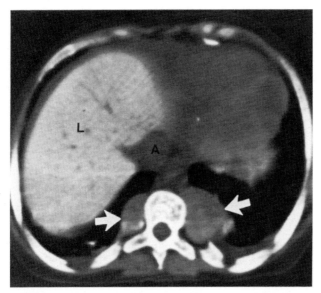

Figure 37.9. Extramedullary hematopoiesis. This young woman with thalassemia major was sent for CT in search of a neurogenic tumor suspected from the chest radiograph. The paravertebral convex extrapulmonary lesions of extramedullary hematopoiesis (*arrows*) are reminiscent of posterior mediastinal lymph node enlargement: CT also shows the elevated density of the liver (*L*), caused by secondary hemochromatosis, anemic hypodensity of the blood (*A*), osseous involvement, and some pleural effusion and ascites.

Extramedullary hematopoiesis is typically located in the thoracic paravertebral area and detected by symmetric extrapulmonary rounded soft tissue masses similar to lymph node enlargement (64) (Fig. 37.9); in epidural location, it may cause spinal cord compression.

In contrast to preexisting *vertebral compression*, acute fracture of a vertebral body is generally accompanied by a localized paravertebral hematoma that displaces pleural reflection lines and may be recognized on portable chest radiographs. The exact extent of the fracture (i.e. the involvement of the dorsal wall of the vertebral body, the dural sac, and spinal canal dimensions) is best evaluated by CT or MRI (65).

Among *inflammatory disorders*, nonspecific bacterial and tuberculous spondylitis remain common. They typically involve an intervertebral disc and destroy adjacent vertebral end-plates. CT scanning can accurately display bone morphology and extravertebral components, and guide aspiration if necessary (66). Paravertebral lymph node enlargement secondary to sarcoidosis can occasionally be seen (67).

Benign neoplasms of the paravertebral soft tissues are mainly neurogenic tumors or meningiomas, with neurofibromatosis being responsible for the majority of multiple lesions (68). Benign tumors of the thoracic vertebrae include hemangiomas, osteoblastomas, osteoid osteomas, aneurysmal bone cysts, and lipomas. Paravertebral neurofibromatosis can degenerate and become malignant, but this area is more often involved by *secondary deposits* from the spine, pleura, or lung or by metastases of malignant lymphoma and retroperitoneal tumors.

Malignant primary tumors of the thoracic spine include Ewing sarcoma, osteosarcoma, chondrosarcoma, and plasmocytoma, whereas metastatic deposits, more common in the dorsal spine, arise mainly from tumors of the breast, lung, prostate, kidney, rectum, and thyroid. MRI is increasingly employed in the study of benign and malignant neoplasms of the thoracic spine (69), demonstrating its ability to clearly identify pathologic lesions and visualize neurovascular, medullary, joint, and soft tissue involvement.

References

1. Kohan JM, Poe RH, Israel RH, et al. (1986) Value of chest ultrasonography versus decubitus roentgenography for thoracentesis. Am Rev Respir Dis 133:1124–1126.
2. Wernecke K (1997) Sonographic features of pleural disease. AJR 168:1061–1066.
3. Kuhlman JE, Singha NK (1997) Complex disease of the pleural space: Radiographic and CT evaluation. Radiographics 17:63–79.
4. Kuhlman JE (1997) Complex disease of the pleural space: 10 questions most frequently asked of the radiologist – new approaches to their answers with CT and MR imaging. Radiographics 17:1043–1050.
5. Patel MC, Flower CDR (1997) Radiology in the management of pleural disease. Eur Radiol 7:1454–1462.
6. Halvorsen RA, Jr, Fedyshin PJ, Korobkin M, et al. (1986) CT differentiation of pleural effusion from ascites: Evaluation of four signs using blinded analysis of 52 cases. Invest Radiol 21:391–395.
7. Vock P, Effmann EL, Hedlund LW, et al. (1984) Analysis of the density of pleural fluid analogs by computed tomography. Invest Radiol 19:10–15.
8. Frola C, Cantoni S, Turtulici I, et al. (1997) Transudative vs. exudative pleural effusions: Differentiation using Gd-DTPA-enhanced MRI. Eur Radiol 7:860–864.
9. Miller BH, Rosado-de-Christenson ML, Mason AC, et al. (1996) From the archives of the AFIP: Malignant pleural mesothelioma: Radiologic–pathologic correlation. Radiographics 16:613–644.
10. Falaschi F, Battolla L, Mascalchi M, et al. (1996) Usefulness of MR signal intensity in distinguishing benign from malignant pleural disease. AJR 166:963–968.
11. Brown JJ, van Sonnenberg E, Gerber KH, et al. (1985) Magnetic resonance relaxation times of percutaneously obtained normal and abnormal body fluids. Radiology 154:727–731.
12. Slasky BS, Siewers RD, Lecky JW, et al. (1982) Catamenial pneumothorax: The roles of diaphragmatic defects and endometriosis. AJR 138:639–643.
13. Tocino IM, Miller MH, Fairfax WR (1985) Distribution of pneumothorax in the supine and semirecumbent critically ill adult. AJR 144:901–905.
14. Choi BG, Park SH, Yun EH, et al. (1998) Pneumothorax size: Correlation of supine anteroposterior with erect posteroanterior chest radiographs. Radiology 209:567–569.
15. Seow A, Kazerooni EA, Cascade PN, et al. (1996) Comparison of upright inspiratory and expiratory chest radiographs for detecting pneumothoraces. AJR 166:313–316.
16. Schramel FM, Golding RP, Haakman CD, et al. (1996) Expiratory chest radiographs do not improve visibility of small apical pneumothoraces by enhanced contrast. Eur Respir J 9:406–409.

17. Wolfman NT, Myers WS, Glauser SJ, et al. (1998) Validity of CT classification on management of occult pneumothorax: Prospective study. AJR 171:317–320.

18. Gobien RP, Reines HD, Schabel SI (1982) Localized tension pneumothorax: Unrecognized form of barotrauma in adult respiratory distress syndrome. Radiology 142:15–19.

19. Visweswaran A, Harris JH, Jr (1996) Identification of tension hemopneumothorax on supine chest radiograph: Value of the visceral pleural line sign. Emerg Radiol 3:158.

20. Raasch BN, Carsky EW, Lane DJ, et al. (1982) Pictorial essay. Pleural effusion: Explanation of some typical appearances. AJR 139:899–904.

21. Blackmore CC, Black WC, Dallas RV, et al. (1996) Pleural fluid volume estimation: Chest radiograph prediction rule. Acad Radiol 3:103–109.

22. Rudikoff JC (1981) The pulmonary ligament and subpulmonic effusion. Chest 80:505–507.

23. Emamian SA, Kaasbol MA, Olsen JF, et al. (1997) Accuracy of the diagnosis of pleural effusion on supine chest X-ray. Eur Radiol 7:57–60.

24. Ruskin JA, Gurney JW, Thorsen MK, et al. (1987) Detection of pleural effusions on supine chest radiographs. AJR 148:681–683.

25. Patz EF, Jr, Goodman PC, Erasmus JJ (1998) Percutaneous drainage of pleural collections. J Thorac Imaging 13:83–92.

26. Park CS, Chung WM, Lim MK, et al. (1996) Transcatheter instillation of urokinase into loculated pleural effusion: Analysis of treatment effect. AJR 167:649–52.

27. van Sonnenberg E, Wittich GR, Goodacre BW, et al. (1998) Percutaneous drainage of thoracic collections. J Thorac Imaging 13:74–82.

28. Wain SL, Roggli VL, Foster WL, Jr, (1984) Parietal pleural plaques, asbestos bodies and neoplasia, a clinical pathological, and roentgenographic correlation of 24 consecutive cases. Chest 86:707–713.

29. Munden RF, Libshitz HI (1998) Rounded atelectasis and mesothelioma. AJR 170:1519–1522.

30. Im J-G, Kang HS, Choi BI, et al. (1987) Pleural endometriosis: CT and sonographic findings. AJR 148:523–524.

31. Labuski MR, Hopper KD (1993) Transmural thoracic lipoma: CT and MR features. Magn Reson Imaging 11:593–594.

32. Ferretti GR, Chiles C, Choplin RH, et al. (1997) Localized benign fibrous tumors of the pleura. AJR 169:683–686.

33. Ferretti GR, Chiles C, Cox JE, et al. (1997) Localized benign fibrous tumors of the pleura: MR appearance. J Comput Assist Tomogr 21:115–120.

34. Knuuttila A, Halme M, Kivisaari L, et al. (1998) The clinical importance of magnetic resonance imaging versus computed tomography in malignant pleural mesothelioma. Lung Cancer 22:215–225.

35. Patz EF, Jr, Rusch VW, Heelan RT (1996) The proposed new international TNM staging sysem for malignant pleural mesothelioma: Application to imaging. AJR 166:323–327.

36. Görg C, Restrepo I, Schwerk WB (1997) Sonography of malignant pleural effusion. Eur Radiol 7:1195–1198.

37. Leung AN, Müller NL, Miller RR (1990) CT in differential diagnosis of diffuse pleural disease. AJR 154:487–492.

38. Bittner RC, Schnoy N, Schonfeld N, et al. (1995) High resolution magnetic resonance tomography of the pleura and thoracic wall: normal findings and pathological changes. RoFo Fortschr Geb Rontgent Neuren Bildgeb Verfahr 162:296–303.

39. Sakai S, Murayama S, Murakami J, et al. (1997) Bronchogenic Carcinoma invasion of the chest wall: Evaluation with dynamic cine MRI during breathing. J Comput Assist Tomogr 21:595–600.

40. Vock P, Hodler J (1986) Cardiophrenic angle adenopathy: Update of causes and significance. Radiology 159:395–399.

41. Mathis G (1997) Thorax sonography – part I: Chest wall and pleura. Ultrasound Med Biol 23:1131–1139.

42. Padhani AR (1998) Spiral CT: Thoracic applications. Eur J Radiol 28:2–17.

43. Vock P, Owens A (1982) Computed tomography of the normal and pathological thoracic inlet. Eur J Radiol 2:187–193.

44. Rémy-Jardin M, Doyen J, Rémy J, et al. (1997) Functional anatomy of the thoracic outlet: Evaluation with spiral CT. Radiology 205:843–851.

45. Takagishi K, Makino K, Takahira N, et al. (1996) Ultrasonography for diagnosis of rotator cuff tear. Skeletal Radiol 25:221–224.

46. Meyer JS, Nicotra JJ (1998) Tumors of the pediatric chest. Semin Roentgenol 33:187–198.

47. Meyer CA, White CS (1998) Cartilaginous disorders of the chest. Radiographics 18:1109–1123.

48. Omell GH, Anderson LS, Bramson RT (1973) Chest wall tumors. Radiol Clin North Am 11:197–214.

49. Press GA, Glazer HS, Wassermann TH, et al. (1985) Thoracic wall involvement by Hodgkin disease and non-Hodgkin lymphoma: CT evaluation. Radiology 157:195–198.

50. Bonomo L, Ciccotosto C, Guidotti A, et al. (1997) Staging of thoracic lymphoma by radiological imaging. Eur Radiol 7:1179–1189.

51. Castellino RA, Hilton S, O'Brien JP, et al. (1996) Non-Hodgkin lymphoma: Contribution of chest CT in the initial staging evaluation. Radiology 199:129–132.

52. Mussurakis S, Buckley DL, Horsman A (1997) Prediction of axillary lymph node status in invasive breast cancer with dynamic contrast-enhanced MR imaging. Radiology 203:317–321.

53. Reede DL (1997) MR imaging of the brachial plexus. MRI Clin North Am 5:897.

54. Hatfield MK, Gross BH, Glazer GM, et al. (1984) Computed tomography of the sternum and its articulations. Skeletal Radiol 11:197–203

55. Stark P (1985) Midline sternal foramen: CT demonstration. J Comput Assist Tomogr 9:489–490.

56. Souba WW, McKenna RJ, Jr, Meis J, et al. (1986) Radiation-induced sarcomas of the chest wall. Cancer 57:610–615.

57. Orel SG (1998) High-resolution MR imaging for the detection, diagnosis, and staging of breast cancer. RadioGraphics 18:903–912.

58. Feig SA (1988) Decreased breast cancer mortality through mammographic screening: Results of clinical trials. Radiology 167:659–665.

59. Waite RJ, Carbonneau RJ, Balikian JP, et al. (1990) Parietal pleural changes in empyema: Appearances at CT. Radiology 175:145–150.

60. Wand A, Gilbert HM, Litvack B, et al. (1996) MRI of thoracic actinomycosis. J Comput Assist Tomogr 20:770–772.

61. Cheon JE, Kim MY, Lee JS, et al. (1998) Thoracic actinomycosis: CT findings. Radiology 209:229–233.

62. Pairolero PC, Arnold PG (1985) Chest wall tumors: Experience with 100 consecutive cases. J Thorac Cardiovasc Surg 90:367–372.

63. Hanson JA, Armstrong P (1997) Staging intrathoracic non small-cell lung cancer. Eur Radiol 7:161–172.

64. Boyacigil S, Ardiç S, Tokoglu F, et al. (1996) Intrathoracic extramedullary haemopoiesis. Australas Radiol 40:179–181.

65. Saifuddin A, Noordeen H, Taylor BA, et al. (1996) The role of imaging in the diagnosis and management of thoracolumbar burst fractures: Current concepts and a review of the literature. Skeletal Radiol 25:603–613.

66. Dagirmanjian A, Schils J, McHenry M, et al. (1996) MR imaging of vertebral osteomyelitis revisited. AJR 167:1539–1543.

67. Miller BH, Rosado-de-Christenson ML, McAdams HP, et al. (1995) From the archives of the AFIP: Thoracic sarcoidosis: Radiologic-pathologic correlation. Radiographics 15:421–437.

68. Murphey MD, Andrews CL, Flemming DJ, et al. (1996) From the archives of the AFIP: Primary tumors of the spine: Radiologic-pathologic correlation. Radiographics 16:1131.

69. Cuénod CA, Laredo JD, Chevret S, et al. (1996) Acute vertebral collapse due to osteoporosis or malignancy: Appearance on unenhanced and gadolinium-enhanced MR images. Radiology 199:541–549.

The Intensive Care Chest

E.M. Marom and P.C. Goodman

Introduction

While portable bedside chest radiography has remained the principle thoracic imaging technique for intensive care unit (ICU) patients, other modalities have gained acceptance in the diagnostic evaluation and treatment of these critically ill individuals. Included among these techniques are bedside ultrasonography and nuclear medicine, as well as computed tomography (CT), magnetic resonance imaging (MRI) and nuclear medicine performed in the radiology department in selected situations. This chapter reviews the efficacy of currently available imaging studies and their latest developments as they apply to the identification of monitoring and therapeutic devices, as well as their value in diagnosing abnormalities of the lungs, heart, mediastinum and pleura.

Efficacy of Studies

The portable chest radiograph is the most commonly used imaging modality in the ICU. In the past, "routine morning portable chest films" were obtained to provide another measure of patient status. Lately, however, this procedure has been subjected to scrutiny as regards its cost, diagnostic capability, and value in changing patient management or outcome (1–11). Results of these studies are not conclusive, not surprisingly, since different study populations and designs were used. For instance, investigations evaluated patients in different ICU settings, the medical and/or surgical ICU; chest films were performed routinely in some studies or following change in patient status, or after line placement in others. Even fundamental interpretation of chest film utility was different. Some

authors considered negative findings of no value others found this important. For these reasons and others, there is no proven consensus as to the worth of a daily ICU chest radiograph, but some observations are worth considering.

New or unsuspected findings are found in 37–65% of ICU chest radiographs (2,10,12,13). Furthermore, Bekemeyer found that 50% of nonroutine chest radiographs and, surprisingly, 39% of routine chest radiographs directed a change in patient management (2). Other authors of course disagree. Silverstein et al. found that in surgical ICU patients, new chest film findings resulted in significant management impact in only 3.4% of individuals (4). Similarly, while one group found that improper positioning of support and monitoring devices was noted in 24–35% of ICU patients (2,14), other authors discovered that only 1.3% of patients required line repositioning (4). Some authors oppose routine chest radiographs to assess complications of central venous line insertion (these can be predicted clinically), but do recommend chest films following endotracheal tube insertion (15). Other authors found that the only independent predictor of a new chest film finding was a newly suspected clinical condition and that only placement of a pulmonary artery catheter would require a follow-up chest film (5). Improper placement of pulmonary artery catheters was more common than improper endotracheal tube positioning, ranging from 24% to 47% and 15% respectively (2,14). In general, unsuspected chest radiographic findings that lead to a management change are much more likely (57%) in patients with pulmonary or unstable heart disease than in patients with stable heart conditions or other miscellaneous diseases (3%) (1).

In conclusion, the practice of obtaining "routine AM chest films" for every ICU patient should be abandoned.

This chapter is dedicated to Charles E. Putman, an extraordinary chest radiologist, compassionate internist, teacher, scientist, and friend, who to our great sorrow passed away before this project was completed.

Instead, chest films should be reserved for those with clinical indication, intubated patients with pulmonary or cardiac disease, and in most cases should be delayed until after support apparatus, especially pulmonary artery catheters and endotracheal tubes, are inserted.

One of the major problems with portable chest radiography in the ICU is film-to-film variation. This creates difficulty in interpretation and thus affects patients' management. Also, poor-quality films secondary to increased scatter radiation, low kilovoltage, inconsistent film density, wide latitude requirements, and difficulties in positioning require repeat exposures leading to an increase in radiation dose to the patient. In the last several years, new techniques in portable film acquisition and display have been developed. Computed radiography (CR) has gained wide acceptance in hospitals as the preferred method of imaging the ICU patient. CR delivers high quality, consistent images when compared with conventional portable technique and offers post-processing flexibility (16–20). Using teleradiology, CR has the capability of being reviewed simultaneously or at convenient times by the treating clinician in the ICU and the radiologist in the radiology department or at a remote site. This latter characteristic facilitates more timely initiation of clinical action due to prompt image display (21) and permits subspecialty expert interpretations after hours (22). Incidentally, ICU teleradiology displays that use CR, rather than film digitizers, offer improved image quality and superior operational efficiency (23). While the diagnostic usefulness of CR is comparable to conventional films in the intensive care unit (23), there are further advantages to CR. CR provides greater edge enhancement, which facilitates detection of indwelling catheter tips and pneumothoraces; CR produces images with consistent lung density enabling recognition of more subtle pulmonary opacity changes from day to day; CR requires fewer repeat examinations (24); and with CR there is higher interobserver agreement for radiologic descriptors (25).

Imaging methods other than bedside portable chest radiography may be indicated in special circumstances or for certain diagnoses. However, if the procedure requires moving the patient from the ICU, then particular consideration regarding the risk of the procedure, the potential benefit to be gained from the diagnosis, and the risk of patient transport must be kept in mind. Transport complication rates ranging from 5.9% to 84% have been reported (26–31). Studies with low diagnostic yields or that will not significantly alter management should not be performed.

For ICU patients with chest disease, CT is the single most effective imaging technique after the bedside radiograph. CT is particularly valuable for detecting pleural disease, mediastinal abnormalities, and in differentiating

pleural from parenchymal processes. In 70–75% of patients, CT provides new information regarding the nature or severity of disease that may alter the diagnosis or treatment (32,33). The majority of significant diagnoses detected by CT involve the mediastinum or pleura. However, the introduction of spiral chest CT has led to protocols for detecting pulmonary emboli that are increasingly replacing ventilation – perfusion radionuclide studies for this purpose. In the therapeutic realm, CT is frequently used as the imaging modality for guidance during thoracocentesis of pleural fluid (95% success rate), or for thoracostomy drainage of empyema (81–88% success rate) (34–36). "Blind" insertion of chest tubes has a success rate of only 47% (34).

MRI for the ICU patient is challenging. Aside from transporting the patient to the scanner and the time spent in the scanner away from the ICU, there is a need for special nonferrous equipment in order to continue physiologic support and monitoring (37–39). Future developments may result in specific indications for the use of this technique for ICU patients but currently, MRI is not recommended.

Ultrasonography, like chest radiography, can be performed at the bedside of an ICU patient. In the chest this modality is principally used to assess pleural space, chest wall, and heart (echocardiography). Diaphragmatic movement can also be accurately assessed by ultrasound and, method can be used instead of fluoroscopy to answer questions regarding paralysis (40–47). Since lung consolidation, atelectasis and peripheral tumors replace alveolar air with tissue or fluid, they can be diagnosed by ultrasonography, but chest films are more reliable for these conditions. Nevertheless, ultrasound has been used to guide transthoracic biopsy when patients could not be transferred to CT (48–52). One study showed that ultrasound could distinguish between pulmonary edema and chronic obstructive pulmonary disease (COPD) exacerbation in ICU patients with 100% sensitivity and 92% specificity (53), however, further studies would be required to see whether this technique should replace chest radiography. Differentiating between parenchymal and pleural disease may be possible with this technique and certainly sonography is very helpful in locating peripheral pleural fluid prior to thoracocentesis.

Monitoring and Support Devices

There are various constantly evolving pulmonary and cardiovascular support devices that contribute significantly to improved management of seriously ill patients. Assessing the correct position of these devices and complications arising from their insertion and use is frequently the task of the chest radiologist (Table 38.1).

Table 38.1. Monitoring and support device position

Device	Feature	Optimal Location
Endotracheal tube	Tip	5 ± 2 cm from carina
	Cuff	$\leqslant$ width of trachea
	Tube	$\frac{1}{2}-\frac{2}{3}$ diameter of trachea
Tracheostomy tube	Cuff	$\leqslant$ width of trachea
	Tube	$\frac{1}{2}-\frac{2}{3}$ diameter of trachea
Chest tubes	Tip	Within area to be drained
	Side holes	Within pleural cavity
	Chest wall entrance site	Angulated
Central venous catheter	Tip	Origin of superior vena cava (medial right anterior intercostal space)
Pulmonary artery catheter	Tip	Right, left or interlobar pulmonary arteries
Intraaortic balloon pump	Tip	Within aorta, just distal to left subclavian artery (projecting over aortic arch or just distal to it)
	Tip shape	Rectangular, parallel to descending aorta
Transvenous pacemaker	Tip	Apex of right ventricle (midpoint between midline of thorax and apex of heart).

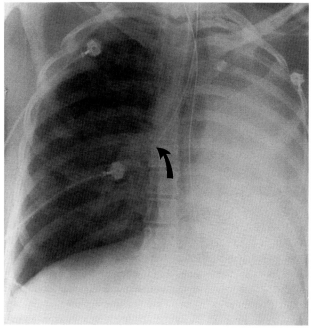

Figure 38.1. Misplaced endotracheal tube. Portable supine chest film demonstrates the tip of the endotracheal tube within the right main bronchus (*curved arrow*) 6 h after abdominal surgery. This resulted in total left lung collapse as demonstrated here with total opacification of the left hemithorax and compensatory hyperinflation of the contralateral right lung.

Endotracheal Tube

Malpositioning of endotracheal tubes occurs in 10–61.9% of patients, with resultant total lung or lobar collapse and occasionally death (9,54–59) (Fig. 38.1) Clinical evaluation fails to detect most misplaced tubes, and therefore chest radiographs are routinely obtained following intubation. Proper tube positioning is based on the relationship of the tip of the tube to the tracheal carina. Since the tip of the endotracheal tube can migrate downward by 2 cm with neck flexion and upwards by 2 cm with neck extension (60), this parameter of the patient's posture should be noted whenever possible. The endotracheal tip should be 5 ± 2 cm from the carina when the neck is in the neutral position. Monitoring this parameter will prevent inadvertent bronchial intubation when the neck is flexed and vocal cord injury or unexpected extubation when the neck is extended. When the carina cannot be identified, a frequently acceptable position for the endotracheal tip is at the level of the T2–T4 vertebral body. With the neck in the neutral position, in over 90% of patients the carina is located at the T6 ± 1 level and the vocal cords at the C5–C6 level (61). A recently described, highly accurate way to estimate the position of the carina is to use the aortic arch tangent line (62). By extending a line rightward from the inferior aspect of the aortic arch, one establishes an inferior position of the carina in 94% of patients. If the tip of an endotracheal tube is 3.4–5.0 cm above this line, proper positioning is assured in 95% of patients. For correct localization one must always check to see that the neck is in the neutral position. This is performed by observing the mandible. In the neutral position, the mandible is over C5–C6; with the neck flexed, it is at T1 or below, and with the neck extended it is above the C3–C4 interspace.

Assessment of features of endotracheal tubes other than position are also important. Ideal tube size should be one half to two thirds the diameter of the trachea. Larger tubes have less resistance to airflow, but are associated with an increased number of laryngeal injuries. Smaller tubes create increased airway resistance. Also, the seal between a small endotracheal balloon cuff and tracheal wall may be poor, allowing air to escape during ventilation. This may

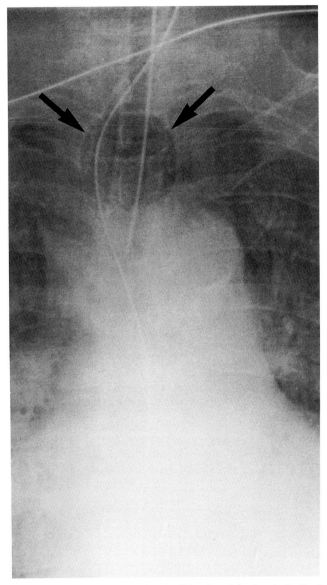

Figure 38.2. Overdistention of endotracheal cuff. Overdistended endotracheal cuff and (*arrows*) causing increase in tracheal diameter three times its normal size.

lead to hyperinflation of the cuff, which can produce pressure on the tracheal mucosa leading to ischemia, necrosis, infection, and eventually tracheomalacia or tracheal stenosis. The cuff should not cause focal distention of the trachea nor should it cause deflection of the tube towards the tracheal wall (Fig. 38.2). Owing to differences in tracheal compliance, however, the portable chest radiograph is not particularly sensitive (56%) nor specific (71%) as a screen for unsafe endotracheal tube cuff hyperinflation (63).

Tracheostomy tubes are governed by the same guidelines as endotracheal tubes. They should be one half to two thirds the diameter of the trachea, several centimeters away from the carina, and parallel to the trachea to avoid tracheal ischemia secondary to tip pressure; tracheostomy

tube cuffs should not be hyperinflated or displace the tracheal wall (Fig. 38.4). They are less influenced by neck motion as they are inserted at the level of the third tracheal cartilage.

Chest Tubes

Ideally, chest tubes should be placed in a specific location of the pleural collection being drained. Thus, for pneumothorax, the tip of the therapeutic catheter is placed cephalad and anterior, whereas, for pleural fluid, thoracostomy tubes are best positioned in the most dependent portion of the pleural space. However, even if the tube is not perfectly located, in most cases it will function adequately if placed somewhere in the collection. However, thoracostomy tubes that are inadvertently placed within the major fissure frequently malfunction (67% of the time) and, in this case, repositioning should be considered (64). In mobile patients, proper chest tube placement is assessed with posteroanterior and lateral chest films; however, lateral chest films are not commonly obtained in ICU patients. Even so, the frontal chest film may provide clues regarding the position of the tube. Correctly placed tubes usually show a focal angulation or sharp curve at their point of entry into the thoracic cavity (Fig. 38.3), whereas tubes in the major fissure lack this angled appearance as they extend instead in a straight line or a gentle curve from the point of entry (64) (Fig. 38.4). A tube placed in the minor fissure may curve gently as it passes directly medially. Finally, since the chest tube outer wall is usually sharply defined by room air, air in the pleural space or aerated lung abutting the tube, when the chest tube wall is indistinct throughtout its entire course, an extrapleural space placement might be suspected (65). These findings of tube malpositioning are unfortunately not consistent enough for accurate assessment based only on the initial frontal chest radiograph (64,66,67), and thus many cases require a lateral film or are detected on CT.

Central Venous Catheter

The tip of the central venous catheter should be central to the venous valves. This prevents interference with direct transmission of right atrial pressure to the catheter. The most proximal of these valves are found in the subclavian and internal jugular veins approximately 2 cm from their junction with their brachiocephalic veins. The origin of the brachiocephalic vein is approximately at the level of the sternoclavicular joint (68) and thus can readily be estimated on a chest radiograph. For correct central venous pressure monitoring, ideally, the tip should be placed even more centrally, at the origin of the superior vena cava,

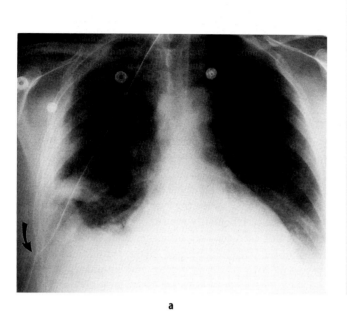

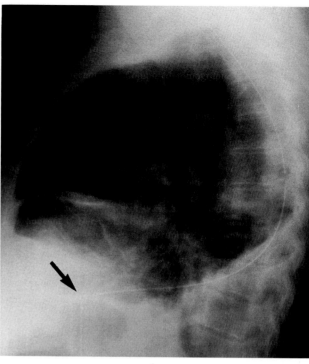

a   b

Figure 38.3. Proper chest tube placement. **a** Posteroanterior chest film demonstrates a chest tube in satisfactory position as indicated by the angulation (*curved arrow*) of the tube at the point of entry into the thoracic cavity. **b** Satisfactory position of the chest tube confirmed by lateral chest film, showing the tube to be located in the posterior pleural space, again with angulation (*arrow*) at the point of entry into the thoracic cavity.

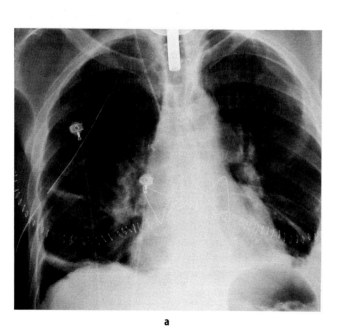

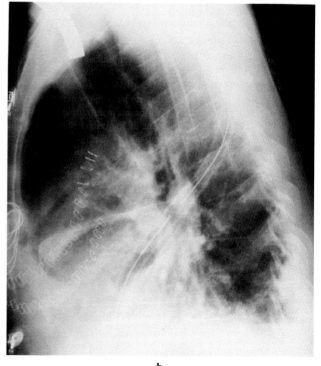

a   b

Figure 38.4. Improper chest tube placement. **a** Posteroanterior chest radiograph status after bilateral lung transplant demonstrates a right chest tube with no angulation throughout its course, signifying its location within the major fissure. Incidental note of the satisfactory position of the tracheostomy tube. **b** The intrafissural course of the chest tube is proven by the lateral chest film, which again demonstrates a smooth, nonangulated course in the expected location of the major fissure.

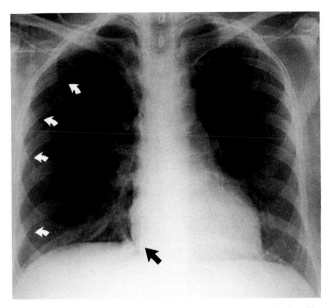

Figure 38.5. Pneumothorax due to central venous line placement. Portable chest film demonstrates central venous line in a low position, coursing through the superior vena cava, right atrium and terminating at the junction of the inferior vena cava and right atrium (*black arrow*). The line insertion was traumatic and resulted in a pneumothorax (*white curved arrows*).

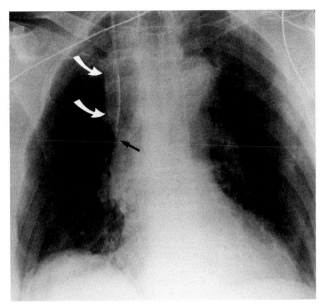

Figure 38.6. Venous perforation by central venous line. Portable chest film demonstrates central venous line at the level of the superior vena cava, as indicated by the tip position (*black arrow*) just below the first anterior intercostal space. However, the tip has a slight lateral angulation and there is right superior mediastinal widening (*white curved arrows*) secondary to acute mediastinal hemorrhage.

which, on a chest radiograph, is near the level of the medial right anterior first intercostal space. Following insertion of a central venous catheter, malposition and complications can be assessed by chest radiography. Aberrant positioning occurs in up to a 47% of cases (69,70). Pneumothorax is seen 6% of patients (71) (Fig. 38.5). Other problems include venous or cardiac perforation (72–75) presenting as a large mediastinum or enlarging pleural effusion or increasing size of the cardiac contour (74–76) (Fig. 38.6). Embolization of broken catheter fragments (77), air embolism (71), and thrombi embolization (78) have also been reported.

Pulmonary Artery Catheter

The ideal location for the tip of a pulmonary artery catheter is wherever inflation of the balloon produces a wedge pressure and deflation of the balloon permits normal flow to resume. Usually this is within the right or left pulmonary arteries or interlobar arteries (79). In theory, the catheter tip should lie at the level of the left atrium with the patient supine. If the tip were ventral to this position, there would be an underestimation of wedge pressure. In practice, the tips of most pulmonary artery catheters are at the appropriate level, only rarely entering the upper, middle (80) or lingular lobes (Fig. 38.7). Inflation of the balloon causes the catheter tip to float downstream into a wedged position, occasionally moving very little before occlusion occurs. The catheter balloon can be recognized as a 1 cm round lucency if air has been injected and the balloon has not deflated.

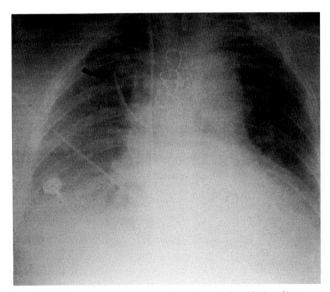

Figure 38.7. Improper pulmonary artery catheter placement. Portable chest film status after coronary artery bypass graft with pulmonary artery catheter tip located in the apical branch of the right upper lobe pulmonary artery (*black curved arrow*). Additional post cardiac surgery findings include enlarged heart and mediastinum, right pleural effusion and bibasilar subsegmental atelectasis.

Since chest films are not obtained while wedge pressures are measured, an inflated balloon seen on chest films indicates a malfunctioning catheter. If the balloon remains inflated too long, or if the tip of the catheter is so distal that it occludes a small vessel, then thrombosis in situ, or prolonged pulmonary artery obstruction, may cause pulmonary infarction (81,82). Redundancy of a pulmonary artery catheter increases the likelihood of complications, which include

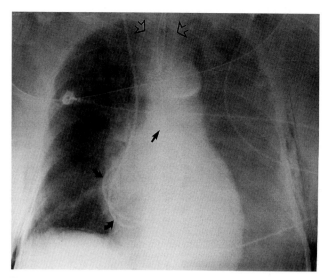

Figure 38.8. Redundant pulmonary artery catheter. Portable chest radiograph shows the pulmonary artery catheter tip to be located in satisfactory position in the right pulmonary artery (*black arrow*; however, the catheter is redundant and coils in the right atrium (*black curved arrow*). Additional findings include an overinflated endotracheal tube balloon cuff (*open black arrows*), and layering left pleural effusion.

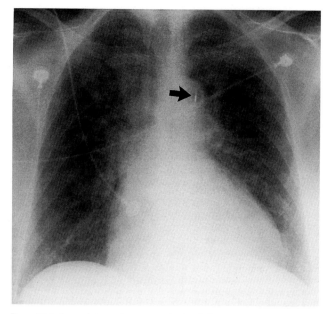

Figure 38.9. Proper intraaortic counterpulsation balloon position. Portable chest radiograph of a 76 year old woman with acute myocardial infarction shows intraaortic counterpulsation balloon tip (*arrow*) in a satisfactory position just at the level of the transverse aorta. Its rectangular shape paralleling the descending aorta confirms its appropriate position.

distal migration resulting in pulmonary infarction, cardiac arrhythmia, knotting, and pulmonary artery rupture (79,83–85) (Fig. 38.8).

Intra aortic Counterpulsation Balloon

The intraaortic counterpulsation balloon inflates during diastole and deflates during systole. The rise in proximal aortic diastolic pressure increases blood flow and thus oxygen delivery through the coronary vessels to the myocardium leading to overall improvement in cardiac function. Ideally, the tip of the catheter is in the aorta just distal to the left subclavian artery branch. This location allows maximal augmentation of the diastolic pressure in the proximal aorta and decreases the risk of obstruction of the left common carotid or left subclavian arteries. If the tip is too low, therapeutic effectiveness is reduced (86). On the chest radiograph the tip of the catheter is seen as a radiopaque rectangle, approximately 3–4 mm long, projecting over or just below the transverse aorta (86,87) (Fig. 38.9). Overadvancement of the tube into the transverse aorta can be recognized on the portable chest film, as, instead of its rectangular shape, the tip acquires a circular shape as it is imaged *en face* (87). When the elongated catheter balloon is inflated, it is seen as an intraaortic lucency on the chest radiograph.

Transvenous Pacemakers

Transvenous pacemakers are ideally placed with their tips in the apex of the right ventricle wedged beneath the cardiac trabeculae to ensure stability and intimate contact with the endocardium. However, modern pacemakers frequently have "screw in" tips, which have a greater tolerance for placement elsewhere in the right ventricle, with less fear of dislodgment. If a dual chamber pacer is used, the atrial lead should deflect upward into the right atrial appendage. For assessment of position both frontal and lateral radiographs are necessary. On the frontal view, the ventricular catheter tip should project over the right ventricular apex, which is located at about the midpoint between the midline of the thorax, and the apex of the heart (88). On the lateral view the tip of the catheter should be 3–4 mm inside the epicardial fat stripe, if this can be seen (89). The catheters should be gently curving, as sharp angulations increase the likelihood for fracture, detachment, and electrode migration. Aberrant catheter positioning into the coronary sinus and its tributaries, the right atrium, and the pulmonary artery have been reported. The majority of these are not clinically significant. Myocardial perforation is perhaps a more dire complication that can lead to pericardial tamponade and death. With the advent of advanced electronic monitoring and the development of cardiac echocardiography, pacemaker problems are less likely to be first detected on chest films, yet they remain a moderately common event. In one recent large series, 11% of patients required an invasive procedure for early or late complications (90).

Acute Pulmonary Disease

The chest radiograph of ICU patients commonly demonstrates pulmonary opacities. Sometimes the abnormalities precede hospitalization and other times the pulmonary disease is acquired in the hospital as a result of nosocomial infection, progression of disease, or complication of therapy. The nature of increased pulmonary opacities is frequently difficult to determine and a broad differential must be entertained. Aside from pneumonia, many noninfectious events are common in the ICU patient, including atelectasis, pulmonary embolus, aspiration, pulmonary edema, and adult respiratory distress syndrome. Preexisting abnormalities such as fibrosis and lung cancer also contribute to the problem of establishing a diagnosis. Nevertheless, the distribution of opacities and, more commonly, the rate of their development and resolution contribute to a correct interpretation.

Atelectasis

Atelectasis is probably the most commonly observed chest radiographic abnormality in ICU patients. Causes include mucus plugging, aspiration, postoperative splinting with reduced inspiratory effort due to pain, malpositioned endotracheal tube, pleural collection compressing the lung, and delayed diagnosis of traumatic bronchial injury. Lobar atelectasis or atelectasis of a major portion of a lobe is confidently diagnosed when signs of volume loss are associated with increased pulmonary opacity (Fig. 38.10). Radiographic signs of volume loss include fissural, medi-

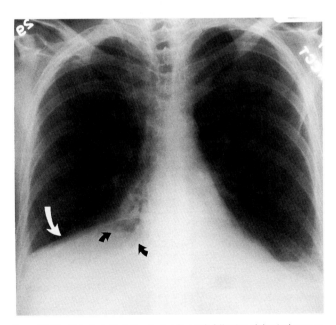

Figure 38.10. Atelectasis. Portable chest radiograph following abdominal surgery. Retrocardiac opacity and left lower lobe volume loss consistent with left lower lobe atelectasis. On the right, there is increased opacity in the right middle and lower lobe obscuring the right heart border and right hemidiaphragm. Volume loss is accompanied by a shift of the minor fissure caudad (*white curved arrow*) and crowding of the right lower lobe bronchi (*black curved arrows*). Atelectasis was due to mucus plugs and the lungs reexpanded the following day after patient mobilization. Incidental note: central venous line too deep within the right atrium.

astinal, hilar, or hemidiaphragmatic shift toward the side of increased opacity, and, to a lesser extent, decreased distance between the ribs on the side of collapse. In addition, compensatory hyperinflation of adjacent lobes or contralateral lung may be observed (Fig. 38.1). Atelectasis may be subsegmental and appear as a mild increase in basilar opacities or as linear bands of opacity, typically horizontally oriented in the basilar portions of the lungs. In some instances it is impossible to know for sure whether atelectasis or pneumonia is the cause of a radiographic abnormality. Either may have an air bronchogram, especially if atelectasis is secondary to lung compression while the major bronchi remain patent. Serial chest radiographs showing rapid clearance or resolution following bronchoscopy will prove the presence of atelectasis and not pneumonia. The absence of air bronchograms in an area of consolidation suggests major airway obstruction, possibly amenable to bronchial toilet through a bronchoscope (91).

Pneumonia

Nosocomial bacterial pneumonia in the ICU complicates the course of 7–42% of patients receiving continuous mechanical ventilation. It is extremely difficult to diagnose as the clinical features of pneumonia (e.g., fever, leukocytosis, sputum production, positive sputum cultures, and radiographic abnormalities) are absent in a significant number of patients with proven disease (92). Also, other etiologies may produce similar findings. As regards the chest radiograph in ICU patients, only 30–40% of pulmonary opacities result from pneumonia (92–94); sensitivity for predicting pneumonia is only 60–64%; and specificity is 27–29% (95). The overall diagnostic yield for pneumonia is low, 52% (96). False-negative interpretations are most likely due to the varying sensitivity (33–100%) of the portable chest radiograph in detecting lung abnormalities in different lung locations (97). False-positive interpretations may be attributed to asymmetric pulmonary edema, retained secretions, blood in the alveoli, aspiration of gastric contents, or atelectasis. Follow-up radiographs of pneumonia generally reveal gradual clearance of opacities over days or weeks, whereas edema, alveolar blood and aspirated material usually clear within 1–3 days, and atelectasis can resolve within hours (98). Pneumococcal pneumonia classically presents as a homogeneous lobar opacity with air bronchograms. Gram-negative pneumonias present typically with several scattered mixed heterogeneous–homogeneous opacities without air bronchograms. Viral pneumonias usually produce a diffuse reticular opacification occasionally with peribronchial thickening. The time of onset of infection and the immune state of the patient may help in determining the causative organism. For example, *Haemophilus influenzae* and *Streptococcus pneumoniae* pneumonias

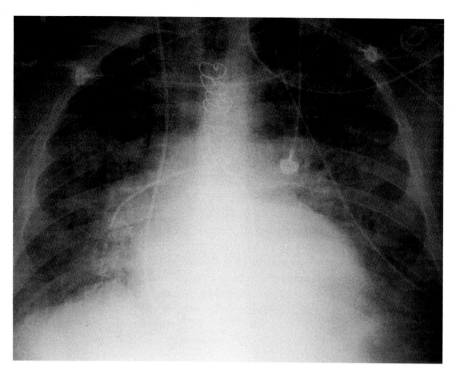

Figure 38.11. Cardiogenic pulmonary edema. Portable chest radiograph of 84 year old man with acute myocardial infarction demonstrates heart size to be the upper limit of normal or slightly enlarged. Sternotomy wires indicate prior coronary bypass grafting. Bilateral symmetric distribution of pulmonary opacities mainly in a perihilar distribution are consistent with cardiogenic pulmonary edema. Incidental note is made of left lower lobe atelectasis and satisfactory position of the pulmonary artery catheter tip in the right interlobar artery.

occur earlier in ICU hospitalizations than methicillin-resistant *Staphylococcus aureus* or Gram-negative pneumonias (94). However, these patterns can overlap. Thus radiographs, although suggestive of a type of pathogen, cannot reliably predict the etiologic agent responsible for pneumonia (99–102). From the described studies, one concludes that a chest radiograph is only a moderate predictor for pulmonary infection, but at least on a par with, if not superior to, many other traditional clinical and laboratory investigations.

Pulmonary Edema

Pulmonary edema is one of the most common problems encountered in the ICU. Patients with edema are typically monitored by placement of a pulmonary artery catheter as well as close observation of daily weight change and assessment of fluid input and output. Generally the etiology of pulmonary edema is designated as being cardiogenic or noncardiogenic, although a combination of causes may exist in the same individual and both can be exacerbated by excess fluid administration. Cardiogenic edema implies a newly discovered or chronic cardiac injury as the cause of heart failure. Discovery of electro-cardiogram abnormalities or echocardiogram abnormalities may also confirm that the source of edema is cardiac. Radiographically this type of edema presents with a large heart, inverted (cephalized) pulmonary blood flow, peribronchial cuffing, symmetric distribution of opacities, pleural effusions and sometimes interlobular septal lines (Fig. 38.11). Non cardiogenic or increased capillary permeability pulmonary edema occurs in a variety of non-heart-related events, including shock, high concentration oxygen ventilation, trauma, and sepsis. The diagnosis is

suspected because of an appropriate history and clinical findings of increasing respiratory distress. Radiographically, this form of edema is distinguished by normal heart size, normal vascular distribution (no cephalization), absence of septal lines, and rare occurrence of peribronchial cuffing and pleural effusions (103) (Fig. 38.12). Differentiating between these two types of edema is made

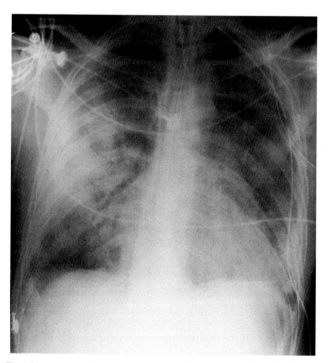

Figure 38.12. Noncardiogenic pulmonary edema. Portable chest radiograph of 32 year old cocaine user found unconscious reveals a normal heart size with bilateral, right greater than left pulmonary opacities. This is consistent with noncardiogenic pulmonary edema. The increased opacity in right lung was thought to be secondary to aspiration or due to dependent edema secondary to the patient's positioning on the right side when found.

Table 38.2. Radiographic criteria for differentiating types of pulmonary edema

Signs	Cardiac	Overhydration	Permeability
Septal thickening	Sometimes	Sometimes	Unusual
Pleural effusions	Present	Present	Unusual
Cardiomegaly	Present	Present	Unusual
Opacities	Diffuse	Central	Scattered, peripheral
Air bronchograms	Rare	Rare	Often present
Peribronchial cuffing	Present	Present	Unusual
Large vascular pedicle	Sometimes	Present	Unusual

difficult for a variety of reasons. Since the majority of portable chest films are obtained in the supine position, pleural effusions are easily missed, pulmonary vessels are cephalized by gravity, and cardiac size is misleading. Furthermore, ventilated patients may have peribronchial cuffing due to bronchial inflammation or inspissated mucus and in the presence of severe interstitial or alveolar fluid, vessel size and distribution is difficult to determine. Other findings used to differentiate cardiogenic from non-cardiogenic pulmonary edema lack high enough sensitivity and specificity to be particularly useful. Some of these include: enlargement of the vascular pedicle (transverse measurement between the superior vena cava and left subclavian artery) and central distribution of edema, indicating cardiogenic origin; and normal vascular pedicle and peripheral distribution of edema, suggesting noncardiogenic etiologies. Determining the types of edema is also hindered by factors such as coexisting chronic obstructive lung disease or pulmonary embolism, which lead to an asymmetric pattern of edema regardless of its cause (104–106). In conclusion, the portable chest radiograph offers an acceptable sensitivity for the detection of pulmonary edema and in some cases, can distinguish between cardiogenic and noncardiogenic pulmonary edema but is not particularly specific for this purpose (Table 38.2).

Adult Respiratory Distress Syndrome (ARDS)

ARDS is a unique form of noncardiogenic pulmonary edema defined as hypoxemia, diffuse pulmonary opacities, and reduced lung compliance (107). It may arise from a variety of direct or indirect insults such as aspiration of gastric contents, near drowning, multiple transfusions, drugs, pneumonia, sepsis, gas inhalation, burns, head trauma, pancreatitis, and more (107). Treatment is supportive. Typically the chest radiograph is normal for the first 12–24 h. Following this period, which is rarely recorded radiographically, patients develop pulmonary edema. Chest films demonstrate bilateral diffuse heterogeneous or homogeneous opacities. Rapidly, within 24 h, the chest film deteriorates to a confluent completely homogeneous alveolar filling pattern. The chest radiograph then remains unchanged for several days, unless altered by

barotrauma or infection. Frequently, when ventilatory support is instituted, chest films may suggest improvement, but this may be secondary to inflation of the lungs rather than resolution of the underlying pathology. Patients who show real improvement on their chest radiographs within 10–14 days have a more favorable prognosis (108). Survivors' chest radiographs either revert to normal or show focal areas of scarring (109).

Hemorrhage

Aspiration of blood into the lungs is usually secondary to trauma to the tracheobronchial tree incurred while suctioning of secretion's is being performed. Chest films demonstrate intralveolar acinar opacities initially. Resolution occurs within days if there is no further bleeding. The distribution of aspirated blood may be localized or diffuse. Occasionally patients in the ICU may bleed within the lung parenchyma and then the chest film will display focal or diffuse homogeneous opacities, which become heterogeneous within days and resolve within 2–4 weeks. Some of the causes of hemorrhage include: aggressive anticoagulation, Goodpasture syndrome, Wegener granulomatosis, Systemic lupus erythematosus, neoplasm, adverse drug reaction (110), pneumonia, infarction or Swan–Ganz catheter tip perforation (111).

Pulmonary Embolism

Pulmonary embolism (PE) is frequently postulated as a cause of sudden chest pain, worsening shortness of breath, or oxygen desaturation in ICU patients. However, the clinical signs and symptoms of PE are neither sensitive nor specific, especially in the critically ill patient who may have infectious or inflammatory causes of respiratory compromise. In evaluating these patients, the chest film is usually the first line of investigation, even though its sensitivity and specificity for the diagnosis of PE are low. In fact, portable chest radiographs primarily screen for other conditions that could mimic PE, such as large effusion, pneumothorax or pneumonia. In patients with documented PE, some of the abnormalities that can be seen on chest radiography include consolidation, atelectasis generally as linear shadows, elevation of a hemidiaphragm, pleural effusion, peripheral wedge-shaped opacities, enlarged hilar pulmonary artery, and focal oligemia. Eight percent of patients with PE have a normal chest film (112). The chest radiographic sensitivity for PE is only 33%, specificity is 59%, and accuracy is only 40%. Since it is unlikely that a diagnosis of PE will be established by chest film alone, other imaging modalities are almost always employed. Further bedside diagnosis is currently limited to ultrasound or nuclear medicine techniques. Noninvasive ultrasound has been used successfully to diagnose deep venous thrombosis of the lower extremities, a condition that may precede PE, especially in postoperative bed-ridden ICU patients. If the examination is positive then patients are treated with anticoagulants just as if they had documented pulmonary emboli. In symptomatic patients with deep vein thrombosis, ultrasound has proven extremely reliable, with sensitivity and specificity above 90% (113–121). Another diagnostic bedside examination for PE is radionuclide ventilation – perfusion scanning (*V/Q* scan). A normal *V/Q* scan virtually excludes the possibility of PE; however, this result is rarely encountered in the ICU (122,123). Occasionally, a high probability scan associated with a high pretest clinical probability of PE will be sufficient for clinicians to initiate therapy. However, in the majority of cases, *V/Q* scanning results in an indeterminate result, which should be clarified with other diagnostic tests.

Pulmonary angiography is minimally invasive but is more difficult to perform in an intubated uncooperative ICU patient. This procedure has a 0.4% risk of complications and a 0.2% risk of death, particularly in patients with right ventricular end-diastolic pressures in excess of 20 mmHg (124). The development of rapid spiral CT over the last decade has provided a better noninvasive alternative for the diagnosis of PE (Fig. 38.13). CT has

proven superior to *V/Q* scanning with sensitivities of 75–92% and specificities of 90–95% as compared with sensitivities of 36–65% and specificities of 74–94% by *V/Q* scan (125–128). In a recent series, the negative predictive value for helical CT in the diagnosis of PE was 99% (123). CT provides greater interobserver agreement than *V/Q* scans for the diagnosis of PE and provides more alternative diagnoses (e.g., pneumonia, pulmonary edema) than the *V/Q* scan does, 93% versus 51%, respectively (125). CT 100% accuracy when assessing central pulmonary emboli (128) and although the technique is inferior to pulmonary angiography for assessing subsegmental clots, these smaller emboli may be of minimal clinical significance. In any case, even pulmonary angiography has difficulty with this level of arterial obstruction, producing a 33% interobserver disagreement for the diagnosis of subsegmental clots (129–131).

Abnormal Air Collections

Abnormal extraalveolar air is one of the common complications of high volume or high pressure ventilation in ICU patients. The principal sites of involvement are the pulmonary interstitium, mediastinum, and pleural space. The collection may remain clinically silent but there is a potential for serious outcomes including death, particularly from large pneumothoraces. Knowledge of the early, subtle radiologic features of extraalveolar air is imperative, in order to alert clinicians of possible problems for their patients. A sudden decline in a patient's respiratory status may then be more quickly explained and treated (132–138).

Pulmonary Interstitial Emphysema

In the ICU, most abnormal air collections are caused by barotrauma or sometimes volutrauma secondary to positive end-expiratory pressure ventilation. When injury occurs, air escapes from an alveolus and dissects along the peribronchovascular interstitium and interlobular septa. This interstitial emphysema then progresses through the hili into the mediastinum, or can travel peripherally to produce a subpleural air collection (139). Radiographic findings of pulmonary interstitial emphysema include lucent streaks radiating from the hili in a disorganized fashion along the parenchymal interstitium, mottled lucencies ("salt and pepper" appearance), and subpleural air-filled cysts measuring 5 mm to several centimeters in diameter (140,141) (Fig. 38.14). Pulmonary interstitial emphysema is infrequently observed but may be easier to see with good-quality chest radiographs and if parenchymal pulmonary opacities coexist. If the condition is noted,

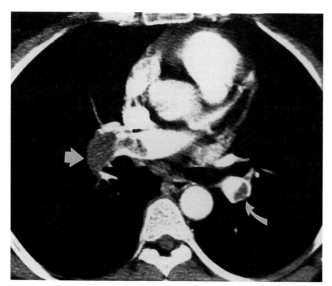

Figure 38.13. Pulmonary embolism. Bedridden woman, 44 years old, with multiple recent pelvic fractures complained of new onset of shortness of breath. Contrast-enhanced spiral chest CT reveals large clots in the right (*white arrow*) and left (*curved white arrow*) pulmonary arteries.

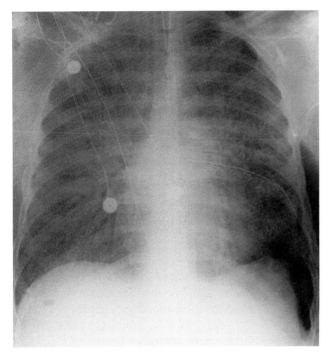

Figure 38.14. ARDS and pulmonary interstitial emphysema. Man, 24 years old, with right lung staphylococcal pneumonia progressed to develop ARDS requiring mechanical ventilation with increasing positive end-expiratory pressures. Portable chest radiograph reveals left perihilar mottled lucencies ("salt and pepper" appearance) and multiple tiny air-filled cysts in the left lung consistent with pulmonary interstitial emphysema. Note is made of the distinct left hemidiaphragm or "deep sulcus sign" signifying a left pneumothorax.

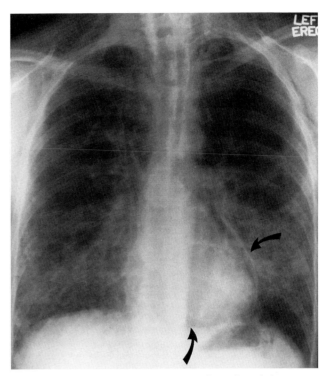

Figure 38.15. Pneumomediastinum. Posteroanterior chest radiograph demonstrates mediastinal lucency outlining the left heart border (*curved black arrows*) consistent with a pneumomediastinum. Subcutaneous air is also seen lateral to ribs and in the soft tissues of the neck.

the clinicians should be informed that evidence of barotrauma is present. Adjustment of ventilator settings, however, should be based on clinical parameters, not the presence of interstitial air.

Pneumomediastinum and Subcutaneous Emphysema

Pneumomediastinum is a common result of pulmonary interstitial emphysema caused by barotrauma; however, other etiologies for air in the mediastinum exist. They include rupture of an airway or esophagus, dissection of air from the retroperitoneum following rupture of an abdominal hollow viscus, or extension of air through the neck secondary to pharyngeal or facial injury. Generally, air in the mediastinum decompresses through the soft tissues of the neck or over the diaphragm to the lateral chest wall. However, pneumothorax arises if the air ruptures through the parietal pleura. Rarely, a large pneumomediastinum can cause vessel compression (142–145). On chest radiographs, pneumomediastinum presents as a lucency outlining mediastinal structures that are not usually in contact with air, such as the central great vessels, or as a well-demarcated lucent stripe parallel to

the lateral margin of the mediastinum (Fig. 38.15). Air seen below the heart and a "continuous diaphragm sign" are the result of pneumomediastinum (146). One should be suspicious of underlying pneumomediastinum if subcutaneous emphysema is seen in the neck.

Subcutaneous emphysema, like pneumomediastinum, may produce a striking radiologic appearance; however, it is usually of no clinical significance but may serve as an indicator of barotrauma, chest tube malfunction, airway or esophageal injury during intubation or feeding tube placement (147,148). When severe, its presence may obscure underlying pneumothorax and lung disease (149). On chest films, linear or mottled lucencies are noted over the lateral chest wall beyond the rib cage, or in the neck lateral to the trachea.

Pneumothorax

The most common cause of pneumothorax in ICU patients is barotrauma or some believe volutrauma. This occurs in up to 25% of mechanically ventilated patients (150). Central line placement may also cause pneumothorax. Radiographically, pneumothorax appears as a lucent crescent of air above the lung apex on upright chest films. However, in the ICU, chest radiography is generally performed with the patient in the supine position. Findings of a pneumothorax on supine chest films

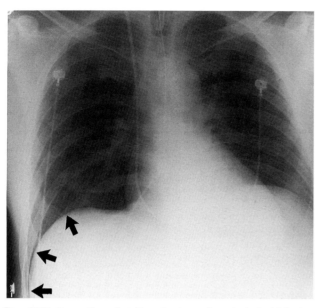

Figure 38.16. Pneumothorax. Portable supine chest radiograph obtained following insertion of a pulmonary artery catheter reveals transradiancy of the right lower hemithorax, increased sharpness of the right hemidiaphragm with a subtle right "deep sulcus sign" (*black arrows*). Upright chest film confirmed the presence of a right small pneumothorax.

include: transradiancy of the lower hemithorax; a deep, large costophrenic recess or "deep sulcus sign" (Figs. 38.14, 38.16); increased sharpness of adjacent mediastinum, heart or diaphragm; air within the minor fissure; sharp definition of the superior pulmonary vein; and irregular heart border due to distorted fat pad (151–155). Patients in the ICU frequently have underlying lung disease and this may produce an unusual distribution of pneumothorax. For example, in the presence of lobar collapse or focal parenchymal disease, air in the pleural space may preferentially accumulate adjacent to the abnormal lung. This may result in a pneumothorax in dependent regions of the chest, delineating posterior structures such as the descending aorta or spine (156). In this particular situation, the pneumothorax has a tubular shape similar to an inferior pulmonary ligament air collection, but unlike the latter, pleural air continues above the level of the hilum (157). If untreated, some cases of pneumothorax in otherwise normal individuals will spontaneously resolve but in patients on positive pressure ventilation, pneumothorax may continue to enlarge and produce tension physiology, which is rapidly fatal (158). In ventilated patients, one cannot necessarily rely on mediastinal shift or total lung atelectasis to indicate a tension pneumothorax. Mediastinal shift may be minimal due to positive airway pressure in the contralateral lung and collapse of lung may not occur secondary to noncompliance (150). Often, inferior displacement of the ipsilateral hemidiaphragm is more useful as a sign of possible tension physiology. In the ventilated patient even small pneumothoraces have the poten-

tial of rapid, unexpected enlargement, so treatment by throacostomy tube should generally be performed (159). Mimics of pneumothorax include overlying tubes, skin folds and pneumopericardium. If necessary, differentiating between these possibilities might be helped by performing an upright or decubitus film or occasionally CT.

Pleural Effusions

Pleural effusions are commonly encountered in the ICU, in 62% of patients in a medical ICU and in 60% of patients in a surgical ICU following upper abdominal operations (160,161). The etiology of pleural fluid is frequently never discovered but most commonly the associated diseases or conditions are congestive heart failure, pneumonia, ARDS, pulmonary embolism, pancreatitis, hypoalbuminemia, malignancy and subdiaphragmatic causes of ascites (139, 160,162). The radiographic appearance of pleural effusion depends on gravity and lung recoil (163,164). In the supine position the most dependent portion of the pleural space is located dorsally, extending from the apices to near the diaphragm. Fluid in the latter location is particularly difficult to detect owing to the common presence of lower lobe parenchymal disease. Nevertheless pleural fluid should be suspected when the supine chest radiograph demonstrates increased lower hemithoracic hazy or homogeneous opacity (Fig. 38.8), loss of sharp definition of a hemidiaphragm, a blunted costophrenic angle, an apical cap, apparent elevation of the hemidiaphragm, and widening of fissures. The accuracy of detecting pleural effusions by portable chest radiographs is good, as shown by correlation with sonography (160). In another study, all moderate to large effusions detected by posteroanterior and lateral films were seen on the portable chest radiographs (165). However, when compared with more sensitive modalities for detection of effusions, such as lateral decubitus chest films and CT, supine chest radiographs do not perform as well (32,33,166–168). In one investigation, the supine chest radiograph was only 67% sensitive, 70% specific, and 67% accurate for the detection of effusion, and the amount of fluid was often underestimated (166). Although, most missed effusions were small, as many as 25% of them were moderate in size. Conversely, some parenchymal disease was misinterpreted as pleural fluid.

Determining the nature of pleural fluid from its CT appearance is at times successful. In trauma ICU patients, low CT density numbers (0–20 Hounsfield units (HU) strongly suggest a transudate or exudate, whereas higher numbers (25–60 HU) are more likely to represent hemorrhage (168). Nevertheless, appearances alone are not sufficient grounds on which to base therapeutic decisions. For example, there is no role for imaging in the differentiation of complicated from noncomplicated parapneumonic effusion. Only pleural fluid analysis can identify patients

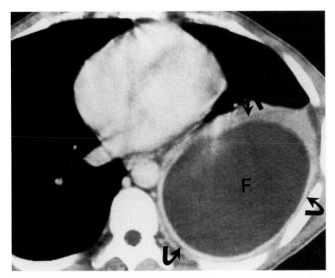

Figure 38.17. Empyema. Contrast-enhanced chest CT demonstrates a lenticular left lower hemithorax fluid collection (*F*), forming obtuse angles with the chest wall, with a uniformly thickened smooth wall. *Curved black arrows* mark the enhancing separated visceral and parietal pleural surfaces ("split pleura sign").

with enough certainty so that therapeutic measures such as tube thoracostomy can be instituted. On the other hand, CT is excellent for solving complex pleuropulmonary issues. For example, patients with pneumonia not responding to antibiotic therapy, who have ambiguous conventional radiographic examinations, may benefit from a chest CT that can distinguish an empyema from a lung abscess. Empyemas form obtuse angles with the chest wall, are lenticular shaped, have uniformly thickened smooth walls, have separated visceral and parietal pleural surfaces ("split pleura sign"), and compress adjacent structures (Fig. 38.17). Lung abscesses are round, irregularly thick walled, form acute angles with the chest wall, have bronchi and pulmonary vessels terminating abruptly at their walls, and do not compress adjacent structures (169).

Acute Mediastinal Abnormalities

The Heart

Assessing heart size on portable chest radiographs may be difficult. The criteria are not as well established as they are for erect posteroanterior films, since there tends to be more variation in diaphragmatic position in supine patients. Also, the focal – film distance may vary more with the portable technique. One study suggests that the upper limit of normal for the cardiac thoracic ratio on posteroanterior chest films is 0.5; on 72 inch focal–film distance anteroposterior chest films it is 0.55; and for 40 inch portable anteroposterior chest films the ratio is 0.57 (170).

Plain film findings associated with pericardial effusions include, "enlarged heart," thickened pericardial stripe seen on lateral chest film, relatively rapid increase in heart size, and predominantly left-sided pleural effusion. An "enlarged heart" is moderately sensitive (71%) but not specific (41%) for detection of pericardial effusions (171). A thickened pericardial stripe is probably more accurate but is visible only on lateral chest films, which are not routinely obtained in the ICU. Therefore, bedside echocardiography is the procedure of choice to diagnose this condition. Alternatively, CT of the chest or upper abdomen obtained for other indications can incidentally but reliably demonstrate pericardial effusions (172,173).

The Mediastinum

Mediastinal enlargement may be indicative of a life-threatening injury, iatrogenic problem, normal postoperative appearance, or infection. Frequently, the medical specialty of the ICU raises awareness as to the correct etiology.

In the traditional medical ICU an abnormal mediastinal contour in the correct clinical setting may indicate an emergency such as aortic dissection. Since the plain chest film findings for an aortic dissection are nonspecific, including mediastinal widening, disparity in size between ascending and descending aorta, indistinct aortic contour, rapid increase in aortic size (174–178), and since a normal chest radiograph does not exclude the possibility of aortic dissection (179), other modalities must be used to make this diagnosis. Spiral chest CT with 96–100% sensitivity and specificity and accuracy as good as angiography is the test of choice (180–182) (Fig. 38.18). Spiral CT is also superior to MRI and transesophageal echo (TEE) in evaluating supraaortic vessel involvement, with sensitivity of 93%, 60%, 67%, and specificity of 97%, 85% and 88%, respectively (182). In unstable patients who cannot be moved from the ICU, TEE is of course, the preferred modality as it can be performed at the bedside and possesses excellent sensitivity and specificity (182).

Other causes of mediastinal enlargement in the medical ICU including thoracic aortic aneurysms; mediastinal fluid collections such as abscess or hematoma should be evaluated by CT.

In the thoracic surgical ICU, mediastinal abnormalities are commonly seen on portable chest films after cardiac surgery. Regardless of the procedure performed (coronary artery bypass grafting (CABG) or valve replacement), postoperative mediastinal appearance is a result of the patient's underlying cardiovascular disease, the use of cardiopulmonary bypass, and the median sternotomy incision. An increase in heart size may be due to perioperative myocardial infarction, hypervolemia, or in fact is most frequently a result of fluid in the pericardial or

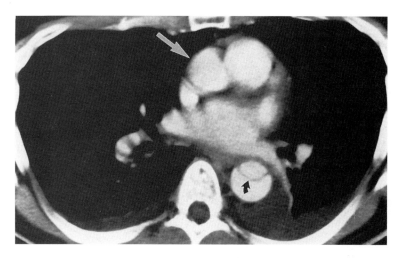

Figure 38.18. Type B aortic dissection. Hypertensive 69 year old male complained of chest pain radiating to the back. Chest radiograph demonstrated small bilateral pleural effusions. However, the clinical presentation prompted an enhanced chest CT that demonstrate a normal ascending aorta (*white arrow*) and an intimal flap (*black arrow*) in the descending aorta consistent with a type B aortic dissection.

mediastinal space (Fig. 38.11). Mild, self-limited bleeding into the mediastinum is frequent after sternotomy and is usually of no consequence (Fig. 38.7). Two percent to 5% of patients' mediastinal hemorrhage leads to surgical exploration (183). However, surgery should not be initiated solely on the basis of the chest film. Acute widening of the mediastinum on the portable radiograph is a secondary indication for reoperation. Clinical judgment is most important, as the width of the mediastinum does not correlate well with the need for surgery (Fig. 38.19). The mediastinum may appear normal on chest radiographs even though serious bleeding has occurred (184); or the

mediastinum may appear erroneously enlarged, since the magnification effect of supine, expiratory radiography may result in a 50% increase in mediastinal width (185). Postoperatively, extrapulmonary air collections, air–fluid levels in the anterior mediastinum, and even abdominal air in asymptomatic patients are considered normal findings and usually disappear within days (186,187).

The complication rate from median sternotomy is low (0.5–5%); however, the mortality from sternal dehiscence, mediastinitis and osteomyelitis is approximately 50% (188–191). Early diagnosis is important as timely aggressive surgical treatment is associated with a decrease in mortality (189–191). However, mediastinitis in the postoperative period is a clinical diagnosis. Radiographs are both insensitive and nonspecific in the postoperative period, with mediastinal widening and air collections normally found in uncomplicated patients. Even with CT one cannot distinguish between mediastinitis and the early normal, noninfected postoperative mediastinum. During the first 3 weeks following surgery, CT of the postoperative mediastinum will exhibit infiltration and indistinctness of the mediastinal fat, fluid collections, small air bubbles, air–fluid levels, and a thickened pericardium (187, 192–195). The use of CT may help to clarify the patient's condition but is not definitive. A negative CT may direct attention elsewhere for the source of sepsis; a positive CT, although nondiagnostic, may be used for guidance in sampling a fluid collection in a febrile patient.

In the trauma ICU, portable chest film demonstration of mediastinal enlargement requires prompt additional imaging to exclude acute thoracic aortic injury or vertebral fracture. The important plain film findings of aortic injury are indistinct aortic arch or descending aorta, left apical cap, tracheal displacement to the right, displacement of the nasogastric tube to the right of the T4 spinous process, mediastinal widening and inferior displacement of the left main-stem bronchus (196–198) (Fig. 38.20). Less specific findings include a left pleural effusion and widened paravertebral stripe (199). These chest

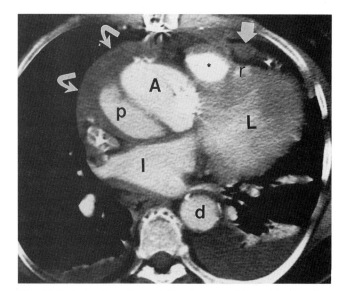

Figure 38.19. Ruptured ascending aortic dissection. Female, 75 years old, presented to the emergency room with a systolic blood pressure of 70, chest pain radiating to the back, 2 weeks after aortic valve replacement. Plain chest film was unchanged since surgery. Contrast-enhanced chest CT revealed a small pericardial effusion (*white arrow*) indenting the right ventricle correlating to her clinical signs of tamponade. Pericardial fluid (*curved white arrows*) also surrounded the dilatated ascending aorta which demonstrated a large pseudoaneurysm. This lesion was presumed to be the result of an intimal injury suffered at surgery. *A*, true lumen of ascending aorta; *p*, pseudoaneurysm; *r*, right ventricle; *l* left atrium; L, left ventricle, *, right atrium; d, descending aorta.

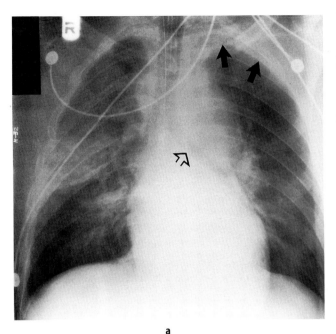

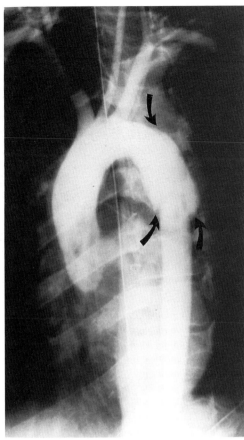

a   b

Figure 38.20. Traumatic aortic rupture. Driver, 23 years old, involved in a motor vehicle accident. **a** Initial portable chest film revealed an indistinct descending aorta, left apical cap (*black arrows*), tracheal displacement to the right, and inferior displacement of the left main-stem bronchus (*open black arrow*). **b** Aortogram confirmed the suspected traumatic aortic rupture revealing contrast extravasation surrounding the descending aorta (*curved black arrows*).

radiographic abnormalities, however, are only suggestive, not indicative of, an aortic injury. In contradistinction, the negative predictive value of a normal chest radiograph for an aortic injury is 94–96% (200,201). Recent advances in CT imaging such as spiral CT with thinner slices and three-dimensional reconstruction have produced results suggesting the appropriate use of CT as the first imaging method for the diagnosis of ruptured aorta (Fig. 38.21). The sensitivity for this technique is 100%, and the specificity ranges from 83% to 99.7% (202–205). The negative predictive value is 100% (202,203). Recent studies have demonstrated that TEE causes unnecessary delays in diagnosing acute thoracic injuries and is subject to artefacts created by air and bone (206,207).

In Conclusion

Despite the lack of sensitivity and specificity of portable chest radiographs in the ICU, they are highly accurate in demonstrating malpositioned tubes and detect significant

unsuspected findings in up to 65% of patients. Daily chest radiographs are still indicated for patients with acute cardiopulmonary problems and for those who are mechanically ventilated. Daily communication between the ICU clinician and the radiologist will lead to better chest film interpretation, and improved patient care.

References

1. Strain DS, Kinasewitz GT, Vereen LE (1985) Value of routine daily chest x-rays in the medical intensive care unit. Crit Care Med 13:534–536.
2. Bekemeyer WB, Crapo RO, Calhoon S, et al. (1985) Efficacy of chest radiography in a respiratory intensive care unit. A prospective study. Chest 88:691–696.
3. Hall JB, White SR, Karrison T (1991) Efficacy of daily routine chest radiographs in intubated, mechanically ventilated patients [see comments]. Crit Care Med 19:689–693.
4. Silverstein DS, Livingston DH, Elcavage J, et al. (1993) The utility of routine daily chest radiography in the surgical intensive care unit. J Trauma 35:643–646.

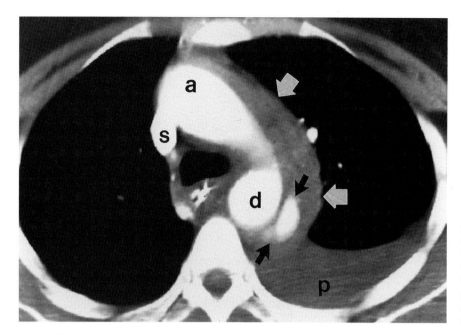

Figure 38.21. Traumatic aortic rupture: CT. Fifty-nine year old involved in a motor vehicle accident. Contrast-enhanced spiral chest CT shows a left pleural effusion, infiltration of the periaortic fat (*white arrows*) consistent with periaortic hematoma, and contrast outside the true lumen of the descending aorta, within a pseudoaneurysm (*black arrows*). *p*, pleural effusion; *a*, ascending aorta; *d*, descending aorta; *s*, superior vena cava.

5. Fong Y, Whalen GF, Hariri RJ, et al. (1995) Utility of routine chest radiographs in the surgical intensive care unit. A prospective study. Arch Surg 130:764–768.

6. Cullinane DC, Parkus DE, Reddy VS, et al. (1998) The futility of chest roentgenograms following routine central venous line changes. Am J Surg 176:283–285.

7. Hornick PI, Harris P, Cousins C, et al. (1995) Assessment of the value of the immediate postoperative chest radiograph after cardiac operation. Ann Thorac Surg 59:1150–1153; discussion 1153–1154.

8. Frassinelli P, Pasquale MD, Cipolle MD, et al. (1998) Utility of chest radiographs after guidewire exchanges of central venous catheters. Crit Care Med 26:611–615.

9. Schwartz DE, Lieberman JA, Cohen NH (1994) Women are at greater risk than men for malpositioning of the endotracheal tube after emergent intubation [see comments]. Crit Care Med 22:1127–1131.

10. Henschke CI, Pasternack GS, Schroeder S, et al. (1983) Bedside chest radiography: Diagnostic efficacy. Radiology 149:23–26.

11. Henschke CI, Yankelevitz DF, Wand A, et al. (1996) Accuracy and efficacy of chest radiography in the intensive care unit. Radiol Clin North Am 34:21–31.

12. Greenbaum DM, Marschall KE (1982) The value of routine daily chest x-rays in intubated patients in the medical intensive care unit. Crit Care Med 10:29–30.

13. Janower ML, Jennas-Nocera Z, Mukai J (1984) Utility and efficacy of portable chest radiographs. AJR 142:265–267.

14. Miller JA, Singireddy S, Maldjian P, et al. (1999) A revaluation of the radiographically detectable complications of percutaneous venous access lines inserted by four subcutaneous approaches. Am Surg 65:125–130.

15. Gray P, Sullivan G, Ostryzniuk P, et al. (1992) Value of postprocedural chest radiographs in the adult intensive care unit. Crit Care Med 20:1513–1518.

16. Schaefer CM, Greene RE, Oestmann JW, et al. (1989) Improved control of image optical density with low-dose digital and conventional radiography in bedside imaging. radiology 173:713–716.

17. Schaefer CM, Greene R, Llewellyn HJ, et al. (1991) Interstitial lung disease: impact of postprocessing in digital storage phosphor imaging. Radiology 178:733–738.

18. Schaefer CM, Greene R, Hall DA, et al. (1991) Mediastinal abnormalities: detection with storage phosphor digital radiography. Radiology 178:169–173.

19. Sagel SS, Jost RG, Glazer HS, et al. (1990) Digital mobile radiography. J Thorac Imaging 5:36–48.

20. MacMahon H, Sanada S, Doi K, et al. (1991) Direct comparison of conventional and computed radiography with a dual-image recording technique. Radiographics 11:259–268.

21. Kundel HL, Seshadri SB, Langlotz CP, et al. (1996) Prospective study of a PACS: information flow and clinical action in a medical intensive care unit. Radiology 199:143–149.

22. Steckel RJ, Batra P, Johnson S, et al. (1997) Chest teleradiology in a teaching hospital emergency practice [see comments]. AJR 168:1409–1413.

23. Huda W, Honeyman JC, Palmer CK, et al. (1996) Computed radiography and film digitizer inputs to an intensive care unit teleradiology system: an image quality comparison. Acad Radiol 3:110–114.

24. Niklason LT, Chan HP, Cascade PN, et al. (1993) Portable chest imaging: comparison of storage phosphor digital, asymmetric screen-film, and conventional screen-film systems [see comments]. Radiology 186:387–393.

25. Maguire WM, Herman PG, Khan A, et al. (1994) Interobserver agreement using computed radiography in the adult intensive care unit. Acad Radiol 1:10–14.

26. Smith I, Fleming S, Cernaianu A (1990) Mishaps during transport from the intensive care unit. Crit Care Med 18:278–281.

27. Stearley HE (1998) Patients' outcomes: Intrahospital transportation and monitoring of critically ill patients by a specially trained ICU nursing staff. Am J Crit Care 7:282–287.

28. Szem JW, Hydo LJ, Fischer E, et al. (1995) High-risk intrahospital transport of critically ill patients: safety and outcome of the necessary "road trip". Crit Care Med 23:1660–1666.

29. Taylor JO, Chulay, Landers CF, et al. (1970) Monitoring high-risk cardiac patients during transportation in hospital. Lancet 2:1205–1208.

30. Waddell G (1975) Movement of critically ill patients within hospital. Br Med J 2:417–419.

31. Braman SS, Dunn SM, Amico CA, et al. (1987) Complications of intrahospital transport in critically ill patients. Ann Intern Med 107:469–473.

32. Mirvis SE, Tobin KD, Kostrubiak I, et al. (1987) Thoracic CT in detecting occult disease in critically ill patients. AJR 148:685–689.

33. Golding RP, Knape P, Strack van Schijndel RJ, et al. (1988) Computed tomography as an adjunct to chest x-rays of intensive care unit patients. Crit Care Med 16:211–216.

34. Ulmer JL, Choplin RH, Reed JC (1991) Image-guided catheter drainage of the infected pleural space. J Thorac Imaging 6:65–73.

35. Reinhold C, Illescas FF, Atri M, et al. (1989) Treatment of pleural effusions and pneumothorax with catheters placed percutaneously under imaging guidance. AJR 152:1189–1191.

36. O'Moore PV, Mueller PR, Simeone JF, et al. (1987) Sonographic guidance in diagnostic and therapeutic interventions in the pleural space. AJR 149:1–5.

37. Rotello LC, Radin EJ, Jastremski MS, et al. (1994) MRI protocol for critically ill patients. Am J Crit Care 3:187–190.

38. Dunn V, Coffman CE, McGowan JE, et al. (1985) Mechanical ventilation during magnetic resonance imaging. Magn Reson Imaging 3:169–172.

39. Barnett GH, Ropper AH, Johnson KA (1988) Physiological support and monitoring of critically ill patients during magnetic resonance imaging. J Neurosurg 68:246–250.

40. Houston JG, Fleet M, Cowan MD, et al. (1995) Comparison of ultrasound with fluoroscopy in the assessment of suspected hemidiaphragmatic movement abnormality. Clin Radiol 50:95–98.

41. Houston JG, Fleet M, McMillan N, et al. (1995) Ultrasonic assessment of hemidiaphragmatic movement: An indirect method of evaluating mediastinal invasion in non-small cell lung cancer. Br J Radiol 68:695–699.

42. Commare MC, Kurstjens SP, Barois A (1994) Diaphragmatic paralysis in children: A review of 11 cases. Pediatr Pulmonol 18:187–193.

43. Balaji S, Kunovsky P, Sullivan I (1990) Ultrasound in the diagnosis of diaphragmatic paralysis after operation for congenital heart disease. Br Heart J 64:20–22.

44. McCauley RG, Labib KB (1984) Diaphragmatic paralysis evaluated by phrenic nerve stimulation during fluoroscopy or real-time ultrasound. Radiology 153:33–36.

45. Park GR, Young GB (1981) Demonstration of phrenic nerve paralysis and its subsequent recovery by ultrasound. Intensive Care Med 7:145–146.

46. Gottesman E, McCool FD (1997) Ultrasound evaluation of the paralyzed diaphragm. Am J Respir Crit Care Med 155:1570–1574.

47. Cohen E, Mier A, Heywood P, et al. (1994) Excursion-volume relation of the right hemidiaphragm measured by ultrasonography and respiratory airflow measurements. Thorax 49:885–889.

48. Yang PC, Luh KT, Chang DB, et al. (1992) Ultrasonographic evaluation of pulmonary consolidation. Am Rev Respir Dis 146:757–762.

49. Versluis PJ, Lamers RJ (1993) Lobar pneumonia: An ultrasound diagnosis. Pediatr Radiol 23:561–562.

50. Hsu WH, Chiang CD, Chen CY, et al. (1997) Ultrasound-guided fine needle aspiration biopsy in the diagnosis of chronic pulmonary infection. Respiration 64:319–325.

51. Anzbock W, Stellamor K, Braun U, et al. (1990) [Sonography of the lungs and pleura]. Rofo Fortschr Geb Rontgenstr Neuen Bildgeb Verfahr 153:278–282.

52. Gehmacher O, Mathis G, Kopf A, et al. (1995) Ultrasound imaging of pneumonia. Ultrasound Med Biol 21:1119–1122.

53. Lichtenstein D, Meziere G (1998) A lung ultrasound sign allowing bedside distinction between pulmonary edema and COPD: The comet-tail artifact. Intensive Care Med 24:1331–1334.

54. Roberts JR, Spadafora M, Cone DC (1995) Proper depth placement of oral endotracheal tubes in adults prior to radiographic confirmation. Acad Emerg Med 2:20–24.

55. Reed DB, Clinton JE (1997) Proper depth of placement of nasotracheal tubes in adults prior to radiographic confirmation. Acad Emerg Med 4:1111–1114.

56. Ong KC, A'Court GD, Eng P, Vol. (1996) Ideal endotracheal tube placement by referencing measurements on the tube. Ann Acad Med Singapore 25:550–552.

57. Bissinger U, Lenz G, Kuhn W (1989) Unrecognized endobronchial intubation of emergency patients. Ann Emerg Med 18:853–855.

58. Brunel W, Coleman DL, Schwartz DE, et al. (1989) Assessment of routine chest roentgenograms and the physical examination to confirm endotracheal tube position [see comments]. Chest 96:1043–1045.

59. Birmingham PK, Cheney FW, Ward RJ (1986) Esophageal intubation: A review of detection techniques. Anesth Analg 65:886–891.

60. Conrardy PA, Goodman LR, Lainge F, et al. (1976) Alteration of endotracheal tube position. Flexion and extension of the neck. Crit Care Med 4:8–12.

61. Goodman LR, Conrardy PA, Laing F, et al. (1976) Radiographic evaluation of endotracheal tube position. AJR 127:433–434.

62. Pappas JN, Goodman PC (1999) Predicting proper endotracheal tube placement in underexposed radiographs: Tangent line of the aortic arch. AJR 173:1357–1359.

63. Valentino J, Myers RK, Baker MD, et al. (1999) Utility of portable chest radiographs as a predictor of endotracheal tube cuff pressure. Otolaryngol Head Neck Surg 120:51–56.

64. Webb WR, LaBerge JM (1984) Radiographic recognition of chest tube malposition in the major fissure. Chest 85:81–83.

65. Webb WR, Godwin JD (1980) The obscured outer edge: a sign of improperly placed pleural drainage tubes. AJR 134:1062–1064.

66. Stark DD, Federle MP, Goodman PC (1983) CT and radiographic assessment of tube thoracostomy. AJR 141:253–258.

67. Maurer JR, Friedman PJ, Wing VW (1982) Thoracostomy tube in an interlobar fissure: radiologic recognition of a potential problem. AJR 139:1155–1161.

68. Ravin CE, Putman CE, McLoud TC (1976) Hazards of the intensive care unit. AJR 126:423–431.

69. Langston CS (1971) The aberrant central venous catheter and its complications. Radiology 100:55–59.

70. McGee WT, Ackerman BL, Rouben LR, et al. (1993) Accurate placement of central venous catheters: A prospective, randomized, multicenter trial [see comments]. Crit Care Med 21:1118–1123.

71. Gibson RN, Hennessy OF, Collier N, et al. (1985) Major complications of central venous catheterisation: a report of five cases and a brief review of the literature. Clin Radiol 36:205–208.

72. Kline IK, Hofman WI (1968) Cardiac tampondade from CVP catheter perforation. JAMA 206:1794–1795.

73. Huyghens L, Sennesael J, Verbeelen D, et al. (1985) Cardiothoracic complications of centrally inserted catheters. Acute Care 11:53–56.

74. Au FC, Badellino M (1988) Significance of a curled central venous catheter tip. Chest 93:890–891.

75. Tocino IM, Watanabe A (1986) Impending catheter perforation of superior vena cava: Radiographic recognition. AJR 146:487–490.

76. Adar R, Mozes M (1970) Hydromediastinum. JAMA 214:372.

77. Blair E, Hunziker R, Flanagan ME (1970) Catheter embolism. Surgery 67:457–461.

78. Bouffard Y, Bouletreau P, Motin J (1985) Deep venous thrombosis with clinical signs after catheterization of the superior vena cava system. Acta Anaesthesiol Scand Suppl 81:65–66.

79. Swan HJ, Ganz W (1975) Use of balloon flotation catheters in critically ill patients. Surg Clin North Am 55:501–509.

80. Kronberg GM, Quan SF, Schlobohm RM, et al. (1979) Anatomic locations of the tips of pulmonary-artery catheters in supine patients. Anesthesiology 51:467–469.

81. Foote GA, Schabel SI, Hodges M (1974) Pulmonary complications of the flow-directed balloon-tipped catheter. N Engl J Med 290:927–931.

82. McLoud TC, Putman CE (1975) Radiology of the Swan-Ganz catheter and associated pulmonary complications. Radiology 116:19–22.

83. Takkunen OS, Kalso EA (1987) Catheter-induced pulmonary artery perforation associated with an unusual wedge pressure tracing. Can J Anaesth 34:168–171.

84. Lipp H, O'Donoghue K, Resnekov L (1971) Intracardiac knotting of a flow-directed balloon catheter. N Engl J Med 284:220.

85. Dieden JD, Friloux LAD, Renner JW (1987) Pulmonary artery false aneurysms secondary to Swan–Ganz pulmonary artery catheters. AJR 149:901–906.

86. Hyson EA, Ravin CE, Kelley MJ, et al. (1977) Intraaortic counter-pulsation balloon: Radiographic considerations. AJR 128:915–915.

87. Chiles C, Vail CM, Coblentz CL, et al. (1991) Intra-aortic balloon pumps: An update on radiographic recognition. Can Assoc Radiol J 42:257–260.

88. Chen JTT (1997) Cardiac pacemakers and prosthetic valves. In: Chen JTT, (ed) Essentials of Cardiac Imaging. Lippincott-Raven, New York, p 309.

89. Ormond RS, Rubenfire M, Anbe DT, et al. (1971) Radiographic demonstration of myocardial penetration by permanent endo-cardial pacemakers. Radiology 98:35–37.

90. Kiviniemi MS, Pirnes MA, Eranen HJ, et al. (1999) Complications related to permanent pacemaker therapy. Pacing Clin Electro-physiol 22:711–720.

91. Marini JJ, Pierson DJ, Hudson LD (1979) Acute lobar atelectasis: A prospective comparison of fiberoptic bronchoscopy and respira-tory therapy. Am Rev Respir Dis 119:971–978.

92. Meduri GU, Mauldin GL, Wunderink RG, et al. (1994) Causes of fever and pulmonary densities in patients with clinical manifesta-tions of ventilator-associated pneumonia. Chest 106:221–235.

93. Louthan FB, Meduri GU (1996) Differential diagnosis of fever and pulmonary densities in mechanically ventilated patients. Semin Respir Infect 11:77–95.

94. Singh N, Falestiny MN, Rogers P, et al. (1998) Pulmonary infiltrates in the surgical ICU: Prospective assessment of predictors of eti-ology and mortality. Chest 114:1129–1136.

95. Lefcoe MS, Fox GA, Leasa DJ, et al. (1994) Accuracy of portable chest radiography in the critical care setting. Diagnosis of pneu-monia based on quantitative cultures obtained from protected brush catheter. Chest 105:885–887.

96. Winer-Muram HT, Rubin SA, Ellis JV, et al. (1993) Pneumonia and ARDS in patients receiving mechanical ventilation: diagnostic accuracy of chest radiography. Radiology 188:479–485.

97. Beydon L, Saada M, Liu N, et al. (1992) Can portable chest x-ray examination accurately diagnose lung consolidation after major abdominal surgery? A comparison with computed tomography scan. Chest 102:1697–1703.

98. Swensen SJ, Peters SG, LeRoy AJ, et al. (1991) Radiology in the intensive-care unit. Mayo Clin Proc 66:396–410.

99. Macfarlane JT, Miller AC, Roderick Smith WH, et al. (1984) Comparative radiographic features of community acquired Legionnaires' disease, pneumococcal pneumonia, mycoplasma pneumonia, and psittacosis. Thorax 39:28–33.

100. Helms CM, Viner JP, Sturm RH, et al. (1979) Comparative features of pneumococcal, mycoplasmal, and Legionnaire's disease pneu-monias. Ann Intern Med 90:543–547.

101. Tew J, Calenoff L, Berlin BS (1977) Bacterial or nonbacterial pneumonia: Accuracy of radiographic diagnosis. Radiology 124:607–612.

102. Moine P, Vercken JP, Chevret S, et al. (1995) Severe community-acquired pneumonia. The French Study Group of Community-Acquired Pneumonia in ICU. Scand J Infect Dis 27:201–206.

103. Milne EN, Pistolesi M, Miniati M, et al. (1985) The radiologic distinction of cardiogenic and noncardiogenic edema. AJR 144:879–894.

104. Fraser RG, Paré JAP (1970) An integrated study based on abnormal roentgenogram. In Fraser RG, Paré JAP, (eds) Diagnosis of diseases of the chest. WB Saunders, Philadelphia pp 199, 855, 958.

105. Heitzman ER (1973) The lung: Radiologic-pathologic correlations. St. Louis, MD, Mosby, p 11.

106. Hublitz UF, Shapiro JH (1969) Atypical pulmonary patterns of congestive failure in chronic lung disease. The influence of pre-existing disease on the appearance and distribution of pulmonary edema. Radiology 93:995–1006.

107. Casty F, Bone RC (1992) Adult respiratory distress syndrome: Clinical perspective. In Goodman LR, Putman CE (eds) Critical care imaging. WB Saunders, Philadelphia, p 129.

108. Wheeler AP, Carroll FE, Bernard GR (1993) Radiographic issues in adult respiratory distress syndrome. New Horiz 1:471–477.

109. Putman CE (1992) Cardiac and noncardiac edema: Radiologic approach. In Goodman LR, Putman CE (eds) Critical care imaging. WB Saunders, Philadelphia, p 83.

110. Brandstetter RD, Tamarin FM, Rangraj MS, et al. (1984) Moxalactam disodium-induced pulmonary hemorrhage. Chest 86:644–645.

111. Brandstetter RD, Alarakhia N, Coli L, et al. (1984) Distal kinking of a pulmonary artery catheter as a cause of fatal hemoptysis. NY State J Med 84:521–522.

112. Stein PD, Alavi A, Gottschalk A, et al. (1991) Usefulness of noninva-sive diagnostic tools for diagnosis of acute pulmonary embolism in patients with a normal chest radiograph. Am J Cardiol 67:1117–1120.

113. Gottlieb RH, Widjaja J, Tian L, et al. (1999) Calf sonography for detecting deep venous thrombosis in symptomatic patients: Experience and review of the literature. J Clin Ultrasound 27:415–420.

114. Atri M, Herba MJ, Reinhold C, et al. (1996) Accuracy of sonography in the evaluation of calf deep vein thrombosis in both postopera-tive surveillance and symptomatic patients [see comments]. AJR 166:1361–1367.

115. Wells PS, Hirsh J, Anderson DR, et al. (1995) Comparison of the accuracy of impedance plethysmography and compression ultra-sonography in outpatients with clinically suspected deep vein thrombosis. A two centre paired-design prospective trial. Thromb Haemost 74:1423–1427.

116. Poppiti R, Papanicolaou G, Perese S, et al. (1995) Limited B-mode venous imaging versus complete color-flow duplex venous scan-ning for detection of proximal deep venous thrombosis. J Vasc Surg 22:553–557.

117. Tan SS, Chong BK, Thoo FL, et al. (1995) Diagnosis of deep venous thrombosis: Accuracy of colour Doppler ultrasound compared with venography. Singapore Med J 36:362–366.

118. Markel A, Weich Y, Gaitini D (1995) Doppler ultrasound in the diagnosis of venous thrombosis. Angiology 46:65–73.

119. Labropoulos N, Leon M, Kalodiki E, et al. (1995) Colour flow duplex scanning in suspected acute deep vein thrombosis: Experience with routine use. Eur J Vasc Endovasc Surg 9:49–52.

120. Lewis BD, James EM, Welch TJ, et al. (1994) Diagnosis of acute deep venous thrombosis of the lower extremities: Prospective evaluation of color Doppler flow imaging versus venography. Radiology 192:651–655.

121. Wester JP, Holtkamp M, Linnebank ER, et al. (1994) Non-invasive detection of deep venous thrombosis: Ultrasonography versus duplex scanning [see comments]. Eur J Vasc Surg 8:357–361.

122. Royal HD (1989) Radionuclide imaging of the lung. Curr Opin Radiol 1:446–459.

123. Garg K, Sieler H, Welsh CH, et al. (1999) Clinical validity of helical CT being interpreted as negative for pulmonary embolism: Implications for patient treatment [see comments]. AJR 172:1627–1631.

124. Mills SR, Jackson DC, Older RA, et al. (1980) The incidence, etiologies, and avoidance of complications of pulmonary angiography in a large series. Radiology 136:295–299.

125. Van Rossum AB, Pattynama PM, Mallens WM, et al. (1998) Can helical CT replace scintigraphy in the diagnostic process in suspected pulmonary embolism? A retrolective–prolective cohort study focusing on total diagnostic yield. Eur Radiol 8:90–96.

126. Mayo JR, Rémy-Jardin M, Müller NL, et al. (1997) Pulmonary embolism: Prospective comparison of spiral CT with ventilation–perfusion scintigraphy. Radiology 205:447–452.

127. Herold C, Rémy-Jardin M, Grenier PH, et al. (1998) Prospective evaluation of pulmonary embolism: Initial results of the European multicenter trial (ESTIPEP). (abstr). Radiology 209:299.

128. Rémy-Jardin M, Rémy J, Deschildre F, et al. (1996) Diagnosis of pulmonary embolism with spiral CT: Comparison with pulmonary angiography and scintigraphy. Radiology 200:699–706.

129. Diffin DC, Leyendecker JR, Johnson SP, et al. (1998) Effect of anatomic distribution of pulmonary emboli on interobserver agreement in the interpretation of pulmonary angiography. AJR 171:1085–1089.

130. Schlueter FJ, Zuckerman DA, Horesh L, et al. (1997) Digital subtraction versus film-screen angiography for detecting acute pulmonary emboli: Evaluation in a porcine model. J Vasc Interv Radiol 8:1015–1024.

131. Stein PD, Henry JW, Gottschalk A (1999) Reassessment of pulmonary angiography for the diagnosis of pulmonary embolism: Relation of interpreter agreement to the order of the involved pulmonary arterial branch. Radiology 210:689–691.

132. Wescott JL, Cole S (1983) Barotrauma. In Herman PG (ed) Iatrogenic thoracic complications. Springer-Verlag, New York p 79

133. Zwillich CW, Pierson DJ, Creagh CE, et al. (1974) Complications of assisted ventilation. A prospective study of 354 consecutive episodes. Am J Med 57:161–176.

134. Bone RC, Francis PB, Pierce AK (1975) Pulmonary barotrauma complicating positive end-expiratory pressure. Am Rev Respir 111:921.

135. Bone RC (1982) Complication of mechanical ventilation and positive end-expiratory expiratory pressure. Resp Care 27:402–407.

136. Leeming BW (1968) Radiological aspects of the pulmonary complications resulting from intermittent positive pressure ventilation (I.P.P.V.). Australas Radiol 12:361–377.

137. Nash G, Blennerhassett JB, Pontoppidan H (1967) Pulmonary lesions associated with oxygen therapy and artifical ventilation. N Engl J Med 276:368–374.

138. Rohlfing BM, Webb WR, Schlobohm RM (1976) Ventilator-related extra-alveolar air in adults. Radiology 121:25–31.

139. Tocino I (1992) Abnormal air and pleural fluid collections. In Goodman LR, Putman CE (eds) Critical care imaging. WB Saunders, Philadelphia, p 137.

140. Unger JM, England DM, Bogust GA (1989) Interstitial emphysema in adults: Recognition and prognostic implications. J Thorac Imaging 4:86–94.

141. Westcott JL, Cole SR (1974) Interstitial pulmonary emphysema in children and adults: roentgenographic features. Radiology 111:367–378.

142. Dondelinger RF, Coulon M, Kurdziel JC, et al. (1992) Tension mediastinal emphysema: Emergency percutaneous drainage with CT guidance. Eur J Radiol 15:7–10.

143. Beg MH, Reyazuddin, Ansari MM (1988) Traumatic tension pneumomediastinum mimicking cardiac tamponade. Thorax 43:576–577.

144. Shennib HF, Barkun AN, Matouk E (1988) Surgical decompression of a tension pneumomediastinum. A ventilatory complication of status asthmaticus. Chest 93:1301–1302.

145. Woodring JH (1985) Pulmonary interstitial emphysema in the adult respiratory distress syndrome. Crit Care Med 13:786–791.

146. Levin B (1973) The continuous diaphragm sign. A newly-recognized sign of pneumomediastinum. Clin Radiol 24:337–338.

147. Kassner EG, Baumstark A, Balsam D, et al. (1977) Passage of feeding catheters into the pleural space: A radiographic sign of trauma to the pharynx and esophagus in the newborn. AJR 128:19–22.

148. Woodall BH, Winfield DF, Bisset GS (1987) Inadvertent tracheobronchial placement of feeding tubes. Radiology 165:727–729.

149. Tocino I, Miller MH (1987) Computed tomography in blunt chest trauma. J Thorac Imaging 2:45–59.

150. Greene R, McLoud TC, Stark P (1977) Pneumothorax. Semin Roentgenol 12:313–325.

151. Tocino IM, Miller MH, Fairfax WR (1985) Distribution of pneumothorax in the supine and semirecumbent critically ill adult. AJR 144:901–905.

152. Rhea JT, van Sonnenberg E, McLoud TC (1979) Basilar pneumothorax in the supine adult. Radiology 133:593–595.

153. Ziter FM, Jr, Westcott JL (1981) Supine subpulmonary pneumothorax. AJR 137:699–701.

154. Gordon R (1980) The deep sulcus sign. Radiology 136:25–27.

155. Chiles C, Ravin CE (1986) Radiographic recognition of pneumothorax in the intensive care unit. Crit Care Med 14:677–680.

156. Proto AV, Tocino I (1980) Radiographic manifestations of lobar collapse. Semin Roentgenol 15:117–173.

157. Elyaderani MK, Gabriele OF (1979) Traumatic para-mediastinal air cysts. Br J Radiol 52:458–460.

158. Kumar A, Pontoppidan H, Falke KJ, et al. (1973) Pulmonary barotrauma during mechanical ventilation. Crit Care Med 1:181–186.

159. Enderson BL, Abdalla R, Frame SB (1993) Tube thoracostomy for occult pneumothorax: A prospective randomized study of its use. J Trauma 35:726–730.

160. Mattison LE, Coppage L, Alderman DF, et al. (1997) Pleural effusions in the medical ICU: Prevalence, causes, and clinical implications. Chest 111:1018–1023.

161. Goodman LR (1980) Postoperative chest radiograph: I. Alterations after abdominal surgery. AJR 134:533–541.

162. Wiener-Kronish JP, Matthay MA (1988) Pleural effusions associated with hydrostatic and increased permeability pulmonary edema. Chest 93:852–858.

163. Fleichner FG (1963) Atypical arrangement of free pleural effusion. Radiol Clin North Am 1:347–362.

164. Raasch BN, Carsky EW, Lane EJ, et al. (1982) Pleural effusion: Explanation of some typical appearances. AJR 139:899–904.

165. Woodring JH (1982) Recognition of pleural effusion on supine radiographs: how much fluid is required? AJR 142:59–64.

166. Ruskin JA, Gurney JW, Thorsen MK, et al. (1987) Detection of pleural effusions on supine chest radiographs. AJR 148:681–683.

167. Baldt MM, Bankier AA, Germann PS, et al. (1995) Complications after emergency tube thoracostomy: Assessment with CT [see comments]. Radiology 195:539–543.

168. Goodman LR, Teplick SK (1983) Computed tomography in acute cardiopulmonary disease. Radiol Clin North Am 21:741–758.

169. Stark DD, Federle MP, Goodman PC, et al. (1983) Differentiating lung abscess and empyema: radiography and computed tomography. AJR 141:163–167.

170. Milne EN (1986) A physiological approach to reading critical care unit films. J Thorac Imaging 1:60–90.

171. Eisenberg MJ, Dunn MM, Kanth N, et al. (1993) Diagnostic value of chest radiography for pericardial effusion [see comments]. J Am Coll Cardiol 22:588–593.

172. Kodolitsch Y, Krause N, Spielmann R, et al. (1999) Diagnostic potential of combined transthoracic echocardiography and x-ray computed tomography in suspected aortic dissection. Clin Cardiol 22:345–352.

173. Nagy KK, Gilkey SH, Roberts RR (1996) Computed tomography screens stable patients at risk for penetrating cardiac injury. Acad Emerg Med 3:1024–1027.

174. Dee P, Martin R, Oudkerk M, et al. (1983) The diagnosis of aortic dissection. Curr Probl Diagn Radiol 12:3–56.

175. Eyler WR, Clark MD (1965) Dissecting aneurysms of the aorta: Roentgen manifestations including a comparison with other types of aneurysms. Radiology 85:1047–1057.

176. Kaufman SL, White RI, Jr (1980) Aortic dissection with "normal" chest roentgenogram. Cardiovasc Intervent Radiol 3:103–106.

177. Smith DC, Jang GC (1983) Radiological diagnosis of aortic dissection. In Doroghazi RM, Slater EE, (eds) Aortic dissection. McGraw-Hill, New York pp.

178. Wyman SM (1957) Dissecting aneurysm of the thoracic aorta: Its Roentgen recognition. AJR 78:247–255.

179. Slater EE, DeSanctis RW (1976) The clinical recognition of dissecting aortic aneurysm. Am J Med 60:625–633.

180. Moncada R, Salinas M, Churchill R, et al. (1981) Diagnosis of dissecting aortic aneurysm by computed tomography. Lancet 1:238–241.

181. Small JH, Dixon AK, Coulden RA, et al. (1996) Fast CT for aortic dissection. Br J Radiol 69:900–905.

182. Sommer T, Fehske W, Holzknecht N, et al. (1996) Aortic dissection: A comparative study of diagnosis with spiral CT, multiplanar transesophageal echocardiography, and MR imaging [see comments]. Radiology 199:347–352.

183. Ikaheimo MJ, Huikuri HV, Airaksinen KE, et al. (1988) Pericardial effusion after cardiac surgery: Incidence, relation to the type of surgery, antithrombotic therapy, and early coronary bypass graft patency. Am Heart J 116:97–102.

184. Katzberg RW, Whitehouse GH, deWeese JA (1978) The early radiologic findings in the adult chest after cardiopulmonary bypass surgery. Cardiovasc Radiol 1:205–215.

185. Harris RS (1980) The pre-operative chest film in relation to postoperative management – some effects of different projection, posture and lung inflation. Br J Radiol 53:196–204.

186. Glanz S, Ravin CE, Deren MM (1978) Benign pneumoperitoneum following median sternotomy incision. AJR 131:267–269.

187. Goodman LR (1992) Imaging after cardiac surgery. In Goodman LR, Putman CE (eds) Critical care imaging, WB Saunders Philadelphia, p 83.

188. Bor DH, Rose RM, Modlin JF, et al. (1983) Mediastinitis after cardiovascular surgery. Rev Infect Dis 5:885–897.

189. Breyer RH, Mills SA, Hudspeth AS, et al. (1984) A prospective study of sternal wound complications. Ann Thorac Surg 37:412–416.

190. Cheung EH, Craver JM, Jones EL, et al. (1985) Mediastinitis after cardiac valve operations. Impact upon survival. J Thorac Cardiovasc Surg 90:517–522.

191. Rutledge R, Applebaum RE, Kim BJ (1985) Mediastinal infection after open heart surgery. Surgery 97:88–92.

192. Goodman LR, Teplick SK, Kay H (1983) Computed tomography of the normal sternum. AJR 141:219–223.

193. Goodman LR, Kay HR, Teplick SK, et al. (1983) Complications of median sternotomy: Computed tomographic evaluation. AJR 141:225–230.

194. Jolles H, Henry DA, Roberson JP, et al. (1996) Mediastinitis following median sternotomy: CT findings. Radiology 201:463–466.

195. Kay HR, Goodman LR, Teplick SK, et al. (1983) Use of computed tomography to assess mediastinal complications after median sternotomy. Ann Thorac Surg 36:706–714.

196. Creasy JD, Chiles C, Routh WD, et al. (1997) Overview of traumatic injury of the thoracic aorta. Radiographics 17:27–45.

197. Stark P, Cook M, Vincent A, et al. (1987) Traumatic rupture of the thoracic aorta. A review of 49 cases. Radiologie 27:402–406.

198. Simeone JF, Deren MM, Cagle F (1981) The value of the left apical cap in the diagnosis of aortic rupture: A prospective and retrospective study. Radiology 139:35–37.

199. Mirvis SE, Bidwell JK, Buddemeyer EU, et al. (1987) Imaging diagnosis of traumatic aortic rupture. A review and experience at a major trauma center. Invest Radiol 22:187–196.

200. Mirvis SE, Bidwell JK, Buddemeyer EU, et al. (1987) Value of chest radiography in excluding traumatic aortic rupture. Radiology 163:487–493.

201. Woodring JH, King JG (1989) The potential effects of radiographic criteria to exclude aortography in patients with blunt chest traucephalic arterial injury. J Thorac Cardiovasc Surg 97:456–460.

202. Fabian TC, Davis KA, Gavant ML, et al. (1998) Prospective study of blunt aortic injury: Helical CT is diagnostic and antihypertensive therapy reduces rupture. Ann Surg 227:666–676; discussion 676–677.

203. Mirvis SE, Shanmuganathan K, Buell J, et al. (1998) Use of spiral computed tomography for the assessment of blunt trauma patients with potential aortic injury. J Trauma 45:922–930.

204. Demetriades D, Gomez H, Velmahos GC, et al. (1998) Routine helical computed tomographic evaluation of the mediastinum in high-risk blunt trauma patients. Arch Surg 133:1084–1088.

205. Wicky S, Capasso P, Meuli R, et al. (1998) Spiral CT aortography: An efficient technique for the diagnosis of traumatic aortic injury. Eur Radiol 8:828–833.

206. Minard G, Schurr MJ, Croce MA, et al. (1996) A prospective analysis of transesophageal echocardiography in the diagnosis of traumatic disruption of the aorta. J Trauma 40:225–230.

207. Saletta S, Lederman E, Fein S, et al. (1995) Transesophageal echocardiography for the initial evaluation of the widened mediastinum in trauma patients. J Trauma 39:137–141; discussion 141–142.

Index